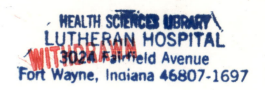

Third Edition

Haimovici's

VASCULAR SURGERY

Principles and Techniques

Third Edition

Haimovici's

VASCULAR SURGERY

Principles and Techniques

Henry Haimovici, M.D.
Clinical Professor Emeritus of Surgery
Albert Einstein College of Medicine
Senior Consultant and Chief Emeritus
Vascular Surgery
Montefiore Medical Center
New York, New York
Foreign Corresponding Member
French National Academy of Medicine
Paris, France

Associate Editors

Allan D. Callow, M.D., Ph.D.
Consultant in Vascular Surgery
Director, Vascular Surgery Research Group
Tufts University School of Medicine
New England Medical Center Hospitals
Boston, Massachusetts

Calvin B. Ernst, M.D.
Clinical Professor of Surgery
University of Michigan Medical School
Ann Arbor, Michigan
Head, Division of Vascular Surgery
Henry Ford Hospital
Detroit, Michigan

Ralph G. DePalma, M.D.
Professor and Chairman
Department of Surgery
George Washington University Hospital
Washington, D.C.

Larry H. Hollier, M.D.
Clinical Professor of Surgery
Tulane University Medical School and
Louisiana State University Medical School
Chairman, Department of Surgery
Ochsner Clinic
New Orleans, Louisiana

APPLETON & LANGE
Norwalk, Connecticut/San Mateo, California

Copyright © 1989 by Appleton & Lange; © 1984, 1976, Appleton–Century–Crofts
A Publishing Division of Prentice Hall

89 90 91 92 93 / 10 9 8 7 6 5 4 3 2 1

Prentice Hall International (UK) Limited, *London*
Prentice Hall of Australia Pty. Limited, *Sydney*
Prentice Hall Canada, Inc., *Toronto*
Prentice Hall Hispanoamericana, S.A., *Mexico*
Prentice Hall of India Private Limited, *New Delhi*
Prentice Hall of Japan, Inc., *Tokyo*
Simon & Schuster Asia Pte. Ltd., *Singapore*
Editora Prentice Hall do Brasil Ltda., *Rio de Janeiro*
Prentice Hall, *Englewood Cliffs, New Jersey*

Library of Congress Cataloging-in-Publication Data

Vascular surgery: principles and techniques/[edited by] Henry
   Haimovici: associate editors, Allan D. Callow . . . [et al.].—3rd
   ed.
     p. cm.
   Includes bibliographies and index.
   ISBN 0–8385–9382–8
   1. Blood-vessels—Surgery. I. Haimovici, Henry, 1907– .
   [DNLM: 1. Vascular Surgery. WG 170 V3317]
RD598.5.V39 1989
617.4' 13—dc20
DNLM/DLC
for Library of Congress   89–6660
                                    CIP

Acquisition Editor: William Schmitt
Managing Editor: Gale Burnick
Designer: Steven Byrum
Production: CRACOM Corporation

PRINTED IN THE UNITED STATES OF AMERICA

*This textbook is dedicated humbly to the pioneers of Vascular Surgery
whose legacy of fundamental contributions is the basis of our specialty.
The present and future generations will owe an everlasting indebtedness to them.*

CONTENTS

PART IV   OCCLUSIVE ARTERIAL DISEASES

Acute Occlusions

Chronic Occlusions

CONTRIBUTORS

Enrico Ascer, M.D.
Associate Professor of Surgery, Albert Einstein College of Medicine; Montefiore Medical Center, New York, New York

Robert W. Barnes, M.D.
Professor and Chairman, Department of Surgery, University of Arkansas for Medical Sciences; Attending Surgeon, McClellan Veterans Administration Medical Center, Little Rock, Arkansas

Arthur E. Baue, M.D.
Vice President for the Medical Center, St. Louis University, St. Louis, Missouri

John J. Bergan, M.D., F.A.C.S., Hon. F.R.C.S. (Eng.)
Magerstadt Professor of Surgery Emeritus, Northwestern University Medical School, Chicago, Illinois; Clinical Professor of Surgery, University of California, San Diego, School of Medicine, San Diego, California

Bruce H. Brennaman, M.D.
Clinical Fellow, Division of Vascular Surgery, Henry Ford Hospital, Detroit, Michigan

David C. Brewster, M.D.
Associate Clinical Professor of Surgery, Harvard Medical School, Massachusetts General Hospital, Boston, Massachusetts

Ronald W. Busuttil, M.D., Ph.D.
Professor of Surgery, Section of Vascular Surgery, Department of Surgery, University of California, Los Angeles, School of Medicine, Los Angeles, California

Allan D. Callow, M.D., Ph.D.
Consultant in Vascular Surgery and Director, Vascular Surgery Research Group, Tufts University School of Medicine, New England Medical Center Hospitals, Boston, Massachusetts

Kenneth J. Cherry, Jr., M.D.
Associate Professor of Surgery, Mayo School of Medicine; Director, Vascular Surgical Training, and Consultant, Section of Vascular Surgery, Department of Surgery, Mayo Clinic and Mayo Foundation, Rochester, Minnesota

Albert K. Chin, M.D.
Cardiovascular Research Staff, Sequoia Hospital, Redwood City, California

Delores F. Cikrit, M.D.
Assistant Professor of Surgery, Indiana University Medical Center, Wishard Memorial Hospital, Indianapolis, Indiana

George J. Collins, Jr., M.D., F.A.C.S., F.C.C.P.
Professor of Surgery, Uniformed Services University of the Health Sciences, Bethesda, Maryland

Daniel P. Connelly, M.D.
Assistant Professor of Surgery, Uniformed Services University of the Health Sciences, Bethesda, Maryland

Joseph S. Coselli, M.D.
Assistant Professor of Surgery, Baylor College of Medicine, Houston, Texas

E. Stanley Crawford, M.D.
Professor of Surgery, Baylor College of Medicine, Houston, Texas

Andrew B. Crummy, M.D.
Professor of Radiology, University of Wisconsin Medical School, Madison, Wisconsin

Ralph G. DePalma, M.D.
Professor and Chairman, Department of Surgery, George Washington University Hospital, Washington, D.C.

Calvin B. Ernst, M.D.
Clinical Professor of Surgery, University of Michigan Medical School, Ann Arbor, Michigan; Head, Division of Vascular Surgery, Henry Ford Hospital, Detroit, Michigan

Thomas J. Fogarty, M.D.
Chief, Cardiac Surgery Section, Sequoia Hospital, Redwood City, California

Julie A. Freischlag, M.D.
Assistant Professor of Surgery, Department of Surgery, University of California, San Diego, School of Medicine, San Diego, California

Peter Gloviczki, M.D.
Assistant Professor of Surgery, Mayo School of Medicine; Director, Vascular Surgical Research, and Consultant, Section of Vascular Surgery, Department of Surgery, Mayo Clinic and Mayo Foundation, Rochester, Minnesota

Jerry Goldstone, M.D.
Professor of Surgery and Chief, Division of Vascular Surgery, University of California, San Francisco, School of Medicine, San Francisco, California

Lazar J. Greenfield, M.D.
Professor and Chairman, Department of Surgery, University of Michigan Medical School, Ann Arbor, Michigan

Warren S. Grundfest, M.D.
Assistant Professor of Surgery, University of California, Los Angeles, School of Medicine; Assistant Director of Surgery and Director of Laser Research, Cedars-Sinai Medical Center, Los Angeles, California

Sushil K. Gupta, M.D.
Associate Professor of Surgery, Albert Einstein College of Medicine; Associate Chief of Vascular Surgery, Montefiore Medical Center, New York, New York

Henry Haimovici, M.D.
Clinical Professor Emeritus of Surgery, Albert Einstein College of Medicine, Senior Consultant and Chief Emeritus Vascular Surgery, Montefiore Medical Center, New York, New York; Foreign Corresponding Member, French National Academy of Medicine, Paris, France

Norman R. Hertzer, M.D.
Department of Vascular Surgery, The Cleveland Clinic Foundation, Cleveland, Ohio

Larry H. Hollier, M.D.
Clinical Professor of Surgery, Tulane University Medical School and Louisiana State University Medical School; Chairman, Department of Surgery, Ochsner Clinic, New Orleans, Louisiana

Barry T. Katzen, M.D.
Professor of Clinical Radiology, University of Miami School of Medicine; Miami Vascular Institute, Baptist Hospital, Miami, Florida

Richard F. Kempczinski, M.D.
Professor of Surgery and Chief, Vascular Surgery, University of Cincinnati Medical Center, Cincinnati, Ohio

Yves E. Langlois, M.D.
Assistant Professor of Surgery, Department of Surgery, University of Montreal, Montreal, Quebec

Robert P. Leather, M.D.
Department of Surgery, Vascular Surgery Section, The Albany Medical College of Union University, Albany, New York

Frank Litvack, M.D.
Assistant Professor of Medicine, University of California, Los Angeles, School of Medicine; Codirector, Cardiac Catheterization Laboratory, Cedars-Sinai Medical Center, Los Angeles, California

Kenneth L. Mattox, M.D.
Professor of Surgery, Baylor College of Medicine, Houston, Texas

Barbara A. Michna, M.D.
Resident in Surgery, Medical College of Virginia, Richmond, Virginia

Yoshio Mishima, M.D.
Professor and Chairman, IInd Department of Surgery, Tokyo Medical and Dental University, Tokyo

Cheryl Montefusco, Ph.D., F.I.C.A., F.A.C.A.
Associate Professor of Surgery, Albert Einstein College of Medicine; Codirector, Noninvasive Vascular Laboratory, Montefiore Medical Center, New York, New York

Wesley S. Moore, M.D.
Professor of Surgery, University of California, Los Angeles, Medical School; Chief, Section of Vascular Surgery, Department of Surgery, The Center for the Health Sciences, Los Angeles, California

Harvey L. Neiman, M.D.
Clinical Professor of Radiology, University of Pittsburgh Medical School; Chairman, Department of Radiology, Western Pennsylvania Hospital, Pittsburgh, Pennsylvania

Thomas F. O'Donnell, Jr., M.D.
Professor of Surgery, Tufts University School of Medicine; Chief of Vascular Surgery, New England Medical Center, Boston, Massachusetts

Pär A. Olofsson, M.D.
Assistant Professor of Surgery, Karolinska Institute, Stockholm

Daniel J. Reddy, M.D.
Clinical Assistant Professor of Surgery, University of Michigan Medical School, Ann Arbor, Michigan; Senior Staff Vascular Surgeon, Henry Ford Hospital, Detroit, Michigan

Ghislaine O. Roederer, M.D.
Senior Research Fellow, Montreal Institute of Clinical Research, Montreal, Quebec

Amiel Z. Rudavsky, M.D.
Associate Clinical Professor of Nuclear Medicine and Medicine, Albert Einstein College of Medicine, Yeshiva University; Attending Physician, Medicine, and Director, Nuclear Medicine, North Central Bronx Hospital; Associate Attending Physician, Montefiore Medical Center, New York, New York

†Allen S. Russek, M.D.

Lester R. Sauvage, M.D.
Clinical Professor, Department of Surgery, University of Washington School of Medicine; Director, Hope Heart Institute, Seattle, Washington

David D. Schmitt, M.D.
Fellow in Vascular Surgery, Medical College of Wisconsin, Milwaukee, Wisconsin

Robert A. Schwartz, M.D.
Assistant Professor of Surgery, State University of New York Health Sciences Center, Syracuse, New York

Donald Silver, M.D.
Professor and Chairman, Department of Surgery, University of Missouri, Columbia, Health Sciences Center, Columbia, Missouri

Seymour Sprayregen, M.D.
Professor of Radiology, Albert Einstein College of Medicine; Acting Chairman, Department of Radiology, Montefiore Medical Center, New York, New York

J. Manly Stallworth, M.D.
Clinical Professor of Surgery, Medical University of South Carolina; Roper Hospital Vascular Laboratory, Charleston, South Carolina

James C. Stanley, M.D.
Professor of Surgery and Head, Section of Vascular Surgery, University of Michigan Medical School, Ann Arbor, Michigan

Jan J. Stokosa, C.P.
Williamston, Michigan

Ronald J. Stoney, M.D.
Professor of Surgery, University of California, San Francisco, Medical School, San Francisco, California

D. Eugene Strandness, Jr., M.D.
Professor and Head, Section of Vascular Surgery, University of Washington School of Medicine, Seattle Washington

David S. Sumner, M.D.
Professor of Surgery and Chief, Section of Peripheral Vascular Surgery, Southern Illinois University; St. John's Hospital, Springfield, Illinois

D. Emerick Szilagyi, M.D.
Chairman of the Department of Surgery Emeritus and Professor of Surgery Emeritus, University of Michigan Medical School, Ann Arbor, Michigan; Editor of the *Journal of Vascular Surgery*; Consultant in Vascular Surgery, Henry Ford Hospital, Detroit, Michigan

Vivian A. Tellis, M.D.
Professor of Surgery, Albert Einstein College of Medicine; Montefiore Medical Center, New York, New York

Brian L. Thiele, M.D., F.R.A.C.S., F.A.C.S.
Professor of Surgery, Pennsylvania State College of Medicine; Chief, Vascular Surgery, University Hospital; Milton S. Hershey Medical Center, Hershey, Pennsylvania

Jonathan B. Towne, M.D.
Department of Vascular Surgery, Medical College of Wisconsin, Milwaukee County Medical Complex, Milwaukee, Wisconsin

† Deceased

Frank J. Veith, M.D.
Professor of Surgery, Albert Einstein College of Medicine; Chief, Vascular Surgery, and Director, Transplant Program, Montefiore Medical Center, New York, New York

Thomas W. Wakefield, M.D.
Assistant Professor of Surgery, Section of Vascular Surgery, University of Michigan Medical School, Ann Arbor, Michigan

James S.T. Yao, M.D.
Professor of Surgery, Department of Surgery, Northwestern University Medical School, Chicago, Illinois

Anson Yeager, M.D.
Formerly Fellow in Vascular Surgery, New England Medical Center; Instructor, Tufts University School of Medicine, Boston, Massachusetts

PREFACE

Keeping abreast of the rapid progress in the field of vascular surgery is often a frustrating, time-consuming task, especially when one is looking for the latest data in textbooks on this topic. A comparison of this edition of *Vascular Surgery* to the first edition, published in 1976, and the second edition, published in 1984, clearly illustrates how soon certain areas require revision and complete updating.

During the relatively short time since the publication of the 1984 text, considerable progress has indeed been made. The Table of Contents reflects both the updating of the chapters from the preceding editions and the additional topics covered. Since publication of the second edition, great strides have been made in the ability to diagnose vascular lesions. These have led to revised concepts in surgical management and to technical improvements. One of the major developments involves the imaging methods used to detect defects. Others involve innovative surgical and nonsurgical procedures for managing many of the vascular lesions encountered today.

Chapters dealing with areas in which there has been recent progress have received greater emphasis. Some examples of this progress may illustrate this point:

1. A better understanding of the biologic interaction between the blood elements and the mural arterial factors has offered a new vision of the atherogenesis concept.
2. How metabolic complications affect acute ischemic tissue syndromes has been clarified.
3. The role of geographic factors in the etiology of atherosclerotic and especially *non*atherosclerotic lesions of the small arteries has been reviewed.
4. The complex cerebrovascular syndromes have received more in-depth discussion.

Since its advent, modern vascular surgery has dealt, on the one hand, primarily with the reconstruction of vessels damaged by disease or trauma and, on the other hand, with their restoration by disobstruction or their replacement by graft materials.

In recent years vascular surgery has evolved from the application of primarily mechanical methods into the application of so-called nonsurgical procedures as well. These consist of management of occlusive arterial lesions by means of transluminal balloon catheters or by use of laser techniques, all of which are mostly part of the field of interventional radiology. Although they may be used solely as substitutes for surgical procedures, not infrequently they may be performed concurrently with reconstructive surgery. Although these interventional radiologic methods may often be significant therapeutically, it should be pointed out that traditional vascular surgery has by no means abdicated its role even in small or medium-size arterial lesions, which are the major areas of interventional radiology. Although indications for vascular surgery may be reduced in certain areas, it remains essential in general as well as in many areas inaccessible to the nonsurgical methods.

The main target of vascular therapy is obviously to relieve tissue ischemia, whether acute or chronic. An in-depth understanding of the biochemistry of ischemic tissue, exclusive of the mechanical modality, is still to be achieved. However, recent studies of the biochemistry of acutely ischemic tissues of brain, myocardium, kidney, and intestine, as well as of skeletal muscle, have begun to provide some insight into the answers of their biochemical complexes. The free radicals in biology, as related to vascular problems, may shed some light on these complex subjects. Recently developed substances, the so-called scavengers, are now available to counteract the noxious effects of the free radicals. These notions are mentioned only in the context of the biology of acute arterial occlusions and future treatment.

With the present edition of *Vascular Surgery*, four seasoned editors joined me in the revision, updating, and planning of this textbook: Allan Callow, Ralph DePalma, Calvin Ernst, and Larry Hollier, all distinguished scholars and renowned masters in vascular surgery. Their role in this endeavor has been most productive and refreshing. Furthermore, their contributions as authors have enhanced the value of this textbook by providing new viewpoints in their areas of expertise for which I am most deeply grateful.

At this stage of proliferation of new developments in the various aspects of vascular surgery, multieditors of such a textbook were unquestionably most appropriate and desirable. Such a formula of editorship provides a solid basis for greater vision of the subject with a net result of excellence. It is hoped that the readers will appreciate its effective, enlightening, and overall up-to-date information.

Henry Haimovici, M.D.

xvii

PREFACE TO THE FIRST EDITION

Almost three decades have now elapsed since the new field of vascular surgery started to assert its individuality. This specialty evolved as a result of significant developments in diagnostic methods and new surgical techniques. Through its often spectacular achievements the modern surgery of blood vessels, along with that of the heart, today occupies a select place in contemporary Medicine. Its increasing role in the treatment of vascular diseases is reflected by the fact that at least 73,000 reconstructions of major arteries are performed in the United States every year, as was recently reported by the Inter-Society Commission for Optimal Resources for Vascular Surgery. These figures illustrate the magnitude of only some of the main problems in vascular surgery.

Recognition of a new field of endeavor, notwithstanding its significance, is always achieved slowly. The history of surgical specialities is replete with such evidence, and vascular surgery is no exception. Within the past few years, however, the leading Vascular Societies, recognizing the need for better education and training of those entering this field, have evolved guidelines for the achievement of standards of excellence. As a result of this concerted effort there is a crescendo movement at present toward fulfilling this goal by establishing a specialty certification board.

Before the advent of the present era, the few surgical approaches available for managing vascular diseases were carried out within the framework of general surgery. But with the introduction of arterial reconstructive procedures progressively encompassing all vessels of the body, it became obvious that the new vascular techniques, though most often achieving spectacular results, do sometimes carry great risks to limb and life. The critical nature of these techniques is abundantly dramatized by the existence of only a narrow margin of error between success and failure when compared to most areas of general surgery. Proficiency in carrying out these exacting procedures requires a broad clinical background and superior technical skill.

While the training programs in other surgical specialties are well standardized today, those in vascular surgery are still far from having received similar implementation. The present-day often fragmentary and limited training in vascular surgery through a rotating general surgical residency does not provide the desired program for acquiring a comprehensive knowledge of this specialty. As in other sur-

gical fields, postgraduate and postresidency vascular fellowship training often represents the main avenue for achieving competency in this discipline.

In his search for more knowledge of a particular aspect of vascular surgical techniques it is often hard for the general surgeon or the surgical resident to know where to begin to look up the most pertinent source of information. To some extent the above considerations prompted this book, which was conceived to provide a comprehensive presentation of all aspects related to vascular diseases and their surgical management.

In the preparation of guidelines for this multiauthored book, one of the major goals was to achieve uniformity in the presentation of the various chapters. Such goals were perhaps best expressed by Joseph Pulitzer, who advised his journalist profession how to present successfully their stories to the public. He said, "Put it before them *briefly* so that they will read it, *clearly* so that they will appreciate it, *picturesquely* so they will remember it and, above all, *accurately* so they will be guided by its light."

The approach for achieving an all-inclusive textbook on this ever-expanding specialty required a large up-to-date survey of all aspects of this field. To do justice to the diversity of the topics and to offer a spectrum of the best available knowledge, it was desirable to entrust some parts of this book to a number of contributors distinguished for their pioneering work and expertise in some specific areas. A multiauthored but well-integrated book should thus offer great advantage to the reader by providing him with the various authoritative options available for a given problem, whether common or uncommon.

The *scope* and the *level* of the contents of this book are designed not only for the experienced vascular and general surgeon, but also for the surgical residents in need of an all-inclusive text and atlas of vascular procedures.

The *contents* of this book are divided into eight parts, some of which include information not usually found in similar textbooks. Besides dealing in detailed fashion with all vascular techniques, it also devotes sizable sections to the basic subjects of the various surgical and biological problems as related to vascular disorders.

Part One on basic considerations includes ten chapters dealing with various aspects ranging from the history of vascular surgery and methods of evaluation of the patient and his vascular disorders to the anesthetic management for the various types of operation. Thus, it reviews the principles of angiography, the biologic behavior of arterial replacements, principles of hemodynamics, thrombogenesis and anticoagulation as related to arterial reconstruction, and many other basic considerations underlying vascular techniques.

Part Two deals with the surgical anatomy of the arteries and the methods for their exposure. This section is designed to fill a serious gap, since most surgical residents and general surgeons, as stated by Daniel Elkin, are "Woefully lacking in anatomic knowledge, particularly as it relates to blood vessels, peripheral nerves and even the musculature of the extremities" (JAMA 132:421, 1946). This situation was true in 1946 and it is even more pertinent at present, as a result of today's more limited curriculum in all medical schools.

Part Three deals with the significant aspects of the biology of atherosclerosis and the angiographic patterns of this process in various arterial locations of the lower extremity. This knowledge is essential to the understanding of the atherosclerotic process, the number one problem in vascular diseases, and to the interpretation of the radiologic patterns.

Part Four deals extensively with the surgical procedures for the various aortic and peripheral arterial lesions (embolism, arteriosclerotic occlusive disease, aneurysms, etc.). The clinical background, indications and contraindications to surgical management, are the object of 23 chapters with an in-depth review of these arterial entities and related complications with specific emphasis on operative procedures.

Part Five deals with the surgery of visceral vessels, including the extracranial arteries and the celiac, mesenteric, and renal arteries. It contains, as well, chapters on kidney transplantation and portal decompression.

Part Six deals with the thoracic outlet compression syndromes, thoracic and lumbar sympathectomy, and sensory nerve crushing in the leg.

Part Seven offers several chapters on the most important aspects of venous disease, including pulmonary embolectomy and the management of lymphedema.

Part Eight presents two comprehensive and practical chapters on the various levels of amputation of the lower extremity and the methods of early rehabilitation of the patient.

In the descriptions of the techniques, great emphasis has been placed not only on the "standard procedures" but also on: (a) the variants with their specific indications, (b) the pitfalls and their avoidance, and (c) the complications and their treatment. These details, so often neglected in textbooks, will add, it is hoped, immeasurably to the practical value of this book. While the accent is placed on the "method of choice," one has to bear in mind that "ideal" methods for reconstruction are not always applicable or feasible in a given case. Variation is often the rule because of the innumerable patterns of occlusive or aneurysmal arterial lesions. In each individual case the method to be preferred must be selected on the basis of clinical and arteriographic data, operative findings, and a surgeon's personal experience. Although the techniques described in this book are mostly those which have stood the test of time, in the years ahead changes, improvements, revisions and variations are to be anticipated.

With few exceptions, statistical data concerning operative results were deliberately omitted, such information being considered outside this book's primary scope. However, should the reader be interested in this aspect, numerous references are available in all chapters.

A particular effort was made to integrate the different chapters by using cross references. Thus repetition or duplication, which is often unavoidable in a textbook so structured, has been kept to a minimum or largely eliminated.

The book is profusely illustrated not only with line drawings for the step-by-step surgical techniques but also with angiograms and operative pictures or pathology specimens. The wide variety of the illustrative material should greatly enhance the value of the text.

Many of the early contributions, basic to the development of the new era of vascular surgery, were revolutionary in their concepts. They introduced innovative procedures which have radically altered our knowledge in vascular replacements and which have long-term implications that we do not yet fully apprehend. What the future holds in terms of further progress is difficult to foresee. But what is certain is that the past three decades have witnessed a phenomenal change in our concepts of vascular diseases and their surgical treatment. The present book has endeavored to record this progress. And so, it is hoped that the scope, contents, and presentation of this book will enhance the knowledge of those interested in the craft of vascular surgery and will provide them with a broad level of information for the optimal performance of this specialty.

Henry Haimovici, M.D.

ACKNOWLEDGMENTS

I am especially grateful to the many contributors for their gracious cooperation in providing their personal experience as well as their critical appraisal of the most pertinent current literature.

I wish, also, to express my appreciation to the illustrators of the various new and older chapters. Their contributions add immensely to the understanding of various texts.

It is a great pleasure to express my appreciation to the staff of Appleton & Lange, who have actively participated in the conception and development of this third edition.

To Lin Paterson, President of Appleton & Lange, I am grateful for her having stimulated and contributed to the initial concept of this edition.

To William Schmitt, Editorial Director, I wish to acknowledge my deep thanks for his graceful way of resolving some thorny problems arising from editiorial differences in the various chapters.

To Gale Burnick, my thanks for the difficult task of managing editor. The attempt to coordinate the chapters for a cohesive approach was ultimately achieved. This facilitated my overall task.

Of all those entrusted with the final production tasks, especially copyediting, Mary Espenschied deserves our indebtedness. She was faced most often with the ungrateful role of clarifying certain areas not entirely accessible to simple linguistics.

In sum, production of this edition from the inception to its final stages required multiple and varied efforts from many individuals endowed with different capacities for handling the many components of a textbook of this nature.

Henry Haimovici, M.D.

Third Edition

Haimovici's

VASCULAR SURGERY

Principles and Techniques

PART I
Basic Considerations

CHAPTER 1

Landmarks and Present Trends in Vascular Surgery

Henry Haimovici

*"If I have seen farther, it is by
standing on the shoulders of giants."**

Isaac Newton

Many of the basic principles and techniques that paved the way for modern vasular surgery were developed at the turn of this century, mostly in the experimental laboratory. The current golden era in vascular surgery began with the brilliant clinically applied contributions made in the 1940s and 1950s.

A brief overview will help the reader to gain a proper perspective of the present state of vascular surgery and its future potentials and to reassess the fundamental contributions of the past, which emerged from both the experimental laboratory and clinical investigations. It will thus offer an appropriate prelude and future vision of the present trends of this ever-expanding field of surgery.

The objectives of this chapter will be limited to a discussion of the major landmarks achieved by the early pioneers. The history of their contributions represents the very basis of vascular surgery. It is beyond the scope of this chapter to cover the entire spectrum of both the early pioneers and later major contributors.

The legacy of the early pathfinders undoubtedly inspired their successors to achieve new and brilliant additions to this field. Illustrating this historical link between our present knowledge and the accomplishments of the pioneers of yesteryear is the old aphorism attributed to Isaac Newton, presented as the lead quotation for this chapter.*

The history of vascular surgery may be divided into the three conventional sections: arterial surgery, venous surgery, and lymphatic surgery.

The overall history will focus primarily on the basic principles, rather than on technologic details of vascular surgery.

ARTERIAL SURGERY

Long before the present era of modern vascular surgery, dating from antiquity to the eighteenth century, occasional reports had dealt with vascular problems, mostly confined to the management of arterial hemorrhage and, less often, to that of aneurysms.

The early surgical attempts to control bleeding from vascular injuries were carried out by a variety of means, ranging from manual compression, to the use of boiling oil for its cauterizing effect, to ligation of the artery. Although ligature for bleeding arteries had been mentioned occasionally from the beginning of the first century, it is Ambroise Paré who is credited with introducing its use for checking arterial hemorrhage and thus with establishing the ligature as an accepted method of treatment.

In the management of aneurysms, ligature of arteries was also introduced during that early era, as is well known through the classic report of Antyllus. His treatment consisted of biterminal ligation of the artery above and below the aneurysm, with incision of the sac and evacuation of its contents, leaving the aneurysmal sac open for spontaneous healing. During the subsequent centuries, sporadic reports describing modifications of the latter method, and other new techniques as well, continued to appear. Anel, in 1710, applied a ligature immediately above the aneurysm without disturbing the sac. Then, in 1785, John Hunter advocated the use of the ligature at a distance well above the aneurysm dilation. Thus, for a popliteal aneurysm, he placed the ligature within the fascial tunnel of the thigh, known since then as "Hunter's canal." When the patient died 15 months later, the aneurysmal sac was thoroughly thrombosed.

In the nineteenth century a notable era of progress was ushered in with the introduction of laboratory-designed

---

* Cited in Merton RK: *On the Shoulders of Giants*. New York, Harcourt, Brace & World, 1965. In his book, Merton attempted to trace the origin of this famous phrase attributed to Sir Isaac Newton. Apparently it appeared originally in Latin, which when translated reads, A dwarf standing on the shoulders of a giant may see farther than a giant himself.

techniques for suturing vascular wounds and anastomosing blood vessels.

Early Problems of Arterial Repair

Improvement in techniques did not occur until the latter part of the nineteenth century, when successful repair of arterial wounds could be accomplished systematically. The technique used by Jassinowsky was a stitch that avoided penetrating the tunica intima. Indeed, one of the early important issues with the technical repair of blood vessels revolved around the proper method of dealing with the intima. Early investigators, as already mentioned, avoided penetrating it completely for fear of injuring its endothelium and thus causing thrombosis. It was not until 1899 that Dörfler adopted the technique of deliberately penetrating all layers of the vessel. The essential feature of this method consisted of the use of fine round needles and fine silk. Dörfler's suture was continuous, embracing all three coats of the vessel. From his experience, he concluded that aseptic silk thread in the lumen of the vessel does not necessarily lead to thrombosis, and therefore the penetration of the intima was not contraindicated. He recommended the same method for repairing veins. This was the first important step in the development of vascular sutures, a technique that is used to this day.

Anastomosis and Grafting of Vessels

In one of the earliest reports of anastomosis between two vessels, Nikolai Eck, in 1877, created an anastomosis between the portal vein and the inferior vena cava. He conducted laboratory experiments of portacaval shunts to clarify some physiologic problems and to determine whether it was possible to treat some cases of mechanical ascites by forming such a fistula. This contribution remained buried for a long time and was discovered with the advent of decompression treatment for portal hypertension. (See Child, 1953).

Toward the end of the nineteenth century, there was a gradually increasing interest in the method of vessel suturing and anastomoses.

Vascular Surgery: Early Contributions

It could be stated that modern vascular surgery started with Matas' contributions (Figs. 1-1 and 1-2). Indeed, Rudolph Matas devised this technique, endoaneurysmorrhaphy, in 1888. "This consisted of repair of a large aneurysm of the brachial artery in the middle third of the arm resulting from a gunshot wound approximately two months earlier [Fig. 1-3]. After opening the sac and removing the clots, three orifices were detected at the bottom of the sac and stitched with fine silk, and thus were sealed completely." Matas states that "this operation was devised as an expedient." He further writes that "the exigencies of the case made it necessary that hemostasis should be obtained and the occlusion by suture appeared to be so easy and plain that it seemed to me that any surgeon similarly situated

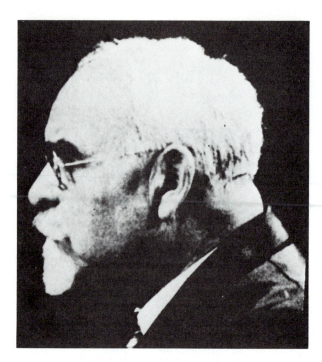

Figure 1-1. Rudolph Matas.

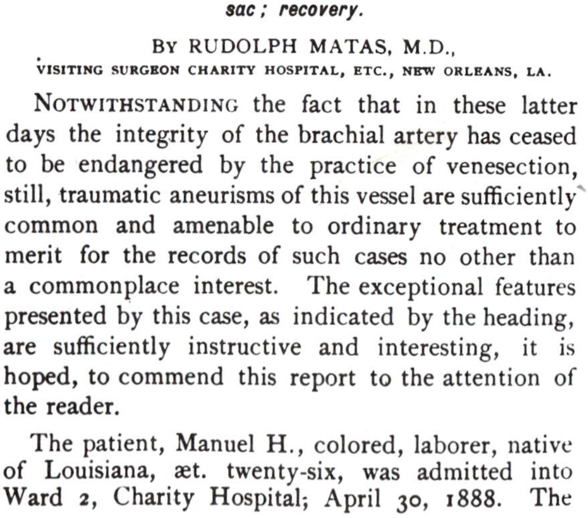

would have instinctively adopted this simple way of getting out of the difficulty." By 1940, Matas reported personal experience with 620 operations for aneurysms. The principles established by Matas in the management of aneurysms

---

ORIGINAL ARTICLES.

TRAUMATIC ANEURISM OF THE LEFT BRACHIAL ARTERY.

Failure of direct and indirect pressure ; ligation of the artery immediately above tumor ; return of pulsation on the tenth day ; ligation immediately below tumor ; failure to arrest pulsation ; incision and partial excision of sac ; recovery.

BY RUDOLPH MATAS, M.D.,
VISITING SURGEON CHARITY HOSPITAL, ETC., NEW ORLEANS, LA.

NOTWITHSTANDING the fact that in these latter days the integrity of the brachial artery has ceased to be endangered by the practice of venesection, still, traumatic aneurisms of this vessel are sufficiently common and amenable to ordinary treatment to merit for the records of such cases no other than a commonplace interest. The exceptional features presented by this case, as indicated by the heading, are sufficiently instructive and interesting, it is hoped, to commend this report to the attention of the reader.

The patient, Manuel H., colored, laborer, native of Louisiana, æt. twenty-six, was admitted into Ward 2, Charity Hospital; April 30, 1888. The

Figure 1-2. First page of Matas's article "Traumatic Aneurysm of the Left Brachial Artery," published in *New York Medical News* (53:412, 1888).

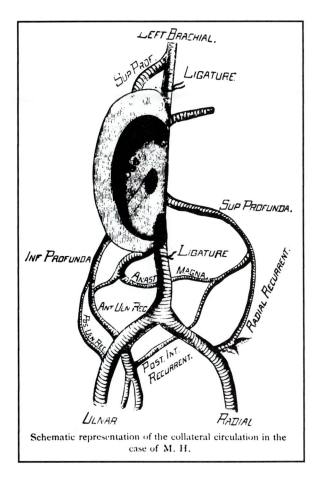

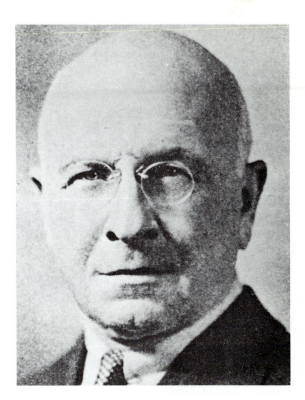

Figure 1-4. Alexis Carrel.

Figure 1-3. Drawing of first endoaneurysmorrhaphy performed by Matas in 1888 for large traumatic aneurysm of brachial artery. Note large collateral circulation. (*From Matas R: NY Med News 53:462, 1988.*)

were destined, however, for several decades of delay, until modern vascular surgery became established.

Experimental Vascular Surgery

At the turn of the century, most of the basic principles and techniques in vascular surgery had been conceived by Alexis Carrel in the experimental laboratory between 1901 and 1910 (Fig. 1-4). In 1902, he published a paper entitled "La Technique Opératoire des Anastomoses Vasculaires et la Transplantation des Viscères," which proved to be a landmark contribution to this field. This brief article, written by Carrel only 2 years after he received his medical degree, marks the beginning of his wide-ranging scientific achievements (Fig. 1-5).

Carrel's biography has been told elsewhere many times. He was born in Lyons, France, in 1873. He went to the Medical School of Lyons, where, after his residency, he devoted himself to experimental vascular surgery.

What led Carrel to devote his lifetime to vascular work? Carrel, as a young intern in 1894, was deeply impressed by the assassination of Sadi Carnot, president of the French Republic. The fatal knife wound had severed the portal vein, and the best surgeons of France were helpless. Carrel

firmly believed that Carnot could have been saved if surgeons had learned to sew up blood vessels just as they sewed together muscle, skin, and other tissues.

Only a few surgeons were then interested in operating on blood vessels. Nevertheless, it was not until Carrel arrived on the surgical scene that vascular sutures and transplantation of vessels achieved a standardized modus operandi.

Carrel started his experimental work in Lyons, France. After coming to the United States, he continued his laboratory work in association with Guthrie, during a period of only 6 months in 1905 and 1906. During this time, their laboratory productivity resulted in 21 coauthored publications.

The importance of Carrel's laboratory findings during these 2 short years in the United States became rapidly known. Carrel was appointed in 1906 at the Rockefeller Institute, where he worked to the end of 1939. During this period his research encompassed cellular aging, intrathoracic surgery, and cellular and organ cultures. In addition, together with Charles Lindbergh, he devised a blood perfusion pump capable of support organs in vitro, culminating in a model of an artificial heart. During the same period, Carrel was the first to study the functional and histologic results of preserved homografts, both arterial and venous.

The clinical significance of the basic principles established by Carrel emerged only much later. It can be truly said that modern vascular grafting, including organ transplantation, stems from the exhaustive investigations of this pioneering work. Sterling Edwards, in the preface to

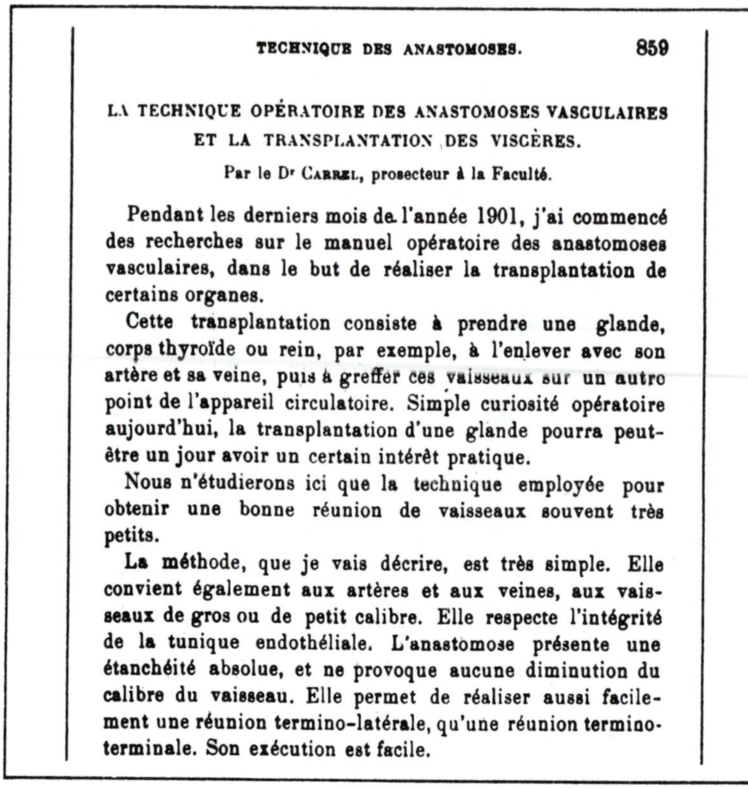

TECHNIQUE DES ANASTOMOSES. 859

LA TECHNIQUE OPÉRATOIRE DES ANASTOMOSES VASCULAIRES ET LA TRANSPLANTATION DES VISCÈRES.

Par le Dr Carrel, prosecteur à la Faculté.

Pendant les derniers mois de l'année 1901, j'ai commencé des recherches sur le manuel opératoire des anastomoses vasculaires, dans le but de réaliser la transplantation de certains organes.

Cette transplantation consiste à prendre une glande, corps thyroïde ou rein, par exemple, à l'enlever avec son artère et sa veine, puis à greffer ces vaisseaux sur un autre point de l'appareil circulatoire. Simple curiosité opératoire aujourd'hui, la transplantation d'une glande pourra peut-être un jour avoir un certain intérêt pratique.

Nous n'étudierons ici que la technique employée pour obtenir une bonne réunion de vaisseaux souvent très petits.

La méthode, que je vais décrire, est très simple. Elle convient également aux artères et aux veines, aux vaisseaux de gros ou de petit calibre. Elle respecte l'intégrité de la tunique endothéliale. L'anastomose présente une étanchéité absolue, et ne provoque aucune diminution du calibre du vaisseau. Elle permet de réaliser aussi facilement une réunion termino-latérale, qu'une réunion termino-terminale. Son exécution est facile.

Figure 1-5. First page of Carrel's original article, which appeared in *Lyon Medical* (98:859, 1902).

his biography on Carrel, mentions advice, given over the past 30 years to young investigators, that illustrates the reputation of the vastness of Carrel's contributions: "If you think you've invented a new technique in heart or blood vessel surgery, you'd better check to see if Dr. Alexis Carrel did not try the same thing 50 years ago."

Not long after his spectacular experiments, as early as 1912, Carrel achieved world acclaim as reflected by a Nobel Prize awarded to him in physiology and medicine "in recognition of his work on vascular suture and the transplantation of blood vessels and organs."

Early Development of Clinical Grafts

Carrel's innovative techniques in vascular surgery helped standardize the procedures of vascular sutures, the anastomoses of vessels and their grafting, and the transplantation of organs. His laboratory work had a tremendous impact on the early clinical applications. Thus in 1906, Goyanes, of Spain, performed a successful interposition of a venous graft for an aneurysmal arterial segment in man. Goyanes was well versed in the experimental work of Jaboulay, Murphy, and others. He credited his mentor, San Martin, with the concept of substituting a venous graft for an excised segment of artery. The case reported by Goyanes was that of a 41-year-old patient who had an aneurysm of the popliteal artery. He used a segment of the popliteal vein as a graft connecting the severed ends of the artery.

At about the same epoch, other surgeons familiar with Carrel's work had also undertaken grafting procedures. Thus Lexer, in 1907, faced a similar problem consisting of a large false aneurysm in the axilla. After excision of some 8 cm between the severed ends of the axillary and brachial arteries, he interposed a segment of the greater saphenous vein, removed from the patient's leg. Thereafter, Lexer did a number of resections with interposition of venous grafts. Several other German surgeons, such as von Bier in 1915, von Haberer in 1916 and 1917, von Bonin in 1917, and Warthmuller in 1917, presented 52 cases of venous transplants. Later, in 1925, Lexer presented 58 cases and published them in the *Archiv for Chirurgie.* Weglowski, from Poland, also in 1925, presented 51 cases of vein transplants primarily for traumatic aneurysms and possibly for two or three cases of interposition for segments of damaged arteries. Also among the early surgeons using venous autogenous grafts was Subbotich, a Yugoslav surgeon.

Pringle, in 1913, reported two cases of vein grafting for arterial reconstruction. In 1915, Bernheim, of Johns Hopkins, removed a 15 cm aneurysm of the popliteal artery and replaced it with a 12 cm segment of the saphenous vein. Later, Bernheim published a monograph entitled *Vascular Surgical Techniques.*

It therefore appears that during World War I and shortly thereafter, a number of surgeons were using vein transplants for repair of arterial lesions. It is astonishing, however, that it took several decades before Kunlin introduced the bypass graft, for which he used a venous segment. It is likely that important ancillary developments for the performance of adequate vascular surgery were missing in the early years, which explains the slow expansion of vascular grafting.

Modern Era

Role of Progress in Other Medical Fields

Although the basic techniques of arterial surgery were fairly well described at the beginning of this century, it was not until the 1940s that the modern era of vascular surgery expanded and flourished. The gap of several decades between the beginning of this century and the modern era was due primarily to the lack of important developments in many other medical disciplines, such as radiology, hematology, and pharmacology (particularly relating to antibiotics). With progress in these disciplines, it became possible for the field of vascular surgery to fulfill its great potential.

Arteriography

Arteriography, an essential diagnostic procedure, had its slow beginnings shortly after Roentgen's discovery in 1895. Indeed, it was not until 1927 that Egaz Moniz, of Lisbon, devised carotid arteriography. Two years later, Reynaldo dos Santos, also of Lisbon, and co-workers developed the technique of translumbar aortography. Although this diagnostic method was adopted by a few surgeons, more time elapsed before it gained greater acceptance. The delay was due primarily to lack of refinements of the radiologic techniques and to inadequate safety of the radiopaque substances. A further step in the progress of angiography was achieved when the technique of percutaneous arterial catheterization was introduced by Seldinger. This allowed a more precise and selective visualization, especially of the visceral vessels.

To the standard Roentgen arteriography, more sophisticated techniques have been recently added, such as digital arteriography (Chapter 6), Doppler ultrasonography (Chapter 7), magnetic resonance imaging (Chapter 8), radionuclide imaging (Chapter 9).

Pharmacologic Agents

Anticoagulants. Heparin, discovered in 1916, became available clinically only in 1936. During the same year, another important development took place in this field, namely, the discovery of dicumarol. The use of these anticoagulants in vascular surgery allowed the handling of blood vessels with relative safety, preventing intraoperative and postoperative thrombosis.

Use of Antiplatelet and Other Antithrombogenic Agents. These agents may be used either prophylactically or postoperatively. Their usefulness is independent of the anticoagulants (see Chapters 4 and 12).

Antibiotics. Discovered at about the same time, antibiotics, by controlling infection, which was a major cause of graft failure, had an important beneficial impact on vascular surgery.

Other Advances

Blood transfusions and substitutes, along with better knowledge of surgery-related metabolic disturbances, were indispensable factors in the successful management of patients undergoing vascular surgery.

New instrumentation and suture materials have greatly contributed to the improvement of vascular diagnostic and treatment techniques. Of the new technologies, noninvasive evaluation of the morphologic and functional characterization of vascular problems provides immediate, safe, and nonexpensive treatment modalities for a host of diseases. In addition, increasing physiologic orientation has occasioned a great demand for accurate monitoring equipment. Simultaneously, the field of bioengineering has come into its own, providing the technical know-how to adapt principles, techniques, and instruments to the needs of today's cardiovascular problems.

From the brief review of these ancillary developments, it is apparent that vascular surgery could not have reached its present state without the backup offered by various medical and scientific achievements since the 1940s.

Progress in Vascular Surgery

The current revival of vascular surgery was ushered in during 1938 by the successful ligation of a patent ductus arteriosus by Gross. That was followed in 1944 by another milestone in this field, when Blalock and Taussig reported their first operation for tetralogy of Fallot, in which they anastomosed the left subclavian to the left pulmonary artery by an end-to-side technique. During the same year, Crafoord and Nylin, of Stockholm, succeeded in correcting a coarctation of the aorta; they published their report in 1945. On July 6, 1945, Gross, working independently, was also successful in correcting the coarctation of the aorta; he reported his first two cases in the same year. These brilliant clinical results were preceded by careful laboratory experiments carried out by Blalock and Park in 1944 and by Gross and Hufnagel in 1945.

These early successes in the management of congenital vascular abnormalities stimulated a great deal of activity throughout the world. A true explosion of various new methods of investigating cardiac and vascular diseases was in the making. New and bold techniques were devised for the treatment of congenital and acquired heart disorders as well as for vascular diseases.

Two major developments, which made possible cardiac and aortic surgery, took place at about this time. One was the use of hypothermia, and the other was the introduction of the heart-lung machine for extracorporeal circulation. Although these two advances, especially the latter, were essential to the current progress in heart surgery, their application was equally basic in handling aortic lesions, more particularly those of the thoracic and thoracicoabdominal segments.

Bigelow et al., in 1950, published their experimental results of the effects of hypothermia on the lowering of oxygen consumption and its impact on blood flow through the heart. After refinement of this technique, hypothermia was applied shortly thereafter in the surgical management of a variety of cardiac lesions. In 1954, DeBakey, working with Pontius and others, published their results of the use of hypothermia to prevent paraplegia after temporary aortic occlusion.

Although hypothermia represented a significant advance for the performance of cardiac and aortic surgery,

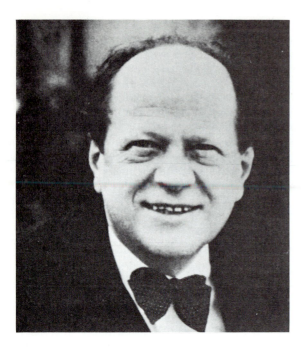

Figure 1-6. René Leriche.

the development of the extracorporeal circulation technique superseded it and offered one of the most dramatic and lasting achievements in the entire field of surgery. Gibbon, in 1937, devised the heart-lung apparatus, which he used in animals. In 1953 he used it to close an atrial septal defect in a young woman. This pioneering effort was followed by numerous contributions that modified, improved, and simplified this technique. In the end, it had completely revolutionized surgery for cardiac and aortic lesions and for pulmonary artery embolism.

Autonomic Physiology and Vascular Surgery. Autonomic surgery played an important role concurrently with arterial surgery. Leriche (Fig. 1-6) was a major advocate of it, and he also devised or influenced the development of many of the pioneering operations for repair of occlusive and aneurysmal lesions.

In 1924, Leriche, as chairman of a major surgical institute in Strasbourg, attracted international attention. Among his many French and foreign assistants, just to name a few, were J. Cid Dos Santos, Michael DeBakey, and Jean Kunlin, all three of whom achieved later pioneering status in their own right through their contributions.

In 1937, Leriche was appointed to the College de France, Paris, where he occupied the prestigious Chair of Claude Bernard. Throughout his career, his interest was focused on the treatment of circulatory problems and related aspects, especially surgery for neurogenic and ischemic pain. Beginning in 1925, he introduced cervical and lumbar sympathectomy, although the latter was reported independently in 1924 by Julio Diez, of Argentina.

Leriche is perhaps best known for his description of the "obliteration of the terminal abdominal aorta," first published in 1923 and again in 1940. It was not until 1950 that Jacques Oudot achieved what Leriche had conceived in 1923: resection of the aortoiliac bifurcation with graft

replacement for the treatment of the syndrome that bears Leriche's name.

Aortic Surgery for Occlusion and Aneurysmal Lesions. Vascular grafting was connected, in a way, with the early phase of surgical correction of congenital cardiac and vascular abnormalities. They are mentioned only as a background to what follows. Indeed, the first arterial transplantation of homografts was carried out for congenital vascular abnormalities by Gross and associates. After extensive laboratory investigation of methods for the preservation and transplantation of arterial grafts, Gross et al., in 1948 and 1949, published the first observations on the use of human arterial grafts in the treatment of coarctation of the aorta and the use of a shunt between the left pulmonary artery and the proximal end of the subclavian artery for tetralogy of Fallot (Fig. 1-7).

The modern phase of vascular grafting truly began with the successful implantation of arterial homografts, as reported by Gross and associates. The impetus provided by these successful applications of grafting procedures led to other, similar innovative uses in other parts of the vascular system.

Jacques Oudot, of Paris, performed the first successful resection of the aortoiliac bifurcation and its replacement with an arterial homograft. As mentioned already, the idea of such a procedure had been conceived by Leriche in 1923. He stated: "The ideal treatment of the thrombosis of the terminal abdominal aorta should consist of resection of the occluded segment and reestablishment of arterial continuity by a graft." Thus the prophecy of 1923 became a reality in 1950.

Dubost, almost concurrently with Oudot's use of homograft replacement for occlusive arterial disease of the aorta, was the first to excise an abdominal aortic aneurysm with

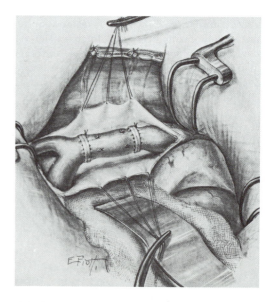

Figure 1-7. Illustration from original article by Gross et al., depicting insertion of human aortic graft after removal of narrowed segment of aorta for treatment of coarctation of the aorta (case 9). (*From Gross RE, et al.: Surg Gynecol Obstet 88:689, 1949.*)

homograft interposition. The excisional technique described by Dubost was subsequently modified by Oscar Creech, who deserves the credit for incorporating some of Matas' principles in dealing with the lumbar vessels and leaving part of the sac to be wrapped around the graft.

Although most of the preceding attempts dealing with peripheral and central aneurysms are of only historic interest today, nevertheless, they provided the impetus and the inspiration to subsequent generations for managing these dreadful conditions. Ultimately, in 1951, excisional therapy for an abdominal aneurysm by Dubost and associates ushered in the current era of curative surgery of aneurysms (Fig. 1-8).

The principle of excisional therapy for abdominal aortic aneurysms was soon to be applied to thoracic aneurysms. Before the use of excisional treatment with graft replacement, there were a few reports of cases of resection of thoracic aneurysms, which consisted of simple saccular aneurysms or aneurysms associated with the coarctation of the aorta. In 1953, DeBakey and Cooley reported the first successful resection of a fusiform thoracic aneurysm with graft replacement. Thereafter, all segments of the thoracic aorta, including the arch, were treated by excision with replacement of homografts. In all these instances, some form of bypass or controlled extracorporeal circulation or hypothermia was used.

Thromboendarterectomy. This procedure, originally designed in 1946 for simple removal of thrombi, turned out to be more than a simple thrombectomy. Because of its impact on the development of vascular surgery, a brief comment on the historical background may provide an insight into how an accidental finding may open a new avenue in scientific thinking.

Disobstruction of occluded arteries by simple thrombectomy was not new at the time. Severeanu in 1880, Jianu in 1909, and Delbet in 1906 and 1911 are credited with attempting thrombectomy for arterial disobliteration. Because these procedures failed almost consistently, the early attempts were relegated to oblivion until 1946, when

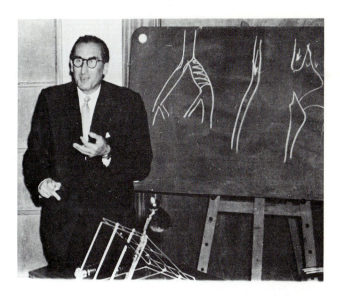

Figure 1-9. J. Cid dos Santos, in Lisbon, 1953, at Second International Cardiovascular Congress, discussing technique of thromboendarterectomy.

J. Cid dos Santos (Fig. 1-9) decided to do this operation under heparin cover, which obviously had been unavailable in earlier attempts. The underlying principles of this technique appeared to be based on a revolutionary idea, since they seemed to negate the prevailing concept, according to which an injured tunica intima leads inevitably to vascular thrombosis. Indeed, unlike embolectomy, in which only the thrombus is removed, in thromboendarterectomy both the thrombus and the endartery (tunica intima and part of the inner tunica media) are excised.

The initial wide usefulness of thromboendarterectomy was displaced by the bypass grafts introduced shortly after the publication of Dos Santos' first cases. More recently, the use of transluminal angioplasty has further encroached on the management of arterial lesions (stenosis or occlusion). However, thromboendarterectomy has certain specific indications, such as for lesions of the carotid artery and visceral arteries and for certain segments of the aorto-iliac system.

Historically, there is little doubt of the impact that thromboendarterectomy provided by originating new concepts in intravascular clotting in the absence of an endothelial lining. Although the procedure, as an operation, seemed to have been displaced by the bypass graft principle, its therapeutic surgical role is valid and useful.

The accidental finding that arterial thrombosis does not necessarily occur after removal of the intimal lining and a portion of the media is a historical landmark and a typical example of serendipity.

The Bypass Principle. Although known only since 1948, the bypass principle was not entirely new. It was first advocated in 1913 by Ernst Jaeger, of Germany, for managing peripheral aneurysms. This principle undoubtedly remained buried in his book (*Die Chirurgie der Blutgeffasse und des Herezens*, p. 262). It was not until 1948 that Jean Kunlin, of Paris, who was an associate of R. Leriche, inde-

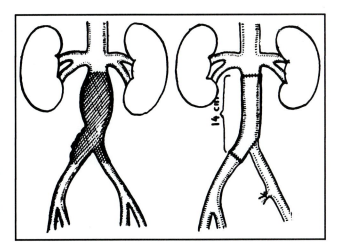

Figure 1-8. Drawing from original article by Dubost, Allary, and Oeconomos, published in 1951, in which they reported first successful resection of abdominal aortic aneurysm and insertion of homograft. (*From Dubost C, et al.: Mem Acad Chir 77:38, 1951.*)

pendently reported this procedure in the management of femoropopliteal occlusive arterial disease (Fig. 1-10).

Until 1948 the conventional technique for managing arterial lesions consisted theoretically of excision of the lesions, with interposition of a graft. The bypass approach was entirely novel and had significant advantages. Its rationale was based on a twofold improvement over the previous techniques: (1) avoidance of operative trauma or damage to adjacent veins or nerves and (2) preservation of collateral vessels. Today, it is widely applied in managing all sorts of arterial lesions, especially those below the groin and those in the coronary arterial location.

Historically, it is of interest to note that the first patient treated by Kunlin with this procedure was a 54-year-old man who had already had an arteriectomy of the superficial femoral artery. The latter procedure was based on Leriche's concept that removal of an occluded arterial segment would result in peripheral vasodilation. The ischemia was not relieved, however, and Kunlin decided to implant a venous graft. Exposure of the previous operative area in the thigh disclosed a tremendous fibrotic reaction around the resected arterial end, thus precluding an end-to-end approach. This left Kunlin with no other alternative but an end-to-side implantation of the venous graft. Thus the bypass procedure was born. This fortuitous decision illustrates another example of a historical landmark in vascular surgery.

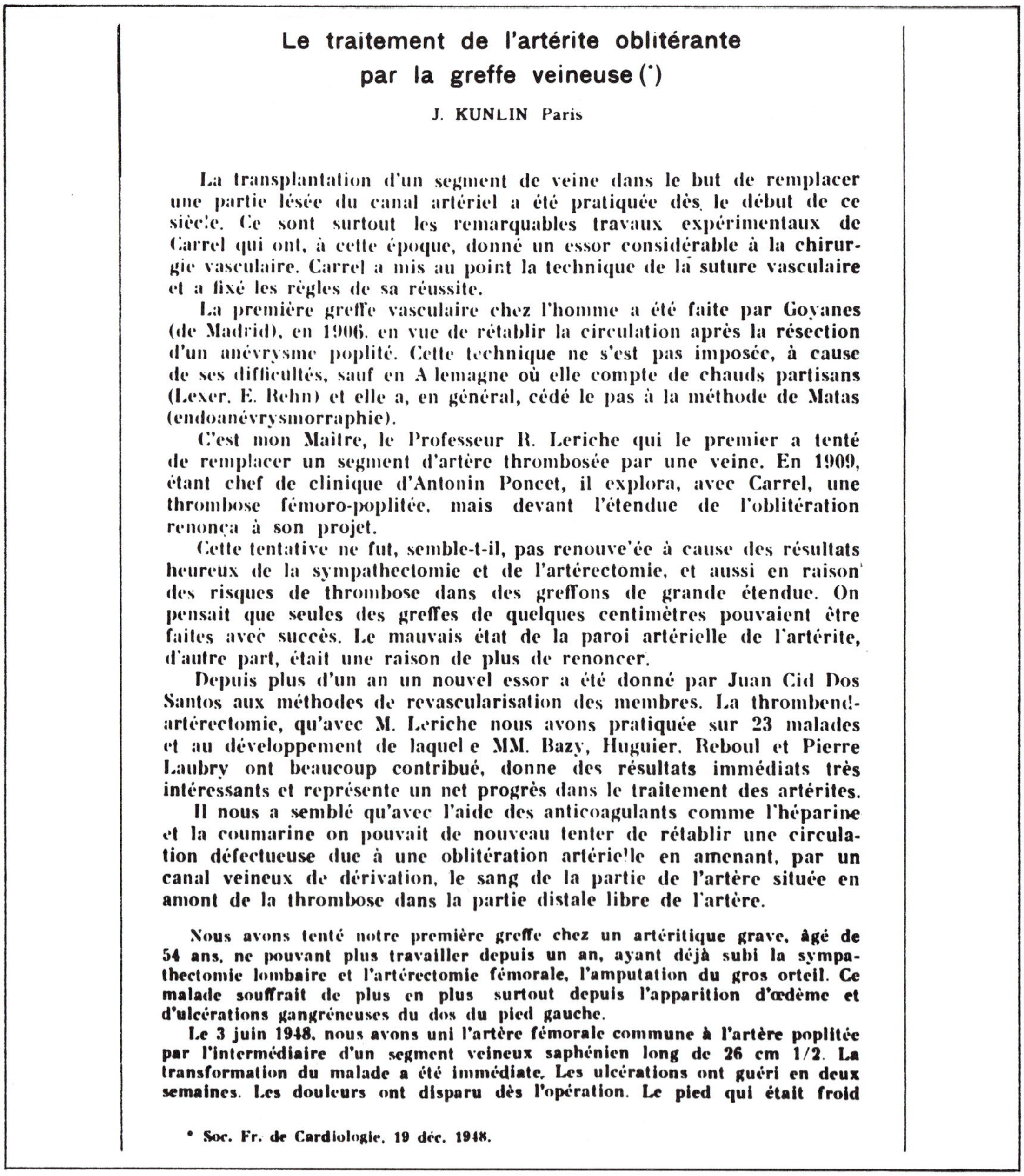

Le traitement de l'artérite oblitérante par la greffe veineuse (*)

J. KUNLIN Paris

La transplantation d'un segment de veine dans le but de remplacer une partie lésée du canal artériel a été pratiquée dès le début de ce siècle. Ce sont surtout les remarquables travaux expérimentaux de Carrel qui ont, à cette époque, donné un essor considérable à la chirurgie vasculaire. Carrel a mis au point la technique de la suture vasculaire et a fixé les règles de sa réussite.

La première greffe vasculaire chez l'homme a été faite par Goyanes (de Madrid), en 1906, en vue de rétablir la circulation après la résection d'un anévrysme poplité. Cette technique ne s'est pas imposée, à cause de ses difficultés, sauf en Alemagne où elle compte de chauds partisans (Lexer, E. Rehn) et elle a, en général, cédé le pas à la méthode de Matas (endoanévrysmorraphie).

C'est mon Maître, le Professeur R. Leriche qui le premier a tenté de remplacer un segment d'artère thrombosée par une veine. En 1909, étant chef de clinique d'Antonin Poncet, il explora, avec Carrel, une thrombose fémoro-poplitée, mais devant l'étendue de l'oblitération renonça à son projet.

Cette tentative ne fut, semble-t-il, pas renouvelée à cause des résultats heureux de la sympathectomie et de l'artérectomie, et aussi en raison des risques de thrombose dans des greffons de grande étendue. On pensait que seules des greffes de quelques centimètres pouvaient être faites avec succès. Le mauvais état de la paroi artérielle de l'artérite, d'autre part, était une raison de plus de renoncer.

Depuis plus d'un an un nouvel essor a été donné par Juan Cid Dos Santos aux méthodes de revascularisation des membres. La thrombendartérectomie, qu'avec M. Leriche nous avons pratiquée sur 23 malades et au développement de laquele MM. Bazy, Huguier, Reboul et Pierre Laubry ont beaucoup contribué, donne des résultats immédiats très intéressants et représente un net progrès dans le traitement des artérites.

Il nous a semblé qu'avec l'aide des anticoagulants comme l'héparine et la coumarine on pouvait de nouveau tenter de rétablir une circulation défectueuse due à une oblitération artérielle en amenant, par un canal veineux de dérivation, le sang de la partie de l'artère située en amont de la thrombose dans la partie distale libre de l'artère.

Nous avons tenté notre première greffe chez un artéritique grave, âgé de 54 ans, ne pouvant plus travailler depuis un an, ayant déjà subi la sympathectomie lombaire et l'artérectomie fémorale, l'amputation du gros orteil. Ce malade souffrait de plus en plus surtout depuis l'apparition d'œdème et d'ulcérations gangréneuses du dos du pied gauche. Le 3 juin 1948, nous avons uni l'artère fémorale commune à l'artère poplitée par l'intermédiaire d'un segment veineux saphénien long de 26 cm 1/2. La transformation du malade a été immédiate. Les ulcérations ont guéri en deux semaines. Les douleurs ont disparu dès l'opération. Le pied qui était froid

* Soc. Fr. de Cardiologie, 19 déc. 1948.

Figure 1-10. First page of original article on bypass graft by Jean Kunlin, published in 1949. (*From Kunlin J: Arch Mal Coeur 42:371, 1949.*)

Dissecting Aneurysms. The first surgical attempt to correct a dissecting aneurysm was made in 1935 by Gurin et al. and the second in 1955 by Shaw. The discovery of the physiopathology of this condition is another example of serendipity. Thus Gurin and colleagues, at operation, found an infiltration of dark blood into the lateral third of the external iliac artery extending as far as could be seen in both directions. When the true lumen of the artery was entered, it was found to be narrowed by dissecting hematoma (aneurysm) and to be completely occluded by an atheromatous mass. The intima and media opposite the atheroma were incised from within the vessel, thus creating an opening into the false lumen of the dissecting aneurysm through which bright arterial blood spurted when the proximal clamp was momentarily released.

This operative maneuver, a purely accidental finding known as "fenestration" of the dissected intima, is performed to allow the blood flow to be rerouted into the normal lumen. After closure of the arteriotomy, pulsations were restored in the extremity. The patient died of renal failure on the sixth postoperative day.

Shaw emphasized the same principle, using the technique of fenestration of the intimal layer of the aneurysm in the abdominal aorta, with establishment of a double-barreled aorta. After repair of the aortotomy, good pulsations were restored in the aorta and peripheral arteries. As in the previous case, the patient died of renal insufficiency on the ninth postoperative day.

The first successful outcome of the surgical management of a dissecting aneurysm was reported during the same year (1955) by DeBakey and associates (Fig. 1-11). Since then, medical management of the arterial hypertension associated with the condition has added a new solution to this problem and is used instead of surgery whenever indicated.

Arterial Embolectomy. Arterial embolectomy, one of the earliest known direct arterial procedures, was first successfully performed in 1911. In spite of the use of anticoagulants and refinement of certain aspects of the technique, it was not until 1963 that arterial embolectomy received its greatest impetus by the introduction of the balloon catheter by Fo-

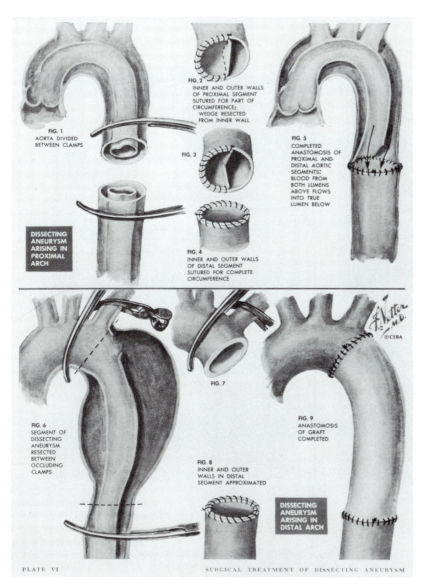

Figure 1-11. Drawings from original article on surgery of aorta by DeBakey, Cooley, and Creech, which appeared in 1956 in the Clinical Symposia series published by CIBA. These illustrations depict two surgical procedures for dissecting aneurysms described by authors in 1955. (*From DeBakey ME, Cooley DA, Creech O Jr: Ann Surg 142:586, 1955.*)

garty. As a result, relief of acute ischemia of the limbs and salvage of life have been greatly enhanced. This instrument is an important part of the surgical armamentarium, and it is widely used in all types of arterial procedures besides embolectomy.

Synthetic Grafts. The shortcomings associated with tissue grafts became readily apparent soon after the introduction of both arterial homografts and autogenous vein grafts. The major difficulties that stood in the way of the large-scale clinical use of tissue grafts were (1) inadequate procurement of homologous arteries, (2) unsuitability of veins in certain vascular areas, and (3) long-term morphologic alteration, sometimes observed in both types of tissue transplants.

It was only natural that when, in 1952, Voorhees, Jaretzki, and Blakemore reported their first observations of successful arterial replacements with synthetic fabric, the prosthetic grafts stimulated an enthusiastic response. In fact, a new phase of vascular surgery was begun, radically altering some of the traditional concepts concerning intravascular thrombogenesis (Fig. 1-12).

Historically, the concept leading to this development was not entirely new. Blood vessel replacement with plastic tubes dates back to the beginnings of experimental vascular surgery. Glass and aluminum tubes lined with paraffin were used by Carrel, and paraffin-coated silver tubes were used by Tuffier in World War I. More recently, many other inert materials, such as Vitallium (Blakemore, Lord, and Stefko), polyethylene, siliconized rubber, steel mesh, and Ivalon, were used either experimentally or clinically for tubing. None of these materials proved entirely acceptable, and the development of prosthetic vessels constructed of synthetic material has subsequently provided the only acceptable nonbiologic graft.

The rationale for the use of plastic prostheses was based on some preliminary observations made by Voorhees et al., who found that, within a few months, a simple strand of silk suture traversing the chamber of the right ventricle of the heart of a dog became coated throughout its length by a glistening film, free of microscopic thrombi. As an outgrowth of this observation, it was conceived that, if arterial defects were bridged by prostheses constructed of fine-mesh cloth, the leaking of blood through the walls of the prosthesis would be terminated by formation of fibrin plugs and would allow the cloth tubes to conduct arterial flow.

These investigators used porous Vinyon "N" cloth tubes implanted in the abdominal aorta of dogs. After 2½ years of laboratory investigation of such grafts, they began

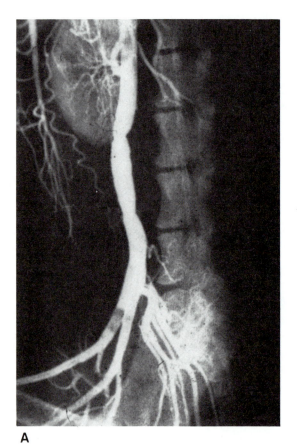

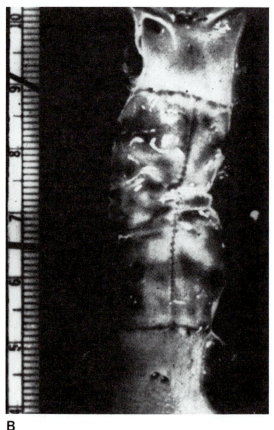

A   B

Figure 1-12. From original article by Voorhees, Jaretzki, and Blakemore, entitled "The Use of Tubes Constructed from Vinyon "N" Cloth in Bridging Arterial Defects," which appeared in 1952. **A.** Retrograde aortogram of cloth tube area; survival time 56 days (prosthesis patent). **B.** Photograph of Vinyon "N" prosthesis on day 115 after implantation in abdominal aorta. Note glistening intimal coat of luminal surface of prosthesis. Longitudinal suture line, made in preparing tube, is visible. (*From Voorhees AB Jr, et al.: Ann Surg 135:332, 1952.*)

to use them clinically in 1953. Thus, in 1954, they reported 18 cases of arteriosclerotic aneurysm (17 abdominal and 1 popliteal) treated by resection and replacement with Vinyon "N" cloth prostheses. They were gratified by the versatility and functional results obtained. A new milestone in vascular surgery had been achieved.

After this report, intensive investigations began in an effort to overcome a number of problems that must be solved before a so-called ideal arterial substitute can be obtained. These investigations are continuing.

Reconstruction of Visceral Arteries. The application of reconstructive arterial procedures in the surgical management of occlusive disease involving the visceral arteries was a natural outgrowth of the experience gained with major peripheral vessels. The specific ischemic manifestations of extracranial cerebral, renal, and mesenteric artery occlusion require special techniques that are usually more complex than those used for vessels of the extremities. The historical background and management of occlusion of visceral arteries will be reviewed in the respective chapters dealing with the various visceral conditions.

Postscript to the History of Arterial Surgery: Perspectives for Tomorrow

The foregoing brief history has attempted to review the pioneering achievements of epoch-making significance that form the basis of what vascular surgery is today. They were spectacular and rewarding in many ways, but they belong already to the past. What are the perspectives for tomorrow? It is best to avoid long-term speculations, but it might be useful to take a closer look at the challenges that will be faced by vascular surgeons in the immediate future.

In the past few years, as a by-product of vascular techniques, interventional radiology using specially designed balloon catheters has been used in the management of stenotic arterial lesions, especially of the coronary, renal, and peripheral vessels. More recently, laser angioplasty has also been attempted for dilation of arteries by the pulverizing of atheromatous plaques. These nonsurgical procedures may offer an alternative to surgery or may be used primarily as adjuncts to the conventional surgical techniques.

The basic challenges of vascular surgery are the problems of arterial abnormalities related to atherogenesis and thrombogenesis, which will continue to be our major biologic concerns for the foreseeable future. Vascular technology will undoubtedly continue to improve and play the major role in the reconstructive modalities of the visceral and peripheral vessels.

The search for better arterial substitutes will remain a top priority. Today, after over four decades, arterial grafts—the centerpiece of vascular surgery—continue to offer a number of challenges that are awaiting solutions. The search for the so-called "ideal" graft has never ceased. Combined massive efforts are being invested in this endeavor by an array of multidisciplinary investigators in the biologic, physicochemical, surgical, and industrial areas. Neverthe-

less, an "ideal" graft seems to have eluded us. Or did it? And if so, why?

It is well known that multiple factors regarding the biologic behavior of grafts and their interplay with the host will determine the long-term fate of any arterial substitute.

Analysis of graft- and host-related factors leaves little doubt that even an "ideal" graft, if available, may not always remain patent for prolonged or indefinite periods, especially because of the intrinsic factors of the host. Unless the atherogenic and other related processes can be controlled, we will have to face the problem of increasing attrition of the integrity of a certain percentage of all types of grafts. Although improved grafts with endothelial cell seeding, providing rapid flow surface and nonthrombogenic lining, may approach the criteria of an ideal arterial conduit, still the overriding question will deal with nonideal host vessels.

Indeed, medicine's greatest challenge, and that of vascular surgery in particular, will be the patient's atherogenic, thrombogenic, and genetic factors. But with better understanding of all the latter elements, and in spite of some limitations, the achievements of vascular surgery will continue to provide the majority of our patients with the means of restoring their body's integrity, improving their life-style, and prolonging their life.

VENOUS SURGERY

Direct reconstructive venous surgery (grafting, thrombectomy), although obeying the basic principles of vascular techniques, is still lagging behind arterial reconstructive procedures. The main reasons reside in fundamental differences in the biologic and hemodynamic characteristics governing the two vascular divisions: arteries and veins. As a result of the morphologic and physiologic differences of veins, long-term venous patency is difficult to achieve. These facts account for the less frequent clinical application of the reconstructive venous procedures.

As mentioned earlier, Eck, in 1877, performed the first successful venovenous anastomosis between the portal vein and the inferior vena cava. This situation was peculiar to this visceral region and does not apply to other areas with different physiopathologic characteristics and demands. Other experimental attempts were reported by another early contribution to venous surgery by Payr in 1904, consisting of a method of uniting divided vessels by invaginating the ends of cylinders of magnesium. Such attempts had rare clinical applications.

In 1902, Carrel published the technique of the circular suture of blood vessels and then, with Guthrie in 1906, reported excellent results with arteriovenous anastomoses in transplantation of organs. However, for a variety of reasons, subsequent reports on vein grafting dealt with either equivocal results or failures.

It was not until the 1940s that renewal of interest in implanting grafts in the venous system was stimulated by the renaissance of arterial grafting. As a result, much experimental work dealt with replacement of all venous segments, including the superior and inferior venae cavae, as well as the peripheral veins. The two major conclusions that emerged from these experimental data were (1) that grafts in the superior vena caval system result in a larger percentage of patency than those in the inferior venae cavae, because of a great tendency in the latter toward thrombosis irrespective of the type of material used, and (2) that autogenous veins appear to be the best graft material in the venous system.

In recent attempts to implant grafts in the venous system, two different concepts have emerged: use of the patient's own vein for bypassing lesions and use of values for transplantation.

1. The use of autogenous veins in the peripheral system seems to have resulted in a more successful outcome in selected cases of postphlebitis syndrome. Crossover saphenous vein grafts, implanted by the technique described by Palma and Esperon, appear to provide relief of venous insufficiency in selected cases of segmental thrombosis of the iliac or femoral veins.

2. In more recent years, in addition to the procedures mentioned above, valvuloplasty or normal vein interposition for chronic venous insufficiency has offered a novel concept of managing insufficiency by replacing the valves themselves. Thus valvular incompetency following deep vein thrombosis is, under certain circumstances, managed directly by dealing with the valvular problem.

In the past decade, several investigators have reported encouraging results with attempts to correct chronic valvular insufficiency. Two methods are being used to that effect: (1) replacement of damaged valves themselves and (2) interposition, as a graft, of a segment of a vein that contains normal valves. Surgical correction of incompetent valves has been reported by several investigators. Kistner and Taheri are the two most active investigators in replacing either valves or segments of veins with normal valves as an interposition segment because of valve incompetence. The results of vein valve transplants, for either acquired postphlebitis syndrome or congenital disorders of valves, appear encouraging, although these procedures are still at an early phase of their application. Further experience is obviously necessary for defining the indications for transplant, the long-term results, and the validity of the conceptual approach to this ubiquitous problem of chronic venous insufficiency.

LYMPHATIC SURGERY

Edema resulting from dysfunction of the lymphatic system is etiologically and clinically distinct from an edema of any other source. Pathologically, it assumes a great variety of forms. As a result, both nonsurgical and surgical treatments are most often elaborate and frustrating.

Lymphedema is characterized by lesions involving the lymphatic vessels of the skin and subcutaneous tissues; the underlying deep tissues, such as muscles, nerves, arteries, and veins, usually remain intact.

In 1952, Kinmonth introduced a method of lymphangiography that helped to establish a more rational classification of the underlying pathologic condition and the corresponding clinical manifestations of lymphedema. Kinmounth thus described aplastic, hypoplastic, hypertrophied or hyperplastic, and varicosed lymphatic vessels.

The original Kinmounth method of lymphography, still reserved for some cases of lymphedema, has been superseded by computed tomography (CT) scanning. It is used primarily to assess the number of pelvic lymph nodes and their size. In addition, CT may offer objective classification of primary lymphedema and may differentiate it from the secondary (neoplastic, inflammatory) type, by the number and size of lymph nodes (O'Donnell).

Thus, because of new concepts regarding the pathophysiology of the lymphatic vessels, newer techniques have evolved, and many of the surgical procedures of the past have been discarded.

When medical measures alone do not suffice to control lymphedema, a surgical approach may be considered. However, in 90% of patients, nonsurgical treatment may be the only management possible. Two basic types of surgical procedures for lymphedema are currently used: (1) the excisional type, in which the markedly edematous subcutaneous tissue is removed and the defects thus created are covered by skin, and (2) the so-called physiologic operations designed to improve lymph drainage. (These procedures are reviewed in Chapter 75.)

Of the new operations based on pathophysiology of the lymphatic vessels, omental transposition, described by Goldsmith and associates, and lymphovenous anastomoses, described by Nielubowicz et al., are rarely applicable (see Chapter 75).

Another recent method of creating lymphovenous anastomoses, described by Degni, consists of implanting lymphatic vessels directly into a vein. This technique seems to offer a better method of lymph drainage.

Unlike the spectacular results obtained with arterial surgery, and to a lesser extent with venous surgery, the procedures devised for the management of lymphedema, because of the complex pathophysiology of this condition, are more elaborate and far less rewarding. If edema and infection can be prevented in the primary lymphedema and also in the secondary inflammatory type, surgical procedures may be rarely necessary.

Many of these operations are still at an experimental stage, and in many instances their results leave much to be desired. For details, see Chapter 75, by O'Donnell and Yeager.

BIBLIOGRAPHY

Barker WF, Cannon JA: An evaluation of endarterectomy. AMA Arch Surg 66:488, 1953.

Bazy L, Huguier J, Reboul H, Laubry P: Techniques des "endarteriectomies" pour arterites obliterantes chroniques des membres inferieurs. J Chir (Paris) 65:196, 1949.

Bernheim BM: The ideal operation for aneurisms of the extremity: Report of a case. Bull Johns Hopkins Hosp 2:7, 93, 1916.

Bernheim BM: Blood-vessel surgery in the war. Surg Gynecol Obstet 30:564, 1920.

Best CH: Heparin and vascular occlusion. Can Med Assoc J 35:621, 1936.

Bier: Chirurgie der gefasse-aneurysmen. Beitr Z Klin Chir 96:556, 1915.

Bigelow WG, Callahan JG, Hopps JA: General hypothermia for experimental intracardiac surgery. Ann Surg 132:531, 1950.

Blakemore A, Lord J: A non-suture method of blood vessel anastomosis. JAMA 127:685, 1945.

Blakemore A, Lord J, Stefko P: The severed primary artery in war wounded: A non-suture method. Surgery 12:488, 1942.

Blakemore A, Voorhees AB Jr: The use of tubes constructed from Vinyon "N" cloth in bridging arterial defects: Experimental and clinical. Ann Surg 140:324, 1954.

Blalock A, Park EA: Surgical treatment of experimental coarctation of aorta. Ann Surg 119:445, 1944.

Blalock A, Taussig HB: The surgical treatment of malformations of the heart where there is a pulmonary atresia. JAMA 128:189, 1945.

Bonin G: Aneurysm durch Schuss-Verletzungen und ihre Behandlung. Beitr Z Klin Chir 97:146, 1915.

Carrel A: La technique opératoire des anastomoses vasculaires et la transplantation des viscères. Lyon Med 98:859, 1902.

Carrel A: The surgery of blood vessels. Bull Johns Hopkins Hosp 18:18, 1907.

Carrel A: Results of the transplantation of blood vessels, organs and limbs. JAMA 51:1662, 1908.

Carrel A: Latent life of arteries. J Exp Med 12:460, 1910.

Carrel A: Resultats Eloignes de la transplantation des veines sur les arteres. Rev Chir 41:987, 1910.

Carrel A: Permanent intubation of the thoracic aorta. J Exp Med 16:17, 1912.

Carrel A, Guthrie GC: Resultats due patching des arteres. C R Soc Biol (Paris) 60:1009, 1906.

Carrel A, Guthrie CC: Anastomosis of blood vessels by the patching method and transplantation of the kidney. JAMA 47:1648, 1906.

Child CG: Eck's fistula. Surg Gynecol Obstet 96:375, 1953.

Clermont G: Suture laterale et circulaire des veines. Presse Med 1:229, 1901.

Cooley DA, DeBakey ME: Surgical considerations of intrathoracic aneurysms of the aorta and great vessels. Ann Surg 135:660, 1952.

Cooley DA, DeBakey ME: Ruptured aneurysms of abdominal aorta: Excision and homograft replacement. Postgrad Med 16:334, 1954.

Cooley DA, DeBakey ME: Resection of entire ascending aorta in fusiform aneurysm using cardiac bypass. JAMA 162:1158, 1956.

Crafoord C, Nylin G: Congenital coarctation of the aorta and its surgical treatment. J Thorac Surg 14:346, 1945.

Crawford ES, DeBakey ME, Fields WS: Roentgenographic diagnosis and surgical treatment of basilar artery insufficiency. JAMA 168:509, 1958.

Davis JB, Grove WJ, Julian OC: Thrombotic occlusion of the branches of the aortic arch, Martorell's syndrome: Report of a case treated surgically. Ann Surg 144:124, 1956.

DeBakey ME, Creech O Jr, Morris GC Jr: Aneurysm of thoracoabdominal aorta involving the celiac, superior mesenteric, and renal arteries: Report of 4 cases treated by resection and homograft replacement. Ann Surg 144:549, 1956.

DeCamp PT, Birchall R: Recognition and treatment of renal arterial stenosis associated with hypertension. Surgery 43:134, 1958.

Degni M: New technique of lymphatic-venous anastomosis for treatment of lymphedema. J Cardiovasc Surg 19:577, 1970.

Delbet P: Chirurgie Arterielle et Veineuse: Les Modernes Acquisitions. Paris, JB Bailiere and fils, 1906, p 104.

Dörfler J: Uber arteriennaht. Beitr Z Klin Chir 25:781, 1899.

Dos Santos JC: Sur la desobstruction des thromboses arterielles anciennes. Mem Acad Chir 73:409, 1947.

Dos Santos R, Lamas A, Pereira CJ: L'arteriographie des membres, de l'aorte et ses branches abdominales. Bull Soc Natl Chir 55:587, 1929.

Dubost C, Allary M, Oeconomos N: A propos du traitement des anevrysmes de l'aorte, ablation de l'anevrysme retablissment de la continuite par greffe d'aorte humaine conserve. Mem Acad Chir 77:381, 1951.

Eastcott HHG, Pickering GW, Rob CG: Reconstruction of internal carotid artery in a patient with intermittent attacks of hemiplegia. Lancet 2:944, 1954.

Eck. Cited in Child CG: Eck's fistula. Surg Gynecol Obstet 96:375, 1953.

Edwards WS: Plastic Arterial Grafts. Springfield, Ill., Charles C Thomas, Publisher, 1957, p 126.

Fogarty TJ, Cranley JJ, et al: A method for extraction of arterial emboli and thrombi. Surg Gynecol Obstet 116:241, 1963.

Gibbon JH Jr: Application of a mechanical heart and lung apparatus to cardiac surgery. Minn Med 37:171, 1954.

Gluck T: Die moderne chirurgie des cirkulationsapparates. Berl Klin 120:1, 1898.

Goyanes J: Nuevos trabajos de chirurgia vascular, substitucion plastica de las arterias por las venas o arterioplastia venosa, applicada, como nuevo metodo, al tratamiento de los aneurismas. El Siglo Med 53:546, 1906.

Gross RE: A surgical approach for ligation of a patient ductus arteriosus. N Engl J Med 220:510, 1939.

Gross RE: Surgical correction for coarctation of the aorta. Surgery 18:673, 1945.

Gross RE: Treatment of certain aortic coarctations by homologous grafts: A report of 19 cases. Ann Surg 134:753, 1951.

Gross RE, Bill AH Jr, Peirce EC II: Methods for preservation and transplantation of arterial grafts: Observations on arterial grafts in dogs—Report of transplantation of preserved arterial grafts in nine human cases. Surg Gynecol Obstet 88:689, 1949.

Gross RE, Hufnagel CH: Coarctation of the aorta: Experimental studies regarding its surgical correction. N Engl J Med 233:287, 1945.

Gurin D, Bulmer JW, Derby R: Dissecting aneurysm of aorta: Diagnosis and operative relief of acute arterial obstruction due to this cause. NY State J Med 35:1200, 1935.

Guthrie CC: Blood vessel surgery and its applications (a reprint), in Harbison SP, Fisher B (eds): Pittsburgh, Pa., University of Pittsburgh Press, 1959, p 360.

Haberer H: Kriegsaneurysmen. Arch Klin Chir 107:611, 1916.

Haimovici H: Ideal arterial graft: An unmet challenge—Scope and limitations [editorial]. Surgery 92:117, 1982.

Haimovici H, Hoffert PW, et al.: An experimental clinical evaluation of grafts in the venous system. Gynecol Obstet 131:1173, 1970.

Haimovici H, Maier N: Experimental evaluation of arterial homografts, in Wesolowsky SA, Dennis C (eds): Fundamentals of Vascular Grafting. New York, McGraw-Hill, 1963, p 212.

Hallowell. In Lambert: Medication Observations and Inquiries, vol II, 1762. Cited by Smith EA: Suture Arteries: An Experimental Research. London, Oxford University Press, 1909.

Hasegawa T, et al.: Use of copolymer graft developed to serve in venous prostheses. Surgery 74:696, 1973.

Herring M, Gardner A, Glover J: A single-staged technique for seeding vascular grafts with autogenous endothelium. Surgery 84:498, 1978.

Howell WH, Holt E: Two new factors in blood coagulation: Heparin and proantithrombin. Am J Physiol 47:328, 1918.

Hurwitt ES, Seidenberg B, Haimovici H, Abelson DS: Splenorenal arterial anastomoses. Circulation 14:532, 1956.

Jaboulay M, Briau E: Recherches experimentales sur la suture et la greffe arterielle. Lyon Med 81:97, 1896.

Jaeger E: Die Chirurgie der Blutgeffasse und des Herzens. Berlin, Hirschwald A, 1931, p 262.

Jassinowsky A: Die arteriennhat: Eine experimentelle studie. Inaug Diss Dorpat, 1889.

Jianu I: Trombectomia arteriala pentru un caz de gangrena uscata a piciorului. Soc de Chirurgie (Bucarest) 27:11, 1912.

Kinmonth JB: Lymphangiography in man: A method outlining lymphatic trunks at operation. Clin Sci 11:13, 1952.

Kistner RL: Surgical repair of the incompetent femoral vein valve. Arch Surg 100:1336, 1975.

Kunlin J: Le traitement de l'arterite obliterante par la greffe veineuse. Arch Mal Coeur Vais 42:371, 1949.

Kunlin J: Letraitement de l'ischemie arteritique par la greffe veineuse longue. Rev Chir 70:206, 1951.

Leriche R: Des obliterations arterielles hautes (obliteration de la terminaison de l'aorte) comme causes des insuffisances circulatoires des membres inferieurs. Bull Mem Soc Chir (Paris) 49:1404, 1923.

Lexer E: Die ideale operation des arteriellen und des arteriovenosen aneurysma. Arch Klin Chir 83:459, 1907.

Lexer E: Zwanzig Jahre transplantationsforschung in der chirurgie. Arch Klin Chir 138:251, 1925.

Malan E: Treatment of chronic obliterative arterial disease with venous autografts. Boll Soc Piemont Chir 22:705, 1952.

Matas R: Traumatic aneurism of the left brachial artery. NY Med News 53:462, 1888.

Matas R: Surgery of the vascular system, in Keen WW, DaCosta JC (eds): Keen's Surgery: Its Principles and Practice, vol 5. Philadelphia, WB Saunders, 1909, p 216.

Merton RK: On the Shoulders of Giants. New York, Harcourt, Brace & World, 1965, p 8.

Moniz E: L'encephalographie arterielle, son importance dans la localisation des tumeurs cerebrales. Rev Neurol (Paris) 2:72, 1927.

Morris GC Jr, DeBakey ME: Abdominal angina: Diagnosis and surgical treatment. JAMA 176:89, 1961.

Murphy JB: Resection of arteries and veins injured in continuity: End-to-end suture—Experimental and clinical research. Med Record 51:73, 1897.

Nielubowicz J, et al.: Surgical lympho-venous shunts. Cardiovasc Surg 9:262, 1968.

Oudot J: La greffe vasculaire dans les thromboses du carrefour aortique. Presse Med 59:234, 1951.

Palma EC, Esperon R: Vein transplants and grafts in the surgical treatment of the postphlebitic syndrome. J Cardiovasc Surg 1:94, 1960.

Payr E: Zur frage der circularen vereinigung von bluntgefassen mit resorbierbaren prothesen. Arch Klin Chir 72:32, 1904.

Seldinger SI: Catheter replacement of the needle in the percutaneous angiography: A new technique. Acta Radiol 39:368, 1953.

Shaw RS: Acute dissecting aortic aneurysm treated by fenestration of the internal wall of the aneurysm. N Engl J Med 25:331, 1955.

Shaw RS, Maynard EP III: Acute and chronic thrombosis of mesenteric arteries associated with malabsorption: Report of 2 cases successfully treated by thromboendarterectomy. N Engl J Med 258:874, 1958.

Shimizu K, Sano K: Pulseless disease. J Neuropathol Clin Neurol 1:37, 1951.

Shumacker HB Jr: Coarctation and aneurysm of the aorta: A case treated by excision and end-to-end anastomosis of the aorta. Ann Surg 127:655, 1948.

Steinman C, Alpert J, Haimovici H: Inferior vena cava bypass grafts. Arch Surg 93:747, 1966.

Stich R, Makkas M, Dowman CE: Beitrage zur gefasschirurgie; cirkulare arteriennaht und gefasstransplantationen. Beitr Klin Chir 53:113, 1907.

Subbotitch V: Kriegchirurgische erfahrungen uber traumatische aneurysmen. Deut Zeitschr Chir 127:446, 1914.

Szilagyi DE, France LC, Smith RF, Witcomb JG: The clinical use of an elastic Dacron prosthesis. AMA Arch Surg 77:538, 1958.

Taheri SA, Lazar L, Elias SM, et al.: Surgical treatment of postphlebitic syndrome with vein valve transplant. Am J Surg 144:221, 1982.

Voorhees AB Jr, Jaretzki A III, Blakemore AH: The use of tubes constructed from Vinyon "N" cloth in bridging arterial defects. Ann Surg 135:332, 1952.

Warthmuller H: Ueber die bisherigen erfolge der gefasstransplantation am menschen. Jena, Diss Neuehahn, 1917.

Wylie EJ: Thromboendarterectomy for arteriosclerotic thrombosis of major arteries. Surgery 32:275, 1952.

CHAPTER 2
Noninvasive Evaluation of Vascular Disease

D. Eugene Strandness, Jr., Yves E. Langlois, and Ghislaine O. Roederer

INSTRUMENTATION

In the last decade, many noninvasive techniques have been developed and used to detect peripheral vascular disease. These techniques permit accurate evaluation of arterial occlusive disease and allow estimation of its physiologic significance. Their use is now an essential part of the evaluation of patients with vascular disease, and physicians who intend to treat these patients should become familiar with these methods. Of all the methods developed, the techniques that employ Doppler ultrasound are the most widely applied and thoroughly evaluated.[1-4]

Doppler Flowmeter

In the assessment of patients with occlusive arterial disease, continuous-wave (C-W) Doppler velocitometers are most commonly used in combination with a blood pressure cuff to measure limb systolic blood pressure. In addition, many laboratories also use C-W Doppler units to record blood flow velocity waveforms from peripheral arteries in the limbs, from extracranial cerebral arteries, and from aortic arch vessels.

Most Doppler ultrasonic instruments used for peripheral arterial studies employ transmitting frequencies in the range of 2 to 10 MHz. Since tissue penetration by ultrasound is inversely related to the transmitting frequency, lower-frequency probes will be best suited for the examination of deep arteries and higher-frequency transducers will be selected for examining superficial vessels.

Doppler ultrasound works on the basic principle that any moving object in the path of the sound beam will shift the frequency of the transmitted signal. The Doppler shift is shown by the following equation:

$$\Delta f = \frac{2f_0 v \cos \theta}{c} \qquad (1)$$

where

$\triangle f$ = frequency shift (hertz)
f_0 = frequency of the transmitted ultrasound (hertz)
v = velocity of the object (cm/sec)
θ = angle of the incident sound beam with the object path (degrees)
c = velocity of the sound in the medium under study (cm/sec)

The simplest commonly used instruments are the pocket-size Doppler units that provide an audio output. These units are satisfactory for simply assessing the presence of arterial or venous flow. For many simple clinical applications, on both the arterial and the venous side of the circulation, audible interpretation of the frequency shift remains adequate. The physician and technician learn to recognize patterns characteristic of normal and diseased states.

Normal peripheral blood velocity waveforms contain forward and reversed flow components. The quantitative assessment of the Doppler signal thus requires a Doppler demodulating scheme that clearly separates these two flow components, even if they coexist.[5] At present, the stereo audible display and the quadrature phase separation are the most commonly used methods to detect the direction of flow.

The pocket-size devices and most of the currently available directional units operate in a C-W mode. Any motion in the path of the beam will produce a frequency shift. Arterial and venous signals are easily distinguished by their different direction and flow characteristics. Venous flow produces low-frequency signals that vary with respiration, whereas arterial flow is associated with relatively high frequency signals that correspond to the cardiac cycle. Superposition of these two signals will result in a summation of the signals and may produce a confusing display.

In the pulsed wave mode, a single transducer may be used as both a transmitter and a receiver. Short bursts of ultrasound are emitted, and a time interval sufficient for the return of the desired echo is allowed before the transducer acts as a receiver. This pulsed mode setup permits the detection of flow from a selected depth along the sound beam, a process called "range gating."[6] The pulsed wave ultrasound devices, therefore, eliminate problems caused by superimposed vessels and permit characterization of flow patterns at specific points within the vessel lumen (Fig. 2–1).

Imaging Systems

The application of ultrasound in vascular imaging can be divided into two large groups: (1) pulsed echo ultrasound and (2) Doppler ultrasound.

B-mode Imaging

The B-mode form of pulsed ultrasound is designed to record characteristics of the reflecting structure under study. The returning echo pulse is shown as a dot on an oscilloscope screen. The strength of the reflection is indicated by its brightness.

In the B-scan method of display, the brightness modulation format of echo presentation is used. The transducer is moved over the surface of the skin in a preselected plane either mechanically or electronically. A two-dimensional cross-sectional picture of the tissue plane can thus be reconstructed on a screen. Real-time ultrasonography recording has been particularly useful in vascular evaluation. In addition to the abdominal aorta and its branches, the inferior vena cava and portal venous system can easily be shown. The method has proved useful also for diagnosing aneurysmal disease of the aortoiliac segment, the common femoral artery, and the popliteal artery[7,8] and allows for the first time an adequate surveillance of these lesions.[9] However, the detection of occlusive disease with B-mode imaging alone has been disappointing.[10]

The Duplex Concept

Blood vessels are easily recognized on a B-mode image by their characteristic prominent wall echoes and dark, sonolucent lumen. Calcified plaques produce bright intraluminal echoes with posterior regions of acoustic shadowing.

Unfortunately, soft noncalcified plaques, thrombi, and flowing blood all have approximately the same acoustic impedance.[11] This limits the gray-scale resolution of B-mode images, making estimation of percent stenosis difficult. It may not even be possible to distinguish between a completely occluded vessel and a patent artery based on the B-mode image alone. Inadequacies of B-mode imaging led to the duplex concept, which combines a pulsed Doppler with a real-time B-mode scanning in one system.[12] The B-mode image is used to localize the artery, recognize anatomic variations, place the pulsed Doppler sample volume within the visualized vessel, and maintain a standard angle of incidence for the sound beam (Fig. 2-2). In this fashion, anatomic and physiologic tests are combined to provide a greater amount of diagnostic information than could be obtained with either one alone.

Doppler Signal Analysis

Two basic analytic methods are most often used to produce a graphic record of the Doppler signal: the zero-crosser system and spectral analysis.

The Zero-Crossing Frequency Meter

The zero-crossing frequency meter is the most commonly used method of processing the Doppler signal because of its low cost and applicability to most clinical situations. It uses a frequency-to-voltage converter that measures the number of zero crossings or cycles in the Doppler signal. This permits the generation of an analog waveform by means of a DC amplifier and a strip chart recorder. However, the system may be affected by errors and artifacts related to signal-to-noise ratio, amplitude dependency, threshold setting, transient responses, and poor directional resolution.[13] Nonetheless, as long as these deficiencies are kept in mind, the zero-crossing detector allows useful qualitative assessment of arterial flow patterns.

Frequency Spectrum Analysis

For effective use of the velocity data acquired with current Doppler devices, it is necessary to employ a method of

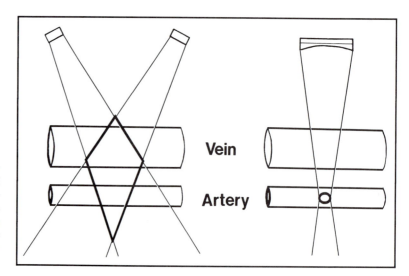

Figure 2-1. A continuous-wave Doppler (*left*) uses two transducers, one emitting and one receiving a continuous mode. The sample volume is the intersection of the two beams (practically all along the emitting beam). In the pulse mode (*right*) only one crystal may be used, and flow is recorded in a more discrete area.

Vein

Artery

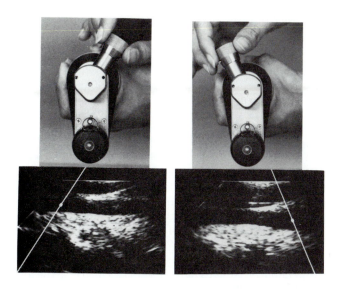

OPERATOR CONTROL OF SAMPLE VOLUME PLACEMENT

Figure 2-2. With a duplex system using a pulsed Doppler unit, it is easy to localize the vessel of interest, place the sample volume in the desired area, and measure the angle of incidence for the Doppler beam. (*From Roederer GO, Langlois YE, Strandness DE Jr: Comprehensive noninvasive evaluation of extracranial cerebrovascular disease, in Hershey FB, Barnes RW, Sumner DS (eds): Noninvasive Diagnosis of Vascular Disease. Pasadena, Calif., Appleton Davies Inc., 1983.*)

signal analysis that displays all information available in the Doppler spectrum. This must include both the absolute frequencies and the amplitudes of the backscattered signals from the moving red blood cells. The simplest and least expensive method uses a zero-crossing detector that provides an envelope of the velocity signal for all times in the pulse cycle. This approach has been widely used but has many practical and theoretical limitations that confine its use to demonstration of the phasic components of arterial flow.

More recently, the fast Fourier transform (FFT) method has been used for accurate portrayal of frequency (velocity), amplitude, and direction of flow. These systems are now a regular component of most ultrasonic systems designed to provide quantitative interrogation of blood flow and information on velocity of blood flow and on the flow pertubations that occur with turbulence.

Plethysmographic Methods

Among the earliest methods devised for measuring blood flow in the extremities, plethysmography remains both useful and accurate.[14,15] In fact, most of our basic knowledge of the physiology and pathophysiology of human arterial and venous disease has been derived from plethysmographic data. This technique also has been widely applied to the diagnostic evaluation of peripheral vascular disease.[16–18]

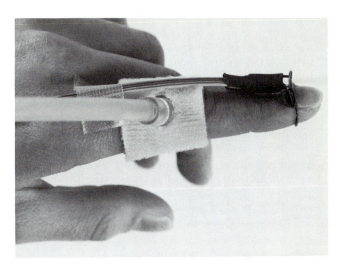

Figure 2-3. A mercury in Silastic strain gauge applied on a finger is used to record the volume pulse. When used in conjunction with a cuff, digital arterial pressure measurements can be made.

Mean blood flow can be measured by recording the rate of increase in volume that occurs as a result of the sudden interruption of venous outflow (venous occlusion plethysmography). Pulsatile information also can be obtained and refers to the transient changes in volume related to the beat-to-beat activity of the left ventricle.

Various plethysmographic instruments exist and can be grouped into five general categories according to their recording characteristics. Some measure volume changes directly by (1) fluid displacement (water filled). Others depend on (2) the compression of air in a closed system (air filled), (3) changes in the circumference of the limbs (strain gauge), (4) changes in electrical resistance (impedance), or (5) the reflection of light from blood cells (photoelectrics).

Plethysmography is particularly recognized as one of the most sensitive available methods for studying digital pressures. Although almost any form of plethysmography can be modified to record digital pulses, the mercury in Silastic strain gauge method is the most appropriate because of its simplicity and high-frequency response (Fig. 2-3).

MEASURING TECHNIQUES AND DATA ANALYSIS IN PERIPHERAL VASCULAR DISEASE

Indirect Arterial Pressure Measurements

In the evaluation of patients with peripheral arterial disease, the noninvasive recording of pressure is the simplest method of assessing functional vascular impairment.[19–23] This technique uses a pneumatic cuff and a flow sensor (a Doppler ultrasonic velocity detector,[24,25] a mercury strain gauge,[16,26] or a photoplethysmograph). Regardless of the type of instrument used, the cuff size applied to the limb is of paramount importance in achieving an accurate reading. A bladder that is too narrow will give erroneously high pressure readings. In general, the bladder size should be 20% wider than the diameter of the limb under study.[27]

Whatever the width of bladder used, one must always be aware of the changes in reading it may cause. In our laboratory, four straight pneumatic cuffs 83 cm long and 11 cm wide with 41 cm long inflatable bladders are used at every level for standardization purposes.

The cuff is placed around the part studied. After the cuff has been inflated above the systolic pressure, it is slowly deflated. The pressure in the cuff when flow reappears is equal to the systolic pressure in the artery underlying the cuff. The resumption of flow is most easily recognized by means of the audio output of a Doppler flowmeter. However, when the Doppler signals are difficult to obtain, it is almost always possible to record a pressure with a mercury in Silastic strain gauge. As the pneumatic cuff is slowly deflated, the digital volume decreases. When systolic pressure is reached, the volume tracing suddenly begins to rise and pulses reappear if they were present before the cuff was inflated.

Ankle Pressure

Ankle pressure measurements provide a simple and reliable means of diagnosing obstructive arterial disease and are easily applicable to follow-up studies. The posterior tibial and dorsalis pedis arteries are readily accessible to Doppler ultrasound. Normally, in the lower limb, peak systolic pressure increases as the pulse wave progresses distally. The finding of an ankle pressure below that of the arm (a difference >10 mm Hg)[28] is good evidence of arterial occlusive disease,[16,21,22,29] and the pressure to which it is reduced is usually proportionate to the severity of the arterial obstruction[20] (Fig. 2-4). The ankle pressure studies can be used to detect operative complications and early failure of an arterial reconstruction and are helpful in predicting healing of ischemic lesions[30] or selecting the optimum site for amputation.[31,32]

Patients with severe arterial occlusive disease and ischemic rest pain usually have resting ankle systolic pressure below 40 mm Hg.[33] Typical ankle-arm pressure gradients, involving superficial femoral artery (SFA) and aorto-iliac (AI) obstruction, are as follows[16]:

Isolated SFA obstruction:	53 ± 10 mm Hg
Isolated AI obstruction:	61 ± 15 mm Hg
Multilevel obstruction:	91 ± 23 mm Hg

Ankle Pressure Index

Since the ankle systolic blood pressure varies with the central aortic pressure, it is most convenient to normalize the value by dividing the ankle pressure by the arm blood pressure.[19,21] This ratio, or ankle pressure index, is normally greater than 1 at rest and averages 1.1 ± 0.10.[19,22,25] Few limbs with hemodynamic significant lesions will have an index greater than 1.0.[19,21,22] In general, limbs with a single occlusive lesion have indexes greater than 0.5, and limbs with multilevel lesions have indexes less than 0.5. The lowest values are obtained when there is impending gangrene, and the highest values are obtained in cases of mild claudication[22] (Fig. 2-5).

Since the ankle pressure index is relatively stable from one examination to the next in the same unchanged individual (SD = 0.06),[34] it provides an effective and precise means of following the patient's course. A consistent decrease in ankle pressure index (>0.15) always indicates a worsening of the arterial disease.[35,36] A spontaneous increase in the

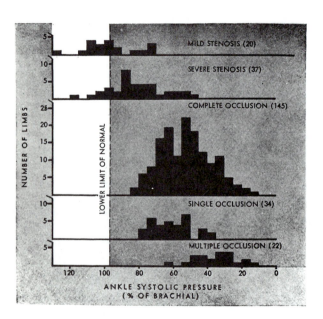

Figure 2-4. Relationship of ankle pressure index to the severity of the occlusive process. (*From Carter SA: JAMA 207:1869, 1969.*)

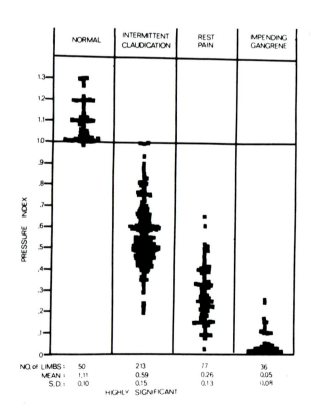

Figure 2-5. When the ankle pressure index is related to the severity of functional impairment, the lowest values are obtained when there is impending gangrene and the highest values in cases of mild claudication. (*From Yao ST: Br J Surg 57:761, 1970.*)

ankle pressure index is usually attributable to the development of collateral vessels.[14,37]

Segmental Pressure

An abnormal ankle pressure index almost invariably indicates the presence of a lesion anywhere proximal to the ankle. Although reduction of the index is proportionate to the severity of the lesion, it cannot determine exact location. This information may best be obtained by studying the systolic pressure at various levels of the limb. These measurements need to be made only when the ankle pressure is abnormal. In our laboratory, four straight pneumatic cuffs 83 cm long and 11 cm wide are applied at high-thigh (HT), above the knee (AK), below the knee (BK), and at ankle level (Fig. 2-6). The systolic pressure is measured at each site by the technique previously described. For all levels of inflation, the Doppler probe is most conveniently placed over the posterior tibial or dorsalis pedis artery. The femoral intraarterial pressure is normally equal to that of the brachial artery.[38] However, in a normal situation, the indirect pressure measurement at the upper part of the thigh exceeds the brachial blood pressure by 30 to 40 mm Hg because of cuff artifacts.[25] A thigh/brachial index exceeding 1.20 indicates that there is no significant aortoiliac occlusive disease.[39] When the index is between 0.8 and 1.2, disease in the aortoiliac segment is usually present but probably not totally occlusive. Indices below 0.8 suggest complete occlusion. Furthermore, the pressure measured in the two thighs should be within 20 mm Hg of each other, and greater differences should raise suspicion of disease proximal to the inguinal ligament.[25,29] Unfortunately, it is now recognized that high-thigh indirect pressure measurements lack the required sensitivity for the detection of aortoiliac disease.[40–43] The simultaneous presence of superficial femoral occlusion with profunda artery disease may give rise to falsely low HT pressures. Other methods using quantitative analysis of the Doppler flow velocity waveform recorded from the common femoral artery can

complement the pressure measurements in assessing the extent of disease in the aortoiliac segment.[44–51]

In the normal leg, the pressure gradient usually does not exceed 20 to 30 mm Hg between any two levels. Gradients greater than 30 mm Hg strongly suggest that a significant degree of arterial obstruction exists in the intervening segment.[16,29] When the artery is completely occluded, the gradient is usually greater than 40 mm Hg (Fig. 2-7).

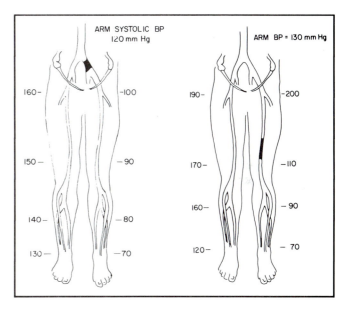

Figure 2-7. A pressure gradient at rest greater than 20 mm Hg between the two thighs indicates a significant stenosis in the iliac artery on the side of the lowest pressure (*left*). Gradients greater than 30 mm Hg at rest suggest a significant stenosis in the intervening segment (*right*). (*From Strandness DE Jr: Peripheral Arterial Disease. Boston, Little, Brown, 1969, p 38.*)

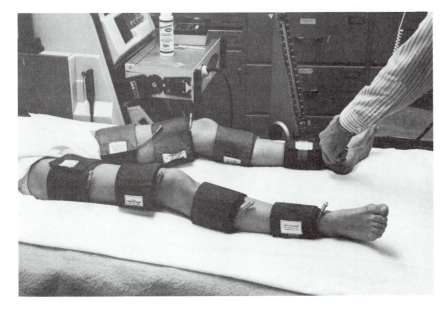

Figure 2-6. Four straight pneumatic cuffs 83 cm long and 11 cm wide are applied at high-thigh, above the knee, below the knee, and at ankle level for measuring segmental arterial systolic pressure. A Doppler flow detector is used over the posterior tibial or dorsalis pedis artery.

Toe Pressure

Toe pressure measurements are used to identify obstructive disease in the digital vessels and in the pedal arch. Normal systolic pressure in the toes is approximately 80 to 90% of brachial artery pressure. A toe/brachial pressure index less than 0.6 is abnormal, and values less than 0.15 are commonly found in patients with rest pain (toe pressure less than 20 mm Hg).[52]

Stress Testing

Reducing the resistance of the peripheral vascular bed by having the patient exercise or by inducing a reactive hyperemia is an effective physiological method for stressing the peripheral circulation.[16] Increasing blood flow in a normal leg creates little or no drop in systolic ankle pressure. However, lesions that may not appear significant at rest can be unmasked during stress testing.[29] When occlusive lesions are present in the main lower limb arteries, blood is diverted through high resistance collateral pathways. Although the collateral vessels may provide adequate flow to the resting extremity with only a modest reduction in ankle pressure, the capacity of these pathways to increase flow during exercise is limited. Pressure gradients that are minimal at rest are accentuated by the stress test, thus providing a good method for detecting less severe degrees of arterial disease.

Treadmill Exercise

Treadmill exercise is the most physiologic method of stressing the arterial circulation. It stimulates the activities responsible for the patient's symptoms and determines the degree of disability under controlled conditions. It also permits an assessment of some nonvascular factors that may affect performance, such as musculoskeletal or cardiopulmonary disease. The ability to perform treadmill exercise is also dependent on the patient's effort, motivation, and pain tolerance.

Walking on a treadmill at 2 miles per hour on a 12% grade is performed for 5 minutes or until symptoms occur and the patient is forced to stop. Both walking time and nature of symptoms are recorded. Arm and ankle systolic pressure are measured before and immediately after exercise. A normal response to exercise is a slight increase or no change in the ankle systolic pressure compared with the resting value. If the ankle pressure is decreased immediately after exercise, the test result is considered positive, and measurements are repeated every 2 minutes for 10 minutes or until the pressure returns to the pretest baseline. The amount of pressure drop and the time of recovery are usually proportionate to the severity of arterial involvement (Fig. 2-8).[23] When a patient is forced to stop walking because of symptoms relative to arterial occlusive disease, the ankle systolic pressure is usually less than 60 mm Hg in the affected side. If symptoms occur without a significant fall in the ankle pressure, a nonvascular cause of leg pain must be considered.[53]

Reactive Hyperemia Testing

Reactive hyperemia is an alternate method for stressing the peripheral circulation.[54] Although less physiologic than the treadmill exercise, it is useful for patients unable to

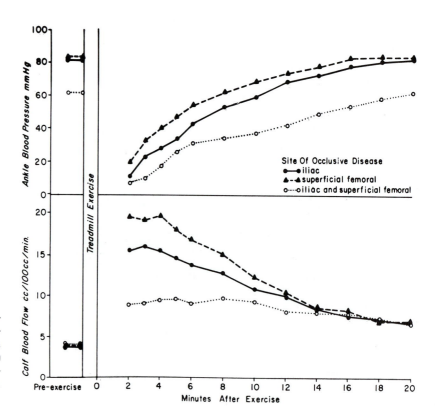

Figure 2-8. Relationship between ankle systolic pressure and calf blood flow after exercise in patients with intermittent claudication. The greatest changes occur in patients with disease at more than one level. (*From Sumner DS, Strandness DE Jr: Surgery 65:763, 1969.*)

walk on the treadmill. Suprasystolic cuff inflation at the thigh level is maintained for 3 to 5 minutes. An ischemic vasodilation ensues, and the resultant changes in ankle pressure can be recorded and interpreted as in the treadmill test.

Doppler Signal Waveform Analysis

A normal velocity waveform in peripheral arteries is characterized by three components (the triphasic response) during each cardiac cycle. The first is a strong, high-frequency signal in the forward direction during systole. It is followed in early diastole by a brief period of reverse flow. Late in diastole, a third small forward-flow component may also be observed. This triphasic flow response can qualitatively be recognized audibly, but a graphic display permits a more objective analysis. These waveforms are characteristic of peripheral arteries that feed vascular beds of relatively high resistance.[3,4,50,51]

It is important to recognize that each organ and vascular bed has its own normal velocity "signature" that characterizes its functional state. For example in all vascular beds of low resistance (brain, kidney, liver), a high-volume flow is required. These can be characterized as low resistance organs. The velocity patterns are quasi steady, and flow normally never reverses at any point during the pulse cycle (Fig. 2-9). On the other hand, organs such as the small intestine will vary their resistance to flow depending on the time the study is done. For example, in the fasting state, flow in the superior mesenteric artery has a prominent reverse-flow component. Within several minutes of eating, the flow to the gut goes up and the reverse-flow component disappears.[55] The importance of these observations will become more evident later in the discussion.

With the availability of both an ultrasonic image and pulsed Doppler in which the angle of insonation is known, it is possible to determine absolute values for velocity parameters. In the normal adult, the peak systolic velocity in the abdominal aorta is in the range of 100 cm/sec. As one moves peripherally, this value gradually decreases to a range of 70 cm/sec in the popliteal artery.[56]

To document the presence of arterial narrowing or occlusion by waveform analysis, one may use several approaches. The first is to examine specific arterial sites, such as the common femoral artery and the popliteal and tibial

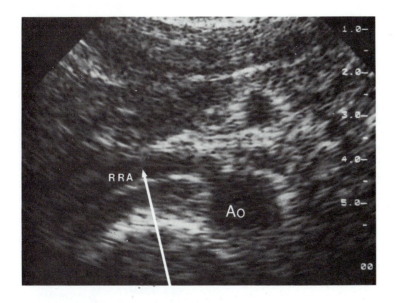

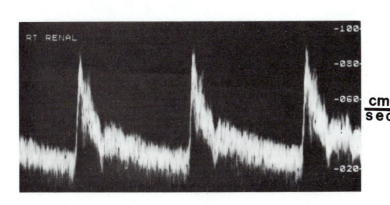

Figure 2-9. For low-resistance organs such as the kidney, flow should never go to zero at any point in the pulse cycle. As shown, the end-diastolic frequency does not return to the baseline (zero flow point). Compare with the triphasic waveform shown in Figure 2–10, which is typical of flow into a high resistance bed such as the lower limb. (*From Taylor DC, Kettler MD, et al.: J. Vasc Surg 7:363, 1988.*)

triphasic   **biphasic**   **monophasic**

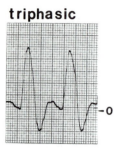 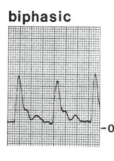 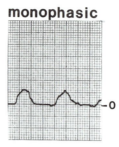

Figure 2-10. The analog waveform of a normal peripheral artery is characterized by a triphasic response (*left*). Biphasic signals (*middle*) are sometimes observed in the absence of disease, especially in distal arteries or in the brachial artery or when the peripheral resistance is low. Distal to a stenosis, the waveform becomes monophasic (*right*).

arteries at the ankle.[22,25,41,45,46] When used in this fashion, the recorded velocity waveforms may tell the observer something about the status of the arteries proximal to the recording site but cannot be used to localize the site precisely (Fig. 2-10). The manner in which this approach is used will be considered next.

Parameters Derived from Doppler Velocity Waveform

It is important to realize that the detected frequency shift cannot be used to calculate the flow velocity unless the angle of the incident sound beam with respect to the flow stream is precisely known. The subjective, qualitative nature of velocity wave interpretation was partially overcome by Gosling et al.,[44,57–59] who introduced a semiquantitative method for the interpretation of velocity waveforms. This method calculates (1) the pulsatility index—the ratio of peak to peak flow velocity over mean forward flow, (2) the damping factor—the ratio of two adjacent pulsatility indices, and (3) the transit time—the time from one velocity pulse to the most distally monitored pulse. As with many other ratios, these indexes have the advantage of being independent of the incident angle of the sound beam relative to the vessel.

Pulsatility Index
The pulsatility index (PI) is calculated by dividing the peak-to-peak frequency difference by the mean forward frequency (Fig. 2-11). This index can be measured on the analog waveform and expressed as the peak-to-peak pulsatility index,[45–51,59–61] as follows:

$$PI = \frac{\text{Peak-to-peak velocity}}{\text{Mean velocity}}$$

The index based on Fourier amplitude of the maximum instantaneous velocity is a more sophisticated approach to quantitate the degree of waveform dampening.[44,59,60] The ratio of the amplitude of each harmonic (An) to the mean amplitude of the wave (Ao) determines the Fourier pulsatility index:

$$PI_f = \frac{An^2}{Ao^2}$$

Today, small microprocessors are available to calculate instantaneously and automatically the Fourier pulsatility index. This method can now be used practically for routine clinical application.

There is a close correlation between the reduction of pulsatility indexes and the severity of peripheral arterial disease, as assessed by standard techniques, such as ankle pressure measurement, arteriography, and limb blood flow.[47,59,62] In a normal femoral artery, the PI is over 4, with a mean of 6.7. More distally, the PI increases to 8 for the popliteal artery and 14.1 for the posterior tibial artery.[58] In the presence of an occlusion or a stenosis, the PI distal to the site of disease decreases.

Damping Factor
The damping factor is the ratio of pulsatility indexes proximal and distal to a stenosis. It can be used to assess the severity of disease, since it increases according to the extent of obstruction in the intervening segment.[45,63]

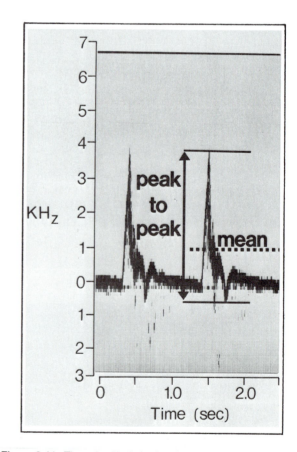

Figure 2-11. The pulsatility index is calculated by dividing the peak-to-peak frequency difference by the mean forward frequency.

Transit Time

This measurement assesses the time taken by a pulse wave to travel from the heart to an artery (e.g., heart to common femoral artery transit time) or through an arterial segment (segmental transit time).[64] The ECG is the time reference used for the transit time calculation. Sensitive to both proximal and distal disease, this method has not proved useful in clinical practice.[65]

Other approaches in the quantitative analysis of the Doppler velocity waveforms seem to hold promise of a better evaluation of arterial disease in the lower limbs.[66–71]

EVALUATION OF EXTRACRANIAL CAROTID DISEASE

Because of limitations with indirect testing, direct testing is now preferred in the assessment of extracranial carotid artery disease. These tests use information obtained directly from the extracranial portion of the carotid artery system and include (1) bruit analysis, (2) Doppler flow imaging, (3) B-mode imaging, both with and without Doppler flow detection, and (4) analysis of Doppler signals by either spectrum analysis or analysis of the velocity waveform.

Bruit Analysis

The stethoscope has always provided interesting clues as to the existence of arterial stenoses. This is particularly true for the carotid and peripheral arteries, where the finding of a bruit has often been the initial sign that serious and potentially dangerous degrees of narrowing might be responsible for the finding.

From a clinical standpoint, a few relevant points about bruits are important to keep in mind. These points are as follows:

1. Bruits represent vibrations of the arterial wall.
2. Whereas turbulence occurring because of arterial narrowing may be the necessary prerequisite for producing a bruit, the sound heard is not from the turbulent flow itself. This is a common misconception!
3. Bruits are transmitted downstream from their origin.
4. Bruits are not transmitted proximal to the site of stenosis.
5. The character of the bruit is not sufficiently distinct to permit a prediction of the degree of stenosis.
6. They should not be used in and of themselves as an indication for arteriography.
7. Bruits—particularly in the carotid arteries—appear to be most predictive of disease in the coronary arteries. However, they have not been useful in predicting the occurrence of ischemic events on the side of the detected bruit. All one can say is that the risk of stroke is higher in patients who are found to have bruits.

Because the stethoscopic evaluation of bruits is inadequate, there have been attempts to quantify these findings to predict the degree of stenosis. One of the most successful was that proposed by Duncan et al.,[72] who used FFT spectral analysis of phonoangiographically detected carotid bruits. The theory predicted that there is a single break frequency beyond which the intensity of the frequencies rapidly declines (Fig. 2-12). Further, this break frequency should be predictive of the residual lumen of the stenotic vessel giving rise to the bruit.[73] The validity of this approach was tested in our laboratory. The size of the residual lumen diameter at the site of the stenosis agreed within 1 mm of the angiography in 85% of the cases studied.[74]

The major problem with this approach is that not all patients with carotid disease have bruits. This is a serious problem that limits the usefulness of the approach. In addition, the expression of residual lumen diameter has very little clinical relevance at the present time. Rightly or wrongly, surgeons are used to thinking in terms of diameter reduction, and it is unlikely that this approach will supersede the time-honored one.

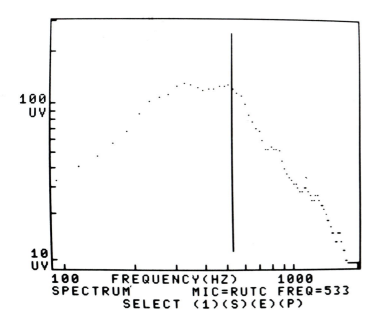

Figure 2-12. A smoothed averaged spectrum of a carotid bruit recorded with a microphone can be used to locate the break frequency. That break frequency can be related to a residual lumen of a stenotic vessel. (*From Roederer GO, Langlois YE, Strandness DE Jr, in Hershey FB, Barnes RW, Sumner DS (eds): Noninvasive Diagnosis of Vascular Disease. Pasadena, Calif., Appleton Davies Inc., 1983.*)

B-mode Imaging

Numerous attempts have been made to apply pulse-echo ultrasound to carotid artery imaging. A real-time, high-resolution B-mode scanner was specially designed for application to the neck at the Stanford Research Institute and clinically tested at the Mayo Clinic.[75] Although interpretable data were obtained in 95% of the cases, agreement with angiography was found in only 6 of the 19 studies (32%). Difficulties were encountered in distinguishing lesions from intraluminal artifacts, in estimating the precent stenosis, and in differentiating between high-grade stenosis and occlusion. Using the same device, Leopold and Bernstein[10] reported a sensitivity of only 27% in predicting more than 50% diameter reducing stenoses. The ability to recognize totally occluded vessels is reported to range from 18 to 29%.[76,77] The most comprehensive study of B-mode imaging alone was that done by Comerata et al.[78] The lesions were subdivided by degree of stenosis (0 to 29%, 40 to 69%, 70 to 99%, occlusion). The predictive value was highest for the early lesions (97%) and poorest for the high-grade stenoses (76%) and total occlusions (84%). Today, most of the commercially available B-mode scanners used in the diagnosis of carotid disease incorporate some form of Doppler detection.

Ultrasonic Duplex Scanner with Spectral Analysis

First introduced by Barber et al.,[12] the duplex scanning concept combines a real-time B-mode scanner and a pulsed Doppler device. The device used in our laboratory employs three fixed-focus 5 MHz transducers imbedded in a rotating wheel, generating a two-dimensional sector image of soft tissue interfaces. The B-mode image is used solely to identify the carotid arteries, localize calcified plaques, recognize anatomic variations, place the sample volume of the pulsed Doppler in the center stream of the vessel, and maintain a standard angle of incidence for the Doppler beam. When the B-mode image is frozen, one of the crystals is used as a pulsed Doppler (Fig. 2-13). The orientation of the Doppler beam and the sample volume location are displayed on the B-mode image. The Doppler velocity pattern can then be recorded from selected points along and across the bifurcation and be analyzed. Correct identification of the common carotid artery and its branches is essential. The study begins low in the neck to identify the common carotid artery. The transducer is then moved cephalad to the level of the carotid bulb and bifurcation. By small adjustments of the scan plane, the origin of the internal and external carotid arteries can be visualized, with the external artery lying anteromedial to the internal. Imaged vessels are identified by their anatomic location and, most importantly, by the characteristics of their Doppler flow signals (Fig. 2-14). In the normal internal carotid, flow is quasi steady and remains above zero throughout the entire cardiac cycle because of the low resistance of the cerebral circulation. This can be easily distinguished from the flow pattern in the external carotid artery, which transiently goes to zero or reverses in early diastole, similar to any other high-resistance periph-

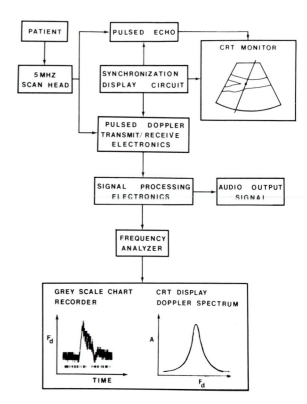

Figure 2-13. Diagram of a duplex scanner. (*From Roederer GO, Langlois YE, Strandness DE Jr, in Hershey FB, Barnes RW, Sumner DS (eds): Noninvasive Diagnosis of Vascular Disease. Pasadena, Calif., Appleton Davies Inc., 1983.*)

eral artery. The common carotid flow pattern normally resembles that of the internal carotid artery.

In addition to the audible interpretation, the directional quadrature outputs are sent to an on-line spectrum analyzer employing a real-time FFT method. The spectrum analyzer provides 400 spectra per second, with a frequency resolution of 100 Hz. A hard copy output of the spectral analysis is obtained on a gray-scale strip chart in the form of frequency-time waveforms, with the amplitude of the backscattered signal expressed in levels of gray. The total frequency is 10 kHz, with 7kHz for forward flow and 3 kHz for reversed flow. The sites from which velocity patterns are routinely recorded for analysis are the low common carotid artery, the high common carotid at the bifurcation, the proximal and distal internal carotid, the external carotid, and, finally, any sites along the bifurcation where high-velocity signals are detected (Fig. 2-15).

Internal Carotid Artery

Clinical validation of this technique was based on five angiographic categories associated with characteristic changes of the pulsed Doppler signal. With a disease classification scheme based on peak systolic frequency and spectral width from the internal carotid spectra, early results of duplex scanning from this laboratory showed a sensitivity of 94%, whereas the ability to detect normalcy (specificity) ranged from 8 to 36%.[79–81]

Two important points emerged from those studies. First, a transducer with a short focal length is more appropriate for arteries, such as the carotid bifurcation, which lies within 2 cm of the skin surface in the majority of subjects. Second, the smaller the size of the sample volume with respect to the diameter of the vessel, the more discrete

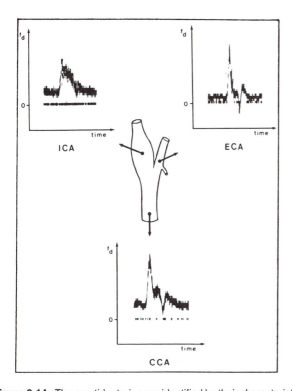

Figure 2-14. The carotid arteries are identified by their characteristic flow patterns. The external carotid artery (ECA) shows a triphasic pattern as with any other peripheral artery. The internal carotid artery (ICA) and common carotid artery (CCA) show a quasi-steady flow with diastolic flow well above the zero baseline. (*From Roederer GO, Langlois YE, Strandness DE Jr, in Hershey FB, Barnes RW, Sumner DS (eds): Noninvasive Diagnosis of Vascular Disease. Pasadena, Calif., Appleton Davies Inc., 1983.*)

will be the range of velocity detected, resulting in a lesser degree of spectral broadening.[81–82] Consequently, the development of a transducer with a focal length of 2 cm and a sample size of 3 mm^3 increased the specificity of the studies to 50%, yet maintaining a sensitivity of 99%.[80–81]

The specificity was further improved by the recognition of the flow patterns that occur in the normal bulb and can be interpreted as abnormal.[83] With increasing experience, we have come to recognize that velocity patterns from the common carotid artery may be important predictors of disease in the internal carotid artery.[84]

The peak systolic maximum frequency (*a*) and the maximum frequency at the point of first zero slope after peak systole (*b*) are measured from the low common carotid velocity waveform (Fig. 2-16). The ratio (*a*−*b*)/*a* thus calculated for each side is used to characterize the low common carotid waveform. A ratio value over 0.5 is associated with a normal internal carotid artery.[84,85] The angiographic categories and the combination of spectral changes used to define them are as follows (Fig. 2-17):

1. Normal: a common carotid artery waveform with a ratio greater than 0.5, an internal carotid artery spectrum with a peak frequency below 4 kHz, and no or minimal spectral broadening during the decelerating phase of systole (Fig. 2-18)
2. Minimal lesion (1 to 15% diameter reduction): a common carotid artery waveform with a ratio (a−b)/a below 0.5, an internal carotid artery spectrum with peak frequency below 4 kHz, with minimal or even no spectral broadening during the decelerating phase of systole (Fig. 2-19)
3. Moderate lesion (16 to 49% diameter reduction): an internal carotid artery spectrum with peak frequency below 4 kHz, with increased spectral broadening during systole until the whole window is filled (Fig. 2-20)
4. Severe lesion (50 to 79% diameter reduction): an internal carotid artery with a peak frequency greater than 4 kHz (corresponding to a velocity of 125 cm/sec) and an end-diastolic frequency of less than 4.5 kHz (corresponding to a velocity of 140 cm/sec) (Fig. 2-21)
5. Preocclusive stenosis (80 to 99% diameter reduction: an end-diastolic frequency exceeding 4.5 kHz (principal di-

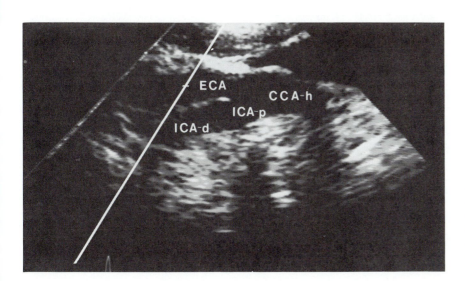

Figure 2-15. Flow is routinely recorded from the low common carotid artery, the proximal internal carotid (p-ICA) and distal internal carotid artery (d-ICA), the external carotid artery (ECA), and, finally, any site along the bifurcation where high-frequency responses are encountered.

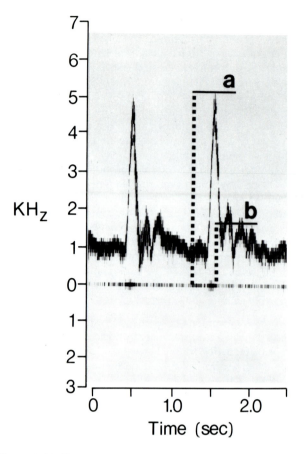

Figure 2-16. The peak systolic frequency (a) and the maximum frequency at the point of first zero slope (b) are used to measure the (a−b)/a ratio from the low common carotid artery waveform.

agnostic feature), representing a greater than 140 cm/sec velocity and establishing the diagnosis (Fig. 2-22)

6. Occlusion: a flow to zero in the common carotid artery and no signal recorded from the internal carotid artery (key elements) (Fig. 2-23).

With the use of these features, a prospective validation of the duplex studies was done in 336 sides.[85] The results obtained by duplex scanning and spectral analysis were compared with biplanar contrast arteriography and are summarized in Table 2-1. Of the 56 normal sides, 47 (84%) were correctly classified. Forty-nine (80%) of the 61 lesions with a 1 to 15% stenosis, 62 (78%) of the 80 lesions with a 16 to 49% stenosis, and 91 (91%) of the 100 sides with a 50 to 99% diameter reduction were correctly classified. All the occluded sides were detected, except one side in which a signal consistent with a 50 to 99% diameter reducing lesion was detected. The specificity of the method increased to 84% and the sensitivity to 99%. Furthermore, spectral analysis correctly classified, in each of the five categories, 287 sides out of 336, for an overall accuracy of 85%, which makes this method the most accurate of all the noninvasive tests developed to evaluate disease at the carotid bifurcation. In addition, spectral analysis of the pulsed Doppler velocity waveform is one of the few noninvasive methods that have shown the capability to discriminate normal arteries from minimal disease, minimal disease from severe disease, and severe disease from occlusion. Spectral analysis is now recognized as a prerequisite for tests intending to diagnose the lesions responsible for cerebral ischemic symptoms, because nearly half of these plaques will reduce the lumen diameter by less than 50%.[86]

In the original studies using duplex scanning, only the 50 to 99% stenosis category was part of the screening classification. However, because it appeared that the higher-grade lesions (>80%) might be the most dangerous clinically, we searched for additional algorithms to make this separation. The simplest appeared to be the end-diastolic frequency (>4.5 kHz—equal to 145 cm/sec).[87] We now use

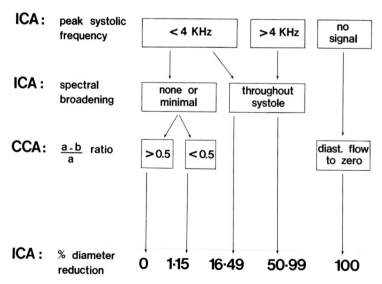

Figure 2-17. Decision algorithm for the disease classification in the internal carotid artery (ICA) with the use of spectra from the ICA and the common carotid artery (CCA).

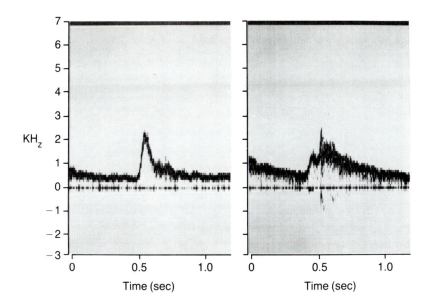

Figure 2-18. Typical normal common carotid artery (*left*) as defined by the (a−b)/a ratio, feeding a normal internal carotid artery (ICA) (*right*). The ICA waveform (*right*) is consistent with a transient flow reversal frequently observed in the normal proximal ICA.

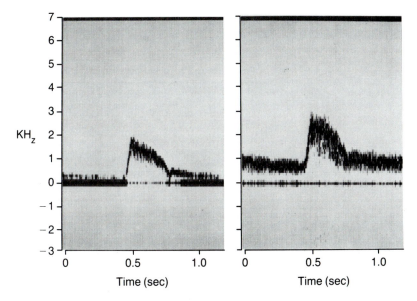

Figure 2-19. Typical abnormal common carotid artery waveform (*left*) feeding an internal carotid artery (*right*) with mild disease (1 to 15% diameter reduction) by angiography.

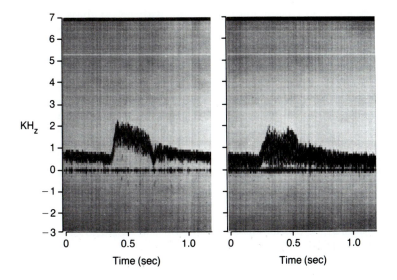

Figure 2-20. Typical abnormal common carotid artery waveform (*left*) feeding an internal carotid artery (*right*) with moderate disease (16 to 49% diameter reduction) by angiography.

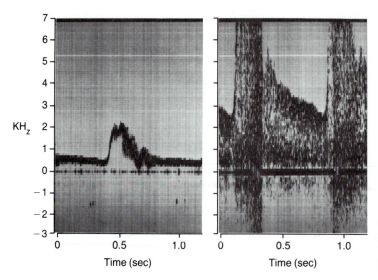

Figure 2-21. Typical abnormal common carotid artery waveform (*left*) feeding an internal carotid artery (*right*) with severe disease (50 to 99% diameter reduction) by angiography.

this routinely and have found it to be useful in selecting those patients who appear to be at greatest risk for the development of transient ischemic attacks, strokes, and total occlusions.[88]

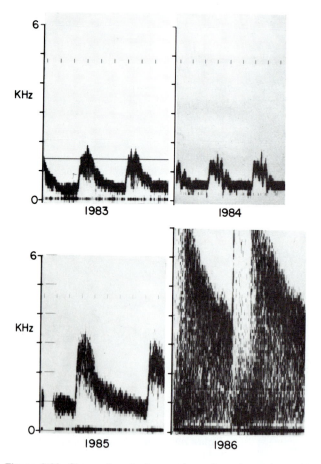

Figure 2-22. Change in velocity waveforms in an internal carotid artery between 1983, when artery was essentially normal, and 1986, when a greater than 80% stenosis was found.

Other Arteries of the Neck

Duplex scanning with spectral analysis of the pulsed Doppler signal also proved to be accurate in estimating the extent of disease at the origin of the external carotid artery. With three categories, 0 to 49%, 50 to 99%, and 100% diameter reduction, the agreement between spectral analysis and angiography is 86%.[89]

The ultrasonic velocity detector can also be helpful with lesions of the vessels at the arch level. It is a simple matter to locate the common carotid artery at the base of the neck and to compare the arterial velocity signals between the two sides. A significant stenosis or occlusion on one side will result in a reduction in the peak velocity that can be readily recognized on the recording. Of course, lesions involving the subclavian or innominate arteries are more easily suspected by physical examination. If the innominate artery is significantly narrowed or occluded, the blood pressure in the right arm will be low and the common carotid pulse will be reduced. Similarly, a subclavian arterial stenosis will create a pressure gradient (>20 mm Hg) between the two arms.

Problems relating to the vertebrobasilar system will occur most commonly with regard to an atherosclerotic process involving the origin of the vertebral artery, shunting of blood away from the basilar artery in cases of subclavian or innominate arterial occlusion, and intermittent obstruction of the vertebral artery as a result of osteophytes in the intervertebral foramina. Once again, noninvasive testing is particularly useful in demonstrating some of the functional changes that are occurring and that may be responsible for the patient's symptoms.

When the posterior circulation is involved, the patient is most likely to have vertigo, visual disturbances, and drop attacks. The first and simplest diagnostic test is to measure blood pressure in both arms. If the blood pressures are normal and equal, it is unlikely that there is reversal of flow in the vertebral artery. When a pressure difference is detected between the arms, it is useful to assess the direction of flow in the vertebral artery by means of a directional ultrasonic velocity detector. Although not essential, the use

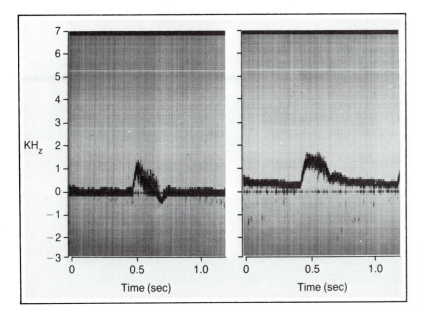

Figure 2-23. Waveforms from a low common carotid artery feeding an occluded internal carotid artery (*left*) and from the contralateral common carotid artery feeding a patent internal carotid (*right*).

of the duplex scanner allows easy localization of the vertebral arteries and discrete sampling of flow at their origin.

The relevance of lesions in the vertebral arteries or of a reversal of flow caused by a subclavian artery occlusion for clinical events has always been a source of confusion. In our studies, we were able to identify 43 patients who were found to have reversal of flow in the vertebral artery at the time of duplex scanning. The patients could be subdivided into four groups based on the following findings: (1) subclavian steal, (2) nonhemispheric symptoms, (3) hemispheric symptoms, and (4) asymptomatic. In this group, 33% were without symptoms, and only 7% had the classic syndrome of nonhemispheric symptoms brought on by exercise of the ipsilateral arm. This is of interest because arm exercise was proposed as the classic method of inducing ischemia of the brain stem on the side of the flow reversal.

An interesting subgroup of patients was termed the "pre-steal" group, in whom both forward flow and reverse flow were found during each cardiac cycle. This phenomenon was found in 21% of the patients studied, mainly in the group with nonhemispheric symptoms. For those patients with hemispheric symptoms and a steal, carotid endarterectomy was successful in reversing the symptoms.

TABLE 2-1. AGREEMENT BETWEEN DUPLEX SCANNING RESULTS AND CONTRAST ANGIOGRAPHY

Angiog- raphy	Duplex					
	A	B	C	D	E	Total
Normal	47	9				56
1–15%	4	49	8			61
16–49%		14	62	4		80
50–99%		1	7	91	1	100
100%				1	38	39
Total	51	73	77	96	39	336

One of the asymptomatic patients with a documented steal developed symptoms. No strokes could be attributed to vertebrobasilar insufficiency. It is clear that retrograde vertebral artery flow, in and of itself, has no clinical relevance in most patients in whom it is detected.

Direct Interrogation of Peripheral Arterial Segments
With the availability of duplex scanners with lower transmitting frequencies, it is possible to assess arterial segments directly from the level of the abdominal aorta to below the knee. This requires adequate sonic penetration to provide both an image and a Doppler signal. It must be emphasized that at greater depths the image quality is not optimal, so the observer must depend entirely on the Doppler velocity information for the detection and grading of stenosis severity.

The accuracy of this approach was studied prospectively in a series of 30 patients (338 arterial segments) to assess the accuracy of duplex scanning against arteriography.[56] In this study, the variability in reading arteriograms was also tested by comparing the results of one angiographer against those of another. The segments evaluated included (1) the iliac, (2) the common femoral, (3) the profunda femoris, (4) the superficial femoral, and (5) the popliteal. The criteria used for disease classification were based on the velocity data obtained from the arterial segments as the pulsed Doppler sample volume was moved along the course of the vessel at the center-stream sites. The criteria tested in this study were as follows:

1. Normal artery: a triphasic waveform without spectral broadening
2. Wall irregularities (1 to 19% stenosis): maintenance of triphasic flow, no increase in peak velocity but with spectral broadening
3. 20 to 49% stenosis: reverse flow maintained, but peak systolic velocity increased by at least 30% of that recorded from an immediately adjacent proximal site

TABLE 2-2. AGREEMENT BETWEEN DUPLEX SCANNING AND ANGIOGRAPHY FOR 338 ARTERIAL SEGMENTS

Sensitivity	Specificity	Positive Predictive Value	Negative Predictive Value
Normal versus abnormal			
96%	81%	92%	91%
<50% versus >50% stenosis			
77%	98%	94%	92%

4. 50 to 99% stenosis: loss of reverse flow with an increase of at least 100% in the peak systolic velocity
5. Occlusion: no flow from a visualized segment

The results from this study in distinguishing lesions that reduce diameter more than 50% from lesser degrees of stenosis are summarized in Table 2-2. The findings of one angiographer compared with those of another for the same arterial segments are shown in Table 2-3. The results of this study suggest that duplex scanning is as accurate as angiography in defining the status of peripheral arterial segments of importance to the vascular surgeon.

Quantitative Spectral Analysis

A sophisticated computer-based velocity waveform pattern recognition method was recently developed to eliminate interpreter bias in the evaluation of the velocity spectra and to expand the diagnostic capabilities of quantitative spectral analysis. This method involves the use of computer-selected waveform parameters that are used in a three-step decision process to classify disease of the internal carotid artery into four categories of stenosis.[90–92]

The pulsed Doppler signals from the common carotid artery and the proximal internal carotid artery at the site of maximal audible disturbance of flow were recorded on audiotape together with a simultaneous recording of the ECG. The recording, consisting of at least 25 consecutive cardiac cycles, is again processed by the FFT spectrum analyzer. The digital output and the ECG timing information are then transferred directly onto digital computer disk storage. The ECG R wave is used as a time reference to synchronize the averaging of Doppler spectra from 20 heart cycles. The mode (maximum amplitude) frequencies and the 3 db and 9 db amplitude levels on both sides of the mode frequency are then computed for each averaged spec-

TABLE 2-3. AGREEMENT BETWEEN TWO ANGIOGRAPHERS READING THE SAME FILMS (338 SEGMENTS)

Sensitivity	Specificity	Positive Predictive Value	Negative Predictive Value
Normal versus abnormal			
98%	68%	89%	92%
<50% versus >50% stenosis			
87%	94%	88%	93%

trum during the heart cycle. These five points are then used to generate a contour plot of five lines that represent the compressed Doppler data for storage, display, and analysis (Fig. 2–24). Basic parameters are then computed from the compressed contour data on the basis of spectral width measurements, time relationships, and frequency decomposition of the first moment waveform. The computer then selects those features that allow classification of the known vessels (training set) with the highest degree of correlation when compared with arteriography. Features are selected and properly weighted to arrive at a discriminant score for each diagnostic step (Fig. 2–25):

1. Normal versus diseased
2. If diseased, decision that stenosis is greater or less than 50%
3. If less than 50%, decision that stenosis is greater or less than 20%

A prospective validation of the method,[92] with 170 carotid sides used as "unknown data," showed an overall agreement of 82% (141/170) between the pattern recognition decision and arteriography (Table 2–4). Of the 29 normal sides, 27 (93%) were correctly classified, and two were classified in the 1 to 20% category. The diagnostic accuracy per category was 82% (44/54) for the 1 to 20% category, 78% (29/37) for the 21 to 50% category, and 82% (41/50) for the 51 to 99% category. Pattern recognition of the pulsed Doppler signal thus appears to be a very accurate method of predicting the extent of disease in the carotid bifurcation. Subsequent efforts will be directed toward developing estimates of confidence in the classification results, making further gradation in the disease state prediction, and to word the implementation of these algorithms in a dedicated microprocessor system for on-line analysis. This approach promises to be a reliable and unbiased method to quantitatively document the natural history of carotid artery disease both before and after a carotid endarterectomy.

Clinical Application of Noninvasive Testing

Screening Tool

The development of noninvasive methods for extracranial carotid artery evaluation over the last decade has led to questions as to their usefulness in daily clinical practice. Currently, patients with ischemic symptoms suggestive of cerebrovascular origin are subjected to contrast arteriography as an essential feature of their evaluation. For this group of patients, many clinicans believe that noninvasive testing is unnecessary and angiography is mandatory. However, contrast arteriography is costly, requires hospitalization and highly trained personnel, and is still associated with significant risks.[93,94] There are several situations in which arteriography might be avoided if the status of the carotid artery could be accurately documented by noninvasive testing. Patients with normal carotid arteries and those with internal carotid artery occlusions are not candidates for endarterectomy and should be spared the contrast study. In a recent study, Thiele et al.[86] reviewed the arteriographic findings of 109 patients with lateralized cerebral ischemic symptoms. Normal internal carotid arteries were found in

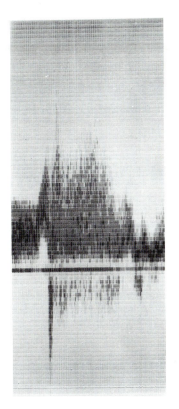

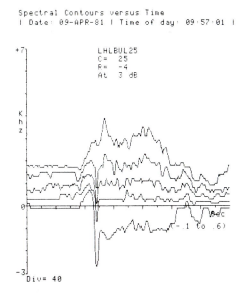

Figure 2-24. Example of an ensemble average waveform from an internal carotid artery. The time axis (horizontal) extends from −100 msec to +600 msec relative to the R wave on the ECG. On the contour plot (*right*), the center line represents the mode of the signal, with the other representing 3 and 9 db above and below the mode frequency. The corresponding gray-scale display is shown in the left frame.

10% of the patients on the symptomatic side and a total occlusion in 7%. Thus, on the basis of this distribution of disease, 17% of the patients (normal and total occlusion) could have potentially been spared an unnecessary angiogram. Routine screening of these patients by means of noninvasive techniques can prove useful and cost efficient.

The Asymptomatic Patient with Carotid Lesion

There is little controversy on the management of patients with transient ischemic attacks (TIAs), but the finding of a carotid lesion in a patient who is completely asymptomatic presents a therapeutic problem that is not yet resolved. With the extraordinary development of noninvasive testing,

Feature Definitions **24-May-82**			
Decision	Definition	Site	Weight
N vs. D	Ln[Early diastolic mean flow/cos(θ)]	CC	−43.8
	Ln[Late diastolic mean flow/cos(θ)]	CC	21.0
	Ln[Mode of mean waveform DFT]	IC	−16.7
	(Post systolic decelleration/cos(θ))**4	CC	15.9
	(1st minimum in mean waveform DFT)**4	IC	10.7
<> 50%	Ln[Lower 3 dB @ systole + 100 msec]	IC	2724
	Ln[1st minima in mean waveform DFT]	IC	−2262
	Ln[Upper 3 dB/cos(θ) @ systole]	IC	2247
	(Post systolic decelleration/cos(θ))**4	IC	1482
	(Maximum overall 9dB frequency)**2	IC	444
<> 20%	Ln[Max overall 9 dB frequency]	IC	25.8
	Ln[Area under systolic peak/cos(θ)]	CC	−23.2
	(Max overall 9 dB frequency)**4	IC	−16.4
	Lower 9 dB width @ systole	CC	5.6
	Ln[Mode of mean waveform DFT]	CC	−3.7

Figure 2-25. Five spectral patterns are used at each decision step. Ln is the natural logarithm, θ is the angle of incidence for the Doppler beam, DFT is discrete Fourier transform, PCCA is proximal common carotid artery, and PICA is proximal internal carotid artery.

TABLE 2.4. AGREEMENT BETWEEN THE COMPUTER PATTERN RECOGNITION RESULTS AND CONTRAST ANGIOGRAPHY

Angiog-raphy	Computer				Total
	Normal	1–20%	21–50%	51–99%	
Normal	27	2			29
1–20%	4	44	6		54
21–50%		5	29	3	37
51–99%		1	8	41	50
Total	31	52	43	44	170

physicians are now increasingly faced with the difficult dilemma of how to deal with these lesions. Several inadequately controlled studies suggested that there may be some benefit from prophylactic endarterectomy, claiming a decline in morbidity and mortality rates because of this procedure. Of major concern, however, is that, even in the best hands, there is definitive risk of stroke and death from both the mandatory angiography and the surgery itself. These concerns have led others to withhold this prophylactic type of surgery until the appearance of the first TIA. Of the 168 patients followed up by Humphries et al.,[95] 111 had undergone carotid endarterectomy on one side. Of the 182 patients with asymptomatic sides thereafter followed up for an average of 32 months, 26 developed TIAs and underwent a successful carotid endarterectomy. Only one patient sustained a stroke without premonitory symptoms.

Although the presence of a bruit correlates with a higher risk of stroke, the site of the bruit and the side of the stroke are not consistently related.[96,97] It has been shown that not all bruits are associated with significant carotid artery disease.[98,99] Of 100 patients with 165 asymptomatic carotid bruits evaluated with duplex scanning and spectral analysis, 12 (7.3%) were normal, 83 (50%) had a less than 50% diameter reducing lesion, 61 (37%) had a 50 to 99% diameter reducing plaque, and 9 (5.5%) had a total occlusion of the internal carotid artery.[100] These results stress (1) the fact that a cervical bruit is a poor indicator of the extent of disease in the internal carotid artery and (2) the need for noninvasive evaluation before considering arteriography.

In our laboratory, asymptomatic patients with bruits were placed into a prospective study to evaluate outcome in relation to degree of stenosis and rate of progression of disease. A total of 167 patients were followed up for up to 36 months with repeat duplex scanning.[88] During the follow-up interval, 10 patients became symptomatic (6 with TIAs and 4 with stroke). The development of symptoms was accompanied by disease progression in 8 patients. The mean annual rate of progression of disease was 8% (for <50% stenosis to a >50% stenosis), which was twice that for the development of symptoms for the entire group.

The most important finding to emerge from this study was the relationship between the degree of stenosis and outcome. The presence of, or progression to, a greater than 80% stenosis was highly correlated with the development of TIAs, stroke, or total occlusion of the internal carotid artery.

There were 10 occlusions of the internal carotid artery, four of which were associated with the development of a stroke. With regard to risk factors, three major findings appeared to be relevant to outcome: (1) age (being less than 65 years of age was more predictive of complications), (2) the presence of diabetes mellitus, which added to the risk, and (3) cigarette smoking. Although cigarette smoking has not been generally considered an important risk factor for stroke in this country, it appeared important in our study.

The role of noninvasive tests in screening patients for cerebrovascular disease before major surgical procedures is also controversial. It has been suggested that certain patients would benefit from both screening and prophylactic carotid endarterectomy before a major surgical procedure.[101–104] Duplex scanning and spectral analysis were used prospectively to study 101 patients before aortocoronary bypass surgery.[102] Of the 24 patients with either a bruit or a history of neurologic symptoms, 11 (46%) had unilateral or bilateral internal carotid stenoses of 50 to 99% diameter reduction, and 2 had a total occlusion on one side. Of the 78 patients without any symptoms or signs, only 5 (6%) had a unilateral or bilateral internal carotid stenosis of more than 50%. Only 2 neurologic complications occurred postoperatively (1 stroke and 1 TIA). Neither of these patients had prior symptoms or signs, and neither had a high-grade stenosis. These findings are consistent with reports by Barnes et al.[103] and by Turnipseed et al.,[104] who failed to relate the incidence of perioperative stroke to the presence of high-grade stenoses, thus questioning the value of prophylactic carotid endarterectomy in these patients before cardiac or any other major surgery.

The only way to determine the benefit of prophylactic carotid surgery will be to conduct properly controlled studies of the problem in which noninvasive testing is expected to play a major role.

Intraoperative Assessment

The need for detecting technical errors during carotid endarterectomy led to the routine use of intraoperative arteriography. This method allows only a single-plane view of the artery, does not provide data on the flow pattern through the endarterectomized segment, and exposes the patient to the risk of arterial puncture and injection of radiographic contrast. Although complications due to operative arteriorapy are rare, their occurrence led some surgeons to stop using this technique routinely.

A new method for intraoperative assessment has been developed that employs a sterile 20 MHz pulsed Doppler probe and a FFT spectrum analyzer.[105] Although a C-W probe would have been adequate for this study, a pulsed Doppler probe was used to assess flow patterns at more discrete points across the bifurcation. The probe is placed directly over the exposed carotid artery and is acoustically coupled with saline solution. An angle of 60 degrees between the probe and the long axis of the vessel is maintained while the sample volume of the pulsed Doppler is positioned in the center of the flow stream. Flow patterns are examined just before the endarterectomy and immediately after restoration of arterial flow. The common carotid artery, the bulb, and the external and internal carotid arteries are successively studied. Flow disturbances can be classified as mild, moderate, or severe depending on the extent of spectral broadening and the presence of increased peak systolic frequencies. When the prethromboendarterectomy (TEA) and post-TEA spectra were compared during 45 carotid endarterectomies, it was noted that, when severe spectral abnormalities were present before the endarterectomy, the majority showed improvement after endarterectomy, although some flow disturbances often persisted. A lack of improvement or deterioration in spectra after endarterectomy may indicate a technical problem and could be used to select patients for operative arteriography. In addition to bringing about more rational use of intraoperative contrast study, these data constitute an important baseline for long-term follow-up studies of these patients, because flow disturbances due to recurrence of stenosis at the carotid bifurcation must be distinguished from those directly attributable to the endarterectomy.

Postoperative Follow-up

Although the clinical effectiveness of carotid endarterectomy in preventing stroke and relieving symptoms is now well established, the hemodynamic and anatomic consequences are poorly documented. Reported rates of recurrent stenosis after endarterectomy range from 1 to 5%.[106-108] The reported cases are predominantly those of patients with recurrent neurologic symptoms, thus warranting the contrast study. Prospective evaluation of patients after endarterectomy is best done by means of noninvasive tests.

Duplex scanning and spectral analysis are routinely done at 3, 6, and 12 months, and then yearly after a carotid endarterectomy. As reported by Roederer et al.,[109] this method is highly accurate when applied postoperatively and has shown a sensitivity of 93% in detecting a more than 50% recurrent stenosis in the internal carotid artery.

Prospective follow-up of 76 patients, with operations performed on a total of 89 sides, was conducted with a mean postoperative follow-up interval of 16 months.[110] Intraoperative technical errors were excluded in every case by routine intraoperative angiograms. Spectral changes indicating a greater than 50% reducing lesion of the internal carotid artery were observed in 32 of the 89 surgically treated sides. Serial follow-up was available for 22 stenotic sides and showed a persistent stenosis in 12 cases, a regression of stenosis in 9, and an internal carotid occlusion in 1. The early appearance of a severe stenosis is known to occur with early proliferative myointimal lesions at the site of the endarterectomy. These lesions may regress with time,[111] which may explain why some high-grade stenoses initially noted became less severe during the follow-up period. The overall incidence of a persistent high-grade stenosis was 19%. If the high incidence of persistent postoperative stenosis reported here is corroborated by other appropriate studies, the use of prophylactic endarterectomy for asymptomatic carotid stenoses will require reconsideration. Since most recurrent stenoses are not associated with recurrent symptoms, the decision to reoperate on the lesion must be made primarily on clinical grounds, and the procedure of choice is usually patch angioplasty without endarterec-

tomy. A more logical approach toward postoperative stenoses will be possible when more information becomes available in further follow-up of these patients.

The use of accurate and reliable noninvasive tests in the evaluation of extracranial arterial disease, both before and after endarterectomy, will improve considerably our understanding of the disease and is expected to change our approaches. Long-term prospective studies using these tests are now feasible and, in addition to clarifying the natural history of carotid disease, will determine the real role of noninvasive testing, arteriography, and surgery in the management of these patients.

THE MESENTERIC ARTERIES

The clinical syndrome of chronic mesenteric ischemia (mesenteric angina) has been a source of confusion in terms of both recognizing it clinically and verifying it by objective tests. The classic clinical presentation is cramping abdominal pain, diarrhea, and weight loss precipitated by eating. After the patient eats, the blood supply to the small bowel cannot increase sufficiently with the resulting ischemia and pain.

The diagnosis is established by the association of the symptoms coupled with involvement of at least two of three of the major inputs to the gut (celiac, superior mesenteric, and inferior mesenteric arteries). In our experience with this disorder, there has been involvement of both the celiac and superior mesenteric arteries in each instance where the diagnosis has been verified by angiography.

Duplex scanning is ideally suited to the study of these vessels. Normally, one finds the following: (1) quasisteady flow in the celiac artery, with no change after a meal, (2) a triphasic velocity pattern in the superior mesenteric artery in the fasting state, and (3) a dramatic and prompt (within minutes) increase in flow in the mesenteric artery, with loss of reverse flow.[112,113] These findings, in association with the appropriate symptoms, are sufficient to make the diagnosis and proceed with selective arteriography and surgical correction.

We have used the same duplex studies postoperatively to assess the success or failure of both angioplasty and surgery. It is clear that a failure of a therapeutic approach which was initially successful can be detected by repeat duplex scanning.

RENAL ARTERIES

The problems associated with renal artery stenosis and its relation to hypertension have largely defied the use of screening procedures other than angiography. The most commonly applied studies have included the urogram and radionuclide scanning. These tests have an unacceptably high incidence of false positive and false negative results, in the range of 20%.[114] This makes them unsuitable for screening and certainly for long-term follow-up studies as well.

For a test to be clinically relevant and useful, it must (1) identify the renal arteries and detect areas of stenosis that are associated with the activation of the renin-angiotensin system, (2) be sufficiently predictive (have a high-enough sensitivity) to warrant the use of selective arteriograms to verify the diagnosis, and (3) be usable for evaluation of the results of both angioplasty and direct arterial surgery, which are designed to correct the problems presented by the renal artery stenosis.

To examine this problem, we used duplex scanning to determine (1) whether a reduction in the renal artery diameter can be reliably detected and quantified by duplex scanning and (2) whether the degree of stenosis as detected could be used to predict the outcome of angiography and, most important, of angioplasty and surgery.[115,116]

The studies that were designed to answer these questions used the ratio of the peak systolic velocity in the renal artery to that in the adjacent aorta (the RAR). In our pilot studies, we noted that for renal artery stenoses that exceeded 60% in terms of diameter reduction, a RAR of greater than 3.5 was predictive of this degree of narrowing. In these studies, a complete examination was possible in 90% of the subjects. Obesity, excess bowel gas, and previous operations were the most common reasons for failure to obtain the necessary data for a diagnosis. If we use a greater than 60% stenosis as that level sufficient for the development of renovascular hypertension, the sensitivity of duplex scanning has proved to be 86%, with a specificity of 93%.[117] The high specificity is particularly important in screening for a disease that has a low prevalence.

REFERENCES

1. Satomura S: Study of flow patterns in peripheral arteries by ultrasonics. J Acoust Soc Jpn 15:151, 1959.
2. Rushmer RF, Baker DW, Stegall HF: Transcutaneous Doppler flow detection as a nondestructive technique. J Appl Physiol 21:554, 1966.
3. Strandness DE Jr, McCutcheon EP, Rushmer RF: Application of a transcutaneous Doppler flowmeter in the evaluation of occlusive arterial disease. Surg Gynecol Obstet 122:1039, 1966.
4. Strandness DE Jr, Schultz RD, et al.: Ultrasonic flow detection: A useful technique in the evaluation of peripheral vascular disease. Am J Surg 113:320, 1967.
5. Nippa JH, Hokanson DE, et al.: Phase rotation for separating forward and reverse blood velocity signals. IEEE Trans Sonics Ultrasonics 22:340, 1975.
6. Baker DW: Pulsed ultrasonic Doppler flow sensing. IEEE Trans Sonics Ultrasonics 17:170, 1970.
7. Leopold GR, Goldberger LE, Bernstein EF: Ultrasonic detection and evaluation of abdominal aortic aneurysms. Surgery 72:939, 1972.
8. Marcus R, Edell SL: Sonographic evaluation of iliac artery aneurysms. Am J Surg 140:666, 1980.
9. Bernstein EF, Dilley RB, et al.: Growth rates of small abdominal aortic aneurysms. Surgery 80:765, 1976.
10. Leopold RG, Bernstein EF: Ultrasonic imaging for occlusive carotid disease, in Bernstein EF (ed): Noninvasive Diagnostic Techniques in Vascular Disease, 2nd ed. St. Louis, Mosby, 1982, pp 265–271.
11. Hartley CJ, Strandness DE Jr: The effects of atherosclerosis on the transmission of ultrasound. J Surg Res 10:575, 1969.
12. Barber FE, Baker DW, et al.: Duplex Scanner II: For simultaneous imaging of artery tissues and flow. Ultrasonic Symposium Proceedings. IEEE No. 74 CHO 896ISU, 1984.
13. Johnston KW, Maruzzo BC, Cobbold RSC: Errors and artifacts of Doppler flowmeters and their solution. Arch Surg 112:135, 1977.
14. Whitney RJ: The measurement of volume changes in human limbs. J Physiol 121:1, 1953.
15. Parrish D, Strandness DE Jr, Bell JW: Dynamic response characteristics of a mercury in Silastic strain gauge. J Appl Physiol 19:363, 1964.
16. Strandness DE Jr, Bell JW: Peripheral vascular disease: Diagnosis and objective evaluation using a mercury strain gauge. Ann Surg 161[Suppl]:1, 1965.
17. Winsor T, Sibley AE, et al: Peripheral pulse contours in arterial occlusive disease. Vasc Dis 5:61, 1968.
18. Strandness DE Jr: Waveform analysis in the diagnosis of arteriosclerosis obliterans, in Peripheral Arterial Disease: A Physiologic Approach. Boston, Little, Brown, 1969, pp 92–112.
19. Carter SA: Indirect systole pressures and pulse waves in arterial occlusive disease of the lower extremities. Circulation 37:624, 1968.
20. Carter SA: Clinical measurements of systolic pressures in limbs with arterial occlusive disease. JAMA 207:1869, 1969.
21. Yao JST, Hobbs JT, Irvine WT: Ankle systolic pressure measurements in arterial diseases affecting the lower extremities. Br J Surg 56:676, 1969.
22. Yao JST: Hemodynamic studies in peripheral arterial disease. Br J Surg 57:761, 1970.
23. Strandness DE Jr: Abnormal exercise response after successful reconstructive arterial surgery. Surgery 59:325, 1966.
24. Stegall HF, Kardon MB, Kemmerer WT: Indirect measurements of arterial blood. Adv Modern Nutr 7:187, 1978.
25. Allen JS, Terry HJK: The evaluation of an ultrasonic flow detector for assessment of peripheral vascular disease. Cardiovasc Res 3:503, 1969.
26. Winsor T: Influence of arterial disease on the systolic blood pressure gradients of the extremity. Am J Med Sci 220:117, 1950.
27. Kirkendall WM, Burton AC, et al.: Recommendations for human blood pressure determinations by sphygmomanometers. Circulation 36:980, 1979.
28. Sanchez SA, Best EB: Correlation of plethysmographic and arteriographic findings in patients with obstructive arterial disease. Angiology 20:684, 1969.
29. Fronek A, Johansen KH, et al.: Noninvasive physiologic tests in the diagnosis and characterization of peripheral arterial occlusive disease. Am J Surg 126:205, 1973.
30. Carter SA: The relationship of distal systolic pressures to healing of skin lesions in limbs with arterial occlusive disease, with special reference to diabetes mellitus. Scand J Clin Lab Invest 31[Suppl 128]:239, 1973.
31. Dean RH, Yao JST, et al.: Prognostic indicators in femoropopliteal reconstructions. Arch Surg 110:1287, 1975.
32. Barnes RW, Shanik GD, Slaymaker EF: An index of healing in below knee amputation: Leg blood pressure by Doppler ultrasound. Surgery 79:13, 1976.
33. Raines JK, Darling RG, et al.: Vascular laboratory criteria for the management of peripheral vascular disease of the lower extremities. Surgery 79:21, 1976.
34. Nielsen PE, Bell G, Larsen NA: Strain gauge studies of distal blood pressure in normal subjects and patients with peripheral arterial disease: Analysis of normal variation and reproducibility and comparison to intra-arterial measurements. Scand J Clin Lab Invest 31[Suppl 128]:103, 1973.
35. Mozersky DJ, Sumner DS, Strandness DE Jr: Long-term results of reconstructive aortoiliac surgery. Am J Surg 123:503, 1972.
36. Mozersky DJ, Sumner DS, Strandness DE Jr: Disease progression after femoropopliteal surgical procedures. Surg Gynecol Obstet 135:700, 1972.

37. Skinner JS, Strandness DE Jr: Exercise and intermittent claudication. II. Effect of physical training. Circulation 36:23, 1967.

38. Pascarelli EF, Bertrand CA: Comparison of blood pressures in the arms and legs. N Engl J Med 270:693, 1964.

39. Cutajar CL, Marston A, Newcombe JF: Value of cuff occlusion pressures in assessment of peripheral vascular disease. Br Med J 2:392, 1973.

40. Flanigan DP, Gray B, et al.: Correlation of Doppler-derived high-thigh pressure and intra-arterial pressure in the assessment of aortoiliac occlusive disease. Br. J Surg 68:423, 1981.

41. Faris IB, Jamieson CW: The diagnosis of aorto-iliac disease: A comparison of thigh pressure measurement and femoral artery flow velocity profile. J Cardiovasc Surg 16:597, 1975.

42. Bone GE, Hayes AC, et al.: Value of segmental limb blood pressure in predicting results of aortofemoral bypass. Am J Surg 132:733, 1976.

43. Sumner DS, Strandness DE Jr: Aortoiliac reconstruction in patients with combined iliac and superficial femoral arterial occlusion. Surgery 84:348, 1978.

44. Gosling RG, King DH: Ultrasonic angiology, in Hareus, Adamson (eds): Arteries and Veins. Edinburgh, Churchill Livingstone, 1975.

45. Johnston KW, Maruzzo BC, Cobbold RSC: Doppler methods for quantitative measurements and localization of peripheral arterial occlusive disease by analysis of the blood flow velocity waveform. Ultrasound Med Biol 4:209, 1978.

46. Johnston KW: Role of Doppler ultrasonography in determining the hemodynamic significance of aortoiliac disease. Am J Surg 21:319, 1978.

47. Harris PH, Taylor LA, et al.: The relationship between Doppler ultrasound assessment and angiography in occlusive arterial disease of the lower limbs. Surg Gynecol Obstet 138:911, 1974.

48. Bone GE: The relationship between aortoiliac hemodynamics and femoral pulsatility index. J Surg Res 32:228, 1982.

49. Flanigan DP, Collins JT, et al.: Hemodynamic and arteriographic evaluation of femoral pulsatility index. J Surg Res 32:234, 1982.

50. Thiele BL, Bandyk DF, et al.: A systematic approach to the assessment of aortoiliac disease. Arch Surg 118:477, 1983.

51. Demorais D, Johnston KW: Assessment of aortoiliac disease by noninvasive quantitative Doppler waveform analysis. Br J Surg 68:789, 1981.

52. Carter SA, Lezack JDF: Digital systolic pressures in the lower limbs in arterial disease. Circulation 43:905, 1971.

53. Strandness DE Jr, Bell JW: An evaluation of the hemodynamic response of the claudicating extremity to exercise. Surg Gynecol Obstet 119:1237, 1964.

54. Fronek A, Johansen KH, et al.: Ultrasonically monitored postocclusive reactive hyperemia in the diagnosis of peripheral arterial occlusive disease. Circulation 48:149, 1973.

55. Jager KA, Fortner GA, et al.: Noninvasive diagnosis of intestinal angina. J Clin Ultrasound 12:588, 1984.

56. Jager KA, Phillips DJ, et al.: Noninvasive mapping of lower limb arterial lesions. Ultrasound Med Biol 11:515, 1985.

57. Gosling RG, King DH, Woodcock JP: Transcutaneous measurement of arterial blood velocity by ultrasound. Ultrasonics in industry. Conference papers 16–23, 1969.

58. Gosling RG, Dunbar G, et al.: The quantitative analysis of occlusive peripheral arterial disease by a noninvasive ultrasonic technique. Angiology 22:52, 1971.

59. Gosling RG, King DH: Continuous wave ultrasound as an alternative and complement to x-rays in vascular examinations, in Reneman R (ed): Cardiovascular Applications of Ultrasound. New York, American Elsevier, 1974.

60. Fitzgerald DE, Carr J: Doppler ultrasound diagnosis and classification as an alternative to arteriography. Angiology 26:283, 1975.

61. Johnston KW, Taraschuk I: Validation of the role of pulsatility index in quantitation of the severity of peripheral arterial occlusive disease. Am J Surg 131:295, 1976.

62. Woodcock JP, Gosling RG, Fitzgerald DE: A new noninvasive technique for assessment of superficial femoral artery obstruction. Br J Surg 59:226, 1972.

63. Skidmore R, Woodcock JP, et al.: Physiologic interpretation of Doppler shift waveforms. III. Clinical results. Ultrasound Med Biol 6:227, 1980.

64. Cranford AD, Chamberlain I: Pulse waveform transit ratios in the assessment of peripheral vascular disease. Br J Surg 64:449, 1977.

65. Gosling RG: Extraction of physiological information from spectrum-analysed Doppler shift continuous wave ultrasound signals obtained noninvasively from the arterial system, in Hill DW, Watson BW (eds): Medical Electronics Monographs, Stevenage, England, Peter Peregrinus, 1976, pp 18–22.

66. Fronek A, Coel M, Bernstein EF: Quantitative ultrasonographic studies of lower extremity flow velocities in health and disease. Circulation 53:957, 1976.

67. Fronek A, Coel M, Bernstein EF: The importance of combined multisegmental pressure and Doppler flow velocity studies in the diagnosis of peripheral arterial occlusive disease. Surgery 84:840, 1978.

68. Blackshear WM Jr, Phillips DH, Strandness DE Jr: Pulsed Doppler assessment of normal human femoral artery velocity patterns. J Surg Res 27:73, 1979.

69. Woodcock JP, Skidmore R: Physiological interpretation of Doppler shift waveforms from the carotid and peripheral circulation, in Woodcock JP, Sequeira RF (eds): Doppler Ultrasound in the Study of Central and Peripheral Circulation. Bristol, England, University of Bristol, 1978.

70. Skidmore R, Woodcock JP: Physiological interpretation of Doppler shift waveforms. I. Theoretical considerations. Ultrasound Med Biol 6:7, 1980.

71. Skidmore R, Woodcock JP: Physiological interpretation of Doppler shift waveforms. II. Validation of the Laplace transform method for characterization of the common femoral blood velocity-time waveform. Ultrasound Med Biol 6:219, 1980.

72. Duncan GW, Gruber JO, et al.: Evaluation of carotid stenosis by phonoangiography. N Engl J Med 293:1124, 1975.

73. Kistler JP, Lees RS, et al.: Correlation of spectral photoangiography and carotid angiography with gross pathology in carotid stenosis. N Engl J Med 305:417, 1981.

74. Knox R, Breslau PJ, Strandness DE Jr.: Quantitative carotid phonoangiography. Stroke 12:798, 1981.

75. Mercier LA, Greenleaf JF, et al.: High-resolution ultrasound arteriography: A comparison with carotid angiography, in Bernstein EF (ed): Noninvasive Techniques in Vascular Disease. St. Louis, Mosby, 1978.

76. Hobson RW II, Berry SM, et al.: Comparison of pulsed Doppler and real-time B-mode echo arteriography for noninvasive imaging of the extracranial carotid arteries. Surgery 87:286, 1980.

77. Katz ML, Comerota JJ: Characterization of athersclerotic plaque by real-time carotid imaging. Bruit 6:17, 1982.

78. Comerata AJ, Cranley JJ, et al.: Real-time B-mode carotid imaging: A three-year multicenter experience. J Vasc Surg 1:84–95, 1984.

79. Fell G, Phillips DJ, et al.: Ultrasonic duplex scanning for disease of the carotid artery. Circulation 64:1191, 1981.

80. Breslau PJ, Knox RA, et al.: The accuracy of ultrasonic duplex scanning as compared with contrast arteriography in extracranial carotid artery disease. Vasc Diagn Ther 3:17, 1982.

81. Langlois YE, Roederer GO, et al.: The concordance between

pulsed Doppler/spectrum analysis and angiography. Ultrasound Med Biol 9:51, 1983.

82. Knox RA, Phillips DJ, et al.: Empirical findings relating sample volume size to diagnostic accuracy in pulsed Doppler cerebrovascular studies. J Clin Ultrasound 10:227, 1982.

83. Phillips DJ, Greene FM, et al.: Flow velocity patterns in the carotid bifurcations of young presumed normals. Ultrasound Med Biol 9:39, 1983.

84. Langlois YE, Roederer GO, et al.: The use of common carotid waveform analysis in the diagnosis of carotid occlusive disease. Angiology 34:679, 1983.

85. Roederer GO, Langlois YE, et al.: Ultrasonic duplex scanning of extracranial carotid arteries: Improved accuracy using new features from the common carotid artery. J Cardiovasc Ultrasonogr 1:373, 1982.

86. Thiele BL, Young JV, et al.: Correlation of arteriographic findings with symptoms in patients with cerebrovascular disease. Neurology 30:1041, 1980.

87. Roederer GO, Langlois YE, et al.: A simple spectral parameter for accurate classification of severe carotid disease. Bruit 3:174, 1984.

88. Roederer GO, Langlois YE, et al.: The natural history of carotid arterial disease in asymptomatic patients with cervical bruits. Stroke 15:605, 1984.

89. Breslau P: Ultrasonic Duplex Scanning in the Evaluation of Carotid Artery Disease, [Thesis]. Maastricht, Holland, University of Maastricht, 1981.

90. Greene FM, Beach K, et al.: Computer-based pattern recognition of carotid arterial disease using pulsed Doppler ultrasound. Ultrasound Med Biol 8:161, 1982.

91. Knox RA, Greene FM, et al.: Computer-based classification of carotid arterial disease: A prospective assessment. Stroke 13:589, 1982.

92. Langlois YE, Greene FM, et al.: Computer-based pattern recognition method for classification of carotid arterial disease: Methodology and results. Proceedings of the San Diego Symposium on Noninvasive Diagnostic Techniques in Vascular Disease, San Diego, Oct. 18–22, 1982.

93. Mani RL, Eisenberg RL: Complications of catheter cerebral angiography: Analysis of 5000 procedures. I. Criteria and incidence. AJR 131:861, 1978.

94. Mani RL, Eisenberg RL, et al.: Complications of catheter cerebral arteriography: Analysis of 5000 procedures. II. Relation of complication rates to clinical and arteriographic diagnosis. AJR 131:867, 1978.

95. Humphries AW, Young JR, et al.: Unoperated asymptomatic significant internal carotid artery stenosis: A review of 182 instances. Surgery 80:695, 1976.

96. Heyman A, Wilkinson WE, et al.: Risk of stroke in asymptomatic persons with cervical bruits. N Engl J Med 302:838, 1980.

97. Wolf PA, Kannel WB, et al.: Asymptomatic carotid bruit and risk of stroke. JAMA 215:1442, 1981.

98. Ziegler DK, Zileli F, et al.: Correlation of bruits over the carotid artery with angiographically demonstrated lesions. Neurology 21:860, 1971.

99. David TE, Humphries AW, et al.: A correlation of neck bruits and arteriosclerotic carotid arteries. Arch Surg 107:729, 1973.

100. Fell G, Breslau PJ, et al.: The impact of noninvasive testing on the evaluation of patients with asymptomatic carotid bruits. Am Heart J 102:221, 1981.

101. Javid H, Ostermiller WE, et al.: Carotid endarterectomy for asymptomatic bruit. Arch Surg 102:389, 1971.

102. Breslau PJ, Fell G, et al: Carotid arterial disease in patients undergoing coronary artery bypass surgery. J Thorac Cardiovasc Surg 82:765, 1981.

103. Barnes RW, Marszalek RN: Asymptomatic carotid disease in the cardiovascular surgical patient: Is prophylactic endarterectomy necessary? Stroke 12:497, 1981.

104. Turnipseed WS, Berkoff HA, Belzer FO: Postoperative stroke in cardiac and peripheral vascular disease. Ann Surg 192:365, 1980.

105. Zierler RE, Bandyk DF, et al.: Intraoperative pulsed Doppler assessment of carotid endarterectomy. Ultrasound Med Biol 9:65, 1983.

106. Stoney RJ, String ST: Recurrent carotid stenosis. Surgery 80:705, 1976.

107. French BN, Rewcastle NB: Recurrent stenosis at site of carotid endarterectomy. Stroke 8:597, 1977.

108. Cossman, Callow AD, et al.: Early restenosis after carotid endarterectomy. Arch Surg 113:275, 1978.

109. Roederer GO, Langlois YE, et al.: Postendarteretomy carotid ultrasonic duplex scanning: Concordance with contrast arteriography. Ultrasound Med Biol 9:73, 1983.

110. Zierler RE, Bandyk DF, et al.: Carotid artery stenosis following endarterectomy. Arch Surg 117:1408, 1982.

111. Diaz FG, Patel S, et al.: Early angiographic changes following carotid endarterectomy. Neurosurgery 10:151, 1982.

112. Jager KA, Bollinger A, et al.: Measurement of mesenteric blood flow by duplex scanning. J Vasc Surg 3:462, 1986.

113. Nicholls SC, Kohler TR, et al.: Use of hemodynamic parameters in the diagnosis of mesenteric insufficiency. J Vasc Surg 3:507, 1986.

114. Treadway KK, Slater EE: Renovascular hypertension. Ann Rev Med 35:665, 1984.

115. Norris CS, Rittgers SE, Barnes RW: A new screening technique for renal artery occlusive disease. Curr Surg March–April 1984, p 83.

116. Kohler TR, Zierler RE, et al.: Noninvasive diagnosis of renal artery stenosis by ultrasonic duplex scanning. J Vasc Surg 4:450, 1986.

117. Taylor DC, Kohler TR, et al.: Duplex ultrasound in the diagnosis of renal artery stenosis. J Vasc Surg 7:363, 1988.

SELECTED BIBLIOGRAPHY

Bernstein EF (ed): Noninvasive Techniques in Vascular Disease, 2nd ed. St. Louis, Mosby, 1982.

Nicolaides AN, Yao JS (eds): Investigation of Vascular Disorders. New York, Churchill Livingstone, 1981.

Strandness DE Jr (ed): Collateral Circulation in Clinical Practice. Philadelphia, Saunders, 1969.

Strandness DE Jr, Sumner DS (eds): Hemodynamics for Surgeons. New York, Grune & Stratton, 1975.

Strandness DE Jr, Thiele BL (eds): Selected Topics in Venous Disorders: Pathophysiology, Diagnosis and Treatment. New York, Futura Publishing, 1981.

CHAPTER 3

Preoperative Evaluation of Vascular Disease

D. Eugene Strandness, Jr., Yves E. Langlois, and Ghislaine O. Roederer

In order to plan the appropriate therapy for a patient with peripheral vascular disease, it is necessary to have as much information as possible concerning the following:

1. Correct diagnosis
2. Effect of the disease on function
3. Exact localization and extent of the process
4. Natural history of the disease with and without operative therapy

The correct diagnosis, or at least a presumptive diagnosis, can usually be made from the initial history and examination. Fairly typical symptoms suggest the diagnosis of arterial occlusive disease affecting the lower limbs. This clinical impression can be further supported and corroborated by a carefully performed physical examination. However, symptoms of ischemia appear very late in the disease process, and the functional effects of arterial disease may be difficult to ascertain accurately by history alone. It is a time-honored method to ask patients with intermittent claudication to relate their walking distance in terms of city blocks. This inexact method of evaluating functional disability is useful, but as experienced clinicians now recognize, it does not in itself take into account walking patterns, elevation, the influence of obesity, and the possible effects of other chronic disorders, such as congestive heart failure and obstructive pulmonary disease. It is also well recognized that patient testimony is often unreliable. Changes in walking habits may mask the presence of disease, and patients may remain unaware of their own limitations, particularly if the occlusive disease occurs gradually. In addition, a variety of disorders produces symptoms in the legs that can simulate true claudication.[1] On the other hand, physical signs of lower limb ischemia, such as the character of the pulses, the presence of bruits, and trophic skin changes, provide only a crude assessment of the location and severity of the arterial occlusion. In a prospective study involving 458 diabetics,[2] 31% of those with no history of claudication and 21% of the group with a normal physical examination had arterial occlusive disease documented by objective noninvasive tests. Conversely, 41% of those who gave a history of intermittent claudication and had an abnormal physical examination presented normal functional studies.

Grossly and microscopically, the complicated plaque appears to be the same regardless of its site of origin. However, there are differences with regard to related risk factors that lead to its development and the different mechanisms involved in the commonly related clinical symptoms. For example, in the extracranial arterial circulation, the clinical expression of disease appears to be more dependent on the biologic behavior of the plaque than on the extent to which it narrows the lumen.[3–5] It is now recognized that the loss of endothelial continuity over the plaque with ulceration is probably the single most important factor in the release of emboli, with the production of transient ischemic attacks and stroke. Conversely, the occurrence of ischemic symptoms in the lower limbs is more directly related to the extent of narrowing in the major vessels.

Awareness of the extreme importance of the biologic behavior of the complicated plaque and the high-grade stenosis is increasing. These lesions tend to thrombose in the coronary circulation, the internal carotid arteries, and the involved arteries of the lower limbs, making them the most dangerous in clinical terms. Why they tend to thrombose is poorly understood.

The introduction of contrast arteriography has been a major factor in bringing the entire field of vascular surgery to its current level of sophistication. It is still the only accepted standard of measuring in vivo the extent of atherosclerosis, and it provides mandatory anatomic information before reconstructive arterial surgery. However, arteriography has limitations, particularly in evaluating the hemodynamic effects of stenoses. Projectional errors with single-plane angiography are now well recognized[5] (Fig. 3–1). Despite the improved accuracy made possible by the addition of oblique and lateral views,[6–9] no physiologic information can be derived from the arteriographic examination. This is especially true in the presence of multilevel occlusive disease, where it is impossible to predict the segment that is most responsible for the symptoms.[10,11] Furthermore, in addition to the variability in the interpretation of angio-

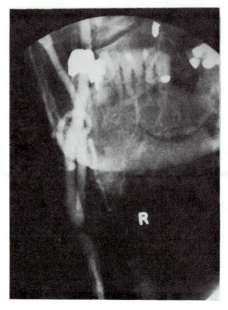 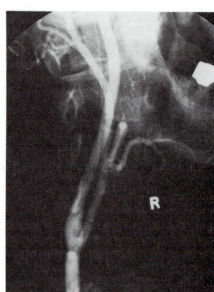

Figure 3-1. Cerebral contrast angiogram. On the AP projection (*left*), a tight stenosis is visible at the origin of the internal carotid artery (ICA). The lesion can hardly be suspected on the lateral projection (*right*). On both projections, there is a confusing overlapping of the ICA and external carotid artery (ECA).

graphic studies, their cost, risk, and poor acceptance by the patient preclude their use for follow-up purposes.

A thorough knowledge of the natural history of the disease is most important in evaluating patients before operation. When available, this knowledge can be balanced against the risk of operation as well as the long-term results with or without operation. The final decision relative to treatment depends on an integration of all the available facts and a reasonable estimate of the patient's ability to survive the proposed reconstruction.

Since duplex scanning can precisely identify the sites of involvement and classify the degree of stenosis, it is also possible to utilize this same method for longitudinal studies. This is true for both the carotid and peripheral arterial segments. Duplex scanning can provide the best data to assess the effect of intervention (surgical, angiographic, pharmacologic) on the natural history of atherosclerosis.

PHYSIOLOGY OF ARTERIAL OCCLUSION

Although arterial occlusion has many causes, the basic physiologic changes that occur and accompany the obstruction are quite similar. The large and medium-sized arteries serve principally as distributing conduits, while their branches and smaller arteries supply the blood to the various nutritive arteriolar and capillary networks. Vessels branching from the major channels assume a critical and somewhat different role when their parent artery becomes narrowed or occluded. Under such circumstances, these distributing branches not only continue to supply their own capillary beds but also redirect the blood around the diseased segments. The function and viability of the ischemic part then become entirely dependent on the ability of this complex hemodynamic network to respond to the tissue requirements for oxygen. It is useful to categorize these collateral channels according to their anatomic location and functional roles.

Longland divided the collateral arteries into three major segments[12] (Fig. 3–2). The stem or exit vessels are those branch arteries located proximal to the narrowed or occluded segment. The direction of flow in these arteries is entirely normal. The stem vessels anastomose with a mesh of smaller intermediate vessels referred to as the "midzone" arteries. Flow through these vessels as they communicate with their distal and third group of arteries is reversed. The midzone arteries unite with arteries of larger size in which the blood flow is reversed. This third and last component has been termed "the reentry channel." It should be clear that, depending on the location of the stenosis or occlusion, a branch vessel may serve either as a stem or a reentry channel to provide blood to the distal limb. These three major components of the collateral artery network are preexisting vessels that are immediately available to assume this new transport role. The stem and reentry channels are the largest of the collateral network, since they communicate directly with the main vessels. The most critical segment in terms of immediate function is located in the midzone and represents the small prearteriolar termination of the branch vessels themselves. In spite of continued expansion of the midzone vessels, the resistance of the collateral bed always exceeds that of the major artery whose function it has replaced. In contrast to the peripheral runoff bed, whose resistance is generally high but quite variable, the resistance of the collateral bed is, for practical purposes, almost fixed.[13–16] With few exceptions, the ultimate effects of both acute and chronic arterial occlusion depend largely upon the resistance to flow offered by these collaterals.

In order to examine some of the known factors that influence the resistance to flow, it is important to define a few elementary concepts. The hemodynamic resistance may be defined simply as the ratio of energy drop between two points along a blood vessel ($E_1 - E_2$) to the mean flow in the vessel (Q):

$$R = \frac{E_1 - E_2}{Q}$$

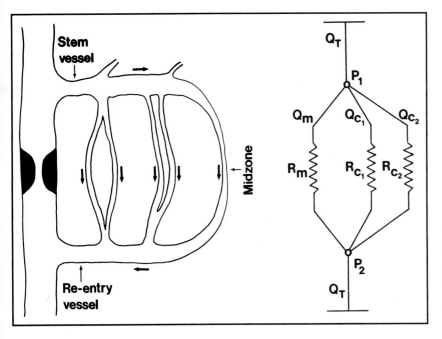

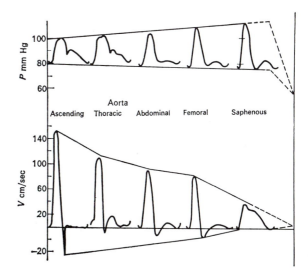

Figure 3-2. Diagram showing a collateral network bypassing a main pathway. Hemodynamically, this network can be illustrated by an electric circuit (*right*) where: Q_t = total flow; Q_m = flow through the main pathway; Q_{c1} and Q_{c2} = flow through the collaterals. In this parallel circuit: (1/total resistance) = $1/R_m + 1/R_{c1} + 1/R_{c2}$.

The kinetic energy ($\frac{1}{2}\,\rho v_2$) seldom contributes appreciably to the total energy, and the gravitational energy (ρgh) is equal to zero when the patient is examined in a supine position. Although this oversimplifies what really happens in human arteries, the resistance to flow can still be approximated by the ratio of the pressure drop ($P_1 - P_2$) to the flow:

$$\text{Resistance to flow} = \frac{\text{Pressure drop from point 1 to point 2}}{\text{Total flow}}$$

$$= \frac{P_1 - P_2}{Q}$$

The factors that contribute to the resistance to flow are expressed in Poiseuille's equation:

$$P_1 - P_2 = \frac{8LQ\eta}{\pi r^4}$$

where

L = length (cm)
r = radius (cm)
Q = volume flow (cm^3/sec)
η = viscosity (dyne-sec-cm^2)
$P_1 - P_2$ = pressure gradient (dynes/cm^2)

The terms of this equation that make up the resistance to flow are ($8L/r^4$) and η. In most situations, the blood behaves like a newtonian fluid, and the viscosity can be considered relatively constant. Thus, the major determinants of resistance are the length and radius of the vessel. Since viscous energy losses within the stenotic segment are inversely proportional to the fourth power of its radius and directly proportional to its length, the radius of a conduit is of much more significance than its length. It should also be noted from the formula that the volume of flow is important in determining the magnitude of the pressure gradient across a narrowed segment.

The mean blood pressure drop across normal arteries from the heart to the ankle is on the order of a few millimeters of mercury. Because of changes in compliance and the reflection of waves originating from the relatively high peripheral resistance, the peak systolic pressure increases as the pulse progresses toward the periphery (Fig. 3–3). Under resting conditions, the systolic pressure at the ankle normally exceeds the brachial systolic pressure by about 10 mm Hg.[17] In a normal extremity, moderate exercise will create an increase in flow, but the peak systolic and mean pressures will be maintained.

Arterial narrowing will affect these parameters. Under resting conditions, a 1 cm long stenosis in the iliac artery

Figure 3-3. As the pulse pressure wave travels from the heart to small peripheral arteries in the dog, the peak blood pressure increases. Conversely, the peak blood velocity decreases. (*Redrawn from McDonald DA: Blood Flow in Arteries. Baltimore, Williams & Wilkins, 1960.*)

of the dog must reduce the cross-sectional area to 20% of its original dimension (about 50% diameter reduction) before a pressure gradient develops.[18] The first pressure change to be noted is a reduction in the systolic pressure. As the stenosis increases further, the pulse pressure diminishes even more, and the mean pressure falls as well. As the resistance to flow increases further and more collaterals are added, the pressure will become nonpulsatile and reach very low levels (<20 mm Hg). With exercise or during reactive hyperemia, flow can be increased by a compensatory decrease in peripheral resistance.[19] However, this will result in a pressure drop distal to the involved area, and a prolonged time interval will be required before the pressure returns to the baseline level. Thus, an increase in flow induced by exercise or reactive hyperemia can create or accentuate a pressure gradient across a lesion and may be used to detect lesser degrees of stenosis.[20]

In contrast to the pressure pulse, there is a gradual reduction in the peak velocity of flow as it travels toward the periphery. Under resting conditions, flow in the peripheral arteries is normally characterized by its triphasic response: a first forward component during systole, followed by a transient reversal of flow in early diastole, and a second forward component in diastole. With exercise, this flow reversal disappears, and flow itself may become quasisteady during the hyperemic phase. Distal to an arterial narrowing, the peak velocity flow is reduced further than usual, and, as flow no longer returns to zero, the triphasic character of the flow pulse is lost.

More discrete changes of flow are present in the vicinity of very mild states of disease. These changes include the appearance of transient flow disturbances distal to a minor plaque, which can be detected by a sophisticated frequency analysis of the Doppler signal.

ACUTE ARTERIAL OCCLUSION

Acute obstruction of the peripheral arterial system is due to either thrombosis, embolism, or trauma. The problem faced by the vascular surgeon is to recognize the existence of the obstruction, determine its location, and plan the appropriate therapy. Although the etiology of the vascular occlusion may be extremely important, the real emergency is to estimate the effects of the obstruction on limb survival and ultimate function. Acute obstruction to the arterial system obviously poses the greatest threat to limb survival, since the midzone segment of the collateral arteries may not be able to respond rapidly enough to maintain distal flow at levels consistent with maintenance of viability. After occlusion occurs, distal pressure falls by an amount proportional to collateral resistance. Pressures less than 40 mm Hg distal to the occlusions are usually insufficient to maintain normal cellular function at rest and often are associated with eventual limb loss.

The cold, pale, pulseless, initially painful and later painless and paralyzed limb presents no problem in diagnosis. It is clear that under these circumstances immediate restoration of flow is mandatory to maintain limb viability. Time is always of the essence when pain, loss of sensation, or paralysis is present. The diagnosis is straightforward, and the time lost in carrying out an arteriography is usually

not justifiable. The ease with which proximal and distal acute occlusions can often be removed, using the common femoral artery as the point of entry for passage of the Fogarty catheter, has greatly simplified and extended the scope and application of this procedure.

Problems in the evaluation of acute arterial occlusion are more apt to occur when the clinical picture is less dramatic and the patient complains only of minimal symptoms. When the diagnosis is suspected, the history and physical examination are first performed in an attempt to estimate the severity of the ischemia and the site of involvement. It is often helpful to have additional information, which may be very useful and includes the distal blood pressure and the quality of the arterial velocity signals.

The peripheral arteries are thus quickly interrogated using a Doppler velocity detector, paying particular attention to the following sites: (1) arm—the axillary, brachial, radial, and ulnar arteries, (2) leg—the common femoral, midsuperficial femoral, popliteal, dorsalis pedis, and posterior tibial arteries at the ankle. Absence of a velocity signal from the arteries at the level of the knee or elbow is sure evidence of an occlusion. If no velocity signals are detected from the pedal arteries or the radial or ulnar arteries at the wrist, the vessels are either obstructed or the flow is so slow that it is not detectable by the instrument. The combination of severe ischemia with absence of velocity signals from the peripheral arteries is an ominous indication of marked compromise of the circulation to the limb. The ankle blood pressure at rest is usually less than 40 mm Hg and the ankle pressure index less than 0.35.

The management of acute arterial occlusions is dependent on several factors, including the general condition of the patient, the severity and duration of the ischemia, the location of the occlusion, and the underlying basis for the obstruction. Although it is always hazardous to generalize about the management of acute arterial occlusion, it is possible to make some suggestions that may be helpful. Indication for operation depends primarily on the location of the occlusions. When the obstruction is at the level of or proximal to the popliteal artery, operative removal of the thrombus or embolus must be done promptly unless there are some pressing contraindications. Since embolectomy in particular can be performed under local anesthesia, the procedure should rarely be withheld when indicated. The procedure should not be terminated until distal flow is assured by the return of normal distal pulses, an improved distal pressure, and, when indicated, an operative angiogram. If the viability of the limb can be reasonably assured, all major reconstructive procedures should be delayed until working conditions are more normal and considerably safer. Occlusions distal to the popliteal trifurcation rarely, unless very extensive, require operation. These patients may do very well without any form of treatment. In a prospective study of 142 patients undergoing cardiac catheterization in our institution, there were 15 patients who sustained embolic complications involving the arteries below the knee.[21] Initially, the ankle pressures were low and the pulses not palpable. Over a period of days, the pressures increased and the pulses returned. This improvement was attributed to the improved collateral function or the spontaneous lysis of the emboli.

While surgical embolectomy is a highly successful approach to the treatment of acute arterial occlusion, there are situations in which the use of a "medical" approach might be worthwhile. The availability of fibrinolytic agents (streptokinase, urokinase, tissue plasminogen activator) that can lyse thrombi has opened a new door for therapy.[22–24] However, in considering the potential role for these agents it is important to establish certain ground rules for their use:

1. They should *never* be used when limb viability is in immediate danger. With acute arterial occlusions, we generally consider any period extending beyond 4 to 6 hours as unwise since irreversible tissue damage and loss begins to occur.
2. If a simple embolectomy can be assured by the location of the occlusion, it is the preferred treatment method.
3. The drugs should never be used when there has been recent trauma or surgery because thrombi will be lysed and may cause severe bleeding.
4. Patients with a history of hypertension and those receiving dialysis should not be offered this therapy because of the risk, particularly for intracranial bleeding.

The ankle and arm pressure measurements provide a good index of the extent of occlusion and its hemodynamic effects and may be used as a method of gauging the improvement that occurs either spontaneously or as a result of therapy. Operative procedures, such as thrombectomy or embolectomy, should succeed in clearing the vessel of the occluding material. Complete removal of the occluding material will result in restoration of the ankle systolic pressure to normal levels. It is our practice to make these measurements in the operating room before and after the completion of the procedure. If the ankle systolic pressure does not increase, the artery is reopened and the embolectomy repeated. If, after the second attempt, the pressure continues to show little or no change, an intraoperative arteriogram is carried out to locate precisely the difficulty. With this type of evaluation procedure, it should rarely be necessary to return the patient to the operating theater for either a missed thrombus or embolus. In all cases, the pressure measurements are performed before closing the wound. The sterile Doppler technique is also used routinely.[25,26] This does not delay the procedure appreciably, and the results can be of great help to the surgeon in planning the subsequent management.

In the immediate postoperative period, arterial flow should be monitored by checking pulses, skin temperature, capillary and venous filling, and, most importantly, serial ankle and arm systolic pressures. In the event of deterioration and only if time permits, an immediate arteriogram is performed. Although major arterial flow can be restored, nutritive flow to the tissues may remain impaired. Since pressure and flow measurements are poor indicators of tissue viability, the evaluation of neuromuscular function is highly recommended as an integral part of postoperative monitoring.

A key, yet unanswered question relates to the issue of fasciotomy: when it should be done and on what to base the decision. The only reason to perform this operation is to prevent muscle necrosis from increased pressure in one of the major compartments of the lower leg. There are no predictive tests to tell the surgeon when and how much to decompress. If there is a delay, one can predict neurologic damage that in some cases will be irreversible as a result of the increase in compartment pressure.

One fact is clear—if a fasciotomy is needed, the sooner it is done the better. There are no firm guidelines other than time after the event. After a 4- to 6-hour interval the need for fasciotomy increases. Although it might appear logical to await the telltale signs of muscle tenderness and neurologic damage, these are late signs and essentially predict that there will be permanent disability due to nerve and muscle damage.

CHRONIC ARTERIAL OCCLUSION

Arteriosclerosis Obliterans

Atherosclerosis is the most common disease responsible for acute and chronic ischemia of the heart, brain, viscera, and lower extremities. The lesion itself results in a progressive narrowing of the involved vessels, with the attendant destruction of normal wall constituents. In later stages of disease, the arteries may become totally occluded or aneurysmal or may be the source of emboli.

There are several peculiarities of the atherosclerotic process that are of importance to the vascular surgeon. Although the process involves multiple levels of the arterial tree, it tends to be a segmental disease with intervening arterial segments remarkably free or minimally involved. The sites most commonly involved include branch points, bifurcations, zones of rapid tapering, and areas where the arteries follow a tortuous course. For unknown reasons, the upper extremity arteries, particularly those distal to the origin of the subclavian artery, are remarkably spared.

The patient with diabetes mellitus presents a unique and difficult problem. It is generally accepted that diabetics and others with abnormal glucose tolerance tests have a higher prevalence of arterial disease than have nondiabetics.[27–29] Approximately 30% of diabetic patients have some evidence of occlusive arterial disease in the legs, as detected by noninvasive vascular testing.[30] Histologically, the atherosclerotic process found in diabetics is indistinguishable from that observed in nondiabetics.[31] However, arteriosclerosis in large and medium-sized arteries not only appears at an earlier age in diabetics but also is more extensive and associated with a higher morbidity and mortality. The Silbert and Zazeela studies on 1198 patients found that in the nondiabetic group, 10% died within 10 years and 33% within 15 years after the onset of vascular symptoms.[32] Patients with diabetes had a much higher mortality, with 38% dying within 10 years and 69% within 15 years.

The amputation rate for nondiabetics is surprisingly low. Boyd[33] reported a 1.4% rate of limb loss per year. Silbert and Zazeela[32] had similar figures, with a rate of 8% in 5 years. This figure increased to 34% in the group with diabetes. The very poor prognosis for the diabetic patient is of great interest to the vascular surgeon who is frequently consulted with regard to the treatment of threatened or actual tissue loss. The diabetic state in itself has not been clearly identified as an independent risk factor for peripheral arterial disease. Other factors, such as a higher prevalence of abnormal lipoprotein metabolism in diabetics, may render them more susceptible to atherosclerosis and tissue loss.[31,34–36]

In an ongoing controlled study, the prevalence of atherosclerosis in diabetics was related to multiple risk factors.[30] Age, hypertension, and cigarette smoking all were found to be prominent independent contributors to atherosclerosis in the lower limbs. No significant correlations were found between fasting plasma glucose or glycosylated hemoglobin values and the presence of atherosclerosis. After accounting for cigarette smoking, the usual sex difference (male greater than female) was no longer observed in diabetics.

At present, it is recognized that the diabetic population must not be considered homogeneous, because there is increasing evidence that the rate of complications among diabetics is different according to the type of therapy. Beach et al. found that among 524 diabetics, those non-insulin-dependent diabetics (NIDDM) treated with an antihyperglycemic drug had a lower prevalence of severe ASO than those on diet therapy only.[37] Among the treated group, the prevalence was even lower in those on insulin therapy than in those on oral sulfonylurea therapy, in spite of similar fasting plasma glucose levels.

The rate of progression of peripheral artery disease is also more rapid among diabetic than among nondiabetic patients. For example, about 50% of patients with arterial disease at the time of entry into our study showed noninvasive laboratory criteria for progression (a decrease of greater than 0.15 in the ankle-arm index) over a two-year follow-up. For those type II patients without arterial disease at the time of entry into the study, 9% developed arterial disease in 2 years. An analysis of these data shows that the risk factors important (cigarette smoking, hypertension, lipid abnormalities) for those patients who develop atherosclerosis are not so for those who simply demonstrate "afferent" progression of disease.

The meaning of these findings is uncertain. For example, if accepted risk factors do not appear to apply to patients with disease progression, what is important? It may be that thrombosis in the vicinity of high-grade stenoses may occur and result in a fall in the ankle-arm index. If this is true, then another strategy might be in order, such as the use of antithrombotic therapy—perhaps aspirin—in treating patients with established disease.

Two other factors may render the diabetic patient more prone to tissue loss: the distribution of atherosclerotic lesions and the presence of peripheral neuropathy. It is generally conceded that there is a difference in the localization of atherosclerotic lesions in the lower extremity of diabetics as compared to the nondiabetic patients.[31] In cases where limbs are amputated, there is a much higher incidence of occlusions in the tibial arteries and peroneal arteries in patients with diabetes mellitus. The distribution of disease in the study reported by Gensler et al.[38] is very similar to that shown in Figure 3–4. These authors also noted a lower incidence of disease in the aortoiliac area in diabetics (13.4%) compared with nondiabetics (25%).

A question that is always raised and is of considerable importance relates to the concept of small vessel disease in the diabetic patient. A distinct and diffuse microangiopathy, characterized by degenerative changes in the arterioles

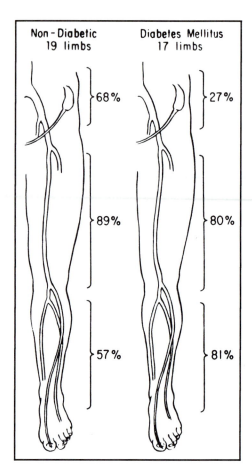

Figure 3-4. Disease distribution in diabetic (17 limbs) (*right*) and nondiabetic patients (19 limbs) (*left*) requiring an amputation.

and thickening of the capillary basement membrane, has been observed in diabetics.[39,40] However, these lesions are not entirely specific to diabetics,[41] and it remains to be proved whether these lesions are sufficient to explain the increased incidence of tissue loss.[42] The disease involving the large and medium-sized arteries is most likely the limiting factor in tissue nutrition.

Strandness and Bell found that approximately 27% of patients with arteriosclerosis obliterans had a peripheral neuropathy manifested by a loss of position sense, a decrease in vibratory sense, absent ankle jerks, and the inability to appreciate deep pain.[42] A neuropathy of this type, even in the absence of occlusive arterial disease, can lead to the development of deep, nonhealing ulcers at pressure points or areas of injury. Its recognition not only is helful in estimating prognosis but also should be taken into account when a lumbar sympathectomy is being considered. A sympathectomy would be of no value in attempting to increase limb blood flow in a leg already autosympathectomized by the neuropathy.

In practice, it is useful to categorize diabetic patients into the following groups:

1. *No arterial disease, no neuropathy.* There is no evidence that patients in this category are at an increased risk for limb loss.

2. *Arterial disease, no neuropathy.* There is a further subdivision of patients that is useful: (a) asymptomatic, (b)

symptomatic with exercise, and (c) symptomatic at rest. The asymptomatic patient requires nothing other than frequent observation and repeat noninvasive testing (every 6 months). The patient with claudication is treated on the basis of need, that is, severity of the pain and occupational-recreational needs. This is not a life-threatening condition, so conservatism must be the order of the day. If surgery or angioplasty is contemplated, one must keep in mind the "usual" distribution of disease in the type II diabetic patient (less aortoiliac disease, greater amount of tibial-peroneal disease). This makes these patients less likely candidates for direct arterial intervention.

Another approach that should be considered is the use of pentoxyfylline—a drug that reduces viscosity and because of this possibly increases tissue perfusion. It is best used for patients with severe claudication. It appears that approximately 80% of the patients get some benefit (either an increase in walking distance or less pain). Approximately half the patients with ischemic rest pain will get some benefit.

3. *No arterial disease, neuropathy present.* These patients present with normal foot pulses, a warm foot, dry skin, and a deep ulcer over pressure points. These lesions will always heal when the pressure is totally removed and there is no underlying joint or bone infection. In some cases it is necessary and possible to do limited excisions of the involved bone and joint to preserve the bulk of the foot, permitting continued use of the foot for walking.

4. *Arterial disease, peripheral neuropathy present.* This combination is particularly difficult to deal with. This is most evident in the patient who appears with an open, nonhealing ulcer. When this combination is present, direct arterial surgery, if feasible, is the only real hope for limb survival. This may be difficult because of the multisegmental disease, particularly the extensive occlusions in the tibial-peroneal segments. In some cases, in-situ saphenous vein graft may be feasible and the last resort in limb salvage.

Anatomically, the lower extremity can be divided into three segments: aortoiliac, femoropopliteal, and below the knee. Those lesions involving only one of the above segments are rarely associated with ischemic rest pain, ulceration, or gangrene. The potential for collateral circulation can usually provide enough blood flow to maintain the needs of the limb, at least under resting conditions.

The problems arise as the circulation is stressed by such events as walking when the nutritional needs of the exercising muscle increase several fold. During exercise, there are basically three factors that determine the extent of ischemia that develops: (1) the oxygen requirement of the muscle, (2) the perfusion pressure, and (3) the resistance of the collaterals. The oxygen requirements, of course, depend upon the workload, i.e., the amount of exercise. The perfusion pressure is countered by the force generated by the contracting muscle. Walder[43] showed that in patients with claudication, the flow may cease entirely during muscle contraction.[43] The higher than normal resistance to flow offered by the collaterals is the key element in the production of ischemia. These smaller alternative channels cannot supply the quantity of blood under the pressure required to prevent ischemia. Rhythmic exercise in the presence of a major artery occlusion initiates a deleterious cycle of events that cannot be reversed until exercise stops. As the ischemia

becomes more profound with each contraction, the resistance to flow during the relaxation phase falls to progressively lower levels, and the perfusion pressure also falls. Blood flow to skin and distal foot is diverted to the exercising muscle, giving rise to the pale white foot so commonly observed after exercise in patients with severe claudication.

A point often not appreciated is that complete occlusion of one large or medium-sized artery may not give rise to symptoms even during exercise. The extent to which an occlusion leads to symptoms is mostly dependent on the location and extent of the disease and the development of the collaterals. Occlusion in the aortoiliac area nearly always produces intermittent claudication with minimal exercise. This is because the entire limb is dependent on the collateral vessels that are bypassing the proximal disease. Isolated obstruction in the superficial femoral or popliteal arteries produces variable degrees of disability, ranging from no restriction in activity to moderately severe claudication. In this case, the thigh muscles are normally supplied, and only the calf muscles are deprived of normal arterial input. The collateral circulation that develops in response to a superficial femoral occlusion is extremely variable and is responsible for the marked difference in symptoms that develops in response to disease in that area.

Intermittent claudication of the lower leg is primarily secondary to ischemia of the gastrocnemius muscle. If the arterial occlusion is distal to the origin of the gastrocnemius, claudication, if it occurs, should be in the other muscle groups of the lower leg. Usually, occlusions in the tibial or peroneal arteries do not produce symptoms until the lesions are very extensive and associated with ischemic rest pain, ulceration, or gangrene.

When more than one arterial segment becomes occluded, an entirely different hemodynamic problem arises. The collateral arteries supplying the limb are now in series, resulting in a situation where the resistances are additive. This situation most commonly causes disabling claudication, ischemic rest pain, nonhealing ulcers, and gangrene. The determination of the hemodynamic and symptomatic significance of each diseased segment then becomes imperative.

Patient Evaluation

A thorough evaluation of the patient with symptoms and signs compatible with the diagnosis of arteriosclerosis obliterans must answer the following questions:

1. Do the symptoms occur at rest or only with exercise?
2. To what extent is the patient disabled?
3. What is the location of the arterial occlusion(s)? If multisegmental, which segment is mostly responsible for the patient's impairment?
4. What is the state of the runoff vessels?
5. Does the patient smoke or have coexisting diseases, such as diabetes mellitus, hypertension, hyperlipemia?
6. Is the patient a candidate for arterial reconstruction?

The history alone will provide many answers to these questions. The patient suffering only from functional limb ischemia will complain of mild to moderate intermittent claudication. At rest, the blood flow to the extremity is normal but cannot be augmented sufficiently to sustain muscular activity. The severity of the claudication is a measure of the capacity of collaterals to meet the demands of the exercising muscle. The location of the discomfort may be helpful in defining the most proximal level of occlusion. However, it must be kept in mind that calf claudication alone may not only be seen with superficial femoral obstruction but may also be the major complaint with aortoiliac disease. The more severe the symptoms, the more suspicious the surgeon must be of more than one level of occlusion.

Limb-threatening ischemia implies a reduction of flow to less than that required for normal resting metabolism of the tissues. It is manifested by pain at rest and/or necrosis. Extremity perfusion is so marginal that minor augmentation of flow, as achieved during limb dependency, usually alleviates ischemic pain. The limb is doomed to amputation unless circulation can be improved.

The physical examination provides additional information on the extent of disease. Pulse examination and arterial bruit auscultation are important parts of the study. However, it must always be remembered that the physical signs are subject to observer subjectivity and provide only a crude assessment of the location of the arterial occlusion. The appearance of the feet is useful only in the presence of advanced disease where the changes are characteristic. Most patients with single segment occlusions will, at the most, have dependent rubor.

After completion of the history and physical examination, the next step is physiologic testing. Many techniques can be used at all stages of diagnosis and follow-up. Because of duplication of effort and the time-consuming nature of these tests, not all are indicated for each patient or at each stage of follow-up. The surgeon must learn to select the modality that best fills the patient's needs. The sequence of noninvasive tests used in our laboratory for routine lower extremity arterial examination is summarized below.

Measurement of blood pressure at the ankle with the Doppler velocity detector is initially performed to rule out peripheral arterial disease. Bilateral brachial pressures are also measured, and the ankle pressure index for each leg is calculated. Stress testing with treadmill exercise can usually be tolerated by most patients who do not have ischemic rest pain and is the most physiologic test for further evaluation. When the ankle pressure is found to be abnormal, segmental pressures are obtained to define the approximate level of disease. The determination of toe pressures by digital plethysmography is performed only when pedal, palmar, or digital artery disease is suspected, when vasospastic phenomena are considered, or in the presence of medial calcification of the arteries at the ankle.

Analog waveforms are often recorded with a directional continuous-wave Doppler and a strip chart recording of Doppler shifted information utilizing the fast Fourier spectrum analyzer. Characteristics of the waveform from the common femoral, superficial femoral artery, dorsalis pedis, and posterior tibial arteries are very useful in the detection of disease. The CFA waveform is routinely recorded, and if the pulsatility index is determined, a value above 4.0 signifies a hemodynamically normal aortoiliac segment.[44,45]

Physiologic testing constitutes a very good screening routine, as shown in Figure 3–5. Patients with abnormal pressure measurements who are candidates for surgery may be submitted to further studies. Symptomatic patients with normal physiologic tests may be spared an unnecessary angiogram, because their symptoms are not likely to be of vascular origin. Abnormal physiologic testing in patients who are not candidates for surgery still constitutes a good baseline for follow-up monitoring. Deterioration often can be recognized before the patient becomes aware of it and can lead to closer surveillance or arteriography and surgery.

Although arteriography remains the final test prior to any intervention, the availability of duplex scanning has made the precise localization of arterial disease possible. In practice, the duplex approach has been helpful for making the following decisions:[46]

1. Is the *aortoiliac segment* normal, are there areas of stenosis, and what is their hemodynamic significance? When the velocity signal recorded from the aorta, the common, and external iliac arteries is triphasic without spectral broadening, it is almost certain that no disease of surgical significance is present. If areas of marked increases in peak systolic velocity are found (greater than 100% from preceding segment), this is almost certain evidence of a high-grade stenosis that cannot be ignored since it contributes to the pressure drop and decrease in flow that is present.

2. *Critical bifurcations.* In some cases, particularly multisegment disease, a critical factor in the success of either surgery or angioplasty may be the profunda femoris artery at and within a few centimeters of the origin.

3. *Femoropopliteal and tibial-peroneal trunks.* For the femoropopliteal segments, the duplex criteria used are the same as for the more proximal arterial inflow. It is possible not only to document the patency but also to estimate the site and magnitude of the hemodynamic derangement. It is possible to document patency of the more distal arteries but we have not yet attempted a more detailed assessment of stenotic lesions.

At the completion of a duplex scan it is possible to define the arterial segments that are diseased and to plan the therapy without resorting to angiography. Angiography is the remaining confirmatory test before direct intervention.

While not as common, lesions of the visceral vessels (mesenteric and renal) continue to be important to the vascular surgeon. The need for angiography and possible intervention has depended on identification of the patient at risk and proceeding directly with angiography. Because duplex scanning is useful for these areas as well, this should be the test to determine the need for angiography.[47,48] Current duplex scanning guidelines follow:

To date, we have not seen a patient with chronic mesenteric ischemia who did not have involvement of both the celiac and superior mesenteric arteries. These arteries are easily studied by duplex scanning. The failure to demonstrate stenoses in these two vessels rules out mesenteric ischemia as the cause of the patient's complaints.

In the renal arteries, a stenosis of 60% or greater (diameter reduction) is necessary to activate the renin-angiotensin system. By comparing the peak systolic velocity in the renal artery (along its course) to the adjacent abdominal aorta, it is possible to calculate the renal-aortic ratio (RAR). If this exceeds 3.5, there is a 90% chance that a high-grade stenosis is present and possibly responsible for the patient's hypertension. If the ratio is less than 3.5, there is a 96% chance that there are no significant lesions in the renal artery.

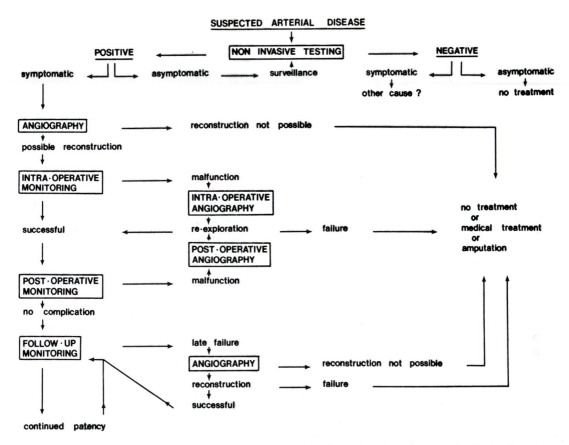

Figure 3-5. Physiologic tests now constitute an important part of the diagnosis and management of patients with peripheral arterial disease.

These same tests are useful after angioplasty or surgery to document both the immediate and long-term results of these approaches. In fact, this appears to be the only method currently available suitable for this purpose.

If surgery is recommended, the preoperative testing establishes the baseline against which improvement must be scaled. Intraoperative studies using the sterile Doppler technique[25,26] or pressure measurements identify operative accidents that can be corrected promptly. Close postoperative surveillance using these same tests permits early recognition of failure of reconstruction and once again prevents delay in necessary correction. Long-term beneficial effects are also best evaluated using these tests (Fig. 3–6).

In general, with single segment disease, direct arterial surgery, if successful, should restore hemodynamic normalcy to the extremity. In terms of pressure and flow, the following should be found: (1) the ankle systolic pressure should be greater than or equal to arm systolic pressure, (2) exercise should not result in a fall in the ankle blood pressure, and (3) the arterial velocity signals recorded from the reconstructed limb should be normal.

Problems with Multisegmental Disease

Extrapolating physiologic meaning from arteriographic data is a frequent error. Arteriography, even when multiple views are used, has a tendency to underestimate the severity of the lesions. When multisegmental disease is present, it becomes impossible to define angiographically which lesion is most responsible for the physiologic impairment.[10] Accurate measurement of the significance of aortoiliac disease is very important for proper management of patients with multisegmental disease. Failure to obtain good results in combined disease is usually due to the fact that the major site of resistance has not been bypassed.[49–51] Determining patients who would be relieved by the more proximal reconstruction is thus very important. The upper thigh pressure measurement and thigh-ankle gradient, even normalized by arm pressure, have little predictive value in that respect.[52–54] Direct intraarterial pressure gradient across the aortoiliac segment is now recognized as the most sensitive method of evaluating hemodynamically significant disease in this segment.[55–57]

Presently there are only two noninvasive tests that may prove useful for estimating the status of the aortoiliac segment. If the common femoral artery waveform is recorded and the pulsatility index (PI) calculated, it is possible to further subdivide patients. For example, if the PI exceeds 4.0, it is possible to rule out the proximal arterial segment as a basis for the production of a reduction in pressure and flow. If it is below 4.0, this is inconclusive because associated femoropopliteal disease may affect the result.[45,58–60]

A more suitable but more complex approach is the use of duplex scanning as previously outlined.[46] Its accuracy is clearly equal to that obtained by arteriography and will

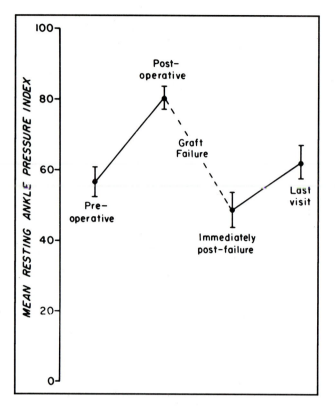

Figure 3-6. Mean resting ankle pressure indexes of 10 claudicants preoperatively (56.8 ± 4.3 SEM), postoperatively (80.7 ± 3.2 SEM), at the time of graft failure (48.9 ± 5.0 SEM), and at last visit (62.4 ± 4.7 SEM). (*From Lye CR, et al.: Ann Surg 183:38, 1976.*)

become more widely used and perhaps the definitive method for assessing patients with multisegment disease.

With multisegmental disease, correction of the proximal obstruction alone would increase the distal pressure, although not to normal levels, since remaining collateral beds would still be operative. Likewise, walking time may be increased, but the ankle blood pressure will still fall after exercise. Conversely, if proper selection of patients is made, as described above, correction of the high resistance lesion in the leg with a nonhemodynamically significant lesion left in the aortoiliac segment should resolve the physiologic abnormalities.

Thromboangiitis Obliterans (Buerger's Disease)

The existence of this disease as a distinct process appeared unquestioned until 1960 when Wessler et al.[61] seriously challenged Buerger's original description. In the ensuing decade, numerous reports were published that not only supported Buerger's original thesis but placed the diagnosis on a more solid base.[62,63] The problem was that the diagnosis was loosely applied to young male smokers with peripheral arterial disease. It is now clear that rigid criteria must be used to properly make this diagnosis.

To appreciate the spectrum of symptoms and signs that develop with this disease, it is necessary to review briefly our current knowledge concerning the pathophysiol-

ogy of thromboangiitis obliterans. The essence of the pathologic picture is widespread thrombosis in small, peripheral arteries and veins with periadventitial scarring that leads to fibrous encasement of the neurovascular bundle. In contrast to arteriosclerosis obliterans, the architecture of the vascular wall remains intact. Presumably, the end-stage organization is preceded, often in terms of years, by an acute lesion that consists of small microabscesses in the freshly organizing thrombus. The abscesses (presumably not bacterial) have a central core of polymorphonuclear leukocytes surrounded by giant cells, whereas the vessels immediately proximal to the involved areas are normal. The disease tends to begin in the smaller peripheral arteries of the legs and, in about 50% of patients, in the hands as well. It is usually confined distal to the knee and the elbow.

The clinical picture in most cases is quite specific, and the diagnosis should not be missed if its many facets are kept clearly in mind. The disease primarily strikes young male smokers. In the carefully studied series reported by McKusick et al.,[62] 4 of the 12 patients had the onset of symptoms before age 20, with another 7 developing the problems prior to age 35. The initial symptoms are quite variable but many include instep claudication, coldness, cold sensitivity, and a history of migratory superficial phlebitis. Late in the disease, severe rest pain, ulceration, and gangrene are common. About 50% of the patients also have hand involvement.

The claudication nearly always involves the instep, a fact of considerable diagnostic importance. The rest pain that occurs is very severe and is rarely helped by any procedure short of amputation. Because the disease involves the distal medium-sized arteries, the femoral, popliteal, and brachial artery pulses are usually normal. Arteriography is useful in documenting the normalcy of the arteries proximal to the involved areas. Although the diagnosis can be strongly suspected on the basis of the above considerations, it is clear that the final confirmation relies on the histologic examination of the neurovascular bundle.

EXTRACRANIAL ARTERIAL DISEASE

Stroke ranks as the second most common cause of death due to vascular disease in the United States and is still a leading cause of permanent disability.[64] It is estimated that between 40 and 70% of all stroke episodes are of vascular origin.[65] Fortunately, the principal site for carotid artery disease is the carotid bifurcation, thus allowing direct access for investigation and surgical correction. Good long-term results after carotid endarterectomy have supported this form of therapy as a good prophylaxis against stroke and increased considerably the need and interest in the evaluation of the carotid arterial system.[66–68]

Stenoses or occlusions involving the neck arteries produce ischemic symptoms by hemispheric flow deprivation that can take place by the following mechanisms: (1) total flow reduction to a hemisphere or region of the brain secondary to the occlusion or marked narrowing of the involved artery, (2) release of small particles of cholesterol, calcium, platelets aggregates, or thrombi originating from ulcerated plaques along the carotid arteries, and (3) diversion of blood away from the brain as an extracranial artery serves as a diverting collateral, usually to the arm (the so-called subclavian steal syndrome).

Clinically, a patient with ischemic cerebrovascular disease may have (1) transient ischemic attacks (TIAs), which are characterized by a sudden, unexpected onset of neurologic symptoms lasting less than 24 hours and resolving completely, usually within minutes, (2) amaurosis fugax or sudden loss of a varying portion of the visual field in one eye with total recovery within minutes also, (3) reversible ischemic neurologic deficits (RINDs) or sudden hemispheric neurologic deficits that may last longer than 24 hours but where there is a gradual improvement until complete recovery, usually within 3 weeks, (4) stroke in evolution, initiating neurologic problems that gradually progress to a fixed state without regression, and (5) complete stroke, defined as a neurologic deficit that appears immediately after the event and remains largely stable. Improvement can occur with time, but the deficit does not completely resolve.

Episodes of transient ischemic attacks are recognized as important precursors of stroke, since 40% of affected patients are likely to develop a cerebral infarction within 5 years after the initial event.[69] Of equal importance for the vascular surgeon are those patients who present with amaurosis fugax and reversible neurologic deficits, since they carry the same risk of developing a stroke after the first event. These patients are prime candidates for a carotid endarterectomy and thus angiography.

While selective contrast arteriography remains the definitive and required diagnostic study prior to carotid surgery, the discomfort, expense, and risk[70,71] associated with this test preclude its use to screen or serially follow patients suspected of having extracranial arterial disease. A variety of safe, quick, and less expensive noninvasive tests have thus been developed to serve as screening methods for this patient population.

These tests can be regarded as either indirect or direct tests. The indirect tests include supraorbital Doppler sonography,[72] oculoplethysmography,[73] and oculopneumoplethysmography.[74] These tests are sensitive only for pressure and flow-reducing lesions and thus will miss any other lesions. In addition, they are unable to distinguish between a high-grade stenosis and a total occlusion, a point of major importance clinically.

A better and more widely used approach is duplex scanning. This permits classifying disease in all stages of development and can also be used to distinguish a stenosis from an occlusion. Furthermore, progress of the disease can also be documented, making duplex scanning the most suitable method for follow-up studies.

ARTERIOVENOUS FISTULA

The development of a communication between a major artery and vein has always been a lesion of considerable interest to the vascular surgeon. The creation of such a lesion may produce problems because of the volume of blood shunted into the venous system and its effect, not only on the heart but on the tissue peripheral to the fistula as well. The simplest representation of an AV fistula is the side-to-side or H-type AV fistula, which comprises a proximal artery and vein, a distal artery and vein, and collateral arteries and veins (Fig. 3–7).

Definite anatomic changes occur in the vicinity of a fistula that are important to recall:

1. The proximal artery undergoes progressive elongation and enlargement to the point where it often becomes very tortuous and aneurysmal.[75–77]
2. Degenerative changes are seen in the proximal artery that are characterized by atrophy of smooth muscle, decrease in elastic tissue, and formation of atheromatous plaque.[78,79]
3. The proximal vein also dilates and becomes tortuous. The wall initially thickens. With time, the internal elastic lamina fragments and tends to disappear. Degenerative changes of the wall and venous aneurysm formation occur.[78,79]
4. The distal vein dilates as well, elongates, and becomes progressively incompetent. With time, the degenerative changes observed are comparable to those seen in the proximal vein.
5. The distal artery remains relatively unchanged.

Hemodynamics

In order to understand the hemodynamics of an AV fistula, it is imperative to review the direction of flow in each of the component branches (Fig. 3–7):

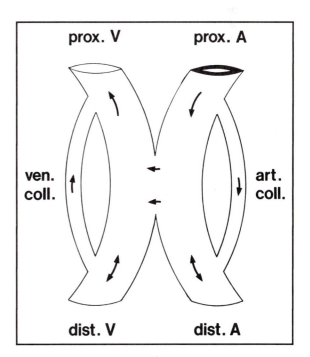

Figure 3-7. Flow in the proximal artery and arterial collateral is always directed distally. Flow in the proximal vein and venous collateral is always directed centrally. Flow in the distal artery or vein can be directed in either direction (see text for explanation).

1. Because the fistula markedly reduces the peripheral resistance, blood flow in the proximal artery loses its triphasic characteristic. Flow will always be increased, particularly during diastole, and no reversed component will be observed. A decreased pulsatility will then ensue.[80–82]
2. Blood flow in the proximal vein increases and shows a dampened pulsatile pattern.
3. The direction of flow in the distal artery and vein can be either toward or away from the fistula. Conversely, flow in the proximal artery and arterial collaterals is always directed toward the periphery, and the flow in the proximal vein and venous collaterals is always directed centrally (Fig. 3–7).
4. In a large chronic fistula, the inverted pressure gradient created will force retrograde flow through the dilated and incompetent distal vein until it reaches a large collateral (Fig. 3–8).[83,84]
5. High resistance in the proximal artery and distal vascular bed, combined with relatively low resistance at the site of the fistula and in the arterial collaterals, will favor a retrograde flow in the distal artery.[81,83,84]

Blood pressures in the arteries and veins contributing to the fistula are important factors that determine the direction and quantity of flow in each branch.

1. Blood pressure in the proximal artery is usually maintained at its normal level or may even increase when the artery becomes dilated.[82]
2. Both the mean and pulse pressures in the distal artery are almost always reduced.[81–84]
3. When the shunt is important, the blood is siphoned by the fistula, lowering the pressure at the arterial side of the fistula. When the collaterals are sufficient to raise the distal pressure, the inverted pressure gradient thus created favors a reversed flow in the distal artery.[83]
4. Pressure levels and pressure gradients are quasinormal in the distal vein when the fistula is small. When the fistula is large, pressure in the distal competent vein may exceed the arterial pressure. When the vein becomes incompetent, pressure levels diminish, and a reversed pressure gradient is created in the distal vein.[80,81]

Acquired AV Fistula

Apart from the angioaccess procedure, which will be dealt with separately, penetrating injuries are by far the most common cause of acquired AV fistula. It can also occur secondary to infection, neoplasm, and aneurysmal erosion. The problem during the evaluation phase can be considered as follows: (1) making the diagnosis, (2) estimating the functional effects of the fistula, (3) deciding upon when therapy should be carried out, and (4) planning the operative approach. The last problem will be discussed in a subsequent chapter and will not be considered further here.

Making the Diagnosis

There should always be a high index of suspicion whenever a patient has a penetrating injury in or adjacent to regions where the major arterial and venous components are likely to be injured. In the acute phase, a hematoma, which is often pulsating, is always present. A palpable thrill and a bruit are always present directly over the site of the fistula. The bruit is continuous, often loud, and very similar to that heard with a patent ductus arteriosus. The diagnosis of an acquired, traumatic AV fistula is rarely missed on the basis of history and physical examination alone and can be confirmed by arteriography. Noninvasive diagnostic procedures will provide invaluable physiologic documentation, critical for the proper management of such patients.

Waveform analysis of the directional Doppler signal is certainly the most useful diagnostic test in this setting. Due to the decreased resistance in periphery, the Doppler velocity waveform of the major inflow artery will show characteristic increases in forward flow with no reversed component. The entire waveform, particularly the diastolic velocities, will be elevated well above the baseline in direct proportion to the decrease in peripheral resistance. The signal heard over the varicose veins draining the fistula will be increased and often pulsatile near the fistula. The directional Doppler probe will best estimate the direction of flow in the various arteries and veins contributing to the fistula and the relative importance of the collateral vessels.

Segmental limb pressure measurements, using the

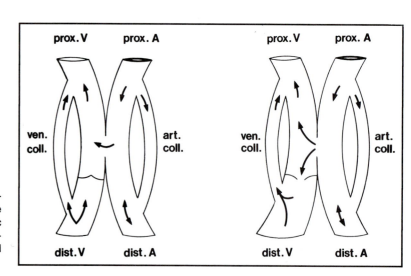

Figure 3-8. In the acute stage (*left*), the distal vein is still competent, and flow in the distal vein is directed centrally. In the chronic phase (*right*), the distal vein dilates and becomes incompetent. Flow can be directed distally until it reaches a large collateral.

Doppler flowmeter or a plethysmographic method, will provide an objective assessment of the functional effects of the fistula. The reduced peripheral resistance associated with the AV fistula and the amount of blood being shunted away from it will result in a decreased arterial pressure distal to the fistula. The arterial pressure gradient across the fistula is particularly increased when the fistula is large, the collaterals are not well developed, and the flow is retrograde in the distal artery, thus creating a significant steal from the distal flow. Proximal to the AV fistula, the segmental pressure is normal or increased as compared to the contralateral side. Of particular diagnostic value is the rise of a lowered peripheral pressure when compression of the suspected lesion or a large proximal or distal vein is done.

Estimating the Functional Effect of an AV Fistula

The amount of blood shunted into the venous system will have an effect not only on the heart but on the tissues peripheral to the fistula as well.

When the peripheral pulse remains intact and the distal systolic pressures are normal, the fistula may be considered relatively small from a hemodynamic standpoint. If the pulses are decreased or absent and the distal pressure is low, this indicates that a large volume shunt is present. In rare instances, the amount of blood siphoned may be large enough to produce peripheral ischemia and gangrene. The best way to evaluate the hemodynamic contribution of the various vessels that make up the fistula is by noting the effect produced by selected compression of each of these branches (Fig. 3-9):

1. Compression of the proximal artery will always cause a decrease in peripheral pressure and pulse. Antegrade flow in the distal artery will be stopped or reversed, but an already reversed flow will be increased in the reverse direction.

2. If compression of the proximal or distal vein increased the distal arterial flow or pressure, it can be assumed that the compressed vein is an important outflow channel to the fistula.

3. Sometimes, the distal pressure is higher than normal, and compression of the distal vein decreases the pressure toward a more normal level. This paradoxical situation indicates that an important venous congestion exists in the distal venous bed, thus leading to a high distal pressure.

4. If compression of a distal artery is followed by a rise in distal pressure, it can be assumed that a distal steal exists. A decrease in distal pressure invariably indicates an antegrade flow in the distal artery.

Selective compression of all the branches contributing to the fistula and the collaterals thus provides a good estimate of their respective roles in the nutrition of peripheral tissues and orients the therapeutic approach.

The cardiac effects have been extensively studied and summarized by Sumner[81] and are as follows:

1. When the fistula is created, the mean systolic blood pressure usually falls but returns to normal within minutes.

2. The heart rate also tends to increase immediately but returns to normal levels unless the volume shunted is excessively large.

3. The cardiac output increases by an amount corresponding to the shunt flow up to approximately 20%. When the volume exceeds this level, the heart is unable to compensate completely for this level of flow. The major change responsible for the increase in cardiac output is in the stroke volume.

4. As the fistula becomes chronic, the blood volume increases.

5. Compression of the fistula results in an immediate decrease in heart rate (Branham's sign), particularly if the

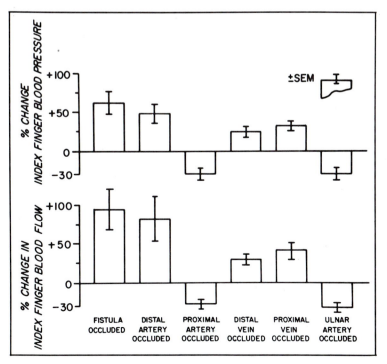

Figure 3-9. These histograms represent the mean and SE of the percent changes in digital blood pressure and flow produced by compressing various portions of the AV fistula circuit in 24 limbs with radial artery–cephalic vein fistulas constructed for hemodialysis. (*From Strandness DE Jr, Sumner DS: Hemodynamics for Surgeons, New York, Grune & Stratton, 1975, p 634.*)

volume shunted is sufficient to result in changes in cardiac performance.

Timing of Therapy

The timing of the operative repair is often dictated largely by the volume of blood being shunted and its effects on the cardiovascular system. The systemic effects are of particular importance in the elderly or in patients who have preexisting cardiac problems. Although it is always difficult to formulate hard and fast rules with regard to this aspect, a few general concepts are in order. In general, the more centrally the fistula is placed, the larger the volume shunted and the earlier the corrective procedure should be done. For example, fistulas between the abdominal aorta and inferior vena cava can be very severe and produce immediate cardiac failure, requiring an emergency operation. If the patient is tolerating well the hemodynamic effects of the shunt, operation can be planned and scheduled in a more leisurely manner.

Congenital AV Fistula

Congenital AV communications are rare lesions that may present serious diagnostic and therapeutic problems for the surgeon. They are developmental anomalies and are present from birth. Szilagyi et al.[85] proposed a simple classification of these lesions that is less confusing than the multitude of terms often used. Because the pathogenesis appears to be similar in most cases, the classification includes: (1) cavernous or simple hemangiomas, (2) microfistulous communications, and (3) macrofistulous communications.

The cavernous or simple hemangioma represents an arrest of the development of the circulation during the stage of an undifferentiated capillary network. If the arrest occurs at a later stage, when differentiation of the main vascular channel is occurring, the intercommunications are then between mature arteries and veins. At this stage, the anomaly produced will result in either microfistulous communications (not visible angiographically) or macrofistulous communications. The extent to which these lesions produce problems is dependent on their location, size, and extent and volume of blood shunted. Although the shunt is rarely important enough to create systemic effects, problems, either cosmetic, hemorrhagic, or secondary to the venous hypertension, may result.

The clues to the existence of underlying arteriovenous communications include unilateral swelling (often out of proportion to the apparent pathology), limb hypertrophy, and varicose veins of atypical location and early onset (Fig. 3-10). The diagnosis can be, in some instances, supported by the finding of arterial signals over the clusters of veins with an ultrasonic velocity detector. Contrast arteriography, using rapid cassette changing technique, is often useful and diagnostic and is mandatory before surgical therapy. However, in nearly 40% of congenital AV fistulas, the communications themselves will not be demonstrated,[86] and the diagnosis will depend solely on indirect evidence[87] (early venous filling, presence of a cluster of anomalous arterial branches in the vicinity of dilated superficial veins, rapid clearance of contrast material). The Doppler velocity detec-

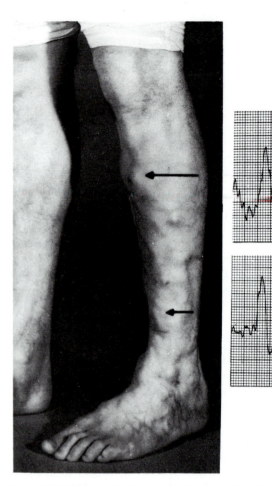

Figure 3-10. Photograph of a patient with congenital arteriovenous fistulas involving the left lower leg. The Doppler flow waveform in the large subcutaneous clumps of veins had an arterial pulsatile pattern (*right*). (*From Strandness DE Jr, Sumner DS: Hemodynamics for Surgeons. New York, Grune & Stratton, 1975, p 634.*)

tor, used both preoperatively and intraoperatively, will provide important documentation of every arterial and venous branch contributing to the lesion. The use of a Doppler probe is particularly useful for postoperative surveillance in searching for residual or recurrent fistulas.

Angioaccess AV Fistula

A carefully performed venous Doppler study is part of the routine preoperative evaluation of patients prior to angioaccess surgery. The venous Doppler signal, its phasicity, and its proximal and distal augmentation are characterized on the course of the major superficial and deep veins of each extremity. To optimize the chance of success and help select the best donor artery, a preoperative survey of the arterial system using Doppler waveform analysis and limb pressure measurements is also done. Careful arterial evaluation is particularly important if distal arteries are being considered as donor arteries. For example, if one considers using the radial or ulnar artery as the donor site, the patency of both vessels should be assured by flow velocity waveform analysis. If only one vessel is patent and is used to create the fistula, one may expect a greater risk of distal steal phenomenon and severe ischemia of the extremity if the fistula thromboses. The patency of the palmar arch is also checked using the Doppler probe and the Allen patency test. Once again, if the palmar arch is found incomplete, the major feeding artery should not be used as the donor artery. The sterilized Doppler probe is also used intraoperatively to document any unrecognized complication.

Strandness and Sumner[82] found that there is a drop in digital pressure in 88% of patients after creation of a radial artery-cephalic vein fistula. With time and the development of collaterals, there will be an improvement in this decreased distal perfusion, and further pressure drop during hemodialysis perfusion rarely occurs.

The noninvasive studies are repeated before the fistula is used and at regular intervals thereafter or at the time of any pain or temperature change, thus permitting early recognition of postoperative complication. Once again, if ischemic pain or swelling develops in the hand, the Doppler study with compression maneuvers previously described will best document the cause of the symptoms and guide the therapeutic approach.

ANTERIOR TIBIAL COMPARTMENT SYNDROME

The development of acute pain, swelling, and a neurologic deficit in and changes in the anterior tibial compartment has long been a source of confusion and concern to the vascular surgeon. In its classic form, the tibial compartment syndrome has been reported following a period of stressful exercise, with local pain, tenderness, weakness of the anterior tibial musculature, and hypoesthesia in the first interdigital cleft. Prompt fasciotomy of this compartment is recommended to minimize the neuromuscular disability that is known to occur if the problem is left untreated or is approached late in the course of the disease.

It is now apparent that besides stressful exercise, there are other causes of the compartment syndrome, which are grouped under the broad classification of traumatic and vascular.[88] Although it is also clear that other compartments of the lower leg can be involved to the extent that fasciotomy is required, the peculiar nature of the anatomy of the anterior compartment make it particularly susceptible to this problem. The anterior compartment is a cylindrical space, with unyielding osteofascial boundaries. Any abrupt change in the size of any of the contents of the space may have pronounced and deleterious effects.

The exact pathophysiology of the compartment syndrome remains incompletely understood, but it is clear that the major factor that ultimately leads to the neuromuscular changes is an increase in pressure within the compartment. Other than the syndrome occurring after an episode of severe exercise, most cases have been associated with either arterial disease or arterial trauma.

The questions relating to timing and indicators for fasciotomy are not clearly definable at present. Although there is little doubt about the patient with a tender, swollen anterior compartment accompanied by hypoesthesia of the first interdigital space, beyond this type of clinical presentation, it is very difficult to draw firm and final conclusions about the indications for fasciotomy. Unfortunately, intracompartmental pressure measurements do not reliably help in that respect. It is clear, however, that when a fasciotomy is indicated, it should be performed immediately, because delays only tend to result in more tissue destruction.

THORACIC OUTLET SYNDROME

Pain in the neck, shoulder, and upper arm, with finger paresthesia is a common disorder that is both confusing and difficult to define precisely. From a diagnostic standpoint, many disorders may create similar symptoms and signs and further complicate an understanding of the pathophysiology involved. The diagnosis of the syndrome is often one of exclusion, and the differential diagnosis should rule out, besides an orthopedic shoulder problem, a cervical disc syndrome or spondylitis of the cervical spine and a carpal tunnel syndrome.

By virtue of its course from the neck and thorax, the neurovascular bundle is subject to compression by both congenitally anomalous fibromuscular bands and skeletal structures.[89,90] Traditionally, the basis for the syndrome has been divided into the underlying anatomic defect(s), which include the scalene, cervical rib, costoclavicular, and hyperabduction syndrome. Disappearance of the radial pulse in a variety of arm positions was considered of diagnostic value in each of these syndromes. It is now generally accepted that alteration of pulses and pressure with the various compression maneuvers has nothing to do with the patient's symptoms. When the symptoms are reproduced at the time of those maneuvers, it is most often caused by the concomitant compression of the brachial plexus. These maneuvers have very limited diagnostic value, since more than 50% of normal subjects will have disappearance of the radial pulse during an Adson test.

The syndrome is mostly seen in young or middle-aged adults, mainly women, who may often present an underlying mechanical susceptibility to this syndrome, such as a congenital anomaly of cervical rib, an elongated transverse process of the seventh cervical vertebra, and congenital fibromuscular bands. Patients with low-lying shoulder girdle on the thorax have a narrow clavicular space that predisposes them to costoclavicular scissor compression of the neurovascular bundle. In addition, fractured clavicle callus, fractured first ribs, exostosis of the first rib or clavicle, or tumors in the outlet make neurovascular compression more likely.

The patient often complains of intermittent aching discomfort felt in the anterior or posterior shoulder region, radiating down the arm, in the medial and lateral brachial area, through the forearm, and into the hand. Paresthesias may be present and accompany the aching pain. Numbness and weakness of the fingers are sometimes observed in severe cases. Raynaud's phenomenon can also develop in some patients. When the symptoms take a dermatomal distribution, it is usually in the C8–T1 dermatomae (ulnar nerve area). Symptoms are induced or aggravated by positional changes, such as elevated use of the hand. Coldness and even pallor of the hand may be part of the neurologic syndrome.

Rarely, compression of the subclavian artery will produce symptoms.[89] When ischemic symptoms of arterial origin occur, they consist of coldness and pallor of the hand, ischemic pain of the arm, and severe cyanosis and pain of the fingertips from arterial emboli. Arterial lesions can develop at the site of compression in the thoracic outlet or from poststenotic aneurysmal dilatation of the subclavian artery, which may further thrombose and give rise to peripheral emboli. When venous problems occur from subclavian vein occlusion, they take the form of a sudden onset of edema of the arm, with dusky cyanosis and limb discomfort. The intermittent subclavian vein compression, with transient edema, heaviness, and discomfort of the arm during exertion or with certain positions, is sometimes observed. Recognition of these premonitory symptoms and proper treatment can prevent certain subclavian thrombosis.[91]

A carefully performed physical examination with specific attention to the neck, shoulder, and upper extremity is the most important factor in making the proper diagnosis and ruling out other causes of the symptoms.

Finger warmth and color are most often normal, sometimes intermittently pale or even cyanotic. There is usually no edema of the fingers. The interosseous muscles are innervated by the ulnar nerve, but their strength is usually normal. The triceps are noticeably weak on the side involved. Percussion of the plexus is painful, and its compression in the supraclavicular fossa may reproduce the symptoms. Reflexes are normal in the thoracic outlet syndrome, but pain sensitivity may be diminished in the territory innervated by the ulnar nerve or sometimes in all areas of the hand. Key diagnostic features in these patients are (1) prompt appearance of paresthesia and numbness with the arm abducted to 90° and externally rotated, (2) appearance of a prominent bruit in the supraclavicular fossa, and (3) immediate disappearance of the symptoms when the arm is returned to the neutral position.

Even with the presence of a certain relationship between arm position and symptoms, it is essential to rule out other causes for the clinical picture, notably, a cervical disc syndrome, a degenerative joint disease, and the carpal tunnel syndrome.

Cervical spine films are routinely taken searching for degenerative cervical spine disease, disc space narrowing, osteophytes, congenital anomalies of the last cervical vertebra, and structural anomalies of the vertebrae, first rib, and clavicle. The shoulder girdle level is determined by counting the number of vertebrae above the clavicle level on the lateral view of a cervical spine series. Cervical myelography is reserved when cervical disc herniation is strongly suspected. X-rays of articulations may be useful when there is a previous history of trauma, collagen disease, or inflammatory process.

Unfortunately, both electromyograms and nerve conduction time studies have been very disappointing in providing objective diagnostic data in the syndrome. Angiography has no value in the diagnosis, because intermittent arterial compression is rarely the cause of the disorder. Its use should be reserved for patients presenting ischemic symptoms of the upper extremity and with a pressure gradient between the arms of more than 20 mm Hg and when an aneurysm or some other source of emboli is suspected.

VASOSPASTIC DISORDERS

In contrast to the situation in the lower limbs, arteriosclerosis obliterans is rarely seen in the upper extremities and is not the main pathologic disturbance leading to hand ischemia. Most commonly, digital ischemia results from inappropriate arterial and arteriolar vasospasm as observed in acrocyanosis, livedo reticularis, drug reaction, nonspecific cold sensitivity, and Raynaud's syndrome.

Acrocyanosis

Constant coolness and persistent bluish discoloration of the hands and feet are conditions sometimes observed in young women. Mild edema is sometimes present. Although cold temperatures may worsen the symptoms, the discoloration and coldness are usually present in warm weather. Good prognosis is expected, and treatment should be conservative.

Livedo Reticularis

The combination of spasm of certain cutaneous arterioles and secondary dilatation of the associated capillaries and venules gives rise to a characteristic persistent bluish mottling of the skin over the lower legs and feet and, occasionally, the hands. Sometimes in association with lupus erythematosus, periarteritis nodosa, or, more rarely, cholesterol embolization, most livedo reticularis cases occur without associated disease. A cold environment does worsen the symptoms, which are often also present in warm temperatures. The condition causes only cosmetic problems, and only avoidance of cold can be recommended.

Raynaud's Syndrome

The patient with episodic digital ischemia secondary to cold exposure often poses a serious dilemma for the physician. The symptomatology is quite specific and consists of the so-called triphasic color response upon exposure to cold. The fingertip(s) initially turn white, then blue, and finally red as the fingers are warmed. During the ischemic phase, the patient usually complains of either pain or numbness or both, which can be very troublesome. The attacks may occur in patients without associated diseases (primary Raynaud's disease) or in patients who have a variety of local or systemic diseases, listed in Table 3-1 (secondary Raynaud's phenomenon). Because the clinical courses of the two entities are different, it is important to make the distinction between the two. Unfortunately, making a determination of an underlying cause is difficult and may often take years after the initial appearance of complaints. Careful adherence to criteria originally described by Allen and

TABLE 3-1. DISEASES ASSOCIATED WITH RAYNAUD'S PHENOMENON

Intravascular
  Cryoglobulinemia
  Cold agglutinins
Vascular
  Thromboangiitis obliterans
  Occupational trauma
  Collagen disorders: Scleroderma; Dermatomyositis; Systemic lupus erythematosus; Polyarteritis
  Frostbite, immersion foot
Extravascular
  Sympathetic hyperactivity
  Thoracic outlet syndrome
  Causalgia

Brown[92] can lead to the correct diagnosis of primary Raynaud's disease in most cases:

1. The attacks can be precipitated by either cold or emotional stimuli.

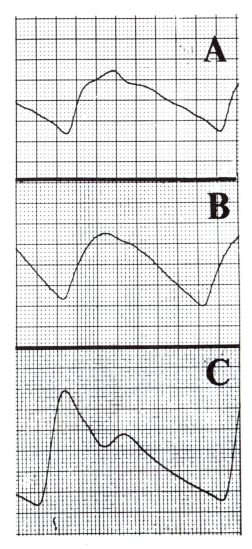

Figure 3-11. Digital volume pulse contour. **A.** Peaked pulse. **B.** Dampened obstructive pulse. **C.** Normal pulse. (*From Sumner DS, Strandness DE Jr: Ann Surg 175:294, 1972.*)

2. The involvement is bilateral and usually symmetric.
3. There is no evidence of occlusive disease of the arm or digital arteries.
4. Gangrene, although rarely present, is always limited to the skin of the tips of the digits.
5. There is a history of symptoms for at least 2 years, preferably longer, during which time none of the conditions associated with Raynaud's phenomenon have been recognized.

Excluding occlusive arterial disease in the hand is the first task of the noninvasive vascular evaluation of a patient presenting with symptoms of cold sensitivity. After the hands have been warmed, Doppler blood flow curves and digit pressure measurements are made. The status of the palmar circulation is also assessed by performing an Allen compression test. Digital strain gauge plethysmography is then used to record pulse waves. Patients with Raynaud's disease will have normal finger pressures. The waveforms recorded with the plethysmograph either will be normal or show a very sharp systolic peak due to the presence of an incisura (the peaked pulse) (Fig. 3-11). Patients with Raynaud's phenomenon will show a reduction in digit pressures and a rounded pulse waveform consistent with digit or palmar artery occlusions. Local cooling of the entire hand or finger[93,94] will result in a fall of the digital pressure when a critical temperature is reached. This finding does not usually occur in normal fingers and is most useful in screening patients suspected of having cold sensitivity. Unfortunately, the cooling test will not permit further separation of those patients with either primary or secondary Raynaud's syndrome. However, the reproducibility of the test (coefficient of variation, 10%)[94] permits useful monitoring of the effect of treatment.

REFERENCES

1. Silver RA, Scherle HL, et al.: Intermittent claudication of neurospinal origin. Arch Surg 98:523, 1969.
2. Marinelli MR, Beach KW, et al.: Noninvasive testing vs clinical evaluation of arterial disease. A prospective study. JAMA 241:2031, 1979.
3. Fisher CM: Observations of the fundus oculi in transient monocular blindness. Neurology 1:333, 1959.
4. Barnett HJM: Platelet and coagulation function in relation to thromboemboli stroke, in Adv in Neurol 15:45, in Thompson RA and Green JR (eds), Raven Press, New York, 1977.
5. Thiele BL, Young IV, et al.: Correlation of arteriographic findings with symptoms in patients with cerebrovascular disease. Neurology 30:1041, 1980.
6. Beales JSM, Adcock FA, et al.: The radiological assessment of disease at the profunda femoris artery. Br J Radiol 44:854, 1971.
7. Sethi GK, Scott SM, Takaro T: Multiple-plane angiography for more precise evaluation of aortoiliac disease. Surgery 78:154, 1975.
8. Crummy AB, Rankin RS, et al.: Biplane arteriography in ischemia of the lower extremity. Radiology 126:111, 1978.
9. Thomas ML, Andrews MR: Value of oblique projections in translumbar aortography. Am J Roentgenol 116:187, 1973.
10. Castaneda-Zuniga Q, Knight L, et al.: Hemodynamic assessment of obstructive aortoiliac disease. Am J Roentgenol 127:559, 1976.

11. Karayannacos PE, Talukder N, et al.: The role of multiple noncritical arterial stenoses in the pathogenesis of ischemia. J Thorac Cardiovasc Surg 73:458, 1977.

12. Longland CJ: The collateral circulation of the limb. Ann R Coll Surg Engl 13:161, 1953.

13. Ludbrook J: Collateral artery resistance in the human lower limb. J Surg Res 6:423, 1966.

14. Skinner JS, Strandness DE Jr: Exercise and intermittent claudication. Effect of repetition and intensity of exercise. Circulation 36:25, 1967.

15. Dornhorst AC, Sharpy-Shafer EP: Collateral resistance in limbs with arterial obstruction: spontaneous changes and effects of sympathectomy. Clin Sci 10:371, 1951.

16. Sumner DS, Strandness DE Jr: The effect of exercise on resistance to blood flow in limbs with an occluded superficial femoral artery. Vasc Surg 4:229, 1979.

17. McDonald DA: Blood flow in arteries. Baltimore, Williams and Wilkins, 1960.

18. May AG, DeWeese JA, Rob CG: Hemodynamic effects of arterial stenosis. Surgery 53:513, 1964.

19. Sumner DS, Strandness DE Jr: The relationship between calf blood flow and ankle blood pressure in patients with intermittent claudication. Surgery 65:763, 1969.

20. Carter SA: Response of ankle systolic pressure to leg exercise in mild or questionable arterial disease. N Engl J Med 287:578, 1972.

21. Barnes RW, Haferman MD, et al.: Noninvasive assessment of altered limb hemodynamics and complications of arterial catheterization. Radiology 107(3):505, 1973.

22. Amery A, Deloof W, et al.: Outcome of recent thromboembolic occlusions of limb arteries treated with streptokinase. Br Med J 4:639, 1974.

23. Katzen BT, Van Breda A: Low dose streptokinase in the treatment of arterial occlusions. Am J Radio 136:1171, 1981.

24. Berni GA, Bandyk DF, et al.: Streptokinase treatment of acute arterial occlusion. Ann Surg 198:185, 1983.

25. Keitzer WF, Fry WJ, et al.: Hemodynamic mechanism for pulse changes seen in occlusive vascular disease. Surgery 57:163, 1965.

26. Mozersky DJ, Sumner DS, et al.: Intraoperative use of a sterile ultrasonic flow probe. Surg Gynecol Obstet 136:279, 1973.

27. Keen H, Rose G, et al.: Blood sugar and arterial disease. Lancet 2:505, 1965.

28. Ostrander LD, Francis T, et al.: The relationship of cardiovascular disease to hyperglycemia. Ann Intern Med 62:1188, 1965.

29. Bierman EL, Brunzell JD: Interrelation of atherosclerosis, abnormal lipid metabolism and diabetes mellitus, in Diabetes, Obesity and Vascular Disease, Advances in Modern Nutrition, vol. VII, Katzen and Mahler (eds). New York, John Wiley, 1978, p 187.

30. Beach KW, Strandness DE Jr: Arteriosclerosis obliterans and associated risk factors in insulin-dependent and non insulin-dependent diabetes. Diabetes 29:882, 1980.

31. Strandness DE Jr, Priest RE, Gibbons GE: Combined clinical and pathologic study of diabetic and nondiabetic peripheral arterial disease. Diabetes 13:366, 1974.

32. Silbert S, Zazeela H: Prognosis in arteriosclerotic peripheral vascular disease. JAMA 166:1816, 1958.

33. Boyd AM: The natural course of arteriosclerosis of the lower extremities. Proc R Col Med 55:591, 1962.

34. Reckless JPD, Betteridge DJ, et al.: High density and low density lipoprotein and prevalence of vascular disease in diabetes mellitus. Br Med J 1:883, 1978.

35. Schonfeld G, Birge C, et al.: Apolipoprotein B levels and altered lipoprotein composition in diabetes. Diabetes 23:287, 1974.

36. Beach KW, Brunzell JD, et al.: The correlation of arteriosclerosis obliterans with lipoproteins in insulin-dependent and non insulin-dependent diabetes. Diabetes 28(9):836, 1979.

37. Beach KW, Brunzell JD, Strandness DE Jr: Prevalence of severe arteriosclerosis obliterans in patients with diabetes mellitus. Relation to smoking and form of therapy. Arteriosclerosis 2(4):275, 1982.

38. Gensler SW, Haimovici H, et al.: Study of vascular lesions in diabetic, non-diabetic patients. Arch Surg 91:617, 1965.

39. Vracko R, Strandness DE Jr: Basal lamina of abdominal skeletal muscle capillaries in diabetics and nondiabetics. Circulation 35:690, 1967.

40. Bloodworth JHMB Jr: Diabetic microangiopathy. Diabetes 12:99, 1963.

41. Vracko R: Skeletal muscle capillaries in nondiabetics. A quantitative analysis. Circulation 41:285, 1970.

42. Strandness DE Jr, Bell JW: A comparative evaluation of peripheral arterial disease in the diabetic and nondiabetic. Rev. Surg. 22:77, 1965.

43. Walder DN: Muscle blood flow during exercise in patients with intermittent claudication. J Physiol (London) 159:70 P, 1961.

44. Gosling RG, Dunbar G, et al.: The quantitative analysis of occlusive peripheral arterial disease by a noninvasive ultrasonic technique. Angiology 22:52, 1971.

45. Thiele BL, Bandyk DF, et al.: A systematic approach to the assessment of aortoiliac disease (submitted to Arch Surg 1982).

46. Jager KA, Phillips DJ, et al.: Noninvasive mapping of lower limb arterial lesions. Ultrasound Med Biol 11:515, 1985.

47. Jager KA, Fortner GA, et al.: Noninvasive diagnosis of intestinal angina. J Clin Ultrasound 12:588, 1984.

48. Kohler TK, Zierler RE, et al.: Noninvasive diagnosis of renal artery stenosis by ultrasonic duplex scanning. J Vasc Surg 4:450, 1986.

49. Sumner DS, Strandness DE Jr: Aortoiliac reconstruction in patients with combined iliac and superficial femoral arterial occlusion. Surgery 84:348, 1978.

50. Flanigan DP, Gray B, et al.: Correlation of Doppler-derived high-thigh pressure and intra-arterial pressure in the assessment of aortoiliac occlusive disease. Br J Surg 68:423, 1981.

51. Faris IB, Jamieson CW: The diagnosis of aorto-iliac: A comparison of thigh pressure measurement and femoral artery flow velocity profile. J Cardiovasc Surg 16:597, 1975.

52. Bone GE, Hayes AC, et al.: Value of segmental limb blood pressure in predicting results of aortofemoral bypass. Am J Surg 132:733, 1976.

53. Sumner DS, Strandness DE Jr: Aortoiliac reconstruction in patients with combined iliac and superficial femoral arterial occlusion. Surgery 84:348, 1978.

54. Harris PH, Taylor LA, et al.: The relationship between Doppler ultrasound assessment and angiography in occlusive arterial disease of the lower limbs. Surg Gynecol Obstet 138:911, 1974.

55. Bone GE: The relationship between aortoiliac hemodynamics and femoral pulsatility index. J Surg Res 32:228, 1982.

56. Flanigan DP, Collins JT, et al.: Hemodynamic and arteriographic evaluation of femoral pulsatility index. J Surg Res 32:234, 1982.

57. Thiele BL, Bandyk DF, et al.: A systematic approach to the assessment of aortoiliac disease. Arch Surg 118:477, 1983.

58. Demorais D, Johnston KW: Assessment of aortoiliac disease by noninvasive quantitative Doppler waveform analysis. Br J Surg 68:789, 1981.

59. Skidmore R, Woodcock JP, et al.: Physiological interpretation of Doppler shift waveforms III. Clinical results. Ultrasound Med Biol 6:227, 1980.

60. Johnson KW, Taraschuk I: Validation of the role of pulsatility index in quantitation of the severity of peripheral arterial occlusive disease. Am J Surg 131:295, 1976.

61. Wessler S, Ming SC, et al.: A critical evaluation of thromboangiitis obliterans: The case against Buerger's disease. N Engl J Med 262:1149, 1960.

62. McKusick VA, Harris WS, et al.: Buerger's disease. A clinical and pathological entity. JAMA 181:5, 1962.

63. Thieme WT, Strandness DE Jr, Bell JW: Buerger's disease: Further support for this entity. Northwest Med 64:264, 1965.

64. Levy RJ: Stroke decline: Implications and prospects. N Engl J Med 300:490, 1979.

65. Hass WK, Fields WS, et al.: Joint study of extracranial arterial occlusion. II. Arteriography techniques, sites and complications. JAMA 203:159, 1968.

66. Thompson JE, Austin DJ, Patman RD: Carotid endarterectomy for cerebrovascular insufficiency: Long term results in 592 patients followed up to thirteen years. Ann Surg 172:663, 1970.

67. Thompson JE: Complication of carotid endarterectomy and their prevention. World J Surg 3:155, 1979.

68. White JS, Sirinek KR, et al.: Morbidity and mortality of carotid endarterectomy. Arch Surg 116:409, 1981.

69. Toole JF: Management of transient ischemic attacks, in Cerebrovascular Disease, Scheinberg P (ed), New York, Raven Press, 1976.

70. Mani RL, Eisenberg RL: Complications of catheter cerebral angiography: Analysis of 5000 procedures. I. Criteria and incidence. Amer J Roentgenol 131:861, 1978.

71. Mani RL, Eisenberg RL, et al.: Complications of catheter cerebral arteriography: Analysis of 5000 procedures. II. Relation of complication rates to clinical and arteriographic diagnosis. AJR 131:867, 1978.

72. Barnes RW, Russell HE, et al.: The Doppler cerebrovascular examination: Improved results with refinements in technique. Stroke 8:468, 1977.

73. Kartchner MM, McRae LP, Morrison FD: Noninvasive detection and evaluation of carotid occlusive disease. Arch Surg 106:528, 1973.

74. Gee W, Oller DW, Wylie EJ: Noninvasive diagnosis of carotid occlusion by ocular plethysmography. Stroke 7:18, 1976.

75. Ingebrigtsen R, Lie M, et al.: Dilatation of the iliofemoral artery following the opening of an experimental arteriovenous fistula in the dog. Scand J Clin Lab Invest 31:255, 1973.

76. Schenk WG Jr, Martin JW, et al.: The regional hemodynamics of chronic experimental arteriovenous fistulas. Surg Gynecol Obstet 110:44, 1960.

77. Shumaker HB Jr: Aneurysms development and degenerative changes in dilated artery proximal to arteriovenous fistula. Surg Gynecol Obstet 130:636, 1970.

78. Stehbens WE: Blood vessel changes in chronic experimental arteriovenous fistulas. Surg Gynecol Obstet 127:372, 1968.

79. Stehbens WE: The ultrastructure of the anastomosed vein of experimental arteriovenous fistulae in sheep. Am J Pathol 76:377, 1974.

80. Schenk WG Jr, Bahn RA, et al.: The regional hemodynamics of experimental acute arteriovenous fistulas. Surg Gynecol Obstet 105:733, 1957.

81. Sumner DS: Arteriovenous fistula, in Strandness DE Jr (ed): Collateral Circulation in Clinical Surgery. Philadelphia, W.B. Saunders, 1969, pp 27–90.

82. Strandness DE Jr, Sumner DS: Arteriovenous fistulas, in Hemodynamics for Surgeons. New York, Grune and Stratton, 1975, pp 621–633.

83. Ingebrigtsen R, Wehn PS: Local blood pressure and direction of flow in experimental arteriovenous fistula. Acta Chir Scand 120:142, 1960.

84. Lough FC, Giordano JM, Hobson RW: Regional hemodynamics of large and small femoral arteriovenous fistulas in dogs. Surgery 79:346, 1976.

85. Szilagyi DE, Elliott JP, et al.: Peripheral congenital arteriovenous fistulas. Surgery 57:61, 1965.

86. Szilagyi DE, Smith RF, et al.: Congenital arteriovenous abnormalities of the limbs. Arch Surg 111:423, 1976.

87. Murphy TO, Margulis AR: Roentgenographic manifestations of congenital peripheral arteriovenous communications. Radiology 67:26, 1956.

88. Bradley EL III: The anterior tibial compartment syndrome. Surg Gynecol Obstet 136:289, 1973.

89. Nelson RM, Davis RW: Thoracic outlet compression syndrome—collective review. Ann Thorac Surg 8:437, 1969.

90. Roos DB: Thoracic outlet syndrome. Rock Mt Med J 64:49, 1967.

91. Tilney NL, Girffiths HJG, Edwards EA: Natural history of major venous thrombosis of the upper extremity. Arch Surg 101:792, 1970.

92. Allen EV, Brown GE: Raynaud's disease: A critical review of minimal requisites for diagnosis. Am J Med Sci 183:187, 1932.

93. Nielsen SL, Lassen NA: Measurement of digital blood pressure after local cooling. J Appl Physiol 43:901, 1977.

94. Nielsen SL: Raynaud's phenomena and finger systolic pressures during cooling. Scand J Clin Lab Invest 38:765, 1978.

CHAPTER 4
Hemodynamics and Rheology of Vascular Disease: Applications to Diagnosis and Treatment

David S. Sumner

The surgeon faced with diagnosis and treatment of vascular disease must make decisions based on an assessment of hemodynamic and rheologic factors. Fluid dynamics is exceedingly complex, even under optimally controlled conditions; therefore, no practical formulas capable of predicting outcomes have been devised. It is possible, however, to use some generally recognized principles to formulate guidelines of value to the surgeon. Although many of these principles are intuitively evident, others are less so and require some insight into the physical behavior of fluids in motion. Moreover, flow disturbances not only affect the immediate supply of blood to the peripheral tissues, but they also directly interact with the wall of the conduit, playing a role—now appreciated as quite important—in the development of atherosclerotic plaques, platelet deposition, and proliferation of fibromuscular tissues, all of which may influence the outcome of any reconstructive procedure.

NORMAL BLOOD FLOW

The fundamental principle governing blood flow is that developed by Bernoulli:

$$P_1 + \tfrac{1}{2}\rho v_1^2 + \rho g h_1 = P_2 + \tfrac{1}{2}\rho v_2^2 + \rho g h_2 + \text{Heat} \qquad (1)$$

This equation simply states that the total fluid energy ($P + \tfrac{1}{2}\rho v^2 + \rho g h$) must be greater upstream than downstream if blood is to move against a resistance, the energy "lost" in the transition being dissipated in the form of heat. Pressure (P)—ordinarily the largest component of total fluid energy—may be segregated into dynamic pressure, derived largely from the contraction of the left ventricle, and hydrostatic pressure ($-\rho g h$), which is equivalent to the weight of a column of blood extending from the point of measurement to the heart. In this expression, ρ is the density of blood (about $1.056\,g/cm^3$); g is the acceleration due to gravity ($980\ cm/sec^2$); and h is the distance in centimeters above the heart. Gravitational potential energy ($+\rho g h$) has the same dimensions as hydrostatic pressure but has the opposite sign. It represents the energy imparted to blood by

virtue of its elevation relative to the earth. Since, in most circumstances, gravitational potential energy is equivalent to hydrostatic pressure, the two cancel out. There are, however, situations in which the two differ—especially on the venous side of the circulation. Finally, kinetic energy, the energy imparted to blood by its motion, is proportional to the product of its density and the square of its velocity ($\tfrac{1}{2}\rho v^2$).

Viscous Energy "Losses"

Heat is generated by the interaction of contiguous particles of fluid in motion. In a long, straight, rigid, cylindrical tube with perfectly steady laminar flow, viscosity accounts for all of the energy losses. Poiseuille's law defines the relationship between the pressure (energy) gradient and flow under these strict conditions.

$$P_1 - P_2 = Q \times \frac{8L\eta}{\pi r^4} = V \times \frac{8L\eta}{\pi r^2} \qquad (2)$$

where η represents the coefficient of viscosity measured in poise, and r, the inside radius of the vessel. This equation states that, given a constant flow, the pressure gradient is directly related to the length of the segment (L) and to the viscosity of blood but is inversely related to the fourth power of the radius. The radius, therefore, has a profound influence on energy losses.

Of the many factors that determine the viscosity of blood, hematocrit is the most important, the viscosity at a hematocrit of 50% being roughly twice that at 35%.[1] Thus, in situations where laminar flow predominates, the hematocrit may have a significant effect on pressure gradient or blood flow. A further complicating feature is the fact that the viscosity of blood, unlike that of water, varies with shear rate (change in velocity between adjacent lamina of blood, dv/dr).[2] Viscosity increases markedly as shear rates drop below $10\ sec^{-1}$; above this level, the viscosity is essentially constant. Although the mean shear rate ($8/3 \cdot v/r$) in all blood vessels is well above this critical level, it may fall below the critical value during those phases of the pulse cycle in which the velocity decreases. These "nonNewtonian" characteristics of blood are probably not too important, producing changes of only 1 or 2% in the pressure gradient.

When flow is laminar, the velocity profile across the lumen of the vessel assumes a parabolic configuration (Fig. 4-1). At the wall, blood is essentially stationary; maximal velocities are in the center of the tube; and the mean velocity is exactly half the maximum. In real life, however, profiles approaching parabolic are found only in the smaller or medium-sized blood vessels and then only during peak systole. Depending on the length, shape, and curvature of the vessel and on the phase of the pulse cycle, the profile may be blunted or severely skewed. Since the adjacent particles of blood are flowing at nearly the same velocity when the profile is blunt, there is little viscous interaction except near the wall; consequently, Poiseuille's law does not hold under these conditions.

Inertial Energy "Losses"

Because velocity is a vector quantity, energy is dissipated every time there is a change in the direction of flow. Directional changes occur in every curve, at every bifurcation or branch point, and whenever the lumen of the vessel narrows or expands. With each pulse cycle, blood accelerates during systole, decelerates and often reverses during diastole, moves toward the wall as the vessel expands, and moves toward the center of the lumen as the vessel contracts. Inertial losses are proportional to the product of the density of blood and the square of the changes in velocity:

$$\Delta P = k \times \tfrac{1}{2} \times \rho dv^2 \tag{3}$$

In many situations, inertial losses are greater than those due to viscous effects.

Resistance

Since the relative contributions of viscosity and inertia vary greatly, it is impossible to characterize blood flow even under normal conditions with a simple formula; however, a general equation incorporating the foregoing concepts is as follows[3]:

$$\Delta P = k_v v + k_i v^2 \tag{4}$$

where k_v represents a constant related to viscosity and k_i, a constant related to inertial losses. These constants vary with many factors, including the viscosity and density of blood, the dimensions and configuration of the vessel, reflection of pulses from the periphery, and heart rate, and are really unique to only a single situation. In all cases, the energy losses will exceed—often by a large amount—those predicted by Poiseuille's law.

Barring the presence of intervening branches, blood flow (Q) is constant in all portions of a continuous vessel, but velocity differs, depending on the cross-sectional area ($A = \pi r^2$):

$$Q = vA = v \times \pi r^2 \tag{5}$$

Since $Q1 = Q2$,

$$v_1 r_1 = v_2 r_2{}^2; \text{ or } V_1/V_2 = (r_2/r_1)^2$$

It is interesting to note that the substitution of equation 5 in equation 4 gives

$$\Delta P = k_v \times Q/r^4 + k_i \times Q^2/r^4 \tag{6}$$

the constants having been appropriately modified. Since the resistance (R) of a blood vessel segment is merely the ratio of the pressure gradient across and the flow through the segment ($\Delta P/Q$), it is clear that resistance is inversely proportional to the fourth power of the radius:

$$R = k_v/r^4 + k_i \times Q/r^4 \tag{7}$$

This formula also shows that resistance is not constant but increases as flow increases.[3] Therefore, unlike an electrical wire, which has a rather constant resistance over a wide

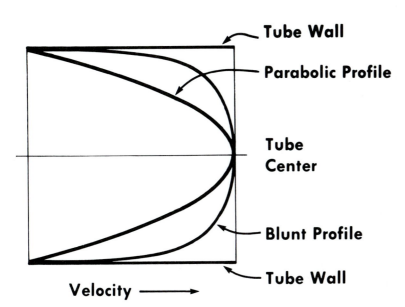

Figure 4-1. Velocity profiles. Parabolic profiles occur only during ideal conditions. Because of entrance effects and flow disturbances, profiles are often blunted. (*From Sumner DS: Hemodynamics and pathophysiology of arterial disease, in Rutherford RB (ed): Vascular Surgery, 2nd ed. Philadelphia, WB Saunders Co, 1984.*)

range of currents, the resistance of a segment of blood vessel can be defined only under precise conditions of flow, pulse rate, and other factors.

Nonetheless, resistance is a very useful concept in thinking about blood flow. Analogous to electrical circuits, the resistance of blood vessels in series are roughly additive:

$$R_T = R_1 + R_2 + \ldots R_n \qquad (8)$$

and the reciprocals of those in parallel are likewise additive:

$$1/R_T = 1/R_1 + 1/R_2 + \ldots 1/R_n \qquad (9)$$

where R_T is the total resistance.

Finally, although we can never say what the actual resistance of a blood vessel or graft is without measuring flow and pressure gradients under defined conditions, we can calculate its *minimal* resistance using Poiseuille's law:

$$R_{min} = (8L\eta)/(\pi r^4) \qquad (10)$$

It must be emphasized that its actual resistance will always exceed this value.

Reynolds Number

Fluids in motion behave similarly when they have the same Reynolds number (*Re*), a dimensionless number that depends on velocity, diameter (2*r*), and the ratio of density to viscosity (ρ/η):

$$Re = v \times 2r \times (\rho/\eta) \qquad (11)$$

Laminar flow tends to break down into turbulence when Reynolds numbers exceed 2,000. Although this breakdown normally occurs only during peak systole in the aortic arch, flow may become unstable in other vessels when stenoses are present—even with Reynolds numbers in the hundreds. Under these circumstances, inertial energy losses are magnified.

ARTERIAL STENOSES

The presence of a stenotic lesion in an artery adds tremendously to the complexities of blood flow. Approaching a stenosis, the particles of blood—both microscopic and ultramicroscopic—must accelerate and change directions to squeeze through an orifice narrower than that of the uninvolved vessel upstream (Fig. 4-2). A pressure drop occurs at this point as potential energy is transformed into kinetic energy. Within the stenosis, the increase in velocity is determined by the reduction in cross-sectional area. At the exit, blood emerges at this same high velocity, forming a jet, which disintegrates into disturbed or turbulent flow as the mean velocity decreases to accommodate the larger cross-sectional area. Once again, an energy transformation occurs—this time from kinetic back to potential. The efficiency of these transformations determines to a large extent the energy gradient across a stenosis (Fig. 4-3).

Inertial losses are greatest at the exit where flow is most disturbed.[4,5] Expressed in terms of pressure gradient, these losses are proportional to the square of the difference

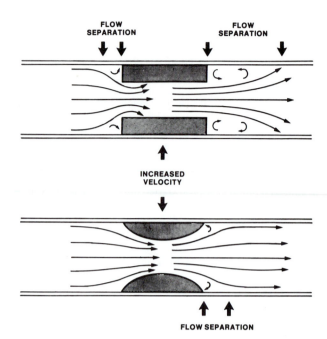

Figure 4-2. Flow patterns through axisymmetrical stenoses. Disturbances of flow are greater when the orifice is abrupt (*upper panel*) than they are when the orifice is smooth and tapered (*lower panel*). Velocities and shear rates are low in areas of flow separation where, near the wall, the direction of flow may be reversed.

between the velocity of blood within the stenosis (V_s) and that in the distal vessel (V_d):

$$\Delta P = \tfrac{1}{2} k(V_s - V_d)^2 \qquad (12)$$

The shape of the exit determines the severity of the flow disorganization, an abrupt orifice causing more disturbance than one that gradually expands (see Fig. 4-2). Reflecting the shape of the orifice, the constant, *k*, varies from about 0.4 (gradual) to 1.0 (abrupt).[6] At the entrance, a similar relationship exists, but flow disturbances and inertial losses are less severe. It is also true that asymmetrical stenoses offer more resistance than axisymmetrical stenoses with the same reduction in cross-sectional area.[7] In part, this may account for the surprisingly high resistance associated with iliac arteries, which do not appear to be significantly obstructed in the anteroposterior arteriographic projection but which are narrowed in the lateral projection.

Velocity profiles are quite blunt at the entrance to a stenosis. The distance (*Le*) required to regain a parabolic profile is a function of the radius of the stenosis and the Reynolds number (*Le* = 0.16 *rRe*). Unless the stenosis is quite long, a fully developed parabolic profile is never established. Although there is little viscous interaction between adjacent lamina in the blunt region of the velocity profile, shear rates (*dv/dr*) near the wall are increased, and viscous losses actually exceed those predicted by Poiseuille's law.

Arteriosclerosis is a diffuse process, and tandem lesions occurring in the same stretch of artery are not uncommon. Because energy losses are greatest at the entrance and exit, two separate lesions will offer more resistance than a single lesion, having a length equal to the combined lengths of the two separate lesions—assuming, of course, that the diameters are the same. The resistance of lesions in series

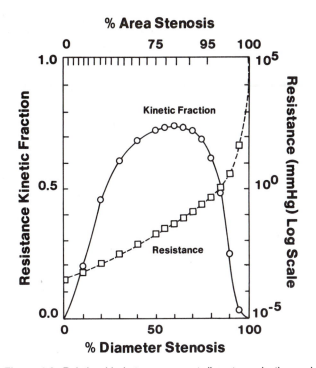

Figure 4-3. Relationship between percent diameter reduction and resistance of a 1 cm long "abrupt" axisymmetrical stenosis in an artery with a diameter of 0.5 cm. Total resistance increases rapidly, becoming infinite at 100% stenosis (total occlusion). Resistance due to inertial factors (kinetic fraction) exceeds that due to viscosity when the diameter stenosis is between 25 and 85%, constituting over 70% of the total resistance when the diameter stenosis is between 50 and 70%. Iterative computer model is based on equations 2, 8, and 12.

Effect on Pressure and Flow

Arterial stenoses must always be considered as part of a larger vascular circuit, consisting not only of the vessels proximal and distal to the stenosis but also of any collateral vessels that bypass the stenotic region.[12] To begin with the most simple case, the resistances distal and proximal to the stenosis are considered to be constant, and collaterals are considered to be absent. Under these conditions, advancing stenosis causes a reduction in flow and an equivalent increase in the pressure gradient (Fig. 4-4).[3] Changes in pressure and flow ordinarily become perceptible only after the cross-sectional area has been reduced by about 75%, which, in an axisymmetrically stenosed vessel, is equivalent to a 50% diameter reduction.[13,14] Beyond this point, which is known as the point of "critical stenosis," the stenosis is said to be "hemodynamically significant." With decreasing peripheral resistance, the curves are shifted to the left, and critical stenosis occurs with less diameter reduction. Thus a lesion that does not compromise blood flow in an artery feeding a high-resistance peripheral vascular bed may do so in an artery supplying a low-resistance bed.[15]

Gradual dilatation of the peripheral arterioles is one of two mechanisms by which the body attempts to compensate for the increased resistance imposed by a stenosis.[16,17,18] Until the arterioles become maximally dilated, flow through the stenosis remains undiminished despite its decreasing diameter. The pressure gradient, however, will increase more precipitously.[19,20] After the ability to dilate has been exhausted, further reductions in lumen area will cause a rapid fall in both pressure and flow (Fig. 4-5).

The development of collaterals is the second major compensatory mechanism. Provided the collaterals are large

are, however, not strictly additive.[8,9] In other words, the total resistance offered by two identical lesions would be less than double their individual resistances. Although there are several reasons for this, the decrease in flow and velocity probably accounts for most of the disparity. Since resistance is a function of velocity, any reduction in velocity would result in a decreased resistance in each of the stenoses.

Pulsatile flow introduces other complexities.[4,10] If flow reversal persists during a portion of the cardiac cycle, the entrance temporarily becomes the exit, and the exit, the entrance. (Usually, however, flow reversal is not maintained in the presence of significant arterial stenosis.) As in normal vessels, the periodic acceleration and deceleration augment inertial losses. Consequently, the resistance of a lesion tends to increase with increasing pulse rate.

To summarize, the energy-depleting effects of a stenosis are inversely proportional to the fourth power of its radius (or the square of its cross-sectional area), are directly proportional to the velocity and to the square of the changes in velocity that occur at the entrance and exit, are more dependent on inertial than viscous effects, are usually greatest at the entrance and exit, and are influenced by the shape and symmetry of the orifices.[5,11] Since resistance is a function of flow and flow, in turn, is a function of resistance, the resistance of a stenosis may vary considerably under different physiologic conditions.

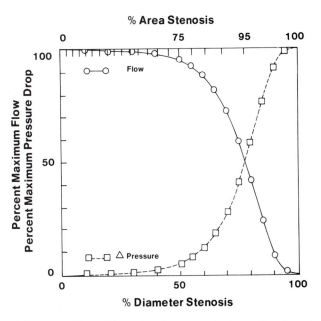

Figure 4-4. Effect of increasing diameter reduction on flow through and pressure drop across an abrupt axisymmetrical stenosis in a circuit with a fixed peripheral resistance. Same model as in Figure 4-3.

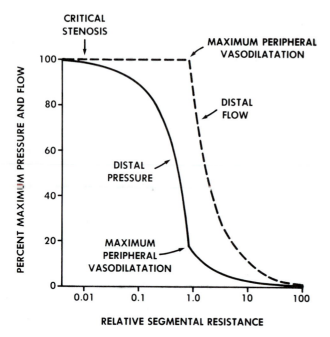

Figure 4-5. Effect of compensatory peripheral arteriolar vasodilation on flow through and pressure drop across a stenosis. Segmental resistance refers to the combined resistances of the stenosis and the parallel collateral bed. (*From Sumner DS: Correlation of lesion configuration with functional significance, in Bond MC, Insull W Jr, et al. (eds): Clinical Diagnosis of Atherosclerosis: Quantitative Methods of Evaluation. New York, Springer-Verlag New York, 1983.*)

enough, the resistance of the vascular segment containing the stenosis may remain unchanged, and peripheral pressure and flow will not be adversely affected. Under these circumstances, there will be no pressure drop across the stenosis, but flow through the stenosis will be severely curtailed. Collaterals capable of such efficiency are the exception rather than the rule; in most clinical situations, therefore, the segmental resistance is increased despite ample time for the collaterals to mature.[18,21] As a result, there is usually some decrease in pressure and some drop in flow across the stenotic lesion, although one of the two may be more affected than the other. This is simply a reflection of the fact that both pressure and flow are manifestations of total fluid energy.

Estimating the resistance of a lesion by measuring only pressure gradient or only flow—as some have done—is likely to provide misleading information. Both must be measured. Even then, the results pertain only to the specific conditions existing at the time.

Effect on Velocity

Unlike the pressure gradient and flow, which are functions of resistance, the ratio of the mean velocity of flow through a stenosis (V_s) to that in the unobstructed vessel (V_0) is determined solely by the relative radii of the stenotic (r_s) and unobstructed segments (r_0):

$$r_s/r_0 = \sqrt{V_0/V_s} \qquad (13)$$

or

$$\% \text{ diameter stenosis} = (1 - \sqrt{V_0/V_s}) \times 100$$

The actual velocity of blood in the stenotic region, however, is determined not only by the relative radii but also by the flow. As a result, velocity increases with progressive narrowing of the lumen until the stenosis becomes quite severe and then drops off very rapidly as the lumen approaches total occlusion (Fig. 4-6).[22,23]

Because the Doppler flow detector can measure velocity percutaneously, it has been used noninvasively to estimate the degree of stenosis. It is evident that this approach is strictly valid only if the mean velocities in the stenotic and unobstructed segments are compared. Nonetheless, when a vascular bed (such as that containing the carotid artery) is well defined and peripheral autoregulation maintains flow at normal levels, velocities above certain arbitrary values have proved to be useful in estimating the degree of stenosis, albeit within broad limits.

Effect on Pulse Wave Contours

A stenosis in an otherwise compliant vessel acts like a low-pass filter in an electrical circuit, attenuating the high-frequency harmonics of the flow or pressure wave (Fig. 4-7).[24] This tends to change the contour of the pulse distal to the stenosis, making it more rounded than that above the stenosis. The upslope becomes less steep, the peak becomes more rounded, and the downslope bows away from the baseline.[25,26] Reversed flow components are less evident and often disappear entirely.[27] Fluctuations around the mean value are decreased, a fact that serves as the basis for the calculation of pulsatility indexes (all of which,

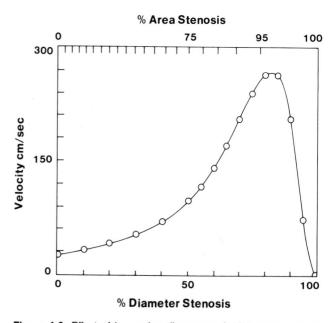

Figure 4-6. Effect of increasing diameter reduction on velocity of flow through a stenosis. Velocity increases even though flow actually decreases until a critical point is reached. Same model as in Figure 4-3.

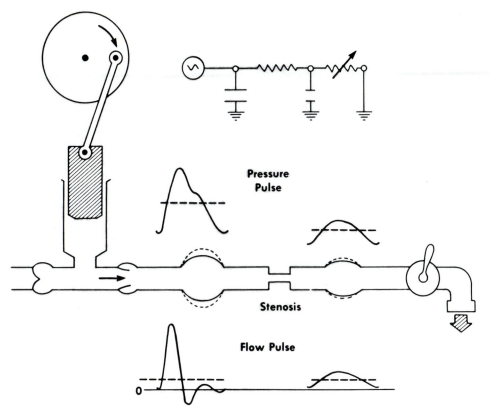

Figure 4-7. Effect of stenosis in a compliant artery on the contour of pressure and flow pulses. Faucet represents the variable resistance of the peripheral vascular bed. Mean pressure (*dashed line*) is reduced, but mean flow (*dashed line*) is unchanged. (*From Sumner DS: Correlation of lesion configuration with functional significance, in Bond MC, Insull W Jr, et al. (eds): Clinical Diagnosis of Atherosclerosis: Quantitative Methods of Evaluation. New York, Springer-Verlag New York, 1983.*)

in one way or another, compare the total excursion of the pulse to its mean value).[28,29] Thus decreases in the pulsatility index over an arterial segment not only predict the presence of a stenosis but also correlate with its severity.[30,31] In contrast, reflections originating from the stenosis may increase the excursion of the pulse wave above a lesion and therefore increase the pulsatility index.[32,33,34] This finding may also have diagnostic value.

Effect on Shear Rate and Atherogenesis

As the jet of blood emerges from the exit of the stenosis, it diverges, coming in contact with the wall downstream (see Fig. 4-2). This creates an area of flow separation, extending from the end of the lesion to the point of reattachment. Within the region of separation, flow is very sluggish and may even be reversed. Shear rates, which are a function of velocity, are therefore correspondingly low and may also be reversed. During the cardiac cycle, shear rates can alternate between forward and reversed orientations.[10] The longitudinal extent of the zone of flow separation varies with Reynolds number and the shape of the orifice. When Reynolds number is low and the orifice angle is gradual, there may be little or no flow separation.[7]

Low shear rates permit the accumulation of platelets and other substances that interact with the vascular wall to foster the development of atherosclerotic plaques, intimal thickening, and fibromuscular hyperplasia.[35,36]

Within the stenosis, shear rates may be quite high and may exceed values demontrated to cause endothelial injury, but there is little evidence that this is conducive to atherogenesis.[37,38] In fact, the endothelium seems to sense the increased shear and transmits this information to the muscular elements of the arterial wall; dilatation occurs, and shear rates return toward prestenotic levels. This has the effect of ameliorating the severity of the stenosis and may be responsible for some of the reported arteriographic observations suggesting plaque resolution.[39,40]

Distal to the stenosis, the vibrations generated in the arterial wall by the disturbed or turbulent flow appear to induce dilatation.[41] This is the apparent cause of the post-stenotic dilatations often seen in conjunction with the thoracic outlet syndrome.

Thus stenoses not only affect pressure and peripheral perfusion, but they may also have local effects that are equally important. Research in this area promises to enhance the understanding of atherogenesis and should provide information of practical value to the surgeon involved in the management of this disease.

STENOSIS AS PART OF A LARGER ARTERIAL CIRCUIT

As mentioned previously, the stenotic artery and its collaterals may be considered as a unit, an arterial segment, in other words, with its own relatively "fixed" resistance (Fig. 4-8). This segment is in series with a peripheral vascular bed, the resistance of which varies extensively in response to stress and other stimuli. Included in this peripheral bed are the arteries distal to the most distal collateral inflow site, the arterioles, capillaries, venules, and veins. Because of their small diameters, their muscular walls, and their copious innervation, most of the peripheral resistance is concentrated in the arterioles. It is the arterioles, therefore, that largely control changes in peripheral resistance.

Although the actual hemodynamic features of such a complex circuit cannot be depicted by simple formulas, simple formulas analogous to Ohm's law do facilitate our understanding of the physiology.[3,12] Blood flow (Q_T) through the peripheral vascular bed is determined not only by the pressure gradient existing between the central arteries (P_a) and the central veins (P_v) but also by the total resistance of the circuit, which is the sum of the segmental resistance (R_{seg}) and the peripheral resistance (R_p):

$$Q_T = (P_a - P_v)/(R_{seg} + R_p) \qquad (14)$$

When there is no arterial obstruction, R_{seg} is quite low, with most of the total resistance residing in the peripheral arterioles. With exercise or other stress that causes arteriolar dilatation and a reduction in R_p, flow is markedly increased—often by as much as five to ten times baseline levels.[20,42,43] In the presence of a proximal arterial obstruction, R_{seg} is almost always increased, despite the development of collaterals. As long as the autoregulatory capacity of the peripheral arterioles has not been exceeded, R_p de-

creases enough to compensate for the increased proximal resistance, total resistance is unchanged, and peripheral blood flow is maintained at normal levels (see Fig. 4-5). During exercise, however, further reduction in R_p is limited; consequently, the fall in total resistance is not sufficient to augment flow to the levels required to sustain the increased demands of the muscles, and claudication is experienced (Fig. 4-9).[20,42-45] In the worst situation, R_{seg} is so high that arteriolar dilatation is unable to reduce the total resistance to normal levels, even at rest. When this situation occurs, peripheral perfusion fails to sustain normal metabolic activities, and rest pain or gangrene may ensue.[46,47,48]

The pressure gradient across a stenotic segment is determined by its resistance and the magnitude of the flow:

$$P_a - P_d = Q \times R_{seg} \text{ or}$$
$$P_d = P_a - Q \times R_{seg} \qquad (15)$$

where P_d is the arterial pressure distal to the stenosis but proximal to the peripheral bed. Normally, R_{seg} is so low that the gradient is only a few mm Hg. (Actually, because of reflected waves, the systolic pressure in the distal artery may exceed that in the proximal artery, but the mean pressure will always be somewhat less.)[49-51] Even though flow is increased manyfold with exercise, the product, $Q \times R_{seg}$, remains low in normal limbs, and the peripheral pressure drop is insignificant. If there is any concomitant rise in the arterial perfusion pressure, the distal pressure may even increase somewhat.

Because compensatory peripheral arteriolar dilatation maintains resting blood flow at normal levels, any increase in segmental resistance causes a similar increase in the pressure gradient across the segment and, provided that the central pressure remains constant, a decrease in peripheral arterial pressure (see Fig. 4-9). Exercise, by augmenting blood flow, causes the peripheral pressure to drop even

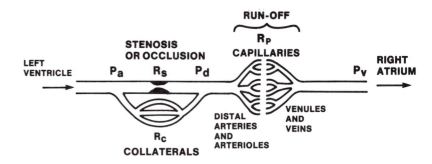

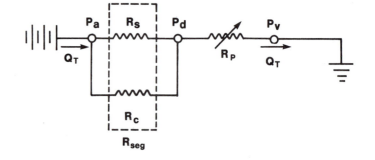

Figure 4-8. *Upper panel.* Components of a vascular circuit containing an arterial stenosis or occlusion. *Lower panel.* An electrical analog, in which the battery represents the left ventricle and the ground potential represents the right atrium. (*From Sumner DS: Hemodynamics of abnormal blood flow, in Wilson SE, Veith FJ, et al. (eds): Vascular Surgery, Principles and Practice. New York, McGraw-Hill Book Co, 1987.*)

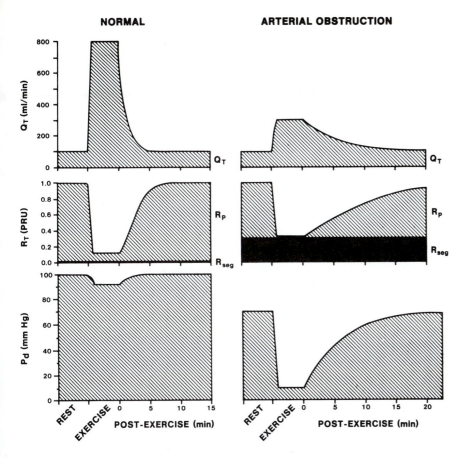

Figure 4-9. Flow (Q_T), segmental resistance (R_{seg}), peripheral resistance (R_p), and distal blood pressure (P_d) in normal limbs and limbs with single-level arterial obstruction before, during, and after exercise. (*From Sumner DS: Hemodynamics of abnormal blood flow, in Wilson SE, Veith FJ, et al. (eds): Vascular Surgery, Principles and Practice. New York, McGraw-Hill Book Co, 1987.*)

further, not infrequently to the point where it can no longer be measured.[20,50,52–54] Following the cessation of exercise, blood flow decreases as the metabolic debt incurred by the exercising muscles is repaid. In normal limbs this debt is minimal, and flow rapidly falls to pre-exercise levels; but in diseased limbs—especially those with the most severely compromised circulation—many minutes may be required before the debt is repaid and flow returns to baseline.[19,50,52–56] As long as flow is increased, the peripheral pressure remains decreased, rising gradually in the postexercise period to pre-exercise levels as flow returns to normal resting values.

The situation becomes more complex when there are multiple levels of obstruction.[3,56,57] In such cases, the physiologic effects are not simply due to the sum of the segmental resistances but involve steal phenomena as well. Since the proximal arterial segment supplies not only the vascular bed fed by the distal segment but also a more proximal bed, exercise will cause some of the blood destined for the distal tissues to be diverted into the more proximal bed. For example, consider a series of obstructions involving the aortoiliac and superficial femoral segments. The arteries comprising the aortoiliac segment feed the tissues of the buttocks, thighs, and calf; while the superficial femoral segment mainly supplies the calf and foot. During exercise, the arterioles in all these muscles are dilated; blood flow through the iliac segment is greatly increased; and the pressure in the common femoral artery falls. Since the common femoral artery supplies the superficial femoral segment, the expected increase in flow through this segment will

not develop despite a profound reduction in the resistance of the arterioles in the calf. In fact, flow may actually fall below resting values in the more peripheral tissues, such as those of the foot.[43,53,58] After exercise, the flow debt to the buttock and thigh muscles is the first to be repaid. As flow through the aortoiliac segment subsides, the common femoral pressure rises, and flow through the superficial femoral segment increases, allowing repayment of the metabolic debt incurred by the calf muscles. During the postexercise period, the pressure in the distal arteries remains severely depressed until the flow through the superficial femoral segment reaches its peak and begins to fall.[53,56,59]

Because blood flow is difficult to determine noninvasively and because there is a wide range of normal resting values and an even wider range of normal exercise values, physiologic assessment, in clinical practice, is usually limited to the measurement of peripheral pressures.[53] Unlike flow, normal values for pressure can be assumed to be close to the central arterial pressure. Moreover, pressure, which represents potential energy, reflects more accurately than flow the capacity of the circulation to accomplish its work.

Collaterals and Segmental Resistance

As mentioned earlier, collateral development is rarely sufficient to maintain normal segmental resistance when the major artery of the segment is severely stenosed or occluded.[18,21] Since collateral resistance parallels that of the diseased artery and since the resistance of each collateral is inversely proportional to the fourth power of its radius, it would take 16 collaterals with a diameter of 0.25 cm or 625 collaterals with a diameter of 0.1 cm to have a resistance as low as that of an unobstructed vessel with a diameter of 0.5 cm. The former would have a total cross-sectional area of 3.1 cm^2, and the latter, a total cross-sectional area of 19.6 cm^2, 4 and 25 times, respectively, that of the unobstructed vessel (0.8 cm^2). Clearly, a few large collaterals are likely to be far more efficient than a large number of small collaterals.

Collaterals, basically, are arteries whose primary function is to supply nutrients to the tissues through which they pass. When recruited to serve as conduits around an arterial obstruction, they dilate in response to the increased shear stress imposed by the augmented blood flow but retain their primary function.[60,61] Thus their effective resistance must exceed that suggested by their lengths and diameters since only a portion of the blood they carry reenters the major arterial system.[12,55] Moreover, during exercise, their effective resistance may rise as more blood is siphoned off to supply the muscular tissues through which they pass.

Thus it may be very difficult to evaluate the capacity of the collateral channels visible on an arteriogram. Segmental resistance, like that of the lesion itself, is best evaluated by physiologic tests.[62]

BYPASS GRAFTS

Because increased segmental resistance is responsible for all the physiologic effects of arterial occlusive disease, the most direct treatment involves reduction of this resistance.

This reduction can be accomplished by endarterectomy if the lesion is well defined and short enough; but in most cases, insertion of a bypass graft is the best approach. In essence, the bypass graft acts as another collateral channel, acting in parallel with the diseased arteries and the existing collateral system. The resistance of the graft is determined not only by its length and diameter but also by the configuration of the proximal and distal anastomoses.

Resistance of the Graft

Poiseuille's law can be used to calculate the minimal resistance of a prosthetic graft. This calculation, of course, neglects energy losses due to inertia, which occur at the entrance and exit and at each curve. These losses can be quite significant.[63,64] Moreover, pulsatile flow also increases the losses over those expected for steady laminar flow. As shown in Table 4-1, a 20 cm long aortofemoral graft with a diameter of 7 mm should be capable of sustaining flows of 3000 ml/min with a minimal pressure drop; but a 5 mm graft would offer an appreciable resistance, even discounting inertial factors. Similarly, 40 cm long femoropopliteal grafts with diameters of 4 mm or greater should function satisfactorily when called on to transmit flows of up to 500 ml/min; but grafts with diameters less than 4 mm would offer an unacceptably high resistance. Long grafts (80 cm) from the femoral to tibial arteries are ordinarily used for the treatment of ischemic symptoms; resting flow rates are not high, and pressure drops of 10 mm Hg may be acceptable. Still, long segments of such grafts with either distal or proximal diameters less than 3 mm are inefficient blood conduits.

TABLE 4-1. PRESSURE GRADIENTS ACROSS GRAFTS (mm Hg) VISCOUS ONLY (VISCOUS + KINETIC)*

Aortofemoral, L = 20 cm Diameter (mm)	Flow (ml/min)			
	300	500	1500	3000
10	0.1 (0.1)	0.2 (0.2)	0.5 (0.9)	1.1 (2.7)
7	0.4 (0.5)	0.7 (0.9)	2.2 (3.9)	4.5 (11.1)
6	0.8 (0.9)	1.4 (1.7)	4.1 (7.2)	8.3 (20.6)
5	1.7 (2.0)	2.9 (3.6)	8.6 (15.0)	17.1 (42.8)

Femoropopliteal, L = 40 cm Diameter (mm)	Flow (ml/min)			
	50	150	300	500
6	0.3 (0.3)	0.8 (0.9)	1.7 (1.8)	2.8 (3.1)
5	0.6 (0.6)	1.7 (1.8)	3.4 (3.7)	5.7 (6.4)
4	1.4 (1.4)	4.2 (4.3)	8.4 (9.0)	13.9 (15.7)
3	4.4 (4.5)	13.2 (13.7)	26.4 (28.4)	44.0 (49.5)

Femorotibial, L = 80 cm Diameter (mm)†	Flow (ml/min)			
	50	100	150	200
6–4	1.3 (1.3)	2.6 (2.6)	3.9 (4.0)	5.2 (5.4)
5–3	3.5 (3.5)	6.9 (7.0)	10.4 (10.5)	13.8 (14.2)
4–2	13.0 (13.1)	26.0 (26.3)	39.0 (39.7)	52.0 (53.3)

* Viscous only, equation 2; viscous + kinetic, equation 6; η = 0.035 poise; ρ = 1.056 g/cm^3.
† Evenly tapered grafts, largest diameter to smallest.

Saphenous veins used for femoropopliteal and femorotibial bypasses contain valves that reduce the cross-sectional area by about 60%.[65,66] Although the length of the obstruction so created is quite short, the intact valves are capable of causing additional inertial losses. Studies have shown that resistance to flow, even in the reversed saphenous vein, is decreased by valve bisection.[67,68]

After implantation, prosthetic grafts develop a pseudointima that further reduces the effective internal diameter. Although a 0.5 mm layer, applied circumferentially, would have little influence on the pressure gradient across a large graft, it might adversely affect the function of a graft with borderline dimensions. Since high velocities are conducive to the formation of a thin, tightly adherent pseudointima, graft diameters should be no larger than necessary to ensure satisfactory flow dynamics. If the diameter of the graft is too large, clots tend to form on the inner walls as the flow stream attempts to mold itself to the diameter of the recipient vessel. These clots are loosely attached and may form an embolus, causing graft failure. As indicated by formula 5, given the same mean flow rate, the velocity in a 7 mm graft would be double that in a 10 mm graft. Because there is little difference in the functional capacity of these two grafts in the iliac region, the smaller diameter is preferred.

Distribution of Flow in Parallel Graft and Stenotic Artery

Surgeons occasionally express concern over the possibility that continued patency of a stenotic artery might lead to thrombosis of a parallel graft. To allay this fear, they either avoid end-to-side anastomoses or ligate the stenotic artery. Theoretical considerations strongly suggest that such concerns are not valid, provided that the arterial segment is sufficiently diseased to merit bypass grafting. As shown in Fig. 4-10, even when the preoperative pressure gradient across a stenosed artery is only 10 mm Hg, over 90% of the flow will be diverted into the graft. The choice of an end-to-side anastomosis should, therefore, be based on other considerations.

Vein Grafts with Double Lumens

Not uncommonly, saphenous veins bifurcate into two separate and parallel channels that rejoin after a variable distance to reconstitute a single lumen. When this situation is encountered, the surgeon must decide whether or not to include both channels in the graft.

Since both of the duplicated channels will have a lumen diameter less than that of the "parent" vein, it is clear that each will offer more resistance than an equal length of undivided vein. If the channels are of the same size, their combined resistance will be greater than that of an equal length of undivided vein (unless their individual diameters exceed 84% of the diameter of the undivided vein). Thus, in most cases, the combined resistance of the two parallel channels exceeds that of the undivided vein. Obviously, the adverse hemodynamic effects are proportional to the relative lengths of the divided and undivided parts; in other words, at a given flow rate, the pressure gradient across a bifurcated graft increases as the length of the divided segment increases.

As shown in Fig. 4-11, at the same flow rate to the thigh and calf muscles, the distal (popliteal) pressure and the flow rate through a bifurcated femoropopliteal graft are higher when both channels are preserved than they are when one channel has been ligated. Although the differences are small at rest, they become appreciable during exercise. Both configurations, however, represent a marked improvement over the nonbypassed situation. The argument that preserving both channels jeopardizes the survival of the graft by decreasing flow velocity through the bifurcated segment is not valid—even when both channels are functional, the velocity in each exceeds that in the undivided part of the vein. From this analysis, one must conclude that preservation of two equal-sized channels is desirable but certainly not mandatory. On the other hand, if one of

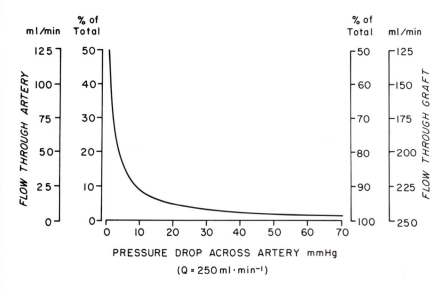

Figure 4-10. Relative flow through bypass graft and stenotic artery. As the preoperative pressure drop across the artery increases (indicating increasingly severe stenosis), the percentage of flow diverted to the graft increases. Lumen of the graft is equal to that of the unobstructed artery. (*From Strandness DE Jr, Sumner DS: Hemodynamics for Surgeons. New York, Grune & Stratton, 1975.*)

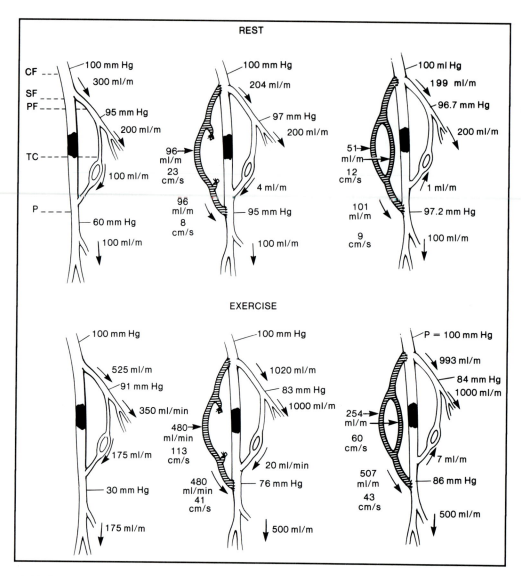

Figure 4-11. Resting and exercise flow and flow velocity through a 40 cm femoropopliteal bypass graft with a 20 cm divided segment. The diameter of the undivided graft is 5 mm and that of each of the divided segments is 3 mm. Arteries are as follows: common femoral (*CF*), superficial femoral (*SF*), profunda femoris (*PF*), popliteal (*P*), and thigh collateral (*TC*). Arrows indicate direction of flow. Thigh and calf resistances are autoregulated to maintain resting flows of 200 and 100 ml/min, respectively. Computer model is based on equations 2, 5, 8, and 9.

the channels is distinctly larger than the other, there is little to be gained by preserving the smaller of the two.

Sequential Grafts

In limbs with combined superficial femoral and below-knee obstructive disease, the surgeon may have the option of performing a bypass to the popliteal segment only, a femorotibial bypass, or a femoropopliteal-tibial sequential graft.[69] Aside from technical and anatomic factors, which frequently dictate the choice, what are the theoretical advantages and disadvantages of each of these approaches?

Limiting the reconstruction to a femoro(blind)popliteal

bypass usually secures only a modest increase in ankle and calf perfusion pressure (Fig. 4-12). If below-knee resistances are quite high, the patient may derive little benefit from this procedure. Although both femorotibial and femoropopliteal-tibial grafts yield significant and virtually equivalent increases in ankle pressure and are capable of relieving foot ischemia, the latter has the advantage of providing a greater increase in popliteal and tibial pressure. Thus sequential grafts are better equipped to cope with the demands of calf muscle exercise (Fig. 4-13).

Flow rates in femorotibial grafts should theoretically be lower than those in the proximal segment of sequential grafts but higher than those in the distal segment (see Figs. 4-12 and 4-13).[70–72] The proximal segment of a sequential graft contributes blood not only to the calf but also, in a

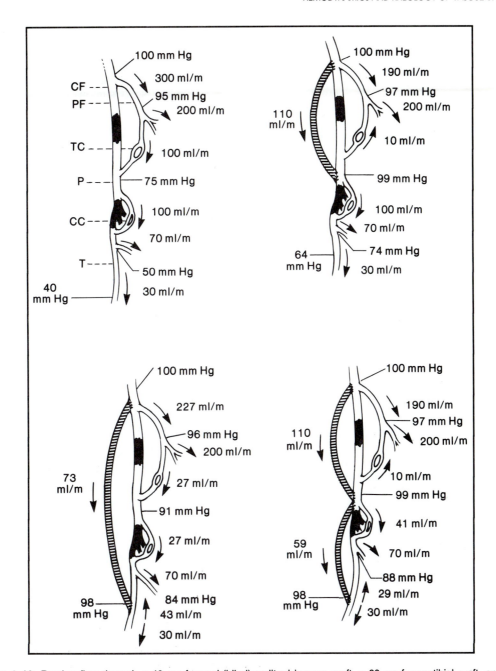

Figure 4–12. Resting flow through a 40 cm femoral-(blind)popliteal bypass graft, a 60 cm femorotibial graft, and a 40 cm proximal, 20 cm distal, sequential femoropopliteal-tibial graft. Diameter of the graft is 5 mm throughout. Symbols not included in Figure 4-11 are calf collateral (*CC*) and tibial arteries (*T*). Resting flows to the thigh muscle, calf muscle, and distal leg and foot are 200, 70, and 30 ml/min, respectively.

retrograde fashion, to the thigh. Having no direct communication with the popliteal artery, femorotibial grafts supply more blood in a retrograde direction to the proximal tissues of the calf than distal segments of sequential grafts do. Because flow velocities are a function of flow rates, distal segments of sequential grafts may be more susceptible than proximal segments to failure.[73] On the other hand, a femorotibial graft may be more likely to fail than the proximal segment of a sequential graft.

Outflow Resistance

Failure of infrainguinal bypass grafts has been correlated with high outflow resistance.[74–76] Since outflow resistance, which is roughly analogous to R_p in equation 14, is in series with graft resistance, blood flow through the graft is inversely proportional to the sum of the two resistances.

Although various methods for estimating outflow resistance have been described, all measure the pressure gener-

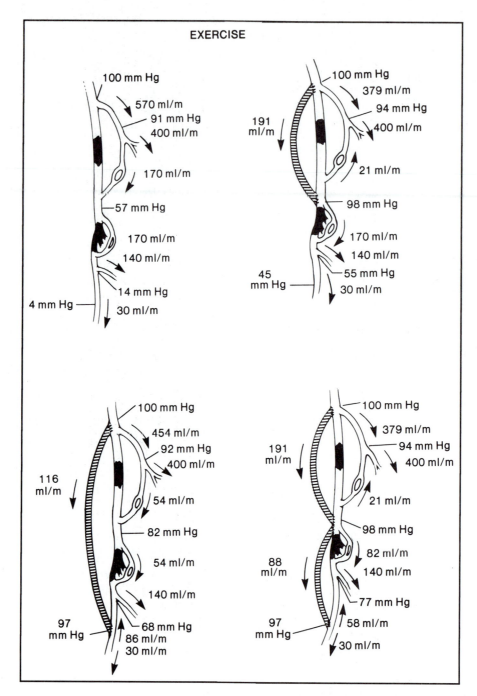

Figure 4-13. Exercise flow through femoral-(blind)popliteal, femorotibial, and sequential femoropopliteal-tibial grafts. Exercise flows to the thigh muscle, calf muscle, and distal leg and foot are 400, 140, and 30 ml/min, respectively.

ated in the distal graft while saline is being infused into the graft at a known rate. Outflow resistance is simply the ratio of the pressure and the flow rate of saline. Measured in this way, outflow resistance reflects both the "true" resistance of the peripheral vascular bed and the resistance of the collateral arteries. At low infusion rates, the pressure developed in the graft does not exceed that at the proximal end of the collaterals; consequently, collateral flow competes with flow from the graft to supply the peripheral vascular bed. On the other hand, at high infusion rates, the pressure developed in the graft is sufficiently high to reverse flow

in the collaterals, which then become a part of the outflow system of the graft (see Fig. 4-11). It turns out, therefore, that the apparent outflow resistance varies with the rate at which saline is being infused, being deceptively high at low rates of infusion and deceptively low at high infusion rates (Table 4-2).[77] Thus, to accurately reflect outflow resistance, measurement should be made at pressures similar to those expected when the graft is functioning.

Although clamping the recipient artery proximal to the distal anastomosis decreases the size of the collateral bed and makes the measurements more reflective of the "true"

TABLE 4-2. RELATIONSHIP OF APPARENT OUTFLOW RESISTANCE TO "TRUE" PERIPHERAL RESISTANCE*

Flow Rates (ml/min)			Input Pressure (mm Hg)	Apparent Outflow Resistance (mm Hg/ml/min)	Apparent/True Resistance Ratio
Graft Infusate	Peripheral Bed	Collateral[†]			
25.0	109.5	+84.5	65.7	2.63	4.38
50.0	118.9	+68.9	71.4	1.43	2.38
75.0	128.4	+53.4	77.1	1.03	1.71
100.0	137.9	+37.9	82.7	0.83	1.38
150.0	156.8	+6.8	94.1	0.63	1.05
200.0	175.8	−24.2	105.5	0.53	0.88
300.0	213.7	−86.3	128.2	0.43	0.71
400.0	251.6	−148.4	150.9	0.38	0.63

* Based on diagram in Figure 4-11, assuming constant resistances (mm Hg/ml/min): true peripheral = 0.6; collateral = 0.35; thigh muscle = 0.475; profunda femoris = 0.017.
[†] + indicates antegrade, and − indicates retrograde collateral flow.

peripheral resistance, it will not affect those collaterals that enter below the anastomosis. Nevertheless, this maneuver does appear to improve the ability of outflow resistance to identify those grafts destined to fail.[75] The fact that saline, which has a viscosity much less than that of blood, is used as the infusate introduces another confounding variable. One would expect the resistance measured with saline to be considerably less than that actually existing when the graft is functioning.

Cross-Over Grafts

Femoral-femoral, axillary-axillary, subclavian-subclavian, axillary-femoral, and other similar grafts all depend for their proper function on the ability of the donor artery to supply an increased blood flow without sustaining an appreciably increased pressure drop. Since the drop in pressure across any arterial segment is a function of the product of its resistance and the flow rate (equation 15), the resistance of the donor artery must be relatively low. When the donor artery is disease free, there ordinarily is no problem; but

when the donor artery contains atherosclerotic plaques (as many do), a steal phenomenon may develop (Table 4-3).[78,79] Questions regarding the resistance of the donor artery are best resolved by hemodynamic measurements. Arteriography may be deceiving. For example, before performing a femoral-femoral bypass, the surgeon who is concerned about the capacity of the donor vessel should measure the common femoral artery pressure on the donor side with the flow rate at least double the resting value. This is most easily accomplished pharmacologically by the administration of papaverine. If the operation is being performed to relieve claudication, there should be relatively little pressure drop; but if the purpose is to alleviate ischemia, a somewhat larger pressure drop may be permissible. In other words, the pressure delivered to the recipient common femoral artery should be high enough to ensure adequate perfusion of the target tissues. One must also consider the effect of the reduced pressure on the donor limb. In most cases this will be minimal, but when stenoses or occlusions of the thigh or calf arteries are present, the fall in pressure may be sufficient to induce symptoms in a previously asymptomatic limb or worsen those in a previously symptomatic limb.

TABLE 4-3. THEORETIC EFFECT OF FEMORAL-FEMORAL GRAFT*

	No Stenosis of Donor Iliac				Stenotic Donor Iliac			
	Rest		Exercise		Rest		Exercise	
	Before Graft	After Graft	Before Graft	After Graft	Before Graft	After Graft	Before Graft	After Graft
Donor								
Iliac flow (ml/min)	250	476	1,266	2,282	250	311	645	730
Common femoral pressure (mm Hg)	99	98	95	91	80	75[†]	48	42[†]
Common femoral flow (ml/min)	250	248	1,266	1,211	250	235[†]	645	554[†]
Recipient								
Iliac collateral flow (ml/min)	250	18	426	84	250	157	426	369
Common femoral pressure (mm Hg)	60	97	32	87	60	75	32	41
Common femoral flow (ml/min)	250	246	426	1,155	250	233	426	545
Cross-pubic graft flow (ml/min)	—	228	—	1,071	—	76	—	176

* Aortic pressure = 100 mm Hg; graft resistance = 0.004 mm Hg/ml/min.
[†] Pressure and flow drops indicative of a "steal."
Data from Sumner DS, Strandness DE Jr: Surg Gynecol Obstet 134:629, 1972.

Anastomotic Configuration

To reduce energy losses due to flow disturbances, the transition from graft to host vessel should be as smooth as possible.[80,81] End-to-end anastomoses, therefore, most closely approximate the ideal. End-to-side or side-to-end anastomoses always result in alterations in flow direction (Fig. 4-14). Tailoring the anastomosis to enter the recipient artery or leave the donor artery at an acute angle will minimize but can never eliminate flow disturbances. Although decreasing the angle will reduce flow disturbances in the antegrade limb of a recipient artery, it will accentuate those in the retrograde limb, where flow vectors are almost completely reversed.[82] Other energy depleting pitfalls to be avoided include marked disparity between the diameters of the graft and the artery to which it is connected and slitlike configurations of the orifice between the two conduits.[83] The latter occurs when the graft lumen is stretched to accommodate an excessively long incision in the artery.

Despite these theoretical considerations, in practice there is usually little difference in the pressure gradients across anastomoses, regardless of their angle or configuration (provided, of course, that the anastomoses have been carefully constructed and that there are no stenoses).[84] There may, however, be important differences that deter-

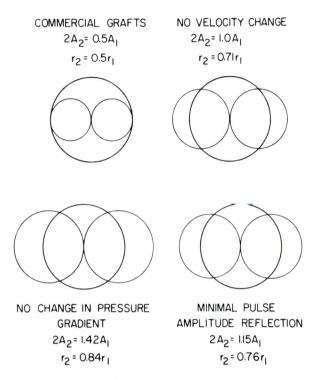

Figure 4-15. Hemodynamic attributes of bifurcation grafts. (r_1, Radius of primary tube; r_2, radius of secondary limbs; A_1, cross-sectional area of primary tube; and A_2, cross-sectional area of secondary tube.) (*From Strandness DE Jr, Sumner DS: Hemodynamics for Surgeons. New York, Grune & Stratton, 1975.*)

mine the longevity of graft function.[85,86] Whenever there are flow disturbances, regions of flow separation are always present.[82,87] Within these regions, shear rates are reduced—a situation that predisposes to the accumulation of thrombi and to the development of fibromuscular dysplasia. Minimizing these flow disturbances by adhering to recognized hemodynamic principles may, therefore, ultimately determine the success of the arterial reconstruction.

Bifurcation Grafts

Although most **Y** grafts used for aorto-biiliac and aorto-bifemoral bypasses have secondary limbs with diameters that are one half that of the primary tube, this is probably not the optimum configuration.[88] Constructed in this way, each of the secondary limbs has 16 times the resistance of the primary tube, and, in parallel, they have eight times the resistance of the primary tube (Fig. 4-15). Flow velocity is doubled, and almost 50% of the incident pulsatile energy is reflected. The reflected energy may contribute to weakening of the proximal suture line in a severely diseased friable aorta, leading to the development of false aneurysms and aorto-enteric fistulas.[89]

No geometric configuration will satisfy all requirements.[12] For example, to maintain a constant flow velocity across the bifurcation, the ratio of the diameter of the secondary tube to that of the primary tube must be 0.71; to maintain the same pressure gradient, the diameter

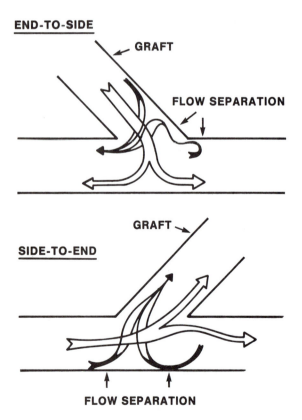

Figure 4-14. Flow patterns at end-to-side and side-to-side anastomoses. Note areas of flow separation. Flow in some areas may reverse and travel circumferentially to reach the recipient artery or graft. (*From Sumner DS: Hemodynamics of abnormal blood flow, in Wilson SE, Veith FJ, et al. (eds): Vascular Surgery, Principles and Practice. New York, McGraw-Hill Book Co., 1987.*)

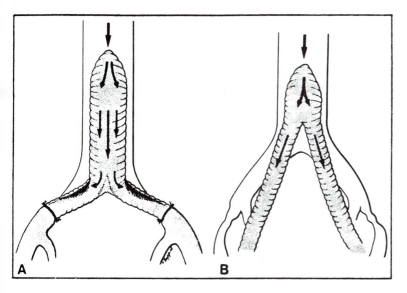

Figure 4-16. Effect of angle between limbs of bifurcation graft on flow disturbances. When the limbs are widely separated, areas of flow separation (indicated by shading) develop. (*From Malan E, Longo T: Principles of qualitative hemodynamics in vascular surgery, in Haimovici H* (ed): *Vascular Surgery, Principles and Techniques, 2nd ed. East Norwalk, Conn, Appleton-Century-Crofts, 1984.*)

ratio must be 0.84; and to achieve minimal pulse reflection, the diameter ratio must be 0.76 (see Fig. 4-15). In animals and in human infants, the ratio is about 0.74 to 0.76, suggesting that the body attempts to minimize reflections at bifurcations. The 16 × 9 mm, 14 × 8 mm, and 12 × 7 mm grafts that are now commercially available have diameter ratios of 0.56, 0.57, and 0.58, respectively. While these ratios represent some improvement over the 0.5 ratio of the older grafts, they still result in increased flow velocity, an increased pressure gradient, and relatively little decrease in the amount of energy reflected (30 vs. 50%). Thus the hemodynamically optimum bifurcation graft has yet to be manufactured.

The angle between the limbs of a bifurcation graft is also of hemodynamic importance. Flow disturbances are minimized when the angle is narrow and are exaggerated when the limbs are widely separated (Fig. 4-16). The latter configuration generates regions of flow separation along the walls opposite the flow divider, encouraging the deposition of a thrombus. By keeping the primary limb short and using longer secondary limbs, the surgeon can reduce the angle.

CONCLUSIONS

Understanding the symptoms of arterial occlusive disease, interpreting the results of physiologic tests, and planning effective surgical therapy are all facilitated by a basic knowledge of hemodynamic and rheologic principles. When predicting the effects of a stenosis, a graft, or other changes in the vascular circuit, one must consider all aspects of the circuit, including collateral input, peripheral resistance, autoregulation, direction of flow, steal phenomena, and inertial factors; otherwise, "armchair" conclusions are apt to be erroneous. This chapter has concentrated on "generic solutions" to various problems commonly encountered in vascular surgery and has based these solutions primarily on models; consequently, the absolute values may differ somewhat from those encountered in real life. Each situation

is different and requires careful physiologic assessment, either by noninvasive or invasive measurement of both pressure and flow. It is hoped that this chapter will stimulate others to make these measurements and that the information presented will aid in their interpretation.

BIBLIOGRAPHY

McDonald DA: Blood Flow in Arteries, 2nd ed. Baltimore, Williams & Wilkins, 1974.

Strandness DE Jr, and Sumner DS: Hemodynamics for Surgeons. New York, Grune & Stratton, 1975.

Patel DJ and Vaishnav RN: Basic Hemodynamics and Its Role in Disease Processes. Baltimore, University Park Press, 1980.

Sumner DS: Hemodynamics and pathophysiology of arterial disease, in Rutherford RB (ed): Vascular Surgery. Philadelphia, W.B. Saunders Co, 1984.

Strandness DE Jr, Didisheim P, et al.: Vascular Disease. Current Research and Clinical Applications. Orlando, Fla., Grune & Stratton, 1987.

REFERENCES

1. Johnson G Jr, Keagy BA, et al.: Viscous factors in peripheral tissue perfusion. J Vasc Surg 2:530, 1985.
2. Litwin MS, Chapman K: Physical factors affecting human blood viscosity. J Surg Res 10:433, 1970.
3. Sumner DS: Hemodynamics and pathophysiology of arterial disease, in Rutherford RB (ed): Vascular Surgery. Philadelphia, W.B. Saunders Co, 1984.
4. Young DF, Tsai FY: Flow characteristics of models of arterial stenosis, II. Unsteady flow. J Biomech 6:547, 1973.
5. Berguer R, Hwang NHC: Critical arterial stenosis: A theoretical and experimental solution. Ann Surg 180:39, 1974.
6. Daugherty HI, Franzini JB: Steady flow of incompressible fluids in pipes, in Fluid Mechanics with Engineering Applications, 4th ed. New York, McGraw-Hill Book Co, 1965, p 191.
7. Young DF, Tsai FY: Flow characteristics in models of arterial stenoses, I. Steady flow. J Biomech 6:395, 1973.

8. Flanigan DP, Tullis JP, et al.: Multiple subcritical arterial stenoses: Effect on poststenotic pressure and flow. Ann Surg 186:663, 1977.

9. Karayannacos PE, Talukder N, et al.: The role of multiple noncritical arterial stenoses in the pathogenesis of ischemia. J Thorac Cardiovasc Surg 73:458, 1977.

10. Cheng LC, Clark ME, Robertson JM: Numerical calculations of oscillating flow in the vicinity of square wall obstacles in plane conduits. J Biomech 5:467, 1972.

11. Byar D, Fiddian RV, et al.: The fallacy of applying Poiseuille equation to segmented arterial stenosis. Am Heart J 70:216, 1965.

12. Strandness DE Jr, Sumner DS: Hemodynamics for Surgeons. New York, Grune & Stratton, Inc, 1975.

13. May AG, Van deBerg L, et al.: Critical arterial stenosis. Surgery 54:250, 1963.

14. Moore WS, Malone JM: Effect of flow rate and vessel calibre on critical arterial stenosis. J Surg Res 26:1, 1979.

15. Moore WS, Hall AD: Unrecognized aorto-iliac stenosis. A physiologic approach to the diagnosis. Arch Surg 103:633, 1971.

16. Jones RD, Berne RM: Intrinsic regulation of skeletal muscle blood flow. Circ Res 14:126, 1964.

17. Kjellmer I: On the competition between metabolic vasodilatation and neurogenic vasoconstriction in skeletal muscle. Acta Physiol Scand 63:450, 1965.

18. Ludbrook J: Collateral artery resistance in the human lower limb. J Surg Res 6:423, 1966.

19. Shepherd JT: Physiology of the Circulation in Human Limbs in Health and Disease, Philadelphia, WB Saunders Co, 1963.

20. Wolf EA Jr, Sumner DS, Strandness DE Jr: Correlation between nutritive blood flow and pressure in limbs of patients with intermittent claudication. Surg Forum 23:238, 1972.

21. Edwards EA: Scope and limitations of collateral circulation. Arch Surg 119:761, 1984.

22. Spencer MP, Reid JM: Quantitation of carotid stenosis with continuous-wave (c-w) Doppler ultrasound. Stroke 10:326, 1979.

23. Russell JB, Miles RD, et al.: Effect of arterial stenosis on Doppler frequency spectrum. Proc 32nd Annu Conf Eng Med Biol 21:45, 1979.

24. Keitzer WF, Fry WJ, et al.: Hemodynamic mechanism for pulse changes seen in occlusive vascular disease. Surgery 57:163, 1965.

25. Strandness DE Jr, Bell JW: Peripheral vascular disease. Diagnosis and objective evaluation using a mercury strain gauge. Ann Surg 161 (suppl):1, 1965.

26. Darling RC, Raines JK, et al.: Quantitative segmental pulse and volume recorder: A clinical tool. Surgery 72:873, 1973.

27. Jager KA, Phillips DJ, et al.: Noninvasive mapping of lower limb arterial lesions. Ultrasound Med Biol 11:515, 1985.

28. Woodcock JP, Gosling RG, Fitzgerald DE: A new non-invasive technique for assessment of superficial femoral artery obstruction. Br J Surg 59:226, 1972.

29. Johnston KW, Maruzzo BC, Cobbold RSC: Doppler methods for quantitative measurement and localization of peripheral arterial occlusive disease by analysis of the blood velocity waveform. Ultrasound Med Biol 4:209, 1978.

30. Evans DH, Barrie WW, et al.: The relationship between ultrasonic pulsatility index and proximal arterial stenoses in a canine model. Circ Res 46:470, 1980.

31. Baird RN, Bird DR, et al.: Upstream stenosis, its diagnosis by Doppler signals from the femoral artery. Arch Surg 115:1316, 1980.

32. Rittenhouse EA, Maxiner W, et al.: Directional arterial flow velocity: A sensitive index of changes in peripheral vascular resistance. Surgery 79:359, 1976.

33. Farrar DJ, Malindzak GS Jr, Johnson G Jr: Large vessel impedance in peripheral atherosclerosis. Circulation 56 (suppl 2):171, 1977.

34. Skidmore R, Woodcock JP: Physiological interpretation of Doppler-shift waveforms, II: Validation of the Laplace transform method for characterization of the common femoral blood-velocity/time waveform. Ultrasound Med Biol 6:219, 1980.

35. Berguer R, Higgins RF, Reddy DJ: Intimal hyperplasia. An experimental study. Arch Surg 115:332, 1980.

36. Zarins CK, Giddens DP, et al.: Carotid bifurcation atherosclerosis: Quantitative correlation of plaque localization with flow velocity profiles and wall shear stress. Circ Res 53:502, 1983.

37. Zarins CK, Bomberger RA, Glagov S: Local effects of stenoses: Increased flow velocity inhibits atherogenesis. Circulation 64 (suppl 2):221, 1981.

38. Vaishnav RM, Patel DJ, et al.: Determination of the local erosion stress of the canine endothelium using a jet impingement method. ASME J Biomech Engr 105:77, 1983.

39. Zarins CK, Zatina MA, et al.: Shear stress regulation of artery lumen diameter in experimental atherogenesis. J Vasc Surg 5:413, 1987.

40. Glagov S, Weisenberg E, et al.: Compensatory enlargement of human atherosclerotic coronary arteries. N Engl J Med 316:1371, 1987.

41. Boughner DR, Roach MR: Effect of low frequency vibration on the arterial wall. Circ Res 29:136, 1971.

42. Pentecost BL: The effect of exercise on the external iliac vein blood flow and local oxygen consumption in normal subjects, and in those with occlusive arterial disease. Clin Sci 27:437, 1964.

43. Lassen NA, Kampp M: Calf muscle blood flow during walking studied by the Xe^{133} method in normals and in patients with intermittent claudication. Scand J Clin Lab Invest 17:447, 1965.

44. Folse, R: Alterations in femoral blood flow and resistance during rhythmic exercise and sustained muscular contractions in patients with arteriosclerosis. Surg Gynecol Obstet 121:767, 1965.

45. Hauser CJ, Shoemaker WC: Use of transcutaneous Po_2 regional perfusion index to quantify tissue perfusion in peripheral vascular disease. Ann Surg 197:337, 1983.

46. Clyne CAC, Ryan J, et al.: Oxygen tension on the skin of ischemic legs. Am J Surg 143:315, 1982.

47. Tonnesen KH, Noer I, et al.: Classification of peripheral occlusive arterial disease based on symptoms, signs, and distal blood pressure measurements. Acta Chir Scand 146:101, 1980.

48. Ramsey DE, Manke DA, Sumner DS: Toe blood pressure—a valuable adjunct to ankle pressure measurement for assessing peripheral arterial disease. J Cardiovasc Surg 24:43, 1983.

49. Remington JW, Wood EH: Formation of peripheral pulse contour in man. J Appl Physiol 9:433, 1956.

50. Yao ST: Haemodynamic studies in peripheral arterial disease. Br J Surg 57:761, 1970.

51. Westerhof N, Sipkema P, et al.: Forward and backward waves in the arterial system. Cardiovasc Res 6:648, 1972.

52. Strandness DE Jr, Bell JW: An evaluation of the hemodynamic response of the claudicating extremity to exericise. Surg Gynecol Obstet 119:1237, 1964.

53. Sumner DS, Strandness DE Jr: The relationship between calf blood flow and ankle blood pressure in patients with intermittent claudication. Surgery 65:763, 1969.

54. Lewis JD, Papathanaiou C, et al.: Simultaneous flow and pressure measurements in intermittent claudication. Br J Surg 59:418, 1972.

55. Sumner DS, Strandness DE Jr: The effect of exercise on resistance to blood flow in limbs with an occluded superficial femoral artery. Vasc Surg 4:229, 1970.

56. Angelides NS, Nicolaides AN, et al.: The mechanism of calf claudication: Studies of simultaneous clearance of ^{99m}Tc from the calf and thigh. Br J Surg 65:204, 1978.

57. Angelides NS, Nicolaides AN: Simultaneous isotope clearance from the muscles of the calf and thigh. Br J Surg 67:220, 1980.

58. Allwood MJ: Redistribution of blood flow in limbs with obstruction of a main artery. Clin Sci 22:279, 1962.

59. Sumner DS: Hemodynamics of abnormal blood flow, in Wilson SE, Veith FJ, et al. (eds): Vascular Surgery, Principles and Practice. New York, McGraw-Hill Book Co, 1987.

60. Rosenthal SL, Guyton AC: Hemodynamics of collateral vasodilatation following femoral artery occlusion in anesthetized dogs. Circ Res 23:239, 1968.

61. Conrad MC, Anderson JL III, Garrett JB Jr: Chronic collateral growth after femoral artery occlusion in the dog. J Appl Physiol 31:550, 1971.

62. Flanigan DP, Ryan TJ, et al.: Aortofemoral or femoropopliteal revascularization? A prospective evaluation of the papaverine test. J Vasc Surg 1:215, 1984.

63. Schultz RD, Hokanson DE, Strandness DE Jr: Pressure-flow relations of the end-side anastomosis. Surgery 62:319, 1967.

64. Sanders RJ, Kempczinski RF, et al.: The significance of graft diameter. Surgery 88:856, 1980.

65. Whitney DG, Kuhn EM, Estes JW: Valvular occlusion of the arterialized saphenous vein. Am Surg 42:879, 1976.

66. McCaughan JJ, Walsh DB, et al.: In vitro observations of greater saphenous vein valves during pulsatile and nonpulsatile flow and following lysis. J Vasc Surg 1:356, 1984.

67. Walsh DB, Downing S, et al.: Valvular obstruction of blood flow through saphenous veins. J Surg Res 42:39, 1987.

68. Ku DN, Klafta JM, et al.: The contributions of valves to saphenous vein graft resistance. J Vasc Surg 6:274, 1987.

69. Brewster DC, Charlesworth PM, et al.: Isolated popliteal segment v. tibial bypass. Comparison of hemodynamic and clinical results. Arch Surg 119:775, 1984.

70. Jarrett F, Perca A, et al.: Hemodynamics of sequential bypass grafts in peripheral arterial occlusions. Surg Gynecol Obstet 150:377, 1980.

71. Jarrett F, Berkoff HA, et al.: Femorotibial bypass grafts with sequential techniques. Arch Surg 116:709, 1981.

72. Hadcock MM, Ubatuba J, et al.: Hemodynamics of sequential grafts. Am J Surg 146:170, 1983.

73. Flinn WR, Flanigan DP, et al.: Sequential femoral-tibial bypass for severe limb ischemia. Surgery 88:357, 1980.

74. Ascer E, Veith FJ, et al.: Components of outflow resistance and their correlation with graft patency in lower extremity arterial reconstructions. J Vasc Surg 1:817, 1984.

75. LaMorte WW, Menzoian JO, et al.: A new method for the prediction of peripheral vascular resistance from the preoperative angiogram. J Vasc Surg 2:703, 1985.

76. Ascer E, Veith FJ, et al.: Intraoperative outflow resistance as a predictor of late patency of femoropopliteal and infrapopliteal arterial bypasses. J Vasc Surg 5:820, 1987.

77. Bliss BP: Peripheral resistance in the leg in arterial occlusive disease. Cardiovasc Res 5:337, 1971.

78. Sumner DS, Strandness DE Jr: The hemodynamics of the femorofemoral shunt. Surg Gynecol Obstet 134:629, 1972.

79. Shin CS, Chaudhry AG: Hemodynamics of extra-anatomical bypass following restriction of inflow and outflow in the donor artery in dogs. World J Surg 4:717, 1980.

80. Malan E, Noseda G, Longt T: Approach to fluid dynamic problems in reconstructive vascular surgery. Surgery 66:994, 1969.

81. Malan E, Longo T: Principles of qualitative hemodynamics in vascular surgery, in Haimovici H: Vascular Surgery, 2nd ed. Norwalk, Conn., Appleton-Century-Crofts, 1984.

82. Crawshaw HM, Quist WC, et al.: Flow disturbance at the distal end-to-side anastomosis. Effect of patency of the proximal outflow segment and angle of anastomosis. Arch Surg 115:1280, 1980.

83. Klimach O, Chapman BLW, et al.: An investigation into how the geometry of an end-to-side arterial anastomosis affects its function. Br J Surg 71:43, 1984.

84. Lye CR, Sumner DS, Strandness DE Jr: The hemodynamics of the retrograde cross-pubic anastomosis. Surg Forum 26:298, 1975.

85. Bond MG, Hostetler JR, et al.: Intimal changes in arteriovenous bypass grafts. Effect of varying the angle of implantation at the proximal anastomosis and of producing stenosis in the distal runoff artery. J Thorac Cardiovasc Surg 71:907, 1976.

86. LoGerfo FW, Quist WC, et al.: Downstream anastomotic hyperplasia. A mechanism of failure in Dacron arterial grafts. Ann Surg 197:479, 1983.

87. LoGerfo FW, Soncrant T, et al.: Boundary layer separation in models of side-to-end arterial anastomoses. Arch Surg 114:1369, 1979.

88. Buxton BF, Wukasch DC, et al.: Practical considerations in fabric vascular grafts. Introduction of a new bifurcated graft. Am J Surg 125:288, 1973.

89. Newman DL, Gosling RG, et al.: Pressure amplitude increase on unmatching the aorto-iliac junction of the dog. Cardiovasc Res 7:6, 1973.

CHAPTER 5
Principles of Arteriography

Harvey L. Neiman

Significant change has occurred in diagnostic arteriography in the last 5 years relating to advancements in instrumentation, contrast material, and techniques. The net result has been to provide safer angiographic studies with an increase in information. The basic principles of arteriography, however, remain the same.

Angiography is a problem-oriented discipline that requires diagnostic acumen, technical skills, and an understanding of the clinical problem. Diagnostic ultrasound, computed tomography, and noninvasive flow studies have decreased the indications for angiographic examinations. Nevertheless, arteriography and venography continue to play a central role in the diagnosis and management of vascular disease. The former two studies delineate arterial and venous anatomy, respectively. Direct physiologic information can also be obtained at the time of examination. Further, interventional radiologic procedures such as angioplasty and embolotherapy play an ever-increasing role in patient management.

HISTORY OF ANGIOGRAPHY

The first angiographic examination was performed by Haschek and Lindenthal in the month following Roentgen's discovery of x-rays. They injected a chalk-containing solution into the blood vessels of an amputated hand.[1] Radiographs of veins were first made by Berberich and Hirsch in 1923 by injecting a radiopaque material, a 20% solution of strontium bromide.[2] In 1928, Moniz and Diaza reported the first attempt to visualize the cerebral circulation by injection of an iodinated solution into a surgically exposed carotid artery.[3] McPheeters and Rice in 1929 used iodized oil (Lipiodol) to visualize lower extremity veins.[4] The emerging techniques of arteriography and venography were seldom used, however, until the introduction of iodinated contrast materials such as diodone by Edwards and Biguria in 1934.[5]

Dos Santos et al. in 1929, utilizing a translumbar approach, were the first to perform abdominal aortography.[6]

Also in 1929, Swick reported the use of an organic iodide for intravenous urography that was much better tolerated than sodium iodide.[7] Forssmann inserted a catheter into his own antecubital vein and obtained a radiograph to confirm his impression that the catheter had reached the right atrium. In 1931, he succeeded in visualizing the right heart and pulmonary vessels of a patient with this technique.[8]

The usefulness of intravenous injection of contrast material for arterial opacification became appreciated as Castellanos et al.[9] in 1937 and Robb and Steinberg[10] in 1939 published results of their experiences. Their examinations focused on diagnosis of many congenital cardiac anomalies. Studies were limited because of the toxicity of contrast materials available at that time and because the density of the images obtained after intravenous injection was frequently inadequate.

In 1934, Zeides des Plantes suggested that photographic image subtraction could be used to separate contrast material densities from those produced by bone or other normal anatomic structures. More recently, these photographic subtraction techniques have become an integral part of arteriography.[11]

Phlebography did not come into routine use until 1938 when Dos Santos described a method of outlining the deep as well as the superficial veins by injecting contrast material into a superficial vein behind the lateral malleolus. A series of films was obtained as the contrast material ascended into the leg and thigh, the technique now known as ascending phlebography.[12]

Retrograde brachial thoracic aortography was described in 1939 by Castellanos and Pereiras.[13] In 1941 Farinas reported the retrograde passage of a catheter from the femoral artery into the abdominal aorta for aortography.[14] The modern era of angiography began with Seldinger's description in 1953 of a percutaneous method of catheter placement over a previously inserted guidewire.[15] Since that time the technique has been refined. Current modifications include incorporation of computer-aided digital subtraction techniques, high-flow catheters with small diameters, and safer contrast materials that are iso-osmolar.

TECHNICAL PRINCIPLES

Angiographic Equipment

The standard angiographic room must contain a high-quality fluoroscopic system with television monitoring. Procedures should never be carried out without fluoroscopic guidance, even when noncatheter techniques are utilized. Safety in placing the needle is assured with fluoroscopic monitoring, and the examination is performed more quickly.

A high capacity three-phase generator of constant load output and a rating of at least 100 kW at 100 kV is also necessary to assure optimum kilovoltage levels at minimum exposure times. Full generator output and voltage stability during the examination require a well-designed power source free of line interference from other hospital equipment. Automatic line voltage compensation should also be integral to the x-ray generator.

Rapid film changers are a further necessity for all types of examinations, whether they be of the carotid or the peripheral vessels. Optimally, biplane filming capabilities should be available, since filming in a single projection often does not give the true picture of the pathologic abnormality. Sequential filming in a second plane is often a satisfactory compromise when biplane equipment is unavailable. This, however, somewhat increases both the time of the procedure and the amount of contrast material used.

For lower extremity arteriography, a programmable, stepping table top should be available. The stepping table top is used in conjunction with a standard changer and specialized computer-driven equipment that allows the table to move at preselected intervals. We have utilized this technique for the past 12 years with excellent results and can perform an efficacious examination quickly.

The angiographic catheterization table should have a floating top to facilitate the performance of procedures. If possible, this table top should be able to move up and down, not only for ease of examination but also to permit magnification filming. X-ray tube and image intensifier should operate independently to increase magnification possibilities. Although angiography can be carried out in a fluoroscopy room without a floating top, this practice should be discouraged unless the volume of procedures is too small to support a dedicated angiographic suite. It is also desirable to be able to produce a single hard copy image quickly. A spot film changer utilizing a 100 or 105 mm camera or the preview film from a digital subtraction system serves this purpose. Cine capability is only necessary if cardiac catheterizations are performed in the same room.

It is obligatory that every angiographic room have ECG monitoring capability and that all patients be so monitored. Pressure monitors are extremely important in peripheral vascular angiography for evaluating significance of stenoses and the results of angioplasty. Pressure measurements are essential in pulmonary angiography before the injection of contrast material.

All contrast medium injections are performed with automatic pressure injectors that provide delivery of a given amount of contrast material at a predetermined rate. Hand injections, however, are utilized for testing the placement of catheters and also during venography. The latter allows for careful monitoring of the injection site during the introduction of contrast material into a vein on the dorsum of the foot.

Finally, a rapid automatic film processor should be in close proximity to the catheterization room for proper management of examinations, since the next "run" often depends on information derived from the previous sequence. Each examination must be tailored to the unique needs of a particular patient.

Modern angiography interweaves conventional filming utilizing cut film placed in a changer with digital subtraction angiographic techniques. The up-to-date angiographic room, therefore, should offer digital subtraction capabilities so that a single examination may include one or two runs filmed with digital subtraction techniques and the remainder utilizing conventional x-ray film.

A well-trained team of angiographic technologists and nurses is invaluable and essential for carrying out high quality examinations with safety. As in the operating room, staff most familiar with the examinations should perform them on a regular basis. Routine rotation of all departmental personnel into the angiographic suite should be discouraged.

To accommodate digital subtraction angiography (DSA), the x-ray tube should have a focal spot combination of at least 0.6 and 1.2 mm and high anode heat storage capacity. For conventional film magnification techniques, bias focal spots of 0.3, 0.2, and 0.15 mm are now commonly used. Thin-window cesium iodide image intensifiers with a thick phosphor are the standard for DSA. Input phosphors with absorption fractions in the range of 0.5 to 0.75 are optimum for DSA. Large intensifiers such as those with a 14-inch diameter are desirable, but 12-inch units are found more commonly. Most frequently a digital matrix 512 by 512 is used to present the information from the video signal. The introduction of high-resolution television systems incorporating 1,000 or more raster lines improves image display. In addition, the video signal should be digitized to at least 256 shades of gray or 8 to 12 bits deep for each pixel.

Contrast Material

All contrast materials are iodinated organic compounds. Iodine compounds are used primarily because of the ability of iodine atoms to absorb x-rays, thus creating the contrast seen on an x-ray. The most commonly used contrast materials are the triple iodine-containing organic compounds: sodium or meglumine diatrizoate, iothalmate, or metrizoate. All are hyperosmolar and cause localized pain on injection in about 60% of patients. The pain is partly related to the sodium content. For these reasons, sodium-free contrast agents such as meglumine diatrizoate or meglumine iothalmate are preferable, at least on the venous side. If the contrast material can be diluted without reducing the diagnostic quality of the study, the discomfort is further reduced.

There has been explosive growth in the use of a new family of drugs, the low-osmolality contrast materials such as metrizamide, iohexol, ioxaglate, and iopamidol[16–18] (Fig. 5-1). It has been well demonstrated that angiography with

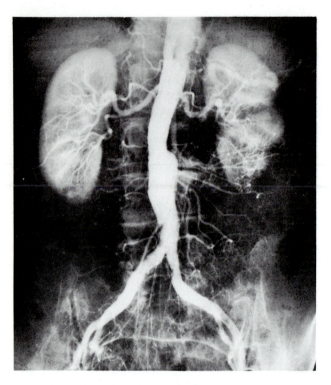

Figure 5-1. Abdominal aortogram performed during a lower extremity arteriogram with a 5 French pigtail catheter and nonionic contrast material. Note the excellent visualization of the major arteries as well as smaller branches.

these agents is painless.[19,20] There is also evidence that these agents are less thrombogenic than conventional contrast material, judged by iodine 125 fibrinogen uptake studies.[21–23] There is also evidence from animal experiments that tissue damage after extravasation is decreased. The use of these low-osmolality, frequently nonionic contrast materials may also increase the safety of the procedure. These agents have been shown to be less nephrotoxic and less injurious to the central nervous system and myocardium.[24–26]

The overall incidence of adverse reactions to conventional hyperosmolar contrast material is 5%. Reactions occur in 10% of patients with an allergic history, and in 15% of patients who have had a reaction to previous contrast injections. Pretesting has been shown to be of no value at predicting these reactions.[27]

Major life-threatening reactions do not tend to recur on reexamination, but minor reactions may be repeated. The nonfatal reaction rate is twice as high for excretory urography as for arterial procedures. This suggests that the lung may be the organ responsible for allergic-type manifestations related to histamine release[28] because the lung has the highest concentration of histamine per gram of tissue. The nonionic contrast agents appear to cause fewer allergic reactions. For patients who have had reactions previously, pretreatment with prednisone, 50 mg, at 13 hours, 7 hours, and 1 hour before the examination and with diphenhydramine (Benadryl), 50 mg, immediately before the study may reduce the incidence of these complications.

Shehadi and Tonioio's survey[29] revealed 18 fatalities in 302,083 examinations (0.006%). An allergic history correlates well with mild and intermediate reactions, but poorly with severe reactions and death.[27] Death correlates with increased age and diminished cardiac reserve. Most reactions occur in the first 5 minutes, but delayed reactions may occur. With most mild reactions, the patient may be reassured and treated with antihistamines (diphenhydramine, 25 to 50 mg IM or IV). With more severe symptoms, 0.1 to 0.2 ml of a 1:1,000 solution of epinephrine may be given intravenously at 1- to 3-minute intervals until the patient responds. With severe reactions, full cardiopulmonary resuscitation may be required.

Contrast material produces vasodilatation of arteries, resulting in increased blood flow. A decrease in systemic pressure is seen with injection of contrast material into the right or left heart, aorta, or peripheral arteries.[30,31]

Other cardiovascular responses to contrast material injection are an increase in cardiac output, heart rate, stroke volume, chamber pressure, and circulating blood volume. When contrast material is injected directly, there is a toxic depressive effect on the myocardium. Ventricular fibrillation or other severe arrhythmias occur in 0.76% of patients undergoing selective coronary arteriography.[32,33] Pulmonary hypertension and systemic hypotension occur with contrast injections into the right heart or pulmonary arteries.

In general, the lower the sodium concentration, the less pronounced are the cardiovascular responses. However, with coronary arteriography, an optimum sodium concentration is required. There is marked increase in the incidence of ventricular fibrillation with sodium concentrations above or below the optimum concentration.[34] The hypertonicity and viscosity of contrast material are also responsible for many of the cardiovascular reactions.[35] Added to the direct cardiovascular responses are indirect effects such as increased vagal activity resulting in slowing of the heart rate.[36]

All angiographic contrast materials are excreted almost entirely by glomerular filtration. Contrast material is not reabsorbed in the tubules and thus produces an osmotic diuresis. The sodium salts produce less diuresis than the meglumine salts.[37] When contrast material reaches the kidney, there is an initial increase in renal blood flow, followed by a decrease in flow, the decrease being the predominant effect.

Acute renal failure may follow contrast studies.[38] Dehydration is often a predisposing factor and is especially significant in diabetics, those with preexisting renal disease, and in patients with multiple myeloma. Swartz et al. found a 12% incidence of postangiographic renal failure in a retrospective review of 109 consecutive patients undergoing angiography.[39] In a prospective study in which an attempt was made to maintain hydration, Eisenberg et al. encountered no cases of renal failure among 537 consecutive patients undergoing angiography.[40] We strongly encourage our patients to be well hydrated and do not restrict fluids before angiography. Intravenous fluids are frequently given to ensure adequate hydration. As a generalization, 300 ml of contrast material is used as the upper limit of dose. This is obviously adjusted downward based on the patient's age, size, and renal status when necessary.[41]

Experimentally, injection of contrast material into the carotid artery alters the blood-brain barrier by increasing endothelial permeability, which allows the contrast material to diffuse into the surrounding tissues.[42] In humans and animals, methylglucamine salts have been shown to cause less neurotoxicity than sodium salts. With cerebral studies, the lower the sodium content, the safer the contrast material. Direct injection of contrast material into the artery of Adamkiewicz may result in paraplegia. Most spinal cord complications, however, are transient and clear within 24 hours.[44]

Patient Preparation

Before the angiography is performed, it is essential that the angiographer discuss the procedure, its risks, benefits, and alternative procedures at length with the patient. Particular note must be made of the patient's hematologic, renal, cardiac, allergic, and neurologic status. Preangiographic orders include no solid foods after midnight, although as noted, liquids are strongly encouraged. Coumadin use is a relative contraindication to performing an elective arteriogram. If clinically possible, patients receiving therapeutic levels of heparin should have this drug stopped several hours before the procedure. Heparin, however, presents no significant problems because its effects can be reversed with protamine sulfate if necessary. Relative contraindications to angiography are listed in Table 5-1.

Almost all catheterizations including translumbar aortograms are performed with local anesthesia. Peripheral arterial injections including lower extremity and hand arteriography (Fig. 5-2) are uncomfortable to quite painful, depending on the patient's tolerance. The pain associated with conventional contrast material can be decreased with the use of intra-arterial lidocaine before or mixed with the contrast material.[45,46] Nonionic contrast material has been shown to markedly reduce pain. Presently, the nonionic contrast materials are not routinely used for all examinations because of their high cost. Specific indications for its use need to be developed in each laboratory.

Improvement in intravenous analgesics has been made in the last several years. Previously, we had used meperi-

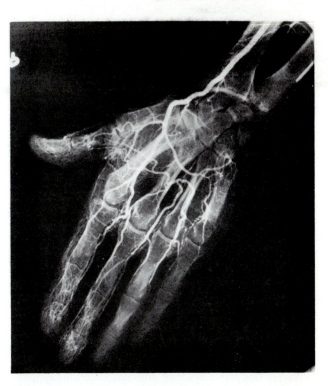

Figure 5-2. Hand arteriogram demonstrates occlusion of the ulnar artery and small vessel disease most prominent in the fourth and fifth digits. Examination was performed with nonionic contrast material, negating the usually painful aspects of this study when performed with conventional ionic contrast material.

dine (Demerol) and sodium secobarbital as our routine preangiographic drugs. We now utilize fentanyl and midazolam (Versed) immediately before the examination. These agents have fewer respiratory and cardiovascular depressant effects, and we have had few complications related to their use. With the exception of children, there is little indication for general anesthesia in angiography. The mild pain associated with diagnostic arteriography or other interventional procedures can be readily alleviated with intravenous agents and local anesthesia. Spinal and epidural anesthesia have been utilized effectively in patients undergoing embolotherapy, with its more significant pain of longer duration.

Routine systemic heparinization is not utilized unless significant disease is encountered during the passage of the guidewire or catheter. Heparin, 3,000 to 4,000 units, may then be given intraarterially. Some have advocated the routine use of systemic heparinization for angiographic procedures.[47] I prefer careful catheter flushing and judicious use of systemic heparinization and have had essentially no thrombotic problems or bleeding at the puncture site.

Catheters and Guidewires

Improvement in catheter and guidewire design has been one of the most significant advances in angiography in the last 5 years. The routine use of 4 and 5 French catheters replacing 6.5 and 7 French catheters has been well established. Wall material has been developed that will allow these smaller diameter catheters to deliver high-flow, high-

TABLE 5-1. RELATIVE CONTRAINDICATIONS TO ARTERIOGRAPHY

1. Recent myocardial infarction or significant arrhythmia
2. History of serious reaction to contrast material
3. Significant hypertension—diastolic pressure greater than 110 mm Hg
4. Bleeding diathesis, e.g., prothrombin time greater than twice the control, platelets less than 50,000
5. Impaired renal function (digital subtraction filming may negate this)
6. Inability to lie supine on angiography table, e.g., congestive heart failure
7. Retained barium from recent examination

From Neiman HL, Yao JST: Angiography of Vascular Disease. New York, Churchill Livingstone, 1985, p 4.

volume injections that are necessary for aortography. The smaller diameter catheters also provide good torque control for selective injection. Multiple manufacturers utilizing slightly different catheter design and polymers have introduced readily available commercial products. Except for select indications, there is little reason to use any catheter larger than 5 French. Similarly, because of advancements in guidewire design, catheterization of extremely tortuous or narrowed vessels is now possible. These guidewires provide greater torque control, greater stiffness (allowing passage of catheters into previously inaccessible positions), and markedly smaller diameter (i.e., 0.16-inch as compared to routine 0.35- and 0.38-inch diameters). These new catheters and guidewires also provide improved safety, being generally flexible yet strong and not likely to break. Further technical developments in equipment include percutaneous angioscopy instruments for direct visualization inside a vessel.

INDICATIONS FOR ANGIOGRAPHY

The indications for the use of angiography have changed dramatically over the last 5 years with the introduction and refinement in noninvasive imaging techniques such as duplex Doppler ultrasound and computed tomography. Magnetic resonance imaging also holds significant promise for noninvasive, noncontrast visualization of the vascular system.[48]

The decision whether to use cut film angiographic techniques or digital subtraction methods is a dynamic one, since these methods should be viewed as variations on a theme rather than as competing modalities. Cut film techniques offer high spatial resolution: small vessel detail is enhanced and sharpness of margination is defined, providing much detail and information for making a specific diag-

nosis (Fig. 5-3). In many situations, however, digital subtraction methods offer comparable visualization and answer the clinical question with a net saving of contrast material and, frequently, of time, since cut film angiographic techniques may take more time to perform (Fig. 5-4). Detail is somewhat less well defined, however. Small but sometimes critical detail such as characterization of plaque in a carotid vessel may not be as well demonstrated with DSA (Fig. 5-5). Contrast resolution is better with digital subtraction techniques than with conventional cut film techniques. This can be invaluable in many situations. Visualization of the dorsalis pedis artery or the pedal arches, for example, may be identified even in cases were the flow is so slow that minimal amounts of contrast material enter these vessels.

In lower extremity arteriography, cut film techniques remain the procedure of choice.[49-51] Large field of view image intensifiers are unable to adequately visualize a large enough area to make DSA a practical technique in runoff studies. Movable, programmable table tops or long leg changers have generally not been developed with digital subtraction techniques.

Digital subtraction and cut film procedures are complimentary and usually are used side by side, with DSA predominating and cut film procedures used in situations where higher spatial resolution is required.

HEAD AND NECK: EXTRACRANIAL VASCULAR DISEASE

Duplex Doppler ultrasound and other noninvasive techniques are the screening methods of choice for extracranial vascular disease.[48] Intravenous DSA has proven to be disappointing. Conversely, intra-arterial DSA studies using 4 and 5 French minicatheters are extremely useful in instances

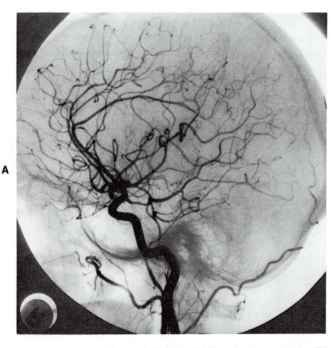
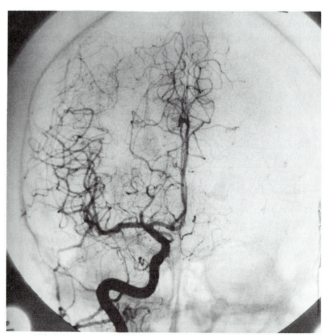

A   B

Figure 5-3. Lateral **(A)** and anteroposterior **(B)** views of an intracranial arteriogram performed for carotid artery disease demonstrate the exquisite visualization obtained with cut film angiography. Outstanding spatial resolution is obtained with this technique.

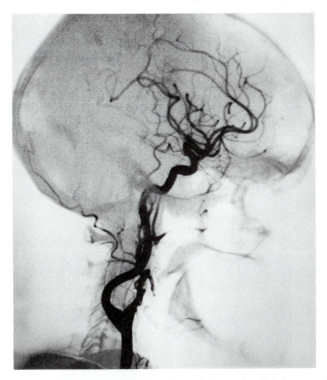
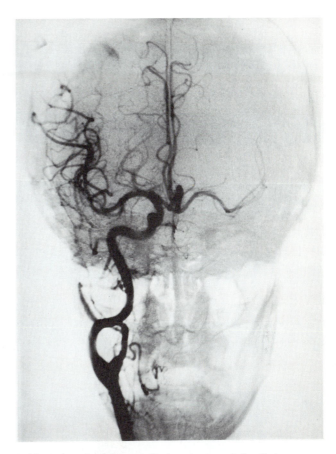

Figure 5-4. Lateral and frontal views of a digital subtraction carotid arteriogram shows excellent contrast resolution that this method provides. Vessel sharpness of margination is slightly less than with cut film techniques, but the excellent ability to differentiate contrast makes this a powerful tool for larger vessel examination.

where direct visualization is required. The examination can be done as an outpatient procedure. Disadvantages compared to standard arteriography are that biplane filming is generally not available and spatial resolution is not quite as good. However, with current equipment, it has for the most part eliminated the need for standard techniques.

Whatever method is used, it is important to stress the need for complete visualization of the arch and neck vessels. A minimum of two views of each carotid bifurcation is essential. More views should be obtained when the bifurcation and course of the vessels are obscured by overlapping adjacent arteries. At least one intracranial view should be obtained during all studies of the neck vessels.

CHEST

Thoracic Aorta

Depending on the clinical indication, the thoracic aorta is best visualized by cut film catheter arteriography or computed tomography. Patients with suspected dissection of the thoracic aorta should be initially evaluated with dynamic CT utilizing a fast (two second or faster) scanner. Dynamic scans obtained at the level of the aortic valve, mid ascending aorta, and aortic arch provide highly sensitive and specific information. Catheter arteriography is then reserved for equivocal cases and selected type I dissections where addi-

tional anatomic detail is required. The routine use of arteriography to diagnose aortic dissection is no longer necessary where appropriate radiologic CT expertise is available. For blunt thoracic trauma, CT is somewhat less sensitive but still remains a useful triage procedure. In cases in which the CT examination is normal, the invasive procedure would not yield additional information. When CT demonstrates a mediastinal abnormality, angiography is required. Differentiation of an aortic laceration (Fig. 5-6) from hemorrhage in the mediastinum secondary to a venous or small arterial rent necessitates cut film catheter arteriography.

Patients suspected of having a thoracic aortic aneurysm should be studied by dynamic computed tomography. This procedure demonstates not only the residual lumen but also the true outer diameter of the aneurysm because the clot-filled segment can be visualized. There is also no magnification with CT, distorting size determinations.

In patients with suspected dissection or laceration requiring angiography, biplane filming must be carried out. A left anterior oblique and an off-axis lateral view are suggested. At times, the contralateral oblique or anteroposterior (AP) view may be useful. Studies of the thoracic aorta for aneurysm and laceration should be performed, preferably via the femoral artery. An axillary artery is used when the femoral pulses are weak or absent. For suspected dissection, the right axillary artery is used to facilitate passage of the catheter directly into the ascending aorta, and to avoid the frequently involved left subclavian artery. This

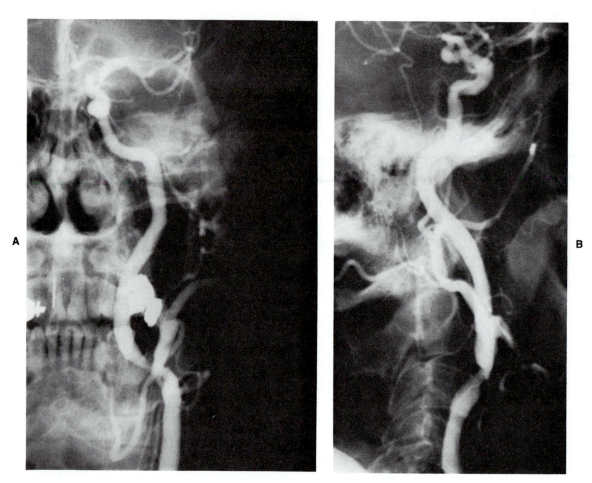

Figure 5-5. Frontal **(A)** and lateral **(B)** views demonstrate a circumferential stenosis of the common carotid artery, with disease extending into the internal carotid artery.

is in contrast to the use of the axillary artery for runoff studies in which the left axillary artery is preferred because of the greater accessibility to the descending thoracic aorta and subsequently abdominal aorta.

Thoracic Outlet Syndromes

Evaluation of the subclavian arteries for thoracic outlet obstruction related to cervical rib, abnormal first rib, or muscular entrapment, can be performed using digital subtraction techniques. The study should be initially performed with the arm in a neutral position, followed by a modified Addison maneuver.

Bronchial Arteriography

Diagnostic bronchial arteriograms are no longer routinely performed because of the possibility of transverse myelitis complicating right bronchial and right fifth intercostal arteriograms.[52] The sole remaining indication for bronchial arteriography is massive hemostasis in which embolotherapy is planned. The speed with which DSA can be utilized in this setting makes it significantly preferable over cut film arteriography.

Pulmonary Arteriography

The cut film technique remains the predominant procedure for filming pulmonary arteriography. The high sensitivity and specificity of this procedure rely on the ability to resolve small vessel detail. Indications for pulmonary arteriography are listed in Table 5-2. Intravenous DSA has proved to be disappointing, and has a lower sensitivity as a screening procedure than radionuclide techniques. Catheters can be introduced via the femoral vein (or less frequently the basilic vein), and selectively placed in the main pulmonary artery, or subselectively on the right or left side, as indicated. With appropriate training, the procedure has a low complication rate even in high-risk patients and is one of the more definitive tests available in medicine.[53]

ABDOMINAL AORTA AND VISCERAL ARTERIES

It is in the abdomen where digital subtraction and cut film techniques are best exemplified as being complimentary and intertwined.[54] Studies frequently involve one to two runs with one recording method and one or two with the other; each is used for its advantages. The format size of

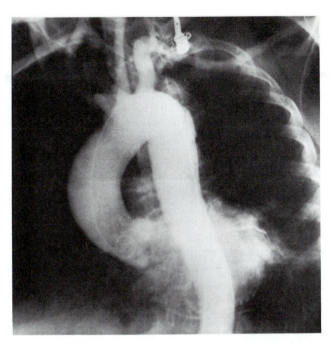

Figure 5-6. Thoracic aortogram performed with a 5 French pigtail catheter demonstrates a laceration distal to the left subclavian artery. Deceleration injury as patient was in automobile accident.

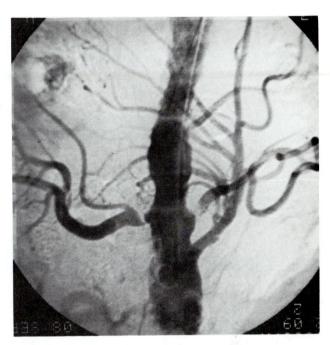

Figure 5-7. Digital subtraction arteriogram demonstrating a very high-grade stenosis of the left main renal artery and short segment occlusion of the right main renal artery. Moderately advanced atherosclerotic disease of the infrarenal abdominal aorta is also present. Examination was performed with a 4 French minicatheter as an outpatient procedure.

14 by 14 inches for cut film is larger than the image intensifiers used for digital subtraction techniques; therefore, the ability to cover a large area is greater with film.

For screening, digital subtraction angiography provides excellent visualization of the abdominal aorta and renal arteries (Fig. 5-7). This can be used as the initial part of a lower extremity arteriogram or as a screening examination for renovascular hypertension. With the use of 4 French catheters, outpatient arteriography can be routinely utilized for work-up of patients with hypertension. However, for suspected segmental renal artery stenosis, cut film detail may be necessary. Similarly, cut film is recommended for evaluation of visceral artery aneurysms (Fig. 5-8), or diagnosis of mesenteric ischemia (both occlusive and nonocclusive

TABLE 5-2. INDICATIONS FOR PULMONARY ANGIOGRAPHY

Diagnosis of pulmonary thromboembolism
  Indeterminate lung scan
  Normal lung scan in the presence of compelling clinical signs
  When absolute diagnosis is mandatory
    Contraindication to anticoagulant therapy
    Treatment with fibrinolytic agents (urokinase, streptokinase)
    Inferior vena caval interruption
    Pulmonary embolectomy
Evaluation of pulmonary vasculature
  Congenital abnormalities
  Acquired abnormalities (trauma, neoplasm, arteritis)
  Pulmonary hypertension
  Presurgical evaluation of functioning lung prior to bullectomy
  Staging of primary lung neoplasm

From Neiman HL, Yao JST: Angiography of Vascular Disease. New York, Churchill Livingstone, 1985, p 496.

varieties) (Fig. 5-9). Hepatic panangiography for portal hypertension can be done entirely with digital filming procedures. Evaluation of renal transplant stenosis can also use the latter.

Diagnosis of abdominal aortic aneurysms should be performed with ultrasound or possibly computed tomography. Ultrasound allows visualization of the residual lumen and the external diameter of the aorta in both the ventrodorsal and transverse planes. Relationship of the aneurysm to the renal arteries can usually be documented, as well as possible extension of the aneurysm into the iliac vessels. Computed tomography can produce the same information, although it generally requires injection of contrast material. It is particularly useful in detection of prosthetic vascular complications.[55] Angiography is reserved for preoperative patients when specific information is required concerning the infrarenal cuff, extension of the aneurysm distally, and status of the mesenteric circulation.

Arteriography provides one essential piece of information that the noninvasive techniques cannot: the status of the mesenteric circulation, specifically the inferior mesenteric artery. Visualization of this vessel provides important data. Its absence may be related to occlusion of the vessel or to nonvisualization because of technical factors such as layering of contrast material and site of injection of the contrast material. Nonvisualization of the inferior mesenteric artery and the presence of collateral vessels (arcade of Riolan and marginal artery of Drummond) are important indicators that it is occluded. It should be stressed that the abdominal aorta should be visualized in anterior and lateral views and that the study should extend from the

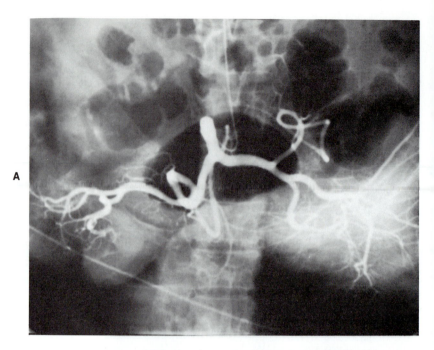

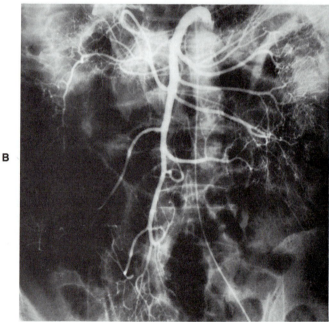

Figure 5-8. Visceral arteriogram of the celiac **(A)** and superior mesenteric **(B)** arteries demonstrates normal vascular anatomy. Patient presented with occult lower gastrointestinal bleeding.

level of the celiac artery to the common femoral vessels (Figs. 5-10 to 5-12). If biplane arteriography is available, this can be done with alternate firing techniques so that the total dose of contrast is no greater than filming with digital subtraction views in a sequential fashion.

PERIPHERAL VASCULAR DISEASE

Lower Extremity

Our general examination for atherosclerotic peripheral vascular disease begins with digital subtraction filming of the abdominal aorta from the level of the celiac artery. Cut films are then obtained beginning at the aortic bifurcation

and ending with the feet (Fig. 5-13). In patients with signs and symptoms referable to aortoiliac disease, at least one oblique view of the pelvis is obtained using digital subtraction. If femoropopliteal disease is suggested or indicated by the arteriogram, lateral views of the feet are obtained using digital subtraction techniques. Oblique views of the iliac, femoropopliteal, or trifurcation vessels are obtained using either information storage method in instances where the anteroposterior view is discordant with clinical symptoms, where there is overlap of vessels obscuring detail, or where there is an unanswered angiographic question. In all cases, lower extremity arteriography is a preoperative or preangioplasty technique (Fig. 5-14). Screening is done using the noninvasive laboratory.

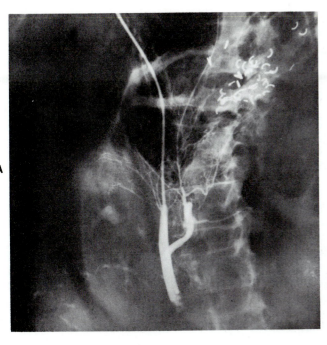
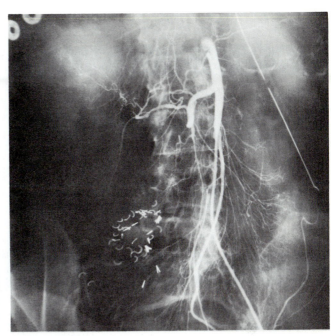

Figure 5-9. A. Oblique view of a superior mesenteric arteriogram demonstrates a marked paucity of jejunal and ileal branches and significant diminution in the caliber of those that are visualized. Nonocclusive mesenteric ischemia. **B.** After 4 hours of intra-arterial papaverine through an indwelling catheter, note the marked interval improvement. Significant disease remains, however.

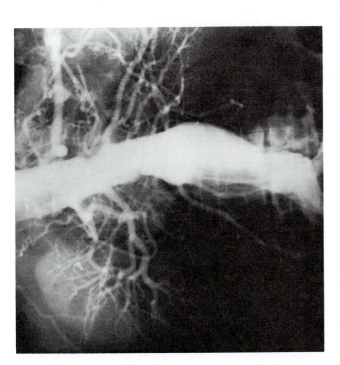
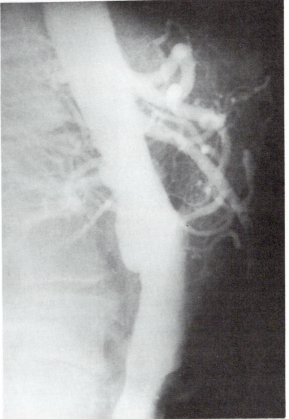

Figure 5-10. Anteroposterior and lateral views of an abdominal aortogram demonstrate the presence of an abdominal aortic aneurysm. The frontal view clearly shows the length of the infrarenal cuff of "normal" aorta. Only the residual lumen of the aorta is demonstrated with the true outer dimension being better evaluated by ultrasound or CT.

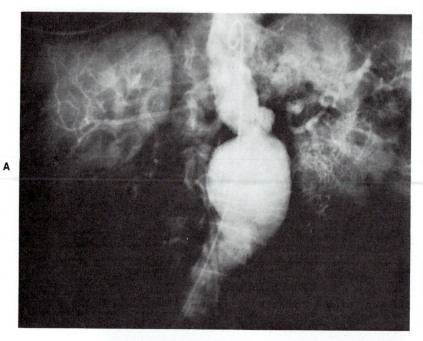

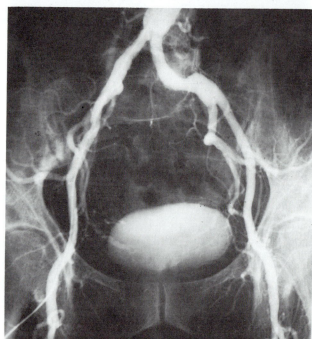

Figure 5-11. (A), Large abdominal aortic aneurysm with slowed velocity of flow in the aorta. Note washout of contrast material in the visceral arteries, but contrast remains in the abdominal aorta. Frontal view of the pelvis **(B)** shows that the aneurysm does not extend into the common iliac arteries but ends at the bifurcation.

The most frequently utilized technique is catheterization of the abdominal aorta by the femoral artery. Entry is always made below the inguinal ligament, generally with the puncture at the inguinal crease. Safety J guidewires as well as pigtail catheters are used routinely, assuring the safety of the examination. I prefer to enter the vascular system by puncturing the better of the femoral arteries, based on examination of the pulses and information provided by the noninvasive examination. I believe that avoiding the more diseased side has diminished our complication rate. The 4 or 5 French pigtail catheter is advanced over the guidewires into the upper abdominal aorta for initiation of the study. The catheter is then moved to the lower abdom-

inal aorta for the lower extremity study. With appropriate techniques, catheterization of the abdominal aorta can almost always be achieved.

In the event that catheterization cannot be achieved, or there are absent pulses, then translumbar aortography using a "high" approach is generally used. Directed translumbar techniques are now possible. The catheter can usually be placed in a position such that the contrast material is injected in an antegrade fashion providing an excellent quality study.[56] Mid and low translumbar aortography should be discouraged. In patients with aortoiliac disease, translumbar aortography is generally very satisfactory. However, for those patients suspected of having distal dis-

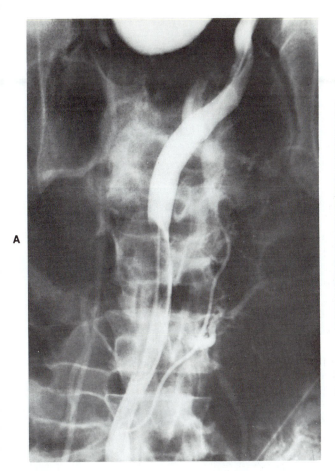

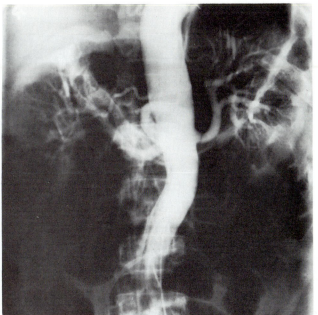

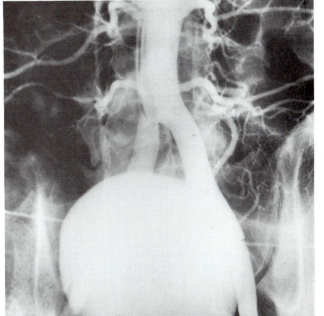

Figure 5-12. Transfemoral arteriogram of an elderly woman with chronic, vague recurrent symptoms of chest and abdominal pain demonstrates aortic dissection. Note in **A** that the catheter has entered the false lumen. In **B**, it has been directed into the true lumen and demonstrates extension of the dissection into the left main renal artery. A transaxillary arteriogram **(C)** was performed, better visualizing the true lumen and line of dissection extending into the left iliac artery.

ease, transaxillary arteriography is carried out with entry into the left axillary artery. In trained hands the complication rates of all three procedures are relatively comparable and acceptable. Transaxillary arteriography provides the potential for selective catheterization of a branch artery, optimizing the study in selected cases.

There is no role for percutaneous needle placement into a femoral artery for unilateral studies using a single film, other than as an intraoperative procedure to answer the specific question of graft patency at an anastomotic site. Too little information is obtained to warrant the risks of inadvertent needle placement, extravasation of contrast material, and contrast reaction and the cost of the procedure,

etc. The importance and incidence of combined aortoiliac and leg artery involvement in the generalized process of atherosclerotic disease was emphasized by Haimovici who showed that aortoiliac lesions were found in 27% of patients with femoropopliteal occlusive disease.[57]

It is virtually impossible to "cookbook" the contrast dose and filming sequence for lower extremity arteriography because it needs to be tailored to each individual patient (Figs. 5-15 and 5-16). In general, we inject 36 ml of contrast material at 18 ml/sec for abdominal aortography utilizing cut film. With digital subtraction techniques the volume and injection rate can be maintained, but the equivalent of half strength contrast can be used. For the lower extremity

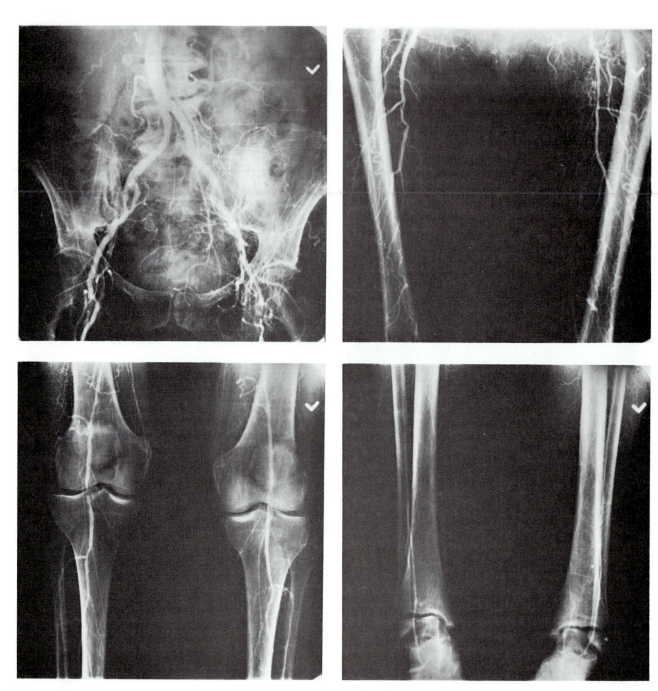

Figure 5-13. Cut film, lower extremity arteriogram extending from the bifurcation of the aorta to the ankles. Extensive atherosclerotic disease is present throughout. Lateral views of the feet were also obtained using digital subtraction techniques, because of the bilateral occlusions of the superficial femoral arteries and of the posterior tibial and peroneal arteries. The low volume of contrast material in the pedal arches is better demonstrated with DSA than with cut film.

portion of the study, 90 to 100 ml of contrast material (Reno-grafin-60 or its equivalent in nonionic contrast) is used at a rate of 8 to 9 ml/sec. Appropriate delay is utilized to allow the contrast column to get ahead of the filming.

Oblique or lateral views may be necessary to fully evaluate the presence of an ulcerated plaque. To evaluate the common iliac bifurcation and the internal iliac artery at its origin, the lateral or ipsilateral posterior oblique view is useful. The profunda femoris artery origin is usually best seen with the ipsilateral anterior oblique view.[58]

Several means are available to evaluate the hemodynamic significance of lesions. Generally, lesions that narrow the diameter of the lumen less than 50% are not hemodynamically significant. Lesions between 50 and 75% are indeterminant, and lesions greater than this are generally of hemodynamic significance. A 50% reduction in luminal diameter corresponds to a narrowing of approximately 75% in the cross-sectional area. Enlarged collateral vessels strongly suggest that a hemodynamically significant stenosis is present. Evaluation of the linear velocity of flow can

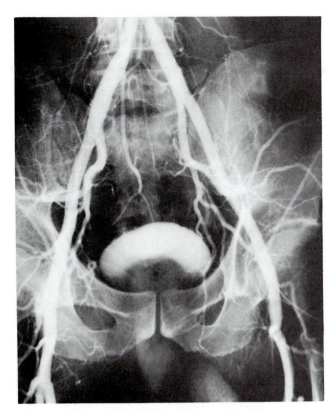

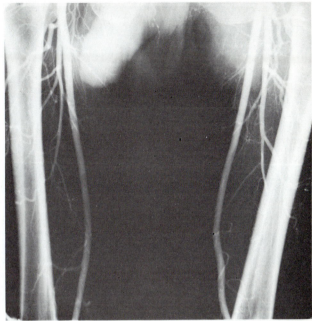

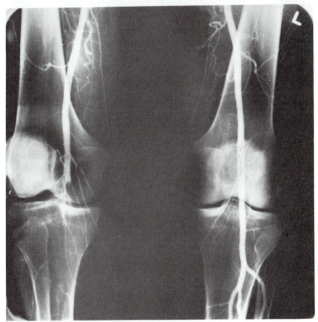

Figure 5-14. Acute onset of right lower extremity ischemic symptoms. The cut film "runoff" study shows occlusion of the right popliteal artery. A meniscus is present, indicating embolus.

also be helpful. For example, the trifurcation vessels are parallel; therefore, flow should be approximately equal. Significant slowing in one branch can be a useful sign of a significant stenosis. Flow in the contralateral vessel (iliac, femoral, or popliteal artery) can be used as a standard against which to measure the flow in its matched pair. Finally, in certain instances pressure gradients can be obtained, particularly in the iliac system and abdominal aorta. Simultaneous pressures across a gradient can be obtained with two catheters: one from the contralateral side, or more commonly using the single angiographic catheter and obtaining continuously running pull-through pressures. In the femoropopliteal system and in the renal arteries, pressure gradients are of no value because the presence of a

catheter across the stenotic segment significantly reduces the blood flow and increases the gradient. This reduction is an unknown since it is dependent on catheter diameter and the variable diameter of the involved vessel.

Hand Arteriography

Selective catheterization of a brachial artery is carried out via percutaneous entry of a femoral artery. This procedure is preferred over direct puncture of a brachial artery, since femoral artery entry has a lower complication rate than entry of the brachial artery. Direct entry of the brachial artery should be reserved for those cases in which the great

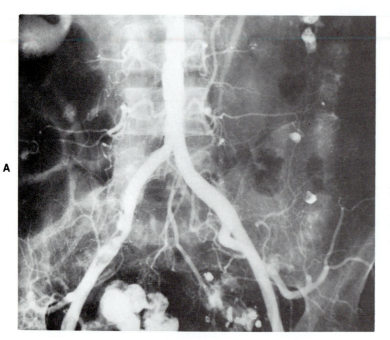

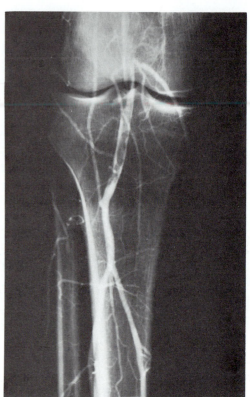

Figure 5-15. Views of the pelvis **(A)** in one patient and of the distal popliteal artery in another **(B)** demonstrate intraluminal filling defects indicative of acute clot. The examinations were tailored to the clinical situations. In **A,** contrast material was injected at the bifurcation of the aorta with a 5 French pigtail catheter. In **B** a 4 French catheter was utilized for subselective injection of contrast material into the superficial femoral artery to optimize visualization of the distal extent of the embolus and to evaluate the status of the trifurcation vessels.

vessels arising from the aortic arch are too tortuous to allow successful catheterization. Studies of the hand vessels should be performed after use of a vasodilator (i.e. tolazoline, nitroglycerine, papaverine). Cut film techniques are preferred over digital subtraction because of the need for visualization of small digital arteries and the ability to note the appropriate filling pattern of these vessels.

TRAUMA

Arteriography plays a significant role in suspected trauma of the abdominal aorta, visceral branches, and upper and lower extremity arteries. In one study, trauma angiography was found to have a sensitivity for detecting major arterial injury of 98.3%, specificity of 98.5%, positive predictive value of 95%, and negative predictive value of 99.5%.[59] Emergency trauma angiography is an excellent technique for determining the presence of direct arterial injury as opposed to extrinsic compression and impingement on the lumen in a closed space. In this setting the principles of arteriography are the same, with cut film being the predomi-

nant imaging technique because of the need for identification of small intimal flaps or punctate areas of extravasation of contrast material.

Interventional Radiology

A host of interventional techniques are currently being utilized on a routine basis (Fig. 5-17) or are under development.[60,61] Digital subtraction angiography is generally the preferred method for recording information because of the need for repeated injections of contrast material to precisely localize catheters. In selected instances, cut film may provide the detail necessary to ensure adequate placement of a balloon, stent, or embolotherapeutic material.

Complications of Angiography

Angiography using transfemoral, translumbar, or transaxillary techniques carries a risk of morbidity and mortality. Therefore, these procedures should be reserved for those

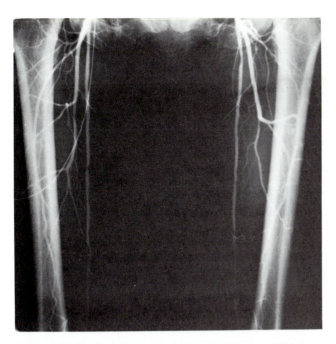

Figure 5-16. Chronic atherosclerotic disease of the superficial femoral arteries is demonstrated bilaterally on this cut film study, performed with a programmable, moving table top and a total of 90 ml of contrast material.

individuals in whom the diagnostic information obtained may significantly aid in the therapeutic approach and in whom the answer cannot be obtained in a noninvasive fashion. Many studies have demonstrated that the complication rate of angiography is directly related to the experience and procedure volume of the individual performing the examination.[62] However, it is difficult to compare complication rates for the various angiographic approaches because type and significance of various complications differ. Additionally, different investigators have recorded or actively searched for various complications.

The mortality from angiographic procedures generally is about 0.05%.[63] In adults, mortality is highest with coronary arteriography. Death due to abdominal aortography or lower extremity arteriography is extremely uncommon.

The incidence of serious complications from catheter techniques has varied from 0.5 to 2.3% in different series.[64,65] In a prospective series of 1,217 consecutive adult patients, serious complications from catheter manipulation were noted in 0.5% of cases. Complications at the puncture site occurred in 0.14% of cases.[64] This corresponds well to another series of 9,200 cases in which there were 15 cases of femoral thrombosis requiring surgical intervention (0.16%).[66] In addition to thrombosis of the femoral artery, potential complications at the percutaneous entry site include intimal flap, pseudoaneurysm, arteriovenous fistulas, infection, and significant hemorrhage. Hematoma formation at the puncture site is the most common minor complication, but it occasionally may be severe, particularly in hypertensive individuals. A diastolic pressure above 110 mm Hg or a wide pulse pressure are relative contraindications to angiography.

Translumbar aortography has a low complication rate in experienced hands. In Szilagyi et al.'s large series of 14,550 patients, there were seven major (0.05%) and two fatal (0.014%) complications.[67] Minor complications that did not require surgical intervention occurred in 7.5% of 500 cases that were evaluated in a separate prospective study. Szilagyi also mentions the use of general anesthesia for

A
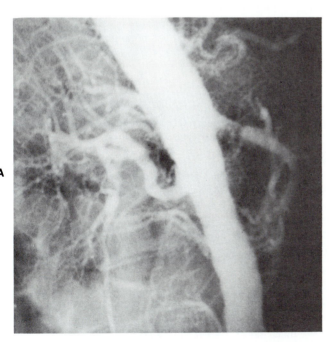
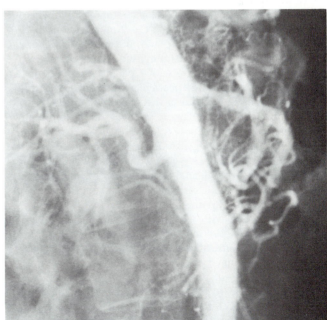
B

Figure 5-17. Preangioplasty **(A)** and postangioplasty **(B)** radiographs of a patient with symptoms suggesting chronic mesenteric ischemia and angiographic evidence of a high-grade stenosis of the superior mesenteric artery. The postangioplasty study shows marked interval improvement, although residual stenosis remains. The patient was asymptomatic after the study.

angiography; however, he fails to mention anesthesia-related complications.

Molnar and Paul reported 37 (2.1%) complications in a series of 1,762 transaxillary arteriographic examinations. Nine (0.5%) of these were major complications.[68] Roy reported a similar major complication rate, although Eriksson and Jorulf reported a somewhat higher rate for brachial and axillary studies.[66,69]

In a multi-institutional series involving 118,591 examinations from 514 institutions, the overall complication rates were transfemoral, 1.73%; translumbar, 2.89%; and transaxillary, 3.29%. Thirty deaths were reported, eight of which were caused by aortic dissection or aneurysm rupture. There were significantly more neurologic complications in the transaxillary group than there were in the other two.[70] Reactions to contrast material were discussed previously.

Rarely, infection is noted secondary to faulty aseptic techniques. This should be rare. Complications that are related to equipment should also be rare, although they have been reported. The breakage of a guidewire can occur. Similarly, knotting of a catheter is a potential risk. The intraventional radiologist must be aware of techniques for retrieval of a foreign body and unknotting of intravascular catheters.[71,72]

Principles of Interpretation

Clearly, an understanding of normal anatomy underlies interpretation of any arteriogram. Further, an appreciation of the normal, sharply marginated smooth wall of a vessel is necessary (see Fig. 5-8). In general, vessels taper proximal to distal and undulate in their course in a rather smooth fashion. Most commonly in vascular surgery, one is dealing with atherosclerotic changes in vessels that may exhibit intimal thickening, stenosis, occlusion, dilatation, aneurysmal changes, and ulcerating plaques. Not infrequently, filling defects indicating the presence of thrombotic material may be present. Characteristically, the arteriosclerotic process is segmental in nature with a patent vessel proximal and distal to the lesion. Stenoses may be single or multiple, depending on the severity of the disease. In chronic ischemia, the presence of collateral pathways are a commonly demonstrated finding; these collateral vessels are often tortuous vessels of varying size depending on the chronicity and level of occlusion. Depending on the level of occlusion, various patterns of collateral pathways have been observed.

Arterial spasm is occasionally seen at the site of a needle insertion or at the tip of a selectively placed catheter. This is more common with women and children. Guidewires that have been placed into branch vessels may also induce spasm. During contrast injection, smooth, tapered narrowing of a vessel may occasionally be seen in children and adults. This has been termed "vascular jet collapse."[73] This is less often seen with multiple side-hole catheters.

Corrugated arteries, accordion-like appearance, stationary waves, standing arterial waves, or arterial ripplings are all terms that describe the unusual appearance of regular, periodic, symmetric transverse striations in the contrast column of an artery. The femoral, popliteal, and tibial arteries may be affected separately or in combination.[74] The

cause is uncertain, and the finding is transient and can frequently be relieved by the use of a vasodilating agent. Circular muscle spasm, a pulse pressure wave phenomenon, and transient arterial spasm due to forceful injection of the contrast material have all been implicated.

Contrast material is generally heavier than blood and may layer dependently producing artifacts such as nonvisualization of the inferior mesenteric artery. Lesions along the anterior wall of a vessel may not be noted because of this posterior layering of contrast material. Overlying vessels may obscure an area of stenosis, and when the arteriogram fails to demonstrate a clinically suspected abnormality, a second or third view, such as an oblique or lateral view perpendicular to the routine frontal examination, should be obtained. In addition, where two contrast-filled vessels cross, there is a linear lucent defect that may be noted in the vessel; this is termed the "mock effect." This may simulate the appearance of a stenosis in one of the vessels.

Arteriovenous anastomoses are known to exist in the human body. The sudden opening of an arteriovenous anastomosis may cause early venous filling during arteriographic examination.[75] Early venous filling, however, bears no relationship to the severity of the arterial occlusive disease, and it tends to be seen more often in patients with varicose veins associated with chronic deep venous insufficiency. Early venous filling also occurs in patients with vasospastic disorders.[72]

Pseudo-obstruction is another artifact that can be noted in arteriograms and is often due to positional factors. For example, forced plantar flexion of the feet during anteroposterior projection views for lower extremity arteriography may cause an apparent obstruction of the anterior tibial artery. This should not be confused with popliteal artery entrapment syndrome.[75] Other causes of pseudo-obstruction include inadequate filling due to insufficient contrast material injection or inappropriate exposure of films, either before or after the contrast has been present.

REFERENCES

1. Haschek E, Lindenthal OT: A contribution to the practical use of photography according to Roentgen. Wien Klin Wochenschr 9:63, 1896.
2. Berberich J, Hirsch S: Die roentgenographische Darstellung der Arterien und Venen am Lebenden. Munch Klin Wochenschr 2:2226, 1923.
3. Moniz E, Diaza A: La radioarteriographic et la topographie cranioencephalique. J Radiol Electrol 12:72, 1928.
4. McPheeters HO, Rice CO: Varicose veins—the circulation and direction of the venous flow. Surg Gynecol Obstet 49:29, 1929.
5. Edwards EA, Biguria F: A comparison of skiodan and diodrast as venographic media, with special reference to their effect on blood pressure. N Engl J Med 211:589, 1934.
6. Dos Santos R, Lamas A, Pereia-Caldas J: Arteriografia da aorta e dos vasos abdominals. Med Contemp 47:93, 1929.
7. Swick N: Darstellung de Niere und Harnwege ein Rontgenbild durch Intravenose ein Bringund eines Neuen Konstrast Stoffes des Uroselectans. J Klin Wochenschr 8:2087, 1929.
8. Forssmann W: Uber Contrastdar Stellung der Hohlen des Levenden Rechten Herzens und der Lungenschlagader. J Munch Med Wochenschr 78:489, 1931.

9. Castellanos A, Pereiras R, Garcia A: Arch Soc Estudios Hubana 31:523, 1937.

10. Robb GP, Steinberg I: Visualization of the chambers of the heart, pulmonary and the great blood vessels. AJR 41:1, 1939.

11. Ziedes des Plantes BGZ: Thesis. Keunik en Zn NV. Utrecht, 1934.

12. Dos Santos JC: Le phlebographic directe. J Int Chir 3:625, 1938.

13. Castellanos A, Pereiras R: Countercurrent aortography. Rev Cuba Cardiol 2:187, 1939.

14. Farinas PL: A new technique for the arteriographic examination of the abdominal aorta and its branches. AJR 46:641, 1941.

15. Seldinger SI: Catheter replacement of the needle in percutaneous arteriography: A new technique. Acta Radiol (Stockh) 39:368, 1953.

16. Nakstad PH, Bakke SJ, et al.: Omnipaque vs. Hexabrix in intravenous DSA of the carotid arteries: Randomized double-blind crossover study. AJNR 7(2):303, Mar-Apr, 1986.

17. Sackett JF, Bergsjordet B, et al.: Digital subtraction angiography. Comparison of meglumine-Na diatrizoate with iohexol. Acta Radiol [Suppl] (Stockh) 366:81, 1983.

18. Wolf GL: Adult peripheral angiography. Results from four North American randomized clinical trials of ionic media versus iohexol. Acta Radiol [Suppl] (Stockh) 366:166, 1983.

19. Dotter CT, Rosch J, et al.: Iopamidol arteriography: Discomfort and Pain. Radiology 155(3):819, 1985.

20. Widrich WC, Beckman CF, et al.: Iopamidol and meglumine diatrizoate: Comparison of effects on patient discomfort during aortofemoral arteriography. Radiology 148:61, 1983.

21. Lea Thomas M, Briggs GM, Kaun BB: Contrast agent-induced thrombophlebitis following leg phlebography: Meglumine loxaglate versus meglumine lothalamate. Radiology 147:399, 1983.

22. Albrechtsson U, Olsson CG: Thrombosis after phlebography: A comparison of two contrast media. Cardiovasc Radiol 2:9, 1979.

23. Walters HL, Clemenson J, et al.: 125 I-fibrinogen uptake following phlebography of the leg. Comparison of ionic and nonionic contrast media. Radiology 135:619, 1980.

24. Bettmann MA, Morris TW: Recent advances in contrast agents. Radiol Clin North Am 24:347, 1986.

25. Gordon IJ, Skoblar, RS, et al.: A comparison of isohexol and conray-60 in peripheral angiography. AJR 142:563, 1984.

26. Higgins CB: Effects of contrast materials on left ventricular function. Invest Radiol 15:S220, 1980.

27. Shehadi WH: Contrast media adverse reactions: Occurrence, recurrence and distribution patterns. Radiology 143:11, 1982.

28. Fischer HW, Morris TW: Possible factors in intravascular contrast media toxicity. Invest Radiol 15:5232, 1980.

29. Shehadi WH, Tonioio G: Adverse reactions to intravascular administered contrast media. Radiology 124:145, 1975.

30. Boijsen E, Dahn I, Hallbrook T: Hemodynamic effect of contrast medium in arteriography of legs. Acta Radiol (Stockh) 11:295, 1971.

31. Higginis CB, Gerber KH, et al.: Evaluation of hemodynamic effects of intravenous contrast materials. Radiology 142:681, 1982.

32. Adams DF, Fraser D, Abrams HL: Hazards of coronary arteriography. Semin Roentgenol 7:357, 1972.

33. Adams DF, Abrams HL: Complications of coronary arteriography: A follow-up report. Cardiovasc Radiol 2:89, 1979.

34. Snyder C, Cramer R, Amplatz K: Isolation of sodium as a cause of ventricular fibrillation. Invest Radiol 6:245, 1971.

35. Fischer HW: Viscosity, solubility and toxicity in the choice of an angiographic contrast medium. Angiology 16:759, 1965.

36. Lindgren P: Hemodynamic responses to contrast media. Invest Radiol 5:424, 1970.

37. Cattell WR: Excretory pathways for contrast media. Invest Radiol 5:473, 1970.

38. Gomes AS, Baker JD, et. al.: Acute renal dysfunction after major arteriography. AJR 145:1249, 1985.

39. Swartz RD, Rubin JE, et al.: Renal failure following major angiography. Am J Med 65:31, 1978.

40. Eisenberg RL, Bank WO, Hedgcock MW: Renal failure after major angiography can be avoided with hydration. AJR 136:859, 1981.

41. Von Sonnenberg E, Neff CC, Pfister RC: Life-threatening hypotensive reactions to contrast media administration: Comparison of pharmacologic and fluid therapy. Radiology 162:15, 1987.

42. Harrington G, Michie C, et al.: Blood-brain barrier changes associated with unilateral cerebral angiography. Invest Radiol 1:431, 1966.

43. Melartin E, Tuohimaa PJ, Daab R: Neurotoxicity of iothalamates and diatrizoates. Significance of concentration and cation. Invest Radiol 5:13, 1970.

44. Djianjian R: Arteriography of the spinal cord. Am J Roentgenol Radium Ther Nucl Med 107:461, 1969.

45. Widrich WC, Singer RJ, Robbins AH: The use of intra-arterial lidocaine to control pain due to aortofemoral arteriography. Radiology 124:37, 1977.

46. Guthaner DF, Silverman JF, et al.: Intra-arterial analgesia in peripheral arteriography. AJR 128:737, 1977.

47. Antonovich R, Rosch J, Dotter CT: The value of systemic arterial heparinization in transfemoral angiography: A prospective study. AJR 127:223, 1976.

48. Jackson VP, Kuehn DS, et al.: Duplex carotid sonography: correlation with digital subtraction angiography and conventional angiography. J Ultrasound Med 4(5):239, 1985.

49. Blakeman BM, Littooy FN, Baker WH: Intra-arterial digital subtraction angiography as a method to study peripheral vascular disease. J Vasc Surg 4(2):168, 1986.

50. Sniderman KW, Morse SS, Strauss EB: Comparison of intra-arterial digital subtraction angiography and conventional filming in peripheral vascular disease. J Can Assoc Radiol 37(2):76, 1986.

51. Walden R, Adar R, et al.: Distribution and symmetry of arteriosclerotic lesions of the lower extremities: An arteriographic study of 200 limbs. Cardiovasc Intervent Radiol 8(4):180, 1985.

52. Kardjiev V, Symeonov A, Chankov I: Etiology, pathogenesis and prevention of spinal cord lesions in selective angiography of the bronchial and intercostal arteries. Radiology 112:81, 1974.

53. Perlmutt LM, Braun SD, et al.: Pulmonary arteriography in the high-risk patient. Radiology 162:187, 1987.

54. Nakagawa N, Takahashi M, et al.: Intra-arterial digital subtraction angiography vs. conventional angiography of abdominal diseases. Comput Radiol 9(3):137, 1985.

55. Vogelzang RL, Limpert JD, Yao JST: Detection of prosthetic vascular complications: Comparison of CT and angiography. AJR 148:819, 1987.

56. Grollman JH Jr, Marcus R: Antegrade translumbar aortography. Radiology 153:249, 1984.

57. Haimovici H: Arteriographic patterns of the lower extremity associated with femoropopliteal arteriosclerotic occlusive disease. J Cardiovasc Surg 2(suppl to No 3):100, 1970.

58. Thomas ML, Andress MR: Value of oblique projections in translumbar aortography. Am J Roentgenol Radium Ther Nucl Med 116:187, 1972.

59. Rose SC, Moore EE: Emergency trauma angiography: Accuracy, safety, and pitfalls. AJR 148:1243, 1987.

60. Lawrence DD Jr, Charnsangavej C, et al.: Percutaneous endovascular graft: Experimental evaluation. Radiology 163:357, 1987.

61. White RI Jr: Interventional radiology: Reflections and expectations. Radiology 162:593, 1987.

62. Bourassi MG, Nobel J: Complication rate of coronary arteriography. Circulation 53:106, 1976.

63. Lang EK: A survey of the complications of percutaneous retrograde arteriography. Radiology 81:257, 1963.

64. Sigstedt B, Lunderquist A: Complications of angiographic examinations. AJR 130:445, 1978.

65. Silverman JF, Wexler L: Complications of percutaneous transfemoral coronary arteriography. Clin Radiol, 27:317, 1976.

66. Eriksson I, Jorulf H: Surgical complications associated with arterial catheterization. Scand J Cardiovascular Surg 4:69–75, 1970.

67. Szilagyi DE, Smith RF, et al.: Translumbar aortography. Arch Surg 112:399, 1977.

68. Molnar W, Paul DJ: Complications of axillary arteriotomies: An analysis of 1,762 consecutive studies. Radiology 104:269, 1972.

69. Roy P: Percutaneous catheterization via the axillary artery: A new approach to some technical roadblocks in selective arteriography. Am J Roentgenol 94:1018, 1965.

70. Hessel SJ, Adams DF, Abrams HL: Complications of angiography. Radiology 138:273, 1981.

71. Cho SR, et al: Percutaneous unknotting of intravascular catheters and retrieval of catheter fragments. AJR 141:397, 1983.

72. Chuang VP, Wallace S, et al.: Complication of coil embolization: Prevention and management. AJR 137:809, 1981.

73. Doumanian HO, Amplatz K: Vascular jet collapse in selective angiocardiography. AJR 100:344, 1967.

74. Wickbom I, Bartley O: Arterial "spasm" in peripheral arteriography using the catheter method. Acta Radiol 47:433, 1957.

75. Milne ENC: The significance of early venous filling during femoral arteriography. Radiology 88:513, 1967.

76. Yao JST, Hobbs JT, Irvine WT: Peripheral arterial insufficiency of the lower extremities unassociated with organic occlusions. Br J Surg 55:859, 1968.

77. Koolpe HA, Embil W, et al.: Pseudo-obstruction of the anterior tibial artery. Am J Roentgenol 134:749, 1980.

CHAPTER 6
Digital Subtraction Arteriography

Andrew B. Crummy

Within 2 months of Roentgen's discovery of the x-ray in 1895, Haschek and Lindenthal published the first arteriogram.[1,2] The arterial system of a cadaver forearm was rendered radiopaque by injecting a chalk solution. In 1910, Franck and Alwens injected an oily solution of bismuth intravenously in dogs and rabbits and studied the blood flow in the veins, right heart, and lungs fluoroscopically.[3] By 1927 Moniz directly introduced thorium dioxide into the carotid arteries to perform a cerebral arteriogram.[4] He is believed to have been the first to perform direct arteriograms in humans. The performance of arteriography gradually improved because of numerous refinements in technique, particularly the introduction of percutaneous catheterization by Seldinger in 1953.[5] The equipment in arteriography became extremely sophisticated, and exquisite delineation of virtually every artery in the body became a practical reality.

During this period the recording of arteriographic data was done in analog format with film or magnetic tape. In the 1970s, digital image processing resulted in a new class of images characterized by moderate contrast resolution and high contrast sensitivity. A good example of such images is computed tomography (CT scanning). Utilization of such techniques in cardiovascular radiology was simultaneously but independently studied at the Universities of Wisconsin and Arizona as well as at the Kinderklinik in Kiel. The application of these techniques in arteriography has come to be known as digital subtraction arteriography (DSA).[6-13] At the University of Wisconsin the first digital subtraction arteriogram was performed in 1977 in a research laboratory. Two years later DSA was first offered clinically.

Our initial DSA studies were done with the contrast agent injected intravenously.[12] The first examinations were performed in a remotely located research laboratory, and the complexity of performing arterial catheterization made it impractical. However, vascular injection into an antecubital vein could be carried out easily. The quality of the initial intravenous studies was sufficient to make us enthusiastic. Nevertheless, definite limitations were recognized. Subsequently DSA capability was installed in our clinical angio-graphic suites, and we were able to employ arterial injection. Many of the problems were solved with arterial injection, and the opportunities for new applications became apparent; however, some distinct disadvantages remained.

After the initial presentations of DSA at the American Roentgen Ray Society meeting in the spring of 1980, considerable enthusiasm for DSA developed. In many quarters this enthusiasm was unbridled, and its shortcomings were minimized. As one would expect in such circumstances, enthusiasm waned and was replaced by some skepticism. Based on more than a decade of experience with DSA, we believe that digital recording of arteriographic data with both intravenous and intra-arterial injection has an important place clinically. In some situations DSA can replace film recordings, in other situations it can complement filming, and in some instances it is clear that DSA is inferior to film. It is apparent that the capability of performing DSA and film recording interchangeably is optimum, and we believe that all angiographic rooms should be equipped to do both.

The view of some, especially nonradiologists, is that DSA is a separate and independent examination. It is important to keep in mind that DSA is a means of recording arteriographic information and that the basic study is an arteriogram. Which method is employed to record the information should be based on which will best address the problem at hand.

ADVANTAGES OF DIGITAL SUBTRACTION ARTERIOGRAPHY

The major advantages of DSA are twofold: increased contrast sensitivity and electronic recording of data, which allows electronic manipulations of the information. The increased contrast sensitivity of DSA results in a decrease in vascular contrast agent requirement when considered relative to film recording under similar circumstances. To study the arteries in an adult with intravenous DSA, we inject 35 ml of a contrast agent that contains 350 to 400 mg iodine per milliliter into the right atrium in less than 2 seconds. A standard film arteriogram performed under similar circumstances would require an injection of 80 to 100 ml. An even greater reduction in contrast agent requirement can be achieved with intraarterial injection. For example, 20 ml of an agent with 270 mg iodine per milliliter is sufficient for a DSA abdominal aortogram, whereas a standard arteriogram would require 50 ml of an agent with 370 mg iodine per milliliter.

With intra-arterial injection, it is advantageous to decrease the concentration of the agent and inject a somewhat larger volume, with the same total amount of iodine. This allows better mixing with unopacified blood. For example, if one wishes to opacify the pelvic arteries, it may be better to have a longer injection with an iodine concentration of 240 mg/ml instead of 370 mg/ml. The total amount of iodine injected is the same. However, utilizing a less dense agent usually results in better mixing and therefore better opacification of the arteries of concern.

The decreased contrast burden results in lessened toxicity, primarily nephrotoxicity, and the patient will have less discomfort. The lessened nephrotoxicity is particularly important when patients with compromised renal function, especially diabetic patients, are examined. The decreased contrast requirement is also advantageous for examining infants. In these circumstances the number of injections can be increased without greater risk of toxicity; therefore, more information may be obtained from the arteriogram.

Patient discomfort is always a major concern. The lessened discomfort afforded by the decrease in the amount of contrast used is of substantial advantage. Patient discomfort is virtually eliminated with the use of nonionic media. However, at the present time the cost of nonionic medium is 10 to 20 times that of standard agents; this represents a substantial disadvantage.

Since images of DSA are recorded electronically, only images of interest for archival purposes need be recorded on film. There is economy in this approach related to decrease in film purchase as well as storage space requirements. With the electronic recording employed with DSA the images are immediately available for study, and the time required to perform a study is reduced. This is a substantial advantage in an emergency situation and can be helpful during procedures such as embolizations when multiple selective catheterizations may be required.

DISADVANTAGES OF DIGITAL SUBTRACTION ARTERIOGRAPHY

DSA has three major disadvantages: decreased spatial resolution, degradation of image quality by patient motion, and bright spots that may result in computer artifacts. Most of these problems can be solved by the simple expedient of case selection. If patients who are unable to remain still are excluded and only those problems in which the spatial resolution of DSA is sufficient are studied, the method can be quite satisfactory. Pixel shifting and hybrid and dual-energy subtraction have been applied to solve the patient motion problem. However, they have not found universal application. Mistretta and associates are working on devel-

opment of a digital beam attenuator that will provide an individual mask for each examination.[13,14] Laboratory experiments suggest that this approach will decrease the problem of bright spots. However, the implementation of digital beam attenuation is being delayed by mechanical problems with the cerium tape used to make the filter.

Spatial Resolution

The limitations of spatial resolution can be obviated by only studying those problems in which DSA, with either intravenous or intra-arterial injection, will provide the requisite detail. The spatial resolution of film arteriography is approximately 10 line pairs per millimeter, compared to 2.5 line pairs per millimeter for DSA. DSA spatial resolution approaches that of film arteriography with the increased contrast density provided with an intra-arterial injection. It is therefore apparent that studies of intraparenchymal arteries, small intracranial vessels, etc. cannot be satisfactorily undertaken with DSA. However, frequently performed studies such as aortography and peripheral arteriography are well suited for DSA study.

Patient Motion

Patient motion is the most serious inherent problem with DSA. This is best approached by selecting patients who are capable of suspending voluntary motion during DSA studies. However, this is difficult if not impossible for some patients, and motion secondary to cardiac contraction, vascular pulsations, and peristalsis can only be eliminated with some difficulty. Presently, two approaches to this problem, both involving some type of energy subtraction, have been described. The first is the hybrid subtraction technique described by Brody.[15] A combination of energy and temporal subtraction is utilized in this technique. This results in degradation of the signal-to-noise ratio, but the image motion artifact is decreased because the mask is temporally closer to the image to be subtracted. We have used this approach in a laboratory but have not found it sufficiently useful to implement it in the clinical angiography suite.

Dual-energy subtraction is currently being investigated. With dual-energy subtraction, the image of the soft tissues is decreased so that the major problem with motion is eliminated. However, the bones remain unsubtracted, just as they do in a standard arteriogram.

Some of our early DSA studies utilized dual-energy k-edge subtraction spectra. The spectra were just above and below the k-edge of iodine.[9] To form these narrow spectra it was necessary to heavily filter the beam with cerium and iodine. This heavy filtration resulted in a very small exit beam, which made it virtually impossible to image subjects greater than 15 cm in diameter. The images tended to be quite noisy, and as the thickness of the subject increased, the noise increased appreciably. The use of spectra above the k-edge of iodine results in a much larger exit dose. Therefore, larger objects can be imaged and more images obtained per second. The use of dual-energy subtraction is being evaluated in the laboratory and may provide a definite advantage in solving the motion artifact problem.

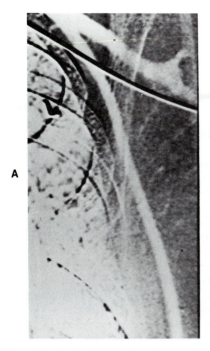

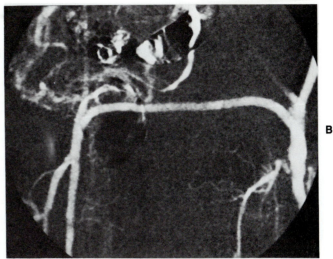

Figure 6-1. A. An IV-DSA shows the proximal end of a left axillobifemoral graft. The proximal anastomosis has a normal appearance, and lumen of the axillary end of the graft is smooth. The study was performed with a catheter passed from the left antecubital fossa into the right atrium. **B.** The distal end of the axillary graft is seen, and the anastomosis is unremarkable. There is excellent delineation of the femorofemoral portion of the bypass with bilateral patent profunda femoral arteries.

INTRAVENOUS DIGITAL SUBTRACTION ARTERIOGRAPHY—CLINICAL APPLICATIONS

Our experience is comparable to that of others in that we find that the number of intravenous DSAs that we are performing has decreased substantially as we have increased the use of DSA with intraarterial injection. Nonetheless, IV-DSA can be useful in studying a number of problems of interest to the vascular surgeon. The preoperative assessments of extracranial carotid artery disease, renal vascular hypertension, the vasculature proximal and distal to abdominal aortic aneurysms, iliac arteries in patients with peripheral vascular disease, and aortic arch anomalies are good examples. IV-DSA is useful in the evaluation of the patency of vascular grafts and percutaneous transluminal angioplasty sites (Fig. 6-1). False aneurysms, which result in the various vascular interventions, also are readily assessed (Fig. 6-2). In these instances the vessels of interest are sizable and therefore are readily delineated with IV-DSA.

Renal Vascular Hypertension

We consider IV-DSA to be the best screening method for the detection of renal vascular hypertension. Hillman, in a study of 89 patients, found diagnostic images in 94% with an accuracy of 92%.[16] If the catheterization is done through a femoral vein when a renal artery stenosis is seen, renin sampling may be done immediately.

Peripheral Vascular Disease

The large area to be studied in a patient with peripheral vascular disease generally would require an inordinately large volume of contrast, if the study were done with IV-DSA. However, in limited examinations that are directed at specific areas, intravenous DSA may be quite satisfactory.[17,18] For example, the study of patients with abdominal aortic aneurysms to note the proximal and distal extent of an aneurysm and its relation to the renal and iliac arteries is readily performed. Evaluation of the iliac arteries in instances of inflow disease is well suited to IV-DSA, as is the study of graft patency and false aneurysms that may arise at anastomoses or arterial puncture sites (Fig. 6-2). Frequently it cannot be determined on the basis of history, physical examination, or noninvasive study whether there has been failure of an intervention or whether progression of the initial disease is a cause of recurring vascular insufficiency. This distinction is usually readily made with intravenous DSA.

Extracranial Carotid Artery Disease

Considerable controversy surrounds the diagnosis and treatment of carotid artery disease. A discussion of this controversy is beyond the scope of this chapter. If the carotid artery is to be imaged, intravenous DSA may yield diagnostic studies in up to 90% of patients, provided the patient can cooperate and has a good cardiac output.[19] Therefore, in patients with asymptomatic bruits or with equivocal symptoms, IV-DSA is considered by many to be the procedure of choice. In patients with definite symptoms, where a detailed outline of the disease is required, use of intra-arterial DSA would probably be more satisfactory.

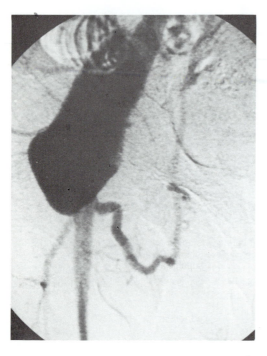

Figure 6-2. An IV-DSA in a patient who had developed a pulsatile mass in the right groin several years after an aortobifemoral bypass graft was placed. The mass is opacified, indicating a false aneurysm. The patent graft proximal to the false aneurysm is visible. The profunda femoral artery fills well, but the superficial femoral artery is obstructed.

INTRAARTERIAL DIGITAL SUBTRACTION ARTERIOGRAPHY

Interest in IA-DSA has rapidly increased. Because the time between the mask and arteriogram image is short in IA-DSA, the problem with patient motion is greatly reduced. The enhanced contrast level present with intra-arterial injection increases spatial resolution to almost that of film arteriography. These circumstances make IA-DSA satisfactory for most arteriographic examination, and its successful use has been reported for virtually every major artery in the body (Figs. 6-3 and 6-4). Our peripheral arteriograms are presently performed exclusively with DSA. In addition, we use IA-DSA for virtually all cerebrovascular examinations, except for patients with subarachnoid hemorrhage or arteriovenous malformations who are going to be embolized or to have surgical treatment. Conversely, some examinations, such as pulmonary arteriograms for the diagnosis of pulmonary embolus, where the patients are likely to be dyspneic and tachypneic, and of cardiac pulsations that result in vascular motion, are done almost exclusively with film. Aortorenal angiograms performed to evaluate the prospective renal donors are also done completely with film. The reason for this is that we do not want to take the chance of missing a small polar artery. As familiarity with the IA-DSA technique develops, those examinations that can be satisfactorily performed with DSA are readily recognized. The decreased contrast agent requirement allows arteriography to be performed with No. 4 or 5 French catheters. The increased safety afforded by such catheters makes outpatient arteriography feasible. This is a major economic advantage.

There are some intrinsic advantages of IA-DSA. A major one is increased contrast detection in evaluation of the runoff in peripheral vascular disease. At times, despite the use of vasodilators or reactive hyperemia to increase flow, it may be impossible to satisfactorily identify runoff vessels.

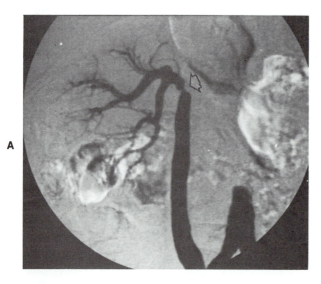

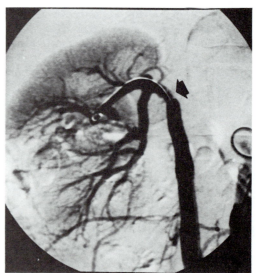

Figure 6-3. A. This patient had transient relief of renovascular hypertension after revascularization with a saphenous vein bypass. The IA-DSA performed with injection into the right common iliac artery showed recurrent stenosis at the distal anastomosis (*open arrow*). **B.** With the guidewire still across the lesion, a DSA was performed to show the appearance of the stenosis after a percutaneous transluminal angioplasty had been performed. No residual stenosis is present.

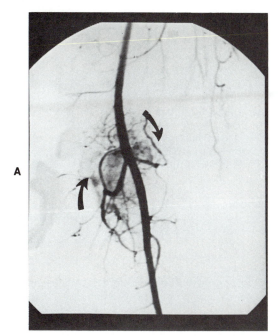 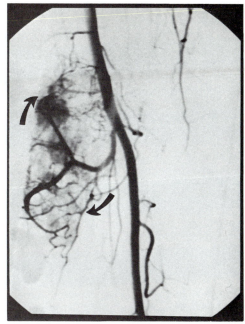

Figure 6-4. This patient had an asymptomatic, readily palpable mass in the anterior aspect of the thigh. CT and MRI scans showed this to be localized and noninfiltrating. Biopsy showed the mass to be a liposarcoma. A localized resection was planned, and an arteriogram was performed to exclude involvement of the superficial femoral artery. **A.** In the frontal projection, neovascularity (*arrows*) extends both medial and lateral to the superficial femoral artery. No evidence of luminal irregularity, which would indicate vascular invasion, is identified. **B.** A lateral projection of the IA-DSA shows neovascularity anterior to and separate from the artery. Again, the lumen appears smooth, suggesting that there has been no invasion of the wall. These findings imply that the mass can be resected, preserving the continuity of the artery; vascular reconstruction will not be necessary.

The runoff may be identified with the increased contrast detection of DSA, even though it cannot be seen on a standard film arteriogram. This is a distinct aid in specific preoperative planning and may obviate the need for an intraoperative arteriogram.[17,18,20]

Another inherent advantage of DSA is "road mapping."[21,22] The continuous mode of digital subtraction arteriography is used in this technique. After the intra-arterial injection of a small quantity of contrast medium, fluoroscopic data are stored in the memory unit. These data then act as a subtraction template, and the real-time fluoroscopic image is continuously subtracted from the stored mask and displayed on the fluoroscopic screen. Structures contained in both images, i.e., soft tissues and bone, are subtracted, and only the iodine-containing structures remain. The resulting combined image is seen on the fluoroscopic monitor, and materials and devices introduced into the fluoroscopic field will be seen in relation to the displayed arterial anatomy. With the use of two side-by-side fluoroscopic monitors, one can view the live fluoroscopy, without the distraction of the superimposed "road map," or the "road map," depending on which is more advantageous at the moment.

Angiographic apparatus such as catheters, dilatation balloons, sheaths, etc. are readily identified and the relation to the anatomy can be determined absolutely. This means that dilatation balloons can be accurately placed in relation to lesions to be dilated. The "road mapping" technique also aids the performance of selective and superselective catheterizations. Embolization of various vessels is greatly facilitated by the use of this technique.

CONCLUSIONS

DSA is a method of recording angiographic data, and of and in itself is not a separate technique. More than a decade of experience with DSA, employing both intravenous and intra-arterial injection, has shown that DSA is extremely useful and a valuable adjunct to standard film arteriography. We believe that all angiographic suites should be equipped to do both DSA and film arteriography interchangeably. When this is possible one can then utilize whichever technique will provide the necessary information in the simplest and safest manner. In addition, some of the advantages unique to DSA, such as the ability to see structures not visible with standard film arteriography, and "road mapping," can be employed as necessary.

REFERENCES

1. Röntgen WC: On a new kind of rays. Erste Mitt Sitzer Phys-Med Ges (Wurzburg) 137, 1895.
2. Haschek E, Lindenthal OT: A contribution to the practical use of the photography according to Röntgen. Wien Klin Wochenschr 9:63, 1896.

3. Franck O, Alwens W: Kreislaufstudien am Rontgenschirm. Munch Med Wochenschr 51:950, 1910.

4. Moniz E, Diaz A, Lima A: La radioarteriographie et la topographie cranioencephalique. J Radiol Electrol Med Nucl 12:72, 1928.

5. Seldinger SI: Catheter replacement of needle in percutaneous arteriography: New technique. Acta Radiol (Stockh) 39:368, 1953.

6. Ovitt T, Capp MP, et al.: Development of digital video subtraction system for intravenous angiography. Soc Photo-optical Instrum Engineers 206:73, 1979.

7. Brennecke R, Brown TK, et al.: Computerized video image processing with application to cardioangiographic Roentgen image series, in Nagel HH (ed): Digital Image Processing. New York: Springer, 1977.

8. Ort MG, Mistretta CA, Kelcz F: An improved technique for enhancing small periodic changes in television fluoroscopy. Optical Eng 12:169, 1973.

9. Crummy AB, Mistretta CA, et al.: Absorption edge fluoroscopy using quasi-monoenergetic x-ray beams. Invest Radiol 8:402, 1973.

10. Kruger RA, Mistretta CA, et al.: A digital video image processor for real-time x-ray subtraction imaging. Optical Engineering 17(6):652, 1978.

11. Kruger RA, Mistretta CA, et al.: Computerized fluoroscopy in real-time for noninvasive visualization of the cardiovascular system: preliminary studies. Radiology 130:49, 1979.

12. Crummy AB, Strother CM, et al.: Computerized fluroroscopy: digital subtraction for intravenous angiocardiography and arteriography. AJR 135:1131, 1980.

13. Mistretta CA, Crummy AB: Diagnosis of cardiovascular disease by digital subtraction angiography. Science 214:761, 1981.

14. Hasegawa BH, Naimuddin S, et al.: Application of a digital beam attenuator to chest radiography. Soc of Photo-instrum Engineers 486:2–7, 1984.

15. Brody WR: Hybrid subtraction, in Digital Radiography. New York, Raven Press, 1984.

16. Hillman BJ: Digital radiology of the kidney. Radio Clin North Am 23:211, 1985.

17. Kubal WS, Crummy AB, Turnipseed WD: The utility of digital subtraction arteriography in peripheral vascular disease. Cardiovasc Intervent Radiol 6:241, 1983.

18. Crummy AB, Strother CM, et al.: Digital video subtraction angiography for evaluation of peripheral vascular disease. Radiology 141(1):33, 1981.

19. Foley WD, Smith DF, et al.: Intravenous DSA examination of patients with suspected cerebral ischemia. Radiology 151:651, 1984.

20. Crummy AB, Stieghorst MF, et al.: Digital subtraction angiography: Current status and use of intra-arterial injection. Radiology 145:303, 1982.

21. Crummy AB, Starck EE, et al.: Digital subtraction angiography "road map" for transluminal angioplasty. Semin Intervent Radiol 1(4):247, 1984.

22. McDermott JC, Starck E, Crummy AB: Road map application to the pulseless common femoral artery. Cardiovasc Intervent Radiol 9:109, 1986.

CHAPTER 7
Duplex Ultrasonography

Brian L. Thiele

In the last decade application of ultrasound as a diagnostic modality has been extended, largely because it can be used noninvasively. Therefore major developments in application occurred in fields in which diagnostic information had usually been obtained by invasive methods, often entailing some morbidity and occasionally mortality. Thus it was natural that one of the areas in which ultrasound was first tested was the diagnosis of arterial disease in an attempt to obviate the difficulties encountered with arteriographic studies, which at the time were associated with a morbidity of approximately 1% and mortality of approximately 0.1%.[1]

The properties of ultrasound make it ideal for examining fluid-filled structures contained by boundaries that reflect ultrasound. Blood (the fluid) and the arterial wall (the barrier) are therefore ideal structures for insonation. The anatomic area of the arterial system initially scrutinized was the region of the carotid bifurcation. These vessels were close to the surface and accessible to scrutiny with ultrasound. The clinically significant disease in this area is usually focal. Current technologies have rapidly developed in the detection of carotid disease and have been applied with increasing accuracy. More recently, the same principles learned in the detection of carotid disease have been widely applied to almost all the peripheral vascular system. Before a detailed discussion of the applications of duplex ultrasonography, it is appropriate to review some basic properties of ultrasound, its interaction with static tissues and moving targets such as blood, and the evolution of the current technology.

BASIC PRINCIPLES

Ultrasound Imaging

The instrumentation used for generating ultrasound-derived images are modifications of early sonar devices. In medical applications, a different transmitting frequency is used, which is determined by the depth of the structures to be visualized. Superficial structures (the carotid and fem-oral arteries) are optimally visualized with high frequencies (e.g., 10 MHz), while deep structures (the aorta) are best studied with lower frequencies (2 to 3 MHz). This feature relates to the fact that the depth of penetration of ultrasound is inversely related to the transmitting frequency. High frequencies have low penetrance, and low frequencies have high penetrance.

The ultrasound beam itself is generated by the passage of a rapidly alternating current through a piezoelectric crystal, resulting in the production of a steady stream of pulses of ultrasound of short duration. These pulses travel through tissue until a change in tissue density or tissue interface is encountered. Then a small component of the signal is reflected back toward the receiver, a small component is absorbed at the interface producing thermal energy, and the largest component continues into the deeper tissues until new interfaces are encountered and the process is repeated. Eventually the strength of the signal in deeper tissues is so weak that no reflected echoes occur. The reflected signal from strong interfaces travels back toward the receiver, where it is received by the same crystal used for generation of the signal during a period when no transmission is occurring. If the interface is at right angles to the ultrasound beam, the major component of the returning signal will be detected by the receiving crystal, but if the beam strikes the interface at an angle, some of the signal will be reflected away from the receiver.

The initial pulsed echo devices electronically processed the returning signal and displayed this information on an oscilloscope screen, from which hard copy reproduction could be made. The strength of the returning echo was depicted by varying the brightness of a white dot on the screen—so-called brightness mode or B-mode. Echo-dense structures such as the arterial wall produced bright echoes which, when coalesced, accurately defined the spatial relationships of the artery and the tissues. This latter capability was obtained by having the transducer oscillate or rotate rapidly through a fixed plane, with progressive accumulation of echo information enabling the compilation of a complete tissue image in the plane being insonated. This process became known as B-scan ultrasonography. This particular technology found early application in the diagnosis of abdominal aortic aneurysms.[2]

The images produced by these early instruments, however, were relatively coarse, and the resolution was not of high quality. The reason for this lack of resolution was that only strong returning echoes triggered the production of a dot on the phosphor-coated oscilloscope screen, resulting in a significant loss of tissue detail that was contained in low intensity echoes. Kossoff developed the concept of gray scale, which enables echoes over a wide range of intensity to be recognized by the receiving and processing system.[3] In this technology, instead of reproduction occurring on an oscilloscope screen, the image is reproduced on a television monitor with a significant improvement in image resolution. The intensity level of the returning echoes is allocated to one of eight shades of gray, with black representing strong signals and white no signal.

The final early phase of pulsed echo imaging came with the development of real-time ultrasonography, accomplished with rapid processing of the returning echoes and display on the monitor at a frame rate that the eye perceived as a continuous phenomenon. Originally this was accomplished with a single transducer moving rapidly over the plane being examined, visualizing a sector of tissue—so-called sector scanning. An alternate approach is used with phased array systems in which the transducer remains stationary and the beam is directed electronically through the tissues. Finally, linear array systems utilize a large number of transducers that are activated sequentially and also receive returning echoes sequentially. These latter systems overcome some of the problems produced by loss of echo information with the sector scanners because of the nonperpendicular angle of the transmitting beam to the tissues in the periphery of the sector. The more recent models of linear array scanners have been associated with a significant improvement in resolution of soft-tissue constituents.

Duplex Ultrasonography

Following early reports of the use of gray scale ultrasonography to identify the abdominal aorta and the carotid arteries,[4] a multidisciplinary research project was launched at the University of Washington by the bioengineering and surgery departments. The purpose of this project was to develop a high resolution ultrasound imaging system to detect carotid atherosclerosis. The early prototype instrument utilized three 5 MHz fixed-focus transducers mounted on a rotating wheel, which produced a gray scale tissue image at a frame rate of 21 per second. A Silastic boot filled with water positioned the transducers 4 cm from the skin surface and provided for a field of examination of vessels within 4 cm of the skin surface. The initial image quality obtained with this instrument was poor by today's standards but was considered excellent at the time. Although initial studies were promising, two major difficulties were encountered. The first was produced by the fact that atherosclerotic plaques at the carotid bifurcation frequently contained large amounts of calcium through which the ultrasound beam could not penetrate. If this calcium was located in the superficial wall of the carotid, no tissue detail was obtained deep to this area and resulted in the production of an acoustic shadow. The second problem became evident when a patient who was thought to have a patent internal carotid artery subsequently underwent arteriography which identified that the artery was thrombosed. With the relatively poor resolution by today's standards, the acoustic density of thrombus was similar to that of flowing blood, and the two could not be differentiated. To facilitate the detection of patent vessels, therefore, an outrigger pulsed Doppler was added to the scan head[5] (Fig. 7-1).

The availability of a pulsed Doppler component enabled the flow stream to be sampled at a precise location in the imaged vessel. The angle of the Doppler beam was represented on the image by a bright white line, and the location

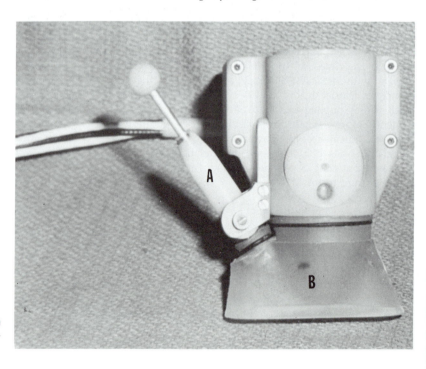

Figure 7-1. Early prototype duplex scan head with outrigger Doppler (*A*) and water-filled Silastic boot (*B*).

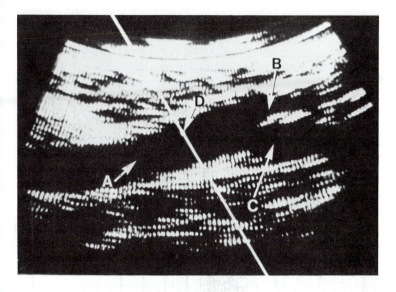

Figure 7-2. Television monitor reproduction of early duplex ultrasonography image showing superimposed cursor angle of Doppler (*A*) and sample volume location depicted by the white dot (*B*).

of the sample volume by a bright white dot (Fig. 7-2). The addition of a Doppler component also necessitated modification of the signal processing system, which was accomplished with a prototype fast Fourier transform (FFT) spectrum analyzer provided by the Honeywell Corporation. The combination of pulsed echo imaging and pulsed Doppler was termed duplex scanning or duplex ultrasonography. Clinical studies soon revealed a close correlation between the severity of the stenosis of the internal carotid artery and the Doppler-derived data depicted by the FFT analyzer.[6] The emphasis of the project rapidly shifted from the imaging priority to a better understanding of the relationships between the severity of disease, changes in blood flow, and signal processing of the Doppler component. A more complete understanding of duplex ultrasonography can be obtained by considering each of these factors separately.

FLOW PATTERNS AND DISEASE

Flow in nondiseased arteries is characterized by the red cell components moving parallel to one another at a uniform velocity (laminar flow). Adjacent to the wall of the artery, however, the velocity of the red blood cells decreases, resulting in a velocity profile that is either parabolic or flat. Thus, if an instrument that detected velocity of red blood cells were used to sample the center stream of such a vessel, it would detect a single velocity, whereas near the wall a range of velocities would be identified.

When the cross-sectional area of the artery is reduced by intramural disease, small perturbations or eddies called vortices are produced immediately beyond the area of narrowing. This process is termed vorticeal shedding. Laminar flow, however, returns rapidly a short distance downstream. The velocity detection instrument sampling this area of disturbed flow would detect a range of velocities rather than a single velocity.

With more severe narrowing of the artery, these perturbations increase in magnitude, and at the point where the stenosis is severe enough to produce a pressure and flow gradient, disturbances become severe; red blood cell movement is quite random, and turbulent flow develops. Sampling in this type of flow stream is associated with the greatest range of velocities. With this severe or hemodynamically significant stenosis, red blood cell velocity within and immediately beyond the stenosis increases dramatically proximal to the development of the turbulent flow zone. With very severe stenosis of a preocclusive type, the pulsatile character of flow is dampened beyond the lesion, and diastolic velocity approaches systolic velocity.

DOPPLER SIGNAL PROCESSING

Analog Display

The application of Doppler analysis to signals returning from moving red blood cells results in the acquisition of information regarding the velocity of these cells as defined by the Doppler equation:

$$\Delta f = \frac{2Vf_0\cos\theta}{C}$$

where Δf = Doppler frequency (kHz)
V = velocity of red blood cells (cm/sec)
f_0 = transmitting frequency (MHz)
θ = angle between Doppler beam and axis of vessel
C = velocity of sound in tissue (cm/sec)

The direction of movement can also be determined using zero crossing or phased quadrature processing. The simplest method of display is accomplished by averaging all the velocities in the returning signal and determining the instantaneous mean value with display as a single line or analog display. In this format, information regarding the direction of flow and the mean velocity of red blood cells at any point in the pulse cycle can be determined. In general terms, however, only severe disease can be detected with this type of display, and features of the pattern of flow in particular (disturbed vs. turbulent) are not readily recognized. The application of fast Fourier transform spectrum analysis enables these abnormalities in the flow pattern to be identified.

Spectrum Analysis

This form of signal processing identifies the individual frequency components in the returning signal and determines the strength of each frequency component. Because it is sound that is being processed, the strength or amplitude is measured in decibels and the frequency shift in kilohertz. The transmitting frequencies used clinically (2 to 10 MHz), when processed through a speaker, produce an audible signal. In the early instrumentation the signal strength was depicted on an oscilloscope screen in real time and simultaneously recorded on a tape recorder. Playback through the Fourier transform analyzer produced a frequency-vs.-time display of each pulse cycle, with the signal strength being depicted by a gray scale representation. The fast Fourier transform refers to the on-line analysis of the Doppler shifted signal with the interim display of the frequency amplitude plot. As noted earlier, in laminar flow conditions red blood cell velocity in the central portion of the vessel is relatively uniform; in fast Fourier transform analysis this is depicted as a single black line. This phenomenon is best seen during the ejection phase of systole. When disturbed flow exists, the backscattered signal contains more than a single frequency because of the range of velocities being detected by the ultrasound beam, and in the gray scale representation the frequency component broadens—so-called spectral broadening. When turbulent flow is being examined, the peak frequencies detected are higher than normal because of the increased red blood cell velocity, and the returning signal contains a broader range of frequencies than is seen under either laminar flow or disturbed flow states. It should be emphasized that these relative changes in frequency in the backscattered signal can only be ascribed to alterations in red blood cell velocity when the angle of the Doppler beam remains constant from one examination to the next. For this reason, all currently available duplex instruments have an angled cursor on the video screen to assist the examiner in maintaining a constant angle. If the speed of ultrasound in tissue is known, as well as the angle, the actual red blood cell velocity can also be calculated. Many of the currently available instruments automatically measure the insonating angle and visually display the peak velocity in centimeters per second.

The early clinical studies of duplex ultrasonography relied on a semiquantitative interpretation of the spectra obtained from an examination utilizing the frequencies detected at peak systole, and a subjective assessment of the magnitude of spectral broadening.[7] Comparison of the spectra with arteriograms on patients tended to confirm the impression that there was a relationship between this parameter and the severity of stenosis, but it was not until a series of control studies was performed that the true relationship was established.[8] In these studies, artificial concentric stenoses were created in the thoracic aorta of dogs, and a computer program was used to measure the degree of spectral broadening throughout the cycle. The results of these studies are depicted in Fig. 7-3, and show that over a stenosis range from 15 to 50% diameter reduction, spectral broadening actually increases linearly, while the time at which the greatest spectral broadening occurs is progressively earlier in the cycle. Thus with minimal degrees of narrowing, this change is seen most conspicuously in diastole and, with severe stenosis, early in systole. Therefore, the parameters available to aid in interpretation and diagnosis are the peak frequency at any point in the cycle and the phenomenon of spectral broadening. Although as noted earlier, quantitative information such as red blood cell velocity can be derived from the frequency data, none of the currently available instruments provides a means of quantifying spectral broadening.

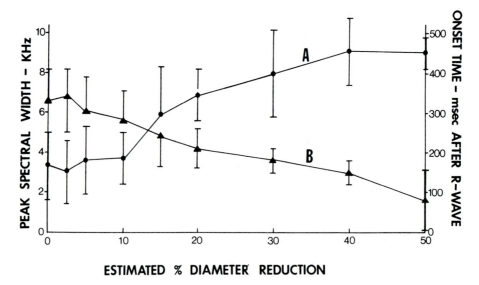

Figure 7-3. Relationship between percent stenosis and computer-measured spectral broadening in a series of animal studies. The peak spectral width increases as the degree of stenosis increases. The time in the cycle at which the peak spectral width is seen occurs earlier in the cycle as the degree of stenosis increases.

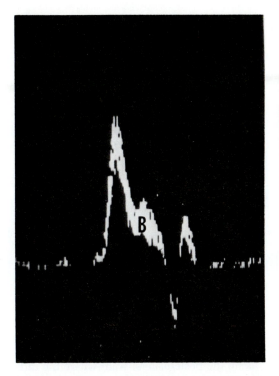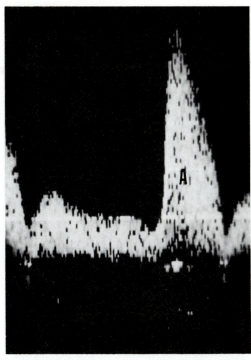

Figure 7-4. Comparison of Doppler signals obtained with a continuous wave **(A)**, and pulsed **(B)** Doppler. Both signals were analyzed with fast Fourier transform and were obtained from the same artery. Note the marked spectral broadening in the signal obtained from the continuous wave compared to that obtained with the pulsed Doppler device.

PULSED DOPPLER vs. CONTINUOUS WAVE DOPPLER

The initial prototype duplex scanners utilized a pulsed Doppler source, although a number of currently available instruments utilize continuous wave ultrasound. The major difference between these two modalities is the fact that the continuous wave systems insonate the entire cross-section of the vessel and therefore are influenced by the red blood cell movement in this zone. The returning signal is very complex, containing a wide range of frequencies even when a laminar flow state exists. If analog processing is used, the continuous and pulsed systems will be comparable, but if FFT analysis is used, the signal from the continuous wave instruments will contain spectral broadening throughout even though flow is laminar (Fig. 7-4). Although this difference is not important if only severe stenosis is being sought, the continuous wave instruments are less proficient in detecting minimal disease and in differentiating between normal arteries and minimal disease.

A deficiency of the pulsed Doppler systems is that the peak frequency detectable is related not only to the transmitting frequency but also to the pulse repetition frequency (PRF) at which the signal is produced. Very high peak systolic frequency shifts are likely to be produced by the jets associated with high-grade stenoses, which may be missed if an inappropriate pulse repetition frequency is used. The problem is readily identified during examination because the systolic peak is amputated (Fig. 7-5). This phenomenon is referred to as aliasing. The true peak systolic frequencies can be detected by recruiting the PRF of the pulsed echo component, which results in loss of the image during the examination, when the operator must rely solely on the quality of the audible signal for sampling purposes. This maneuver doubles the operating PRF of the Doppler mode and usually overcomes the difficulty. When very high frequencies are expected in the returning signal, however, as is seen with cardiac valvular stenosis, continuous wave systems may be more reliable, particularly when this information is used to directly estimate the degree of stenosis.

With the preceding knowledge of the capabilities of current duplex instrumentation to detect occlusive disease, it is now appropriate to consider the current clinical applications.

CAROTID DISEASE DETECTION

The extracranial vascular system is ideally suited to examination by ultrasound devices because these vessels are located a short distance beneath the skin surface and atherosclerosis in these vessels is usually focal. The examination consists primarily of visualizing the common, internal and external carotid arteries, and then sampling the flow stream in each of these vessels at locations where disease is suspected. The cerebrovascular bed is relatively low resistance, and flow is characterized by a significant component occurring in diastole. Because the majority of flow in the common carotid eventually courses to the brain via the internal carotid artery, the velocity pattern in these two vessels is similar.

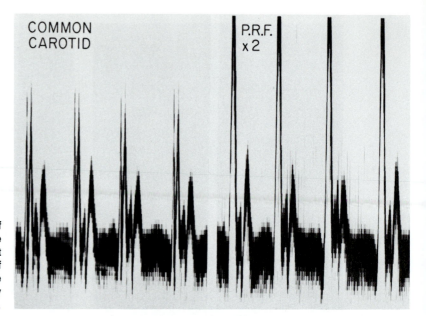

Figure 7-5. Phenomenon of aliasing of Doppler signal due to use of inappropriate pulse repetition frequency (PRF). Correct display is obtained by recruiting the PRF of the pulsed echo component, doubling the available PRF of the Doppler. The previously cut-off signal is now normal in appearance.

Before consideration of the diagnostic features associated with disease, the normal flow patterns will be reviewed. The important characteristics of the spectra obtained from a normal internal carotid artery are shown in Fig. 7-6. These include laminar flow during the acceleration phase of systole (A), mild spectral broadening during the early deceleration phase of systole (B), with more marked broadening in diastole (C). The peak systolic frequency is less than 3 kHz, and diastolic flow is always in the forward direction.

In the external carotid artery, which supplies the facial musculature, a high resistance waveform is seen that differs from that of the internal carotid artery because of the flow reversal that occurs in diastole.

Recently it has been recognized that if sampling of the flow stream is performed in the bulb, unusual spectra will be obtained[9] (Fig. 7-7). This pattern of forward followed by reverse flow is produced by the presence of vortices along the posterolateral wall, where the direction of flow rapidly changes. The change in velocity and direction of red blood cells in this region is responsible for the spectral broadening present as well as the forward-reverse feature. The presence of this phenomenon has served as a useful marker for detecting a nondiseased carotid bulb. It should be emphasized, however, that inadvertent sampling in this region may be responsible for difficulties in interpretation.

As occlusive lesions develop in the proximal internal carotid artery, the spectral patterns seen in Figure 7-6 change,[10] the most notable feature being an accentuation of the spectral broadening in diastole (Fig. 7-8). This change is consistent with the observations of the previously described animal studies and is due to vorticeal shedding

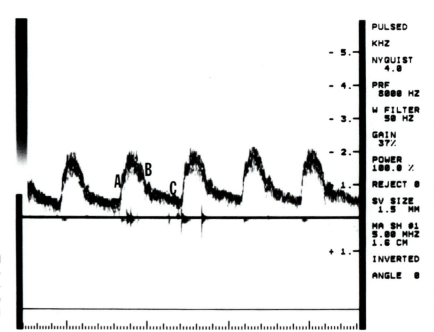

Figure 7-6. Spectra obtained from normal internal carotid artery. Note laminar flow representation in the acceleration phase of systole (A), mild spectral broadening during the early deceleration phase of systole (B), and the broadening in diastole (C).

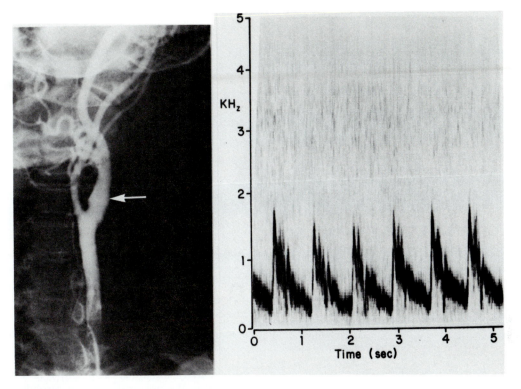

Figure 7-7. Spectra obtained from within the bulb of the normal internal carotid artery show forward flow immediately followed by reverse flow, and spectral broadening associated with vorticeal shedding in this region.

immediately distal to the area of stenosis. It should be emphasized that these changes are detectable for only a short distance distal to the lesion, which requires careful multiple sampling.

In the presence of lesions approaching a 50% diameter reduction, the velocity of blood flow through and immediately beyond the lesion increases. This is detected by the Doppler as a rise in the peak systolic frequency compared to that seen in the proximal common carotid artery. The frequencies encountered with such lesions range from 3.5 kHz to 4.5 kHz and are accompanied by spectral broadening throughout the whole cycle (Fig. 7-9).

The development of severe stenosis is characterized by the presence of a high velocity jet, which is represented in the Doppler mode by a significant increase in peak systolic frequency and turbulent flow, depicted as marked spectral

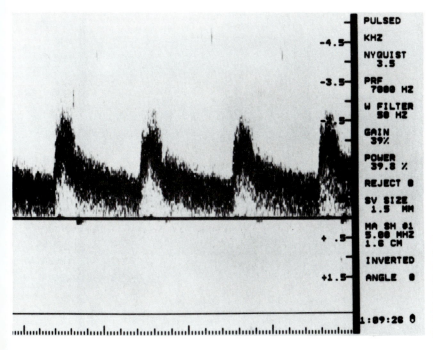

Figure 7-8. Spectra obtained from internal carotid artery with diameter reduction of 20 to 40%. Salient features include the relatively low peak systolic frequency and the accentuation of broadening into the deceleration phase of systole. Diastolic spectral broadening is more marked than that seen in the normal carotid.

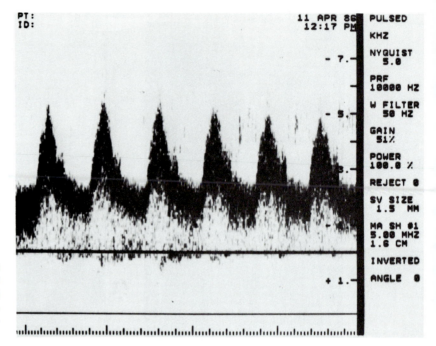

Figure 7-9. Spectra obtained from lesions approaching hemodynamic significance (40 to 60% diameter reduction). Peak systolic frequency has increased to the region of 4 kHz; spectral broadening is even further accentuated.

broadening (Fig. 7-10). Both of these flow changes are propagated for some distance distal to the stenosis. The frequency elevation is greatest within the stenosis, and the flow disturbance is maximal two to three vessel diameters distally.

The preocclusive lesion (80 to 99% diameter reduction) is often associated with peak frequencies so high they cannot be detected by the pulsed Doppler because of the technical factors discussed previously. A diastolic frequency that exceeds 4.5 kHz, however, is diagnostic for this critical lesion (Fig. 7-11).

Occlusion of the internal carotid artery is characterized by the absence of a flow signal in the visualized internal carotid artery and the development of flow to zero or even reversal in the proximal common carotid artery[11] (Fig. 7-12). The detection of internal carotid artery occlusion may be difficult if the external carotid artery becomes a major source of collateral flow to the brain. When this occurs, the external carotid artery assumes the flow characteristics of the normal internal carotid and there is no flow reversal in the common carotid. This difficulty can be overcome by the competent examiner searching for branches of the artery being examined; this would immediately identify the vessel as the external carotid. Also, digital compression of the facial or superficial temporal arteries produces a transient increase in the resistance of the distal vascular bed,

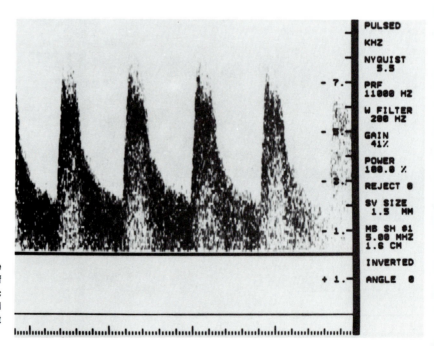

Figure 7-10. Spectra obtained from severe stenosis (60 to 80% diameter reduction) of the internal carotid artery. The peak systolic frequency is now greater than 4.5 kHz, and spectral broadening is marked throughout the whole cycle.

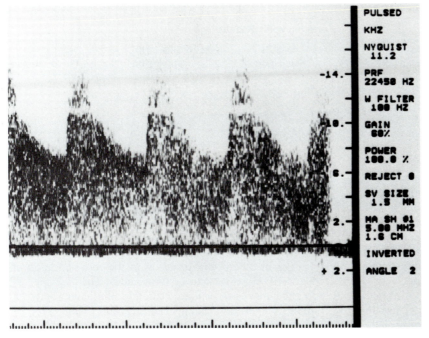

PULSED
KHZ
NYQUIST
11.2
-14.- PRF
22450 HZ
W FILTER
100 HZ
10.- GAIN
60%
POWER
100.0 %
6.- REJECT 0
SV SIZE
1.5 MM
2.- MA SH #1
5.00 MHZ
1.6 CM
INVERTED
+ 2.- ANGLE 2

Figure 7-11. Spectra obtained from preocclusive lesion (80 to 99% diameter reduction) of the internal carotid artery. Peak systolic frequency cannot be determined, but the end-diastolic frequency has shifted to the 4.5 kHz range.

resulting in oscillations of the signal obtained from the artery being insonated.

The recognition and characterization of the above features has resulted in the widespread acceptance of duplex ultrasonography as an accurate means of detecting the severity of internal carotid artery disease. This capability has been documented by comparative studies of this technique with cerebral arteriography.[12] Our laboratory results are shown in Table 7-1. The greatest discrepancies occur in the differentiation of normal and completely occluded arteries. While the difficulties encountered in detecting the latter are largely technical as well as physiologic, a significant source of conflicting results is the now-recognized difficulty associated with the accurate interpretation of even standard contrast arteriograms. This factor is highlighted by the determination of observer variability of interpretation, which is greatest for the differentiation of normal from abnormal and the decision for greater or less than 50% diameter reduction.[13] Comparative studies between duplex ultrasonography and arteriographic lesions have become even more difficult as arterial digital subtraction studies, with slightly poorer resolution than contrast arteriograms, have become more widely utilized in this field.

Physiologic changes occurring in response to disease may also be a source of true error in estimating the severity or location of disease, as noted in the diagnosis of internal

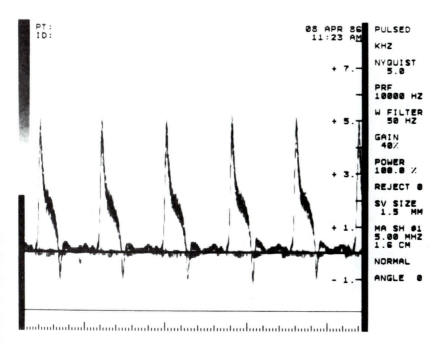

PT:
ID:
08 APR 86
11:23 AM
PULSED
KHZ
NYQUIST
5.0
+ 7.- PRF
10000 HZ
W FILTER
50 HZ
+ 5.- GAIN
40%
POWER
100.0 %
+ 3.- REJECT 0
SV SIZE
1.5 MM
+ 1.- MA SH #1
5.00 MHZ
1.6 CM
NORMAL
- 1.- ANGLE 0

Figure 7-12. Spectra obtained from the common carotid artery of a patient with internal carotid artery occlusion. Note flow reversal in early diastole.

TABLE 7-1. DUPLEX ULTRASONOGRAPHY vs. ARTERIOGRAPHY

Duplex Results	Arteriographic Results				
	Normal	15–40% Occlusion	40–60% Occlusion	60–99% Occlusion	Occlusion
Normal	62	3			
15–40%	8	55	1		
40–60%		3	54		
60–99%			2	88	
Occlusion				1	40

carotid artery occlusion. This is frequently seen in patients with bilateral disease, when there may be a compensatory increase in flow through the less-diseased carotid artery. For example, when the internal carotid artery on one side is occluded, the flow rate and therefore velocity increase in the contralateral carotid and may result in overestimation of the severity of disease in this vessel because of the changes in the baseline frequency parameters. Cato et al. have recently documented that the greatest errors in estimation of degree of stenosis occur in patients with bilateral severe disease.[14]

In addition to the evaluation of the carotid arteries, duplex ultrasonography has been extended to examination of all the extracranial vessels, including the first part of the vertebral arteries and the second and third segments of the subclavian arteries. Disease at the origins of the vertebral artery can readily be detected by increases in peak systolic frequency in the presence of spectral broadening. Flow reversal in these arteries, as occurs with subclavian steal, is also readily diagnosable.

Disease Progression

Because of the ease of repetitive study and the lack of morbidity, serial studies of carotid artery disease with duplex ultrasonography have yielded important information regarding the natural history of patients with asymptomatic lesions. Although the natural history of asymptomatic ca-

rotid artery disease remains controversial, duplex ultrasonography can provide important data regarding the stability of identifiable lesions. When serial examinations are made, the technique must be standardized to ensure comparability. Evidence of disease progression is provided by major changes in the spectra resulting in the reclassification of disease severity up one or two grades. For example, although it may be difficult to accurately differentiate between studies suggesting a change from 20 to 40% diameter reduction to 40 to 60% diameter reduction, it is relatively easy to differentiate between 20 to 40% diameter reduction and 60 to 80% diameter reduction because of the major spectral changes between the two. In this area the change of greatest clinical significance appears to be the progression of disease to the preocclusive stage (80 to 99% diameter reduction), a change which can be readily appreciated because of the characteristic spectral changes associated with this lesion (Fig. 7-13). A number of studies suggest that this lesion in particular is prone to progress to occlusion and may be associated with the development of symptoms of either transient or permanent cerebral ischemia.[15]

Recurrent Carotid Stenosis

An ideal result from carotid endarterectomy includes not only the prevention of future symptoms, but also minimization of recurrent stenosis. Although the incidence of symp-

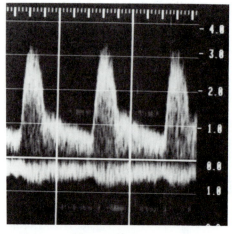

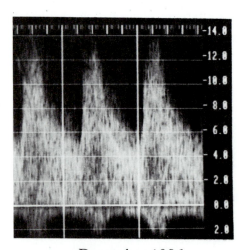

May 1986   December 1986

Figure 7-13. Serial spectra obtained from the same patient show accentuation of the spectra with gradual development of preocclusive type spectra.

tomatic recurrent stenosis is small,[16] the development of recurrent stenosis, particularly in patients with contralateral severe disease, creates a therapeutic dilemma. Duplex ultrasonography after carotid endarterectomy has shown that the incidence of recurrent stenosis is significantly higher than previously thought and varies in different reported series from 10 to 20%.[17,18] Studies following carotid endarterectomy have also documented that the spectra rarely return to normal but are usually similar to those seen in patients with mild disease in which there is mild spectral broadening without significant increases in peak systolic frequency. It has also become apparent that flow abnormalities may decrease over time, probably due to remodeling of the endarterectomized segment. Knowledge obtained from such serial studies has focused attention on the factors responsible for this process, with the subsequent observation that it may be minimized by restoring the anatomy of the bifurcation as closely as possible to a normal configuration with either meticulous arteriotomy closure or, if so indicated, patch angioplasty.[19]

The recognition that occlusive lesions in any artery are associated with characteristic changes in the flow pattern that are detectable by pulsed Doppler in particular, and the development of scan heads with deep focusing capabilities, has recently resulted in the application of this technology to examine arteries not previously accessible. The major contributions in the field of deep Doppler ultrasonography have occurred in the detection of lesions of the mesenteric vascular system and renal artery lesions. It is now possible to scan the aortoiliac system in selected patients; more recently this technology has provided a valuable means of serially following the changes that occur in renal transplants. Each of these applications is discussed in the following sections.

MESENTERIC VASCULAR DISEASE DETECTION

Before the availability of duplex ultrasonography, arteriography was the only reliable means of assessing the status of the mesenteric vascular system. The diagnosis of mesenteric ischemia in particular was extremely difficult; the guidelines stated that this syndrome was likely to be present if there was severe disease in two of the three major mesenteric vessels. A means of identifying such patients, who usually have obscure symptoms and signs, without necessitating arteriography is urgently needed.

The frequency spectra obtained from the celiac artery are characterized by features similar to those seen in the internal carotid artery, with a high resting flow component during diastole. This is probably related to the fact that the major organs supplied, that is, the liver and spleen, have low resistance vascular beds. Furthermore, this pattern persists after the ingestion of a test meal, again probably related to the fact that the metabolic rate of these major organs remains relatively static throughout a 24-hour period. By contrast, the velocity pattern of the superior mesenteric artery is dependent on the time at which the study is performed. In the fasting state, the spectra are similar to those seen in a peripheral artery with a flow reversal component during diastole, signifying a moderately high

peripheral resistance. With the ingestion of a test meal, however, there is a major change in the shape of the waveform associated with the increase in flow into the superior mesenteric system, and loss of the reverse flow component with the imposition of a major forward flow component[20] (Fig. 7-14). The development of severe stenosis in these vessels is usually seen at the origins, and is associated with marked shifts in the peak systolic frequency and the development of spectral broadening throughout the whole cycle[21] (Fig. 7-15).

It is essential that examination of patients in whom this diagnosis is suspected be performed while they are in the fasting state; even then the examination is quite tedious. Ongoing studies in numerous institutions are addressing the accuracy of duplex ultrasonography in the diagnosis of this problem and will also help to provide important information regarding the natural history of asymptomatic disease in the mesenteric vascular system.

RENAL ARTERY STENOSIS

The detection of hemodynamically significant stenosis of the renal artery remains a major diagnostic dilemma. Currently this involves the use of arteriography to identify a lesion, and the performance of a functional study (renal vein renin ratios) to document the functional significance. Clearly, if a test were available that could identify hemodynamically significant lesions in one step, it would have a major positive impact on our ability to detect such lesions. This particular application of duplex ultrasonography is in an early phase, but already several important observations have been made. It is essential that low transmitting frequencies (3.5 MHz) be used for the evaluation, and that patients also be fasted to avoid the difficulties encountered with large amounts of bowel gas. Multiple approaches to the renal artery may be necessary, including the transxiphoid and lateral approach. Very frequently it is impossible to image the origins of the renal arteries; reliance for sampling is placed solely on the use of the pulsed Doppler and recognition of the characteristic renal artery signals. Currently in our laboratory, approximately 90% of patients can be adequately examined and a definitive decision made regarding the status of the renal arteries.

The characteristic features of flow in the renal arteries are similar to those seen in the internal carotid and celiac vessels. Under normal circumstances, flow during diastole is high without any reversal pattern. Diffuse spectral broadening is a normal component of these spectra. Scanning is also continued into the parenchyma of the kidney, which provides important information regarding the presence of primarily parenchymal disease. Standardization of the signals obtained from the renal arteries is accomplished by expressing the peak systolic frequency as a ratio of the peak systolic frequency in the abdominal aorta immediately proximal to the take-off of the renal arteries. A normal ratio of these parameters has been identified as 1.1 ± 0.3.[22]

The changes produced by high-grade stenosis include elevations of the peak systolic frequency associated with severe diffuse spectral broadening (Fig. 7-16). Sampling in the region of the orifice of the renal artery should be avoided because of the flow disturbances generated by the angle

112

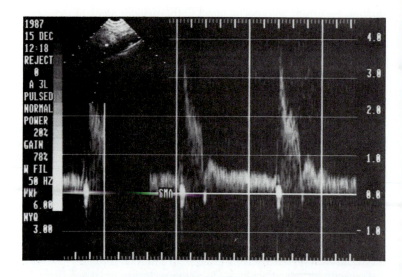

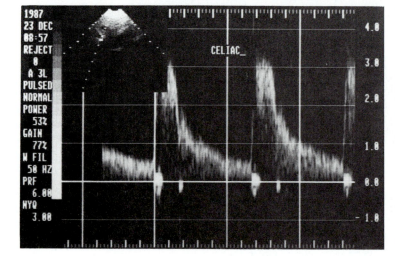

Figure 7-14. Spectra obtained from the normal celiac and superior mesenteric arteries. Note the pattern in the celiac artery with the high diastolic flow component. The superior mesenteric artery has a spectral pattern similar to that seen in a peripheral artery. After ingestion of a test meal (2) the celiac signal remains unchanged but the superior mesenteric artery spectra change dramatically, with a shift in the diastolic forward flow component.

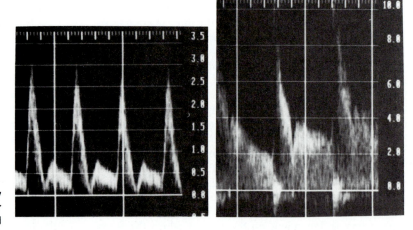

SMA — Fasting   **SMA — Stenosis**

Figure 7-15. Spectra obtained immediately distal to a severe stenosis of the superior mesenteric artery. Note diffuse spectral broadening throughout the cycle and the high peak systolic frequencies. Reverse flow component has also been lost.

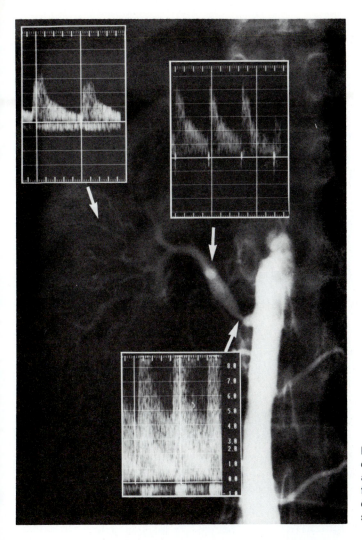

Figure 7-16. Spectra obtained immediately distal to a high-grade stenosis of the renal artery depicted. Note the increase in peak frequency associated with elevation of the diastolic flow component and the diffuse spectral broadening.

of take-off. When present, flow disturbances are usually propagated for some distance along the renal artery, and this is associated with a reduction in the amplitude of the signal in this region. A full examination should involve sampling within the renal parenchyma and estimation of the pole-to-pole length of the kidney.

Preliminary studies comparing duplex ultrasonography to arteriography have documented a diagnostic accuracy of approximately 90% in detecting renal artery stenosis greater than 60% diameter reduction. Because of the difficulty associated with the arteriographic interpretation of disease in these arteries, further studies to measure renin production to establish the relationship between this parameter and the spectral changes outlined above are warranted. Despite the relatively early stage of the application in this area, it has achieved widespread acceptance.

AORTOILIAC OCCLUSIVE DISEASE

Assessment of the hemodynamic significance of atherosclerotic lesions in the aortoiliac segment remains a problem, largely because of the diffuse nature of disease in this loca-

tion. Currently, femoral artery pressures or parameters derived from the femoral velocity waveform have been applied, but both of these methods of assessment have their deficiencies. Preliminary results obtained with duplex scanning of the aortoiliac segment have determined that this technique can be useful and may provide additional information in certain circumstances.

The instrumentation used to assess the aortoiliac segment is similar to that used for the renal and mesenteric vessels. Waveforms are obtained from the distal abdominal aorta, the common iliac, and the external iliac arteries. Normal waveforms are characterized by a triphasic pattern with little or no spectral broadening (Fig. 7-17). Immediately distal to severe stenoses, the waveform becomes monophasic, while the systolic peak is increased by 100% over the resting value,[23] and marked spectral broadening is present (Fig. 7-18). Proximal to these severe stenoses, the peak frequency is reduced. Occlusions are identified by absence of flow in the segment; proximal to the occlusion a characteristic thump is usually audible. Depending on the anatomic status of the collateral circulation, a Doppler signal is usually detectable beyond the area of occlusion, characterized by a very low peak systolic frequency and diffuse spectral

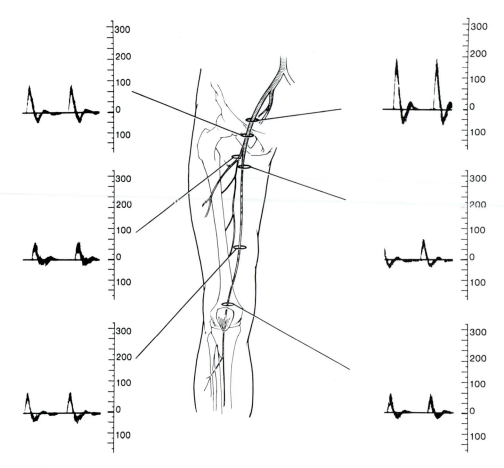

Figure 7-17. Spectra obtained from a normal aortoiliac system. Note the absence of spectral broadening and the reverse flow component in all segments, with a gradual reduction in peak systolic frequency from proximal to distal.

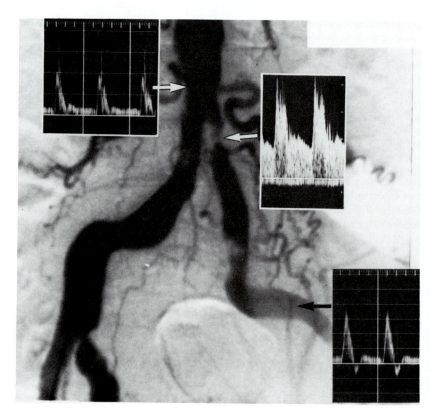

Figure 7-18. Spectra obtained immediately distal to a high-grade stenosis in the iliac artery.

broadening. More distally, the peak frequency may increase due to augmentation of collateral flow, while the spectral broadening may become less apparent. Jager et al.[23] have developed detailed spectral criteria for diagnosing varying degrees of stenosis, and reported good initial results compared to arteriography.

Significant difficulties remain with this method of assessing the aortoiliac segment. Whereas disease in the renal and mesenteric arteries is focal, the aortoiliac involvement is usually diffuse and confuses the interpretation when stenoses in series are present. Access to these vessels is also difficult because of bowel gas, despite having patients fast before studies. Wall calcification is also a major problem in these patients, and further limits the applicability of the technique. The ideal patients for scanning are those with mild claudication, who are likely to have focal stenotic le-

sions that may be suitable for dilatation. Although duplex ultrasonography will have a major impact on the detection of visceral artery lesions, its role in assessing the aortoiliac segment is likely to have only limited application.

RENAL TRANSPLANTATION

Oliguria following renal transplantation poses a diagnostic problem of determining whether this is a consequence of acute tubular necrosis or early rejection. Accurate diagnosis is important because of the different therapies required for each problem. Currently, renal biopsy is the only technique of establishing the diagnosis, but carries with it the attendant risks of potentially severe structural damage to the transplanted kidney. Recent studies in our institution[24] have

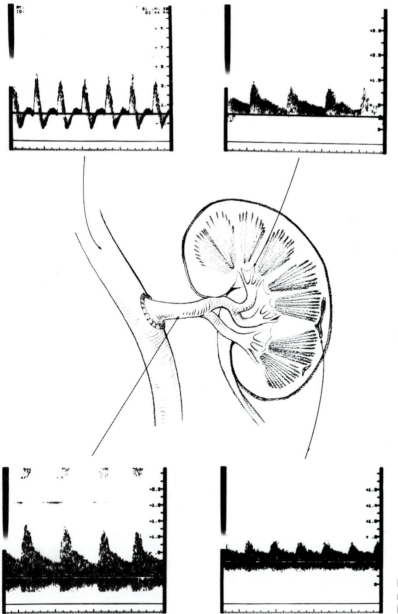

Figure 7-19. Spectra obtained from a normal renal transplant with no rejection or tubular necrosis.

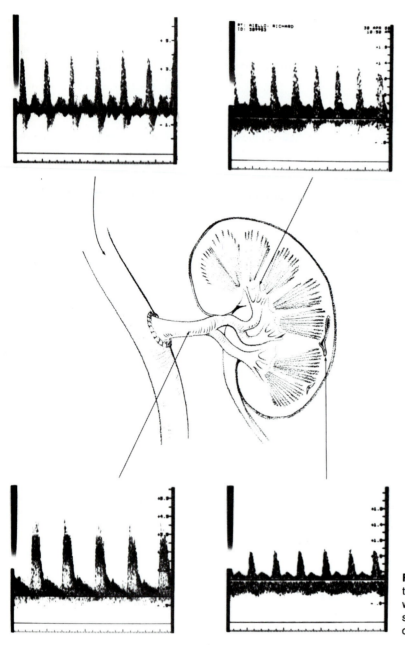

Figure 7-20. Spectra obtained from a renal transplant patient in whom cellular rejection was confirmed by needle biopsy. Note absence of diastolic flow and the intermittent character of the signal.

documented the utility of duplex ultrasonography as a means of differentiating between these two conditions.

The basis for differentiation relates to the pathophysiology of these complications, with renal vascular resistance being increased in cellular rejection and unchanged in tubular necrosis. In the normal kidney, a high diastolic flow component is present (Fig. 7-19), which is lost in cases of rejection and replaced by an abrupt intermittent blunted signal. This change is also detectable into the parenchymal vessels and substantiates the diagnosis (Fig. 7-20). Spectral broadening is usually present throughout because of the small size of the vessels compared to the sample volume size of the Doppler instrumentation. Conversely, in patients in whom the oliguria is produced by acute tubular necrosis, the normal spectral patterns are identifiable in the main renal artery and into the renal cortex. The accuracy of duplex ultrasonography in differentiating between these two conditions may soon make renal biopsy unwarranted.

CONCLUSIONS

Although initially developed as a diagnostic technique for the detection of carotid artery atherosclerosis, duplex ultrasonography is undergoing widespread application for the diagnosis of both arterial and parenchymal disease throughout the body. Although the characteristic flow patterns produced by occlusive disease in the arterial system are now well recognized and are being applied, the interaction between parenchymal disease and alterations in blood flow patterns is only now being explored. This chapter has focused on the applications of this technology, primarily in the areas of arterial disease of most interest to vascular surgeons, but it should be noted that this technology is being widely applied in such diverse areas as the detection of venous thrombosis, evaluation of the portal venous system, particularly in patients with liver disease, and the effect of chemotherapy on solid tissue tumors. The major initial impact of this technology has been in the diagnosis of focal arterial lesions, but the lack of morbidity and the ease of serial examination provide us with a powerful tool to study the natural history of atherosclerosis in multiple areas of the arterial and venous systems.

REFERENCES

1. Hessel SJ, Adams DF, Abrams R: Complications of angiography. Diag Radiol 138:273, 1981.
2. Leopold G: Ultrasonic abdominal aortography. Radiology 96:9, 1970.
3. Kossoff: Gray scale echography in obstetrics and gynecology. Report No. 60, Sydney, Australia, April 1973. Commonwealth Acoustic Laboratories.
4. Olinger CP: Ultrasonic carotid echoarteriography. AJR 106:282, 1969.
5. Barber FE, Baker DW, et al.: Duplex scanner II: For simultaneous imaging of artery tissues and flow. Ultrasonic Symp. Proc. IEEE, No. 74, CHO 8961SU, 1974.
6. Blackshear WM, Phillips DJ, et al.: Detection of carotid occlusive disease by ultrasound imaging and pulsed Doppler spectrum analysis. Surgery 86:698, 1979.
7. Blackshear WM, Phillips DJ, et al.: Carotid artery velocity patterns in normal and stenotic vessels. Stroke 11:67, 1980.
8. Thiele BL, Hutchison KJ, et al.: Pulsed Doppler waveform patterns produced by smooth stenosis in the dog thoracic aorta, in Taylor DEM, Stevens AL (eds): Blood Theory and Practice. New York, Academic Press, 1983.
9. Phillips DJ, Greene FM Jr, et al.: Flow velocity patterns in the carotid bifurcations of young, presumed normal subjects. Ultrasound Med Biol 9:39, 1983.
10. Bodily KC, Zierler RE, et al.: Spectral analysis of Doppler velocity patterns in normals and patients with carotid artery stenosis. Clin Physiol 1:365, 1981.
11. Bodily KC, Phillips DJ, et al.: Noninvasive detection of internal carotid artery occlusion. Angiology 32:517, 1981.
12. Breslau PJ, Knox RA, et al.: Ultrasonic duplex scanning with spectral analysis in extracranial carotid artery disease: Comparison with contrast arteriography. J Appl Radiol 12:81, 1983.
13. Chikos PM, Fischer L, et al.: Observer variability in evaluating extracranial carotid artery stenosis. Stroke 14:885, 1983.
14. Cato RF, Bandyk DF, et al.: Carotid collateral circulation decreases the diagnostic accuracy of duplex scanning. Bruit 10:68, 1986.
15. Roederer GO, Langlois YE, et al.: The natural history of carotid arterial disease in asymptomatic patients with cervical bruits. Stroke 15:605, 1984.
16. Callow AD: Recurrent stenosis after carotid endarterectomy. Arch Surg 117:1082, 1982.
17. Zierler RE, Bandyk DF, et al.: Carotid artery stenosis following endarterectomy. Arch Surg 117:1408, 1982.
18. Thomas M, Otis SM, et al.: Recurrent carotid stenosis following endarterectomy. Ann Surg 200:74, 1984.
19. Stewart GW, Bandyk DF, et al.: Influence of vein patch angioplasty on carotid endarterectomy healing. Arch Surg 122:364, 1987.
20. Jager KA, Bollinger A, et al.: Measurement of mesenteric blood flow by duplex scanning. J Vasc Surg 3:462, 1986.
21. Jager KA, Fortner GA, et al.: Noninvasive diagnosis of intestinal angina. J Clin Ultrasound 12:588, 1984.
22. Kohler TR, Zierler RE, et al.: Noninvasive diagnosis of renal artery stenosis by ultrasonic duplex scanning. J Vasc Surg 4:450, 1986.
23. Jager KA, Phillips DJ, et al.: Noninvasive mapping of lower limb arterial lesions. Ultrasound Med Biol 11:515, 1985.
24. Neumyer MM, Gifford RRM, Thiele BL: Identification of early rejection in renal allografts with duplex ultrasonography. J Vasc Technol J Vasc Technol 12:19, 1988.

CHAPTER 8
Magnetic Resonance Imaging and the Vascular Surgeon

David D. Schmitt and Jonathan B. Towne

The past decade has seen significant growth in noninvasive modalities that evaluate vessel morphology and measure blood flow. New applications of magnetic resonance imaging (MRI) to the arterial system offer the ability to study vessel wall characteristics and measure blood flow velocity, and by MRI spectroscopy, the possibility to study the metabolic environment of the vessel wall. Although MRI images are similar to those obtained by conventional computed axial tomography (CAT) scans, the methods used to obtain the magnetic resonance images are entirely different from those of x-rays. This chapter reviews the principles on which MRI is based and discusses current and proposed clinical applications.

PRINCIPLES OF MRI

Atomic nuclei consist of protons and neutrons that give each atom an intrinsic magnetic movement, with the exception of hydrogen (^{1}H), which has only a single proton. However, when paired particles are present their spins cancel each other, so that a "net" spin is present only when a nucleus contains an odd number of protons, neutrons, or both. In the absence of a magnetic field the axes of these spins are in random directions. When these nuclei are placed in a magnetic field, they act like small bar magnets and become aligned within that field (Fig. 8-1). The space of the magnetic field is usually described in a three-dimensional coordinate system with the Z axis parallel to the magnetic lines of force, and the X and Y axes perpendicular both to the Z axis and to each other. Once aligned in the static magnetic field, the spin alignment of the atoms can be altered, termed *precession*, by applying short bursts of low-level radiofrequency energy from a coil or magnet surrounding the sample. These low-level radiofrequency bursts result in a second magnetic field of lesser strength being applied to the small bar magnets, causing rotation out of the Z axis in the X and Y plane, similar to a spinning gyroscope.

In a static magnetic field of a specific strength the nuclei of a particular element will only respond to certain radio frequencies, termed the *magnetic resonance* or *Lamor frequency* (Fig. 8-2). When the low-level radiofrequency energy is withdrawn, the nuclei realign to the static magnetic field, termed *relaxation*. This results in emission of radiofrequency energy dependent on the strength of the static magnetic field, the density of the atom, and two relaxation parameters: T1 (longitudinal realignment time) and T2 (transverse realignment time). T1 and T2 are also dependent on local chemical and physical factors, including molecular structure, elemental composition, temperature, and viscosity. In summary, MRI is based on the ability to induce and measure radiofrequency energy emitted from atomic nuclei placed in a magnetic field.[1–4]

Many elements are found in high enough concentrations in the body to be studied with MRI. These include hydrogen, sodium, phosphorus, calcium, oxygen, carbon, chlorine, and potassium. Hydrogen is the element most often studied with MRI because it has both the greatest sensitivity for alignment in a static magnetic field and greatest sensitivity for altering that alignment with precession. It is also easy to study because it is the most abundant element in the body. The other elements have lower inherent MRI sensitivity and lower physical concentration than hydrogen, making it difficult to use these nuclei in clinical imaging. Two elements other than hydrogen that are used to study the vascular system are calcium and phosphorus. The presence of calcium in arterial plaques and phosphorus in the form of AMP (adenosine monophosphate), ADP (adenosine diphosphate), and ATP (adenosine triphosphate) may make these elements important in the future of vessel imaging and in the study of vessel wall and tissue metabolism using MRI.

Magnet strengths currently used in imaging are in the range of 0.3 to 1.5 Tesla (T)* whereas magnets used only to measure flow are smaller, ranging from 0.1 to 0.15 T.

---

*Tesla: unit of magnetic flux density in the meter-kilogram-second system (equivalent to 1 weber per square meter).

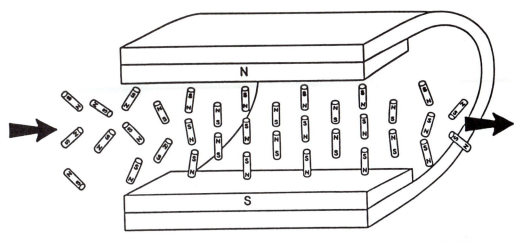

Figure 8-1. Nuclei in blood represented as small bar magnets align with the magnetic field.

Because phosphorus and carbon, the elements used for spectroscopy, have only a fraction of the magnetic sensitivity of hydrogen (phosphorus 6.7% and carbon 1.6%), larger magnets are needed, which only recently have become available.[5]

CLINICAL APPLICATIONS OF MRI

The use of MRI in assessment of the vascular surgery patient is twofold: quantitating blood flow and evaluating the arterial system architecture.

Blood Flow Scanning Using MRI

More than a decade before MRI was first used to obtain images in patients, Lauterbur[6] and Singer[7] demonstrated the ability to measure blood flow using magnetic resonance. This type of imaging system has two components: the main MR unit and the computer work station. The combined weight of the system is 3500 pounds, necessitating that the floor have sufficient concentrating load capabilities. The room must be at least 15 by 15 feet and located 50 feet

from elevators, vehicular traffic, and loading docks, or concurrently operated ultrasound systems to prevent interference. Magnet size for this type of scanner is approximately 0.1 T. Several scanners for quantitative blood flow have been developed (Fig. 8-3).

The physics principles on which MRI blood flow scanners are based differ slightly from MRI scanners used for angiographic evaluation.[4,8,9] Precession of hydrogen atoms in flowing blood results in the release of small amounts of energy detected in the scanner's central sensing region. The strength of the signal is directly proportional to the number of hydrogen atoms traversing the region being scanned. This signal strength correlates with the flow of blood through the area. Precession in blood flow scanners is achieved with continuous 8 kHz pulsations rather than short intermittent burst of radiofrequency energy.

The limb is initially scanned in two dimensions and the vessels identified and localized (Fig. 8-4). Only pulsed forward flow is evaluated by filtering out venous flow data with the computer software program. The sensory region, or voxel, can then be adjusted from scanning the entire limb to looking at an individual artery. The smallest area that can be examined currently is a cylinder 7.5 mm in diameter and 5 cm in length. The initial scanning provides

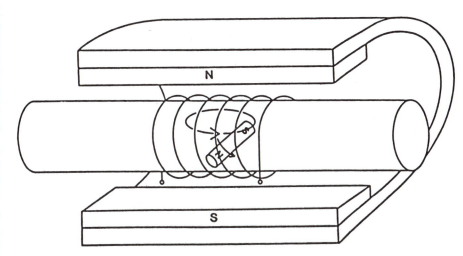

Figure 8-2. Precession of nuclei at the Lamor frequency.

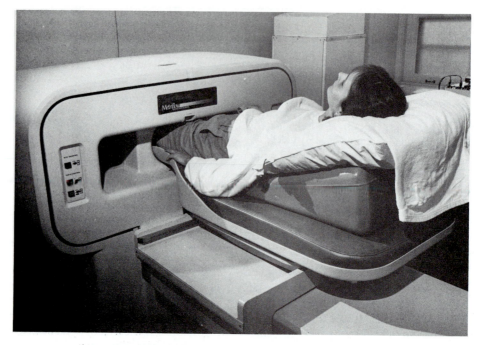

Figure 8-3. Metriflow Medical System Scanner at Medical College of Wisconsin.

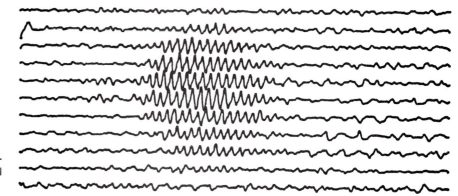

Figure 8-4. Raw flow scanning data generated by a system scan of a normal popliteal artery.

a display of arteries in a cross-section of the limb and identifies sources of flow within the limb. The computer generates a color-coded image to aid in vessel localization (Fig. 8-5). A pulsed flow wave can then be obtained by summation of peak frequency disturbances occurring within the area being scanned (Fig. 8-6). From this waveform, peak systolic flow is determined in milliliters per minute. The computer software allows for filtering of frequency disturbances from nonpulsed sources such as vasa vasorum and veins.

The potential clinical applications are numerous, ranging from evaluation of patients with lower limb occlusive disease to surveillance of leg grafts postoperatively for the development of lesions that would result in graft thrombosis if not corrected.

At the Medical College of Wisconsin, we use a Metriflow Medical Systems AMF 100 MR Blood Flow Scanner. Before applying this scanner to clinical work, it was tested in normal controls and correlated to strain-gauge plethys-

mography (SGP) (venous occlusion technique).[*] Limb blood flow was measured in both legs of 10 normal volunteers on 5 different days. Limb flow rates were 101 ± 35 ml/min (SGP) and 93 ± 21 ml/min (MR). The coefficients of variance (standard deviation/mean) were 34% (SGP) and 21% (MR). Although the measurements were similar, the variability of the MR flows were less.

We use the MR Blood Flow Scanner to follow patients who have had in situ saphenous vein bypass grafts for lower extremity ischemia. Patients are studied preoperatively for baseline flow, and then serially postoperatively. The results of five patients who have been followed postoperatively are shown in Table 8-1. We use flow data from the MRI scanner in conjunction with other noninvasive

---

[*]Salles-Cunha S, Tolan D: Evaluation of a magnetic resonance scanner (submitted abstract).

Angiographic Evaluation

Clinical angiographic evaluation of the vascular system using MRI is still in the experimental stages and is only available at a few research centers.[2,5] Nevertheless, this appears to be one of the most impressive advancements in noninvasive diagnostic imaging. Magnets for angiographic evaluation are usually 1.5 T and weigh more than 6 tons. This is a magnet strength 10 times that used for evaluation in blood flow scanning. Because of the magnet's strength, all metal objects must be kept more than 50 feet away, or they become missiles directed toward the magnet when the magnet is activated. MRI can visualize the anatomic detail of vessels because the contrast between flowing blood and vessel walls is precisely defined along luminal contours. Plaques are easily imaged because they project into the lumen and contain lipids and calcium that produce specific signals that allow for image enhancement.

To date experimental work has primarily centered on evaluation of the carotid-vertebral and aortoiliac systems (Fig. 8-7). Abdominal aortic aneurysms can easily be imaged. The ability to identify intraluminal, noncalcified thrombus, as well as vessel wall thickness and extent of disease (either aneurysmal or occlusive) in secondary visceral vessels remains to be developed.

Venous imaging is also possible with MRI and has allowed the evaluation of the vena cava and mesenteric veins. With refinement of the technology, it should be possible to use MRI to diagnose thrombosis of the subclavian, iliofemoral system, and to determine patency of portasystemic shunts.

The use of MRI for cardiac evaluation has been complicated by the intrinsic motion of the heart. Gating the images with cardiac and respiratory cycles has enhanced the imaging ability; however, presently only 30 to 50% of patients can have either their coronary arteries or vein bypass grafts visualized using the current techniques.[5]

Compared to conventional angiography, MRI does not require irradiation or contrast material, eliminating the very

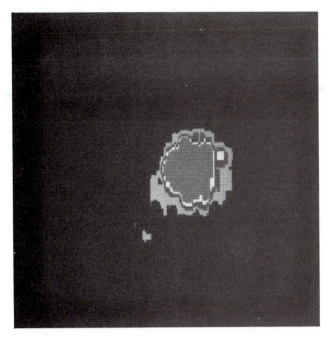

Figure 8-5. Computer-generated, color-coded image to represent the volume blood flow rate.

modalities including spectral analysis, ankle-brachial indexes, and toe pressures to establish the patient's baseline for following graft patency and to determine the accuracy of MRI compared to these other noninvasive measurements.

The potential advantages of MRI are the ease with which the exam is performed, and the noninvasive nature of the study. Patients need only lay supine while the extremity is being scanned. The examination takes approximately 45 minutes to complete. Technical error is greatly reduced because scanning is computerized. However, a technician is responsible for calibration before scanning and for voxel determination.

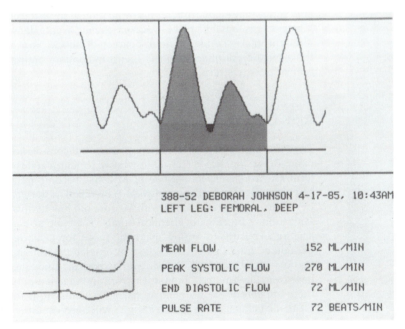

388-52 DEBORAH JOHNSON 4-17-85, 10:43AM
LEFT LEG: FEMORAL, DEEP

MEAN FLOW	152 ML/MIN
PEAK SYSTOLIC FLOW	270 ML/MIN
END DIASTOLIC FLOW	72 ML/MIN
PULSE RATE	72 BEATS/MIN

Figure 8-6. Waveform obtained from summation of peak frequency disturbances, enabling determination of peak systolic flow.

TABLE 8-1. CLINICAL RESULTS OF MRI FOLLOWING IN SITU BYPASS

Patient	Type of Bypass Performed	ABI	Toe Pressure (mm/Hg)	Spectral Analysis* Graft Velocity (cm/sec)	MRI Flow (ml/min) Whole Limb	Graft
1	Right femoropopliteal	1.01	80	AK—52	BK—57	BK—45
2	Left femoroperoneal	0.96	80	AK—51 K—51 BK—50	BK—62	BK—42
3	Left femoroperoneal	1.17	90	AK—52 BK—48	BK—94	BK—60
4	Right femoropopliteal	1.03	90	AK—60 BK—64	BK—65	BK—52
5	Right femoropopliteal	0.94	120	AK—60	BK—62	BK—49

* All triphasic waveforms.
ABI, ankle-brachial index; AK, above knee; BK, below knee; K, knee.

real risks of nephrotoxicity and allergic reactions. The noninvasive nature of the process significantly decreases patient discomfort and thereby increases patient compliance when repeated examinations are needed. The method of examination also allows images to be obtained in the transverse, sagittal, and coronal planes. There are, however, drawbacks to the use of MRI in anatomical imaging: the tortuous path followed by most vessels usually requires obtaining several different views to demonstrate the entire length of a vessel. Image resolution is also limited because images are obtained in 1.0 to 1.5 cm thick slices, resulting in loss of detail due to considerable computer averaging. Finally, the expense

of this technique may be a limiting factor. The MRI machine itself costs approximately two million dollars, and requires construction of a special building with a limited amount of metal material. Also, personnel required to operate the system will need to be trained. The cost of an examination will probably exceed 1000 dollars.

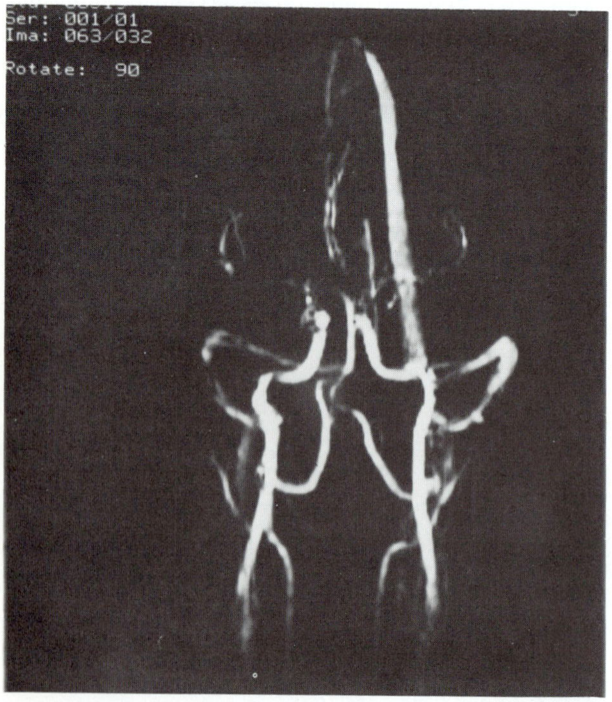

Spectroscopy

A third clinical application of MRI is the use of spectroscopy to study the metabolism of the vessel wall and the surrounding tissue environment and its effect on the evolution of vascular diseases. As previously noted, calcium and phosphorus are the two elements other than hydrogen that hold the most potential in MRI spectroscopy. Spectroscopy not only can identify and quantitate these elements in the tissues being studied but also can detect changes in concentration over time. MRI evaluation of the phosphorus spectrum allows for quantitative analysis of AMP, ADP, and ATP, and other organic an inorganic compounds.[1,5] This ability to quantitatively determine changing concentrations of energy stores may enable differential evaluation of the intracellular changes that take place in acute ischemic events, long-term chronic ischemia, various degrees of shock, and in the evaluation of pharmacologic agents in relation to intracellular energy stores.

Figure 8-7. Combined arterial and venous phase cerebral image. (*Courtesy General Electric Corporate Research and Development Center.*)

RISK OF MRI

The term *nuclear magnetic resonance* carries the connotation of anything "nuclear." Hence, to waylay patient fears, the term *magnetic resonance imaging* or MRI has become more popular, since no ionizing radiation is involved in the process. The energies associated with MRI are too low to cause ionization or breaking of chemical bonds. The biologic hazards of exposure to strong magnetic fields for extended periods of time has been studied by England's National Radiological Protection Board, and exposure guidelines have been determined.[3] From their work and that of others, there appears to be no biologic risk to patients from the magnetic fields used to date. This area will need continued evaluation as larger, more powerful magnets become commercially available.

Specific patient limitations presently deal primarily with indwelling metal devices. Patients with pacemakers are not imaged because the magnetic field may reprogram or shut off the pacemaker. Patients who have had prior surgery with the insertion of intracerebral metal clips or intraspinal nerve-stimulating devices are not imaged for fear of causing damage from migration of the metal in the magnetic field. However, the presence of intra-abdominal metal clips, metal prostheses in extremities, or even metal cardiac valves is not felt to be a contraindication to MRI.

FUTURE APPLICATIONS

The future clinical applications of MRI appear encouraging. As software programs become more advanced, imaging resolution should increase. The current limitation of flow detection is flow 10 to 15 cm/sec. In the future, even slower flows may be discernible, permitting more detailed evaluation of both arterial and venous flow patterns. Postoperative flow determination in grafts and endarterectomized vessels will be done with greater ease. By being able to determine the flow rates in various runoff vessels, MRI may be useful in vessel selection for distal bypasses. MRI may also be used to determine whether lesions seen on arteriography are truly flow-limiting. Magnets for digital flow are being developed that may allow evaluation of vasospastic disorders such as Raynaud's syndrome.

CONCLUSIONS

Magnetic resonance imaging techniques are being applied to clinical situations in many areas of medicine. From the demonstration of vascular structures, including evaluation of vessel wall composition, to quantitative flow determinations, MRI is beginning to play an increasing role in the therapeutic decision making involving the vascular surgery patient. This role is likely to be even more prominent in the future.

REFERENCES

1. Pylcett IL, Newhouse JH, et al.: Principles of nuclear magnetic resonance imaging. Radiology 143:152, 1982.
2. Dumoulin CL, Hart HR: Magnetic resonance angiography. Radiology 161:717, 1986.
3. James AE, Partain CL, et al.: Nuclear magnetic resonance imaging: The current state. AJR 138:201, 1982.
4. Mills CM, Brant-Zawadcki M, et al.: Nuclear magnetic resonance: Principles of blood flow imaging. AJR 142:165, 1984.
5. Rhodes RS, Cohen AM: Magnetic resonance imaging and spectroscopy in the study of cardiovascular disease. J Vasc Surg 2:354, 1985.
6. Lauterbur PC: Image formation by induced local interactions: Examples employing NMR. Nature 242:190, 1973.
7. Singer JR: Blood flow rates by NMR measurements. Science 130:1652, 1959.
8. Kaufman L, Crooks L, et al.: The potential impact of nuclear magnetic resonance imaging on cardiovascular diagnosis. Circulation 67:251, 1983.
9. Battocletti JH. Blood flow measurement by NMR. CRC Crit Rev Bioeng 13:(4)311, 1986.

CHAPTER 9
Isotope Angiography in Evaluation of Peripheral Vascular Disease

Amiel Z. Rudavsky

Until the recent introduction of minimally invasive techniques, the accurate evaluation of the integrity of native, transplanted, or surgically repaired arteries and veins required invasive procedures. Thus, isotope angiography, ultrasonography, digital intravenous angiography, computed tomography, and plethysmography have supplemented and even supplanted contrast angiography in many instances. The accuracy, safety, ease, and relative patient comfort of these procedures have popularized their use as diagnostic and screening procedures and for periodic evaluation of vessels and vascular segments.

Isotope angiography is one of the simplest, least invasive, quickest, and most reliable of the commonly available imaging techniques. It utilizes equipment and radiopharmaceuticals available in virtually every hospital, requires no special patient preparation, takes little time to perform and interpret, is virtually painless (except for venipuncture), carries a low radiation burden, is extremely safe, and is relatively inexpensive. Its accuracy and reproducibility have been validated in studies of over 800 arterial segments. Isotope angiography is capable of visualizing flow in vessels as large as the aorta and as small as the digital arteries of the hand. It has been effectively used for the diagnosis and evaluation of vascular trauma, vascular occlusion and stenosis, bypass and shunt integrity, and false and true aneurysms. It has been accepted as a reliable diagnostic procedure in many institutions throughout the world.

HISTORY

Isotope angiography became feasible with the development of the modern gamma camera in the late 1960s. Several authors described the application of this instrument to visualize flow in various parts of the vascular tree after the injection of the then newly available radiopharmaceutical technetium-99m pertechnetate.[1-4] Freeman and Mindelzun were among the first to describe a group of patients studied for a particular vascular problem (aortic aneurysms) using isotope angiography.[5] These authors, as well as Dibos et al.,[6] Meindok,[7] Kappert and Rosler,[8] Hurlow et al.,[9-11] and Diamond et al.[12] demonstrated the excellent correlation of isotope angiograms with established modalities such as contrast arteriography and direct visualization at surgery.

In 1974 a surgical colleague (Charles M. Moss, M.D.) and I were reviewing the dynamic phase of a renal scan performed following the insertion of an aortorenal bypass graft. We noted the clear demonstration of the patent bypass graft as well as excellent perfusion of the involved kidney. This study called to mind the capability of radionuclides to provide excellent visualization of the aorta and iliac and femoral arteries in studies performed for the evaluation of blood flow and viability of renal transplants.[13,14] Because we were working in a municipal hospital with severely limited facilities for radiographic arteriography and which served an inner-city population with a high incidence of vascular trauma, we wondered whether we could develop an accurate scintigraphic technique to evaluate the integrity of the major arteries of the limbs and trunk. We were fortunate in being able to refine isotope angiography to visualize arteries as peripheral as the digital vessels of the fingers. We were able to show that isotope angiography is useful in the demonstration and evaluation of various forms of vascular disease, including stenoses, obstructions, injuries, grafts, and repairs.[15-30]

VALIDATION

Acceptance of a new procedure is predicated on demonstration of its safety, ease of performance, patient acceptability, and most importantly, its accuracy and reliability. Several million patients undergo isotopic imaging studies each year. Because of their noninvasive nature, these studies are essentially free of morbidity and mortality except for extremely rare instances of allergic reactions to the nonradioactive moieties of the injected radiopharmaceuticals. Virtually all allergic reactions have been reported in studies using radiopharmaceuticals containing albumin, dextrans, or sulfur colloid; these substances are rarely used in isotope angiography.

The accuracy and reliability of isotope arteriography have been evaluated in 555 patient studies in which 867 arterial segments were visualized.[29] Contrast arteriography, or surgery, or both were performed in 192 of these patients. In 104 instances the positive findings of the isotope arteriograms were confirmed; in 88 cases the negative interpretation of the nuclear technique was corroborated. In only five instances in this group of 192 patients was there a discrepancy between the results of isotope arteriography and contrast angiography or surgery. These five isotope studies were false positives rather than false negatives; thus no abnormalities were missed by the isotope arteriogram. Four of the five false positives occurred before we had become experienced in the interpretation of the studies. In each of these four cases the false-positive interpretation was due to an abnormality noted on the static phase (see Techniques below) of an isotope study performed more than 24 hours after arterial trauma was sustained. We have subsequently learned that such abnormalities may be artifactual (see p 126). The results of 358 additional isotope arteriograms were compared to the results of long-term (greater than 3 months) clinical follow-up. Ninety-four studies revealed abnormalities that were determined to be relatively minor; although confirmed by clinical examination, they were not considered serious enough to require contrast angiography or surgical intervention. The remaining 264 isotope arteriograms was interpreted as normal, and this impression was confirmed by clinical follow-up in every instance. Thus, our experience with these 555 isotope arteriograms validates the accuracy and reliability of the technique. In this group of isotope arteriograms, the sensitivity (defined as the number of true-positive studies divided by the total number of true-positive and false-negative studies) was 100%. Likewise, the specificity (defined as the number of true-negative studies divided by the total number of true-negative and false-positive studies) was between 95 and 99%.

TECHNIQUE

Arterial Studies

Isotope angiography is easily performed utilizing radiopharmaceuticals and instruments commonly available in virtually every nuclear medicine facility. Any technetium-99m preparation that has a significant intravascular residence time is suitable. Thus technetium-99m pertechnetate, glucoheptonate, or diethylenetriaminepentaacetic acid are all suitable agents for isotope angiography. However, either in vivo or in vitro tagged red blood cells yield the best quality static images, and it is suggested that this preparation be used whenever possible. Adequate tagging of red blood cells may be achieved by injecting the patient with a "cold" stannous phosphate compound about 20 minutes before to the intravenous administration of technetium-99m pertechnetate in a dose of 10 to 25 mCi.[31] When it is anticipated that two discrete regions will be imaged within a short time of each other, as may occur in instances of multiple trauma or when several vascular grafts have been inserted in the same patient, either technetium-99m macroaggregated serum albumin or technetium-99m sulfur colloid are the preferred imaging agents. Because these agents are rapidly sequestered in the lungs and liver, respectively, background radioactivity outside these areas is minimal, allowing almost immediate reinjection and reimaging with the same or another agent. Because of the rapid selective organ uptake of these radiopharmaceuticals, satisfactory static images cannot be obtained when they are used but adequate dynamic isotope angiograms can be obtained when 5 to 10 mCi of either agent is administered.

To obtain a satisfactory dynamic isotope angiogram, the radioactivity must be administered as a relatively intact bolus. A modification of the Oldendorf injection technique is effective in delivering a satisfactory bolus of radioactivity.[32] After carefully positioning the patient under the gamma camera detector, a blood pressure cuff with a hook or Velcro closure is applied to the patient's arm and inflated above the systolic pressure. Venipuncture of an appropriate vein in the medial aspect of the antecubital fossa is performed and injection of the entire bolus of the radiopharmaceutical (preferably in a volume of 1 ml or less) is completed before the rapid release of the sphygomomanometer cuff. The needle is removed from the vein after the cuff is released. The gamma camera and (when available) the dedicated computer or data recorder are activated coincident with release of the cuff, and serial images of the flow of activity are obtained for the first 100 seconds after the appearance of radioactivity in the field of view. Acquisition of one or more 300,000-count static images starting about 5 minutes after injection completes the study. After the study the images are replayed and reframed, if necessary, to optimize image quality. Framing rates between 1 and 6 seconds are used, depending on the flow characteristics of the visualized arterial tree and the administered dose of radioactivity. Creating a closed-loop movie of the dynamic phase of the study (analogous to the cine mode employed in multiple gated cardiac studies) often facilitates interpretation of the isotope angiogram.

Venous Studies

Performing isotope venography is similar to acquiring isotope arteriograms. Although several agents have been used for isotope venography, technetium-99m-tagged red blood cells are preferred.[33] This radiopharmaceutical preferentially remains within the high-volume venous circulation after injection and redistribution. The injection is made into a vein distal to the site of the suspected venous occlusion whenever possible, using a modified Oldendorf technique. Both dynamic and static images are acquired. An important advantage of using technetium-99m-tagged red blood cells is the possibility of subsequently visualizing radioactivity in veins distant from the initially imaged region, thus detecting occlusions in more than one part of the venous system with a single injection. This can be achieved by acquiring additional static images after the initial study.

INTERPRETATION

Arterial Studies

Interpretation of the dynamic phase of isotope arteriograms is relatively easy and straightforward. In a normal study there is smooth, uninterrupted flow of the column of radioactivity within the major arterial channels in the field of view. Any accumulation of radioactivity outside the vessel indicates extravasation and is suggestive of disruption of the arterial wall. Localized widening of the column of radioactivity may indicate true or false aneurysmal dilatation of the vessel, whereas narrowing of the column is compatible with stenosis. Either a delay or "hang-up" in the flow of activity from one part of the visualized vessel to a contiguous section or a localized decrease in activity suggests significant stenoses or occlusion. An abrupt "cut-off" of the column of activity indicates vessel occlusion or disruption. Deviation of the flow of radioactivity from the normal course of the artery may be due to extrinsic pressure on the vessel from a hematoma, abscess, clot, tumor, or area of inflammation. These lesions may also give rise to focal regions of decreased activity on static images.

The normal static image of the isotope arteriogram shows the larger vessels of the arterial tree against a relatively homogenous background of activity. When both the static and dynamic phases of the isotope arteriogram are normal, the study can confidently be interpreted as negative, irrespective of any temporal relation to surgery or possible vessel trauma. However, the situation is complicated in instances when the dynamic phase of the study appears normal but the static images reveal a localized accumulation of activity outside established vascular channels. In our experience the appearance of such extravascular activity on the static image reliably indicates extravasation or false aneurysm formation if the study has been obtained within 24 hours of surgery, or possible vascular trauma. Isotope arteriograms performed more than 24 hours after such an event may display an accumulation of activity on the static phase due to inflammation or infection rather than to any actual disruption in vessel integrity. Thus, isotope arteriograms with a normal dynamic phase but abnormal static phase may be "false positives" and must be interpreted with caution. This pitfall in interpretation was not recognized in our early experience with isotope angiography and caused four of the five false-positive studies mentioned in the Validation discussion on p 124.

Venous Studies

Interpretation of the dynamic phase of venous studies is based on the criteria outlined for arterial studies. Often collateral veins may be demonstrated, especially when there has been long-standing stenosis or occlusion of major venous channels.

Static venous images delineate the distribution of activity in the major veins of the trunk and limbs following equilibration of the tagged red blood cells in the circulation because most intravascular blood resides in the venous system. Thus, static venous images may reveal the absence of a normal venous pattern as well as the establishment of alternate venous channels, either due to collateralization or graft insertion. Because tagged red blood cells preferentially remain within the venous system, multiple images of the veins of various parts of the body may be obtained.

APPLICATIONS

Isotope angiography is a useful modality for the diagnosis and evaluation of the integrity of major vascular channels in the body. It is often used as the primary screening procedure in suspected vascular disease and, if positive, usually leads to the performance of an invasive, but more definitive, diagnostic procedure such as contrast angiography. When negative, it frequently obviates the need for further investigation.

Isotopic brain scans were common procedures until the introduction of computed tomography. The dynamic phase of the brain scan is capable of demonstrating patency of the carotid arteries. With a modification of this routine technique, extravasation due to carotid artery trauma can be clearly demonstrated by isotope angiography (Fig. 9-1). Images of the normal brachial artery and its division into the radial and ulnar arteries (Fig. 9-2) contrast sharply with those obtained in studies of antecubital trauma (Fig. 9-3) and brachial artery fistulas (Fig. 9-4). Decreased perfusion of portions of the hand because of obstruction at the level of the distal radial or ulnar artery may be clearly demonstrated (Fig. 9-5). Isotope angiograms obtained in cases of digital reimplantation following trauma have shown that patent digital arteries are not a prerequisite for a successful outcome (Fig. 9-6). Aortic and peripheral artery aneurysms may be diagnosed preoperatively, and the results of surgery evaluated (Fig. 9-7). Occlusion of the iliac system (Fig.

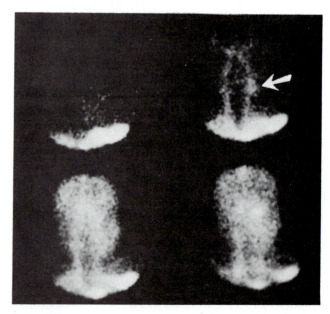

Figure 9-1. Serial 5-second images from a dynamic isotope angiogram demonstrating extravasation (*arrow*) from the left carotid artery of a 63-year-old man with a stab wound to the left neck.

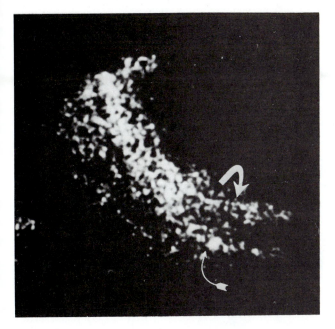

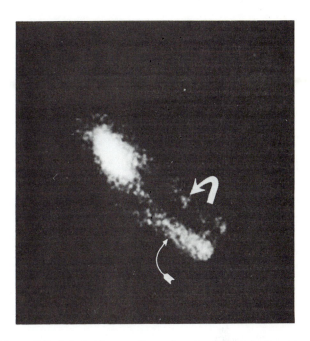

Figure 9-2. Selected 3-second image from the normal dynamic iso-tope arteriogram of the antecubital region of a 33-year-old woman. Note the brachial artery bifurcating into the radial artery (*large arrow*) and ulnar artery (*small arrow*).

Figure 9-3. Selected 3-second image from the dynamic isotope arte-riogram of a man with a stab wound to the antecubital fossa. Note the presence of a false aneurysm at the brachial artery bifurcation, with adequate flow in the ulnar artery (*small arrow*) but poor visualiza-tion of the radial artery (*large arrow*).

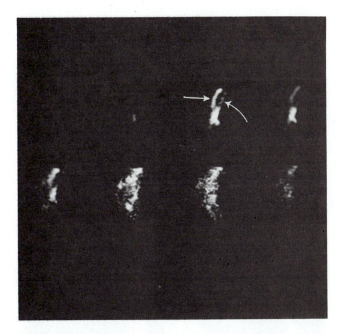

Figure 9-4. Serial 2-second images from the dynamic isotope angio-gram of a 23-year-old man with a stab wound to the left antecubital fossa with development of a false aneurysm that was repaired at another facility. The patient was first seen with a pulsatile antecubital fossa mass that proved to be a postsurgical arteriovenous fistula between the brachial artery (*straight arrow*) and the cephalic vein (*curved arrow*).

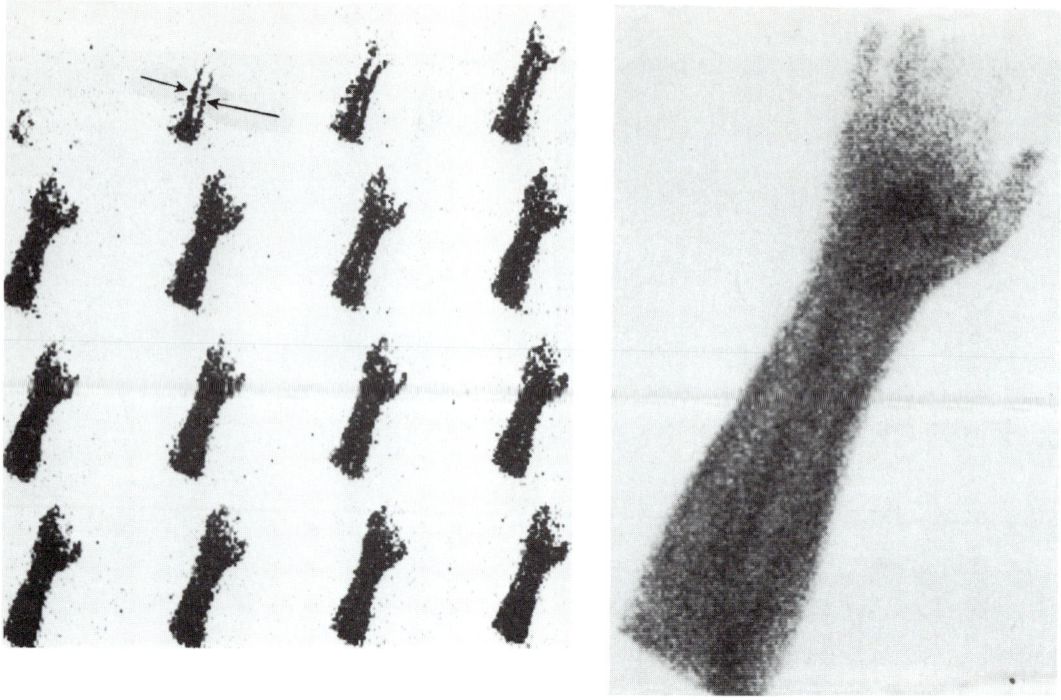

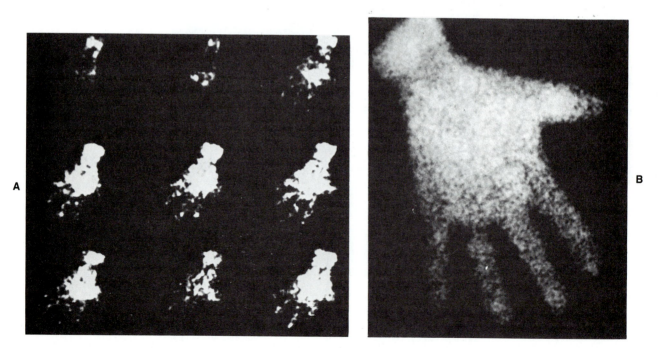

Figure 9-5. Isotope arteriogram of the right wrist and hand of a 30-year-old man obtained about 1 year after he sustained a laceration of his right wrist. He was noted to have a cool hand and fingers. **A.** Serial dynamic 3-second images show adequate activity in both the radial (*large arrow*) and ulnar (*small arrow*) arteries to the level of the wrist laceration. Distal activity in the distribution of the ulnar artery appears adequate but there is little activity in the radial artery and its distribution distal to the wrist, suggesting occlusion of that vessel, confirmed by contrast arteriography. **B.** Static image from the same study demonstrates markedly decreased perfusion of the radial artery distribution in the hand.

Figure 9-6. Isotope angiogram of the hand of a middle-aged dentist obtained after microsurgical reimplantation of his left thumb, which was traumatically amputated. At the time of the study the patient had returned to his dental practice and had fairly good use of the reimplanted thumb. **A.** Serial 5-second dynamic images show essentially absent perfusion of the thumb in all images. **B.** Static image shows that activity in the thumb at equilibrium is comparable to that of the four digits not operated on. Note the photon-deficient band on the ring finger representing photon attenuation by the patient's wedding ring. Capillary and collateral circulation was apparently sufficient to sustain the viability of the reimplanted thumb, suggesting that digital artery patency is not a prerequisite for the survival of reimplanted digits.

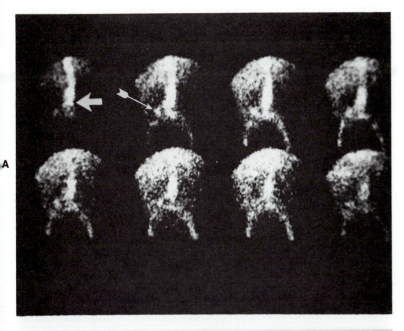

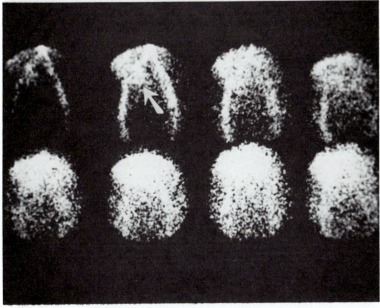

Figure 9-7. Dynamic isotope arteriograms of a 77-year-old man who was admitted because of a pulsatile abdominal mass. **A.** Serial 2½-second images demonstrate accumulation and outpouching of activity just proximal to the aortic bifurcation, suggesting an aortic aneurysm (*large arrow*) with probable extension into the right iliac system (*small arrow*). **B.** Serial 5-second images obtained after placement of an aortic bypass graft. Note extravasation of radioactivity at the level of the anastamosis between the graft and the right iliac system, (*arrow*) and decreased activity in the left iliac system. These findings were corroborated at surgery.

9-8) and traumatic iliac artery disruption (Fig. 9-9) can be clearly differentiated from the normal iliofemoral system (Fig. 9-10). The development of a femoral artery false aneurysm after cardiac catheterization may be documented without performing an additional invasive procedure (Fig. 9-11). Periodic confirmation of the continued patency of vascular grafts can be confirmed (Figs. 9-12 and 9-13). Bleeding into and clotting within aneurysms of peripheral vessels may often be accurately diagnosed (Fig. 9-14). Lower limb

arteries as distal as the anterior tibial vessel may easily be imaged (Fig. 9-15). Thrombosis within the venous system (Fig. 9-16) and patency of venous bypass grafts (Fig. 9-17) may be demonstrated.

These illustrations represent a less than comprehensive listing of the indications for isotope angiography in the evaluation of vascular integrity. The imaginative physician will find may applications for this procedure besides those discussed here and in the literature.

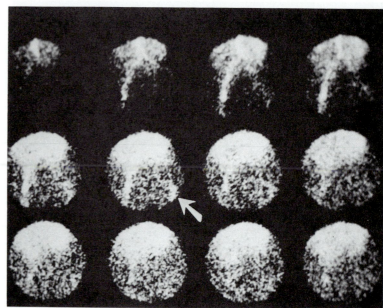

Figure 9-8. Dynamic isotope angiogram of an 84-year-old man who had bounding right femoral pulses but faint to absent pulses in the left groin. The patient's clinical diagnosis was a possible right femoral artery aneurysm. The serial 2-second images show normal flow of activity in the right iliac artery but significantly decreased activity in the left iliac system. Distal reconstitution of the left iliac system (*arrow*) is apparent. High-grade stenosis of the left iliac system was confirmed at surgery.

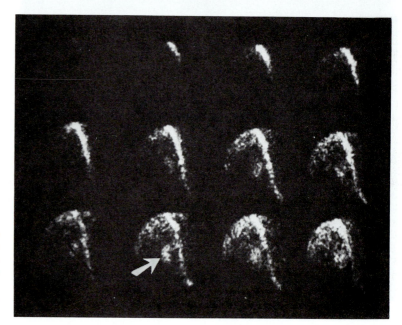

Figure 9-9. Serial 2-second images from the dynamic isotope angiogram of a 52-year-old man with a gunshot wound to the left thigh 4 days before examination. Extravasation of activity from the femoral vessels is demonstrated (*arrow*). The vessel laceration was surgically repaired.

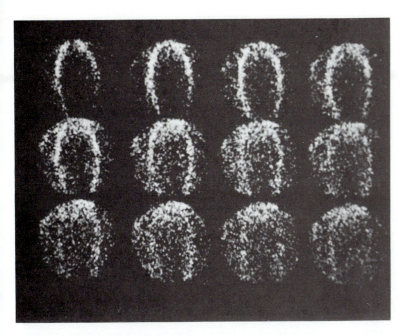

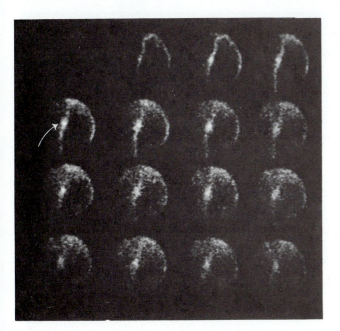

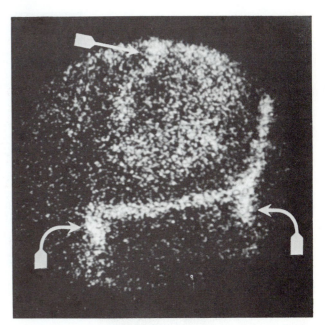

Figure 9-10. Serial 3-second images from the normal dynamic isotope angiogram of the groins and thighs of a 30-year-old man with a superficial grazing gunshot wound to the right groin. Note symmetrical, smooth, and uninterrupted flow of activity in the major vessels bilaterally. Only background activity is noted outside the borders of the major arteries.

Figure 9-11. Dynamic isotope angiogram obtained in a 48-year-old man 4 days after he had cardiac catheterization via the right femoral route. A pulsatile mass was noted at the site of the arterial puncture (*arrow*). Serial 2-second images show a discrete area of increased activity consistent with a false aneurysm; the patient subsequently had successful surgical repair of the false aneurysm.

Figure 9-12. Selected 3-second image from the dynamic isotope angiogram of the lower abdomen and groin of a 72-year-old man performed 2 weeks after insertion of a axillary bifemoral bypass graft because of aortic occlusion. This image shows patency of the distal limbs of the graft (*curved arrows*) and, by inference, its patency over its entire length. The distal stub of the occluded aorta is also seen (*straight arrow*).

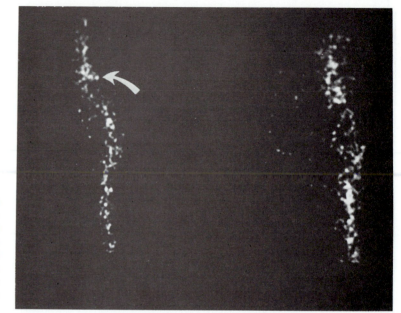

Figure 9-13. Serial 4-second images from the dynamic isotope angiogram of a 61-year-old woman with a right femoral to small vessel bypass graft. Note patency of graft with some displacement of the column of activity distal to the site of anastamosis of the graft with the native vessel (*arrow*) but without evidence of extravasation or aneurysm formation.

Figure 9-14. Isotope angiogram of the left popliteal region of a 73-year-old man with a history of aneurysms of the aorta and both femoral arteries who was initially seen with a soft-tissue mass proximal to the knee. **A.** Selected 4-second dynamic image shows a focal area of markedly increased activity in the proximal portion of the palpable mass (*arrow*), with draping of the major arterial channel around the mass. **B.** Static image shows a large halo of decreased activity surrounding the area of increased activity; the mass corresponded to the areas of abnormal activity demonstrated on the isotope study. At surgery a popliteal aneurysm surrounded by clot was found, corroborating the isotope angiogram.

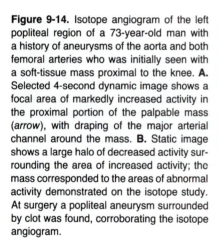

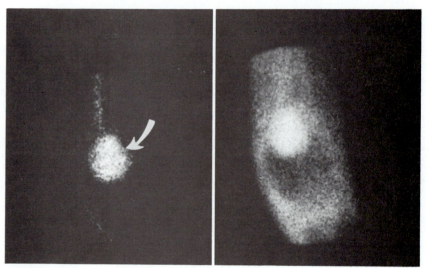

A   B

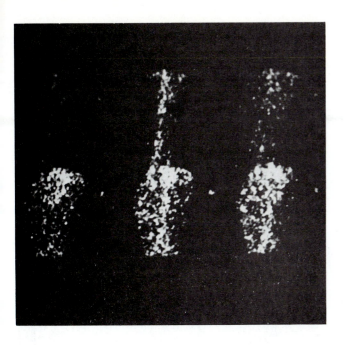

Figure 9-15. Serial 4-second images from the normal dynamic isotope angiogram of the anterior tibial artery of a 24-year-old man with a gunshot wound to the left leg that caused a tibial fracture. Note demonstration of the patent, intact arterial channel.

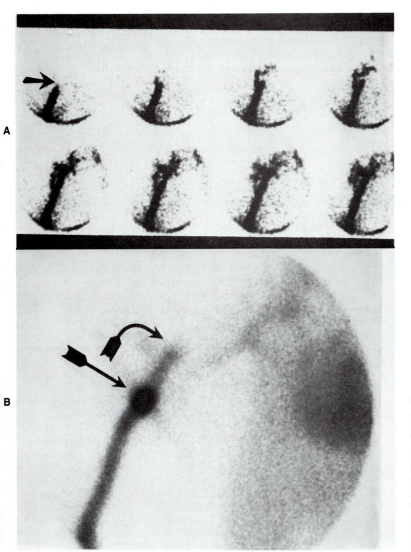

Figure 9-16. Isotope venogram of the right axillary region of a 26-year-old man suspected to have thrombosis of the axillary vein. The isotope was injected into a vein in the right hand. **A.** Serial 2-second dynamic images show a "cut-off" of activity in the axillary vein (*arrow*) with extensive collateralization. **B.** Static image. Note abrupt interruption in the flow of activity (*curved arrow*) in the axillary vein and a focal area of increased activity distally (*straight arrow*), probably representing the distal extent of the clot.

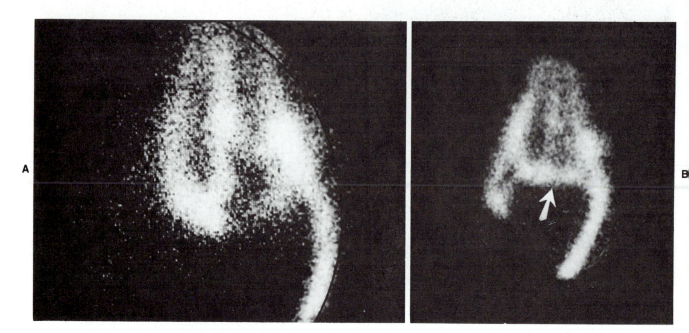

Figure 9-17. Dynamic isotope venograms of the pubic region of a young man who had insertion of a left-to-right crosspubic venous bypass graft because of left iliac vein occlusion. The isotope was injected into a vein in the left foot. **A.** Selected 3-second image from a study performed shortly after surgical insertion of the bypass graft. At this time, the bypass is apparently not the major channel of flow of venous blood; the flow of activity appears to be primarily via collateral venous channels. **B.** Selected 3-second image from a study performed about 6 months after insertion of the bypass graft. The crosspubic bypass (*arrow*) now is clearly the major conduit of venous drainage from the left lower extremity; some collaterals remain visible. Studies obtained 3 years after surgery (not shown) showed the essentially complete disappearance of venous flow in collateral vessels.

ACKNOWLEDGMENTS

This work would not have been possible without the encouragement and cooperation of Charles M. Moss, M.D., Frank J. Veith, M.D., Harry M. Delany, M.D., Berish Strauch, M.D., and the late Robert Jason, M.D. Conscientious and expert technical assistance was provided by the staffs of the Nuclear Medicine Laboratory of North Central Bronx Hospital and the now defunct Morrisania City Hospital.

REFERENCES

1. Anger HO, VanDyke DC, et al.: Gamma camera offers a simple method of visualizing blood flow through vessels and organs. Nucleonics 23:57, 1965.
2. Rosenthall L: Application of gamma scintillation camera to dynamic studies in man. Radiology 86:634, 1966.
3. Powell MR, Anger HO: Blood flow visualization with the scintillation camera. J Nucl Med 7:729, 1966.
4. Rosenthall L: Radionuclide angiography as a method for detecting relative differences in renal blood flow—Preliminary report. J Can Assoc Radiol 19:8, 1968.
5. Freeman LM, Mindelzun R: Diagnosis of aortic aneurysm with radionuclide angiography. Am J Surg 116:433, 1968.
6. Dibos PE, Muhltaler C, Natarajin TK: Intravenous radionuclide arteriography in peripheral vascular occlusive disease. Radiology 102:181, 1972.
7. Meindok H: Visualization of arterial and arterial graft patency by intravenous radionuclide angiography. Can Med Assoc J 106:1180, 1972.
8. Kappert A, Rosler H: Nuclear medicine analysis of peripheral blood circulation by means of 99m-technetium. Schweiz Med Wochenschr 103:1087, 1119, 1973.
9. Hurlow, RA, Chandler ST, Strachan CJ: The assessment of aortoiliac disease by isotope angiology. Br J Surg 65:263, 1978.
10. Hurlow RA, Strachan CJ: The clinical scope and potential of isotope angiology. Br J Surg 65:688, 1978.
11. Hurlow RA, Chandler ST, et al.: Intravenous isotope calf scanning in the assessment of intermittent claudication. Br J Surg 65:619, 1978.
12. Diamond AB, Meng CH, et al.: Radionuclide demonstration of traumatic arterial injury. Radiology 109:623, 1973.
13. Nirmul G, Rudavsky AZ, et al.: 99m-Tc dynamic scintiscanning as a diagnostic aid in post-transplant oliguria. Eur Dialyzis Trans Assn 272:1972.
14. Nirmul G, Rudavsky AZ, Burrows L: Dynamic scintiscanning with technetium-99m as a diagnostic aid in oliguria after renal transplantation. S Afr Med J 50:1614, 1976.
15. Rudavsky AZ, Moss CM: Peripheral vascular scintiangiography. Appl Radiol 4:165, 1975.
16. Moss CM, Delany HM, Rudavsky AZ: Isotope angiography for the detection of embolic arterial occlusion. Surg Gynecol Obstet 142:57, 1976.
17. Moss CM, Rudavsky AZ, Veith FJ: Isotope angiography: Technique, validation and value in the assessment of arterial reconstruction. Ann Surg 184:116, 1976.
18. Moss CM, Rudavsky AZ, Veith FJ: The value of scintiangiography in arterial disease. Arch Surg 111:1235, 1976.
19. Rudavsky AZ, Strauch B, Moss CM: Scintiangiographic demonstration of bleeding into a wrist ganglion. Hand 9:28, 1977.
20. Moss CM, Rudavsky AZ, Veith FJ: Value of scintiangiography in arterial surgery. J Cardiovasc Surg 18:87, 1987.

21. Moss CM, Rudavsky AZ, Veith FJ: Arterial visualization by isotope angiography, in Dietrich EB (ed): Proceedings, Non-Invasive Cardiovascular Diagnosis I. Baltimore, Md., University Park Press, 1978.

22. Moss CM, Veith FJ, Byer A, Rudavsky AZ: Isotope angiography for arterial surgery. Cont Surg 16:47, 1980.

23. Moss CM, Rudavsky AZ, et al.: The diagnosis of arterial injury by isotope angiography, in Dietrich EB (ed): Proceedings, Non-Invasive Cardiovascular Diagnosis II. Littleton, Mass., PSG Publishing, 1981.

24. Moss CM, Veith FJ, et al.: Isotope angiography in arterial trauma. Surgery 86:881, 1979.

25. Moss CM: Veith FJ, Rudavsky AZ: Isotope angiography for the diagnosis of arterial injury. NY State J Med 80:1688, 1980.

26. Rudavsky AZ, Moss CN: Emission angiography for the evaluation of trauma. J Nucl Med 21:403, 1980.

27. Rudavsky AZ, Strauch B, et al.: The use of isotope angiography to assess the blood supply to reimplanted digits. J Nucl Med 20:674, 1979.

28. Rudavsky AZ, Moss CM: Radionuclide angiography for the evaluation of peripheral vascular injuries, in Freeman LM, Weissmann HS (eds): Nuclear Medicine Annual 1981. New York, NY, Raven Press, 1981.

29. Rudavsky AZ, Moss CM: Emission angiography in the detection of vascular integrity, in Raynaud C (ed): Proceedings, Third World Congress, World Federation of Nuclear Medicine and Biology. Paris, Pergamon Press, 1982.

30. Rudavsky AZ, Moss CM: Radionuclide evaluation of peripheral vascular injuries. Semin Nucl Med 13:142, 1983.

31. Pavel DG, Zimmer AN, Patterson VN: In-vivo labeling of red blood cells with 99m-Tc: A new approach to blood pool visualization. J Nucl Med 18:305, 1977.

32. Oldendorf WH, Kitano M, Shimuzio S: Evaluation of a simple technique for abrupt intravenous injection of radioisotope. J Nucl Med 6:205, 1965.

33. Lisbona R, Derbekyan V, et al.: Tc-99m red blood cell venography in deep venous thrombosis of the lower limbs. Clin Nuc Med 10:208, 1985.

CHAPTER 10
Biologic Behavior of Grafts in Arterial System

Lester R. Sauvage

The biologic behavior of arterial grafts based on the morphologic, healing, and patency characteristics of their walls is discussed in this chapter. These data provide an information base on which to assess the design features and compositional characteristics of the graft wall and to make recommendations regarding their clinical use. These assessments have led me to propose a subdivision of the arterial system into four zones based on the graft types that I believe are best suited for use in these zones (Fig. 10-1):

Division 1: to encompass only the coronaries and to be identified as the *arterial (internal mammary artery) zone*

Division 2: to extend upward from the heart to the neck and downward to the groin and to be identified as the *prosthetic zone*

Division 3: to include the neck and the region from the groin to the knees and to be identified as the *optional venoprosthetic zone*

Division 4: to include the entire upper extremity and the distal lower extremity beyond the knee joint and to be identified as the *venous zone*

The saphenous autograft is a moderately satisfactory backup for the internal mammary artery autograft in the coronary zone. However, synthetic and biologic prostheses are less satisfactory backups for the autogenous saphenous vein in the venous zone and become less satisfactory the farther they extend distally.

We will discuss the important design features and host factors that influence the biologic behavior of arterial grafts and, based on these considerations, make clinical recommendations regarding graft selection and techniques of implantation. However, we will first consider a structural classification of arterial grafts based on framework porosity and wall substance characteristics that may assist our understanding of the biologic behavior of arterial grafts.

STRUCTURAL CLASSIFICATION OF ARTERIAL GRAFTS

All arterial grafts are composed of a porous support framework and of a material to close the framework of the interstices if they are large enough to allow blood to escape.

Thus, arterial grafts may be classified according to the size of the interstices and what type of material is used to close those that are not initially impervious to blood.

The support framework is classified as microporous if the interstices are so small that the viscosity and surface tension of the blood prevents bleeding, and as macroporous if these factors cannot prevent bleeding through the interstices. A microporous framework requires no material to close its tiny interstices and can be used without preclotting; for example, a tightly-woven Dacron or a PTFE (*polytetrafluoroethylene*) prosthesis. On the other hand, a macroporous framework requires a material to close its interstices before use to prevent serious transinterstitial hemorrhage.

The macroporous interstices of vascular autografts and of biologic prostheses are closed by nature with a cellular parenchyma, which is viable in autografts and preserved in a nonviable state by aldehyde processing in prostheses. The macroporous frameworks of knitted and of loosely woven prostheses are closed by the surgeon with a fibrin matrix deposited in preclotting.

Polymeric fibrin matrices have been used in millions of patients since Blakemore and Voorhees introduced the first fabric graft, constructed of macroporous Vinyon "N," in 1952.[1,2] Cross-linked fibrin is a highly elastic compound of considerable strength. When freed of thrombin, the procoagulant enzyme which catalyzes its formation, it is a hypothrombogenic material capable of forming a stable flow surface suitable for successful long-term use in aortic, axillofemoral, and above-knee femoropopliteal Dacron grafts.[3,4] The fibrin flow surface is less suitable for below-knee femoropopliteal grafts and much less suitable for femorotibial grafts. Despite the wide utility of fibrin as a matrix for prostheses used in the prosthetic and venoprosthetic zones, the time required to preclot a graft properly (about 15 minutes) and the possibility of the rare occurrence of a marked fibrinolytic reaction with uncontrollable hemorrhage (about 1 in 250 patients) have spurred efforts to close the interstices of knitted grafts in manufacture with materials that are both hypothrombogenic and resistant to accelerated lysis. Two proteins prepared as aldehyde compounds, allogeneic albumin and xenogeneic bovine dermal collagen, are now being evaluated for this purpose.

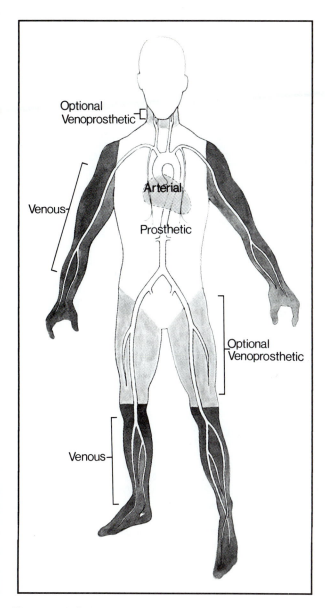

Figure 10-1. Subdivisions of the arterial system into four zones according to recommended graft types.

Table 10-1 classifies arterial grafts into four broad categories based on the porosity of their support framework and the presence or absence of a cellular parenchyma or protein matrix. Representative grafts from each of these categories are shown in Figure 10-2.

In this chapter we will consider the influence of design and host factors that impact on the biologic behavior of arterial grafts and, lastly, consider clinical graft selection.

DESIGN CONSIDERATIONS THAT INFLUENCE THE BIOLOGIC BEHAVIOR OF ARTERIAL GRAFTS

In designing an arterial prosthesis, prime consideration must be given to each of the following characteristics: suturability, imperviousness, thrombogenicity, healability, and

dimensional stability. These characteristics are considered in relation to their effect on the biologic behavior of the graft after implantation into the arterial system of the patient.

Suturability

The first requirement of an arterial graft is that its physical characteristics allow satisfactory suturing to the host artery. The prime determinant of suturability is the ease with which a needle can penetrate its wall. The secondary determinant is the ability of the wall to conform to the arterial stoma. Both characteristics are determined largely by the thickness and compaction of the support framework and by its interaction with the parenchymal or matrical component of the wall.

Knitted grafts with an average wall thickness of about 600 μm (0.6 mm) are approximately three times thicker

TABLE 10-1. STRUCTURAL CLASSIFICATION OF ARTERIAL GRAFTS WITH REFERENCE TO FRAMEWORK POROSITY AND WALL SUBSTANCE CHARACTERISTICS

I. Vascular autografts (composed of macroporous framework and a viable parenchyma that renders the wall impervious)
   A. Venous autografts
      1. Saphenous vein[18]
         a. Greater[75–79]
         b. Lesser[80]
      2. Arm vein[81]
   B. Arterial autografts
      1. Internal mammary artery[20–26]
      2. Radial artery[34–36]
      3. Internal iliac artery[37]

II. Biologic prostheses of allogeneic or xenogeneic origin (composed of a chemically fixed, macroporous framework and a fixed, nonviable parenchyma that renders the wall impervious)
   A. Allogeneic venous grafts
      1. Umbilical vein[42–47;71,74]
      2. Saphenous vein[82]
   B. Xenogeneic arterial grafts
      1. Bovine carotid artery[83–35]
      2. Canine carotid artery[86–88]

III. Composite biosynthetic macroporous prostheses (composed of a knitted or loosely woven Dacron framework with macroporous interstices closed by a protein matrix)
   A. Knitted or loosely woven Dacron prostheses combined with autogeneic fibrin deposited in preclotting for interstices closure[4,6,8–10;31,39,40,48–52;59,66,68,71,89,90]
   B. Knitted Dacron prostheses combined with allogenic albumin-glutaraldehyde gel deposited in manufacture for interstices closure[91–93]
   C. Knitted Dacron prostheses combined with a xenogeneic collagen-formalin compound deposited in manufacture for interstices closure[94,95]

IV. Microporous synthetic prostheses (composed of a synthetic framework with tiny air-filled interstices that are so small that blood will not pass through them)
   A. Fabric (tightly-woven Dacron)[40,48,66,72,88,96,97]
   B. Nonfabric
      1. Expanded PTFE (Teflon)[28–31;40,41,53–56;59,67,72–74;98]
      2. Polyurethane[99]

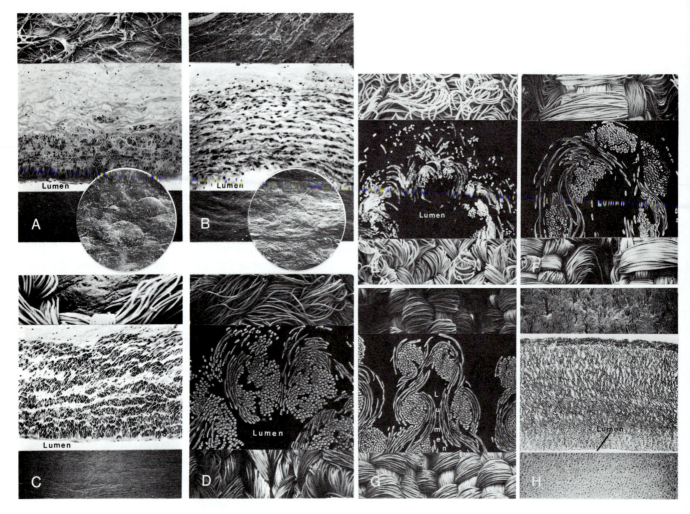

Figure 10-2: Eight different graft types (Table 10-1), shown in comparative three-panel manner. *Upper panels*: SEM of outer surfaces (×50). *Middle panels*: Light microscopy of longitudinal sections of wall (×50). *Lower panels*: SEM of outer surfaces (×50). Endothelium of saphenous vein and internal mammary artery is shown in circles at higher magnification (×1110 and ×472, respectively). **A.** Saphenous vein. **B.** Internal mammary artery. **C.** "Biograft" human umbilical vein. Meadox Medicals, Inc. **D.** "Bionit II," Bard Cardiosurgery Division, C.R. Bard, Inc. **E.** "Microvel," Meadox Medicals, Inc. **F.** Woven Double Velour, Meadox Medicals, Inc. **G.** DeBakey woven "Soft Crimp," Bard Cardiosurgery Division, C.R. Bard, Inc. **H.** "Gore-Tex" PTFE, W.L. Gore and Associates, Inc. (*A C G H from Sauvage LR: Opportunities and responsibilities in the use of arterial grafts, in Nyhus LM (ed): Surgery Annual 1984. Norwalk, Conn., Appleton-Century-Crofts, 1984, pp 229, 96, 97, 102. D from Sauvage LR, Davis CC, et al.: Development and clincal use of porous Dacron arterial prostheses, in Sawyer PN (ed): Modern vascular grafts. New York, McGraw-Hill Book Co., 1987, P 244.*)

than woven grafts, which have an average wall thickness of about 200 μm (0.2 mm). Despite this greater thickness, knitted grafts, by virtue of looser construction (Figs. 10-2D and 10-2E), are easier to penetrate with a needle and are more conformable than tightly-woven grafts (Fig. 10-2G).

There is a stark comparison between the excellent suturing characteristics of vascular autografts for coronary or tibial anastomoses and the grosser characteristics of fabrics, especially woven, and of PTFE prostheses. However, the fine suturability of the vascular autograft, which is best adapted to delicate anastomoses, would be poorly suited for anastomosis to the diseased aorta or iliac arteries, even if the autograft were of adequate caliber. The coarser but sturdier suturing characteristics of synthetic prostheses are better suited for anastomosis to these markedly diseased large-caliber vessels. Biologic prostheses are better adapted than synthetic prostheses to the suturing requirements of smaller caliber anastomoses. However, successful end-to-side anastomosis of a biologic prosthesis to a fragile, small-caliber artery is made difficult by the marked loss of elasticity that results from aldehyde fixation.

Imperviousness

The second requirement of an arterial graft is that its wall must be impervious to blood loss. Vascular autografts have impervious walls because of their confluent cellular parenchymas. Aldehyde-processed allogeneic veins and xenogeneic arteries are impervious because their nonviable architecture is preserved from a point in time, as if in a wax museum. Viable grafts have a regenerative capacity, but chemically processed grafts must depend on ingrowth from the perigraft tissues into their outer walls for reinforcement.

When received from the manufacturer, knitted and loosely woven prostheses are but fiber frameworks that lack a matrix to close their macroporous interstices (Figs.

10-2D and 10-2E). Profuse hemorrhage will occur through their porous walls if they are implanted without preclotting. Thus preclotting must be regarded as the essential final sequence of the definitive construction of these biosynthetic composite prostheses and should be performed in a precise manner. In 1978 we described a functional three-step preclotting technique for the porous Dacron graft (Fig. 10-3) to complete its construction as a biosynthetic composite

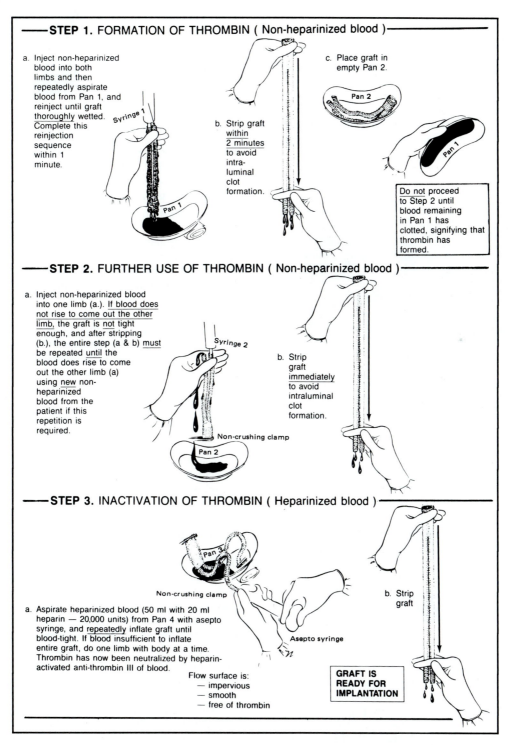

Figure 10-3. Three-step method of preclotting porous fabric prostheses.

of fibrin and Dacron with impervious walls and a hypo-thrombogenic flow surface (Fig. 10-4).[3]

We have observed that a filamentous wall enhances the ease of preclotting a knitted prosthesis.[5] However, we have further observed that a filamentous inner wall increases the thrombogenicity of the flow surface and therefore advise that the filamentousness be confined to the outer surface of a knitted prosthesis.[6,7]

The wall of the microporous prosthesis is impervious because the cohesive forces of the blood (viscosity and surface tension) are stronger than the intraluminal pressure acting to force blood outward through the tiny interstices of the wall. The microporous, tightly woven fabric graft is impervious for the nonheparinized patient, usually adequately impervious for the patient in whom heparin can be quickly reversed, but often inadequate for the patient on cardiopulmonary bypass who requires reconstruction of the ascending or descending thoracic aorta and in whom precise heparin reversal is more difficult. For this reason a type of preclotting for tightly woven grafts was developed

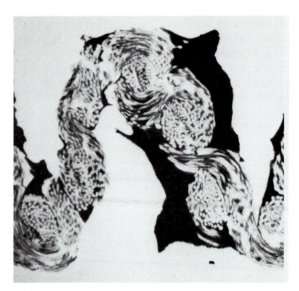

Figure 10-5. Cooley woven Dacron prosthesis after albumin soaking and autoclave treatment at 132° C for 3 minutes.

by Bethea and Reemtsma and further modified and popularized by Cooley in which the prosthesis is soaked in an albumin solution and then autoclaved to deposit a heat-denatured protein matrix on the surface and in the tiny interstices of the graft, rendering it completely impervious (Fig. 10-5).[8-10] I believe that this need of the tightly woven graft for a hemostatic protein matrix when used with cardiopulmonary bypass is a reflection of the shortness (about 100 μm) of the narrow central portion of the interstitial channel (Fig. 10-6), rather than of its caliber (10 to 20 μm) at this central point. The thinness of the woven prosthesis (ca. 200 μm) is pertinent to this discussion because its wall is only one third the thickness of the knitted prosthesis (ca. 600 μm) and only one fourth that of the PTFE prosthesis (ca. 800 μm).

The wall of the PTFE prosthesis, despite being 85% air, is impervious to blood, probably due more to the substantial depth of its interstitial labyrinth (ca. 800 μm) than to the small caliber of its channels (ca. 15 to 30 μm), which are actually larger than the narrowest portion (ca. 10 to 20 μm) of the interstice of the woven prosthesis.

Thrombogenicity

The third requirement of an arterial graft is that its inner surface does not provoke a significant thrombotic reaction by the blood that flows over it. The thrombotic response is initiated by the contact activation of platelets, white blood cells, or factor XII, either singly or in combination. If the flow surface has little contact-activating capacity, it is said to be passive. If the flow surface also has the capacity to deactivate platelets, neutralize thrombin, and lyse fibrin, it is said to possess antithrombotic capacities.

The confluent, functioning endothelial flow surface of a vascular autograft, when harvested properly and protected from injury before implantation, has enormous advantage over the flow surface of any synthetic or biosynthetic prosthesis because of its powerful antithrombotic

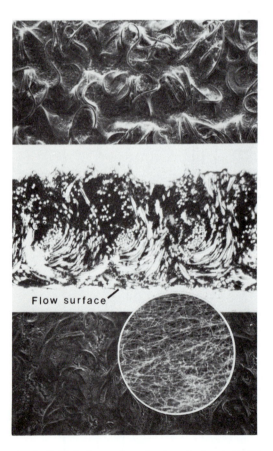

Flow surface

Figure 10-4. Preclotted, noncrimped, external velour knitted Dacron prosthesis. *Upper panel*: SEM of outer surface (×51). *Middle panel*: Light microscopy of longitudinal section (×50). *Lower panel*: SEM of fibrin flow surface (×47). Fibrin surface shown in circle of higher magnification (×206). Proper preclotting transforms the fabric skeleton into a biosynthetic composite of fibrin over Dacron. (*From Sauvage LR: Opportunities and responsibilities in the use of arterial grafts, in Nyhus LM, (ed): Surgery Annual 1984. Norwalk, Conn., Appleton-Century-Crofts, 1984, P 105.*)

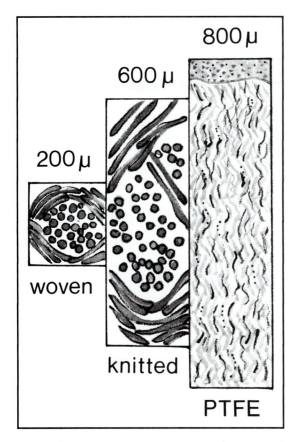

Figure 10-6. Schematic depiction of wall structure showing comparative thickness of woven, knitted, and PTFE prostheses.

capabilities. These antithrombotic characteristics of endothelium result from secretory capacities that produce cell-surface heparan sulfate and heparin-like molecules, thrombomodulin, prostacyclin, plasminogen activators, α_2 macroglobulin, and antithrombin III.[11–17] To assist comparison of any known synthetic surface to a confluent, functioning endothelial flow surface, recall that the endothelial surface maintains patency of human capillaries at a caliber of 4 μm, smaller than the caliber of the red blood cells that must elongate to traverse them. In contrast to this is the fact that there is no truly satisfactory synthetic prosthesis below a caliber of 6,000 μm (6 mm).

Unfortunately, after implantation in the arterial system, the venous autograft is influenced adversely by the high pressure, which causes not only major structural change in the wall but also loss of confluence of its endothelial flow surface during the early postimplant period.[18–20] Regaining confluence of the endothelial flow surface requires days, weeks, or even months (Fig. 10-7A and B).

In contrast, the thin-walled structure of the arterial autograft, including its confluent endothelial flow surface, is unaffected by transplantation within the arterial system (Fig. 10-7C and D). The nutrition by luminal diffusion of the transplanted wall and the pressures to which it is subjected are unchanged from those of its native site. The outstanding long-term success of the internal mammary artery autograft used for coronary bypass is a reflection both of the remarkable stability of its wall and the potent

antithrombotic capability of its confluent endothelial flow surface from the time of implantation onward.[21–26]

The flow surfaces of the allogeneic and xenogeneic biologic prostheses are probably more hypothrombogenic, that is, passive, than those of any synthetic prosthesis. However, these passive surfaces cannot defend themselves against activated platelets extending from contiguous surfaces or arising from distant sources.

The mechanisms by which the platelet activation and the fibrin formation systems interact in response to contact with a prosthetic surface are shown in Figure 10-8. The release of chemical substances by "activated" platelets can trigger the cascade reaction of plasma coagulants to produce thrombin, a strong stimulator of platelets.

The first response of blood to a thrombogenic synthetic surface is to cover it with fibrinogen within seconds, to a depth of about 20 nm. Platelets adhere within minutes and rapidly become activated, releasing adenosine diphosphate and thromboxane A_2.[27] These active compounds cause aggregation and activation of other platelets and deposition of leukocytes and lead to activation of the intrinsic coagulation system with deposition of fibrin (Fig. 10-8).

Unfortunately, all known synthetic materials suitable from a manufacturing standpoint for construction of an arterial prosthesis are capable of activating the platelet and fibrin defense systems of the blood. At present only Dacron and Teflon (PTFE) are used for graft construction, Dacron in fabric form and Teflon in an expanded nonfabric form. Both have a reduced activating capacity, Teflon being more passive than Dacron.[28–30]

The somewhat less passive surface of Dacron has little relevance to the macroporous knitted graft, because the flow surface of the macroporous knitted graft, in its completed biosynthetic form after proper preclotting (Figs. 10-3 and 10-4), is formed by dethrombinated, hypothrombogenic, crosslinked, adherent, elastic fibrin. Furthermore, after implantation the passage of high-velocity laminar blood flow further decreases the thrombogenicity of the fibrin flow surface by the poorly understood passivation process. However, if thrombin is not inactivated in the last step of preclotting by heparin-activated antithrombin III, the flow surface, by virtue of its residual enzymatic contamination, is exceedingly thrombogenic and may remain so after implantation. Thrombin should be regarded as a dangerous contaminant that must be removed once the wall has been rendered impervious by deposition of the fibrin matrix in the preclotting process. Unfortunately, the time required for proper preclotting is a serious obstacle for many busy surgeons, with the result that inactivation of thrombin is often incomplete.

It would be advantageous for most surgeons if the manufacturer could complete the construction of the knitted prosthesis into a finished biosynthetic product ready for surgical use. The progress that is currently being achieved in this area with both allogeneic albumin and xenogeneic collagen holds promise of not only a healable, impervious matrix deposited in manufacture but also of a medicated matrix having antithrombogenic capability.

The microporous PTFE or woven Dacron wall possesses the significant advantage over the macroporous knitted Dacron wall of not requiring preclotting, thus not requiring

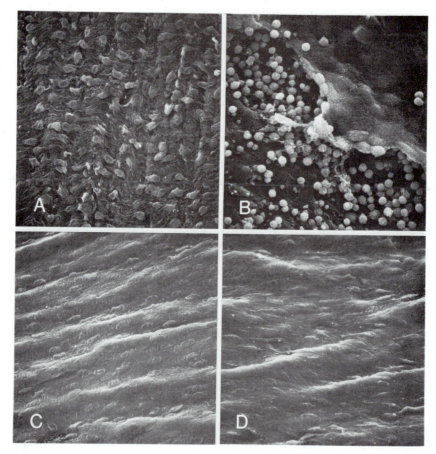

Figure 10-7. SEMs showing effect on endothelial surface of experimental implantation in the canine carotid artery. **A.** Control external jugular vein (×510). **B.** Appearance of external jugular vein flow surface after 21-day implantation (×533). **C.** Control carotid artery (×480). **D.** Appearance of carotid artery flow surface after 21-day implantation (×523). (*From Sauvage LR, Wu H-D, et al.: Ann Thorac Surg 42:452, 1986.*)

the neutralization of the thrombin formed in this process. The initial reduced thrombogenicity of the PTFE flow surface accounts for the minimal early reaction of the blood to this surface. Unfortunately, the thrombogenicity of the PTFE surface increases substantially in the early hours after implantation because blood gradually seeps into the wall as the air (85% by volume) is absorbed from it. The intrinsic coagulation system of this blood trapped within the wall is activated to form thrombin, which permeates back to the luminal surface to increase its thrombogenicity.[31]

Theoretically, a tightly woven microporous fabric graft of Teflon should be less vulnerable to the deleterious influence of intramural thrombin formation because its wall is much thinner (ca. one fourth as thick) than that of the PTFE prosthesis. However, this question cannot be answered by experimental study because fabric grafts of Teflon are no longer manufactured, having been replaced by Dacron.

Healability

Healing of an arterial graft in man is the cellular response by which the host attempts to incorporate the graft. There are two components to the incorporation process: an arterial

component, limited closely to the area of the anastomotic union, and a perigraft areolar tissue component along the entire outer surface of the graft. The arterial component, termed pannus ingrowth, consists of smooth muscle cells arising from the media and of endothelial cells arising from the intima. Pannus ingrowth is true arterial healing and may extend across the anastomosis to cover the inner surface of a prosthesis for as much as 10 mm. In contrast, the perigraft component consists of vascularized fibrous tissue that rapidly invades the outer wall of a porous prosthesis but seldom penetrates beyond the midwall depth. The perigraft reaction is the response of the areolar tissue to the presence of a foreign body. In essence, it is an encapsulation reaction.

On the basis of my studies, I believe that healing in man will never be better than that observed in the dog. Thus, a graft that heals poorly in the dog will heal no better in man. Likewise, if a porous prosthetic graft heals completely by 2 months in the descending thoracic aorta of the dog, as exemplified by uniform full-wall transinterstices fibrous tissue ingrowth with confluent flow surface endothelialization, good healing may be expected in man. However, in man the degree of healing that may be expected in this time period is less complete, being limited to outerwall fibrous tissue ingrowth to about the midportion of

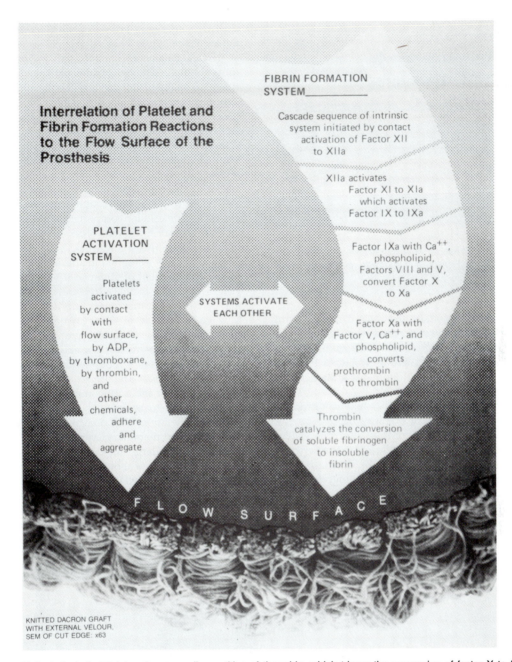

Figure 10-8. Activated platelets release small quantities of thrombin, which trigger the conversion of factor X to factor X_a, "short-circuiting" the cascade reaction of the intrinsic system and leading to formation of more thrombin and fibrin. Thrombin formed by the intrinsic system in turn activates platelets. This self-perpetuating vicious cycle will progress to occlusive thrombosis, if not counteracted by adequate blood flow velocity. (*From Sauvage LR, Berger K, et al.: Grafts for the '80s. Seattle, Bob Hope International Heart Research Institute, 1980, P 13.*)

the wall, with little progression likely beyond this point in most cases. The flow surface of such favorable clinical grafts is formed of translucent, compacted fibrin, except closely adjacent to the suture lines where endothelialization by pannus ingrowth occurs. Except for this perianastomotic zone, fibrin forms the definitive flow surface of both macroporous and microporous prostheses in man. However, this is not to imply that the more limited outer-wall healing that may be anticipated in man is of no value. On the contrary, this tissue ingrowth into the outer wall, even when limited, is vitally important because it abolishes the capillary space along the outside of the graft and thus essentially eliminates the risk of seroma formation and of perigraft infection.

Vascular Autografts

Healing of a vascular autograft differs from the healing of nonviable graft types because the cells of the autograft, being viable, participate actively in the healing reaction. All other graft types are nonviable (Table 10-1) and can

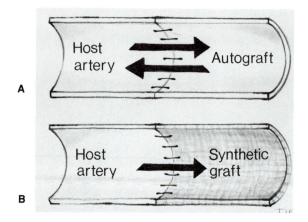

Figure 10-9. Anastomotic healing. **A.** Autograft healing to host artery is a two-way process. **B.** Healing of a synthetic graft joined to the host artery is a one-way process.

serve only as a trellis to assist the inward migration of cells arising from the proliferative response of the perigraft areolar tissue. The healability of nonviable grafts can be judged on the ability of their support structures to serve as a trellis for healing. We have found that a filamentous design is best for this purpose.[32]

Whereas healing of viable grafts is a two-way process, healing of nonviable grafts is a one-way process by the host artery (Fig. 10-9). The autograft, because it is viable, heals to the artery at the anastomotic site and to the perigraft tissues throughout its length, and at the same time the artery and the perigraft tissues heal to the autograft. Integrity of the anastomoses of a vascular autograft to the host artery becomes independent of the continued presence of the sutures within a few weeks, but the anastomotic integ-

rity of all other graft types depends forever on the holding power of the suture lines.

Healing of a venous autograft in the arterial system presents the additional features of the adaptations that a tissue accustomed to low intravascular pressure must undergo when it is suddenly thrust into a high-pressure pulsatile environment. Experimentally, scattered endothelial cell loss occurs in the early days following implantation of the venous autograft into this hostile environment;[18–20] these same changes may be expected clinically. Healing of the injured flow surface occurs by endothelial proliferation over weeks to months. Following this early endothelial loss, the venous wall adapts by a rapid and profound proliferative reaction of its cellular components that leads to a marked increase in wall thickness, often as much as a six- to ten-fold increase within a few weeks (Fig. 10-10).

The venous autograft in the arterial system is prone to the development of atherosclerotic degeneration after 5 years, especially in the aortocoronary position. Approximately 50% of aortocoronary saphenous grafts are closed by 7 years because of these changes, and most of those that are still open show angiographic evidence of atherosclerotic degeneration that portends their closure within an additional few years.[21–26] Saphenous autografts in the femoropopliteal position are subject to the same degenerative changes seen in the aortocoronary position, but the incidence appears to be less.[18,33] In contrast to the marked histologic alterations that occur in venous autografts, thin-walled internal mammary artery autografts used for coronary bypass undergo little histologic change and have a patency at 10 years of about 90%.[21–26] This is understandable because the entire wall of this thin-walled arterial graft continues to be nourished by luminal diffusion and is subjected to the same pressures in its new environment as it was in its native location. Furthermore, endothelial cells

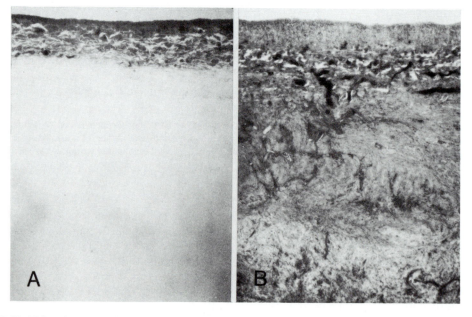

Figure 10-10. Light microscopy showing effect on wall thickness and structure after experimental external jugular vein implantation in the canine carotid artery. **A.** Longitudinal section of canine external jugular vein control (×41). **B.** Longitudinal section of devascularized reversed canine external jugular vein autograft implanted in the carotid artery for 21 days (×39; H & E). (*From Sauvage LR, Wu H-D, et al.: Ann Thorac Surg 42:454, 1986.*)

of the internal mammary artery have been shown to have a higher rate of prostacyclin production than those of autogenous veins.[26]

The phenomenal long-term success of the internal mammary artery autograft for coronary bypass has been heeded by surgeons the world over with a concomitant marked increase in their use of this procedure. The real challenge, however, is not to use the left internal mammary for a convenient left anterior descending coronary artery anastomosis and two or three veins for the rest of the heart, but rather to revascularize the entire left ventricle with only the internal mammary arteries.[20] This may be accomplished as shown in Figure 10-11. However, the true value of these more time-consuming and technically more difficult procedures remains to be ascertained by careful clinical follow-up.

The radial artery was used as an aortocoronary graft years ago but was discarded because of poor long-term patency.[34-36] Except for the frequent use of the internal mammary artery for coronary bypass and the infrequent use of the internal iliac artery for replacement of the fibromuscular dysplastic renal artery in young patients,[37] there is little opportunity to use this true gold-standard graft because of lack of other suitable autogenous donor arteries.

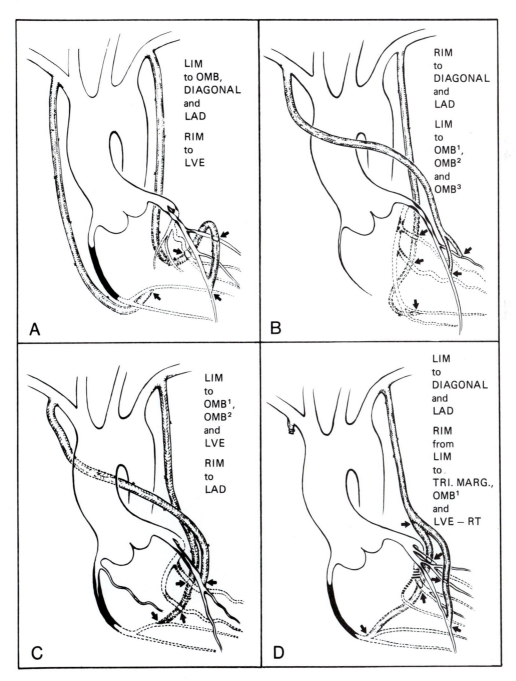

Figure 10-11. Four variations of operative technique for complete revascularization of the left ventricle using only the internal mammary artery. (*From Sauvage LR, Wu H-D, et al.: Ann Thorac Surg 42:461, 1986.*)

Biologic Prostheses

Chemically fixed veins or arteries may be considered biologic prostheses. Like vascular autografts, these grafts of allogeneic or xenogeneic origin (Table 10-1) are formed of a macroporous framework and a parenchyma that renders the wall impervious; the difference being that the biologic prosthesis has been chemically processed with loss of both its viability and immunologic identity. Aldehyde fixation, either of the more unstable formaldehyde or the more stable glutaraldehyde type, converts degradable organic material into a chemically-fixed structure that possesses little ability to activate white blood cells, platelets, or factor XII.

Tissue ingrowth from the perigraft areolar tissue into the biologic prostheses is limited to the loose structure of the adventitia. The impervious fixed parenchyma that forms the substance of the wall prevents further ingrowth. Pannus ingrowth at the anastomotic site is limited to the immediate vicinity of the suture line. Pannus ingrowth beyond this point requires a positive chemotactic stimulus that is not provided by the glutaraldehyde-fixed endothelial surface.

Composite Biosynthetic Macroporous Prostheses

We shall next consider the healing in man of preclotted knitted Dacron prostheses and how design features influence this process. The avascular pannus ingrowth arising from the arterial wall is generally completed by 2 months and seldom extends inward to cover the flow surface for more than a centimeter (Fig. 10-12A). The highly vascularized areolar tissue response arising from the perigraft tissue invades the interstices of the outer wall of the entire graft, usually reaching to about the middepth of the knitted wall (ca. 300 µm) by 2 months (Fig. 10-12B). There is often no healing beyond this point, although on occasion we have seen full-wall fibrous tissue invasion (Fig. 10-12C), and in one patient apparent endothelialization (Fig. 10-12D) based on silver nitrate staining features, which are now recognized to be inadequate documentation.[38] However, except for this single instance, neither we nor anyone else has reported the presence of endothelium in a vascular graft in man beyond the point that could be explained by pannus ingrowth. In a satisfactory knitted graft, the flow surface beyond this limited perianastomotic zone is formed of compacted, crosslined, hypothrombogenic fibrin.

Our studies indicate that tissue ingrowth from the perigraft areolar tissue response into a knitted prosthesis will be enhanced in both experimental animals and man by an external velour surface.[32] Thus, for reasons of healing and preclotting efficiency we advise that the external surface of a knitted prosthesis be as filamentous as possible and, for reasons of thrombogenicity, that the flow surface be as smooth as possible. We also advise that the porosity of the graft be as low as is consistent with excellent surgical-handling characteristics because we have observed that porosity can be decreased to levels far below that consistent

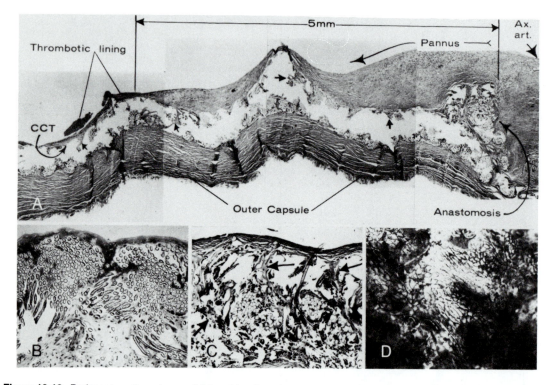

Figure 10-12. Perianastomotic and more distal graft healing of arterial prostheses in man. **A.** Pannus healing of Wesolowski Weavenit graft (Meadox Medicals, Inc.) (×35; H & E). **B.** Central portion of aortofemoral Bionit II graft at 56 days (×100; H & E). **C.** Central portion of right iliac limb of external velour, weft-knit Dacron prosthesis at 182 days (×45; H & E). The luminal aspect of the graft is a thin tissue layer with complete tissue tufts through the interstices (*arrows*). **D.** Central portion of axillofemoral graft at 21 months showing endothelial-like cells as demonstrated by silver nitrate staining (×250, approximately). (**A** *from Sauvage LR, Rao AM, Wood SJ: Ann Surg 175:123, 1972.* **C** *from Sauvage LR, Berger K, et al.: Surgery 70:951, 1971.* **D** *from Sauvage LR, Berger K, et al.: Ann Surg 182:752, 1975.*)

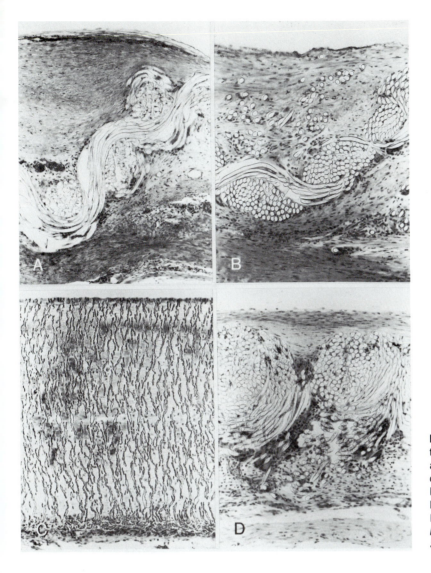

Figure 10-13. Light microscopy of sections taken from midportion of grafts 6 cm long and 8 mm in diameter implanted in canine descending thoracic aorta for 56 days (×110; H & E). **A.** DeBakey woven graft. **B.** Woven Double Velour. **C.** Gore-Tex PTFE. **D.** Bionit II warp-knit external velour prosthesis. (*A and D from Mathisen Sr, Wu H-D, et al.: J Vasc Surg 4:40, 1986.*)

with acceptable needle penetrability and wall conformability and still not impair healing to any appreciable extent.[39]

Microporous Synthetic Prostheses

Because I have little experience with microporous grafts in man but have studied these grafts carefully in the descending thoracic aorta of the dog, I will summarize our experimental findings and relate them to published clinical observations. Additionally, for comparative purposes I will also include the healing of a knitted prosthesis in the descending thoracic aorta of the dog.

The tightly woven, thin-walled grafts, with and without velour surfaces, become well healed in the descending thoracic aorta of most dogs by 8 weeks (Figs. 10-13A and B), whereas the much thicker walled Gore-Tex PTFE prostheses (Fig. 10-13C) do not.[40] In fact, little tissue grows into the PTFE wall even at 6 months.[41] Endothelialization is restricted to pannus ingrowth in the PTFE prosthesis, but it is found throughout the woven prosthesis in association with full-wall transinterstices healing. The healing of woven prostheses approaches, but does not equal, that of knitted prostheses (Fig. 10-13D).

Dimensional Stability

Internal mammary artery autografts used for coronary bypass show no thickening and no dilation, reflecting the fact that this graft does not recognize its relocation in the arterial system as foreign.

Venous autografts in the arterial system are surprisingly resistant to aneurysm formation. This resistance is probably due to the violent early proliferative response of the wall to arterial implantation. In the dog, this response is associated with a six- to ten-fold increase in wall thickness within the first 3 weeks (Fig. 10-10), with maintenance of stable luminal dimensions.[20] Saphenous aortocoronary autografts in man also develop markedly thickened walls and maintain stable luminal dimensions, but over time are prone to the development of degenerative change (Fig. 10-14).[20]

In contrast to the stability of both arterial and venous autografts in the arterial system, the high incidence of aneurysm formation in the glutaraldehyde-processed umbilical vein Biograft after 2 to 3 years has become a factor limiting its use.[42–47] This development results from breakdown of the graft structure and has occurred despite a wide-mesh

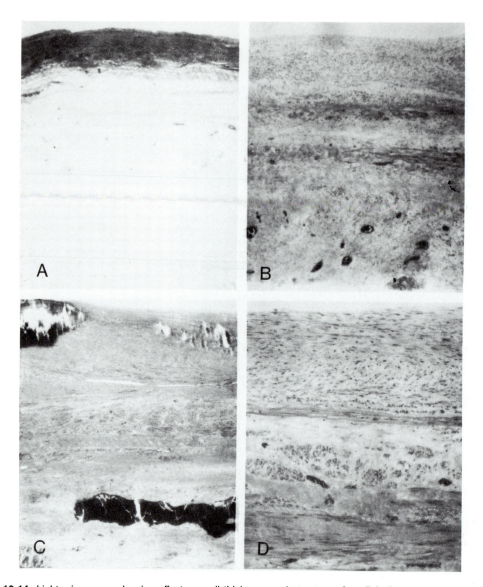

Figure 10-14. Light microscopy showing effect on wall thickness and structure after clinical aortocoronary implantation (&38: H & E). **A.** Longitudinal section of human greater saphenous vein control. **B.** Longitudinal section of well-functioning 4-month reversed greater saphenous vein aortocoronary sequential autograph to diagonals 1, 2, and 3 and the left anterior descending coronary artery shows marked thickening. **C.** Longitudinal section of well-functioning 9-year reversed greater saphenous vein aortocoronary autograph to distal right coronary in same patient shows widespread degenerative calcific change. **D.** Longitudinal section of different area of the graft in **C** shows no calcific and minimal degenerative change. (*From Sauvage LR, Wu H-D, et al.: Ann Thorac Surg 42:457, 1986.*)

Dacron sleeve that is placed in manufacture to support the fragile biologic wall.

The long-term maintenance of dimensional stability of a prosthetic graft depends on the continued integrity of its support framework. The fibrous capsule that forms around a prosthesis lacks the intrinsic strength necessary to contain the intraluminal pressure and would, if unsupported by the Dacron fiber framework, undergo progressive aneurysmal dilation.[48–50] A few years ago, we reported a series of Dacron grafts from three different manufacturers that had undergone fiber breakdown and false aneurysm formation.[51] Use of excessively high temperatures to shrink

Dacron prostheses to reduce their porosities appeared to be the common denominator responsible for these occurrences. Recognition of this etiology and avoidance of such temperatures has essentially eliminated this complication in current Dacron grafts. A weft-knit Dacron aortic bifurcation graft with stable dimensions and intact structure after 25 years of implantation has been recently reported by Guidoin et al.[52] This supports the contention that Dacron, a polymer and ethyl terephthalate, has adequate strength for indefinite dimensional stability when properly processed.

Pourdehymi and Wagner have pointed out the impor-

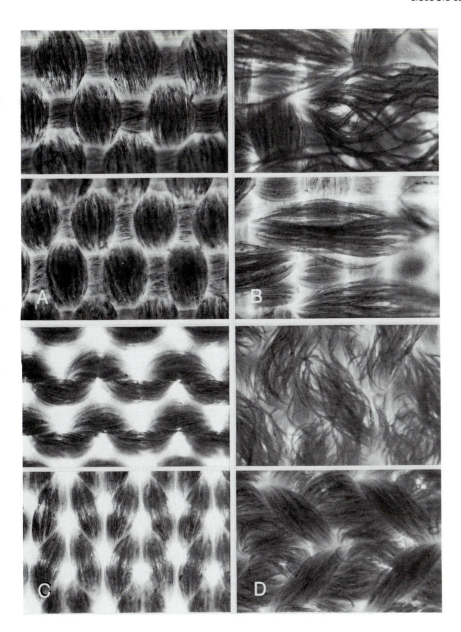

Figure 10-15. Transilluminated photomicrographs show wall construction of different grafts (*upper panels* show outer surface; *lower panels* show inner surface). **A.** DeBakey woven (×44). **B.** Woven Double Velour (×55). **C.** Milliknit (weft-knit; Golaski Laboratories, Inc.) (×55). **D.** Bionit II (warp-knit) (×48).

tance of graft structure to the long-term dimensional stability of fabric grafts.[48] Tightly-woven prostheses, constructed of two sets of yarn interlaced at right angles to each other, are the strongest synthetic grafts (Fig. 10-15A). This is true even though their wall structure (200 μm) is only about one third that of the current velour warp-knit prostheses. The tight compaction and the interlaced relationship of the yarn bundles account for the relative imperviousness of these grafts and also for their poor compliance, difficult suturing, and tendency to fray. The yarn bundles of tightly woven grafts have little mobility except at the cut edge.

An innovation of the woven graft that has improved its suturability and healability is the addition of a velour component, achieved by less frequent interlacing of some of the yarn bundles that allows them to "float" on both surfaces and spread their filaments, giving the graft a soft feel and a high-density, spotty type of filamentousness (Fig.

10-15B). The strength of the woven velour is still high despite the greater mobility of some of its yarn bundles. The disadvantages of this fabrication are its increased porosity which may require preclotting, and the marked tendency of the cut edge to fray, possibly necessitating cautery to seal the edges.

Knitted grafts are constructed of interlooped yarn bundles rather than the right-angle interlacing used in woven grafts. There are two basic types of knitted grafts, weft-knit and warp-knit. The weft-knit graft is formed from one set of yarns that interlock in a circular manner (Fig. 10-15C). The warp-knit graft is formed of several sets of yarn that are interlooped in a zigzag pattern throughout the fabric (Fig. 10-15D). In general, I believe that warp-knit grafts are superior to both weft-knit and woven grafts. They are more compliant than woven grafts but less compliant than weft-knit grafts. Warp-knit grafts do not run, unravel,

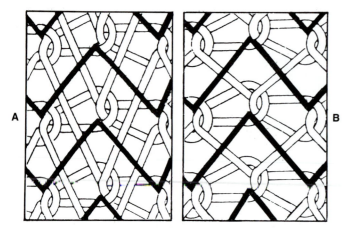

Figure 10-16. Loop diagrams showing internal surface of **A**, Bionit two-bar, and **B**, Microvel half tricot construction. (*Drawings by the late Sig Titone, 1923–1984.*)

curl up, or fray at the cut edges. The loop diagrams of two common types of warp-knit prostheses are shown in Figure 10-16, the Bionit two-bar locknit and the Microvel half tricot. The latter configuration is dimensionally unstable in contrast to the former.[48]

The dimensional stability of the Gore-Tex PTFE graft is assured by a transverse outer wrap of the same material (Fig. 10-2H). Marked dilation was seen in some early PTFE grafts that lacked this support.[53–56]

HOST FACTORS THAT INFLUENCE THE BIOLOGIC BEHAVIOR OF BLOOD TO THE FLOW SURFACE OF THE GRAFT

In this section we consider the thrombotic potential of the blood, the velocity of blood flow through the graft, and the influence of antithrombotic, anticoagulant, and fibrinolytic therapies on the ability of the blood to react against the flow surface of a graft. The atherogenic factors that especially predispose venous autografts to development of a peculiar type of accelerated atherosclerosis will also be discussed.

Thrombotic Potential

We have demonstrated experimentally the critical influence of the inherent thrombotic potential of blood on small-caliber graft performance.[57] This work allowed us to select a battery of tests that describes the blood's inherent predisposition to thrombotic events. Our data suggest that thrombotic potential can be determined by platelet aggregability and prostaglandin metabolite levels, namely proaggregatory thromboxane A_2 (TxA_2) and antiaggregatory prostacyclin. Although the ratio of these metabolites varies in value, reflecting the source of TxA_2 generation, it runs parallel in terms of assigning responder types to high-, middle- and low-risk study groups. Another test that has proved to be of value in identifying high- and low-responder types

is the malondialdehyde (MDA) assay that also can be used as an index of overall platelet prostaglandin activity. The hypothesis that evaluation of thrombotic potential indicates a systemic expression of a predisposition to thrombosis, or the lack of it, was validated by observing the 3-week fate of Dacron grafts 4 mm in diameter and 6 cm long implanted in the carotid arteries of dogs. The disparity in graft patency figures for low- and for high-risk subjects (100% and 10%, respectively) substantiated the proposed theory.

Although the early protective effect of aspirin on small-caliber graft patency is widely accepted, it has been our experience that the degree and duration of this beneficial effect is dependent on each subject's inherent thrombotic potential. With respect to long-term patency, aspirin was found to be inadequate therapy for high-risk subjects, unnecessary for low-risk subjects, and beneficial only for subjects in the intermediate risk group.[58] We then evaluated the antithrombotic strength of a combination of aspirin and thromboxane synthetase inhibitor as a means of medicinally altering the prostaglandin metabolite balance and reducing platelet aggregability in high-risk subjects. With this effective antithrombotic combination, 100% patency was maintained in those subjects who had been inherently predisposed to graft occlusion.

The clinical significance of our experimental data remains to be determined. The importance of this subject is apparent. If we could, by whatever means, establish the thrombotic potentials of our patients, we would better know what type of grafts to choose for them and when we should administer anticoagulant, antithrombotic, and fibrinolytic medications.

Velocity of Blood Flow

Regardless of its thrombotic potential, the faster the blood flows through a graft, the less the opportunity for platelet aggregation and fibrin formation to occur on the flow surface. Conceptually I believe that there is a specific thrombotic threshold velocity for each type of flow surface. In other words, there is a velocity above which thrombosis does not occur and below which it does. I have termed the velocity where thrombosis begins the thrombotic threshold velocity (TTV).[59] The lower the thrombogenicity of a surface, the lower the TTV, and the higher the thrombogenicity, the higher the TTV.

When the TTV is reached, thrombus deposition occurs until the lumen caliber is reduced sufficiently to raise the velocity to just above threshold, thereby stopping further deposition. This new equilibrium is, however, tenuous, with little reserve, leaving the graft in danger of sudden thrombotic closure if cardiac output falls or flow is compromised by peripheral vasoconstriction or positional change.

With progressive decrease of the luminal caliber by cyclic deposition of thrombus, the point is eventually reached in the critical 2 to 3 mm size where further decrease in the flow channel cannot increase the velocity of flow due to loss of pressure head. At that point, occlusive thrombosis occurs.

These velocity relationships to thrombus formation in

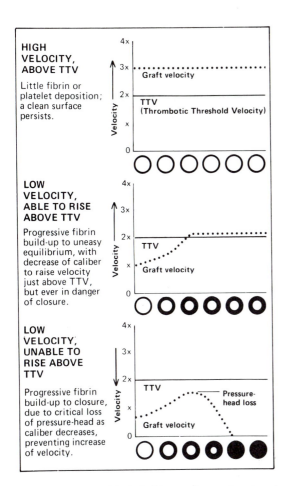

HIGH VELOCITY, ABOVE TTV

Little fibrin or platelet deposition; a clean surface persists.

LOW VELOCITY, ABLE TO RISE ABOVE TTV

Progressive fibrin build-up to uneasy equilibrium, with decrease of caliber to raise velocity just above TTV, but ever in danger of closure.

LOW VELOCITY, UNABLE TO RISE ABOVE TTV

Progressive fibrin build-up to closure, due to critical loss of pressure-head as caliber decreases, preventing increase of velocity.

Figure 10-17. Relation of fibrin buildup on flow surface to velocity of blood flow through graft. If the velocity is above the thrombotic threshold of the surface, buildup does not occur. If velocity is below the threshold, buildup results, with progressively diminishing caliber. (*From Sauvage LR, Berger K, et al.: Grafts for the '80s. Seattle, Bob Hope International Heart Research Institute, 1980, P 12.*)

arterial grafts are shown in Figure 10-17. The TTV of the flow surface of a given graft depends on both the characteristics of the surface and the thrombotic potential of the blood. Patency of the graft in a given flow environment depends on whether the distal bed will accept a volume of flow that will keep the velocity above threshold. If it does, the outlook for patency of the graft is good. If it does not, but circumferential fibrin deposition narrows the lumen and raises the velocity to just above threshold, the graft may remain patent for a long period, although it will always be in danger of sudden closure. If the velocity at implantation is so low that fibrin deposition cannot raise it above threshold, acute thrombosis must occur.

Antithrombotic, Anticoagulant, and Fibrinolytic Activities

When concerned about the patency of a peripheral graft in a small-capacity bed, I prescribe low-dose warfarin (Coumadin) (to raise the prothrombin time only 3 to 4 seconds), one aspirin per day (to block thromboxane A_2 forma-

tion, even though there is an accompanying impairment of prostacyclin production), and stanozolol, 2 mg t.i.d. (to enhance the activity of the patient's fibrinolytic system). The value of stanozolol is under continuing evaluation.[60–61] A suitable agent to enhance prostacyclin production is not yet available.

Atherogenic Factors

Prosthetic grafts rarely are affected by atherosclerotic change, possibly because their flow surface is composed of passivated fibrin, which has a low reactive capacity. Venous autografts, on the contrary, especially in the coronaries of hyperlipidemic patients, are prone to the development after 5 years of a soft, amorphous atherosclerotic inner-wall lesion that is prone to embolization and is often progressive, leading to graft occlusion.[62–65] There is strong but incomplete evidence to implicate other presumed important factors such as smoking, obesity, hypercholesterolemia, hypertension, diabetes, gout, and hypothyroidism to the development of atherosclerotic change in arterial grafts. An unexplained but remarkable attribute to the internal mammary artery when used as a coronary bypass graft is its relative freedom from atherosclerotic degenerative change, even after long periods of implantation.

HOST FACTORS INFLUENCING BIOLOGIC BEHAVIOR OF PERIGRAFT TISSUES TOWARD OUTER WALL OF GRAFT

Proper Positioning of Graft In Areolar Tissue Bed

The most suitable position for a graft is in an areolar tissue bed because the optimal perigraft healing response arises from this source. Specifically, the graft should not be placed within the fat layer because this tissue has inferior healing capacity. Proper positioning of a graft is especially important for axillofemoral, femorofemoral, and lower-extremity bypass grafts. These grafts should be positioned beneath the fatty layer in the areolar tissue atop the deep fascia, or positioned in the areolar tissue between muscle groups.

Perigraft Hematoma Formation

The importance of avoiding perigraft hematoma formation cannot be overemphasized because the perigraft areolar tissue response in man is seldom able to organize more than the outer half of the fibrin matrix of a knitted prosthesis with a wall thickness of about 600 μm. Even when a graft is positioned in the proper areolar tissue bed, if these tissues are prevented from contact with the graft by hematoma formation, healing of the outer graft wall will be prevented (Fig. 10-18). The capacity of the human to heal a porous synthetic arterial graft is limited at best, and if this restricted healing capacity is expended in an endeavor to organize a perigraft hematoma, the replicative capacity of the perihematomatous response will be exhausted before the outer wall of the graft can be invaded. Placing a drain is not a

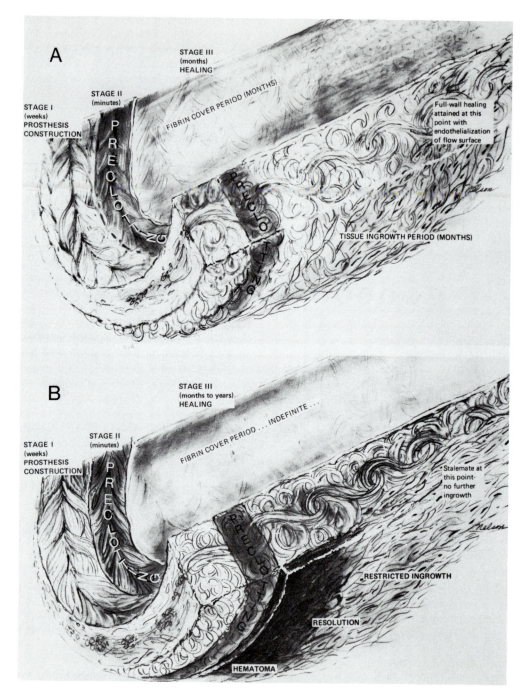

Figure 10-18. A. The three separate stages in attainment of a healed synthetic arterial prosthesis. The initial step involves the manufacture of a bare skeleton or framework (the tubular prosthesis) designed for optimal tissue penetration. The second step involves careful preclotting, which converts the bare framework to an impervious fabric-fibrin conduit ready for implantation. The third stage (healing) occurs following implantation and involves ingrowth of perigraft tissues into the fabric. Under ideal circumstances, full-wall transinterstices healing occurs, with an intact endothelial flow surface ultimately formed as a consequence. This ideal endothelialization, although common and complete in many animal species, has never been conclusively proven to occur in man. In fact, tissue ingrowth seldom occurs beyond the midwall. **B.** The healing processes shown in **A** may be slowed or completely halted by hematoma, seroma, or lymph accumulation around the graft. These barriers retard the ingrowth of tissues, which apparently lose their invasive capabilities when their inward progress is arrested or delayed. (*From Sauvage LR: Graft complications in relation to vascular healing, in Haimovici H (ed): Vascular Emergencies. New York, Appleton-Century-Crofts, 1982, p 435.*)

substitute for gentle handling of tissues and achievement of precise hemostasis. Furthermore, if there is blood in the wound, the drain will soon become obstructed by thrombus and will be rendered functionless. If a hematoma is recognized after surgery, the patient should be returned promptly to the operating room for evacuation of the hematoma so that the perigraft tissues can contact the wall and heal at least the outer portion.

Lymph Collection

Lymph collections at the groin are especially prone to occur after reoperations. These collections are a deterrent to healing, although not as severe as perigraft hematoma. I suspect that a graft implanted in a wound that develops a lymph leak tends to lie on the bottom of the "pool," with at least its back wall in contact with the tissue. Although lymph has a bacteriostatic action, I am nonetheless concerned when the patient has a lymph collection around a graft in a groin wound. I am hesitant to send such a patient home, especially if he lives a long distance away, preferring instead to keep him under close observation until the lymph leak has sealed because I fear that healing will be impaired and infection may develop.

Prevention of lymph collections at the groin is preferable to becoming proficient in aspirating them. Approaching the femoral artery from the lateral side and lifting the fatty layer bearing the lymph channels and nodes medially is the best way to prevent this troublesome complication.

Infection

Synthetic grafts that have been secured by outer-wall healing are relatively immune to infection. However, if this outer-wall healing does not occur, the graft remains a nonhealed foreign body susceptible to infection. Thus, the best defense against infection is to do all that is possible to facilitate outer-wall healing. Because perigraft hematoma formation is the most common cause of nonhealing, it is also the most common cause of graft infection. The hematoma not only prevents the perigraft areolar tissue response from healing the outer wall, but also provides an ideal culture medium for bacterial growth.

The most feared complication of arterial grafts is anastomotic hemorrhage, which is nearly always due to perigraft infection that lyses the vessel wall at the anastomotic site. Conventional teaching dictates that the graft should be removed if infection involves this area.

I have had several instances of graft infection in patients over the years and have evolved a plan that appears effective for handling these infrequent occurrences. At the first sign of infection involving an axillofemoral, femorofemoral, or lower-extremity bypass, I return the patient to the operating room. With the patient under general anesthesia, I reopen the wound, obtain a culture, debride as needed, and lavage the wound copiously with a solution of equal parts of povidoneiodine (Betadine), saline solution, and hydrogen peroxide. I then preplace through-and-through monofilament sutures, again thoroughly lavage the wound, place a dependent Jackson-Pratt suction drain, and, when the wound

is meticulously dry, close it loosely by tying the sutures. The patient is returned to the operating room at 2- to 3-day intervals until the wound culture becomes negative. Usually this is achieved by the fourth treatment. The drain is removed when drainage, which has become serous, ceases. Intravenous antibiotics are continued for a week after the culture has become negative and the drain removed. The patient is then discharged and continued on oral antibiotics for several months.

Perigraft Seroma Formation

This is a rare occurrence, developing about once in every 200 to 300 patients. This condition occurs as a consequence of lack of outer-wall healing. Graft placement in fat, perigraft hematoma formation, and lymph collection all predispose to this complication. I also believe that a few patients react to Dacron (and still fewer to Teflon) in an "allergic" manner with the development of a perigraft seroma. Fortunately, the seroma fluid is bacteriostatic and seldom becomes infected. Open drainage of a chronic perigraft seroma will likely lead to a persistent draining sinus and should be avoided if possible. If the graft must be replaced, the new graft should be of a different material. Under these circumstances, if the graft is Dacron it should be replaced by PTFE, and if PTFE, by a Dacron prosthesis, because crossreactions are rare.

INFLUENCE OF GEOMETRIC AND ANASTOMOTIC FACTORS ON BIOLOGIC BEHAVIOR OF ARTERIAL GRAFTS

Geometric Factors

Arterial grafts may have a conduit or patch graft configuration. If synthetic, the graft's length has a major influence on man's ability to achieve complete healing. Porous synthetic grafts up to 2 to 3 cm long can heal completely through the union of the outgrowth arising from the internal arterial pannus layer with the ingrowth arising from the perigraft areolar tissue reaction. However, grafts over 3 cm in length seldom attain inner-wall healing beyond the pannus zone. The flow surface in these longer grafts is composed of compacted, crosslinked fibrin because the perigraft ingrowth is unable to reach the flow surface, and pannus healing seldom extends into the graft from the anastomoses for more than 10 to 15 mm. These relationships between the degree of healing and the length of a synthetic conduit are shown in Figure 10-19.

The healing of a patch graft is similar, but the width, rather than the length, of the patch is the major influence on its biologic behavior. For this reason, arterial patch grafts heal completely within a few weeks because the healing distance for the pannus ingrowth is only half the width. For example, a 10 cm long, 10 mm wide Dacron patch graft used in a profundaplasty has a healing distance of only 5 mm. Similarly, a 6 cm long, 8 mm wide Dacron patch graft used in a carotid repair has a healing distance of only 4 mm (Fig. 10-20A and B). In essence, arterial patches

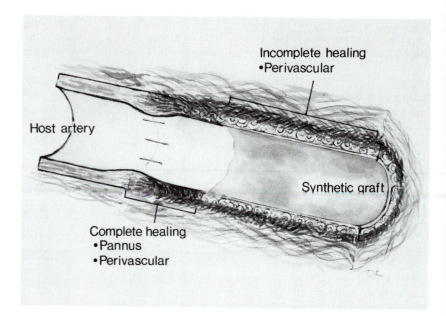

Figure 10-19. Healing mechanism of arterial conduits. Full-wall perianastomotic healing occurs by a combination of pannus and areolar tissue reactions, the former from the arterial wall and the latter from the perigraft tissues. Beyond this point, healing depends solely on ingrowth from perigraft tissues.

heal by a combination of pannus extension from the arterial wall and by ingrowth from the perigraft tissues, being analogous to the perianastomotic healing of an arterial conduit (Fig. 10-19). In contradistinction to an arterial patch graft, which is seldom wide enough to be beyond the range of complete inner-wall healing by pannus ingrowth, a circular patch graft in areas of the heart such as the atrial septum may be so wide that the central portion will remain unhealed

because pannus ingrowth cannot extend that far (Fig. 10-20C and D).

Anastomotic Factors

Regardless of the superb design and fabrication attributes of a given graft, the surgeon has an important influence

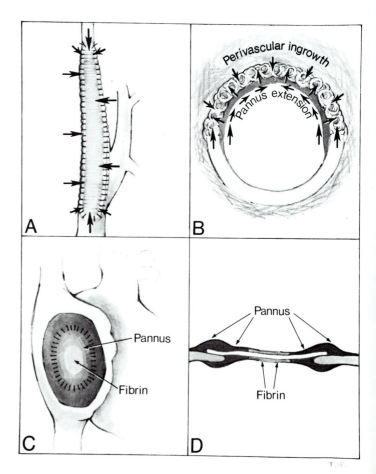

Figure 10-20. Healing mechanism of arterial and intracardiac patches. **A.** Carotid patch graft. **B.** Transverse section shows complete healing of patch graft repair by pannus and areolar tissue reactions with the same mechanisms involved in the perianastomotic healing of an arterial conduit (Fig. 10-19). **C.** Repair of large atrial septal defect with patch graft. **D.** Transverse section of atrial patch graft shows incomplete healing solely by pannus extension. Here there is no perigraft tissue, only blood. Healing of the patch in this totally hemic environment depends solely on pannus ingrowth. The central portion of a large patch may remain unhealed, because it is too far from adjacent tissues to be healed by the pannus ingrowth mechanism.

on its biologic fate. If the anastomotic process is flawed, the graft may be lost. However, if the anastomotic process is perfect, the success of the graft depends on whether the capacity of the distal bed is adequate to keep the velocity of flow through the graft above the thrombotic threshold.[59] The anastomotic process is influenced by surgical technique in a generic sense, by specific techniques in a restricted sense, and by the degree of longitudinal tension acting on an anastomosis.

Surgical techniques. The accuracy and perfection of our work is what should distinguish our specialty. If we can also perform our procedures quickly, so much the better. However, poorly done work performed rapidly is seldom of lasting value to our patients. The blood, when confronted with an irregular anastomotic union with graft edges protruding into the flow path, is seldom forgiving.

Anastomotic techniques. There are two basic types of anastomoses: end-to-end and end-to-side. Most anastomoses of grafts to the aorta and common iliacs are performed by end-to-end technique. On the contrary, the anastomoses of layer-sized grafts to small arteries and of small-caliber grafts to large arteries are performed by the end-to-side technique.

There is always some degree of intimal thickening at the point of anastomotic healing of the host artery to the graft. This is of little consequence with a large-caliber artery, but it is of major concern with a small artery. The impact of this intimal thickening is of special importance to small-caliber, vertical, end-to-end anastomoses. The reason for this is obvious when one considers the effects of 100, 500, and 1,000 μm circumferential inner-wall anastomotic thickenings on the cross-sectional area of a vertical end-to-end anastomosis of a vessel 4 mm in diameter, in comparison to the effects of the same anastomotic thickenings on the cross-sectional area of a vessel 2 mm in diameter (Fig. 10-21). The problem with the vertical end-to-end anastomo-

sis is that the intimal thickening at every point of the anastomotic circle faces directly into a comparable area of intimal thickening, forming a concentric ring. Because of this spatial relationship, end-to-end anastomoses of small- and medium-caliber vessels should be performed in an oblique manner for the reasons shown in Figure 10-22. The advantage of the oblique end-to-end anastomosis is that the healing reaction in any vertical plane results in only two localized points of anastomotic thickening that face each other, leaving uninjured arterial wall above and below, except at the heel and toe of the anastomosis where these points meet.

End-to-side anastomoses to small-caliber arteries are less vulnerable to complete closure by intimal thickening because at least the central portion of the anastomosis is spread widely enough that the circular thickening located in the horizontal plane does not narrow the lumen to as critical a degree in this wider central area. However, the narrowing of the ends of an originally long end-to-side anastomosis to a small-caliber artery may be explained on the basis of crosschannel bridging of the anastomotic inner wall thickening. Further narrowing of the channel to "round" the ends probably occurs as a result of hemodynamic forces that are not yet understood (Fig. 10-23).

Longitudinal tension. Excessive longitudinal tension on an anastomosis tends to avulse the graft from the host artery, forming a false aneurysm. I have learned by experience that it is far better to leave a graft a little too loose than too tight. The graft that is tight at implantation will become far too tight over time from the contraction caused by the healing reaction. On the other hand, a graft can be placed so loosely that it is in danger of kinking. There is a happy medium.

False aneurysms are most common at the groin with aortofemoral grafts and generally do not appear for several years. I believe that excessive tension is an important, preventable cause of these late occurrences and may be both axial and intraanastomotic (Fig. 10-24).

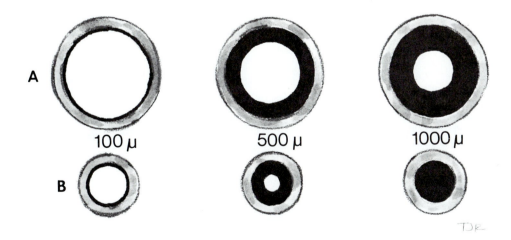

Figure 10-21. Comparative effect of 100, 500, and 1,000 μm anastomotic intimal thickening on residual luminal area of a 4 and a 2 mm artery. **A.** 4 mm artery. The reductions are 10%, 44%, and 75% respectively. **B.** 2 mm artery. The reductions are 19%, 75%, and 100% respectively.

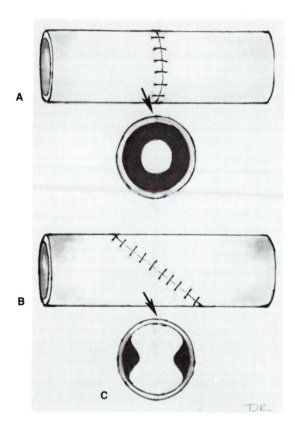

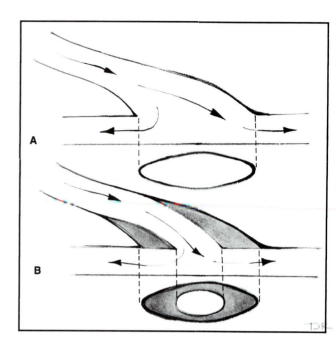

Figure 10-23. Luminal reduction of long end-to-side anastomosis of small caliber arteries by annastomotic healing reaction. **A.** Luminal configuration at implantation. **B.** In time the intimal thickening that occurs with healing tends to decrease the anastomotic opening to the caliber of the inflow channel.

Figure 10-22. Effect of anastomotic technique on lumen encroachment by a 1,000 μm thick healing reaction at the suture line of an artery 4 mm in diameter. **A.** Vertical end-to-end anastomosis with universally opposing suture line shows 75% compromise. **B.** Oblique end-to-end anastomosis shows limited encroachment because only two points are opposed in any transverse section. Luminal configuration at implantation. **C.** In time the intimal thickening that occurs with healing tends to decrease the anastomotic opening to the caliber of the inflow channel.

Figure 10-24. Proper and improper tension relationships between grafts and arteries joined by end-to-side anastomoses. Excessive tension predisposes to the late development of false aneurysms in large arteries and occlusions in small ones. **A.** Correct graft-to-common femoral artery tension relationships. **B.** Anastomosis elevated from its bed by excessive axial tension. **C.** Anastomosis distorted by suture of a small graft lumen to a larger arterial lumen, producing excessive intraanastomotic tension. (*From Sauvage LR: Graft complications in relation to vascular healing, in Haimovici H (ed): Vascular Emergencies. New York, Appleton-Century-Crofts, 1982, P 434.*)

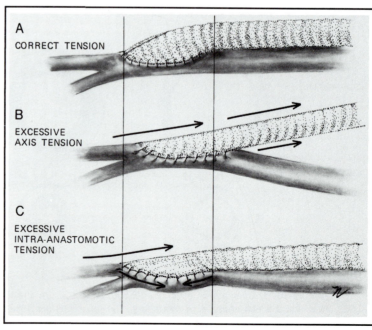

CLINICAL RECOMMENDATIONS (Fig. 10-25)

The thin-walled internal mammary artery has clearly emerged as a superior graft for coronary bypass. These grafts at 10 years have approximately 90% patency and have shown an amazing resistance to atheromatous degeneration.[21-26] These results are in marked contrast to the approximately 50% patency of saphenous aortocoronary grafts at 7 years, which is due primarily to the development of severe atherosclerotic degenerative change.[21-26,62-65] Innovative techniques have been devised that, in most instances, enable complete revascularization of the entire left ventricle with the internal mammary artery.[20] The alarming frequency of delayed closure of aortocoronary saphenous autografts after 5 to 7 years clearly suggests that these grafts should be reserved as a backup to the internal mammary for myocardial revascularization.

Woven grafts are an appropriate choice for use in the thoracic aorta. The Cooley autoclaving technique for grafts soaked in plasma is a wise precaution to assure complete imperviousness.[8-10] The long-term patency and dimensional stability of woven grafts in the thoracic aorta have been excellent despite limited tissue ingrowth. The chief drawbacks of these grafts in this location are their relatively poor surgical-handling characteristics, their tendency to fray, and their lack of complete imperviousness without auxiliary treatment.

Knitted grafts are the choice of many surgeons for aortoiliac replacement or bypass and for femorofemoral bypass because they are superior to woven prostheses in their handling and healing characteristics. The long-term results of these prostheses in this region have been excellent.[66] For knitted prostheses we recommend a filamentous outer wall, a smooth inner wall, and as low a water permeability as is possible without sacrificing desirable surgical handling characteristics (Table 10-2). Tissue ingrowth into approximately the outer half of the wall is attained within 2 months, with little inward progression beyond that time. However, despite their inferior surgical-handling and healing characteristics, the convenience of being able to use woven

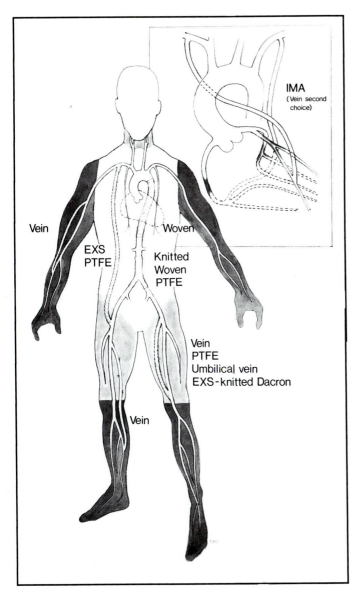

Figure 10-25. Appropriate graft types for use in the four zones of the arterial system.

TABLE 10-2. INTERRELATIONSHIPS OF STRUCTURAL FEATURES OF FABRIC PROSTHESES TO PERFORMANCE CHARACTERISTICS

	Preclotting Efficiency	Suturability	Healing
Increasing outer wall filamentousness	Positive effect	No effect	Positive effect
Increasing inner wall filamentousness	Positive effect	No effect	Negative effect
Increasing yarn denier*	Positive effect	Negative effect	Minimal effect
Decreasing water permeability	Positive effect	Negative effect	Minimal effect

* Denier is a unit of weight; the heavier the individual fiber, the higher the denier.

prostheses without preclotting has made these grafts the choice for the aortoiliac region of an approximately equal number of surgeons. If warp-knit Dacron grafts can be manufactured with an impervious, hypothrombogenic and healable matrix, this type of graft could find extended usefulness in the prosthetic zone, and possibly the venoprosthetic zone as well.

PTFE prostheses have obtained results equivalent to those of crimped knitted Dacron in the axillofemoral area; noncrimped knitted Dacron grafts supported by an external coil of polypropylene have shown superior results.[66–70]

PTFE, umbilical vein, and externally supported, noncrimped knitted Dacron prostheses all give results for above-knee femoropopliteal bypass that are sufficiently close to those obtained by the saphenous autograft to justify their use in their location, enabling the vein to be preserved for the more demanding areas below the knee joint or in the coronaries.[66–71] However, there is no prosthesis that is competitive with the venous autograft for bypass beyond the knee.[66–74]

REFERENCES

1. Voorhees AB, Jaretski AA, Blakemore AH: The use of tubes constructed from Vinyon "N" cloth in bridging arterial defects. Ann Surg 135:332, 1952.
2. Blakemore A, Voorhees AB Jr.: The use of tubes constructed of vinyon-N cloth in bridging arterial defects: Experimental and clinical. Ann Surg 140:324, 1954.
3. Yates SG, Barros D'Sa AAB, et al.: The preclotting of porous arterial prostheses. Ann Surg 188:611, 1978.
4. Savastianov VI, Tseytlina EA, et al.: Importance of absorption-desorption processes of plasma proteins in biomaterials hemocompatibility. Trans Am Soc Artif Intern Organs 30:137, 1984.
5. Sauvage LR, Berger K, et al.: The USCI-Sauvage filamentous vascular prosthesis: rationale, clinical results, and healing in man, in Sawyer PN, Kaplitt MJ (eds): Vascular Grafts. New York, Appleton-Century-Crofts, 1977, p 185.
6. Wu H-D, Zammit M, et al.: The influence of inner wall filamentousness on the performance of small-and large-caliber arterial grafts. J Vasc Surg 2:255, 1985.
7. Zammit M, Wu H-D, Sauvage LR: A comparison of external velour and double velour Dacron grafts in the canine thoracic aorta. Am Surgeon 51:637, 1985.
8. Bethea MC, Reemtsma K: Graft hemostasis: an alternative to preclotting. Ann Thorac Surg 27:374, 1979.
9. Cooley DA, Romagnoli A, et al.: A method of preparing woven Dacron aortic grafts to prevent interstitial hemorrhage. Cardiovasc Dis: Bull Texas Heart Inst 8:49, 1981.
10. Rumisek JD, Wade CE, et al.: Heat-denatured albumin-coated Dacron vascular grafts: Physical characteristics and in vivo performance. J Vasc Surg 4:136, 1986.
11. Shimada K, Ozawa T: Evidence that cell surface heparan sulfate is involved in the high affinity thrombin binding to cultured porcine aortic endothelial cells. J Clin Invest 75:1308, 1985.
12. Esmon CT, Owen WG: Identification of an endothelial cell cofactor for thrombin-catalyzed activation of protein C. Proc Natl Acad Sci USA 78:2249, 1981.
13. Weksler BB, Ley CW, Jaffe EA: Stimulation of endothelial cell prostacyclin production by thrombin, trypsin and ionophore A 23187. J Clin Invest 62:923, 1978.
14. Loskutoff DJ, Edgington TS: Synthesis of a fibrinolytic activator and inhibitor by endothelial cells. Proc Natl Acad Sci USA 74:3903, 1977.
15. Becker CG, Harpel PC: α_2-macroglobulin on human vascular endothelium. J Exp Med 144:1, 1976.
16. Donati MB, Dejana E, Enedatta LM: Pharmocologic intervention and events at the endothelium, in Cryer A (ed): Biochemical Interaction at the Endothelium. Amsterdam, Elsevier, 1983, P 406.
17. Chan TK, Chan V: Antithrombin III, the major modulator of intravascular coagulation is synthesized by human endothelial cells. Thromb Haemost 46:504, 1981.
18. Szilagyi DE, Elliott JP, et al.: Biologic fate of autogenous vein implants as arterial substitutes: clinical, angiographic and histopathologic observations in femoro-popliteal operations for atherosclerosis. Ann Surg 178:232, 1973.
19. Henderson VJ, Mitchell RS, et al.: Biochemical (functional) adaptation of "arterialized" vein grafts. Ann Surg 203:339, 1986.
20. Sauvage LR, Wu H-D, et al.: Healing basis and surgical techniques for complete revascularization of the left ventricle using only the internal mammary arteries. Ann Thorac Surg 42:449, 1986.
21. Singh RN, Sosa JA, Green GE: Long-term fate of the internal mammary artery and saphenous vein grafts. J Thorac Cardiovasc Surg 86:359, 1983.
22. Grondin CM, Campeau L, et al.: Comparison of late changes in internal mammary artery and saphenous vein grafts in two consecutive series of patients 10 years after operation. Circulation 70 (suppl 1):I-208, 1984.
23. Barner HB, Standeven JW, Reese J: Twelve-year experience with internal mammary artery for coronary bypass. J Thorac Cardiovasc Surg 90:668, 1985.
24. Lytle BW, Loop FD, et al.: Long-term (5–12 year) studies of internal mammary artery and saphenous vein coronary bypass grafts. J Thorac Cardiovasc Surg 89:248, 1985.
25. Cameron A, Kemp HG Jr, Green GE: Bypass surgery with the internal mammary artery graft: 15 year followup. Circulation 74 (suppl III):III-30, 1986.
26. Subramanian VA, Hernandez Y, et al.: Prostacyclin production by internal mammary artery as a factor in coronary artery bypass grafts. Surgery 100:376, 1986.
27. Sauvage LR: Graft complications in relation to prosthesis healing, in Haimovici H (ed): Vascular Emergencies. New York, Appleton-Century-Crofts, 1982, p 427.
28. Clagett GP, Graeber GM, et al.: Differentiation of vascular prostheses in dogs with serial tests of in vivo platelet reactivity. Surgery 95:331, 1984.

29. Wesolowski SA: Teflon, glass, and mysticism. Surgery 54:287, 1962.
30. Campbell CD, Brooks DH, Bahnson HT: Expanded microporous polytetrafluoroethylene (Gore-Tex) as a vascular conduit, in Sawyer PN, Kaplitt MJ (eds): Vascular Grafts. New York, Appleton-Century-Crofts, 1978, P 336.
31. Kenny DA, Berger K, et al.: Experimental comparison of the thrombogenicity of fibrin and PTFE flow surfaces. Ann Surg 191:355, 1980.
32. Sauvage LR, Berger KE, et al.: Future directions in the development of arterial prostheses for small and medium caliber arteries. Surg Clin North Am 54:213, 1974.
33. DePalma R: Atherosclerosis in vascular grafts, in Gotto AM, Paoletti R (eds): Atherosclerosis Review. New York, Raven Press, 1979, p 147.
34. Grondin P: Small diameter arteries in the aortocoronary position, in Sawyer PN, Kaplitt MJ (eds): Vascular Grafts. New York, Appleton-Century-Crofts, 1978, P 375.
35. Loop FD: Experience with grafts of biologic origin, in Sawyer PN, Kaplitt MJ (eds): Vascular Grafts. New York, Appleton-Century-Crofts, 1978, P 390.
36. Piccone VA: Alternative techniques in coronary artery reconstruction, in Sawyer PN (ed): Modern Vascular Grafts. New York, McGraw-Hill, 1987, P 263.
37. Ehrenfeld WK, Stoney RJ, Wylie EJ: Autogenous arterial grafts, in Stanley JC (ed): Biologic and synthetic vascular prostheses. New York, Grune & Stratton, 1982, P 295.
38. Sauvage LR, Berger K, et al.: Presence of endothelium in an axillary-femoral graft of knitted Dacron with an external velour surface. Ann Surg 182:749, 1975.
39. Mathisen SR, Wu H-D, et al.: The influence of denier and porosity on performance of a warp-knit Dacron arterial prosthesis. Ann Surg 203:382, 1986.
40. Mathisen SR, Wu H-D, et al.: An experimental study of eight current arterial prostheses. J Vasc Surg 4:33, 1986.
41. Camilleri J-P, Phat VN, et al.: Surface healing and histologic maturation of patent polytetrafluoroethylene grafts implanted in patients for up to 60 months. Arch Pathol Lab Med 109:833, 1985.
42. Dardik H, Ibrahim IM, et al.: Biodegradation and aneurysm formation in umbilical vein grafts. Ann Surg 199:61, 1984.
43. Guidoin R, Noel H-P, et al.: The fate of human umbilical vein grafts as an infrarenal aortic substitute in monkeys. J Vasc Surg 2:715, 1985.
44. Boontje AH: Aneurysm formation in human umbilical vein grafts used as arterial substitutes. J Vasc Surg 2:524, 1985.
45. Hasson JE, Newton WD, et al.: Mural degeneration in the glutaraldehyde-tanned umbilical vein graft: incidence and implications. J Vasc Surg 4:243, 1986.
46. Karkow WS, Cranley JJ, et al.: Extended study of aneurysm formation in umbilical vein grafts. J Vasc Surg 4:486, 1986.
47. Guidoin R, Gagnon Y, et al.: Pathologic features of surgically excised human umbilical vein grafts. J Vasc Surg 3:146, 1986.
48. Pourdehymi B, Wagner D: On the correlation between the failure of vascular grafts and their structural and material properties: a critical analysis. J Biomed Mater Res 20:375, 1986.
49. Trippestad A: Late rupture of knitted Dacron double velour arterial prostheses. Report on four cases. Acta Chir Scand 151:391, 1985.
50. Sladen JG, Gerein AN, Miyagishima RT: Late rupture of prosthetic aortic grafts. Presentation and management. Am J Surg 153:453, 1987.
51. Berger, K, Sauvage LR: Late fiber deterioration in Dacron arterial grafts. Ann Surg 193:477, 1981.
52. Guidoin R, Downs A, et al.: Anastomotic false aneurysms with aortic Dacron graft after 25 years. Ann Surg 1:369, 1986.
53. Campbell CD, Brooks DH, et al.: Aneurysm formation in expanded polytetrafluoroethylene prostheses. Surgery 79:491, 1976.
54. Roberts AK, Johnson N: Aneurysm formation in an expanded microporous polytetrafluoroethylene graft. Arch Surg 113:211, 1978.
55. Mohr LL, Smith LK: Polytetrafluoroethylene graft aneurysms. A report of five aneurysms. Arch Surg 115:1467, 1980.
56. Graham LM, Bergan JJ: Expanded polytetrafluoroethylene vascular grafts: clinical and experimental observations, in Stanley JC (ed): Biologic and synthetic vascular prostheses. New York, Grune & Stratton, 1982, P 576.
57. Kaplan S, Marcoe KG, et al.: The effect of predetermined thrombotic potential of the recipient on small-caliber graft performance. J Vasc Surg 3:311, 1986.
58. Zammit M, Kaplan S, et al.: Aspirin therapy in small-caliber arterial prostheses: long-term experimental observations. J Vasc Surg 1:839, 1984.
59. Sauvage LR, Walker MW, et al.: Current arterial prostheses. Experimental evaluation by implantation in the carotid and circumflex coronary arteries of the dog. Arch Surg 114:687, 1979.
60. Noll G, Lammle B, Duckert F: Treatment with stanozolol before thrombolysis in patients with arterial occlusions. Thromb Res 37:529, 1985.
61. Sue-Ling HM, Davies JA, et al.: Effects of oral stanozolol used in the prevention of postoperative deep vein thrombosis on fibrinolytic activity. Throm Haemost 53:141, 1985.
62. Campeau L, Enjalbert M, et al.: The relation of risk factors to the development of atherosclerosis in saphenous-vein bypass grafts and the progression of disease in the native circulation. A study 10 years after aortocoronary bypass surgery. N Engl J Med 311:1329, 1984.
63. Grondin CM: Graft disease in patients with coronary bypass grafting. Why does it start? Where do we stop? J Thorac Cardiovasc Surg 92:323, 1986.
64. FitzGibbon GM, Leach AJ, et al.: Coronary bypass graft fate. Angiographic study of 1,179 vein grafts early, one year, and five years after operation. J Thorac Cardiovasc Surg 91:773, 1986.
65. Fox MH, Gruchow HW, et al.: Risk factors among patients undergoing repeat aorta-coronary bypass procedures. J Thorac Cardiovasc Surg 93:56, 1987.
66. Sauvage LR, Smith JC, et al.: Dacron arterial grafts: comparative structures and basis for successful use of current prostheses, in Kambic HE, Kantrowitz A, Sung P (eds): Vascular Graft Update: Safety and Performance, ASTM, STP 898. Philadelphia, American Society for Testing and Materials, 1986, P 16.
67. Gupta SK, Ascer E, Veith FJ: Expanded polytetrafluoroethylene arterial grafts: an eight-year experience, in Sawyer PN (ed): Modern Vascular Grafts. New York, McGraw-Hill Book Co., 1987, P 181.
68. Kremen AF, Mendez-Fernandez MA, et al.: The dacron EXS graft: patency in femoropopliteal and femorotibial surgery. J Cardiovasc Surg 27:125, 1986.
69. Schultz GA, Sauvage LR, et al.: A five- to seven-year experience with externally-supported Dacron prostheses in axillofemoral and femoropopliteal bypass. Ann Vasc Surg 1:214, 1986.
70. Sauvage LR, Davis CC, et al.: Development and clinical use of porous Dacron arterial prostheses, in Sawyer PN (ed): Modern Vascular Grafts. New York, McGraw-Hill Book Co., 1987, P 225.
71. Dardik H: Long-term experience with the glutaraldehyde-stabilized human umbilical cord vein graft in lower extremity revascularization, in Sawyer PN (ed): Modern Vascular Grafts. New York, McGraw-Hill Book Co., 1987, P 153.
72. Callow AD: Current status of vascular grafts. Surg Clin North Am 62:501, 1982.

73. Veith FJ, Gupta SK, et al.: Six-year prospective multicenter randomized comparison of autologous saphenous vein and expanded polytetrafluoroethylene grafts in infrainguinal arterial reconstructions. J Vasc Surg 3:104, 1986.

74. Esquivel CO, Blaisdell FW: Why small caliber vascular grafts fail: a review of clinical and experimental experience and the significance of the interaction of blood at the interface. J Surg Res 41:1, 1986.

75. Edwards WH, Mulherin JL Jr: The role of graft material in femorotibial bypass grafts. Ann Surg 191:721, 1980.

76. Leather RP, Karmody AM, et al.: The saphenous vein as a graft and as an in situ arterial bypass, in Sawyer PN (ed): Modern Vascular Grafts. New York, McGraw-Hill Book Co., 1987, P 133.

77. Porter JM: In situ versus reversed vein graft: Is one superior? J Vasc Surg 5:779, 1987.

78. Taylor LM Jr, Phinney ES, Porter JM: Present status of reversed vein bypass for lower extremity revascularization. J Vasc Surg 3:288, 1986.

79. Taylor LM Jr, Edwards JM, et al.: Reversed vein bypass to infrapopliteal arteries: modern results are superior to or equivalent to in-situ bypass for patency and for vein utilization. Ann Surg 205:90, 1987.

80. Weaver FA, Barlow R, et al.: The lesser saphenous vein: autogenous tissue for lower extremity revascularization. J Vasc Surg 5:687, 1987.

81. Andros G, Harris RW, et al.: Arm veins for arterial revascularization of the leg: arteriographic and clinical observations. J Vasc Surg 4:416, 1985.

82. Ochsner JL, Lawson JD, et al.: Homologous veins as an arterial substitute: long-term results. J Vasc Surg 1:306, 1984.

83. Sawyer PN, O'Shaughnessy AM, Sophie Z: Development and performance characteristics of a new vascular graft. J Biomed Mat Res 19:991, 1985.

84. Ramasamy N: Physical chemistry of the blood-vascular interface, in Sawyer PN (ed): Modern Vascular Grafts. New York, McGraw-Hill Book Co., 1987, P 56.

85. Sawyer PN, O'Shaughnessy, Sophie Z: Patency of small-diameter negatively charged glutaraldehyde-tanned (St. Jude medical biopolymeric) grafts, in Sawyer PN (ed): Modern Vascular Grafts. New York, McGraw-Hill Book Co., 1987, P 163.

86. Malone JM, Brendel K, et al.: Detergent-extracted small-diameter vascular prostheses. J Vasc Surg 1:181, 1984.

87. Wu H-D, Kaplan S, et al.: The carotid artery as a coronary bioprosthesis: five potential donor species. Vasc Surg 19:163, 1985.

88. Kaplan S, Wu H-D, et al.: Glutaraldehyde preparation of coronary artery bypass bioprostheses. J Surg Res 38:45, 1985.

89. Cooley DA, Subram A, Houchin DP: Clinical experience in 1040 patients with double-velour knitted Dacron vascular prostheses: with particular reference to dilatation and aneurysm formation. Cardiovasc Dis: Bull Texas Heart Inst 8:320, 1981.

90. King MW, Guidoin RG, et al.: Designing polyester vascular prostheses for the future. Med Progr Technol 9:217, 1983.

91. Domurado D, Thomas D, Broun G: A new method for producing proteic coatings. J Biomed Mater Res 9:109, 1975.

92. Guidoin R, Snyder R, et al.: Albumin coating of a knitted polyester vascular prosthesis: an alternative to preclotting. Ann Thorac Surg 37:457, 1984.

93. Guidoin R, Martin L, et al.: Polyester prostheses as substitutes in the thoracic aorta of dogs. II. Evaluation of albuminated polyester grafts stored in ethanol. J Biomed Mat Res 18:1059, 1984.

94. Maurer PC (ed): Collagen-impregnated grafts for vascular surgery: Experimental and clinical status. Proceedings of a colloquium held in Zürich, Switzerland, May 3, 1985. Angio Archiv band 9, Grafelfing, Demeter Verlag, 1985.

95. Quinones-Baldrich WJ, Moore WS, et al.: Development of a "leak-proof," knitted Dacron vascular prosthesis. J Vasc Surg 3:895, 1986.

96. Abbott WM, Cambria RP. Control of physical characteristics (elasticity and compliance) of vascular grafts, in Stanley JC, Burkel WE, et al. (eds): Biologic and synthetic vascular prostheses. New York, Grune & Stratton, 1982, P 208.

97. Scott SM, Hoffman H, et al.: A new woven double velour vascular prosthesis. J Cardiovasc Surg 26:175, 1985.

98. Hanel KC, McCabe C, et al.: Current PTFE grafts. A biomechanical, scanning electron, and light microscopic evaluation. Ann Surg 195:456, 1982.

99. Wright CB, White RA, et al.: Small caliber vascular grafts—alternatives, in Kambic HE, Kantrowitz A, Sung P (eds): Vascular graft update; safety and performance ASTM STP 898. Philadelphia, American Society for Testing and Materials, 1986, P 60.

CHAPTER 11
Atherosclerosis: Biologic and Surgical Considerations

Henry Haimovici and Ralph G. DePalma

Atherosclerosis, the most common cause of arterial diseases, today occupies a position of heightened interest. It is the most frequently lethal disease of modern Western society, although within the last 2 decades cardiovascular mortality in the United States has decreased dramatically. During the 2 decades before 1983, cardiovascular mortality in this country declined about 36% nationwide.[1,2] Recognition of the importance of atherosclerosis as a major cause of serious disability and death in Western society led to research that has generated better understanding of this disease,[3] although many questions remain to be answered.[4-6]

The most common terms applied to this process, *arteriosclerosis*, *atheroma*, and *atherosclerosis*, reflect a wide divergence in the implications of these terms for different workers.

Lobstein,[7] in 1829, introduced the term *arteriosclerosis* to describe any disease of the arteries in which there was thickening of the wall and induration. Medial calcification, described by Monckeberg,[8] could be put into the general category of arteriosclerosis, although it appeared to be unrelated to other quite dissimilar processes also grouped therein.

The term *atheroma* was applied to arterial lesions by von Haller in 1755 to denote the common type of plaque that, during sectioning, exudes its yellow, pultaceous contents. The use of the word *atheroma* has been preserved and was redefined by the World Health Organization in 1958. WHO suggested that it should be applied to plaques in which fatty softening is predominant.[9]

In 1904, Marchand[10] proposed the term *atherosclerosis*, which was intended to include all lesions of all coats and to emphasize the importance of the fatty element. It is well recognized that atherosclerosis, at least at its onset, is a focal process affecting several arterial segments in the same individual but in which the tempo of development of the lesions in different parts of the arterial tree may vary greatly.

These three terms are those most commonly applied to this arterial disease and are often used interchangeably without regard to the exact morphologic picture. Perhaps atherosclerosis, usually employed by pathologists and experimentalists, is the most applicable of the three terms, provided one bears in mind the above morphologic and biochemical definitions.

Modern considerations of atherosclerosis and the detailed examination of atheromas in man and experimental animals show that these lesions contain three major components: cholesterol, mainly in the form of cholesterol esters; cells, mainly smooth muscle cells, as well as macrophages and other cell types; and fibrous proteins. Proportions of all these components can vary widely. Smooth muscle proliferation is a hallmark of almost all lesions, and within most plaques modified smooth muscle cells tend to form large amounts of connective tissue matrix, mainly collagen, elastic fibers, and proteoglycans. Thus, although lesion variability is common, the term *atherosclerosis* has evolved to its current meaning of lesions exhibiting these characteristics in varying degrees.

MORPHOLOGY OF NORMAL ARTERIAL WALL

Morphologic features vary with the location and function of the arteries, and their variables are reflected in the arteries' three coats; the intima, media, and adventitia (Fig. 11-1). Arteries are generally divided into muscular and elastic arteries; the distinctive structures of muscular and elastic arteries are contrasted in Figure 11-1. These three layers react differently to the various factors leading to the pathologic changes. Some of them are initially affected by the pathologic process, and then changes spread to the other coats in a later phase.

The *intima* of the large and medium-sized arteries consists of an endothelial lining resting on a layer of connective tissue that separates it from the internal elastic membrane and the media. Throughout life, the intima of the human aorta and of the medium-sized arteries progressively thickens because of proliferation of connective tissue in the subendothelial region. This intimal thickening is usually not regarded as atherosclerosis.

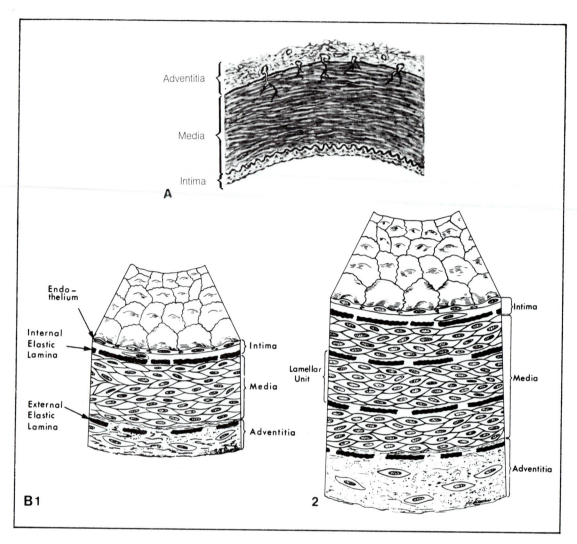

Figure 11-1. A. Diagram of the cross section of an arterial wall. **B 1.** Structure of normal muscular artery. **2.** Structure of normal elastic artery. (*From Ross R, Glomset JA: Atherosclerosis. N Engl J Med 295:369, 420, 1976.*)

The *endothelium* of arteries consists of flattened cells with a slightly bulging center arranged in a squamous pattern. Through this layer pass the substances required for the metabolism of that portion of the vessel that is not dependent on the vasa vasorum. Normal endothelial cells tend to exhibit a continuous monolayer when vessels are fixed while distended and without prior manipulation.[11] The fibrillar layer beneath the endothelium is called the basal lamina; it bonds the endothelial cells and the subendothelial connective tissue matrix. The subendothelial layer is a thin but complex loose connective tissue containing fine elastic and collagen fibers. In certain arteries, there are some plain muscle fibers and a ground substance that reacts weakly to mucopolysaccharides.

Changes in endothelial cells have been described in an almost endless number of situations. Wilens,[12] as well as other investigators,[11] stressed the fact that the capacity of the endothelial lining to withstand damage differs in various areas of the body and that abnormal characteristics tend to develop in particular sites, as seen on electron micrographs.

When injured, endothelial cells react in a unique fashion. The depth of arterial injury apparently modulates reendothelialization as the cells respond to the connective tissue matrix to which they have been exposed. Endothelial cells preferentially attach to type 4 collagen via laminin, a ubiquitous protein of the basement membranes and the internal elastic lamina.[13]

The *internal elastic membrane* usually appears as a single, corrugated, homogenous, and generally unbroken band around the vessel, separating the intima from the media. When the vessel has been fixed in a distended state, the undulations are lost, and it appears as a flat membrane. It is to be noted that the elastic membrane lies well within the zone of diffusion of nutrients from the lumen. Recently, electron microscopy has revealed fenestrations or gaps in it. These fenestrations appear to be the main pathway for transfer of fluids from the intima to the media.

The *media*, in which elastic tissue is diffusely found throughout the aorta, owes its distinctive characteristics to the proportion of muscle fibers and elastic tissue. Thus the amount of elastic tissue in the media progressively decreases from the thoracic aorta (elastic artery) until it reaches the medium-sized arteries, such as the femoral or carotid artery (muscular artery). The thoracic aorta and arch vessels exhibit more of a lamellar architecture than do the peripheral muscular vessels. In the human aorta, there are 58 lamellar units total; 29, or only the outer 50%, are supplied by vasa. It is believed that the human abdominal aorta is peculiar in that it has fewer and thicker lamellar units than would be predicted solely on the basis of average radius.[14] This discrepancy is thought to make the human abdominal aorta more prone to aneurysm formation.

The media in the muscular arteries is formed primarily of plain muscle cells, with a relatively small number of fine elastic fibers. These fibers disappear in the smaller vessels, in which the media is almost entirely made up of circularly oriented muscle cells. In addition to the circular fibers, many arteries contain a number of longitudinal ones.

The *external elastic membrane,* which separates the media from the adventitia, is variably developed according to the arteries. In the coronary artery, in addition to the internal elastic membrane, there is a moderately developed external elastic lamina outside the medial coat. In contrast, in the arteries of the lower limb, the external elastic membrane is poorly developed; but there is a readily identifiable thick layer of many longitudinal elastic fibers forming a double-edge around the outside of the media.

The *adventitia* is best developed in vessels of medium size with a predominantly muscular structure such as those of the leg. Its thickness may equal or even exceed that of the media. It should be pointed out that the adventitia, besides containing the vasa vasorum, is an important element in the strength of the vessel wall and plays an important role in reconstructive arterial procedures.

Vasa Vasorum

The arterial wall, like any tissue, is provided with a system of blood vessels known as the vasa vasorum. They consist of afferent arterioles, a capillary plexus, and efferent venules and veins. The arterial system is also complemented by a system of efferent lymphatic capillaries and vessels.

The vasa vasorum appear to play a significant role not only in the normal state of the arterial wall but also in its pathologic state, both as a cause or as a reflection of the changes in the arterial tissue. Physiologically, the vasa vasorum are considered the nutrient vessels, since they provide oxygen and the elements for the cellular metabolism of the arterial tissue. Evidence has been presented for more than 3 decades that degenerative changes in these vasa vasorum may play a significant role in the etiology of atherosclerosis.

Vasa Vasorum in Normal Arterial Wall

The origin, distribution, and extent of the vasa vasorum display individual variations. The vasa vasorum differ also according to the size of the arterial segment. Usually, they arise from proximal portions of branches of the arteries whose walls they vascularize and form an extensive adventitial plexus around the latter. Branches from this plexus supply a superficial and a more deeply situated, more dense

plexus of smaller vessels at the junction of the adventitia and media. The depth of penetration into the media by portions of this deeper plexus lying at the medioadventitial junction is quite variable. It is not always the same in all the arteries of an individual, and it may vary from place to place in the same artery.

The inner portions of the media and the intima in non-diseased human aortas and coronary arteries do not have any vasa vasorum (avascular zone). Although in some animals these two layers may have vasa arising directly from the lumen and passing outward without branching but having an extensive capillary plexus confined mostly to the adventitia, in the human arteries such vessels are rare or, most often, absent. In brief, the circulation provided by the vasa vasorum is limited to the outer wall of the vessel and has no direct connection with the circulation in the lumen. The intima and approximately the inner half of the media receive their nutrients from the circulating blood by diffusion. The point at which these two sources of nutrient supplies meet represents a watershed. There is still much controversy about the exact location of the meeting of these two sources. In healthy aortas and other vessels of larger size, the intima and the inner third or inner half of the media are avascular layers, receiving their oxygen and nutrition by diffusion through the endothelium. Capillaries are practically never present in these tissues unless some pathologic change such as atherosclerosis has developed.

In arteries with a caliber of less than 1 mm, there are no known vasa vasorum. These vessels can subsist without them.

Pathologic Vascularization of Arterial Wall

Winternitz, Thomas, and Le Compte,[15] in their study of arteriosclerosis, demonstrated extensive vascular networks in the walls of the larger atherosclerotic vessels (Fig. 11-2). The source of the vascularization of the atherosclerotic plaques has been a source of controversy. The vascularization of intimal thickenings would come in the main from the vasa vasorum, although to some extent it would also come from the lumen, especially in patients with atheroma.

The role of the vascularization of intimal thickenings is variously interpreted. According to Wilens,[12] the vascularity of atheroma influences the fate of the lesions. If the blood supply is adequate and there are no vascular accidents, the plaques undergo fibrosis; otherwise, hyalinization occurs. Vascularization of plaques is regarded in a less favorable light by other investigators.[15] The poorly supported capillaries in the plaques may rupture, resulting in intramural hemorrhage and subsequent occlusion of the lumen of the vessel.

From a review of the reports on the vascularization of the arterial wall, it is apparent that much is still unknown regarding the morphology and function of the vasa vasorum in health and disease.

Studies in experimental subhuman primates have shown atherogenesis to promote ingrowth of new and thinner-walled vasa vasora into the coronary arteries.[16] In human coronary and carotid arteries, such vasa vasora are

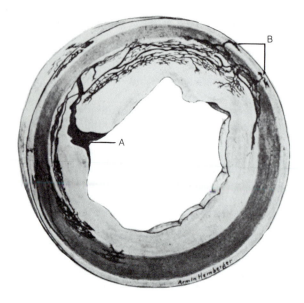

Figure 11-2. Injected and cleared block of a femoral artery showing a plexus derived from an intimal vessel (A) and adventitial vessels (B). The adventitia has been removed. (*From Winternitz MC, Thomas RM, et al.: The Biology of Arteriosclerosis. Springfield, Ill, Charles C Thomas, Publisher, 1938.*)

thought by some to rupture and cause intraplaque hemorrhage.[17] The instability of carotid bifurcation plaques has been repeatedly documented. Ulcerated carotid plaques in particular suddenly expand, with rupture of porridgelike material into the arterial lumen.[18,19]

NATURAL AGE-RELATED CHANGES IN THE ARTERIAL WALL

The natural age-related structural changes in the arteries, from birth onward, are important in relation to the evolution of atheromatous lesions. Studies were performed on arteries of fetuses, as well as in people ages 1 month to 95 years, excluding those with hypertension. Robertson[20] found mural cushions of thickening of the media and intima, containing longitudinal muscle and elastic fibers, in the lower end of the brachial artery, in the popliteal arteries, and at the mouths of their branches. He found no cushions in the fetal aorta and only small scattered cushions in the coronary arteries.

The progressive intimal thickening of that proceeds from infancy to old age is diffuse and is more prominent in arteries that develop severe atherosclerosis.

With advancing age, the internal elastic membrane of the aorta and other large arteries becomes segmented and reduplicated, whereas the rest of the elastic tissue of the media atrophies, undergoes progressive calcification, and loses much of its elasticity. The atrophic changes in the media are usually associated with atherosclerosis of the intima. This association may be either causal or merely a reflection of the simultaneous occurrence of two separate aspects of the aging process in the arterial wall.

Obviously, their presence raises the questions as to whether the changes have any effect on the dynamics of the circulation and whether they predispose the vessel to atheromatous changes. Whether the age-related changes represent a preatheromatous lesion or a favorable condition for the development of atheroma is difficult to state. Since both conditions occur at an advancing age and are associated with hypertension, some overlap must be inevitable.

With aging, arteries tend to increase in diameter and become longer. This process of diffuse ectasia involves the aorta and larger arteries and is accompanied by a relative overall increase in collagen content, a decrease in elastin, calcification of elastic fibers, and decreased arterial wall compliance.[21] Complications of the ectatic process possibly include aortic aneurysm formation, which tends to occur a decade later than occlusive aortic disease.

MORPHOGENESIS OF ATHEROSCLEROTIC LESIONS

On the basis of their gross appearance and morphologic characteristics, atherosclerotic lesions have been classified into several evolutionary phases. From a clinicopathologic point of view, the atherosclerotic process may be divided into three major stages: (1) asymptomatic, or latent, characterized initially by fatty streaks and later by fibrous plaques; (2) potentially symptomatic, characterized by complicated lesions such as calcification, hemorrhage, ulceration, and thrombosis; and (3) ischemic or terminal process, characterized by occlusive thrombosis, which may result in myocardial or cerebral infarction, ischemic damage to other organs, or gangrene, of extremities (Fig. 11-3).

The chronologic relationship between these various stages is still uncertain. However, one fact appears certain—this process begins in childhood but does not become apparent until middle age.

Fatty streaks appear soon after birth, as seen in the aortas of most people over the age of 3 years. Holman et al.,[22] in 1958, found that the surface area involved with fatty streaks gradually increases with age. These streaks are found with increasing frequency from the thoracic to the abdominal aorta in children between the ages of 8 and 18, with the most rapid rise near puberty. Histologically, masses of lipid are found in the intima, with some of it in macrophages (foam cells). Fraying of elastic fibers adjacent to the intimal foamy layer is often noted, together with proliferation of plain muscle fibers in the intima.

Some but not all fatty lesions become fibrous plaques. Whether or not all fibrous plaques must evolve through a fatty streak stage is uncertain.[22]

Fibrous plaques may take many years to develop and so do not appear until the second decade at the earliest. However, they do not increase in number very much until the fourth decade. Holman estimated that they lagged about 15 years behind fatty streaks and that only about 20% of them had converted to fibrous plaques by the age of 40 years. This process, it should be noted, is progressively more marked toward aortic bifurcation, in which the more severe atheromatous lesions are usually found. Histologically, lipids are seen beneath a thick fibrous elastic cap that is often associated with medial thinning beneath the

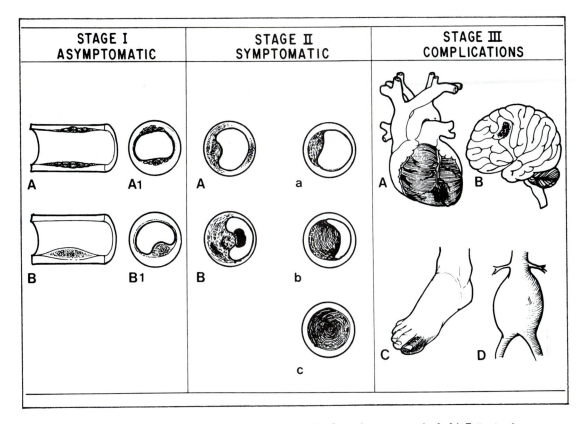

Figure 11-3. Diagram of natural history of atherosclerosis. *Stage I*, asymptomatic: **A, A1.** Fatty streaks. **B, B1.** Fibrous plaque. *Stage II*, symptomatic: **A.** Fibrous plaque and medial calcification. **B.** Enlarged fibrous plaque with thrombus formation. **a.** Asymptomatic arterial stenosis. **b.** Significant hemodynamic stenosis. **c.** Complete occlusion. *Stage III*, complications: **A.** Myocardial infarct. **B.** Brain infarct. **C.** Gangrene. **D.** Aneurysm.

plaque. In addition, there is splitting of the internal elastic layer adjacent to the lipid deposits that may be near the media. However, very little lipid penetrates the media at this stage. In some atheromatous plaques, cholesterol clefts are found under the fibrous layer that encapsulates the lesion. Some fibrous plaques can arise through other pathways, as, for example, the evolution of a thrombotic lesion into an atheroma, a sequence illustrated by chronic intra-arterial catheter implantation.[23] This mechanism illustrates the Duguid thesis[24] that atherosclerosis might also be an end result of organization of mural thrombi.

The thickened intima overlying the plaque is nourished by the blood from the lumen until it grows too thick. It then becomes vascularized on its deep surface from the adventitial vessels that traverse the media. It appears then as a zone in a very thick intima that is not adequately vascularized from either side and in which lipids continue to accumulate.

Fatty streaks and many fibrous plaques are strictly pathologic findings without any clinical manifestation. However, should these plaques become ulcerated or the site of other complications, these lesions may assume important clinical significance. In addition, an important adaptive response in atherosclerotic arteries has been described recently by Glagov et al.[25] It is believed that certain of these arteries may enlarge to compensate for disease progression;

however, the general nature and extent of this adaptation needs further elaboration.

Complicated Lesions

Calcium Deposits in Atheromatous Plaque
Calcification of the normal artery or of plaques can occur independently of other factors affecting atheromatous growth and development. Calcification of atheromatous plaques can have important hemodynamic consequences by altering the elastic properties of the lesions (Fig. 11-4). This effect is not widely recognized, possibly because most significant calcific atheromatous plaques occur in the aorta, a vessel with a wide lumen in which blood flow is not greatly altered by change in elasticity of the wall. However, in arteries with thicker walls and smaller lumina, calcification of the atheromatous plaque may severely impede the blood flow.

The essential difference between plaques and normal vessel wall is that plaques have a great capacity to bind much larger amounts of calcium. In normal vessel wall, the tissue-binding calcium is probably elastin, whereas in plaques, collagen is the more likely tissue involved. Calcification of plaques may begin as diffuse calcium deposition and proceed to its end stage without the intervention of

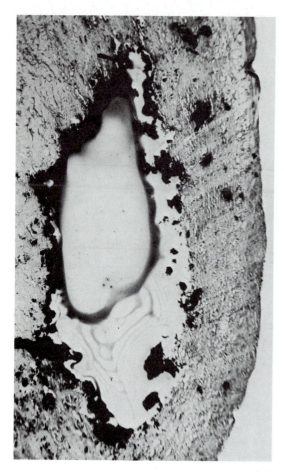

Figure 11-4. Patchy calcification of the media of the arterial wall.

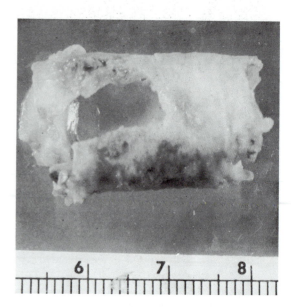

Figure 11-5. Cylinder shape of calcification of the media removed from the neck of an infrarenal abdominal aortic aneurysm in a 70-year-old woman.

local factors. However, local hemorrhage or ischemic necrosis of the plaque may be more likely to calcify the plaque in aortas, especially with large amounts of diffuse aortic atheromas.

Occasionally, ossification occurs in calcified plaques. Its significance as a complicating local factor in reconstructive arterial surgery is obvious, particularly when the process involves the media and adventitia (Fig. 11-5).

Medial calcification or calcinosis, also known as Mönckeberg's sclerosis, is found in the aorta and in the large arteries of the extremities in middle-aged or, mostly, elderly persons. This process is not necessarily associated with atheroma and is of little clinical significance. It may be noted in young and middle-aged persons who have severe diabetes mellitus. The medial calcification in diabetes is often associated with atherosclerotic and thrombotic lesions.

Ulceration of and Embolization from Atheromas
Ulcerated atheromatous plaques are a complication of advanced intimal disease and, like the calcific ones, are sites of increased thrombogenesis (Fig. 11-6).

Factors in the development of ulcerations are mechanical stress, ischemic necrosis, and hemorrhage. If there is thinning and weakening of the media, aneurysm formation

results. Release of atheromatous debris into the circulation as emboli may occlude small arteries in various organs or extremities. The frequency of atheromatous emboli varies with the extent of the ulcerated lesions. These emboli are most commonly observed in the kidney, spleen, and pancreas. Coronary atheroemboli, by comparison, rarely seem to be involved. By contrast, cerebral atheroemboli have been more often implicated in the causation of cerebral ischemia. Considering the usual severity of atherosclerosis of the abdominal aorta, involvement of the lower extremities seemed, in the past, relatively uncommon. This apparent lack of involvement is due, in part at least, to the infrequency with which the legs are examined at autopsy. Recent publications indicate that atheroembolism is more common than previously reported.[26]

Thrombotic Occlusion and Atheromatous Plaque
A discrete atheromatous plaque may induce little or no narrowing of the lumen of the artery (Fig. 11-7). By contrast, in severely stenotic lesions, superimposed thrombosis occurs, leading to complete occlusion of the artery. In the early stages, fibrinous encrustations and platelet aggregations may be deposited as delicate fibers and small clumps. However, as stenosis develops, larger deposits form, and they have been demonstrated in various stages of incorporation into the intima (Figs. 11-8 to 11-10). As a rule, when the cross-sectional area of an artery is reduced to one third or less of its original size, the remainder of the lumen is usually occluded by a thrombus. The buildup of the severe stenosis that precedes the occlusion involves recurrent thrombosis, with incorporation of these successive mural thrombi into the wall. As a result, the occlusive plug is composed of two or more zones of differing ages. Thus, if the buildup of stenosis and the final occlusion are considered together, it is evident that in a high proportion of

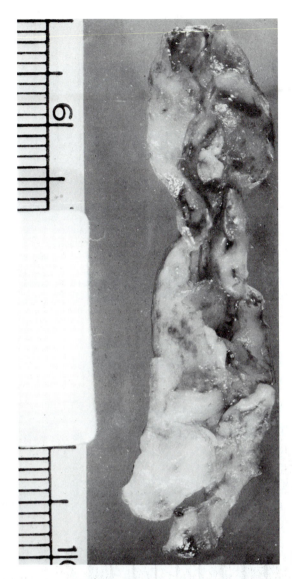

Figure 11-6. Ulcerated atheromatous plaque removed from a common femoral artery where it produced marked stenosis of the vessel.

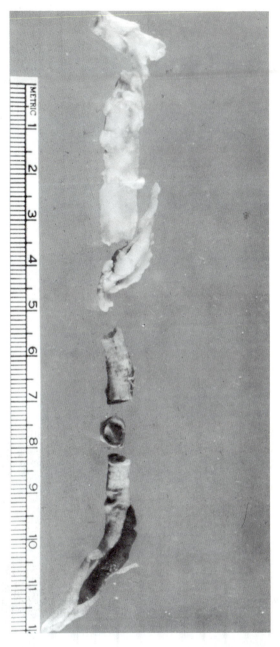

Figure 11-7. Specimen of thromboendarterectomy removed from the common and superficial femoral arteries. Note the proximal segment is composed only of a thick plaque, which almost completely occluded the origin of the superficial femoral; the latter was occluded by a recently organized thrombus.

these patients, recurrent thrombotic episodes have been occurring over a considerable time, perhaps extending over many months or even years. At a late stage, the thrombus may or may not be recanalized.

In contrast to the progressive or chronic mural thrombi formation, there are instances of acute occurrence of thrombosis, which are often mistaken for arterial emboli.

RISK FACTORS: ETIOLOGY

Atherosclerotic lesions go through the several evolutionary stages mentioned previously. The initiating factors responsible for the early lesions are undoubtedly the prime movers in the development of this process. The subsequent lesions, although related to the early changes, may be induced by different and more complex pathogenic factors.[27]

Role of Dietary Fat and Serum Cholesterol

Based on data currently available, serum cholesterol appears to be the key lipid measurement for assessing risk of premature atherosclerotic disease. In the management of hypercholesterolemic patients, fasting serum triglycerides and lipoprotein determinations seem to have an important predictive value (see Pathogenesis).

Epidemiologic studies have shown that the severity

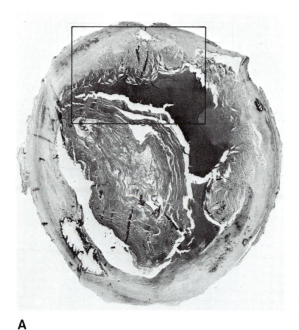

A

Figure 11-8. A. Cross section of an occluded abdominal aorta in a 66-year-old diabetic patient. The section displays marked mural changes, with calcification, atheromatous and fibrotic plaques, and a freshly organized thrombus, all of which represent typical stage III of the evolution of atherosclerosis (elastica–Van Gieson's stain ×5). **B.** Enlarged section (×15) of the microphotograph indicated by the square in **A.** Note cholesterol clefts in the atheromatous plaque. The thrombus is located between the latter in the fibrotic plaque.

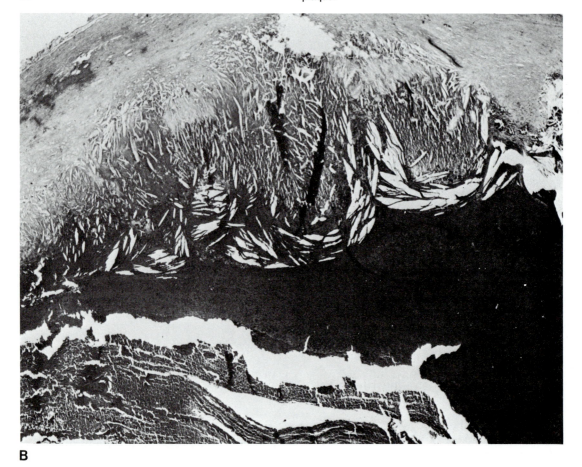

B

of atherosclerosis is closely associated proportionately with the total calories derived from fat and with serum cholesterol concentration. These findings are consistent with a large body of experimental and clinical evidence relating atherosclerosis to fat consumption and serum cholesterol.

A report, "Primary Prevention of the Atherosclerotic Diseases," published by the Inter-Society Commission for Heart Disease Resources,[28] emphasized two key generalizations on this matter:

1. Of central importance is the finding that arterial lesions cannot generally be produced experimentally in animals

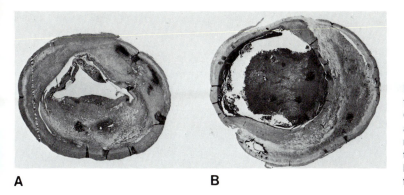

Figure 11-9. Specimen removed during a thromboendarterectomy of an iliac artery. **A.** Cross section markedly stenosed by a mixed atheromatous and fibrotic plaque and a markedly narrowed lumen. **B.** Different section from the same specimen in which the lumen is almost completely occluded by a freshly organized thrombus.

without a substantial modification of the diet that involves increased intake of cholesterol and fat, leading to elevation of serum lipid levels.

2. Similarly, with very few exceptions, human populations consuming diets high in saturated fat and cholesterol have high mean serum cholesterol levels and high incidence and mortality rates from premature coronary heart disease. Conversely, human populations consuming diets low in cholesterol and saturated fat have low mean serum cholesterol levels and low incidence and mortality rates from premature coronary heart disease.

The major risk factors for atherosclerosis include hyperlipidemia (mainly elevation of low-density lipoprotein [LDL] cholesterol, hypertension, diabetes mellitus, and cigarette smoking. The epidemiologic studies done by the Framingham group relate quantitatively the intensity and duration of these risk factors to the frequency of the clinical disorders that signal atherosclerotic disease. At the present, it is not possible to relate each of these risk factors to particular pathogenetic mechanisms within the arterial wall.

Hyperlipidemia

Various hyperlipidemic states have been classified on the basis of plasma lipid concentrations or of their response to high dietary carbohydrate or fat. Their classification, as described by Frederickson and Lees,[29] was based on the electrophoretic pattern of the lipoproteins in the fasting state.

Hyperlipidemias are divided into two categories, primary and secondary. Primary hyperlipidemia may be associated with a genetic defect or a lipase deficiency, usually exaggerated by dietary intake. Its defective lipid metabolism is due either to overproduction of lipoprotein or to insufficient clearance of lipoprotein from the plasma. Secondary hyperlipidemia is associated with hypothyroidism, nephrotic syndrome, diabetes mellitus, and biliary obstruction (see Pathogenesis).

Hypertension

Autopsy data of the International Atherosclerosis Project and observations of others show that atherosclerosis in the aorta, coronary arteries, cerebral arteries, and other major vessels is more extensive and more severe in hypertensive than in normotensive subjects. The data on prospective studies demonstrate, at least for affluent populations, that hypertension is related to risk of premature atherosclerotic disease independently of other major risk factors such as hypercholesterolemia and cigarette smoking.[30,31] Hypertension probably predisposes to continued hemodynamic injury, thereby accelerating plaque complications.

Diabetes Mellitus

It is a well-known clinicopathologic fact that diabetes mellitus of the maturity-onset type represents an enhanced risk of premature atherosclerotic disease involving the coronary, cerebral, and peripheral vessels. This relationship has been extensively documented in retrospective and autopsy studies. These investigations have shown that diabetics have atherosclerotic disease more often, more severely, and more prematurely than do nondiabetics.[32]

Several studies have indicated that patients with manifestation of atherosclerotic disease exhibit abnormalities in glucose tolerance more frequently than do clinical controls. Furthermore, it is known through prospective studies on population groups in the United States that not only clinical diabetes but also asymptomatic hyperglycemia (so-called subclinical, preclinical, or chemical diabetes) are important factors in atherosclerotic disease of coronary, cerebral, and peripheral arteries. The Framingham data on this subject indicated that glucose intolerance, although a significant factor to all three atherosclerotic events, is more strikingly related to the incidence of intermittent claudication. The importance of glucose intolerance for the peripheral vascular manifestations is comparable in significance to such factors as blood pressure and serum cholesterol for the other vascular lesions. Currently, diabetologists emphasize rigorous control of blood glucose levels without the use of oral agents. The pathogenetic mechanisms by which diabetes promotes atherosclerosis are poorly understood. Insulin therapy, for example, controls hyperlipidemia associated with diabetes and decreases total cholesterol synthesis.[33] Studies in wound healing show that insulin treatment may restore impaired collagen formation in diabetic laboratory animals.[34]

Cigarette Smoking

Vast amounts of international and national data have shown that cigarette smoking is related to risk of premature atherosclerotic disease independent of and in addition to such other major risk factors as hypercholesterolemia and hyper-

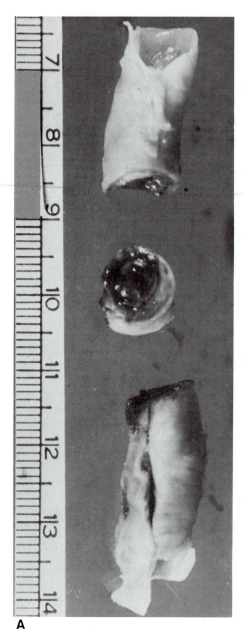

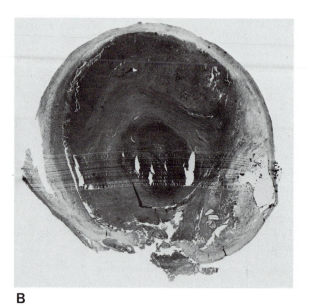

B

Figure 11-10. A. Specimen removed during thromboendarterectomy of the right common iliac artery, extending from the aorta to the bifurcation of the iliac. The middle and proximal segments contained a recently organized thrombus; the distal one contained an old fibrotic organized lesion. **B.** Cross section of the proximal iliac containing an organized thrombus, a portion of the media, and hypertrophied intima (elastica–Van Gieson stain ×6.75). **C.** Magnification of a segment of microphotograph **(D)** as indicated by the box (×40). **D.** Cross section of the iliac near its bifurcation, which is completely occluded by an organized thrombus represented by fibroblastic infiltration and minimal iron deposition. Note large fibrous plaques of the intima and portion of the media (elastica–Van Gieson's stain ×8).

A

tension. The younger the age group, the higher is the relative risk associated with cigarette smoking. Absolute risk, however, is increased with age. Risk of cerebral vascular disease is also greater for men and women who smoke cigarettes compared with nonsmokers up to age 70. Similar data are available about cigarette smoking as a major risk factor for premature atherosclerotic disease of the lower extremities.[35]

The exact mechanisms by which cigarette smoking promotes atherosclerosis are incompletely understood. Intermittent carbon monoxidemia possibly predisposes the arterial wall to endothelial injury, leading to increased plasma flux and increased LDL entry into the arterial wall. Cigarette smoking also causes increased platelet reactivity, promotes

peripheral vasoconstriction, and is associated with reduced high-density lipoprotein (HDL) levels.

Other Factors

Hereditary influences are thought to play a significant role in the development of atherosclerosis. Little, however, is known about the underlying biochemical, physiologic, and hemodynamic factors that identify the genetic characteristics of an individual prone to develop atherosclerosis.

Age, sex, and race have been extensively evaluated for their effects on atherosclerotic disease. The relative importance of each in clinical settings is widely debated and has been the subject of numerous statistical analyses.

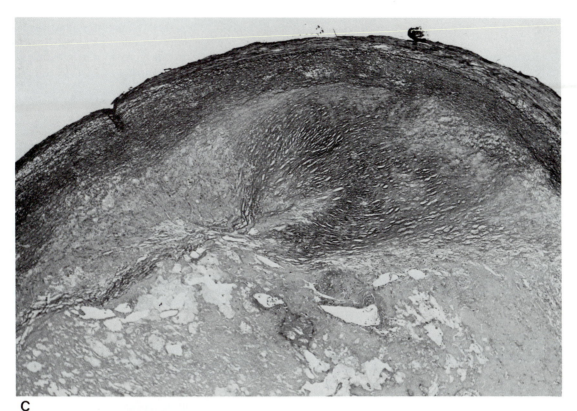

C

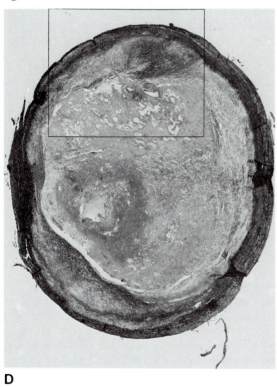

D

Figure 11-10, cont'd. For legend see opposite page.

PATHOGENESIS

It is now widely recognized that the pathogenesis of athero-sclerosis is a multifactorial process.[36] One thing that appears clear from the vast amount of studies is that this process is rarely, if ever, induced by one single factor. Several mechanisms, some of which are interrelated, are involved in its causation. It is thus not surprising that a great number of theories have been formulated to explain the origin, distribution, and ultimate fate of atherosclerotic lesions.

The initial phase of atherogenesis should be distinguished from the subsequent evolution of the lesions to understand clearly the overall complex process. The factors involved in the initial stage may be entirely different from those responsible for the later phases because they reflect the complications of this process.

Thrombogenic Theory

The thrombogenic theory, first suggested by von Rokitansky[37] in the nineteenth century, postulated that fibrinous substances deposited from the lumen on the arterial surface undergo metamorphosis into a mass composed of large numbers of cholesterol crystals and of fatty globules. This theory was revived by Duguid[24] in 1946, but a number of debatable objections exist about its initiating pathogenic mechanism.[38,39] Although there is little doubt that the thrombogenic mechanism is operative during the complicated plaque stage, its role during the inception of the fatty streaks remains controversial.

Although primarily related to the thrombogenic mechanism, recent new facets have been added to this concept. Indeed, it was shown experimentally that the platelets and prostaglandins, particularly thromboxane A_2 and prostacyclin, may play a role in the initiation of atherosclerosis. Their participation in clinical atherogenesis remains to be further confirmed.

Physical and Pressure-Flow Factors

A number of clinical and experimental studies have shown that increases in arterial pressure can enhance the accumulation of cholesterol in the vessel wall.[40] Attention has been called by several investigators to the application of Laplace's law, which correlates the factors influencing circumferential stretching as applied to arteries and the localization of atherosclerosis. Thus increases in hydrostatic pressure, in curvature of the vessel, and in the radius of the lumen radius would predispose to the local formation of atherosclerosis. There also seems to be also a close correlation between sites where turbulent blood flow occurs or is likely to occur and the prevalence of raised plaques. Fatty streaks do not show this correlation. Mitchell and Schwartz[39] suggested that different mechanical and hemodynamic factors may be of importance in localizing the two types of plaques—namely, that raised plaques commonly occur in areas of turbulent blood flow, whereas flat fatty streaks occur in areas where the shearing strain on the arterial wall is likely

to be high.[41] Although these pressure-flow relations may help us to understand to some extent the localization of the plaques, they do not represent the initiating factors of the atheromatous process.

Role of Lipid Metabolism: The Cholesterol Connection

The Early Investigations

The presence of cholesterol and other lipid complexes in atheromatous lesions, as demonstrated by pathologic and biochemical studies, is the basis for the pathogenesis implicating these substances in the causation of atherosclerosis. Following Anitschkow's production of atheromatous lesions in the rabbit by cholesterol feeding,[42,43] a large body of clinical and experimental evidence has been accumulated, suggesting that this arterial disease is the result of an abnormal lipid metabolism.

Anitschkow attributed this disorder either to excessive consumption of lipids or impaired control of lipid metabolism by endocrine organs. Among the lipids involved, cholesterol assumed the most important role. He reasoned that the increased blood lipoproteins had a tendency to settle in avascular connective tissue (intima) by transmural filtration, with the resulting changes typical of atherosclerosis, whereas all other factors (mechanism, chemical, and pharmacologic) were only of a contributing nature. Ever since that time, the lipid theory has almost monopolized the field of atherosclerosis.

Although in certain experimental animals, such as the rabbit, cholesterol feeding is almost always followed by atherosclerotic lesions, in other animals such lesions do not develop following cholesterol feeding alone. For such lesions to develop in the dog, for instance, in addition to the diet, thyroid function must be suppressed by either a pharmacologic or a surgical procedure. It is apparent, therefore, that besides cholesterol intake there must be other determining factors in atherogenesis.

In the human being, particularly in the population groups, there is substantial evidence that there is a relationship between the amount and the composition of dietary fats and various manifestations of atherosclerosis, although the correlation is not absolute.

Biochemical Studies: Role of Lipoproteins

Lipid analysis of plasma and atherosclerotic lesions shows that the cholesterol in the latter is derived from the former, but phospholipids may be synthesized in the intima.[44] This observation is important because it draws attention to the fact that not all lipids in the lesions are derived from blood and that the arterial wall determines in some ways the atherosclerotic process.

Based on the current status, it can be said that the lipid theory, which evolved through various stages from a past simplistic view to today's sophisticated biochemical status, retains a central importance in the pathogenesis of atherosclerosis.

Of considerable interest are the more recent biochemical studies of blood lipoproteins. It is known that virtually all the lipid material in the blood is transported in the form of lipoproteins. Seventy percent of the cholesterol in lipoproteins is present as esterase. The free, or nonesterified, cholesterol is on the surface of the lipoproteins. There are four main types of lipoproteins, which are classified according to their size and density: (1) chylomicrons, (2) the very low-density lipoproteins (VLDL), (3) the low-density lipoproteins (LDL), and (4) the high-density lipoproteins (HDL). Of the four main types of lipoproteins, LDL is the most atherogenic component. HDL is considered, on the other hand, to protect against the development of atherosclerotic lesions.[6,45]

LDL Cholesterol Receptors

Based on data currently available, measurements of total serum cholesterol, LDL cholesterol, and HDL cholesterols are the key lipid measurements for assessing the risk of premature atherosclerotic disease. Lipoproteins are large complexes containing cholesterol, cholesterol esters, triglyceride, phospholipid, and protein in varying quantities. Although a high level of LDL cholesterol is a major risk factor promoting atherosclerosis, a high level of HDL cholesterol is a negative risk factor. It is believed that HDL is responsible for transporting lipid out of the artery. At all ages in the United States, the total cholesterol level tends to mirror the LDL level.[39,46,47] Measurements of LDL cholesterol and HDL cholesterol provide refined measures. Estimates of levels that constitute an abnormally elevated cholesterol level have been changing. Generally, cross-sectional data in middle-aged men with total cholesterols of 185 mg/dl with an LDL level of 140 mg/dl or lower and an HDL level of 45 mg/dl are considered favorable. An additional factor—whether the lipid will enter the arterial wall—is believed to depend on the apoprotein moiety or the protein constituent of the lipoprotein molecule. Apoprotein B is associated with LDL and has a tendency to enter the arterial wall, whereas apoprotein A is a main constituent of HDL ("helper lipoprotein"). Hyperapobetaliproteinemia also identifies patients with hypertriglyceridemia who are more prone to atherosclerotic disease.

Abnormally elevated levels of LDL cholesterol or triglycerides can be controlled dietarily or with drug therapy. Disorders of plasma lipoproteins have been reviewed recently.[39] Severe genetic hyperlipidemia such as occurs in familial hypercholesterolemia type II is due to the lack of LDL receptors on hepatocytes and the inability to internalize and thus metabolize LDL within the liver.[46,47] This condition has been treated by portacaval shunting[48] and more recently by liver transplantation. Experiments by Brown and Goldstein,[47] identifying the negative-feedback system regulating cellular cholesterol synthesis in response to extra cellular LDL levels, were pivotal in understanding cholesterol metabolism and resulted in a recent Nobel award for these investigators. Brown and Goldstein discovered and purified the LDL receptors, crucial elements in the regulation of blood cholesterol levels. They also demonstrated that familial hypercholesterolemia was caused by genetic defects in the LDL receptor. Through a combination of studies of isolated cell systems, experimental animals, and living patients, they outlined the role of this receptor in body cholesterol metabolism (Fig. 11-11).[49]

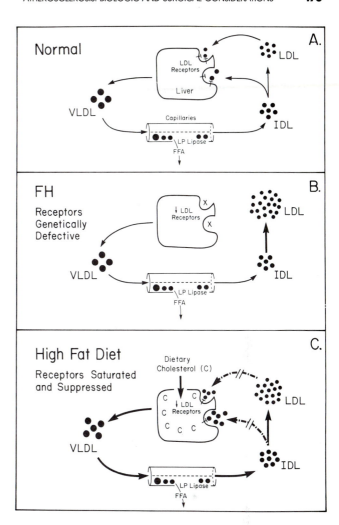

Figure 11-11. Schematic model of the mechanism by which LDL receptors in the liver control both the production and catabolism of plasma LDL in normal human subjects (**A**), in individuals with familial hypercholesterolemia (**B**), and in individuals consuming a diet rich in saturated fats and cholesterol (**C**), VLDL, very low density lipoprotein; IDL, intermediate density lipoprotein; LP, lipoprotein lipase; FFA, free fatty acids. (*From Brown MS, Goldstein JL: Science 232:34–47, 1986.*)

Early Events of Atheroma Formation

The events initiating early atheroma formation and localizing particular arterial sites are incompletely understood. The initial process appears associated with increased endothelial permeability resulting from altered endothelial cell function or from actual endothelial cell injury. The earliest lesion of atherosclerosis, or the fatty streak, occurs because of the entry of LDL into the artery through the intima and subintima of the arterial wall. This mechanism is most likely because the lipids of the early plaque are chemically similar to those of the plasma. It was believed that LDL entry stimulated arterial smooth muscle to form foam cells. However, a significant fraction of foam cells is also derived from the circulating macrophages and monocytes, which have been observed in recent studies of early atherosclerotic lesions of subhuman primates after only 12 days of hypercholesterolemia.[45]

Simultaneously, the plaque is enlarged by medial smooth muscle cells' migrating through the internal elastic lamina into the intima and proliferating. These cells then also accumulate lipid. Medial smooth muscle cells subsequently change into fibroblast-like cells capable of collagen production.

The overwhelming body of data that implicates the plasma lipoproteins, particularly LDL, suggests that metabolic changes that result from the interaction of lipoproteins with the arterial tissue may play a key role in the initiation of the atherosclerotic lesions. Recent studies of smooth muscle cells in tissue culture responding to the influence of hyperlipemic serum have demonstrated the growth-promoting activity associated with LDL and not with other serum fractions. The results of these studies underscore again the significance of LDL as an atherogenic factor.

The Response-to-Injury Hypothesis

In certain circumstances, focal desquamation of the endothelium exposes the underlying subendothelial connective tissue to platelets and other elements in the circulation. The platelets adhere to subendothelial collagen, aggregate, and release the contents of their granules. The massive infiltration of platelet factors, plasma lipoproteins, and other constituents at these sites of injury usually leads to focal proliferation or arterial smooth muscle cells and deposition of lipids within both the cells and their surrounding connective tissue matrix. Based on such observations, recent investigators[45] formulated the hypothesis that the sequence of events involved in atheroma formation begins with injury to the endothelium and exposure of the subendothelial tissue to plasma constituents, including lipoproteins, hormones, and platelet factors. According to this hypothesis, the various known risk factors in atherogenesis, such as hypertension, hyperlipidemia, smoking, diabetes, and genetic factors, actually can be explained on the basis of endothelial changes or the subsequent smooth muscle response to this injury.[45] Although this hypothesis may remotely evoke some similarity with the physical and pressure-flow factors, several factors of this concept require further elucidation. To date, this hypothesis rests solely on animal experimentation, and it is difficult to extend it to spontaneous human atherogenesis.

Role of Arterial Wall

Local Metabolic Factors

It is generally assumed that the chemical composition of the arterial wall is largely a reflection of the components of the plasma environment as propounded by the filtration concept of atherosclerosis.[50] Although filtration may play an important role by enhancing the passage of lipids through the endothelium of the arterial wall, it is also most likely that the endothelial permeability is not a passive phenomenon. Experimental evidence indicates that arterial tissue is indeed a metabolically active organ.[51–55]

Our own studies on the oxidative activity of aortic tissue in man, dog, and rabbit, with special reference ot succinic oxidase, cytochrome oxidase systems, and esterase, have shown that (1) a species difference was present, (2) the oxidative capacity of the succinic oxidase system was lower in the abdominal aorta of the dog than in its thoracic segment, and (3) of the three species, human aortic tissue exhibited the lowest oxidative capacity.[56,57]

The mechanism governing arterial tissue metabolism is a complex one. It is dependent on both local and systemic influences. Of these influences, hormonal and enzymatic factors may play an important role, as indicated by work done in the senior author's laboratory.[58–60]

Cellular Events in Atherogenesis

The endothelial cells, macrophages, and smooth muscle cells are capable of producing chemotactic and growth factors similar to platelet-derived growth factor (PDGF). These are the most striking characteristics of all the cells connected with the arterial wall. The human PDGF is a mitogen, which is a heat-stable cationic polypeptide derived from the alpha granules of platelets.[61] All cellular growth factors that exist in the arterial wall potentially contribute to plaque growth.

As a result of experimental and deductive reasoning, Ross[45] postulated two pathways for the initial events that might promote early atheroma formation. In the first pathway (e.g., in patients with hypercholesterolemia), monocytes and macrophages migrate into the arterial wall without endothelial denudation. At times, there might also be endothelial loss, with platelet carpeting of their areas. In such an event, platelets would stimulate proliferation of smooth muscle by PDGF release. In the second pathway, endothelium itself is postulated to release growth factors, which also stimulate smooth muscle proliferation. There is experimental evidence to indicate that regrowing endothelium induces myointimal proliferation beneath its advancing edge, with resulting collagen and glycosaminoglycan accumulation. Stimulated smooth muscle itself, in turn, releases growth factors that might lead to an autocrine proliferative response. The second pathogenetic pathway is considered relevant in atheromas that are possibly stimulated by diabetes, cigarette smoking, or hypertension.

Although hypertension has been recognized as causing endothelial injury and accelerating atherosclerosis, striking differences exist between the behavior of smooth muscle cells as a result of atherosclerosis vs. hypertension. In atherosclerosis there is overt smooth muscle proliferative response; in hypertension, thickening of the arterial wall occurs in most instances by virtue of increased protein synthesis without an increase in cell number.[61]

The growth factor of the PDGF is extremely potent; it causes the proliferation of all susceptible cells in culture at levels of 5 ng/ml of culture medium. In whole blood serum, PDGF is the principal mitogen to which cells characteristically respond with cell proliferation.

Based on their studies, Ross and associates stated that exposure of the PDGF could trigger the initiation of all the components of a proliferative lesion. The function of platelets in inducing experimental atherosclerosis in vivo seems to be proven. The role of the PDGF in stimulating mitogenesis in cell culture is clear; however, the question remains whether this factor is active in vivo.

In addition to the PDGF, there are other growth factors such as the endothelial-derived factor, which is capable of forming a mitogen or growth factor in culture. This substance, termed endothelial-derived growth factor, appears to be a potent molecule in terms of its capacity to stimulate cells such as fibroblasts in smooth muscle cells to proliferate. Indeed, smooth muscle proliferation has long been recognized as possessing a number of features important to normal arterial function, including their capacity to contract, to maintain arterial tone, and to synthesize connective tissue proteins.

It should be pointed out that many of these factors have been demonstrated, particularly in experimental studies, but have not yet been demonstrated conclusively in vivo to human pathology.

Concurrent with the newer developments pertaining to platelet and endothelium related to vascular function, there is recent interest in omega-3 fatty acids, which may produce effects that potentially can ameliorate or prevent atherosclerosis. Experimentally, eicosapentaenoic acid (EPA) has inhibited vein-graft atherosclerosis in an experimental animal.[62] A cellular mechanism for the action of omega-3 fatty acids is postulated to be reduction of leukocyte interleukin-1 production, a cytokine that also might stimulate the proliferation of vessel wall cells.[63] As discussed previously, intense proliferation of smooth muscle is a characteristic feature of atherosclerotic plaques. Interventions based on particular cellular events require long-term prospective clinical controlled studies to demonstrate actual beneficial effects in the arterial wall and on clinical outcomes. The question of whether interleukin-1 contributes to atherogenesis or whether EPA might reduce the risk of heart disease (e.g., in the Eskimo population) remains to be answered.

In brief, based on the foregoing data, it is clear that in our present state of knowledge of atherogenesis, the arterial wall has evolved from the original concept of a simplistic morphologic structure into a new biologic role. Recent understanding of cellular events and molecular aspects of this tissue may help unravel its true function in atherogenesis.

Role of Arterial Susceptibility

It is well known that some arteries are more vulnerable or susceptible to atherosclerosis than others and, moreover, that in the same artery, such as the aorta, certain sites are more susceptible than others. Thus in the dog, as well as in the human being, the abdominal aorta is more susceptible to atherosclerosis than is the thoracic aorta (Fig. 11-12). Although mechanical factors have been advanced for explaining the difference between these two aortic segments, our studies on the fate of canine aortic homografts suggested that a biologic difference may account for it.[64-67]

In these experiments, fresh thoracic and abdominal aortic homografts were implanted into the abdominal and thoracic aorta of dogs subsequently put on an atherogenic regimen. The thoracic aortic implants exhibited minimal or no atheromatous changes in contrast to the abdominal implants, which always developed marked lesions, regardless of the site of implantation into the aorta (Figs. 11-13 to 11-15). These studies strongly suggest that the aortic segments maintained their original behavior, namely, greater susceptibility to atherosclerosis of the abdominal as compared with the thoracic segment. These and other of our results further suggest that the arterial tissue itself may be a determining factor in atherogenesis rather than the location in the vascular tree as propounded by the hemodynamic theory. Our metabolic studies of the various aortic segments have disclosed a difference in the enzymatic makeup in the normal and in atherosclerotic arterial tissue.[57-60]

Architectural differences between various arterial segments may also play a significant role in the degree of

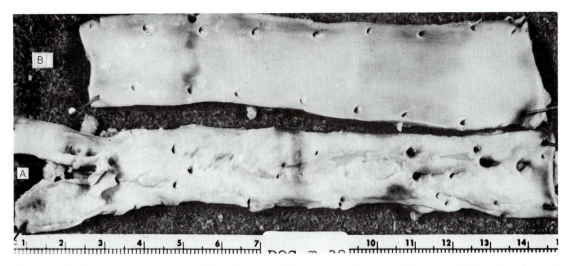

Figure 11-12. Photograph of abdominal **(A)** and thoracic **(B)** aorta of a dog on an atherogenic diet for 14 months, with an average serum cholesterol of 1037 mg/dl (range 721 to 1340). Note the massive atheromatous involvement of the abdominal aorta in contrast to absent thoracic lesions except in the ostia of the intercostal arteries.

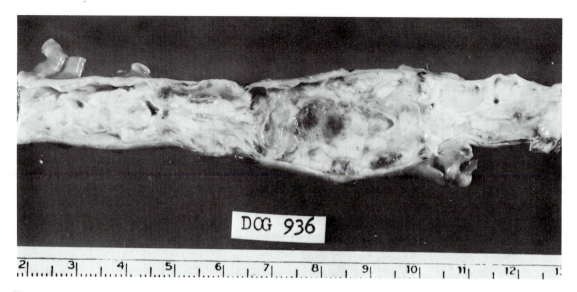

Figure 11-13. Abdominal aortic homograft implanted into an abdominal aorta, resulting in massive atheromatous involvement of both host and graft. Note ulceration in the center of the graft. Duration of the graft implantation was 9¾ months, and duration of the atherogenic regimen 8¾ months. Average serum cholesterol level was 1441 mg/dl.

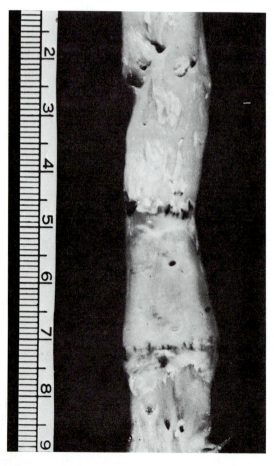

Figure 11-14. Thoracic aorta homograft implanted into the abdominal aorta for 24 months and after 20 months on atherogenic diet. Note marked atheromatous plaques on the host abdominal aorta in contrast to the absence of such lesions in the thoracic segment.

vulnerability to atherosclerosis. Wolinsky and Glagov[68] demonstrated differences of structure and vasal supply between normal thoracic and abdominal aortic segments that may be related to differences in susceptibility to atherosclerotic involvement. Similar architectural characteristics of other arteries, i.e., the coronary, may also explain their greater propensity to develop atherosclerosis more often than other arteries of similar size. However, the fact that the medium-sized arteries (circle of Willis, peripheral arteries of the limbs) are the most severely involved strongly indicates that, among the important factors, the diameter of the artery may also play a determining role in the incidence, degree, and pattern of atherosclerosis.

From this brief review of the major pathogenic factors, it is obvious that atherosclerosis is a complex dynamic process resulting from an interaction between components of the blood lipids, hemodynamic forces, and the structure and function of the arterial wall.

Atherosclerosis is, therefore, the summation resulting from an interplay of the aforementioned pathogenic factors.

Atherogenesis in Veins Used as Arterial Substitutes

Veins in their normal location, in human beings and in experimental animals, do not develop atheromatous changes even in the presence of prolonged and severe hypercholesterolemia. The venous tissue resistance to atherosclerosis, a fact in marked contrast to the arterial tissue susceptibility to this process, has raised obvious questions concerning its pathogenesis.

Recently, clinical reports indicate that atherosclerotic changes do occur in an autogenous vein graft implanted into an artery.[69–71] (See also Chapter 10.) Concern has been

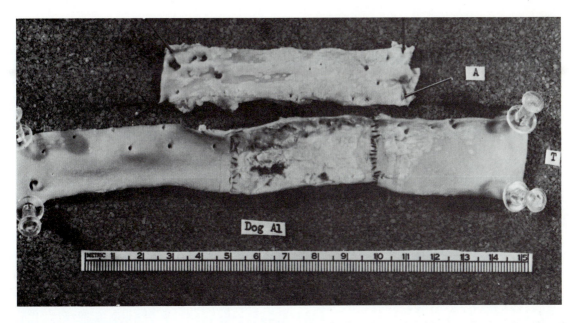

Figure 11-15. Host abdominal aorta and abdominal aortic homograft after 12 months of implantation into the thoracic aorta of a dog on cholesterol-thiuracil regimen for 10¼ months. The average serum cholesterol concentration was 1588 mg/dl. Marked atheromatous lesions of the graft are comparable to those found in the host abdominal aorta (A). In the host thoracic (T) proximal to the graft there are atheromatous plaques along the clamp marks, whereas none are present in the distal segment.

expressed that vein grafts in the arterial system of patients with atherosclerosis may be subject to degenerative changes due to this process. With the widespread use of vein grafts in the management of atherosclerotic occlusive disease of the peripheral arteries and of the coronary vessels, the study of potential vulnerability of venous tissue to the host atherogenic factors has received further impetus. To provide an answer to this question, we, as well as a number of other investigators, have studied the behavior of vein grafts in the arterial system in animals exposed to an atherogenic regimen.[72] Similarly, studies were carried out on grafts removed during surgery or at postmortem from patients having had venous bypass grafts.[69,71]

Based on these findings, three groups of data are available for evaluating the fate of vein grafts and their behavior when implanted into the arterial system: (1) data from normal animals, (2) data from animals subjected to a hypercholesterolemic diet, and (3) clinical and pathologic observations of veins used as femoropopliteal or aortocoronary bypass grafts.

Autogenous vein grafts implanted into the arterial system, in the absence of atherogenic diet, undergo morphologic changes noted by several investigators.[73,74] Jones et al.[75] studied the behavior of such grafts in canine femoral and aortocoronary arterial bypass that were implanted from 2 to 365 days. Shortly after implantation, the femoral grafts showed focal endothelial disruption, mural fibrin deposition, and medial edema with inflammatory infiltrates. Later, there was loss of medial smooth muscle cells and focal subendothelial lesions. In coronary grafts studied at 6, 9, and 12 months postoperatively, medial fibrosis and extensive intimal proliferation (hyperplasia) causing up to 90% luminal narrowing were found. Extension of the intimal

hyperplastic process into the coronary artery distal to the bypass graft also compromised the arterial lumen. These same investigators found similar subendothelial proliferation in coronary grafts obtained from human beings dying 17 and 57 days after graft insertion.

The study of vein grafts in hypercholesterolemic dogs investigated by us[72] dealt with autogenous vein grafts inserted into the abdominal aorta and peripheral arteries. The grafts in the abdominal aorta developed atherosclerotic changes, became dilated, and in most instances were surrounded by moderate to severe fibrous reaction. Microscopically all three coats of the vein were involved to variable degrees, with characteristic morphologic and lipid degenerative changes (Figs. 11-16, 11-17). The grafts implanted by end-to-side anastomosis into peripheral arteries (femoral, carotid) displayed minimal or no atheromatous changes, whereas those implanted by end-to-end anastomosis became stenosed or occluded by organized thrombi.

Clinical experience has shown that atherosclerotic changes may occur in autogenous vein grafts implanted into an artery.[69,70] Szilagyi et al., in a comprehensive study based upon 377 femoropopliteal autogenous vein bypasses, found that in 64% after 5 years and in 44% after 10 years of observation the vein graft was structurally sound and functionally unimpaired.[71] However, structural defects developed in 32.7% of the grafts as a result of technical mishaps (stenosis due to improper suturing and to instrumental trauma) and intrinsic tissue changes (subendothelial hypertrophy, layering of intimal thrombi, fibrosis of venous valves, and atherosclerosis). All these changes were found to be progressive and may have led to loss of patency of the graft. Szilagyi concluded that atheroslcerosis and intimal thickening, such as subendothelial hypertrophy and fibrin

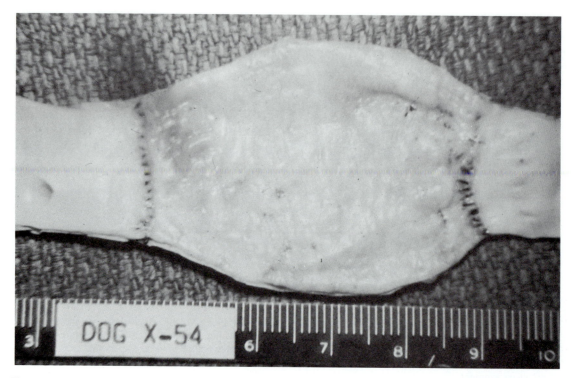

Figure 11-16. Jugular vein graft in the abdominal aorta after 16 months of implantation and 12¾ months on an atherogenic diet. Average serum cholesterol level was 1337 mg/dl. Note marked diameter disparity between graft and host aorta. Atheromatous lesions were disseminated throughout the graft, and only a few focal raised lesions were visible in adjacent aorta at the site of cross-clamping during surgery. (*From Haimovici H, Maier N: Arch Surg 109:95, 1974.*)

layering, are not remediable and may continue to be a major cause of loss of graft function.

Morphologic changes in coronary bypass vein grafts have also been reported by several investigators.[76–78] The lesions consisted of intimal fibrous proliferative changes that appeared primarily due to an arterial pressure response within the segment of the vein. Obstructive atherosclerosis in the artery beyond the anastomosis with its graft may favor the development of intimal lesions. Although these lesions in the coronary bypass grafts were not reported as being specifically due to lipid infiltration, had the grafts remained patent for longer periods of time, atheromatous changes might have occurred. Rossiter et al.[79] have reported that vein grafts as aortocoronary bypass also develop atheromatous degenerative changes, as demonstrated in dogs on an atherogenic diet. The problem of aortocoronary bypass grafts and atherogenesis has received confirmation in recent publications. These observations are similar to those of the peripheral vessels in which the bypass grafts were observed for periods ranging from 2 to over 10 years. In Chapter 10 the advantages of internal mammary artery grafts over vein grafts for coronary revascularization have been emphasized.

The pathogenesis of venous atheroma is rather complex. Among the factors contributing to venous atherogenesis in the veins used as arterial substitutes are the morphologic changes, turbulence, increased pressure, and filtration factors. It should be pointed out that when veins are placed into the arterial tree, factors other than the tissue itself appear responsible for the morphologic and lipid degenerative changes.[72]

SURGICAL CONSIDERATIONS

Distribution of Atherosclerotic Lesions

The atherosclerotic process usually involves in the same individual somatic as well as visceral arteries in variable degrees. The relative incidence of distribution of arterial lesions differs widely, according to the available statistical clinical studies. An overall correlative study of degree and distribution of human atherosclerotic lesions is largely lacking. Most of the studies have focused attention either on the peripheral arterial tree or on individual visceral arteries, such as the cerebral, renal, and coronary, and have mentioned only incidentally the involvement of the other arterial systems. Human necropsy studies dealing with the entire arterial system are also rather meager. A correlative study dealing with patterns of distribution, severity, and incidence of lesions affecting the various arterial beds may provide significant information concerning the natural history and prognosis of the disease process.

Experimental Data

In an experimental study in the dog, we have been able to correlate the degree of coronary atherosclerosis with that of cerebral atherosclerosis and atherosclerosis of the major systemic arteries.[80] A comparison of the incidence of ath-

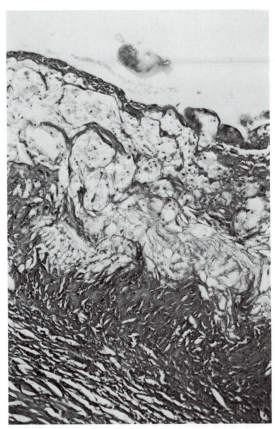

Figure 11-17. Vein graft of a dog. Note the thickened intimal layer with lipid-laden macrophages in the superficial intima and cholesterol clefts in the deeper layer (Verhoeff-Van Gieson stain ×72.5). (*From Haimovici H, Maier N: Arch Surg 109:95, 1974.*)

erosclerotic lesions found in the coronary vessels with those in the abdominal aorta and its major limb arteries (Figs. 11-18, 11-19). disclosed that the coronaries are less prone to develop this process (63.2%) than are the peripheral arteries (92.7%), with the abdominal aorta occupying an intermediate position (71.6%). Although these percentages indicate the overall involvement of these arterial beds, the percentage of the lesions displaying grade 3+ and 4+ was much higher in the peripheral arteries (68.5%) and aorta (43.1%) than in the coronary arteries (34.7%). Whether the experimental findings in the dog parallel the distribution and incidence of atherosclerosis in man remains undetermined.

Clinical Data

The clinical findings of Singer and Rob[81] and of Bloor[82] suggest that the presence of atherosclerosis in any one artery implies arterial disease elsewhere. Robertson,[83] in a similar study, emphasized, however, the lack of correlation between the extent and severity of atherosclerosis from one arterial bed to another. In contrast, according to Mitchell and Schwartz,[84] there is a tendency for atherosclerosis to develop in parallel in the different arterial systems. Young et al.[85] reported significant correlations between coronary and cerebral lesions in 37 autopsy cases. The coronary lesions usually were more advanced, however, than those in the cerebral vessels within a given age group. According

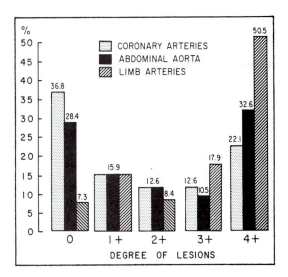

Figure 11-18. Relative incidence of atherosclerotic lesions in the coronary arteries, abdominal aorta, and limb arteries. (*From Haimovici H, Maier N: J Cardiovasc Surg 14:1, 1973.*)

to Holman and Moosy,[86] aortic lesions are already evident in the first decade, coronary lesions appear in the second, and cerebrovascular lesions appear in the third. In each decade, the aortic lesions are, on the average, quantitatively the greatest, the coronary arteries coming second, and the cerebral arteries last.

This account deals essentially with the distribution of the lesions in the lower extremities, although it alludes also to the cerebrovascular and other visceral arteries.

The atherosclerotic lesions of the lower extremities are classified into three main groups: the aortoiliac, the femoropopliteal, and the tibioperoneal.[87]

Some of the reports dealing with purely clinical data, without the support of arteriography or operative findings, fail to provide information concerning the anatomic distribution and classification of the arterial lesions. Therefore,

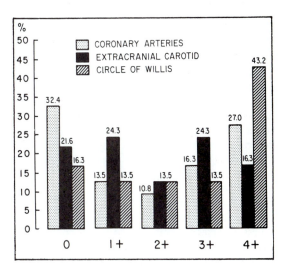

Figure 11-19. Relative incidence of atherosclerotic lesions in the coronary, extracranial carotid, and circle of Willis. (*From Haimovici H, Maier N: J Cardiovasc Surg 14:1, 1973.*)

the relative incidence of the three groups of arteries is difficult to ascertain from such studies.

The same pitfalls, to a lesser degree, are found in studies in which, despite the use of arteriography, the extent, location, and distribution of the arterial lesions were not always clearly defined. Thus, Humphries et al.,[88] in a study of 1850 patients, reported 513 having aortoiliac disease, 473 having combined aortoiliac and femoropopliteal disease, and 864 having femoropopliteal disease alone. Likewise, Valdoni and Venturini,[89] reporting the incidence of atherosclerotic occlusive disease in 600 patients with a total of 830 obstructions, showed that the aortoiliac segment was involved in 24%, iliofemoral in 4%, the femoropopliteal in 50%, the popliteal alone in 5%, and the tibial vessels in 17%. This classification is based on the arterial location of reconstructive procedures, without mentioning the combined arterial patterns. In other studies in which groups of selected patients with surgical procedures were reported, the relative incidence of the arterial locations varies widely. Fontaine et al.,[90] studying a group of 1125 operated cases, reported 68 involving the abdominal aorta, 321 the iliac arteries, 613 the femoral artery, and 123 the popliteal artery. By contrast, DeBakey et al.[91] reported 2029 aortoiliac lesions and only 1523 femoropopliteal lesions in a total of 3522 cases. This series, because of the greater percentage of the aortoiliac as compared with the femoropopliteal, would suggest a highly selected group of patients.

Our own studies have shown that atherosclerotic lesions are more prevalent in the femoropopliteal and tibial vessels than in the aortoiliac segment (75.4% versus 24.6%). One possible explanation for this peripheral preponderance may be the large number (40.6%) of diabetics in our series.[87,92]

Thus, excluding the report by DeBakey et al.,[91] it would appear from most statistical studies that the femoropopliteal and tibial vessels are predominantly involved in the occlusive atherosclerotic process (stage (III) in comparison with the aortoiliac segment.

Clinical correlation between peripheral arterial disease and death rate from cerebrovascular disease and cardiac infarction has been found to be much higher than in the general population of comparable age. Schwartz and Mitchell,[93] using a necropsy survey in an unselected group of patients, studied the relationship among coronary, carotid, and iliac artery lesions. They found a strong correlation between the degree of carotid and iliac stenosis and the severity of coronary stenosis. In patients with large cardiac lesions, the severity of aortic disease increases earlier than in unselected cases. This correlation appears even much more striking at a more advanced stage of the atherosclerotic process. Thus, clinical opinion supported by pathologic studies favors the concept that occlusive arterial disease in any site is but one manifestation of a widespread disorder. The study by Schwartz and Mitchell emphasizes the close association in individual patients among coronary, carotid, vertebral, and iliac artery lesions. Another point of considerable clinical significance is the bilateral nature of the lesions, which must be taken into account especially when reconstructive surgery is considered. This point is fairly well documented by clinical and necropsy findings.

NATURAL HISTORY, PROGRESSION OF DISEASE, AND PROGNOSIS

Clinical Data

The concept of the natural history of atherosclerosis, beginning in childhood and progressing through various stages and leading to ischemic complications in later years, although a somewhat oversimplified classification, is nevertheless justified in a wide percentage of cases.

The interrelationships of the different anatomic stages are not always entirely clear. However, it has been suggested that morphologically these three stages (fatty streaks, fibrous plaques, and complicated lesions) are age-sequence-related.[22]

The natural course of the complicated lesions, as expressed in terms of clinical manifestations, is perhaps easier to define.

Data limited to either clinical or necropsy surveys alone are not sufficient to provide a clinicopathologic comprehensive correlative study. A brief review of a few clinical or necropsy reports may, nevertheless, be helpful in attempting to define the natural course, progression, or regression, and prognosis of the atherosclerotic process in the major arterial regions.

Juergens et al.[94] reviewed a group of 520 nondiabetic patients, less than 60 years of age, whose major clinical diagnosis was that of atherosclerosis of the lower extremities. The ratio of male to female was 11:1. The incidence of smoking and arterial hypertension was higher than in a control group, the latter condition being present about three times as often. The survival rate of patients with atherosclerosis obliterans was less favorable than that of a normal population of a similar age and sex distribution. The survival rate for patients with atherosclerotic aortoiliac occlusion was significantly less favorable than that of patients with atherosclerotic occlusion of the femoral artery. In approximately three fourths of the patients who died, the cause of death was attributed to coronary artery disease. Four percent of the patients required amputation of the leg shortly after the diagnosis was made, and an additional 5% subsequently required amputation during the 5-year period following the initial examination. Only 3% with intermittent claudication as the only symptom of their disease required an amputation during this period. This study was carried out before the advent of reconstructive arterial surgery and thus may be used as a possible basis for comparative evaluation of results in patients subjected to direct arterial surgery.

In a somewhat similar study, Silbert and Zazeela[95] reported a survey designed to determine the prognosis for life and limb in patients with atherosclerotic peripheral vascular disease as related to diabetes, tobacco smoking, hypertension, age at onset of symptoms, and sex. Like the previous one, this study was a restrospective investigation that concerned itself during a 15-year period with 1198 patients having only peripheral arterial disease. Those with evidence of coronary or cerebral vascular disease were excluded from this survey. Furthermore, their selection was based on the presence of uncomplicated atherosclerotic peripheral vascular disease at the time of the first visit. They were followed for at least 3 years after onset of symptoms and extended up to the time of death or amputation.

The diabetic patients were found to have a 10-year mortality rate of 38% compared to 11% for nondiabetics. They also had a much higher rate of amputations (34%) than did nondiabetics (8%). As in the previous series, severe hypertension was associated with shortening of life expectancy. Its relation to frequency of amputation was dominated by smoking. Thus, amputation rate was lower in patients who stopped smoking than in those who continued to do so.

In another study also based on clinical evaluation, Gordon and Kannel,[35] in a 16-year follow-up survey of 5209 Framingham adults, showed that blood pressure, serum cholesterol, cigarette smoking, electrocardiographic evidence of left ventricular hypertrophy, and glucose intolerance are precursors common to all three major atherosclerotic events: atherosclerotic brain infarction (ABI), coronary heart disease (CHD), and intermittent claudication (IC). From this study, they concluded that the dominant factor predisposing to brain infarction was high blood pressure. None of the five factors mentioned above was clearly dominant for coronary heart disease. Of interest was the fact that glucose intolerance was only weakly related to coronary heart disease, and cigarette smoking was relevant weakly if at all to angina pectoris. With regard to peripheral vascular disease, all five factors seem to play an important role. This finding is in close agreement with the two preceding surveys. When all five variables were considered jointly, they had a closer relationship with brain infarction and intermittent claudication than with coronary heart disease. Basically, however, the most striking conclusion of this study was that all three atherosclerotic diseases appear to share a common set of precursors and that this was true in either sex.

The three preceding studies were based primarily on clinical criteria without the benefit of arteriography or other means of precise anatomic evaluation of the arterial involvement. The value of such surveys is, therefore, somewhat limited in terms of location and extent of lesions.

Imparato et al.,[96] in an arteriographic study of 104 patients with intermittent claudication as the only presenting symptom, found that the prognosis was determined by the severity of below knee arterial involvement. Thus, the overall amputation rate in this group was 5.8% in a 2.5-year mean follow-up and was only 12.5% in those with the most pronounced involvement of the leg arteries. Imparato failed to make a distinction between diabetic and nondiabetic patients. By contrast, in an arteriographic survey of 305 patients,[92] we found diffuse lesions involving the superficial femoral, popliteal, and tibial arteries more often in diabetics (75.4%) than in nondiabetics (42.6%). Involvement of the aortoiliac segment was found to be approximately twice as common among nondiabetics. The overall good results with revascularization procedures were significantly higher in nondiabetics (77%) than in diabetics (54%).

From our study as well as from those of others, it is concluded that the main factors accounting for the difference observed between the diabetic and nondiabetic patients

stem from the difference in the site, extent, and rate of progression of the atherosclerotic process in both the limbs and vital organs.

Coronary Atherosclerosis

The clinical assessment of coronary artery disease is based on the clinical presence or absence of angina pectoris, myocardial infarction, or congestive heart failure. Pathologic correlation of the coronary artery lesions with the clinical manifestations has been carried out by a number of studies. Allison et al.[97] reported a study based on 430 patients in which postmortem coronary angiography was used for comparison with a meticulous exploration of the coronary arteries and of the myocardium. This survey showed that coronary artery disease was present in 82% of the hearts examined and was severe in 43%. The gradations of severity, from none to occlusive, were approximately equal in incidence (none, mild, moderate, severe, occlusion). One or more occlusions of a major coronary artery were present in 24% (103 hearts), with a total of 227 occlusions.

Mitchell and Schwartz reported in some detail[41] on the distribution and prevalence of coronary stenosis and occlusion as determined by necropsy studies alone. They have shown that the pattern of arterial stenosis in the various groups and sites offered three important features: (1) severe coronary stenosis is associated with large myocardial lesions, (2) the coronary stenosis is more severe in men than in women, and (3) the left coronary arterial branches are more severely affected than those of the right.

The site of occlusion in the coronary arteries was the left coronary artery in two thirds of our patients. The majority of these, namely, half of the whole group of occlusions, were found in the anterior descending artery and its branches.

Vlodaver and Edwards reported that the segment of artery in which severe disease is most common is the segment of the right coronary artery that lies between the marginal and posterior descending branches of that artery, which they call the intermediate segment.[98] The second most common site in their study, is the proximal one half of the anterior descending artery. The third most common site for severe disease is the anterior segment of the right coronary artery, that segment that lies between the origin of the vessel and its marginal branch. These findings are somewhat at variance with those reported by Mitchell and Schwartz.

It is well known that in a given patient with coronary heart disease there are multiple lesions with involvement of more than one artery.

Diethrich and associates, in a study of 313 selective coronary cinearteriograms in patients with angina pectoris, found that significant involvement of only one vessel occurred in 23%, involvement of two vessels was seen in 40%, three vessels in 29%, and four vessels including the main left coronary artery in 9% of the patients.[99]

It should be pointed out that classification of the prevalence and multiplicity of coronary artery lesions based on angiography should be tempered by the fact that pathologic examination tends to show more significantly obstructed lesions than are portrayed in the arteriogram.[100–103] In addition, there is great variability in the analysis of coronary arteriograms, a fact that has been stressed by several angiographers and heart surgeons.[104]

Carotid and Vertebral Arteries

Although the possible clinical significance of stenosis or occlusion of the extracranial arteries in the causation of strokes was recognized a long time ago, it was not until 1957 that Hutchinson and Yates[105] stressed the importance of considering the carotid and vertebral arteries in the pathogenesis of cerebral vascular disease. Angiographic and pathologic studies have since demonstrated that there are certain anatomic sites of predilection for severe atherosclerotic lesions that lead to clinical disease. In a recent study of 961 autopsy subjects, Solberg and Eggen[106] showed that the topographic distribution of carotid and vertebral atherosclerotic lesions does not vary appreciably with geographic residence, sex, or age. Early lesions in younger age groups occur in the same topographic sites which, in later life, are the usual locations for stenotic and occlusive lesions. These results suggest that the lesions that begin as fatty streaks may progress gradually to the occlusive lesions that produce clinical disease. This close topographic association is consistent with the hypothesis that fibrous plaques are derived from fatty streaks. The early atherosclerotic lesions appear to be located at the same sites where stenotic and occlusive lesions are reported later. Thus, it is likely that the early atherosclerotic lesions and the stenotic or occlusive lesions are pathogenically closely associated with each other.

Prevalence of Lesions by Artery

Atherosclerotic lesions do not develop at the same rate in all parts of the neck arteries. The prevalence of lesions by segments has a characteristic pattern for each artery regardless of geographic location, sex, or age. In the carotid arteries, the maximum prevalence occurs at the bifurcation, sinus portion, and siphon region, and the minimum prevalence occurs at the second segment of the internal carotid. In the vertebral artery, lesions develop more uniformly along its axis, although the prevalence tends to be somewhat greater in the proximal and distal segments than in the intermediate. These patterns in the carotid and vertebral arteries are similar for males and females.

The question of relationship of fatty streaks to fibrous plaques has been the subject of some controversy and disagreement. Mitchell and Schwartz[41] found that the distribution of fatty streaks is different from that of raised lesions and thus consider that the fatty streaks should be regarded as separate processes from the fibrous lesions and not as the first stage of the raised plaque formation. Solberg and Eggen,[106] as well as other investigators, consider that a close association exists between these two lesions and suggest a pathogenic relationship between the fatty streak and the advanced lesions.

Caroticovertebral lesions are often associated with aortic disease or other peripheral arterial lesions. Indeed the International Atherosclerosis Project shows that coronary heart disease and cerebral vascular disease are associated with increased frequency of atherosclerotic lesions elsewhere. The association of these various lesions, as stated previously, emphasizes the widespread nature of the arterial disease.

Plaque ulceration, unlike similar lesions in other anatomic areas, assumes great significance in the carotid and vertebral arteries. Mitchell and Schwartz[41] found ulcerated plaques in 13 patients of 93 in whom caroticovertebral systems were examined, a prevalence of 14%. The possible significance of plaque ulceration in the neck arteries as a source of emboli to the brain is widely recognized today in the relationship between these lesions and strokes.[18]

Plaque Detection and Quantification

Delineation of the atherosclerotic lesions preferably depends on quantifiable assessments. A recent symposium was devoted to the problem of quantifying atherosclerosis.[107] Arteriosclerotic plaque measurements are needed to assess intervention end points. Asymptomatic, nonhemodynamically significant lesions are characterized mainly by abnormalities within the arterial wall rather than in its lumen. Not all plaques intrude into the arterial lumen; therefore the capability of angiography in early lesion detection is limited. Although angiography is a useful clinical tool, alternative techniques are being developed to track changes in plaques and in arterial wall morphology, size, and composition. To assess the effect of treatment or the improved effects in diseased vessels, there should be less luminal intrusion, less arterial wall involvement, and a more stable plaque. Ideally, beneficial treatment effects could be documented in the arterial wall itself and also would correlate with enhanced patient survival.

Past clinical studies of medical treatment for atherosclerosis have commonly used surrogate end points such as reduced lipid levels or mortality rates over time in large scale epidemiologic trials. The outcome of such studies are vulnerable to variables extrinsic to arterial pathology. An improving technology now exists that allows a minute focus on the arterial wall to assess evolving or regressing lesions.

Serial angiography and ultrasound imaging are conventional tools for the study of arterial wall dynamics. Angiography, however, lacks sensitivity for early lesion detection.[108] Refined B-mode imaging and computerized axial tomography have become more useful tools for arterial wall examination. A recent B-mode ultrasound study[109] of atherosclerosis in cynomolgus monkeys was capable of detecting lesions as small as 0.4 mm in arteries with lumen diameters of 2 mm. Clinical studies with B-mode ultrasonography suggest that morphologic variants of carotid plaques might be defined[110] and that B-mode ultrasonic sensitivity for ulcerated carotid plaques exceeds that of conventional angiography.[111]

The quantification of dilating or aneurysmal disease by angiography is flawed in many instances because of a laminated clot. Ultrasonic examination or computerized axial tomography are preferred methods for measuring aneurysmal size. Recent research using proton nuclear magnetic resonance (NMR) imaging in vivo and in vitro shows that the intensity of NMR signals from atherosclerotic plaques differs from that of the normal vascular wall.[112] This unique characteristic of NMR permits detection of a fat-containing plaque in its early stages before it intrudes into the arterial lumen. NMR is a highly promising clinical tool; when used with cardiac gating to correct for artifacts due to pulsatile arterial wall motion, it is capable of imaging a 3 mm slice thickness in large vessels. (See Chapter 8.)

Plaque Regression or Arrest

Atherosclerotic plaques in experimental animals regress as plaque bulk is reduced, mainly by lipid egress[113–116]; connective tissue accumulation in plaques also regresses slowly.[117] Experiments employing serial biopsy, gross observation, and angiography to follow single lesions in individual animals show conclusively that lesion intrusion and plaque bulk are lessened by drastic reduction of serum cholesterol below certain levels.[118,119] Conversely, serum cholesterol levels exist above which lesions inevitably progress.[119,120] This critical level of cholesterol in man may approximate a total serum cholesterol of 140 to 150 mg/dl or an LDL level of 100 mg/dl. Above these levels progression tends to occur, whereas below these levels regression or arrest is possible. It is likely that an increased level of HDL is required to transport lipids from the arterial wall. A recent trial used serial coronary angiography[121]; lesion arrest correlated with ratios of total cholesterol to HDL of less than 6.9. A confounding variable in experimental quantitative studies to follow plaques exists: arterial luminal diameter might increase during early atherogenesis, a phase that precedes the stenotic disease stage.

In spite of operational limitations, as a result of animal studies, human plaque regression with dramatic lipid reduction has been sought and has been clearly documented.[122–125] Plaque regression in humans occurs in instances of partially intrusive luminal lesions. Such lesions are usually not hemodynamically dramatic; plaque regression in human symptomatic lesions overall is not a common clinical response. Among 143 arteriograms, 32 convincing instances of regression were collected by Malinow up to 1981.[126] Recently, Duffield et al.,[127] in a controlled randomized study, showed arrest of femoral artery atherosclerosis and improvement of twice as many arterial segments with the reduction of LDL cholesterol by 28% and of plasma triglycerides by 45%. Others[128] have shown failure to control plaque progression with medical treatment. These failures probably relate to the inability to control the multiple risk factors promoting human disease, the failure to achieve threshold lipid reduction as can be done in laboratory animals, and the more advanced state of human plaques when intervention therapy begins.

Quantifiable methods of evaluating plaque change should demonstrate favorable or unfavorable change over time. One strategy tests the efficacy of atherosclerosis with measurement of the rate of plaque change in tests in control groups. This discipline of arterial wall lesion measurement has been called auxometry by Blankenhorn.[125] Current auxometric studies in progress evolve serial measurements using angiography of both femoral and coronary arteries and ultrasound imaging of carotid arteries. These investigations track lesion changes with a technology now capable of increasingly precise quantification.

To date, the only manipulations found to alter human atherosclerotic lesions toward arrest or regression use serum-lipid reduction and cessation of cigarette smoking. Antiplatelet therapy has not been shown to produce a favorable effect on directly observed human lesions. Experimentally, in a test using relatively large doses of aspirin and dipyridamole and serial morphologic and angiographic studies, combination antiplatelet therapy was noted to be deleterious in dietarily induced atherosclerosis in a rhesus monkey model.[129] Hollander et al.[130] reported a similar effect in cynomolgus monkeys.

Antiplatelet agents continue to be used empirically to treat atherosclerosis. It has been hoped that antiplatelet treatment would alter disease progression, based on suppositions that these drugs might negate abnormal platelet kinetics or inhibit the action of PDGF. These hopes have not yet materialized. However, anticoagulant actions of antiplatelet agents could be beneficial. A voluminous literature regarding the optimal dose of aspirin has been reviewed recently by Wechsler and others.[131–132] Smaller doses of aspirin are now considered advantageous; however, clinical trials must be performed. In the case of dipyridamole, Morisaki and associates[133] showed experimentally that this drug was an antioxidant promoting the proliferation of cultured aortic smooth muscle cells. Experiments using hypercholesterolemic rabbits showed that dipyridamole enhanced plaque formation[134] and exhibited similar effects when combined with aspirin. Such results may raise serious questions. Further studies are obviously indicated.

Experimental human trials with surrogate end points do not provide direct information about dynamic changes in the arterial wall or in atherosclerotic plaques themselves. Progress in devising treatment strategies might also be estimated from quantitative real-time serial studies of plaques combined with the analysis of clinical events as they occur. Given more accurate means of imaging arteries, arterial wall improvement and patient survival would prove the efficacy of the particular interventions. It should be recognized, however, that one of the most effective means of improving arterial dynamics is surgical intervention, as illustrated abundantly by the results of bypass surgery, endarterectomy, patch angioplasty, and recent balloon dilatation procedures.[4,135] Clearly, life expectancy is increased after abdominal aortic reconstruction for aneurysm[136,137] or after bypass of obstructed left main coronary arteries.[138] In the future, combined surgical and medical approaches to atherosclerosis will likely further enhance the efficacy of current treatment.

CONCLUSIONS

Atherosclerosis, the most common cause of arterial diseases, is the result of a complex pathogenesis

Causes and mechanisms responsible for the early lesions are undoubtedly the prime movers in the development of this process. Of these, the central pathogenic factor appears related to a disturbance of the lipid metabolism, one factor that is widely accepted as playing an essential initiating role.

Whether the thrombogenic concept, assigning to small mural thrombi the initial step in the development of atherosclerotic lesions, offers any valid basis is still highly debatable. Even the supporters of the thrombogenic theory admit that other mechanisms must operate in the inception of the majority of fatty streaks.

The response-to-injury and pressure-flow relations, which to some extent further understanding of the localization of the lesions, are based more on animal experimentation than on data about humans.

The arterial wall, considered to be a passive tissue in this process, appears to play an active part in the development of atherosclerosis as a result of an interplay between exogenous and endogenous factors.

Arterial tissue is indeed a metabolically active tissue. In addition to these endogenous factors, recent studies of exogenous cellular events, such as the platelet-derived growth factor (PDGF) and those of endothelial cells, macrophages, and smooth muscle cells, have provided a new dimension to our understanding of the role of arterial tissue in atherogenesis.

Although transmural filtration may play a significant role by allowing the lipids to pass through the endothelium of the arterial wall, it is also most likely that the endothelial permeability it not a passive phenomenon. The activity of the arterial tissue depends on hormonal and enzymatic factors that determine the degree of participation of the arterial tissue in this process. Among other factors that may determine whether atherosclerosis will develop is the degree of susceptibility of the specific artery or a segment of it to this process, which is largely an intrinsic characteristic of the tissue or is due to the individual's genetic inheritance.

The study of the fate of canine abdominal and thoracic aortic segments (the former susceptible, the latter largely refractory to atherosclerosis) when a segment thereof is transposed into sites of predilection or refractoriness in the aorta has disclosed unequivocally that some segments remain susceptible whereas others are refractory, irrespective of the location of the segment. This transposition method offers an invaluable model for assessing the role of the intrinsic mural factors and dissociating them from mechanical factors due to hydrostatic pressure and filtration.

The long-term fate of vein grafts used as arterial substitutes is of great practical significance. Current evidence has disclosed that a number of these vein segments implanted as bypass grafts into the peripheral vessels or into the aortocoronary location will eventually show degenerative changes due to both hydrostatic influence and atherogenic factors.

From a clinicopathologic point of view, the atherosclerotic process may be divided into three major stages: (1) asymptomatic or latent, characterized initially by fatty streaks and later by fibrous plaques that occur in childhood and early adult life, (2) potentially symptomatic, characterized by complicated lesions, such as calcification, hemorrhage, ulceration, and thrombosis, that occur later in life and may be responsible for several functional changes, and (3) ischemic or terminal, characterized by an occlusive process that may result in myocardial or cerebral infarction, ischemic damage to other organs, gangrene of the extremities, or aneurysms. Although the chronological relationship between these various stages is not always certain, there is enough evidence to indicate that they are age related. From a number of careful pathologic studies, it appears that the process begins in childhood but does not become apparent until middle age or later life. *To understand clearly the atherogenic process, a sharp line of distinction must be drawn between the initial phase of atherogenesis and the subsequent evolution of the lesions that may or may not precipitate symptomatic disease, for the factors involved in the initial stage may be entirely different from the factors responsible for later lesions.*

The atherosclerotic process usually involves somatic as well as visceral arteries in variable degrees. The relative incidence of distribution of arterial lesions differs widely from individual to individual, although a definite tendency for atherosclerosis to develop in different arterial systems in the same individual is well established.

The natural history, progression of the disease, and the prognosis appear complex and sometimes difficult to identify. However, the overall problem of assessing these factors requires not only careful clinical and angiographic evaluations but also a detailed anatomic knowledge of the site and extent of the atherosclerotic lesions.

Reversibility of the lesions may be achieved in the first stages of the process, when fatty streaks and fibrous plaques are present. However, during the second and, especially, the third stages of the process, complicated lesions may be arrested but can no longer be reversed. As a result, surgical management may often be required in these stages. In the future, combined surgical and medical approaches will likely enhance the efficacy of current treatment.

REFERENCES

1. Kannel WB, Thom IJ: Declining cardiovascular mortality. Circulation 70:331, 1984.
2. Levy RA, Moskowitz J: Cardiovascular research: Decades of progress, a decade of promise. Science 217:121, 1982.
3. Ross R: The pathogenesis of atherosclerosis—an update. N Engl J Med 314:488, 1986.
4. Haimovici H (ed): Atherosclerosis: Recent Advances. New York, New York Academy of Sciences, 1968.
5. Paoletti R, Gotto AM Jr: Atherosclerosis Reviews, New York, Raven Press, 1976, vol. 1.
6. Davignon J: Current views on the etiology and pathogenesis of atherosclerosis, in Genest J, Koiw, E, Kurchel O (eds): Hypertension. New York, McGraw-Hill Book Co, 1977, p 961.
7. Lobstein J: Traite d'Anatomie pathologique. Paris, Levrault, 1829.
8. Monckeberg JG: Uber die reine Mediaverkalkung der Extremitatenarterien und ihr Verhalten zur Arteriosklerose. Virchows Arch [A] 171:141, 1903.
9. World Health Organization: Report of a study group: Classification of atherosclerotic lesions. WHO Tech Rep Ser 143, 1958.
10. Marchand F: Uber Arteriosklerose. Verh Dtsch Kongr Inn Med 21:23, 1904.
11. Duff GL, McMillan GC, Lautsch EV: The uptake of colloidal thorium dioxide by the arterial lesions of cholesterol atherosclerosis in the rabbit. Am J Pathol 30:941, 1954.
12. Wilens SL: The experimental production of lipid deposition in excised arteries. Science 114:389, 1951.
13. Madri JA, Pratt BM: Endothelial cell-matrix interactions: In

vitro models of angiogenesis. J Histochem Cytochem 34:85, 1986.

14. Wolinsky H, Glagov S: Lamellar units of aortic medial structure and function in mammals. Circ Res 20:99, 1967.

15. Winternitz MC, Thomas RM, LeCompte PM: The Biology of Arteriosclerosis. Springfield, Ill, Charles C Thomas, Publisher, 1938.

16. Heistad DD, Armstrong ML: Blood flow through vasa vasorum of coronary arteries in atherosclerotic monkeys. Arteriosclerosis 6:326, 1968.

17. Glagov S: Hemodynamic risk factors: Mechanical stress, mutual architecture, medial nutrition and the vulnerability of arteries to atherosclerosis, in Wissler RW, Geer JC, and Kaufman N (eds): The Pathogenesis of Atherosclerosis. Baltimore, The Williams and Wilkins Co, 1972, p 164.

18. Lusby RJ, Ferrell LD, et al.: Carotid plaque hemorrhage. Arch Surg 117:1479, 1982.

19. Imparato AM: Presidential address: The carotid bifurcation plaque—a model for the study of atherosclerosis. J Vasc Surg 3:249, 1986.

20. Robertson JH: Stress zones in fetal arteries. J Clin Pathol 13:133, 1960.

21. Mendez J, Tejada C: Chemical composition of aortas from Guatemalans and North Americans. Am J Clin Pathol 51:598, 1969.

22. Holman RL, McGill HC, et al.: Natural history of atherosclerosis. Am J Pathol 34:209, 1958.

23. Moore S: Thromboatherosclerosis in normolipemic rabbits. A result of continued endothelial damage. Lab Invest 29:478, 1973.

24. Duguid JB: Thrombosis as a factor in the pathogenesis of coronary atherosclerosis. J Pathol 58:207, 1946.

25. Glagov G, Weisenberg E, et al.: Compensatory enlargement of human atherosclerotic coronary arteries prevents narrowing of the lumen. Fed Proc 45:583, 1986.

26. Haimovici H: Atheroembolism, in Haimovici H (ed): Vascular Emergencies. New York, Appleton-Century-Crofts, 1982, p 205.

27. Holman RL, McGill HC Jr, et al.: Arteriosclerosis—the lesion. Am J Clin Nutr 8:85, 1960.

28. Inter-Society Commission for Heart Disease Resources: Atherosclerosis Study Group and Epidemiology Study Group: Primary prevention of the atherosclerotic diseases. Circulation 42[A]:55, 1970.

29. Fredrickson DS, Lees RS: A system for phenotyping hyperlipoproteinemia. Circulation 31:321, 1965.

30. Kannel WB: Importance of hypertension as a major risk factor in carviovascular disease, in Genest J, Koiw E, Kurchel O (eds): Hypertension. New York, McGraw-Hill, Chap 29, p 888.

31. Hollander W: Biochemical pathology of atherosclerosis and relationship to hypertension, in Genest J, Koiw E, Kurchel O (eds): Hypertension. New York, McGraw-Hill, 1977, Chap 30.2, p 945.

32. Haimovici H: Peripheral arterial disease in diabetes. NY State J Med 61:2988, 1961.

33. Bennion LJ, Grundy JM: Effects of diabetes mellitus on cholesterol metabolism in man. N Engl J Med 296:1365, 1977.

34. Goodson WH III, Hunt TK: Studies of wound healing in experimental diabetes mellitus. J Surg Res 22:221, 1977.

35. Gordon T, Kannel WB: Predisposition to atherosclerosis in the head, heart, and legs: The Framingham study. JAMA 221:661, 1972.

36. Haimovici H: Atherosclerosis: A multifaceted challenge, in Haimovici H (ed): Atherosclerosis: Recent Advances. New York, New York Academy of Sciences, 1968, 588.

37. Rokitansky C von: A Manual of Pathological Anatomy (trans-

lated by GE Day). London, Sydenham Society, 1852, vol 4.

38. Virchow R: Cellular Pathology. As Based upon Physiological and Pathological Histology (translated from the second German edition originally published by JB Lippincott Co, Philadelphia, 1863). New York, Dover Publications, 1971.

39. Levy RI: Cholesterol, lipoproteins, apoproteins and coronary heart disease: Present status and future prospects. Clin Chem 27:653, 1981.

40. Werthessen NT, Nyman MA, et al.: In vitro study of cholesterol metabolism in calf aorta. Circ Res 4:586, 1956.

41. Mitchell JRA, Schwartz CJ: Arterial Disease. Philadelphia, FA Davis Co, 1965, p 64.

42. Anitschkow N: Uber die veranderungen der kaninchenaorta bei experimentaller cholesterinsteatose. Beitr Pathol 56:379, 1913.

43. Anitschkow N: In Cowdry EV (ed): Arteriosclerosis. New York, Macmillan, Inc, 1933.

44. Zilversmit DB: Phospholipid turnover in atheromatous lesions, in Hormones and Atherosclerosis. New York, Academic Press, Inc, 1959, p 145.

45. Ross R, Glomset JA: The pathogenesis of atherosclerosis—an update. N Engl J Med 314:488, 1986.

46. Brown MS, Goldstein JL: Lipoprotein receptors in the liver: Control signals for plasma cholesterol traffic. J Clin Invest 72:743, 1983.

47. Brown MS, Goldstein JL: How LDL receptors influence cholesterol and atherosclerosis. Sci Am 251:58, 1984.

48. Starzl TE, Chase HP et al.: Portacaval shunt in patients with familial hypercholesterolemia. Ann Surg 198:173, 1983.

49. Brown MS, Goldstein JL: A receptor-mediated pathway for cholesterol homeostatis. Science 232:34, 1986.

50. Wilens SL: Comparative vascularity of cutaneous xanthomas and atheromatous plaques of arteries. Am J Med Sci 233:4, 1957.

51. Haimovici H, Maier N: Role of the arterial wall in atherogenesis. Arch Surg 82:1, 1961.

52. Holman RI, McGill HC Jr, et al.: Filtration versus local formation of lipids in pathogenesis of atherosclerosis. JAMA 170:416, 1959.

53. Chernick S, Srere PA, Chaikoff LL: The metabolism of arterial tissue, II: Lipid synthesis: The formation in vitro of fatty acids and phospholipids by rat aorta with C^1 and p^1 as indicators. J Biol Chem 179:113, 1949.

54. Siperstein MD, Chaikoff LI, Chernick S: Significance of endogenous cholesterol in arteriosclerosis: Synthesis in arterial tissue. Science 113:747, 1951.

55. Whereat AF: Lipid biosynthesis in aortic intima from normal and cholesterol-fed rabbits. J Atheroscler Res 4:272, 1964.

56. Maier, N, Haimovici H: Metabolism of arterial tissue, oxidative capacity of intact arterial tissue. Proc Soc Exp Biol Med 95:425, 1957.

57. Maier N, Haimovici H: Oxidative activity of aortic tissue of man, the rabbit and the dog, with special reference to succinic dehydrogenase and cytochrome oxidase. Am J Physiol 195:282, 1958.

58. Maier N, Haimovici H: Oxidative capacity of atherosclerotic tissue of rabbit and dog, with special reference to succinic dehydrogenase and cytochrome oxidase. Am J Physiol 195:282, 1958.

59. Maier N, Haimovici H: Metabolism of arterial tissue with special reference to esterase and lipase. Proc Soc Exp Biol Med 118:258, 1965.

60. Maier N, Rubinstein LJ, Haimovici H: Enzyme histochemistry in normal and atherosclerotic canine aorta. J Cardiovasc Surg, Dec 1969.

61. Schwartz SM, Ross R: Cellular proliferation in atherosclerosis and hypertension. Prog Cardiovasc Dis 26:355, 1984.

62. Cahill PD, Mitchell RS, Miller DC: Diet and biochemistry in atherogenesis, in Bergan JJ, Yao JST (eds): Arterial Surgery: New Diagnostic and Operative Techniques. Orlando, Fla, Grune & Stratton, Inc, 1988, p 3.

63. Report from International Workshop on Monokines and Other Non-Lymphocytic Cytokines: Cytokines are two-edged swords in disease, research news. Science 239:258, 1988.

64. Haimovici H, Maier N, Strauss L: Fate of aortic homografts in experimental canine atherosclerosis I. Study of fresh thoracic implants into abdominal aorta. Arch Surg 76:282, 1958.

65. Haimovici H, Maier N, Strauss L: Fate of aortic homografts in experimental canine atherosclerosis. II. Study of fresh abdominal aortic implants into abdominal aorta. Arch Surg 78:239, 1959.

66. Haimovici H, Maier N: Fate of aortic homografts in experimental canine atherosclerosis. III. Study of fresh abdominal and thoracic aortic implants into thoracic aorta. Role of tissue susceptibility in atherogenesis. Arch Surg 89:961, 1964.

67. Haimovici H, Maier N: Experimental canine atherosclerosis in autogenous abdominal aortic grafts implanted into the jugular vein. Atherosclerosis 13:373, 1971.

68. Wolinsky H, Glagov S: Comparison of abdominal and thoracic aortic medial structure in mammals: Deviation of man from the usual pattern. Circ Res 25:677, 1969.

69. Beebe HG, Clark WF, DeWeese JA: Atherosclerotic change occurring in an autogenous venous arterial graft. Arch Surg 101:85, 1970.

70. Ejrup B, Hiertonn T, Moberg A: Atheromatous changes in autogenous venous grafts: Functional and anatomical aspects: Case report. Acta Chir Scand 121:211, 1961.

71. Szilagyi DE, et al: Biologic fate of autogenous vein implants as arterial substitutes: Clinical, angiographic and histopathologic observations in femoropopliteal operations for atherosclerosis. Ann Surg 178:232, 1973.

72. Haimovici H, Maier N: Autogenous vein grafts in experimental canine atherosclerosis: Their fate in the abdominal aorta and peripheral arteries. Arch Surg 109:95, 1974.

73. Carrel A, Guthrie CC: Uniterminal and biterminal venous transplantations. Surg Gynecol Obstet 2:266, 1906.

74. Chatterjee KN, Warren R, Gore I: Long-term functional and histologic fate of arteriotomy patches of autogenous arterial and venous tissue: Observations on "arterialization." J Surg Res 4:106, 1964.

75. Jones M, et al: Lesions observed in arterial autogenous vein grafts: Light and electron microscopic evaluation. Circulation 48 (suppl 3): 198, 1973.

76. Grondin CM, Meere C, et al: Progressive and late obstruction of an aorto-coronary venous bypass graft: A case report. Circulation 43:698, 1971.

77. Johnson WD, Auer JE, Tector AJ: Late changes in coronary vein grafts (abstract). Am J Cardiol 26:640, 1970.

78. Vlodaver Z, Edwards JE: Pathologic changes in aortic-coronary arterial saphenous vein grafts. Circulation 44:719, 1971.

79. Rossiter SJ, Brody WR, et al: Internal mammary artery versus autogenous vein for coronary artery bypass graft. Circulation 50:1236, 1974.

80. Haimovici H, Maier N: Correlative study of degree of canine experimental coronary atherosclerosis with that of other visceral and major systemic arteries. J Cardiovasc Surg 14:463, 1973.

81. Singer A, Rob C: The fate of the claudicator. Br Med J 2:633, 1960.

82. Bloor K: Natural history of arteriosclerosis of the lower extremities. Ann R Coll Surg Engl 28:36, 1961.

83. Robertson WB: Atherosclerosis and ischaemic heart disease. Lancet 1:444, 1959.

84. Mitchell JRA, Schwartz CJ: Relationships between arterial diseases in different sites. Br Med J 1:1293, 1962.

85. Young W, Gofman JW, et al: Interrelationships between cerebral and coronary atherosclerosis. Geriatrics 2:413, 1956.

86. Holman RL, Moosy J: Natural History of Aortic, Coronary and Cerebral Atherosclerosis. Symposium on Cerebrovascular Disease, Houston Neurological Society, Houston, Texas, March 12, 1959.

87. Haimovici H: Patterns of arteriosclerotic lesions of the lower extremity. Arch Surg 95:918, 1967.

88. Humphries AW, DeWolfe VG, et al: Evaluation of the natural history and the results of treatment involving the lower extremities in 1,850 patients, in Wesolowski SA, Dennis CA (eds): Fundamentals of Vascular Grafting, New York, McGraw-Hill Book Co., 1963.

89. Valdoni P, Venturini A: Considerations on late results of vascular prostheses for reconstructive surgery in congenital and acquired arterial disease. J Cardiovasc Surg 5:519, 1964.

90. Fontaine R, Kieny JM, et al: Long-term results of restorative arterial surgery in obstructive diseases of the arteries. J Cardiovasc Surg 5:463, 1964.

91. DeBakey ME, Crawford ES, et al: Late results of vascular surgery in the treatment of arteriosclerosis. J Cardiovasc Surg 5:473, 1964.

92. Gensler SW, Haimovici H, et al: Study of vascular lesions in diabetic, nondiabetic patients. Arch Surg 91:617, 1965.

93. Schwartz CJ, Mitchell JRA: Observations on localization of arterial plaques. Circ Res 11:63, 1962.

94. Juergens JL, Barker NW, Hines EA Jr: Arteriosclerosis obliterans: Review of 520 cases with special reference to pathogenic and prognostic factors. Circulation 21:188, 1960.

95. Silbert S, Zazeela H: Prognosis in arteriosclerotic vascular disease. JAMA 166:1816, 1958.

96. Imparato AM, Kim GE, et al: Intermittent claudication: Its natural course. Surgery 78:795, 1975.

97. Allison RB, Rodriguez FL, et al: Clinicopathologic correlations in coronary atherosclerosis: 430 patients studied with postmorten coronary angiography. Circulation 27:170, 1963.

98. Vlodaver Z, Edwards JE: Pathology of coronary atherosclerosis. Prog Cardiovasc Dis 14:256, 1971.

99. Diethrich EB, Liddicoat JE, et al: Surgical significance of angiographic patterns in coronary arterial disease. Circulation 35, 36 (suppl 1):155, 1967.

100. Schwartz JN, Kong Y, et al: Comparison of angiographic and postmortem findings in patients with coronary artery disease. Am J Cardiol 36:174, 1975.

101. Humphries JP, Kuller L, et al: Natural history of ischemic heart disease in relation to arteriographic findings: A twelve year study of 224 patients. Circulation 49:489, 1974.

102. Webster JS, Moberg C, Rincon G: Natural history of severe proximal coronary artery disease as documented by coronary cineangiography. Am J Cardiol 33:195, 1974.

103. Grondin CM, Dyrda I, et al: Discrepancies between cineangiographic and postmortem findings in patients with coronary artery disease and recent myocardial revascularization. Circulation 49:703, 1974.

104. DeRouen TA, Murray JA, Owen W: Variability in the analysis of coronary arteriograms. Circulation 55:324, 1977.

105. Hutchinson EC, Yates PO: Carotico-vertebral stenosis. Lancet 1:2, 1957.

106. Solberg LA, Eggen DA: Localization and sequence of development of atherosclerotic lesions in the carotid and vertebral arteries. Circulation 43:711, 1971.

107. Bond MG, Insull W Jr, et al. (eds): Clinical Diagnosis of Atherosclerosis: Quantitative Methods of Evaluation. New York, Springer-Verlag New York, Inc, 1982.

108. DePalma RG: Angiography in experimental atherosclerosis: Advantages and limitations, in Bond JG, Insull S Jr, et al. (eds): Clinical Diagnosis of Atherosclerotic Lesions: Quantitative Methods of Evaluation. New York, Springer-Verlag New York, 1983, p 99.

109. Bond MG, Gordin JF, et al.: Noninvasive high resolution B mode ultrasound imaging of arteries, in Hegyeli RJ (ed): Atherosclerosis Reviews: Endpoints for Cardiovascular Studies. New York, Raven Press, 1984, p 155.

110. Katz ML, Comerota AJ, Cranley JJ: Characterization of atherosclerotic plaque by real-time B mode carotid imaging. Bruit 4:17, 1982.

111. O'Donnell TF Jr, Erdoes L, et al.: Correlation of B-mode ultrasound imaging and arteriography with pathologic findings at carotid endarterectomy. Arch Surg 120:443, 1985.

112. Soila K, Nummi P, et al.: Proton relaxation times in arterial wall and atheromatous lesions in man. Invest Radiol 20:411, 1986.

113. Schettler E, Stange E, Wissler RW: Atherosclerosis—Is It Reversible? New York, Springer-Verlag New York, Inc, 1978.

114. Armstrong ML, Megan MB: Lipid depletion in atheromatous coronary arteries after regression diets. Circ Res 30:675, 1972.

115. Wissler RW, Vessilinovitch D: Studies of regression of advanced atherosclerosis in experimental animals and man. Ann NY Acad Sci 275:363, 1976.

116. DePalma RG, Bellon EM, et al.: Approaches to evaluating regression of experimental atherosclerosis, in Manning GW, Haust MD (eds): Atherosclerosis: Metabolic Morphologic and Clinical Aspects. New York, Plenum Publishing Corp, 1977, p 459.

117. Armstrong ML, Megan MB: Arterial fibrous proteins in cynomolgus monkeys after atherogenic and regression diets. Circ Res 36:265, 1975.

118. DePalma RG, Bellon EM, et al.: Atherosclerotic plaque regression in rhesus monkeys induced by bile acid sequestrant. Exp Mol Pathol 31:423, 1979.

119. DePalma RG, Klein L, et al.: Regression of atherosclerotic plaques in rhesus monkeys. Arch Surg 115:1268, 1980.

120. DePalma RG, Koletsky S, et al.: Failure of regression of atherosclerosis in dogs with moderate cholesterolemia. Atherosclerosis 27:297, 1977.

121. Arztzenius AC, Kromhout D, et al.: Diet, lipoproteins, and the progression of coronary atherosclerosis. N Engl J Med 312:805, 1985.

122. Blankenhorn DH, Brooks SH, et al.: The rate of atherosclerosis change during treatment of hyperlipoproteinemia. Circulation 57:355, 1978.

123. DePalma RG: Control and regression of atherosclerotic plaques, a commentary, in Dale WA (ed): Management of Arterial Occlusive Disease. Chicago, Year Book, 1971, p 63.

124. Brooks SH, Le Croissette DH, Blankenhorn DH: Determinants of atherosclerosis progression and regression. Arch Surg 113:75, 1978.

125. Blankenhorn DH, Sanmarco ME: Angiography for study of lipid-lowering therapy (editorial). Circulation 59:212, 1979.

126. Malinow MR: Regression of atherosclerosis in humans: Fact or myth? Circulation 64:1, 1981.

127. Duffield RGM, Miller NE, et al.: Treatment of hyperlipidaemia retards progression of symptomatic femoral atherosclerosis: A randomised controlled trial. Lancet 2:639, 1983.

128. Barmeyer J, Buchwalsky R, et al.: Clinical course of arteriosclerosis of coronary and lower limb arteries. Deutsch Med Wochenschr 101:443, 1976.

129. DePalma RG, Bellon EM, et al.: Failure of antiplatelet treatment in dietary atherosclerosis: A serial intervention study, in Gallo LL Vahouny GV (eds): Cardiovascular Disease: Molecular and Cellular Mechanisms, Prevention, Treatment. New York, Plenum Publishing Corp, 1986.

130. Hollander W, Kirkpatrick B, et al.: Studies on the progression and regression of coronary and peripheral atherosclerosis in the cynomolgus monkey, I: Effects of dipyridamole and aspirin. Exp Mol Pathol 30:55, 1979.

131. Wecksler BB: Arterial thrombosis, atherosclerosis and platelet activity: A reassessment of antiplatelet therapy, in Hegyeli RJ (ed): Atherosclerosis Reviews. New York, Raven Press, 1984, p 39.

132. Wecksler BB, Kent JJ, et al.: Effect of low dose aspirin on platelet function in patients with recent cerebral ischemia. Stroke 16:5, 1985.

133. Morisaki N, Stitts JM, et al.: Dipyridamole: An antioxidant that promotes the proliferation of aorta smooth muscle cells. Artery 11:88, 1982.

134. Koster JK Jr, Tryka AF, et al.: The effect of low dose aspirin and dipyridamole in the rabbit. Artery 9:405, 1981.

135. DeBakey ME, Lawrie GM, Glaeser DH: Patterns of atherosclerosis and their surgical significance. Ann Surg 201:115, 1985.

136. Steinberg I, Tobier N: Study of 200 consecutive patients with abdominal aneurysms diagnosed by intravenous aortography, comparative longevity with and without aneurysmectomy. Circulation 35:530, 1965.

137. Szilagyi DE, Smith RF, et al.: Contribution of abdominal aortic aneurysmectomy to prolongation of life. Ann Surg 164:678, 1966.

138. Takaro T, Hultgren HN, et al.: The V.A. cooperative randomized study of surgery for coronary arterial occlusive disease, II: Subgroup with significant left main lesions. Circulation 54:107, 1976.

CHAPTER 12
Thrombogenesis and Thrombolysis

Donald Silver and Dolores F. Cikrit

Twenty years ago blood coagulation was considered difficult because little was known about the system; today it is considered difficult because so much is known.[1]

Surgeons who operate on the cardiovascular system have an added challenge to those encountered during other types of surgery. The cardiovascular surgeon must render blood noncoagulable during times of total or local circulatory arrest and later must achieve sufficient hemostasis to prevent wound complications and exsanguinating hemorrhages. In addition, the ability to lyse unwanted thromboemboli should be part of the cardiovascular surgeons armamentarium. Thus the cardiovascular surgeon must be intimately familiar with the physiology and the methods for ensuring and inhibiting thrombogenesis and thrombolysis.

THROMBOGENESIS

Hemostasis

The many complex reactions that lead to hemostasis have been divided into the vasoconstriction and platelet plug formation stages (i.e., primary hemostasis) and into thrombus formation and stabilization (i.e., secondary hemostasis). Vasoconstriction, occurring within seconds, is the earliest event following vessel injury, with the muscular elements contracting in response to neurogenic and myogenic influences. Platelets subsequently adhere to the injured vessel and secrete epinephrine, serotonin, adenosine triphosphate (ATP), adenosine diphosphate (ADP), and thromboxane, which contribute to the vasoconstriction. The substances released by the platelets, in addition to aiding vasoconstriction, contribute to additional platelet aggregation and the development of the platelet plug.

Secondary hemostasis, the formation of a fibrin network, occurs to maintain the hemostasis begun by the initial two events. The fibrin monomers polymerize into insoluble strands of fibrin. The stable thrombus provides long-term hemostasis.

Platelets

Platelets are small, anuclear, disc-shaped fragments of megakaryocytes that have a circulating life of approximately 8 to 12 days. There are usually 200,000 to 400,000 platelets/mm³ in human blood. Coagulation factors I, V, VIII, IX, XII, and XIII adhere to the mucopolysaccharide coat that surrounds platelets. This same mucopolysaccharide coat contributes to platelet adhesion. Platelets contain surface receptors for fibrinogen, thrombin, ADP, epinephrine, serotonin, collagen, and immune complexes. The platelet is also a rich source of phospholipid, which becomes, when released, a clot-promoting phospholipid (platelet factor III). Platelets contain three types of granules: alpha granules contain platelet factor IV, beta thromboglobulin, mitogenic factor, fibronectin, factor VIII–related antigen, and fibrinogen; the dense bodies contain calcium, serotonin, ADP, and ATP; and the lysosome-like granules contain numerous acidic hydrolases.

Platelets usually do not adhere to each other or to normal vascular endothelium. However, within seconds after vascular injury, platelets adhere to the injured vessel, especially to exposed basement membrane and collagen. After adhesion, platelets undergo a change in shape and secrete bioactive substances such as ADP, ATP, and serotonin that cause additional changes in the platelet surface that are conducive to platelets adhering to each other (i.e., platelet aggregation). The adhesion and aggregation contribute to the formation of the platelet plug. The platelets supply procoagulant activity as platelet factor III and release coagulation factors (i.e., fibrinogen and factors III and V) in the early stages of aggregation. The release of these substances activates the coagulation system. The thrombin that is produced promotes more platelet aggregation and also the establishment of the fibrin network that stabilizes the platelet hemostatic plug.

Platelet membrane phospholipase may be activated by ADP, thrombin, catecholamines, and other agents with a release of arachidonic acid. The arachidonic acid is converted by cyclo-oxygenase to prostaglandin cyclic endoperoxides, which can be converted to thromboxane A_2. Thromboxane A_2 causes additional platelet aggregation and contributes to the constriction of small vessels. Aspirin inhibits platelet aggregation and release by irreversibly preventing the formation of thromboxane A_2 by the affected platelets. Aspirin also temporarily blocks endothelial synthesis of prostacyclin, a potent vasodilator. Other nonsteroidal anti-inflammatory agents such as ibuprofen, indomethacin, and phenylbutazone reversibly inhibit cyclo-oxygenase. Dipyridamole inhibits platelet phosphodiesterase, leading to increases of platelet cyclic adenosine monophosphate (AMP) and inhibition of platelet aggregation. Dipyridamole also inhibits thromboxane production and augments prostacyclin production; thus it functions as both a vasodilator and a platelet function inhibitor.

Defects in platelet function can be quantitative or qualitative and congenital or acquired. Qualitative platelet disorders should be suspected when the bleeding occurs in the presence of normal coagulation test results and normal platelet count results. The qualitative platelet disorders contribute to spontaneous bleeding less frequently than do the quantitative ones. Abnormal platelet function is rarely the cause of bleeding but may exacerbate existing bleeding such as the bleeding occurring with trauma or surgery. Acquired qualitative abnormalities are commonly related to the ingestion of drugs such as aspirin, dipyridamole, indomethacin, and ibuprofen. Other acquired causes of platelet malfunction include cirrhosis, uremia, and macroglobulinemias. Patients with acquired qualitative platelet function abnormalities usually have normal platelet counts but prolonged bleeding times secondary to defects in aggregation. Congenital qualitative platelet disorders include von Willebrand's disease, "storage pool disease," and other thrombocytopathias. These patients have normal platelet counts, may have large platelets or abnormally shaped platelets, and always have abnormal platelet function. Von Willebrand's disease, which is one of the more common hereditary abnormalities of hemostasis, is associated with a deficiency of plasma factor VIII–relating antigen (VIIIR:Ag) and the von Willebrand factor (VIII-WF). Patients with von Willebrand's disease have prolonged bleeding times due to poor platelet adhesion and aggregation.

Quantitative platelet disorders are usually detected through the platelet count. Prolonged thrombocytopenia in the 20,000 to 30,000/mm^3 range is frequently associated with increased vascular fragility and permeability, with extravascular accumulation of fluid and blood cells (i.e., petechiae). Bleeding may be associated with platelet counts less than 30,000/mm^3 but rarely occurs in the presence of counts greater than 100,000/mm^3 of normal platelets. Spontaneous bleeding usually does not occur with platelet counts greater than 30,000/mm^3. Surgery associated with limited blood loss can frequently be accomplished safely in patients with platelet counts as low as 30,000/mm^3. An excessive number of platelets is more often associated with thrombosis than with bleeding. However, a patient with sustained thrombocytosis may experience bleeding from the mucous membranes or the gastrointestinal tract. The platelet count of such a patient is often greater than 1,000,000/mm^3.

Correction of coagulation defects resulting from congenital qualitative defects in platelet function requires platelet transfusions. Acquired defects of platelet function are usually corrected by eliminating the inciting drug or illness. However, platelet transfusion occasionally is required for these patients also. When quantitative defects are present, platelet transfusions are necessary to increase the platelet count to greater than 50,000 platelets/mm^3 to obtain intraoperative hemostasis. Usually 10 units, or 0.1 U/kg, of platelets will increase the platelet count to more than 50,000/mm^3.

Coagulation Mechanism

Blood coagulation is the result of a series of complex interrelated enzymatic reactions that involve the plasma coagulation factors. Twelve clotting factors have been identified and are numbered I through XIII. The original factor VI proved to be an activated form of another clotting factor. Table 12-1 lists the clotting factors, their synonyms, plasma half-lives, vitamin K dependency, and the disorders associated with deficiencies of the factors. Four of the clotting factors are vitamin K dependent (i.e., II, VII, IX, and X). All factors except III and VIII are synthesized in the liver. The large glycoprotein component of factor VIII, the factor VIII–related protein (VIIIR) is synthesized in vascular endothelial cells and megakaryocytes. The origin of the synthesis of the coagulant activity of factor VIII (VIII:C) is unknown.

The activation of factor X leads to the final pathway of coagulation, which includes the conversion of prothrombin to thrombin and the subsequent conversion of fibrinogen to fibrin. Factor X activation may occur through the activation of the intrinsic or extrinsic or both pathways of coagulation (Fig. 12-1). Surgery and other forms of trauma activate either or both pathways. Injured tissues release thromboplastin into the blood to form a complex with factor VII and calcium to activate factor X (the extrinsic system). The prothrombin time tests the efficiency of the extrinsic system of coagulation. The intrinsic coagulation sequence begins when factor XII is activated through contact with foreign surfaces (e.g., collagen or basement membranes). Factor XIII, prekallikrein, and high-molecular-weight kininogen contribute to the activation of the intrinsic system with the production of activated factor XII (XIIa). The partial thromboplastin time is a good monitor of the extrinsic system. The conversion of thrombin to prothrombin by Xa is augmented by factor V, calcium ions, and phospholipids. Thrombin cleaves fibrinogen into fibrin monomers and also activates factors XIII and VII. Furthermore, fibrin augments the action of factors VIII and V and causes platelet aggregation.

The initial fibrin that is produced is soluble. However, the cross-link induced by activated factor XIII increases its stability and reduces its solubility. The two pathways of coagulation are not distinct but are linked by the activation of factor IX by factor VIIa.

Disorders of coagulation may be caused by congenital or acquired deficiencies of the coagulation factors, inadequate replacement of coagulation factors during times of bleeding or consumption of coagulation factors, or during clotting at a faster rate than they can be replaced. Congenital deficiencies have been described for all the factors except

TABLE 12-1. COAGULATION FACTORS

Factor	Synonym	Plasma Half-life (Hours)	Vitamin K Dependent	Congenital Coagulation Disorders	
				Manifestations of Deficiency	Inheritance
I	Fibrinogen	90	No	Serious neonatal and early bleeding	Autosomal recessive
II	Prothrombin	65	Yes	Serious neonatal and early bleeding	Autosomal recessive
III	Tissue thromboplastin	—	No	—	—
IV	Calcium	—	No	—	—
V	Proaccelerin	15	No	Mild, excessive bleeding early in life	Highly penetrant autosomal recessive
VII	Preconvertin	6	Yes	Mild to moderate bleeding or purpura	Autosomal recessive
VIII	Antihemophiliac factor A	12	No	Bleeding during infancy; excessive bleeding after minor trauma, dental procedures, and minor surgery	Sex-linked recessive
IX	Antihemophiliac factor B	25	Yes	Excessive bleeding after trauma or surgery	Sex-linked recessive
X	Stuart-Prower	40	Yes	Mild bleeding in later life	Autosomal recessive
XI	Plasma thromboplastin antecedent	45	No	Excessive bleeding after trauma or surgery; bleeding may be delayed	Autosomal recessive
XII	Hageman factor	50	No	Rarely associated with significant bleeding	Autosomal recessive
XIII	Fibrin-stabilizing factor	120	No	Neonatal bleeding is common, with cord hemorrhage, ecchymoses, and hematomas	Autosomal recessive
	von Willebrand's disease	—	No	Spontaneous gastrointestinal bleeding and easily bruised	Autosomal dominant and recessive

factors III and IV (see Table 12-1). The congenital coagulation disorders usually involve a single factor deficiency, whereas acquired deficiency disorders frequently have deficiencies of several factors. Patients with a congenital deficiency of a clotting factor usually bleed only when stressed by surgery or trauma since only 5 to 10% of factor activity is needed to maintain hemostasis under normal conditions.

The most common congenital bleeding disorders are hemophilia and Christmas disease (hemophilias A and B).

These disorders are caused by deficient or defective production of factors VIII and IX, respectively. Von Willebrand's disease is another relatively common congenital disorder of hemostasis. Patients with this disease have reduced levels of factor VIII coagulant activity and the von Willebrand factor, which has an important role in initial adherence of platelets to surfaces and to the subsequent aggregation of platelets.

Acquired disorders of coagulation are due to deficient

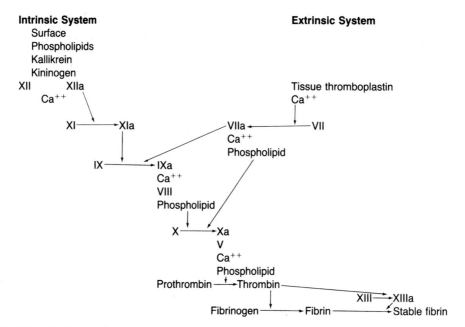

Figure 12-1. The intrinsic or extrinsic system of coagulation, or both, are activated by surgery and other forms of trauma. The two pathways are interrelated.

production, deficient replacement or excessive consumption of coagulation factors, or to anticoagulant therapy. Because all of the coagulation factors except III and VIII are produced in the liver, impaired hepatic function can lead to significant decreases in coagulation factor concentration. Patients with vitamin K deficiency and patients receiving warfarin may produce insufficient amounts of functional factors II, VII, IX, and X. Massive blood transfusions may cause bleeding through dilution of clotting factors, especially the labile factors V and VIII. Excessive intravascular coagulation may occur with sepsis, amniotic fluid embolism, and incompatible blood transfusions and may deplete fibrinogen, prothrombin, and factors V, VIII, IX, X, XII, and XIII and platelets so that a consumptive coagulopathy ensues.

Inhibitors of Coagulation

The natural inhibitors of coagulation are proteins that dampen the activity of the various procoagulants. These inhibitors are either inhibitors of the serine proteases or inhibitors of activated cofactors such as activated protein C.[2] Human plasma contains two heparin-dependent inhibitors of coagulation, antithrombin III (ATIII) and heparin cofactor II. In addition, there are a number of non-heparin-dependent inhibitors (e.g., α_2-macroglobulin and α_1-antitrypsin). Of these inhibitors, ATIII provides at least 70% of the activity and apparently is the major circulating anticoagulant.

Deficiencies of ATIII are associated with a high risk of thrombosis. ATIII is a glycoprotein that is synthesized by the liver and possibly by the endothelial cells. ATIII inhibits all of the activated serine enzymes except activated protein C. ATIII binds to heparin. This binding is mediated by ionic interactions and induces conformational changes in ATIII so that it is readily recognized by the serine enzymes. Heparin accelerates the formation of a complex of ATIII and the serine enzymes. After the formation of the ATIII-serine complex, heparin dissociates from ATIII and acts as a catalyst for the formation of other ATIII-serine enzyme complexes.

Congenital and acquired deficiencies of ATIII have been reported. ATIII deficiency should be suspected in a person with a family history of thromboembolic disorders, in a person under 30 with a thromboembolic disorder, in women with thromboembolic disorders during pregnancy, in a person with recurrences of thrombosis during heparin therapy, and in patients requiring very high doses of heparin to achieve therapeutic prolongation of the partial thromboplastin time. Inherited ATIII deficiency apparently is a causative factor in approximately 2% of patients who are initially seen with venous thrombosis.[3] Acquired ATIII deficiencies may occur in patients with liver disorders and active thromboses. The diagnosis of ATIII deficiency is difficult to substantiate when the patient is initially seen with active thrombosis since ATIII is consumed during clot formation. A low level of ATIII at this time is nondiagnostic, whereas a normal level rules out the possibility of an inherited ATIII deficiency. ATIII levels are also reduced during heparin administration—especially in the first 7 to 10 days. Patients with ATIII deficiencies are usually treated for prolonged periods with warfarin or other vitamin K antagonists. Warfarin acts primarily by reducing the vitamin K coagulation

factors and thus reducing intravascular coagulation. Warfarin also increases, through an unknown mechanism, ATIII levels. ATIII concentrates are available and may be of use with heparin during the early management of thrombosis in patients with ATIII deficiencies and during the management of a patient with disseminated intravascular coagulation (DIC).

Heparin cofactor II is activated by higher concentrations of heparin and seems to selectively inhibit thrombin. Patients with reduced levels of heparin cofactor II also suffer from recurrent venous thromboses.

Protein C is a vitamin K–dependent plasma proenzyme that is produced in the liver. Thrombin is the only known circulating enzyme capable of activating protein C. Activated protein C (APC) inactivates factors Va and VIIIa and thus interferes with the activation of factor X. The anticoagulant effect of APC is very rapid, with prompt decreases of the activity of V and VIII. APC inactivates platelet-bound and free-factor Va. Hereditary deficiencies of protein C exist and are transmitted as an autosomal dominant trait. Patients with protein C deficiency are at risk for recurring thromboembolism and are usually treated with warfarin. However, they should receive heparin for the first few days of warfarin therapy because protein C levels are depressed more rapidly than are the coagulation factor levels. After 3 or 4 days, when factors II, VII, IX, and X are reduced sufficiently, the heparin can be stopped, and the patient is maintained on warfarin indefinitely. The full expression of the anticoagulant potential of APC is dependent on the availability of a second glycoprotein known as protein S. Protein S acts as a cofactor protein (with APC) in the inactivation of Va. Deficiencies of protein S are also inherited as an autosomal dominant trait.

Predictors of Coagulation Abnormalities

The patient's history is invaluable for detecting latent hemorrhagic disorders and for defining active ones. A careful history of bleeding or thromboembolic events in the patient or his family should alert the physician to the possibility of an inherited bleeding disorder and should help distinguish a congenital disorder from an acquired one. When excessive bleeding occurs with umbilical cord separation, with circumcision, or with the minor traumas of childhood, an inherited bleeding disorder should be suspected. Most of the acquired hemorrhagic disorders appear later in life. Excessive bleeding after tonsillectomy, minor trauma, tooth extraction, and surgical procedures requires careful laboratory evaluation. The bleeding associated with platelet or vascular disorders is eventually controlled, whereas the bleeding associated with coagulation defects is poorly controlled and is usually associated with hemarthrosis, hematuria, and retroperitoneal hematomas. The physical examination should include a search for petechiae, purpura, ecchymoses, hemangiomas, tumors, jaundice, hematomas, and hemarthroses. This examination is useful in detecting disorders that accompany or cause coagulation problems (e.g., enlarged spleen, malignancies, hepatic insufficiency, jaundice, lupus erythematosus, and other collagen disorders).

A complete history and physical examination provide an adequate ''screen'' for most bleeding disorders. The history must include questions about drugs that inhibit platelet function or inhibit the production of coagulation factors. Although their yields are low, screening tests are used by many surgeons to raise the level of assurance that their patients will be hemostatically competent intraoperatively. The most commonly used screening tests include the prothrombin time (PT), the activated partial thromboplastin time (aPTT), thrombin time (TT), platelet count, and the template bleeding time. These tests help the surgeon detect, preoperatively, most patients with hemostatic defects. When the screening tests are abnormal, tests of coagulation, platelet function, and fibrinolytic activity may be required to determine and correct specific defects of hemostasis. A patient with a negative history and physical examination and normal screening tests who bleeds intraoperatively most likely has an acquired defect of hemostasis. The acquired defects include the thrombocytopenia or factor deficiency that occurs during the replacement of brisk blood loss with large quantities of older bank blood. The other common cause of acquired surgical bleeding is a consumptive coagulopathy and at times the accompanying secondary hyperfibrinolysis.

THROMBOLYSIS

The fibrinolytic system, like the coagulation system, is one of the body's defense mechanisms, with its role that of reducing and eliminating fibrin deposits through fibrinolysis. Although the most dramatic effect of fibrinolysis noted by vascular surgeons will be in the vascular system, fibrinolysis has important roles in other body systems (e.g., mesothelial fibrinolysis helps with the removal of pleural and peritoneal hematomas). Fibrinolytic activity is determined by the action of plasminogen activators on the available plasminogen, the effect of fibrinolytic inhibitors, and the affinity of these substances for fibrin. The vascular surgeon should be knowledgeable about the fibrinolytic mechanism with its many activators and inhibitors, the recognition and control of excessive fibrinolysis, and ways to safely induce thrombolysis.

Physiology

Plasmin, a serine protease, has an affinity for fibrin and is primarily responsible for fibrinolysis. Plasmin also digests multiple other plasma proteins (e.g., fibrinogen, factors V and VIII, and components of the complement system). Plasmin is usually formed in immediate contact with its substrate, fibrin, and in this location is somewhat protected from circulating inhibitors. Free plasmin is rapidly and strongly bound to its specific inhibitor, α_2-plasmin inhibitor. Another inhibitor, α_2-macroglobulin, has a substantially lesser role in inhibiting the activity of plasmin. Minute amounts of free plasmin accelerate the activating process.

Plasminogen (profibrinolysin), found in all mammals, is a plasma zymogen of the protease plasmin. Plasminogen is synthesized in the liver and is widely distributed in body fluids. It is converted (activated) to plasmin by a variety of activators. Plasminogen activators are also widely distributed, being found in vascular endothelium, epithelial cells,

urine, seminal fluid, and tissue. There are two major categories of activators: activators with a high affinity for the plasminogen in fibrin (e.g., tissue activator) and those activators with a low affinity for the fibrin-bound plasminogen (e.g., streptokinase-plasminogen complex). Blood plasminogen activator comes predominantly from the endothelium.

Activators
Although there are many activators of plasminogen, four have clinical applicability. *Streptokinase* (SK) combines with plasminogen to form an activator complex, which then converts additional plasminogen to plasmin. The SK-plasminogen activator has a low affinity for the plasminogen bound to fibrin and is therefore predominantly a producer of systemic fibrinolysis. Since SK is of bacterial origin, its administration may be associated with allergic reactions, sensitization, and the production of antibodies.

The administration of human *urokinase* (UK) has been relatively free of sensitivity complications and antibody production. UK is a direct plasminogen activator. UK is also considered a low fibrin-affinity plasminogen activator, although it has a higher affinity for fibrin-bound plasminogen than does the SK-plasminogen activator.

Tissue-plasminogen activator (t-PA) is synthesized in endothelial cells and is released, in the presence of fibrin and many other stimuli, into the circulation. t-PA is a direct activator of plasminogen. t-PA has a high affinity for fibrin and binds, almost quantitatively, to any clot to which it has access. This adsorption of circulating t-PA to blood clots greatly contributes to their lysis while markedly reducing the possibility of inducing systemic lysis. Recombinant human t-PA is being tested (thus far with promising results) in clinical trials.

Pro-urokinase (Pro-UK), an inactive zymogen of urokinase, also has a high affinity for fibrin-bound plasminogen. Pro-UK has a longer half-life than t-PA and is believed to activate only fibrin-bound plasminogen. Clinical trials with Pro-UK are beginning.

Inhibitors
Fortunately, several mechanisms exist to modulate fibrinolysis and thus prevent or control the potential destructive effects of uncontrolled proteolysis. Five of the plasma proteases that inhibit fibrinolysis are α_1 protease inhibitor, antithrombin III, α_2-macroglobulin, C1 inhibitor, and α_2 plasmin inhibitor (α_2PI). The most important inhibitor of plasmin-induced fibrinolysis is α_2PI (also called α_2-antiplasmin). α_2PI interferes with the adsorption of plasminogen to fibrin and rapidly inhibits plasmin's activity. α_2PI also inhibits plasminogen activators such as UK and t-PA. The concentration of α_2PI in the plasma is approximately 7 mg/100ml. Minute amounts of α_2PI are transported by platelets.

Synthetic fibrinolytic inhibitors (e.g., epsilon-amino caproic acid [EACA] and tranexamic acid) are potent antifibrinolytic agents. They inhibit the activity of plasmin and of plasminogen activators. They also inhibit the adsorption of plasminogen to fibrin, further contributing to the inhibition of fibrinolysis.

EACA is the inhibitor most often used to control excessive fibrinolysis. The usual dose for an adult with excessive, fibrinolytic activity is 5 g, intravenously or orally, followed by 1 g/hr until the excessive lysis is controlled. If EACA is administered intravenously, it should be given slowly because hypotension, brachycardia, and arrhythmias have been associated with rapid infusions.

Hyperfibrinolysis

Fibrinolytic activity maintains vessel patency by removing unwanted fibrin deposits. Excessive fibrinolytic activity frequently is associated with bleeding and, unless controlled, may lead to exsanguinating hemorrhage. Increased fibrinolytic activity usually falls into one of three categories: primary fibrinolysis; secondary fibrinolysis; and systemic or locally induced fibrinolysis.

Primary fibrinolysis refers to the fibrinolytic activity that is not associated with intravascular coagulation and is not induced by infusion of activators or plasmin. Primary fibrinolysis results from excessive plasminogen activation caused by a variety of pathologic conditions (e.g., electric shock, leukemia, hepatic failure, extracorporeal circulation, sudden profound hypotension, and ulcerative colitis). Management of primary fibrinolysis is directed toward eliminating or controlling the underlying cause and using EACA to control the lytic state.

Secondary fibrinolysis refers to the fibrinolysis that accompanies clotting. Most often the lysis is limited to the thrombus being lysed and is of no consequence. However, during times of extensive intravascular coagulation such as occurs during disseminated intravascular coagulation (DIC), the release of large amounts of activators may result in the excessive activation of circulating plasminogen. When this situation occurs, the inhibitors are frequently overwhelmed, and an intense lytic state is produced, contributing to the bleeding by lysing thromboses and digesting the coagulation proteins, which frequently are being consumed more rapidly than they can be replaced.

Although primary fibrinolysis is quite rare, secondary fibrinolysis always is present during intravascular coagulation. The platelet count helps differentiate between primary and secondary fibrinolysis. The platelet count is normal during primary fibrinolysis and is low, secondary to the intravascular coagulation, during secondary fibrinolysis. The hyperfibrinolysis that accompanies DIC must be treated cautiously because the lytic state is important in maintaining patency of the microcirculation. Consequently, the DIC must be controlled first; then, if the excessive lytic state persists, the lysis is controlled with EACA.

Induced fibrinolysis began with the intravenous injection of SK into patients in 1955.[4] Systemic fibrinolytic activity was produced by infusions of first SK and then UK in attempts to lyse venous thromboemboli and, later, arterial thromboemboli. Since 1955, there has been a constant evolution of indications, protocols, and agents for inducing thrombolysis. Successful thrombolysis is affected by the age and the texture of the thrombus. Cross-linked fibrin is less susceptible to lysis than non-cross-linked fibrin. The binding of α_2PI to fibrin by XIIIa adversely inhibits thrombolysis. The thrombolytic state is directly dependent on the concentrations and interactions of plasminogen, plasminogen activators, plasmin, and plasmin inhibitors with fibrin and fibrinogen.

SK has a proven beneficial effect on the management of massive pulmonary embolisms[5] and acute myocardial thromboses[6] when given systemically. Systemic SK has had varied results in the management of a deep venous thrombosis, with up to 44% complete clearance of the thrombosis being reported.[7] The standard systemic dose of SK is 250,000 units as the initial dose and a 100,000/hr maintenance dose for 3 to 5 days. In recent years SK has been infused into, or adjacent to, intravenous and intra-arterial thromboses at doses that range from 1,000 to 10,000 U/hr up to 1.5 × 10^6 U/hr. Intracoronary injections at 1,000 to 6,000 units of SK per minute have been quite successful in lysing acute coronary thromboses and preserving myocardial function while preparing the patient for successful angioplasty or bypass. SK has been used intraoperatively by the authors in doses of 3,000 to 15,000 units injected intra-arterially to lyse successfully arterial thromboses distal to bypass grafts. The antigenicity of SK precludes its being administered for more than 4 or 5 days or at frequent intervals.

Urokinase has had systemic and local applications similar to those of SK, with similar results. UK is not antigenic and can be administered for prolonged periods of time and as often as needed. It is rarely associated with sensitivity reactions. A disadvantage of UK is its cost, which is approximately 10 times that of SK. The standard systemic dose of UK is 2,000 to 4,000 U/kg as a loading dose and hourly for 12 to 48, or more, hours or until lysis has occurred. The amount of UK infused locally has not been determined but has varied between one tenth to one twentieth of the systemic dose. High doses of urokinase have been infused locally, with 84% improvement in blood flow.[8]

Tissue-plasminogen activator has a greater potential (up to 5 to 10 times greater) for inducing thrombolysis than SK or UK has.[9] It has been used to lyse iliofemoral thromboses,[10] coronary thromboses,[11] and thromboses of peripheral arteries and grafts.[12] The results obtained with t-PA have been quite good, with 92% lysis of the peripheral arterial and graft thromboses. The duration, dose, and cost of t-PA therapy remain to be determined.

Pro-UK is a fibrin-specific thrombolytic agent that has successfully induced thrombolysis in animals and, recently, in humans.[13] There may be major differences in the natural and the recombinant pro-UK preparations.[14] Additional animal and clinical trials with pro-UK are needed before it can be recommended for general use.

Other thrombolytic agents such as brinase[15] and SK-plasminogen complex have had limited clinical application.[16,17] More extensive clinical trials are needed before these agents can be recommended.

Heparin is occasionally administered during and almost always following the fibrinolytic therapy used to reduce the incidence of recurring thrombosis. After thrombolysis is achieved, the causes of the thromboses must be eliminated or reduced. Long-term anticoagulation therapy is required for those patients with persistent uncontrolled risk factors for recurrent thromboses.

REFERENCES

1. Ban NU: Biochemistry and in vitro diagnosis of thrombosis, in Ban NU, Glover JL, et al. (eds): Thrombosis and Atherosclerosis. Chicago, Year Book Medical Publishers, Inc, 1982, p 87.

2. Salem HH: The natural anticoagulants. Clin Haematol 15(2):371, 1986.

3. Thaler E, Lechner K: Antithrombin III deficiency and thromboembolism. Clin Haematol 10(2):369, 1981.

4. Tillett WS, Johnson AJ, McCarty WR: The intravenous infusion of the streptococcal fibrinolytic principle (streptokinase) into patients. J Clin Invest 34(2):169, 1955.

5. Urokinase-streptokinase embolism trial: Phase 2 results, a cooperative study. JAMA 229(12):1606, 1974.

6. The European Cooperative Study Group: Streptokinase in acute myocardial infarction. Extended report of the European cooperative trial. Acta Med Scand (suppl) 648:7, 1981.

7. Watz R, Savidge GF: Rapid thrombolysis and preservation of valvular venous function of high deep vein thrombosis. Acta Med Scand 205:293, 1979.

8. McNamara TO, Fischer JR: Thrombolysis of peripheral arterial and graft occlusions: Improved results using high-dose urokinase. AJR 144:769, 1985.

9. Hoylaerts M, Rijken DC, et al.: Kinetics of the activation of plasminogen by human tissue plasminogen activator: Role of fibrin. J Biol Chem 257(6):2912, 1982.

10. Weimar W, Stibbe J, et al.: Specific lysis of an iliofemoral thrombus by administration of extrinsic (tissue-type) plasminogen activator. Lancet 2(8254):1018, 1981.

11. Goldsmith MF: Recombinant plasminogen agent continues to show promise in trials. JAMA 253(12):1693, 1985.

12. Risius B, Graor RA, et al.: Recombinant human tissue-type plasminogen activator for thrombolysis in peripheral arteries and bypass grafts. Radiology 160:183, 1986.

13. Van de Werf F, Nobuhara M, Collene D: Coronary thrombolysis with human single-chain, urokinase-type plasminogen activator (pro-urokinase) in patients with acute myocardial infarction. Ann Intern Med 104:345, 1986.

14. Gurewich V, Pannell R: Biological properties of recombinant and of natural pro-urokinase. Thromb Haemost 54(2):558, 1985.

15. FitzGerald DE, Frisch EP, Miliken JC: Relief of chronic arterial obstruction using intravenous brinase. Scand J Thorac Cardiovasc Surg 13:327, 1979.

16. Duckert F: Thrombocytic therapy. Semin Thromb Hemost 10(1):87, 1984.

17. Walker ID, Davidson JF, et al.: Acylated streptokinase-plasminogen complex in patients with acute myocardial infarction. Thromb Haemost 51(2):204, 1984.

CHAPTER 13
Cardiopulmonary Assessment for Major Vascular Reconstructive Procedures

James C. Stanley and Thomas W. Wakefield

Careful preoperative assessment of cardiopulmonary function is essential in the planning of major arterial reconstructive surgery. In fact, recognition and treatment of underlying cardiac or pulmonary disease may be of greater importance in some patients than performance of a technically successful vascular surgical procedure. Coronary artery disease causes many, if not the majority, of immediate and late postoperative deaths following peripheral vascular surgical procedures. Although the role of impaired pulmonary function in contributing to operative mortality with peripheral vascular procedures is not as well defined as is that of cardiac disease, postoperative morbidity accompanying severe pulmonary disease is well recognized by all clinicians.

Coronary artery disease is clearly an important factor in determining the eventual outcome of surgical therapy in patients with vascular disease. For example, cardiac complications after carotid endarterectomy, abdominal aortic aneurysm resection, and lower-extremity revascularization at the Cleveland Clinic were responsible for 43% of early deaths, and fatal myocardial infarctions occurred in 20% of the survivors during an 8-year follow-up.[1] In this later experience, 5- and 10-year actuarial survival rates were 82% and 49% among patients without antecedent indications of coronary artery disease, compared to 67% and 31% during these same time periods in those patients suspected of having coronary artery disease. Myocardial infarction at this same institution accounted for 37% of early postoperative deaths among 343 patients undergoing operations for abdominal aortic aneurysm and for 52% among 273 patients undergoing operations for lower-extremity ischemia.[2,3] Others have encountered similar mortality and morbidity rates, a clear reflection that patients with peripheral vascular disease are likely to have life-threatening coronary artery disease.[4]

PREOPERATIVE CARDIAC ASSESSMENT

The value of screening studies for patients with coronary artery disease depends, in part, on the incidence of angiographically confirmed disease among patients undergoing peripheral vascular surgical reconstructions. Among 1,000 patients subjected to mandatory coronary arteriography before undergoing aortic reconstruction, lower-extremity revascularization, or carotid artery surgery between 1978 and 1982 at the Cleveland Clinic, 8% had normal coronary arteries, and coronary artery disease was mild to moderate in 32%, advanced but compensated in 29%, severe but surgically correctable in 25%, and inoperable in 6%.[5] Severe coronary artery disease was present in 36% of patients with abdominal aortic aneurysms, in 32% of patients with cerebrovascular disease, and in 28% of patients with lower-extremity ischemia. Surgically correctable severe coronary artery disease affected 34% of patients having a positive cardiac history or an abnormal electrocardiogram (ECG) and affected a surprising 14% of patients with a negative history and normal ECG. Thus neither the specificity or sensitivity of the patient's history and a routine ECG appear adequate for screening purposes.

In a classic study published a little more than a decade ago, cardiac risk in surgery patients was assessed by Goldman and his colleagues[6] who evaluated 1,001 patients undergoing noncardiac procedures. Nine independent factors were found to represent significant cardiac risks:

1. An S_3 gallop or jugulovenous distention
2. Myocardial infarction during the 6 months before surgery
3. Rhythm other than sinus or premature arterial contractions
4. Premature ventricular contractions greater than five per minute
5. Intraperitoneal, intrathoracic, or aortic operations
6. Age greater than 70 years
7. Significant aortic stenosis
8. Emergency surgical procedures
9. Poor general health evidenced by hypoxemia, hypercarbia, hypokalemia, chronic liver disease, or impaired renal function

With multivariant analysis, these cardiac risk factors correctly predicted and classified 81% of subsequent cardiac outcomes and became known as the Goldman index. Unfor-

TABLE 13-1. PREOPERATIVE CARDIAC ASSESSMENT

	Low Risk	Minimal Risk	High Risk
Stress ECG	Normal ECG, >85% predicted maximal heart rate	Abnormal ECG, 75–85% predicted maximal heart rate	Abnormal ECG, <75% predicted maximal heart rate
Radionuclide angiocardiography	Ejection fraction >55%	Ejection fraction 36–55%	Ejection fraction <35%
Dipyridamole-thallium scan	No defect or redistribution	Fixed defect without redistribution (scar from prior infarction)	Thallium redistribution, especially with congestive heart failure, angina, prior infarction, or diabetes mellitus.
Coronary angiography	No disease, mild compensated disease, or corrected disease	Advanced but compensated disease	Severe uncorrected or inoperable disease

tunately, this index was not particularly useful in assessing patients undergoing vascular surgery.[7,8]

Classification by Evans[9] of cardiac risk factors in 566 patients subjected to peripheral vascular procedures revealed six variables that had significant individual association with cardiovascular complications:

1. Presence of congestive heart failure
2. Prior myocardial infarction
3. Prior stroke
4. Arrhythmias
5. Abnormal electrocardiogram
6. Angina

By applying these factors to an equation-defining risk, postoperative cardiac complications occurred in a predictable fashion, affecting 1.3% of low-risk patients vs. 23.2% of high-risk patients.

The role of prior myocardial infarction is well established as a dominant risk factor for perioperative myocardial events in all surgical patients. In a Mayo Clinic study, patients undergoing operation within 3 months of a transmural myocardial infarction experienced a 27% reinfarction rate.[10] This rate decreased to 11% within 6 months and to a relatively stable 4 to 5% reinfarction rate thereafter. The recommendation that at least 6 months elapse between occurence of myocardial infarction and subsequent elective surgery was firmly advanced by this data. In a more recent study, perioperative reinfarction occurred 0 to 3 and 4 to 6 months after myocardial infarction in 36% and 26% of patients during 1973 to 1976 but in only 5.7% and 2.3% of patients during the same time periods after myocardial infarction when studied from 1977 to 1982.[11] This difference suggests that contemporary perioperative monitoring and cardiac support have caused a decrease in reinfarction rates. A number of basic tests are available for preoperative cardiac assessment (Table 13-1) and their use in practice deserves individualized discussion.

Stress Electrocardiography

Stress electrocardiography was one of the earlier means of screening for cardiac disease.[12–15] Findings that correlated with physiologically important stenoses included the following[16]:

1. Typical angina pectoris and a positive exercise test with more than 1 mm of ST-segment depression in three or more leads
2. A positive exercise test and an abnormal thallium scan
3. A positive exercise test with 2 mm of ST-segment depression in three or more leads

However, in a recent study of 100 patients requiring arterial reconstructive surgery, using either treadmill testing or arm ergometry, the degree of ST-segment depression was not a good predictor of cardiac complications unless the patient failed to achieve 85% of the predicted maximum heart rate.[17] Those patients with ST-segment depression of more than 1 mm and with less than 85% of the predicted maximum heart rate had a 33% myocardial complication rate, whereas those patients with a positive stress test who were able to achieve greater than 85% of their predicted maximum heart rate had a 0% complication rate ($P < 0.5$).

Unfortunately, many surgical patients are unable to participate in exercise-related stress testing. Gage and his colleagues[12] reported that only 76% of such patients were able to undergo adequate stress for testing purposes. In their experience, among 38 of 50 patients in whom the stress studies were complete, 25 were abnormal, but only 15 were confirmed truly positive through coronary arteriography. Just as important was the fact that a third of the patients without cardiac symptoms and a normal ECG exhibited an abnormal stress test, indicating once again that silent coronary artery disease is common. Further concern regarding screening with exercise-stress ECGs has been expressed by Weiner,[15] who noted that 65% of men and 33% of women with angina and significant coronary artery disease had negative studies. Finally, the actual predictive value of these tests also depends on the disease prevalence, a factor that further lessens their screening potential.

An attempt to better quantitate exercise stress testing evolved from a recent evaluation of 2,842 patients undergoing exercise electrocardiography within 6 weeks of cardiac catheterization.[18] This study described a treadmill score, defined as exercise time minus (5 × ST deviation) − (4 × treadmill angina index). Patients with three-vessel disease and a score of −11 or less had a 5-year survival rate of 67% vs. a 5-year survival rate of 93% with a score of +7 or more. The value of such a system to predict operative complications in patients undergoing peripheral vascular surgical procedures remains to be determined.

Radionuclide Ventriculography

Radionuclide ventriculography also serves as a screening test for coronary artery disease.[19] This test is relatively precise, with correlations between dye dilution and technetium-99m pertechnetate–determined cardiac output being 0.94 in healthy individuals and 0.89 in patients with a history of coronary artery disease. Nuclide scanning defines the volumes of the heart during end-diastole and end-systole, allowing, with analysis of 300 to 400 cardiac cycles, accurate quantification of the ventricular-ejection fraction. Such gated-pool radionuclide ventriculograms (MUGA scans) are used to provide quantitative data about cardiac function.

At the New York University Medical Center, among patients who were undergoing major abdominal aortic reconstructions and who had preoperative radionuclide ventriculography, perioperative myocardial infarction was 0% with a MUGA-determined ejection fraction of 56 to 85%, 20% with an ejection fraction of 36 to 55%, and 80% with an ejection fraction of less than 35%.[20] In a British study of patients undergoing aortic surgery, ejection fractions greater than and less than 30% were associated with cardiac-related deaths in 2.7% and 75%, respectively.[21] Similar experiences have been reported in patients undergoing extremity revascularizations.[22] The effect of exercise on the ejection fraction provides further prognostic information about the severity of the underlying coronary artery disease.[23]

Radionuclide Myocardial Imaging

Thallium-201 chloride provides a marker of myocardial blood flow and allows recognition of decreased or redistributed flow during increased cardiac activity, a finding suggesting that the cardiac muscle is at risk (Fig. 13-1). In this regard, a fixed defect observed during both stress and rest thallium scanning (such as would occur in the region of prior myocardial infarction and fibrosis) represents a less hazardous situation than would occur with redistribution. Such fixed defects represent a nonreactive ventricular scar.

Thallium studies using maximal coronary vasodilation with intravenous administration of dipyridamole were an outgrowth of difficulties in achieving adequate stress using treadmill exercise during both electrocardiographic and radionuclide studies.[24–29] These new testing methods have shown great promise and have overcome difficulties in testing patients with extremity vascular disease who cannot adequately exercise, as well as those patients receiving beta blockers who are unable to increase their heart rate and generate an acceptable increase in rate-pressure products. An early evaluation of thallium-dipyridamole studies was performed by Brewster and his colleagues[27] at Massachusetts General Hospital on 54 patients whose treatments were nearly equally divided between aortic and peripheral arterial reconstructive procedures. In this experience, 22 patients, including five who had evidence on ECG of an old myocardial infarction, exhibited a normal test, and none developed postoperative cardiac ischemic events. Persistent defects were demonstrated in 10 patients, none of whom developed postoperative cardiac ischemic complications.

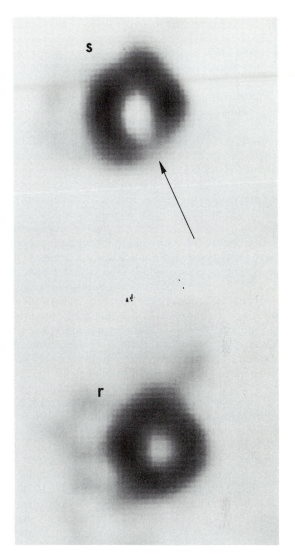

Figure 13-1. Radionuclide myocardial imaging with thallium-201 chloride. Perfusion defect during stress (s) in the inferolateral left ventricle (arrow) is not present 3 hours later during recovery (r). Such redistribution of myocardial blood flow establishes the existence of tissue vulnerable to further ischemic injury.

Among the 22 patients who demonstrated thallium redistribution, seven patients had their vascular operation deferred after coronary arteriography demonstrated significant coronary artery disease, and 15 patients underwent vascular operation, with seven exhibiting definite myocardial ischemia postoperatively, including one death, three nonfatal transmural myocardial infarctions, and four instances in which unstable angina developed. In this study perioperative myocardial ischemia did not correlate with age greater than 70 years, a history of angina pectoris, the type of operation performed, or anginal discomfort and ST-segment changes accompanying administration of dipyridamole. Most importantly, a previous myocardial infarction in this study was not predictive of operatively related ischemic events unless accompanied by thallium redistribution.

Cutler[28] reported on 116 patients undergoing dipyridamole stress-thallium studies, of whom 60 had normal preoperative scans with no myocardial infarctions after surgery for abdominal aortic aneurysm, and 31 had abnormal preoperative scans, eight of whom had myocardial infarctions. The risks of developing a myocardial infarction were 12 times greater for a patient with an abnormal scan. Abnormal scans occurred with similar frequencies in this series among patients with clinically asymptomatic, as well as symptomatic, coronary artery disease.

Another recently published study on dipyridamole stress-thallium testing from the Massachusetts General Hospital involved a total of 111 patients.[29] In the first 61 patients studied, myocardial events occurred in eight of 18 patients with preoperative thallium redistribution compared to no events in 43 patients without thallium redistribution. In a subsequent portion of this study, patients were categorized as those without evidence of congestive heart failure, angina pectoris, prior myocardial infarction, or diabetes mellitus vs. those with one or more of these factors. None of the 23 patients in whom these clinical conditions were absent had adverse outcomes, despite the fact that six exhibited thallium redistribution. On the other hand, 27 patients had more than one of these clinical risk factors, and of 18 patients with redistribution, eight experienced postoperative ischemic events, compared to only two such events among the nine patients without redistribution. Thus dipyridamole-thallium scanning may be useful in stratifying patients at risk for myocardial ischemia when one or more clinical markers of cardiac disease or diabetes exist. The overall incidence of perioperative ischemic events in this series was 45% with thallium redistribution, compared to 7% without thallium redistribution.

A cautionary note regarding thallium-stress images is warranted for hypertensive patients with a low likelihood of coronary artery disease who have had diastolic pressures exceeding 90 mm Hg for at least 2 years. These patients are more likely to have abnormal scans than are normotensive patients, perhaps as a reflection of limited coronary reserve due to hypertension-related myocardial hypertrophy.[30] Such findings may lessen the specificity of these tests. A second word of caution relates to the potential for dipyridamole-induced myocardial ischemia, allegedly caused by coronary "steal" in the presence of epicardial coronary collateral vessels.[31] This potential hazard has received little attention because of the large number of useful studies performed without occurrence of this complication.

Arteriography

Arteriography is the most accurate means of identifying surgically correctable coronary artery disease in patients who are candidates for peripheral vascular surgery. However, its use as a screening test in all patients has been questioned by many, including surgeons from the Mayo Clinic, where routine coronary artery bypass plus aortic aneurysmectomy in certain subgroups carries a risk exceeding that of aneurysm resection alone.[32,33] Mortality at the Mayo Clinic among patients who had not undergone prior coronary artery bypass in the 50- to 69-year age group was due to a cardiac cause 70% of the time, compared to 50% for patients 70 to 79 years old, and 33% among patients older than 80 years. The Mayo group now recommends

that treatment of younger patients should include the liberal performance of coronary artery bypass surgery before peripheral vascular procedures.

In summary, current practice standards support the performance of stress-thallium scans, preferably with intravenous dipyridamole, in all patients who are to undergo peripheral vascular surgical reconstructions, regardless of whether a significant cardiac history does or does not exist. Patients exhibiting redistribution of myocardial blood flow should undergo coronary arteriography, and if correctable lesions are found, coronary artery revascularization should be undertaken before the peripheral vascular surgical procedure. In the absence of dipyridamole-thallium scanning less specific and sensitive means of testing must be accepted. Under such circumstances it would seem reasonable to follow closely the Cleveland Clinic recommendations wherein patients having a positive cardiac history, as well as physical examination or electrocardiographic evidence of coronary artery disease, should undergo preoperative coronary arteriography. Patients without these clues of coronary artery disease should undergo noninvasive studies such as stress electrocardiography or exercise stress-thallium scanning. If the latter studies are positive, the patient should undergo coronary arteriography; if they are negative, the patient may proceed with the anticipated vascular surgical procedure.

INTRAOPERATIVE CARDIAC MANAGEMENT

Intraoperative risk analysis based on anesthetic classification has allowed definition of a system of overall operative mortality rates. For example, the mortality in class I ASA (American Society of Anesthesiologists) risk patients is 0.08%, whereas the mortality in class V ASA risk patients is 9.4%.[34] However, this classification does not distinguish the treatable factors contributing to myocardial infarction, which may affect 50 to 60% of patients undergoing certain major vascular procedures. Surgeons should be familiar with the intraoperative maneuvers that decrease the cardiac risks of peripheral vascular reconstructions.

Clearly, use of the Swan-Ganz catheter has allowed more optimal fluid administration during performance of vascular procedures. The Brigham group[35] used Swan-Ganz catheter monitoring preoperatively to determine Starling responses to incremental infusions of salt-poor albumin and lactated Ringer's solution, with subsequent pulmonary capillary wedge pressures maintained intraoperatively and postoperatively at levels consistent with optimal left-ventricular performance as predicted by their preoperative studies. They reported 110 consecutive patients who had elective or urgent repair of abdominal aortic aneurysms with no 30-day mortality, only a 0.9% in-hospital mortality, and a 5-year cumulative survival rate of 84%. Increased arterial pressures were treated with sodium nitroprusside as a vasodilator, but monitoring of the cardiac index and pulmonary capillary wedge pressures suggested that this treatment was seldom necessary and at times hazardous. In fact, the Brigham group does not now use vasodilators during aortic cross clamping. Others have had similar experiences and have reported the optimal fluid management with aortic reconstruction includes administration of balanced salt solutions rather than hypotonic solutions.[36]

Maintenance of pulmonary capillary wedge pressures with volume expansion is often supplemented with both inotropic drugs and afterload-reducing drugs.[37] These agents become important in that the diastolic compliance or relationship between the wedge pressure and the end-diastolic volume index may decrease after aortic declamping.[38] This is probably a reflection of early myocardial ischemia, and under such circumstances the wedge pressure may need to be restored to higher levels to return the cardiac index to acceptable levels.

Other types of intraoperative monitoring contribute to improved myocardial performance and to detection of early myocardial ischemia. One such technique includes on-line computerized monitoring of systolic time intervals, left ventricular preejection times, left ventricular ejection times, and ratios of left ventricular preejection time to ejection time.[39] Experience with this type of monitoring revealed systolic time intervals to be sensitive indexes for titration of anesthetic and vasoactive drugs, whereas pulmonary artery diastolic pressures apparently were more specific for alterations in blood and fluid volume management.

Perhaps a more direct approach for assessing intraoperative cardiac function and myocardial ischemia is two-dimensional transesophageal echocardiography as advocated by Roizen and his colleagues.[40,41] In a study of 24 ASA class III and IV patients, half underwent supraceliac clamping and half underwent suprarenal-infraceliac or infrarenal-aortic cross clamping, with a special 3.5 MHz two-dimensional electrocardiographic transducer placed in the esophagus to provide a cross-sectional view of the left ventricle through the base of the papillary muscle.[40] Supraceliac-aortic occlusion caused major increases in left ventricular end-systolic and end-diastolic areas, decreases in ejection fraction, and frequent wall-motion abnormalities. Suprarenal clamping caused similar but less pronounced effects, whereas infrarenal clamping caused minimal changes. Wedge pressure changes did not correlate with the findings of two-dimensional electrocardiography. For example, with supraceliac-aortic cross clamping, wedge pressures and systemic pressures were normal in 10 of 12 patients, whereas 11 of 12 developed wall-motion abnormalities indicative of ischemia. Two-dimensional echocardiography, in another study of 50 patients, revealed 24 individuals who developed segmental wall-motion abnormalities, but only six exhibited concomitant ST-segment changes on the ECG.[41] Thus intraoperative two-dimensional transesophageal echocardiography apparently is a sensitive means for identifying segmental wall-motion abnormalities indicative of early myocardial ischemia that occur before either ST-segment changes or abnormal wedge pressures develop.

Vasodilators have been administered during aortic cross clamping to decrease the systemic arterial blood pressure and afterload against which the heart must pump. Nitroglycerin and nitroprusside are the most common agents used to achieve this effect. Nitroglycerin is a potent venous vasodilator and a mild arterial vasodilator. It decreases myocardial oxygen demand, lessens myocardial ischemia by reducing diastolic volume, and may increase oxygen delivery to ischemic myocardium by dilating coronary arteries and collateral vessels. Nitroprusside, on the other hand, is a relatively balanced arterial and venous vasodilator. It has greater relaxing effects on coronary resistance vessels and less influence on coronary collateral vessels. In this regard, nitroprusside decreases blood flow in the ischemic myocardium of patients with stable angina and increases ST-segment elevations in those patients with acute myocardial infarction, supporting the suggestion by Fremes and his colleagues[42] that it may cause reduction of myocardial oxygen supply in patients with significant cardiac disease. In a related study by this group, 33 hypertensive patients undergoing coronary bypass procedures had their arterial pressure decreased to 85 mm Hg through the use of both nitroglycerin and nitroprusside, but only nitroglycerin improved myocardial metabolism as assessed by myocardial lactate flux.[43]

Volume loading may be an important adjunct to the use of vasodilators. The Brigham group[44] reported on 50 patients who had an abdominal aortic aneurysm resection, of whom 10 received customary preoperative maintenance fluids, 23 received 1,500 ml of balanced salt solution in the 12 hours before the operation to keep the pulmonary capillary wedge pressure at 10 to 13 mm Hg, and 17 received the same fluid regimen with the addition of vasodilators. Fourteen of the latter patients received nitroprusside at a rate of 1.5 to 6.0 µg/kg/min, and three received nitroglycerin at a rate of 0.5 to 3.5 µg/kg/min. Both vasodilators were administered after aortic cross clamping to control afterload, and additional volume expansion was used to maintain a constant preload, but the mean arterial blood pressure and cardiac index fell, and furthermore the cardiac index remained depressed after aortic declamping. These events occurred concurrently with increased pulmonary capillary wedge pressures without corresponding increases in cardiac index, suggesting myocardial depression. In this setting vasodilators did not appear useful.

The combined administration of inotropic and vasodilator agents in patients after coronary artery bypass grafting has been advocated by the Stanford group.[45] Volume loading with the addition of vasodilators and dopamine increased the cardiac index 45%, increased left ventricular stroke work index 30%, decreased systemic vascular resistance 41%, and only decreased mean arterial pressure 10%. In comparison to dopamine alone, addition of vasodilators and volume infusion increased the cardiac index 14% and decreased systemic vascular resistance 24%, without a significant change in left ventricular stroke work index. This form of combined therapy appears to facilitate beneficial responses from both drugs while minimizing their individual disadvantages. In this regard the usefulness of dopamine is limited when the preload is decreased because its enhanced inotropic activity may actually increase myocardial oxygen demand and consumption. Similarly, nitroprusside alone is contraindicated in patients with left ventricular failure complicated by hypotension because it may also decrease cardiac output if the preload is inadequate. The usefulness of vasodilators in cardiac surgical procedures may relate to the severe vasoconstriction known to occur after coronary artery grafting and cardiopulmonary bypass.[45] In addition, cardiac output with ventricular failure is more sensitive to afterload than preload, and patients with severe ventricular failure would more likely benefit from nitroprusside afterload reduction.

Another important issue regarding vasodilators is their effect on regional blood flow in ischemic tissue. For example, vasodilator therapy should be most useful in patients requiring high thoracic-aortic cross clamping. However, as noted in canine experiments, thoracic-aortic cross clamping and infusion of nitroprusside cause the mean arterial blood pressure below the occlusion to decrease, causing further reductions in renal and spinal cord blood flow, factors that may negate any cardiac protection afforded by the vasodilator.[46,47] Nitroprusside, on the other hand, administered during infrarenal cross clamping in similar laboratory studies, decreased arterial pressure by 30%, brought cardiac output back down to baseline, and appeared to normalize hepatic and intrarenal blood flow.[48] Thus, with infrarenal aortic occlusion, renal and splanchnic blood flow do not appear to be adversely affected by the administration of nitroprusside. In summary, vasodilator and inotropic drug use during aortic cross clamping is controversial. Those patients with the poorest myocardial function and most dependent on afterload reduction would appear to benefit the greatest from use of vasodilators, but perfusion pressure below the level of high aortic cross clamping in such patients must be closely monitored to ensure adequate regional blood flow to vital organs.

PREOPERATIVE PULMONARY ASSESSMENT

Adequate pulmonary assessment is dependent on acquisition of a detailed history, the presence or absence of specific physical findings, measurement of arterial blood gases, and performance of certain pulmonary function tests using spirometric techniques.

Historically, the number of pack-years of smoking becomes important, with 20 pack-years appearing to be the level at which significant pulmonary risks become apparent.[49] The presence or extent of shortness of breath during activity, prior episodes of respiratory failure, existence of asthma, and exposure to noxious environmental agents are all relevant in assessing the pulmonary status. The quantity and nature of sputum production are particularly important in patients with long-standing lung disease, since it is this information that allows one to distinguish chronic bronchitis from emphysema.

The physical examination easily detects hypoventilation in weak or debilitated patients, and hyperinflation in patients with chronic obstructive pulmonary disease. The ability to climb one or two flights of stairs at a steady pace without dyspnea is a practical test, and if such cannot be done, further tests are mandatory before operative intervention occurs. Chest radiographs augment the findings of the routine physical examination.

Arterial blood gases should be measured preoperatively on all patients identified as high risk by history, physical examination or spirometric testing. Oxygenation is assessed by measuring Pa_{O_2} during room-air breathing and is dependent on the appropriate matching of alveolar gas to pulmonary blood flow. Ventilation is assessed by measuring Pa_{CO_2}, inasmuch as CO_2 removal is dependent entirely on alveolar ventilation. Arterial blood gas values define both alveolar hypoventilation ($Pa_{CO_2} > 45$ mm Hg) and significant right-to-left shunting, diffusion block, and ventilation-perfusion mismatch ($Pa_{O_2} < 70$ mm Hg).

Definitions of normal pulmonary function tests (Table 13-2) are useful in assessing the preoperative status of vascular surgery patients. Tidal volume (TV) is the amount of air exchanged during a normal resting ventilatory cycle. Vital capacity (VC), also known as forced expiratory volume (FEV) or forced vital capacity (FVC), is the volume of air expelled with maximal exhalation after a maximal inspiration. Functional residual capacity (FRC) is the volume of air remaining in the lungs after TV exhalation. Typical normal values for these volumes are TV of 7 to 8 cc/kg body weight, VC of 30 to 50 cc/kg body weight, and FRC of 15 to 30 cc/kg body weight. Volume measurements are reported as the percent of predicted, with 80 to 120% being considered within the normal range.

Expiratory flow rates are commonly expressed as volume per time, such as $FEV_{0.5}$, which defines the volume of forced expiration during a half second. This measure is dependent on patient effort and reveals the existence or absence of obstructive airway disease. Flow measurements are also expressed as a percentage of the expected value for the individual patient being studied FEV_1 is a similar measure except that it assesses volume exhaled over 1 second. The $FEF_{25\%-75\%}$ (MMFR or maximal midexpiratory flow rate) is most sensitive to disease in smaller airways and is considered normal when greater than 80% of the amount predicted or when 150 to 200 L/min. The maximal voluntary ventilation (MVV) an individual can generate is highly dependent on patient effort, the dead space to tidal volume ratio, and lung compliance. MVV usually ranges from 150 to 500 L/min. MVV is one of the more sensitive tests for predicting pulmonary complications because an abnormal value (less than 80% predicted) may be caused by general patient weakness, as well as by pulmonary disease.

Static compliance is defined as the TV divided by the peak inspiratory pressure and is normally 100 to 200 cc/

TABLE 13-2. PREOPERATIVE PULMONARY ASSESSMENT

	Normal	High Risk
Vital capacity (VC)	30–50 cc/kg; >80% predicted	<30–50%
Forced expiratory volume, 1 second (FEV₁)	>80% predicted	<40–50%
Maximal midexpiratory flow (FEF₂₅%–₇₅%)	150–200 L/min; >80% predicted	<35–50%
Maximal voluntary ventilation (MVV)	150–500 L/min; >80% predicted	<35–50%
Pa$_{O_2}$, room air	85 ± 5 mm Hg	<50–55 mm Hg
Pa$_{CO_2}$, room air	40 ± 4 mm Hg	>45–55 mm Hg

cm H_2O. An esophageal balloon is required to measure compliance. Effective compliance is the TV per plateau pressure on a ventilator, with normal being greater than 50 cc/cm H_2O. Inspiratory force (IF) is defined as the maximal subatmospheric pressure that can be exerted on a closed airway. A normal IF is −100 cm H_2O, with −20 cm H_2O being the lower limit of acceptability.

Patients with obstructive defects have an essentially normal VC but have abnormal expiratory air flows such as FEV_1, $FEV_{0.5}$, and $FEF_{25\%-75\%}$, whereas patients with restrictive defects have a low VC but have normal expiratory air flows. Some have suggested that the MVV, as measured directly or as approximated by the $FEV_1 \times 30$, is the best test to predict postoperative pulmonary complications. With an MVV less than 50% of predicted, respiratory complications developed in a high portion of patients undergoing thoracotomy, and in the majority of the patients, multiple complications ensued.[50] Other more detailed tests such as measurement of FRC using helium dilution or nitrogen wash out, diffusing capacity, or response of arterial Pa_{O_2} to breathing 100% oxygen are rarely necessary in these preoperative assessments.

Variations in pulmonary function studies during a 24-hour period for patients with normal lungs were 5% for FEV_1, 5% for FVC, and 13% for $FEF_{25\%-75\%}$. Similar variations in patients with chronic obstructive pulmonary disease were 13%, 11%, and 23%, respectively.[51] Thus, with interventions such as the use of bronchodilators, these percentages represent the minimal changes necessary to assume that a significant therapeutic effect has occurred.

Attesting to the importance of blood gas analysis and spirometrically derived pulmonary function tests was a pulmonary complication rate of 3% in patients with chronic obstructive pulmonary disease who had normal preoperative tests compared to a complication rate of 70% of those patients with abnormal tests; the most important predictors were a Pa_{CO_2} greater than 45 mm Hg and a Pa_{O_2} less than 60 mm Hg.[52] However, even patients at increased risk with seemingly prohibitive test data (e.g., an MVV less than 50 L/min and an $FEF_{25\%-75\%}$ less than 50 L/min) can undergo major operative procedures with a low mortality rate and an acceptable pulmonary complication rate.[53] Poor performance on spirometric testing is not a contraindication to a major vascular procedure but rather is a means of identifying those patients who will require special preoperative preparation and careful attention to postoperative mechanical ventilation.

For patients with chronic obstructive pulmonary disease, asthma, or chronic bronchitis, respiratory flow measurements should be obtained before and after the use of bronchodilators. Intensive preoperative preparation using these agents and respiratory exercises until pulmonary function is optimal (as documented by spirometry) has reduced by more than half the pulmonary complication rate associated with chronic obstructive pulmonary disease.[54]

In a small series of patients at Duke who were undergoing abdominal aortic aneurysm resection and who had severe preoperative pulmonary compromise, there was no mortality, and only 20% required prolonged ventilatory support.[55] Preoperatively all patients stopped smoking for at least 1 month, pulmonary infection was treated with antibiotics, nebulized bronchodilators and humidified air were administered, and exercises were instituted that stressed improved inspiratory effort. Intraoperatively, blood filters were used for all blood transfusions, minimizing anesthetic time was emphasized, blood use was minimized, and the pulmonary capillary wedge pressure was used as a guide for fluid administration. Postoperatively, these patients were mechanically ventilated and extubated as soon as possible but were reintubated early if necessary. The amount of narcotics usually given was reduced and patients were ambulated early. All these factors lessened operative mortality and morbidity in vascular surgery patients whose preoperative pulmonary function was marginal.

CONCLUSIONS

The objectives of perioperative cardiopulmonary assessments and intervention in patients who are candidates for vascular surgery are twofold. First is performance of the surgical procedure with minimal morbidity and mortality. Second is an improved long-term survival of the patient, in particular by reducing late cardiac mortality. Patients undergoing preoperative coronary artery bypass before peripheral vascular reconstructions have had excellent outcomes, with operative mortality reported as low as 0.2% in one large experience.[56] Even severely ill patients have been able to undergo abdominal aortic aneurysm resection with a mortality rate less than 6%, despite such factors as the use of home oxygen, a Pa_{O_2} less than 50 mm Hg or an $FEF_{25\%-75\%}$ less than 25%, NYHA (New York Heart Association) Classification III or IV, active angina pectoris, an ejection fraction less than 30%, recent congestive heart failure, complex ventricular ectopy, large left ventricular aneurysms, severe valvular heart disease, or unreconstructable coronary artery disease.[57] The late 43% mortality from heart disease reported by Crawford and his colleagues[58] among 949 patients undergoing treatment for aortoiliac occlusive disease should be reduced with present management programs. For instance, greater than a 90% 5-year survival may be expected after coronary artery reconstruction, even in patients with multiple vessel disease.[59-61]

One of the first long-term studies of an aggressive preoperative cardiac assessment and management approach to patients undergoing peripheral vascular surgery involved 246 patients with infrarenal abdominal aortic aneurysms treated at the Cleveland Clinic.[62] Severe coronary artery disease was documented in 32% of the patients, 28% of whom underwent myocardial revascularization with a mortality rate of 5.7%. A total of 56 patients in this subset underwent staged aneurysm repair with an accompanying 1.8% mortality rate. During the follow-up interval, 25% of the patients in this group died, leaving a 5-year survival rate of 75%, but there was only a 5% cardiac mortality rate. This survival was nearly identical to that for patients having both trivial coronary lesions and severe coronary involvement without an aneurysm who underwent coronary revascularization and was much better than the 5-year survival rate of only 29% for patients with uncorrected or inoperable coronary artery disease. More attention to early treatment of correctable coronary artery disease in vascular surgery patients seems appropriate.

REFERENCES

1. Hertzer NR: Clinical experience with preoperative coronary angiography. J Vasc Surg 2:510, 1985.
2. Hertzer NR: Fatal myocardial infarction following abdominal aortic aneurysm resection. Three hundred forty-three patients followed 6–11 years postoperatively. Ann Surg 192:667, 1980.
3. Hertzer NR: Fatal myocardial infarction following lower extremity revascularization. Two hundred seventy-three patients followed six to eleven postoperative years. Ann Surg 193:492, 1981.
4. Nicolaides AN: The diagnosis and assessment of coronary artery disease in vascular patients. J Vasc Surg 2:501, 1985.
5. Beven EG: Routine coronary angiography in patients undergoing surgery for abdominal aortic aneurysm and lower extremity occlusive disease. J Vasc Surg 3:682, 1986.
6. Goldman L, Caldera DL, et al.: Multifactorial index of cardiac risk in noncardiac surgical procedures. N Engl J Med 297:845, 1977.
7. Calvin JE, Kieser TM, et al.: Cardiac mortality and morbidity after vascular surgery. Can J Surg 29:93, 1986.
8. Jeffrey CC, Kunsman J, et al.: A prospective evaluation of cardiac risk index. Anesthesiology 58:462, 1983.
9. Cooperman M, Pflug B, et al.: Cardiovascular risk factors in patients with peripheral vascular disease. Surgery 84:505, 1978.
10. Steen PA, Tinker JH, Tarhan S: Myocardial reinfarction after anesthesia and surgery. JAMA 239:2566, 1978.
11. Rao TLK, Jacobs KH: Reinfarction following anesthesia in patients with myocardial infarction. Anesthesiology 59:499, 1983.
12. Gage AA, Bhayana JN, et al.: Assessment of cardiac risk in surgical patients. Arch Surg 112:1488, 1977.
13. Cutler BS, Wheeler HB, et al.: Assessment of operative risk with electrocardiographic exercise testing in patients with peripheral vascular disease. Am J Surg 137:484, 1979.
14. Cutler BS, Wheeler HB, et al.: Applicability and interpretation of electrocardiographic stress testing in patients with peripheral vascular disease. Am J Surg 141:501, 1981.
15. Weiner DA, Ryan TJ, et al.: Exercise stress testing. Correlations among history of angina, ST-segment response and prevalence of coronary-artery disease in the coronary artery surgery study (CASS). N Engl J Med 301:230, 1979.
16. Selwyn AP: The value of Holter monitoring in managing patients with coronary artery disease. Circulation 75 (suppl 2):31, 1987.
17. McPhail N, Calvin JE, et al.: The use of preoperative exercise testing to predict cardiac complications after arterial reconstruction. J Vasc Surg 7:60, 1988.
18. Mark DB, Hlatky MA, et al.: Exercise treadmill score for predicting prognosis in coronary artery disease. Ann Intern Med 106:793, 1987.
19. Jones RH, Douglas JM, et al.: Noninvasive radionuclide assessment of cardiac function in patients with peripheral vascular disease. Surgery 85:59, 1979.
20. Pasternack PF, Imparato AM, et al.: The value of radionuclide angiography as a predictor of perioperative myocardial infarction in patients undergoing abdominal aortic aneurysm resection. J Vasc Surg 1:320, 1984.
21. Mosley JG, Clarke JMF, et al.: Assessment of myocardial function before aortic surgery by radionuclide angiocardiography. Br J Surg 72:886, 1985.
22. Pasternack PF, Imparato AM, et al.: The value of the radionuclide angiogram in the prediction of perioperative myocardial

infarction in patients undergoing lower extremity revascularization procedures. Circulation 72(suppl II):213, 1985.
23. Bonow RD: Exercise testing and radionuclide procedures in high-risk populations. Circulation 75:(suppl 2):18, 1987.
24. Albro PC, Gould KL, et al.: Noninvasive assessment of coronary stenoses by myocardial imaging during pharmacologic coronary vasodilation, III: Clinical trials. Am J Cardiol 42:751, 1978.
25. Leppo J, Boucher CA, et al.: Serial thallium-201 myocardial imaging after dipyridamole infusion: Diagnostic utility in detecting coronary stenoses and relationship to regional wall motion. Circulation 66:649, 1982.
26. Boucher CA, Brewster DC, et al.: Determination of cardiac risk by dipyridamole-thallium imaging before peripheral vascular surgery. N Engl J Med 312:389, 1985.
27. Brewster DC, Okada RD, et al.: Selection of patients for preoperative coronary angiography: Use of dipyridamole-stress-thallium myocardial imaging. J Vasc Surg 2:504, 1985.
28. Cutler BS, Leppo JA: Dipyridamole thallium 201 scintigraphy to detect coronary artery disease before abdominal aortic surgery. J Vasc Surg 5:91, 1987.
29. Eagle KA, Singer DE, et al.: Dipyridamole-thallium scanning in patients undergoing vascular surgery. Optimizing preoperative evaluation of cardiac risk. JAMA 257:2185, 1987.
30. Schulman DS, Francis CK, et al.: Thallium-201 stress imaging in hypertensive patients. Hypertension 10:16, 1987.
31. Keltz TN, Innerfield M, et al.: Dipyridamole-induced myocardial ischemia. JAMA 257:1515, 1987.
32. Brown OW, Hollier LH, et al.: Abdominal aortic aneurysm and coronary artery disease. A reassessment. Arch Surg 116:1484, 1981.
33. Reigel MM, Hollier LH, et al.: Late survival in abdominal aortic aneurysm patients: The role of selected myocardial revascularization on the basis of clinical symptoms. J Vasc Surg 5:222, 1987.
34. Vacanti CJ, VanHouten RJ, Hill RC: A statistical analysis of the relationship of physical status to postoperative mortality in 68,388 cases. Anesth Analg 49:564, 1970.
35. Whittemore AD, Clowes AW, et al.: Aortic aneurysm repair. Reduced operative mortality associated with maintenance of optimal cardiac performance. Ann Surg 192:414, 1980.
36. Bomberger RA, McGregor B, DePalma RG: Optimal fluid management after aortic reconstruction: A prospective study of two crystalloid solutions. J Vasc Surg 4:164, 1986.
37. Babu SC, Sharma PVP, et al.: Monitor-guided responses. Operability with safety is increased in patients with peripheral vascular diseases. Arch Surg 115:1384, 1980.
38. Kalman PG, Wellwood MR, et al.: Cardiac dysfunction during abdominal aortic operation: The limitations of pulmonary wedge pressures. J Vasc Surg 3:773, 1986.
39. Dauchot PJ, DePalma R, et al.: Detection and prevention of cardiac dysfunction during aortic surgery. J Surg Res 26:574, 1979.
40. Roizen MF, Beaupre PN, et al.: Monitoring with two-dimensional transesophageal echocardiography. Comparison of myocardial function in patients undergoing supraceliac, suprarenal-infraceliac, or infrarenal aortic occlusion. J Vasc Surg 1:300, 1984.
41. Smith JS, Cahalan MK, et al.: Intraoperative detection of myocardial ischemia in high-risk patients: Electrocardiography versus two-dimensional transesophageal echocardiography. Circulation 72:1015, 1985.
42. Fremes SE, Weisel RD, et al.: A comparison of nitroglycerin and nitroprusside, II: The effects of volume loading. Ann Thorac Surg 39:61, 1985.
43. Fremes SE, Weisel RD, et al.: A comparison of nitroglycerin and nitroprusside, I: Treatment of postoperative hypertension. Ann Thorac Surg 39:53, 1985.

44. Grindlinger GA, Vegas AM, et al.: Volume loading and vasodilators in abdominal aortic aneurysmectomy. Am J Surg 139:480, 1980.
45. Miller DC, Stinson EB, et al.: Postoperative enhancement of left ventricular performance by combined inotropic-vasodilator therapy with preload control. Surgery 88:108, 1980.
46. Gelman S, Reves JG, et al.: Regional blood flow during cross-clamping of the thoracic aorta and infusion of sodium nitroprusside. J Thorac Cardiovasc Surg 85:287, 1983.
47. Laschinger JC, Owen J, et al.: Detrimental effects of sodium nitroprusside on spinal cord motor tract perfusion during thoracic aortic cross-clamping. Surg Forum 38:195, 1987.
48. Gelman S, Petel K, et al.: Renal and splanchnic circulation during infrarenal aortic cross-clamping. Arch Surg 119:1394, 1984.
49. Auchincloss JH: Preoperative evaluation of pulmonary function. Surg Clin North Am 54:1015, 1974.
50. Boysen PG, Block AJ, Moulder PV: Relationship between preoperative pulmonary function tests and complications after thoracotomy. Surg Gynecol Obstet 152:813, 1981.
51. Pennock BE, Rogers RM, McCaffree DR: Changes in measured spirometric indices. What is significant? Chest 80:97, 1981.
52. Gaensler EA, Weisel RD: The risks in abdominal and thoracic surgery in COPD. Postgrad Med 54:183, 1973.
53. Williams CD, Brenowitz JB: ''Prohibitive'' lung function and major surgical procedures. Am J Surg 132:763, 1976.
54. Gracey DR, Divertie MB, Didier EP: Preoperative pulmonary preparation of patients with chronic obstructive pulmonary disease. A prospective study. Chest 76:123, 1979.
55. Smith PK, Fuchs JCA, Sabiston DC: Surgical management of aortic abdominal aneurysms in patients with severe pulmonary insufficiency. Surg Gynecol Obstet 151:407, 1980.
56. Reul GJ Jr, Cooley DA, et al.: The effect of coronary bypass on the outcome of peripheral vascular operations in 1093 patients. J Vasc Surg 3:788, 1986.
57. Hollier LH, Reigel MM, et al.: Conventional repair of abdominal aortic aneurysm in the high-risk patient: A plea for abandonment of nonresective treatment. J Vasc Surg 3:712, 1986.
58. Crawford ES, Bomberger RA, et al.: Aortoiliac occlusive disease: Factors influencing survival and function following reconstructive operation over a 25 year period. Surgery 90:1055, 1981.
59. Crawford ES, Morris GC Jr, et al.: Operative risk in patients with previous coronary artery bypass. Ann Thorac Surg 26:215, 1978.
60. Loop FD, Cosgrove DM, et al.: An 11 year evolution of coronary arterial surgery (1967–1978). Ann Surg 190:444, 1979.
61. Mahar LJ, Steen PA, et al.: Perioperative myocardial infarction in patients with coronary artery disease with and without aorta-coronary artery bypass grafts. J Thorac Cardiovasc Surg 76:533, 1978.
62. Hertzer NR, Young JR, et al.: Late results of coronary bypass in patients with infrarenal aortic aneurysms. The Cleveland Clinic Study. Ann Surg 205:360, 1987.

PART II
Procedures for Exposure of Vessels

CHAPTER 14
The Upper Extremity and the Neck

Henry Haimovici

EXPOSURE OF SUBCLAVIAN ARTERY

Anatomic Review

The anatomic structures surrounding the subclavian artery are the supraclavicular region and the suprasternal fossa.

The *supraclavicular region* is a depressible space above the clavicle. Its base rests on the dome of the pleura and is in broad communication with the sternomastoid, mediastinal, and axillary regions. The anterior wall of the supraclavicular region is composed of a fairly loose aponeurosis, which passes over and is adherent to the clavicle, from where it extends into the thoracic region as the pectoral fascia. The posterior wall is composed of groups of muscles that extend downward and outward from the cervical column. The scalenus medius and posterior muscles, although fused in their upper portions, form most of the anterior segment of the floor of the region and are attached to the first and second ribs. The subclavian artery and the trunks of the brachial plexus, as they emerge from the cleft between the anterior and middle scalene muscles, lie on the floor of the region. The anterior scalene muscle arises from the transverse processes to the third, fourth, fifth, and sixth cervical vertebrae and runs downward and laterally to insert on the scalene tubercle and ridge on the medial margin of the first rib. The subclavian vein lies between the anterior scalene muscle and the clavicle and grooves the upper portion of the first rib. Behind this muscle lie the subclavian artery and the large nerve trunks of the brachial plexus.

The *right subclavian artery* is a subdivision of the innominate, whereas the *left subclavian artery* arises directly from the arch of the aorta. The right artery begins at the point deep to the sternoclavicular joint. The left, the longer of the two, arises within the thorax on the left side of the trachea. Both arteries run lateralward in an arching course across the root of the neck, grooving the pleural dome. Each artery is conveniently divided into three segments: medial, posterior, and lateral to the anterior scalene muscle. Unlike the neighboring common carotid, the subclavian artery gives off a considerable number of widely distributed branches.

The *subclavian vein* is a direct continuation of the axillary, or main, vein of the upper extremity.

The individual nerves that make up the *brachial plexus* derive from the anterior roots or primary divisions of the fifth, sixth, seventh, and eighth cervical and first thoracic spinal nerves. These roots emerge between the anterior and middle scalene muscles and appear in the lower part of the posterior triangle of the neck.

The *skeletal* structures in this region are the clavicle and the first rib. The sternal extremity of the clavicle has posterior relations with the innominate vein. On the right, it is related to the bifurcation of the innominate artery and, on the left, to the common carotid artery.

The body of the first rib is placed so that its superior surface is almost flat. In its middle portion, it presents two transverse grooves, one for the artery and the other for the vein.

Exposure of Cervical Segment of Subclavian Artery

The cervical portion of the subclavian artery is situated deeply in the supraclavicular region and is in direct contact with the first rib. Because of the different origins of the subclavian on the right and left, a description of the exposure will deal separately with each side.

Exposure of Left Subclavian Artery

The left cervical segment of the subclavian artery (Fig. 14-1) is somewhat deeper than on the right. In this region, the thoracic duct empties into the left innominate vein at the angle of the union of the left internal jugular and subclavian veins.

The patient is placed in the supine position, with the shoulders elevated in the usual fashion and the head turned to the opposite side. The upper extremity is in adduction close to the body.

The skin incision is made 1 cm above the clavicle and extends from the sternoclavicular joint to the lateral portion of the supraclavicular region for about 8 to 10 cm (Fig. 14-1A). The cutaneous incision extends through the subcu-

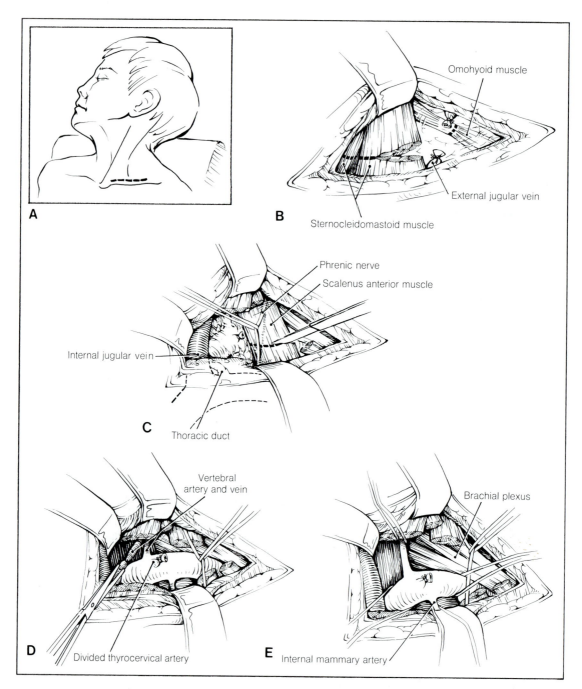

Figure 14-1. Exposure of the left subclavian artery. **A.** Position of the head and the line of skin incision. **B.** Lines of incision of sternocleidomastoid and omohyoid muscles and divided external jugular vein. **C.** Dissection of the second deep layer, showing the line of anterior scalene muscle transection and protection of the phrenic nerve. Note, in front, the thoracic duct at the subclavian-jugular angle and, in the background behind the scalene muscle, the subclavian artery. **D.** Subclavian artery freed, with the phrenic nerve retracted laterally. **E.** Further cephalad retraction of divided muscles, allowing better exposure and mobilization of the subclavian artery.

taneous tissue, the platysma, and the superficial cervical fascia. Laterally, the external jugular vein is exposed, divided, and ligated. Medially, the posterior border of the sternocleidomastoid muscle is exposed, and the clavicular head is divided about 1 cm above its insertion on the clavicle (Fig. 14-1B). If medial extension is necessary, the sternal head may be divided subsequently during the procedure.

The middle cervical fascia behind the sternocleidomastoid is divided, and the anterior scalene muscle is exposed behind the latter muscle. The adipose mass in front of the anterior scalene is identified. The subclavian vein that crosses in front of this muscle should be carefully mobilized, since the thoracic duct enters the junction between the internal jugular and the subclavian at that level. To expose the retroscalene portion of the subclavian artery, the muscle is divided after the subclavian and internal jugular are gently retracted downward and medially. As the muscle is transected, its proximal portion retracts spontaneously. The phrenic nerve, which crosses the scalene muscle from above downward and from lateral to medial side, must be identified before section of the muscle and preserved (Fig. 14-1C). A rubber vessel loop is passed around it and retracted upward and laterally. The subclavian artery is then exposed in its third portion. Should the medial portion of the subclavian have to be mobilized for the purpose of exposing the vertebral artery, division of the sternal head of the sternocleidomastoid muscle would have to be done by transection at the same level as the clavicular head. To achieve this,

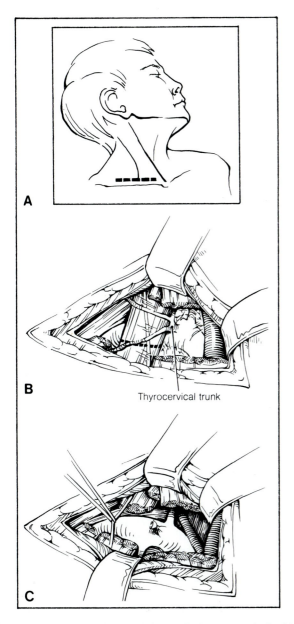

Figure 14-2. Exposure of the right subclavian artery. **A.** Position of the head and the line of skin incision. **B.** Note the thyrocervical trunk emerging from the subclavian artery medially to the scalene muscle and coursing anterior to the latter. **C.** Exposure of the subclavian artery, similar to Figure 14-1E.

the dissection of the branches of the subclavian at this level is mandatory (Fig. 14-1D). The posterior scapular, the thyrocervical, and the internal mammary arteries must be identified and mobilized and tapes placed about them (Fig. 14-1E).

If further exposure is hampered by the adjacent structures, resection of the clavicle may be necessary (see below).

Exposure of Right Subclavian Artery

The prescalene segment of the right subclavian is short, the bifurcation of the brachiocephalic being behind the sternoclavicular joint. Exposure of the right subclavian artery can be achieved almost completely in most instances through the cervical approach. If a wide exposure of the initial segment of the right subclavian is necessary, a thoracocervical exposure is indicated (see Chapter 16).

Figure 14-2A depicts the position of the patient and the skin incision above the clavicle. Figure 14-2B shows the exposure of the subclavian before the anterior scalene muscle has been divided. Figure 14-2C shows the retraction of the internal jugular medially and the phrenic nerve laterally. The vertebral and the internal mammary arteries are seen in the prescalene portion of the subclavian.

Variant Techniques of Subclavian Exposure

Exposure of the intrathoracic portion of the left subclavian artery and of the left common carotid is best approached through a *left-sided thoracotomy* in the third or fourth intercostal space.

For lesions of the innominate, of the first portion of the right subclavian, and of the intrathoracic portion of the common carotid arteries, surgery is best carried out by a longitudinal sternotomy through the anterior mediastinum. This approach allows a less traumatic dissection and a smoother postoperative convalescence than does partial median sternotomy with extension of the incision into the third intercostal space. (See Chapter 16 for more detail.)

Exposure of Subclavian Artery with Resection of the Clavicle

The approach to the subclavian artery may be greatly facilitated by the resection of a portion of the clavicle, especially if a combined subclavian and axillary exposure is indicated.

The incision is made over the portion of the clavicle to be excised and is then extended into the axillary region, as indicated in Figure 14-3. After the skin incision and its retraction, the periosteum of the medial two thirds of the clavicle is incised and stripped. The portion of the clavicle to be excised is divided with a Gigli saw and removed subperiosteally. The transverse scapular vessels run close to its posterior surface and may be easily injured if the layer of periosteum is torn. The sternal end of the incision allows exposure of the innominate and carotid vessels. Its central portion allows exposure of the subclavian vessels and brachial plexus. The scalene anterior muscle is transected, thereby facilitating the exposure of the subclavian artery as well as that of the origin of the vertebral and thyrocervical trunk. If the axillary vessels are to be exposed, the incision is extended into the axillary region (see below).

As is well known, excision of a portion of the clavicle does not interfere with motion of the shoulder and produces

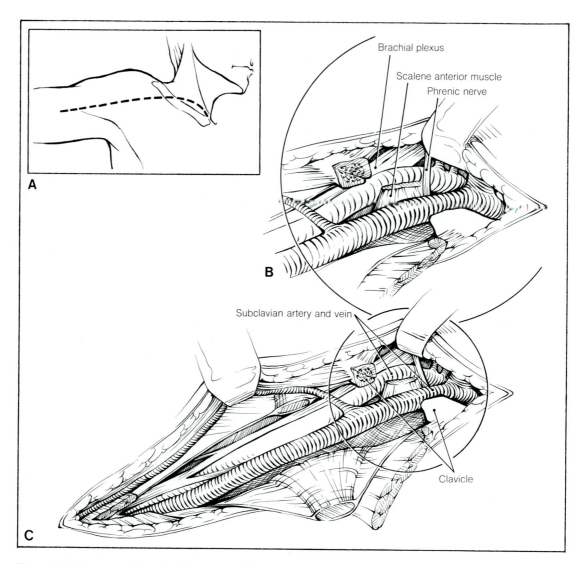

Figure 14-3. Exposure of the subclavian artery with resection of the clavicle. **A.** Line of skin incision for the subclavian-axillary approach. **B.** Exposure of the subclavian and proximal axillary vessels after resection of the clavicle. **C.** Exposure of the subclavian artery and of the entire length of the axillary vessels after transection of pectoralis major and minor vessels.

no noticeable deformity. Replacement of the resected segment is, therefore, not necessary. (See Chapter 60 for more detail.)

EXPOSURE OF AXILLARY ARTERY

Anatomic Review

The axillary region is the space situated between the upper lateral aspect of the chest wall and the proximal part of the upper limb. The apex of the pyramid-shaped region transmits the large vessels and nerves from the root of the neck to the upper extremity.

The anterior wall consists of two main layers. The pectoralis major muscle with its enveloping fascia forms the outer layer, and the pectoralis minor muscle with the costocora-

coid membrane of the clavipectoral fascia forms the deeper layer. The pectoral fascia attaches above to the clavicle and medially to the sternum. It closes the superficial deltopectoral triangle laterally and is continuous below with a fascial covering of the serratus anterior and external oblique muscles. The medial or costal wall of the space corresponds to the five upper ribs and their intervening spaces.

The lateral wall of the space, to which the important axillary vessels and nerves are related, is formed by the coracobrachialis and biceps muscles, the proximal part of the shaft of the humerus, and the medial aspect of the shoulder joint.

The axillary artery is the direct continuation of the subclavian artery. It extends from the outer margin of the first rib to the lower border of the teres major muscle, beyond which it is known as the brachial artery. Throughout its course, it is accompanied closely by the axillary vein and has intimate, although changing, relations with the nerves of the brachial plexus. The artery is divided into three segments corresponding to the part of the vessel situated proximal, behind, and inferior to the pectoralis minor muscle.

The axillary vein is formed from the union of the basilic and the two brachial veins. Its principal affluent is the cephalic vein, which enters a short distance below the clavicle through the crease between the pectoralis major and deltoid muscles.

The various nerves of the brachial plexus surround the third segment of the axillary artery. The median nerve is recognized by its great size and its two heads of origin. The ulnar nerve may be difficult to distinguish from the medial cutaneous nerve of the forearm, since both arise from the median cord and are overlaid by the axillary vein at their origin. The ulnar nerve is the larger and more posterior. The radial nerve is the direct continuation of the posterior cord and differs from the ulnar nerve in its posterior position and greater size. Axillary lymph nodes are embedded in the areolar adipose tissue occupying the axillary space.

Technique of Exposure of Axillary Artery

The approach for the exposure of the axillary artery can be through the anterior wall or through the base of the axillary space.

Anterior Exposure
The anterior approach to the axillary artery allows one to expose the artery either at its origin or in its entirety from the apex to the base of the axillary space.

Subclavicular Horizontal Approach
The skin incision, 8 to 10 cm long, is parallel to the inferior border of the clavicle, corresponding to its middle portion (Fig. 14-4).

The pectoralis major muscle is transected progressively until the clavipectoral axillary fascia is exposed. Incision of its anterior sheath and of the subclavius muscle is done along its entire length.

Retraction of the subclavius muscle proximally allows incision of the posterior sheath of the clavipectoral axillary fascia. At this point, the nerve of the pectoralis major crossing the anterior surface of the artery must be identified.

This approach affords the exposure and mobilization of only the initial segment of the axillary artery above the origin of its collateral branches. The exposure is most suitable for ligation of the vessel in the event of its injury but is less suitable if arterial reconstructive surgery is to be carried out at this level.

Deltopectoral Approach
The patient is placed in the supine position, with the upper extremity in slight abduction and external rotation.

The technique of this exposure (Fig. 14-5) is based on the simple anatomic landmarks indicated by the deltopectoral groove extending from the middle of the clavicle down to the junction of the pectoralis major and deltoid, at its lowest segment.

The skin incision extends from the clavicle down to the distal edge of the pectoralis major along the deltopectoral groove. In the upper part of the groove, the cephalic vein is present and must be dissected out and preserved. The pectoralis major is retracted medially, which allows exposure of the pectoralis minor and its pectoral axillary fascia.

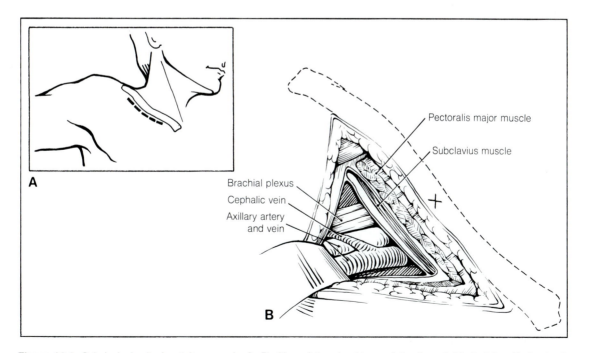

Figure 14-4. Subclavicular horizontal approach. **A.** Position of the shoulder and the line of skin incision. **B.** Anatomic structures to be divided for exposing the proximal segment of the axillary artery and the adjacent vein and brachial plexus.

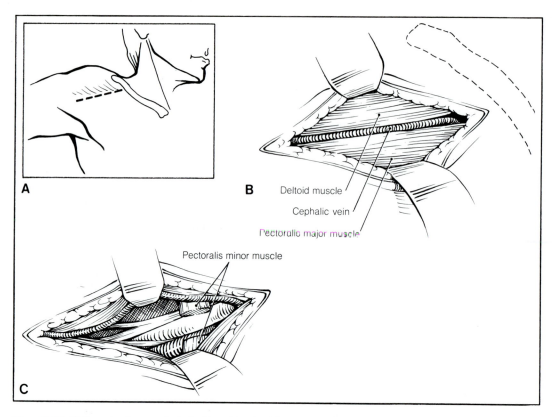

Figure 14-5. Deltopectoral approach. **A.** Position of the shoulder and the line of skin incision. **B.** Exposure of the deltopectoral groove and cephalic vein. **C.** Retraction of the deltoid and pectoralis major muscles, transection of the pectoralis minor, and exposure of axillary vessels and the brachial plexus.

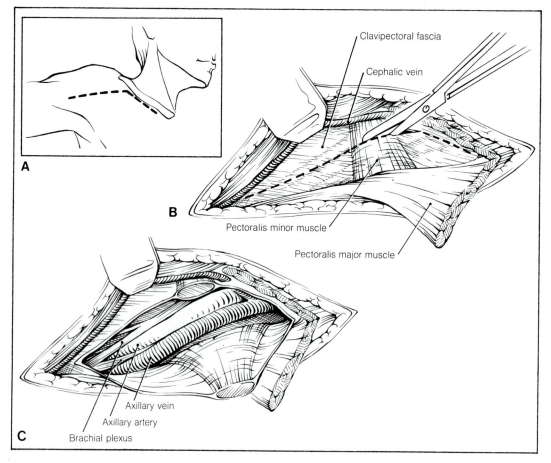

Figure 14-6. Combined deltopectoral-subclavicular approach. **A.** Position of the shoulder and the line of skin incision. **B.** After division of the clavicular portion of the pectoralis major, the tendon of the pectoralis minor is transected. **C.** The clavipectoral fascia is opened, thus exposing the neurovascular structures.

The latter is incised vertically close to the coracobrachial inner edge on the coracoid process. At this point, the tendon of the pectoralis minor is transected and retracted medially. The neurovascular bundle appears in view and is surrounded by cellular adipose tissue. The artery is the central structure with its collateral branches. The vein, somewhat larger, is medial to the artery. The brachial plexus is divided in its terminal branches at this level.

This approach allows exposure of all the neurovascular structures of the axillary region. However, retraction of the muscles is somewhat limited, making it difficult to obtain an adequate exposure. Should it be necessary because of extensive vascular lesions, the deltopectoral approach can be extended, as indicated in Figure 14-6.

Combined Approach: Deltopectoral-Subclavicular

This approach is a combined procedure of the two previously described techniques. It can be carried out either as a secondary enlargement of the previous procedure, or it can be done deliberately as a primary exposure, as indicated in Figure 14-6. The skin incision, as indicated in Figure 14-6A, is both subclavicular and deltopectoral, using a hockey-stick incision. After the pectoralis major has been transected below the clavicle, the rest of the exposure is similar to the one in the deltopectoral approach.

Transpectoral Approach

The transpectoral approach (Fig. 14-7) is used for limited access to the vessels for the purpose of exposure of the axillary artery and vein.

The patient is placed in the supine position, with the shoulder slightly elevated and the upper extremity in a horizontal position at a 90-degree angle with the body.

The skin incision extends from the middle of the clavicle to the anterior axillary line in the direction of its apex. The pectoralis major is divided along its fibers near its inser-

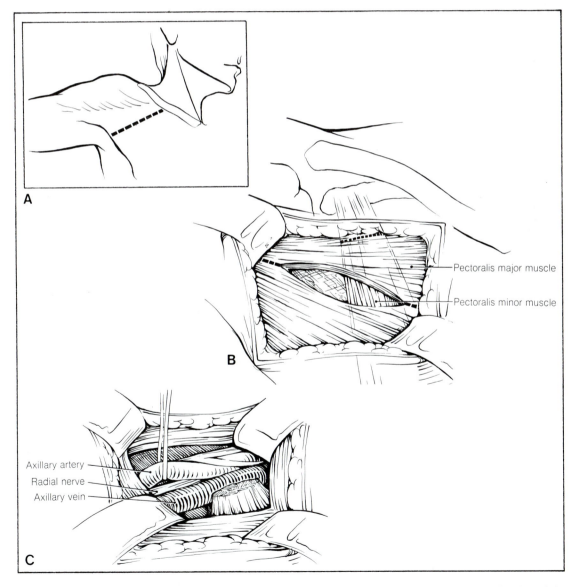

Figure 14-7. Transpectoral approach. **A.** Line of skin incision medial to the deltopectoral groove. **B.** Division of the pectoralis major along its fibers and the line of transection of the pectoralis minor. **C.** Exposure of the axillary neurovascular structures.

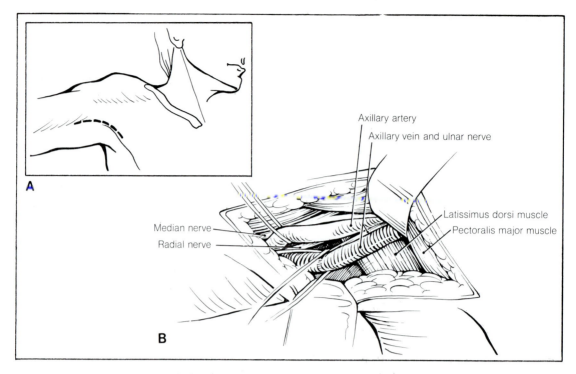

Figure 14-8. Subpectoral-axillary approach. **A.** Line of skin incision just at the distal edge of the pectoralis major. **B.** Exposure of axillary-brachial vessels and their relations with the adjacent structures.

tion on the humerus. The vessels are exposed after the pectoralis minor is divided near its insertion on the coracoid process.

Subpectoral-Axillary Approach

This exposure (Fig. 14-8) leads to the distal axillary artery and affords an easy extension toward the brachial artery without having to divide the pectoralis major.

The patient is placed in the supine position, with the shoulder slightly elevated and the arm in abduction at 90 degrees with the body. The skin incision follows the inferior border of the pectoralis major and is 8 to 10 cm in length. The pectoralis major is then retracted upward and medially. The sheath of the coracobiceps is opened at its medial border, and the muscle is retracted laterally. The median nerve is then encountered. It is mobilized and placed under the protection of a rubber or umbilical tape. The artery is then exposed. It is surrounded by collateral veins coursing its surface from the satellite veins, and other structures of the brachial plexus are situated posteriorly and laterally.

This exposure is fairly simple—requiring little dissection, being rather atraumatic, and having few disadvantages. Its main indication, however, is as an approach for proximal control of the brachial artery and less as a routine exposure of the axillary vessels. The incision usually results in an invisible scar, although it may be troublesome if a keloid develops.

EXPOSURE OF BRACHIAL ARTERY

Anatomic Review

The brachial is the main artery of the arm and is part of the neurovascular bundle situated on the medial aspect of the bicipital sulcus. The latter begins in front of the posterior axillary fold and descends along the inner aspect of the arm as far as the lower third, where it inclines obliquely forward, terminating at the center of the bend of the elbow. It separates the coracobrachialis and biceps muscles in front from the triceps muscle behind. The sulcus indicates the course of the basilic vein toward the brachial vein and is the superficial guide to the brachial vessels and the median nerve.

The deep fascia of the arm furnishes its complete investment and is continuous with the deep fascia of the forearm. From the deep surface of this ensheathing layer are derived the lateral and the medial intermuscular septa, dividing the arm into anterior and posterior osseoaponeurotic compartments (Fig. 14-9). The medial intermuscular septum extends from the epicondyle to the insertion of the coracobrachialis muscle. The neurovascular bundle is situated in this compartment.

The brachial artery, a continuation of the axillary, extends from the lower border of the teres major muscle to the antecubital fossa, just distal to the skin crease at the bend of the elbow. The artery is divided into three segments. The proximal third is beneath the deep fascia, bounded laterally by the coracobrachialis muscle and partly separated from it by the median nerve, the medial (internal) cutaneous nerve of the forearm, and the ulnar nerve separated from the basilic vein. The middle third inclines gradually forward and outward and is overlapped by the medial border of the biceps muscle. It is overlaid by the median nerve, which crosses it obliquely. The distal third is overlapped by the medial border of the biceps muscle, but near its termination it lies medial to its tendon, overlaid by the bicipital fascia. Medial to it lies the median nerve.

The brachial artery is accompanied by two satellite veins

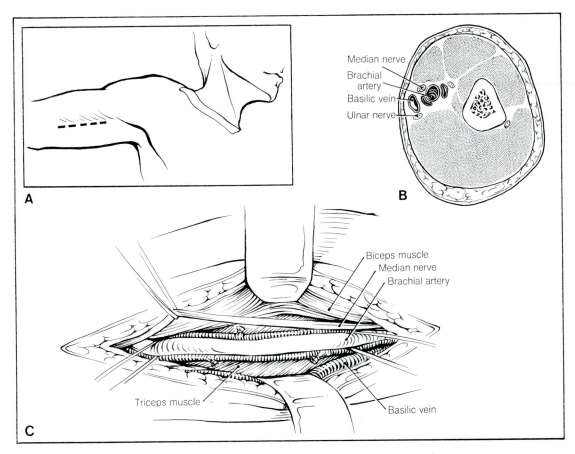

Figure 14-9. Exposure of the proximal brachial artery. **A.** Position of the arm and the line of skin incision along the bicipital groove. **B.** Cross-section of the arm, upper third. **C.** Exposure of the neurovascular structures in the groove formed by the biceps and triceps muscles.

that receive the basilic vein at their upper segment. The latter vein is extrafascial in the lower half of the arm but becomes subfascial in its upper segment.

Exposure of Upper Half of Brachial Artery

The patient is placed in the supine position, with the upper extremity in abduction and slight external rotation. A medial longitudinal incision is made along the bicipital groove (Fig. 14-9A). The incision follows the medial border of the biceps along its groove, which separates the biceps anteriorly from the triceps posteriorly. A 6 to 8 cm long incision is adequate for exposure of the artery. If necessary, proximal or distal extension of the incision can be easily achieved.

The skin incision should be made anterior to the basilic vein. The incision is carried down to the fascia of the biceps after identifying its medial border. The muscle is then retracted laterally, and with the elbow slightly flexed, the neurovascular bundle appears under a thin aponeurotic sheath, which is then opened.

The median nerve is exposed, mobilized, and placed under slight traction on a rubber strip and is retracted laterally, thus exposing the artery (Fig. 14-9C). Sometimes the brachial artery bifurcates quite high, in which case two arteries are found at this level. The cubital nerve is separated from the artery by the intermuscular septum. At this level,

the artery is surrounded by two satellite veins and their communicating branches. The basilic enters into one of the brachial veins at its proximal end.

Exposure of Distal Brachial Artery and Its Bifurcation

The arm is positioned in abduction at 90 degrees, with the forearm in extension and in supination. The antecubital fossa is delineated by flexing the elbow joint and by identifying the medial border of the bicipital tendon.

A longitudinal incision of the skin should be avoided because of possible keloid scarring and subsequent retraction of the skin. Instead, an S-shaped or Z-shaped incision is recommended, as indicated in Figure 14-10A. The subcutaneous incision should preserve the veins and, as much as possible, the nerve fibers. The basilic vein should be avoided and retracted posteriorly, but it may sometimes be necessary to ligate it at its extrafascial level.

The aponeurotic extension of the biceps (bicipital aponeurosis) is then divided, thereby exposing the brachial artery and its two branches, the radial and ulnar arteries (Fig. 14-10C). Like the proximal segment, the artery is surrounded by two satellite veins, with a plexus of communicating branches surrounding it anteriorly. The median nerve is located medial to the vascular bundle and should be retracted medially under the protection of a rubber band.

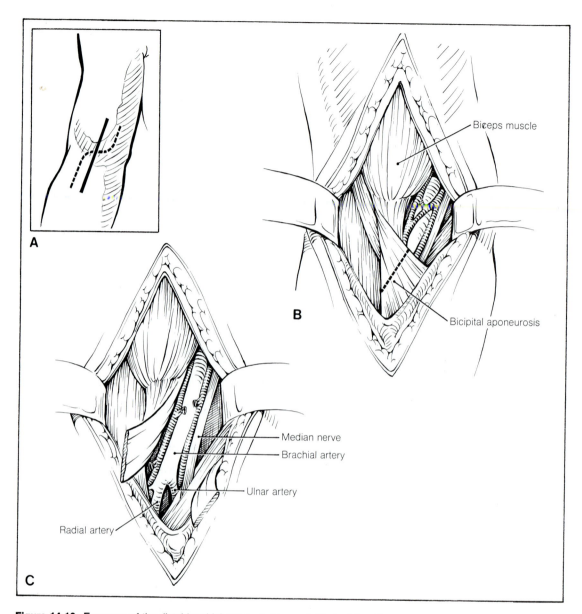

Figure 14-10. Exposure of the distal brachial artery. **A.** Lines of skin incision; S-shaped incision is preferable to straight incision. **B.** Exposure of the biceps muscle and the bicipital aponeurosis. **C.** After section of the bicipital aponeurosis, exposure of the distal brachial artery and its bifurcation is easily achieved.

The radial and ulnar divisions of the brachial artery are found at the distal angle of the exposure, with the radial being along the axis of the brachial and the ulnar plunging deeply under the median nerve and under the pronator muscle.

Extension proximally or distally of this exposure can be easily achieved, depending on the necessities of the surgical procedure.

EXPOSURE OF RADIAL AND ULNAR ARTERIES

Anatomic Review

The forearm, containing the radial and ulnar arteries, extends three fingerbreadths below the level of the elbow to the bend of the wrist. In terms of arterial exposures, the forearm is placed in the supine position, with the palm of the hand facing forward.

The deep antebrachial fascia invests the forearm completely and is continuous with a deep fascia of the arm and hand. The deep fascia is reinforced anteriorly by the bicipital fascia, which is an extension from the biceps tendon. At the wrist, the deep fascia is continuous with the transverse, carpal, or annular ligaments. From its deep surface, the fascia furnishes attachment to several muscles and sends intermuscular septa to the radius and ulna.

The radial artery runs a fairly straight course through the forearm. In its upper two thirds, it lies under cover of the brachioradialis muscle and crosses the supinator muscle. In the distal third, the artery is subcutaneous and lies on the radius and on the flexor pollicis longus muscle.

The ulnar artery is the larger of the two terminal trunks of the brachial artery. From its origin, it descends through the anterior surface of the forearm and crosses the transverse carpal ligament on the radial side of the pisiform bone. In the lower two thirds of the forearm, the course of the artery is straight and is indicated by a line drawn from the front of the medial epicondyle to the radial surface of the pisiform bone with the forearm in full supination. The artery lies on the flexor digitorum profundus muscle between the flexor carpi ulnaris muscle medially and the flexor digitorum sublimis muscle laterally. It gradually becomes superficial toward the wrist. In the upper third of the forearm, the vessel is placed deeply between the superficial and deep layers of the anterointernal musculature.

The nerves of the forearm are the median, the ulnar, and the radial with its superficial and deep branches.

Each artery is accompanied by two satellite veins, which send communicating branches across the artery, as in the vessels previously described.

Exposure of Radial Artery

The radial artery may be exposed in its upper or lower third. The line of skin incision (Fig. 14-11A) is an extension of the antecubital one for the lower third of the brachial artery along the edges and the groove of the pronator teres muscle and the brachioradialis muscle (Fig. 14-11B). After incision of the deep fascia, these two muscles are retracted. A thin fascial layer is then incised over the vascular bundle, and the artery is identified and separated from the adjacent two satellite veins.

The lower third of the radial artery is more superficial, although subfascial, and is situated laterally to the flexor carpi radialis tendon (Fig. 14-11C).

Exposure of Ulnar Artery

As is true for the radial artery, exposure of the ulnar artery (Fig. 14-12) can be carried out proximally or distally. The

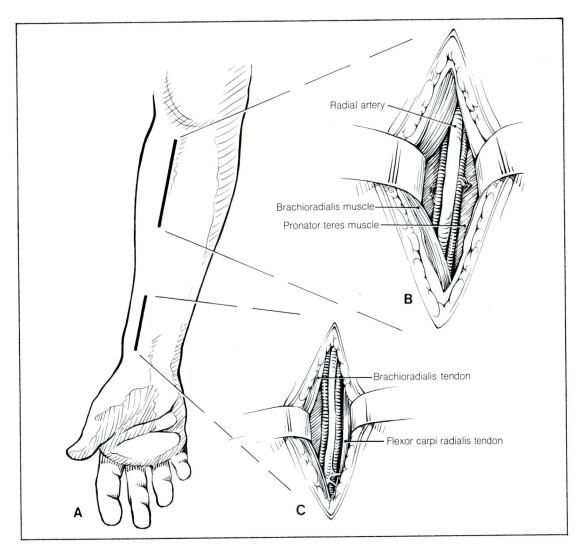

Figure 14-11. Exposure of the radial artery. **A.** Lines of skin incision for exposure of the radial artery. **B.** Proximal exposure. **C.** Distal exposure.

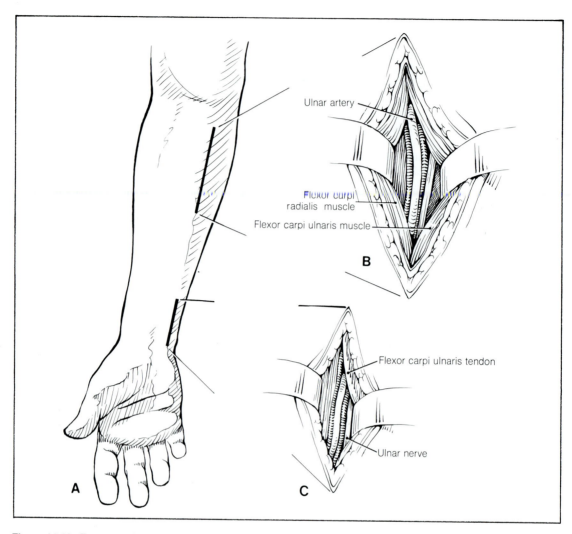

Figure 14-12. Exposure of the ulnar artery. **A.** Lines of skin incision for exposure of the ulnar artery. **B.** Proximal exposure. **C.** Distal exposure.

patient is placed in the supine position, with the arm in abduction and slight external rotation. The forearm is in supination, with slight flexion for relaxing the flexor muscles and with the hand in hyperextension and abduction.

The anteromedial approach to the ulnar artery offers good access to this vessel on the line that extends from the epicondyles to the lateral border of the pisiform bone.

The proximal third exposure is carried out through an 8 to 10 cm skin incision that begins three to four fingerbreadths below the epicondyle. After incision of the deep fascia, the flexor carpi ulnaris muscle is exposed. The ulnar nerve is medial to the vessels, and the artery is surrounded by two satellite veins.

In the lower third of the forearm the ulnar artery is more superficial. The approach to it is carried out by the same incision about 4 to 5 cm distal to the previous one. After incision of the fascia and the retraction of the tendons of the flexor carpi ulnaris and of the flexor carpi radialis, the exposure of the vessel and the ulnar nerve is achieved (Fig. 14-12).

The radial artery, the interosseous branch, and espe-

cially the ulnar artery above the wrist are often used for shunts in dialysis.

EXPOSURE OF CAROTID ARTERY

Anatomic Review

The carotid artery is located in the lateral region of the neck, bounded by the broad sternocleidomastoid muscle laterally, by the mastoid process above, and by the clavicle and upper sternum below.

The major landmark that stands out in bold relief is the sternocleidomastoid muscle, which courses from the mastoid process to the medial end of the clavicle. Anterior to the muscle is the vascular groove, which separates the muscle from the anterior neck region.

The superficial structures, running into a duplication of the superficial cervical fascia, are the external jugular vein and a few superficial branches of the cervical plexus. These structures are covered by the platysma muscle.

The sternocleidomastoid muscle is held securely in place by duplication of the enveloping fascia of the neck. Its sternal and clavicular heads are separated by a triangular interval. The outer covering of the deep fascia is thick and fibrous above. The deep fascial covering separating the muscle from the subadjacent structures is thin.

When the sternocleidomastoid muscle is retracted laterally, the internal jugular vein can be distinguished in the upper half or two thirds of the exposed area. The lymph nodes disposed between the muscle and the vein adhere more or less intimately to both structures. Adhesions caused by pathologic changes above the glands may be so dense as to require removal of the sternocleidomastoid muscle and internal jugular vein during lymph gland dissection.

The carotid sheath is the tubular investment of the deep cervical fascia, which encloses the common and internal carotid arteries, internal jugular vein, and the vagus nerve. Above the common carotid artery, the structure of the sheath is somewhat attenuated. Its posterior wall is adherent to the prevertebral fascia. The anterior wall fuses with and, to some extent, is derived from the pretracheal fascia. It is tenuous over the internal jugular vein but is thick and dense over the common carotid artery.

The latter arises from the innominate trunk on the right and from the arch of the aorta on the left. It emerges from behind the sternoclavicular joint and ascends obliquely in the direction of the angle of the mandible. At the superior margin of the thyroid cartilage, the artery, after forming the carotid bulb, divides into its two terminal branches, the internal and external carotid arteries. The internal carotid continues in the direction of the common trunk.

The common carotid artery has posterior relations with the sympathetic ganglia and its chain, the prevertebral fascia, underlying prevertebral muscles and the anterior surface of the transverse processes. Anteriorly, the common carotid is in relation with the areolar tissue of the neck in the upper two thirds of its course and with the pretracheal fascia in the lower third.

The internal carotid artery that begins at the level of the superior margin of the thyroid cartilage is situated a little posterolateral to the external carotid, but, as it ascends, it passes to its medial side toward the lateral wall of the pharynx. The external carotid artery is directed upward and backward to the angle of the jaw. Its branches supply the upper neck and extracranial soft parts of the head.

The internal jugular vein is the principal venous trunk of the neck and is the direct downward continuation of the transverse lateral sinus. The vessel is rarely seen surgically in its upper portion, which lies deep to the styloid process and the parotid compartment. It descends in the carotid sheath and may be recognized easily by its bluish gray color. It runs to a point a little lateral to the sternoclavicular joint, where it unites with the subclavian vein to form the innominate vein.

The common facial vein is the most important contributing branch of the internal jugular. The trunk is formed at about the level of the submaxillary gland by the union of the anterior and posterior facial veins. It passes backward and downward to pierce the carotid sheath and enter the internal jugular vein opposite the great horn of the hyoid bone. It receives the thyroid and lingual veins and might be termed the thyrolingual-facial trunk.

The vagus nerve lies between the internal jugular vein and common carotid artery and passes through the neck to its terminations in the thorax and abdomen.

The hypoglossal or motor nerve to the tongue is an occupant of this region only in its proximal portion, where it lies deep to the parotid gland and descends between the internal carotid artery and the internal jugular vein.

Technique of Carotid Exposure

Position
The patient is placed in the supine position, with the head turned slightly away from the side to be operated on. The head is in slight hyperextension to expose the carotid groove. An inflatable pillow is placed under the shoulders. Marked hyperextension of the head and neck should be avoided if there is associated basilar arterial insufficiency (Fig. 14-13).

Skin Incision
The classic line of incision extends from the tip of the mastoid and is directed obliquely to the sternoclavicular joint. The skin incision for the exposure of the common carotid artery and its bifurcation is made only in the upper half of this line (Fig. 14-13A).

The incision is carried down through the subcutaneous tissue and the platysma. After the division of the external jugular vein, the sternocleidomastoid fascia is opened anteriorly and longitudinally, and the muscle is retracted laterally, thus exposing the neurovascular bundle.

Exposure of Carotid
The carotid sheath is opened near the bulb after having infiltrated the bifurcation with a local anesthetic (Fig. 14-13B).

The internal jugular vein is dissected carefully from the artery. The common facial vein is ligated and divided. The internal jugular vein is then retracted laterally. Similarly the ansa hypoglossi nerve is retracted laterally (Fig. 14-13C).

The common carotid artery is exposed and mobilized for about 2 to 3 cm below its bifurcation. The artery is carefully dissected from the vein and the vagus nerve. A tape is passed around the carotid below the bifurcation. The dissection is then continued distally to expose the hypoglossal nerve, which courses over the internal and external carotid arteries. As this is the motor nerve to the tongue, it should be dissected free, and its injury is to be avoided. The superior thyroid artery is freed and mobilized. Dissection is then carried to the internal and external carotid arteries.

Exposure of Carotid Artery at Its Origin on Aortic Arch
This exposure may require a sternotomy or a left thoracotomy. (For details, see Chapter 16.)

(See Bibliography at the end of Chapter 20.)

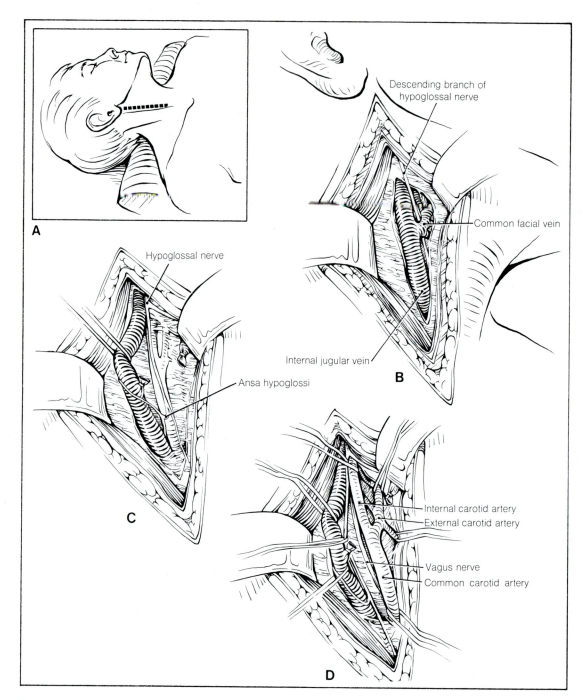

Figure 14-13. A. Exposure of carotid artery. Position of the head and shoulders and the line of skin incision in the neck. **B.** Lateral retraction of the sternocleidomastoid muscle, exposing the carotid sheath. Note the descending branch of the hypoglossal nerve entering the carotid sheath and its relation with the common facial vein and its tributaries. **C.** Lateral retraction of the internal jugular vein after division of the facial vein, thereby exposing the carotid artery and the ansa hypoglossi nerve. **D.** Further mobilization of the common, internal, and external carotid (see text for further details).

CHAPTER 15

Extrathoracic Exposure for Distal Revascularization of Brachiocephalic Branches

Henry Haimovici

HISTORICAL BACKGROUND

Surgical correction of the arterial lesions involving the branches of the aortic arch was originally carried out by direct transthoracic arterial reconstructions.[1] After introduction of extra-anatomic bypasses for the management of aortoiliac lesions, similar principles were applied for the brachiocephalic lesions. Thus extrathoracic approaches were devised for lesions in the proximal segments of the brachiocephalic arterial systems. The carotid-subclavian bypass was introduced as the first extrathoracic procedure.[2,3] Although it obviates a thoracotomy and is easier to perform, it is applicable only for subclavian lesions but not when the occlusion is in the innominate artery. In addition, although carotid-subclavian bypass had found a wide degree of acceptance, theoretical concerns of possible compromise of the carotid flow led to the search for alternative extrathoracic approaches. Subclavian-subclavian[4,5] and axillary-axillary[6–8] bypasses appeared to offer greater ease of anatomic exposure with no concern of interfering with the carotid circulation. These approaches have gained greater acceptance in management of this condition.

CLINICAL BACKGROUND

Subclavian steal syndrome was first noted in 1960 by Contorni, an Italian radiologist, who called attention to the occluded proximal subclavian artery as a cause of reversal flow from the vertebral artery into the subclavian.[9] Reivich et al., in 1961, demonstrated this reversal blood flow through the vertebral artery and described its effects on cerebral circulation.[10] An editorial in the *New England Journal of Medicine*, in the same issue as Reivich's paper, called attention to this new entity and called it "the subclavian steal syndrome."[11] Although North et al., in 1962, described the same syndrome under the name of "brachial-basilar insufficiency," the steal stigma attached to it prevailed.[12]

Stenosis or complete occlusion of the subclavian or innominate arteries is due in almost all instances to an atheromatous plaque. However, a congenital cause and an embolic occlusion have been reported in a few rare instances.[13–15] The left subclavian artery was involved in 72% of reported cases, whereas the right was found to be the cause in 16%, with the innominate the cause in 10 to 12%.[2,3] The lesion of the affected arteries is located proximal to the vertebral artery and is accompanied by vertebral-basilar transient ischemic attacks or ischemic manifestations of the upper extremity or both (Fig. 15-1).

The cerebral symptoms are usually characterized by headaches, dizziness, and blurring of vision, often occurring during all sorts of activities of the involved upper extremity. The upper extremity manifestations are those of intermittent claudication characterized by weakness, numbness, and paresthesias. Each of the two syndromes may occur alone or together, the cerebral symptoms being by far the more common.

CAROTID-SUBCLAVIAN BYPASS TECHNIQUE (FIG. 15-2)

The patient is placed in the supine position, with the shoulders being elevated in the usual fashion and the head rotated slightly to the opposite side. The upper extremity is kept in adduction, close to the body.

The cervical segment of the subclavian artery is somewhat deeper on the left than the right. In the left region, the thoracic duct empties into the left innominate vein at the angle of the union of the internal jugular and subclavian veins.

The skin incision is made 1 cm above the clavicle and extends from the sternoclavicular joint to the lateral portion of the supraclavicular region for about 8 to 10 cm (Fig. 15-2A). The cutaneous incision extends through the subcutaneous tissue, the platysma, and the superficial cervical fascia.

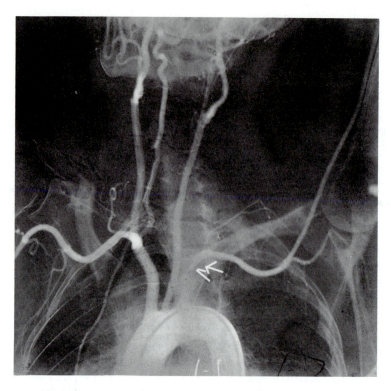

Figure 15-1. Transfemoral arch aortogram of a 50-year-old woman who developed ischemia of the left hand with no cerebral manifestations. The atherosclerotic stenosing plaque of the subclavian artery was located proximal to the origin of the vertebral artery. A 6 mm segment of Gore-Tex graft was used for the bypass.

Laterally, the external jugular vein is exposed, divided, and ligated.

Medially, the posterior border of the sternocleidomastoid muscle is exposed, and the clavicular head is divided about 1 cm above its insertion on the clavicle. If medial extension is necessary, the sternal head may be divided subsequently during the procedure.

The middle cervical fascia behind the sternocleidomastoid is divided, and the anterior scalene muscle is exposed behind the latter muscle. The adipose mass in front of the anterior scalene is identified. The subclavian vein that crosses in front of this muscle should be carefully mobilized, since the thoracic duct enters the junction between the internal jugular and the subclavian veins at that level. To expose the retroscalene portion of the subclavian artery, the muscle is divided after the subclavian and internal jugular veins are retracted gently downward and medially. As the muscle is transected, its proximal portion retracts spontaneously.

The phrenic nerve, which crosses the scalene muscle from above downward and from the lateral to the medial side, must be identified before section of the muscle so it can be preserved. A siliconized vessel loop is passed around it and retracted upward and laterally.

The subclavian artery is then exposed in its third portion. Because the medial portion of the subclavian has to be mobilized for the purpose of exposing the vertebral ar-

tery, the sternal head of the sternocleidomastoid muscle must be divided at the same level as the clavicular head. To achieve this, the dissection of the branches of the subclavian at this level is mandatory. The posterior scapular, the thyrocervical, and the internal mammary arteries must be identified and mobilized, and tapes placed around them.

Exposure of the carotid artery is then carried out. The carotid sheath is opened near and above the subclavian artery. The internal jugular vein is dissected carefully from the artery and is retracted laterally. Similarly, the vagus nerve is carefully handled and kept out of the area of carotid mobilization. The carotid artery is then isolated and surrounded with vessel loops. A segment of satisfactory length and caliber for the bypass is exposed.

At this point, temporary occlusion of the carotid artery is carried out. Two methods are available for handling the sharp hemodynamic alterations of the distal carotid artery after its clamping: (1) monitoring the electroencephalogram (EEG) changes and measuring the systolic, diastolic, and mean pressures distal to the occlusion—a mean pressure near 50 mm Hg or above is acceptable for maintaining adequate intracerebral function—and (2) use of an internal carotid shunt for continuous cerebral perfusion during graft implantation. This second method is, of course, mandatory if the EEG or the mean arterial pressure appears to be below a safe level.

The graft material used for the bypass may be a saphe-

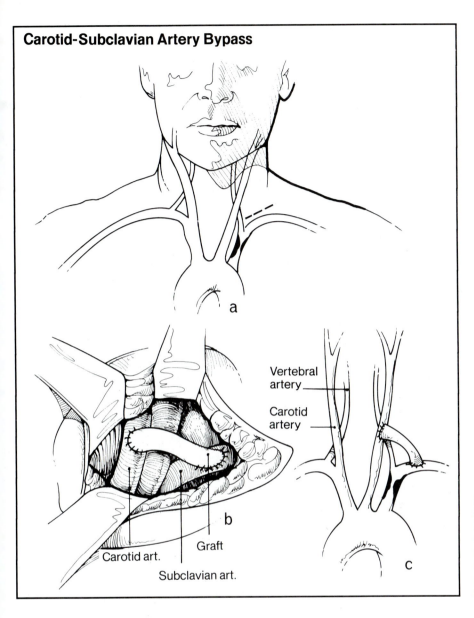

Carotid-Subclavian Artery Bypass

a

Vertebral artery

Carotid artery

b

Graft

Carotid art.

Subclavian art.

c

Figure 15-2. A left carotid to subclavian graft bypass. **A.** The arch with its brachiocephalic branches. **B.** Exposure of the subclavian and carotid areas (for details, see text). Note that the graft crosses the jugular vein anteriorly. **C.** Diagram indicating the position of the bypass graft in relation to the supraclavicular region.

nous vein or any commonly available synthetic graft; my preference is PTFE (Gore-Tex) graft.

The implantation of the graft is first carried out in the subclavian artery through an end-to-side anastomosis using 6-0 suture material. After completion of the end-to-side routine anastomosis in the subclavian, the graft is tunneled toward the carotid artery. The carotid graft anastomosis is similarly carried out by end-to-side anastomosis using the 6-0 suture material (Fig. 15-2C). Before completion of the anastomosis into the carotid, flushing of the carotid as well as of the subclavian is carried out to remove any possible thrombi that might have occurred during the procedure. Heparin is administered to the patient before and throughout the completion of the bypass (Fig. 15-3).

The wound is closed in layers in the usual fashion. The divided muscles are reattached except for the scalene.

Careful handling of the phrenic nerve is essential to avoid any paralysis of the diaphragm.

Correction of the subclavian lesion by carotid-subclavian bypass has raised the possibility of a theoretical risk of siphoning blood from the distal common carotid artery, which would then constitute a carotid steal induced by the procedure. Several investigators have shown that no carotid steal was detected during controlled experiments.[16]

AXILLARY-AXILLARY BYPASS GRAFT TECHNIQUE (FIG. 15-4)

The axillary artery is divided into three segments. The first extends from the outer border of the first rib to the medial border of the pectoralis minor muscle. This segment of

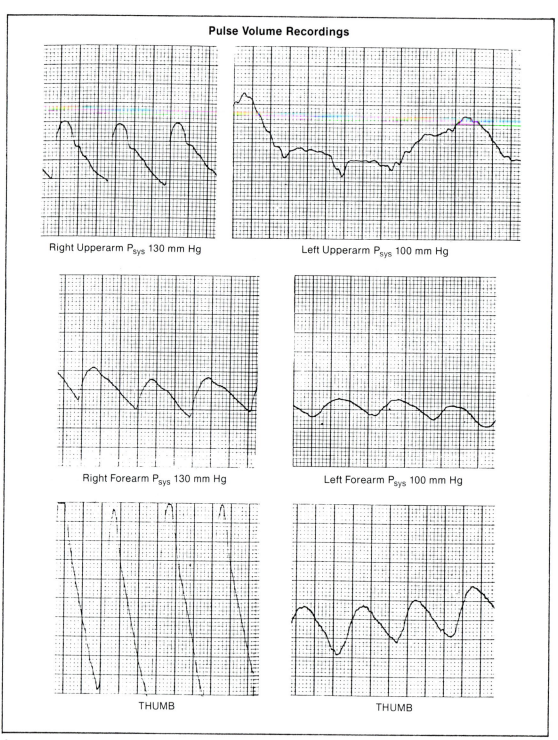

Right Upperarm P_{sys} 130 mm Hg

Left Upperarm P_{sys} 100 mm Hg

Right Forearm P_{sys} 130 mm Hg

Left Forearm P_{sys} 100 mm Hg

THUMB

THUMB

A

Figure 15-3. For legend see opposite page.

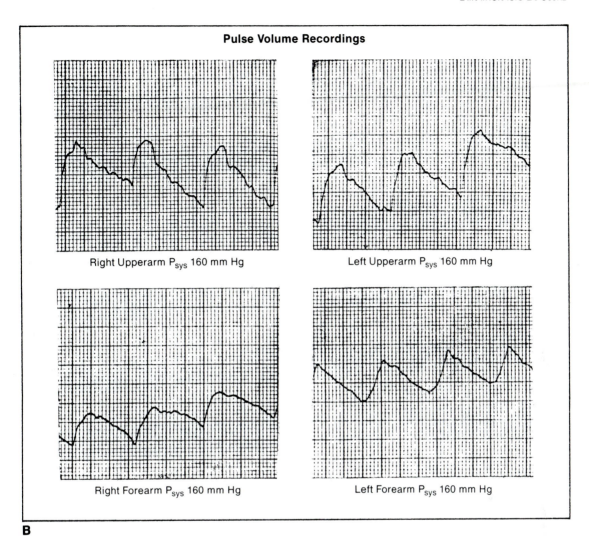

B

Figure 15-3. Pulse volume recording tracings taken before and after the bypass graft. **A.** Before the carotid-subclavian bypass. Note abnormal and decreased amplitude of pulse waves on the left side and lower systolic pressure at the arm and forearm. **B.** Postoperative recordings (day 7 after the bypass) indicate return to normal systolic pressure of upper arm and forearm with normal pulse waves.

the axillary artery is free of major branches and is the most desirable for the use of graft implantation. The second segment lies behind the pectoralis minor muscle and provides the thoracoacromial trunk and lateral thoracic branches. The third segment extends from the lateral border of the pectoralis minor to the lower border of the teres major.

A subclavicular horizontal approach is used for exposure of the first segment. A skin incision 8 to 10 cm long is made parallel to the inferior border of the clavicle corresponding to its middle portion (Fig. 15-4A).

The pectoralis major muscle is transected progressively until the clavipectoral axillary fascia is exposed. Incision of its anterior sheath and of the subclavius muscle is done along its entire length.

Retraction of the subclavius muscle proximally allows incision of the posterior sheath of the clavipectoral axillary fascia. At this point, the nerve of the pectoralis major crossing the anterior surface of the artery must be identified.

This approach affords exposure and mobilization of the initial segment of the axillary artery, which is above the origin of its main collateral branches. The axillary vein, which is also free of tributaries at this level, is retracted upward. The exposure is most suitable for the anastomosis of the axillary-axillary bypass, as well as for the axillo-femoral.

After exposure of both axillary arteries, a subcutaneous tunnel is developed between the two areas. The tunnel is anterior to the sternal region.

Implantation of the graft starts in the recipient site. After the axillary vein is mobilized by dividing several inferior tributaries, it is greatly elevated, revealing the underlying axillary artery. An autogenous saphenous vein or PTFE (Gore-Tex) graft 6 mm in diameter is sutured end-to-side into the recipient artery. The graft is then passed through the tunnel and across anteriorly to the sternum for the donor anastomosis, also carried out in an end-to-side fash-

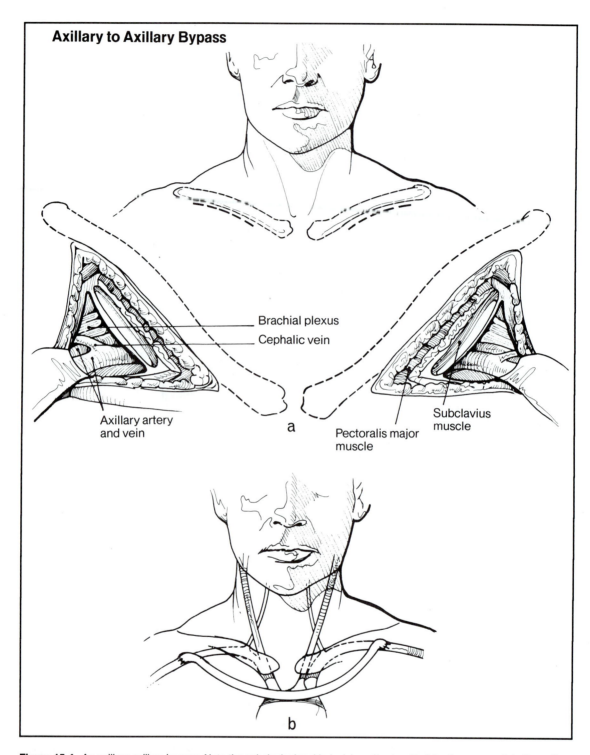

Axillary to Axillary Bypass

Brachial plexus
Cephalic vein

Axillary artery
and vein

a

Subclavius
muscle

Pectoralis major
muscle

b

Figure 15-4. An axillary-axillary bypass. Note the subclavicular skin incisions (*broken line*) for the approach to the axillary arteries. **A.** *Below*, bilateral exposure of the axillary regions. Note the major structures from lateral to medial: brachial plexus, axillary artery hidden by axillary vein and its cephalic tributary. **B.** Diagram of the bypass.

ion (Fig. 15-4C). Care is taken to flush the proximal ends of the recipient artery back through the graft to remove any clots or atheromatous debris that may have accumulated during the procedure. The patient, as mentioned already, is heparinized systemically during the entire period of clamping.

SUBCLAVIAN-SUBCLAVIAN BYPASS (FIG. 15-5)

The procedure is carried out through bilateral supraclavicular incisions. The operative exposure is achieved through a 3-inch incision, one fingerbreadth above the clavicle and extending posteriorly from the sternocleidomastoid muscle

Subclavian to Subclavian Bypass

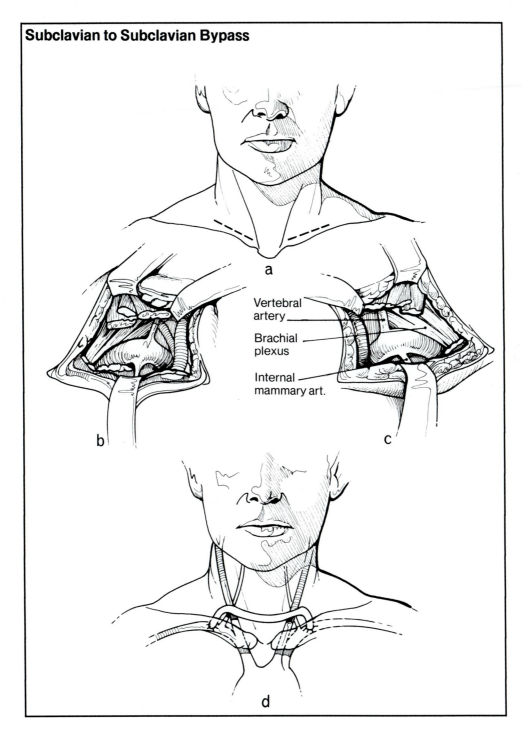

Figure 15-5. A subclavian to subclavian artery bypass. **A.** Note the supraclavicular skin incisions (*broken line*). **B** and **C.** Right and left exposures of the subclavian arteries in the supraclavicular region. Note the brachial plexus laterally, the vertebral and internal mammary branches, the divided muscles and jugular vein (medially). **D.** Diagram of the position of the subclavian-subclavian bypass.

(Fig. 15-5A). The external jugular vein is divided, the sterno-cleidomastoid muscle is retracted anteriorly, and the phrenic nerve is isolated. The scalenus anticus muscle is divided, allowing more complete inspection of the vessel and the thoracic outlet. After systemic heparinization is achieved, one subclavian artery is crossclamped, and a vein graft or PTFE (Gore-Tex) tube 6 mm in diameter is anastomosed to the vessels with a running fine 6-0 suture material. After the graft has been anastomosed to the recipient vessel, the graft is tunneled subcutaneously into the anterior tissues of the neck, and the donor anastomosis is carried out (Fig. 15-5C). The divided scalenus anticus muscle is not reapproximated. The graft pulsation is visible and palpable above the manubrium.

CONCLUSIONS

In recent years, the extrathoracic procedures have gained in popularity and, in most cases, have superseded the earlier direct approach of the intrathoracic procedure. Although the latter may still be indicated for innominate arterial lesions and may produce excellent hemodynamic results, thoracotomy is fraught with greater risk, especially in patients with mild or chronic chest disease or cardiovascular problems. Extrathoracic bypasses are technically much simpler and more expeditious than are the intrathoracic procedures. The type of bypass to be used in a given case will depend on the individual circumstances. Carotid-subclavian bypass may not be applicable on the right side if the innominate artery is involved. In addition, if there is stenosis or complete occlusion of one carotid, the carotid-subclavian bypass may be hazardous without first correcting the internal carotid lesion. Under those circumstances, any decrease in carotid blood flow may be totally undesirable. The axillary-axillary bypass is indicated in the majority of cases for revascularizing the upper extremity and correcting the vertebrobasilar insufficiency.[17] Variants of the axillary-axillary bypass have also been reported.[18-20]

Potential disadvantages of the superficial subcutaneous bypasses may be related to cosmetic and mechanical problems. Since the bypasses are at the base of the neck or just at the upper portion of the chest, they may not really interfere with the cosmetic appearance of these anatomic regions. On the other hand, mechanically they are less prone to compression than the axillofemoral or femorofemoral bypasses, which are proven to this date not to be subjected to much mechanical stress. The long-term results accumulated in the past 10 years are encouraging and have established these procedures as the most appropriate ones for the management of the occlusive process of the brachiocephalic branches.

REFERENCES

1. Crawford ES, DeBakey ME, et al.: Thrombo-obliterative disease of the great vessels arising from the aortic arch. J Thorac Cardiovasc Surg 43:38, 1962.
2. Diethrich EB, Garrett HE, et al.: Occlusive disease of the common carotid and subclavian arteries treated by carotid-subclavian bypass. Analysis of 125 cases. Am J Surg 114:800, 1967.
3. Hafner CD: Subclavian steal syndrome—a 12-year experience. Arch Surg 111:1074, 1976.
4. Finkelstein NM, Byer A, Rush BR: Subclavian-subclavian bypass for the subclavian steal syndrome. Surgery 71:142, 1972.
5. Forrestner JE, et al.: Subclavian-subclavian bypass for correction of the subclavian steal syndrome. Surgery 71:136, 1972.
6. Myers WO, Lawton BR, Sautter RD: Axillo-axillary bypass graft. JAMA 217:826, 1971.
7. Mozersky DJ, Sumner DS, et al.: Subclavian revascularization by means of a subcutaneous axillary-axillary graft. Arch Surg 106:20, 1973.
8. Jacobson JH, Mozersky DJ, et al.: Axillary-axillary bypass for the "subclavian steal" syndrome. Arch Surg 106:24, 1973.
9. Contorni L: Il circolo collaterale vertebrale nella obliterazione dell'arteria succlavia alla sue origine. Minerva Chir 15:268, 1960.
10. Reivich M, et al.: Reversal of blood flow through the vertebral artery and its effect on cerebral circulation. N Engl J Med 265:878, 1961.
11. A new vascular syndrome: The subclavian steal (editorial). N Engl J Med 265:912, 1961.
12. North RR, Fields WS, et al.: Brachial-basilar insufficiency syndrome. Neurology 12:810, 1962.
13. Massumi RA: The congenital variety of the "subclavian steal" syndrome. Circulation 28:1149, 1963.
14. Levine S, Serfas LS, Rusinko A: A right aortic arch with subclavian steal syndrome (atresia of left common carotid and left subclavian arteries). Am J Surg 111:632, 1966.
15. Dardik H, Gensler S, et al.: Subclavian steal syndrome secondary to embolism: First reported case. Ann Surg 164:171, 1966.
16. Lord RSA, Ehrenfeld WK: Carotid-subclavian bypass: A hemodynamic study. Surgery 66:521, 1969.
17. Mozersky DJ, Sumner DS, et al.: The hemodynamics of the axillary-axillary bypass. Surg Gynecol Obstet 135:925, 1972.
18. Sproul G: Femoral-axillary bypass for cerebral vascular insufficiency. Arch Surg 103:746, 1971.
19. Moseley HS, Porter JM: Femoral-axillary bypass for arm ischemia. Arch Surg 106:347, 1973.
20. Jacobson JH, Baron MG: Axillary-contralateral brachial artery bypass for arm ischemia. Ann Surg 179:827, 1974.

CHAPTER 16
Transthoracic Exposure of Great Vessels of Aortic Arch

Calvin B. Ernst

Adoption of extrathoracic arterial reconstructive procedures for treatment of symptomatic occlusive arterial disease of the vessels from the aortic arch evolved because of the perceived greater morbidity and mortality accompanying transthoracic arterial reconstruction.[1] Extrathoracic extraanatomic procedures such as carotid subclavian bypass, subclavian-subclavian bypass, and axillary-axillary bypass may be preferred, especially when thoracotomy or mediastinotomy and exposure of the origins of the innominate, subclavian, and common carotid vessels pose undue risk to the patient. However, exposure of the great vessels from the aortic arch may occasionally be required when managing proximal arteriosclerotic lesions when no brachiocephalic inflow source is adequate for extrathoracic reconstruction.

Although arterial reconstruction for severe arm ischemia may represent only 2% of all vascular surgical procedures,[2] revascularization by intrathoracic exposure of the arch vessels is by no means outdated and continues to be an important part of the armamentarium of the vascular surgeon. Transthoracic reconstructive procedures may be required for approximately 30% of patients with multiple great vessel involvement.[3] Knowledge and techniques of such exposure is mandatory when managing injuries to the great vessels. The great vessels arising from the aortic arch are relatively inaccessible, not only because they are obscured by bone but also because most surgeons have not had experience with, or need to expose them. Although arterial reconstruction for the various lesions encountered may require innovative bypass and endarterectomy technical maneuvers, the common denominator to successful outcome is adequate exposure of inflow and outflow vessels.

EXPOSURE OF LEFT SUBCLAVIAN ARTERY

The most common reason demanding exposure of the left subclavian artery is trauma. Aneurysmal and occlusive lesions are less frequent.

Various techniques for gaining exposure to the left subclavian artery have been provided during this century since Halsted[4] performed the first successful excision of a subclavian arterial aneurysm on May 10, 1892. In that operation, Halsted resected the medial two thirds of the clavicle. Since that time, other alternatives to clavicular resection have been advocated, including anterior third-interspace left thoracotomy as well as standard fifth-interspace posterolateral thoracotomy, with or without combined supraclavicular subclavian artery exposure.[5,6]

Management of brachiocephalic occlusive disease rarely requires exposure of the intrathoracic left subclavian artery because priority is given to reconstructing the innominate and left common carotid vessels, and the left subclavian is left alone. If left subclavian reconstruction is required, exposure of its supraclavicular segment is usually adequate for a bypass graft originating from an innominate bypass graft or for subsequent carotid subclavian bypass. Therefore, intrathoracic left subclavian artery exposure is almost wholly reserved for management of traumatic lesions.

Depending on the arterial segment injured (distal or proximal), the left subclavian artery may be exposed through a supraclavicular incision for distal lesions or through an anterior third-interspace thoracotomy for proximal lesions (Figs. 16-1 and 16-2). Because the left subclavian artery arises posterolaterally from the aortic arch, median sternotomy does not provide adequate exposure from its aortic origin to its exit from the thorax at the first rib. An anterolateral third-interspace thoracotomy is required (Fig. 16-2). For exsanguinating hemorrhage from penetrating subclavian trauma, this third-interspace incision can be made in the emergency ward to achieve proximal arterial control, either with a vascular clamp or by manual pressure tamponade (Fig. 16-1).

Although third-interspace thoracotomy provides exposure of the intrathoracic left subclavian artery for expeditious proximal occlusion, it is not adequate for repair of distal intrathoracic traumatic lesions, particularly those immediately proximal to the first rib. To expose the distal subclavian artery, an additional left supraclavicular incision is necessary. Division of the clavicular head of the sternocleidomastoid muscle and the anterior scalene muscle is required,

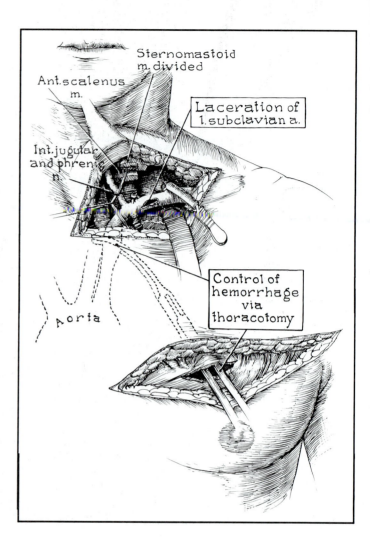

Figure 16-1. Anterolateral third-interspace limited thoracotomy through which proximal occlusion of a lacerated left subclavian artery is obtained. Exposure of the distal subclavian artery is obtained through a separate transverse supraclavicular incision. The sternocleidomastoid and anterior scalene muscles are divided. The internal mammary and thyrocervical arteries are ligated and divided but the vertebral artery is preserved. The phrenic nerve is retracted medially. (*From Ernst CB: Surg Rounds 8:21, 1985.*)

taking care to identify and protect the phrenic nerve and thoracic duct. Through both incisions, after ligating and dividing the internal mammary and thyrocervical branches, sufficient length of subclavian artery may be mobilized to deliver it into the supraclavicular wound for repair. The vertebral artery must be identified and preserved (Fig. 16-1).

Blunt injuries or nonexsanguinating left subclavian injuries are best exposed through a standard left posterolateral fifth-interspace thoracotomy. It is important to widely prepare and drape the left arm free so it may be maneuvered if supraclavicular exposure is also required. Dual incision exposure may be necessary, particularly for injuries immediately proximal to the first rib.

Proximal left subclavian and juxtaaortic exposure require fifth-interspace, left posterolateral thoracotomy (Fig. 16-3). An anterior third-interspace incision is not appropriate, except under the most extreme circumstances requiring immediate proximal control to prevent exsanguination, because it compromises exposure for subsequent arterial repair. Under such circumstances when optimal posterolateral thoracotomy is precluded by urgency of the situation, retroclavicular subclavian exposure may be facilitated by dividing

and excising a segment of the clavicle (Fig. 16-4). The medial one third of the clavicle may be removed subperiosteally. The transverse scapular vessels lie close to its undersurface and may be injured, if the periosteum is disrupted. After clavicular excision, the subclavian artery, as it emerges from the chest, is easily exposed, with care taken to protect the phrenic nerve and thoracic duct.

INNOMINATE, RIGHT SUBCLAVIAN, AND COMMON CAROTID RECONSTRUCTION

Whereas atherosclerotic occlusive lesions involving the origin of the left subclavian artery are left undisturbed, intrathoracic exposure and reconstruction of the innominate and left common carotid vessels provide viable options to extrathoracic reconstruction for occlusive disease involving these vessels. Morbidity and mortality, among appropriately selected patients and in expert hands, are comparable to extrathoracic reconstruction, and durability of direct transthoracic reconstruction is superior to extraanatomic methods.[3,7–9]

Indications for transthoracic exposure of the innomi-

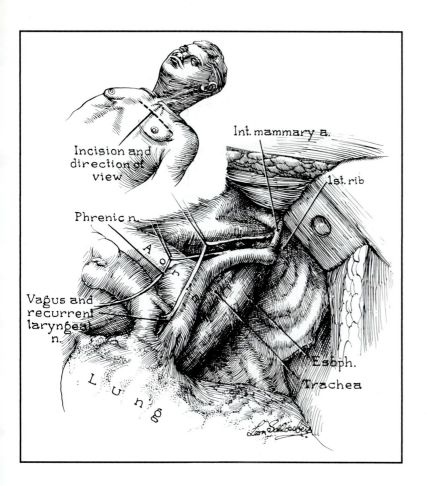

Figure 16-2. Exposure of the proximal left subclavian artery through a full third-interspace anterior thoracotomy. Vagus and phrenic nerves are retracted medially with elastic loops. The subclavian artery distal to the internal mammary branch is obscured by the first rib. View is from the left side looking up into the apex of the chest as the internal mammary branches from the inferior surface of the subclavian artery. (*From Ernst CB: Surg Rounds 8:21, 1985.*)

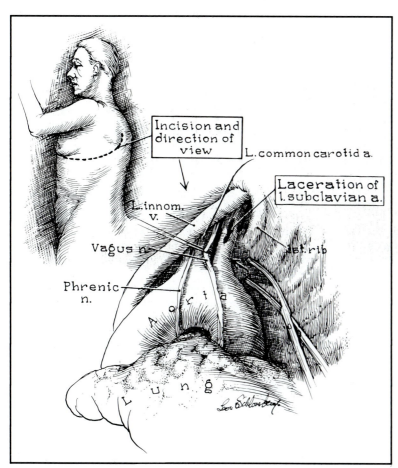

Figure 16-3. Exposure of the proximal lacerated left subclavian artery and distal aortic arch through a fifth-interspace posterolateral thoracotomy. The left innominate vein and the vagus and phrenic nerves are retracted with elastic loops. The left arm is draped free to facilitate access to the supraclavicular region if the distal subclavian artery exposure is required. (*From Ernst CB: Surg Rounds 8:21, 1985.*)

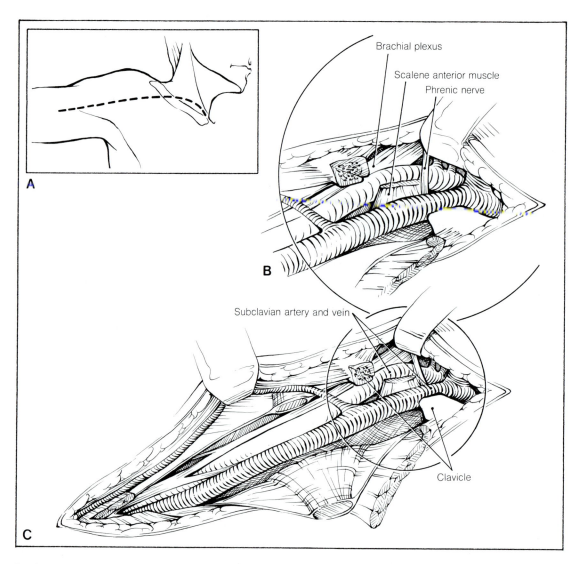

Figure 16-4. A. Incision for exposure of right subclavian artery employing clavicular resection. This is equally applicable for left retroclavicular subclavian exposure. **B.** Exposure of the subclavian artery after subperiosteal resection of the medial one third of the clavicle. **C.** The pectoralis minor is transected to expose the underlying second portion of the axillary artery.

nate, right subclavian, and both common carotid vessels are similar to those requiring left subclavian exposure, with trauma the predominating indication. Optimal exposure of these vessels is obtained through a full-length median sternotomy extended transversely into the supraclavicular area just above and parallel to the right clavicle (Fig. 16-5). Following sternotomy and placement of a standard self-retaining sternal retractor, the anterior mediastinum is widely exposed (Fig. 16-5). The contents of the upper mediastinum must be carefully dissected from the posterior surface of the sternum to allow atraumatic and expeditious median sternotomy by use of a power saw. Periosteal bleeding is minimized by using electrocautery to score a vertical line down the center of the sternum. Bleeding from the divided sternum is not usually a problem but may be controlled by placing thin strips of thrombin-soaked absorbable

gelatin sponge along the cut edges. Foreign materials such as bone wax are rarely used. The thymic remnant is divided, and by blunt dissection the anterior edges of the pleura are swept laterally.

The innominate vein may be divided with impunity, particularly if urgent proximal control for traumatic injury is necessary. However, when possible, and depending on the location of the occlusive lesion being treated, the innominate vein may be preserved and appropriately mobilized and retracted cephalad. When the prosthesis originates from the ascending aortic arch, it is tunneled behind the innominate vein. The vagus and recurrent laryngeal nerves must be identified at the innominate bifurcation and protected (Fig. 16-5). Lateral extension of the supraclavicular incision with division of the origin of the sternocleidomastoid, anterior scalene, and strap muscles provides excellent exposure

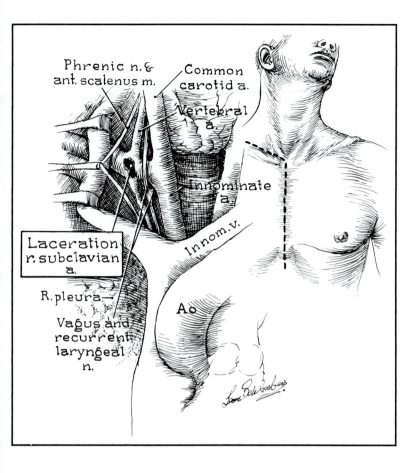

Figure 16-5. Exposure of the innominate, right subclavian, and common carotid arteries through a full median sternotomy. Extending the skin incision transversely and parallel to the clavicle provides additional exposure of the distal subclavian artery. The clavicle is not resected but retracted laterally with the sternum. The vagus, recurrent laryngeal, and phrenic nerves must be identified and protected. The innominate vein may be mobilized to expose the origins of the innominate and left common carotid arteries. (*From Ernst CB: Surg Rounds 8:21, 1985.*)

of the right subclavian to the point where it passes over the first rib. The clavicle is not transected but is retracted laterally as a unit attached to the manubrium. The phrenic nerve, as it courses over the anterior scalene muscle from lateral to medial, must be identified and protected.

For management of traumatic injuries, median sternotomy not only provides excellent exposure of the innominate, proximal common carotid, and proximal right subclavian arteries but also avoids the chest wall morbidity associated with other approaches, such as the trap door or book thoracotomy originally described by Sencert and popularized by Steenburg and Ravitch.[10] Variations on the book thoracotomy theme, which have no advantages over median sternotomy, include resection of the medial one third of the clavicle along with a median sternotomy to the third or fourth interspace.

Management of traumatic lesions usually requires innominate exposure for proximal arterial control rather than reconstruction. However, occasionally the origin of the innominate artery is injured, requiring prosthetic graft replacement[11] (Fig. 16-6). Under these circumstances, the distal innominate artery is exposed just proximal to its bifurcation into the subclavian and common carotid arteries. For repair of such injuries, protective shunting of the cerebral circulation is not necessary.

Elective transthoracic exposure for reconstruction of occlusive lesions, although less hurried than for the management of traumatic lesions, is no less demanding of meticulous technique. The innominate vein may be divided or retracted, as seems appropriate, for adequate exposure of the arteries in question.

Innominate endarterectomy is preferred, if the occlusive process extends to the bifurcation but does not involve its origin.[12] It must be noted that endarterectomy of the innominate osteum requires side-biting clamp occlusion of the innominate origin with the occasional requirement (3 to 5% of cases) of occluding the adjacent left common carotid artery or interrupting blood flow in the left common carotid because it originates from a common brachiocephalic trunk (10 to 20% of cases).[13] Furthermore, endarterectomy of the innominate osteum requires extending the arteriotomy and endarterectomy into the aortic arch, with the attendant hazard of development of an aortic dissection. Consequently, when the osteum of the innominate is involved, most surgeons prefer prosthetic tube aortobrachiocephalic grafting or a bifurcation graft aorto-subclavian-common carotid bypass, as first described in 1958 by DeBakey et al.[14] The bypass should originate from as undiseased a segment of the ascending aorta as possible. This is best accomplished by opening the pericardium at the aortic root for a short distance and using the intrapericardial segment of the aortic arch for the proximal anastomosis. Any deep-troughed side-biting aortic clamp provides adequate inflow occlusion during the proximal anastomosis and also permits uninterrupted aortic blood flow.

Varieties of bypass reconstruction are limited only by

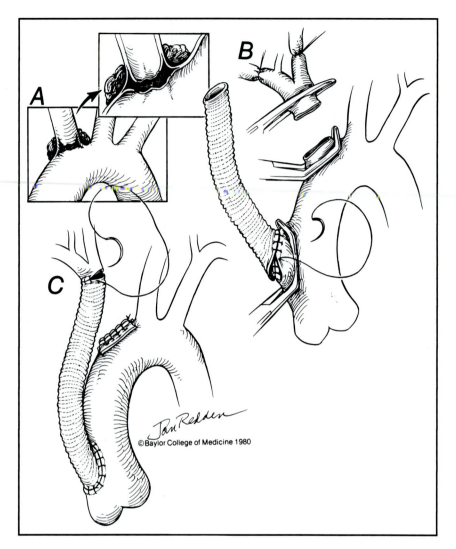

Figure 16-6. Aortoinnominate interposition graft for traumatic lesion at the innominate origin. The proximal innominate artery is oversewn and the graft is anastomosed to the intrapericardial segment of the ascending aorta. (*From Mattox KL: Aortic arch and proximal brachiocephalic penetrating injury, in Ernst CB, Stanley JC (eds): Current Therapy in Vascular Surgery. Philadelphia, BC Decker, 1987, p 262.*)

the surgeon's imagination and the extent of occlusive disease being treated (Figs. 16-7 and 16-8). It is important to avoid too great a bulk of prosthesis, which may occur with a bifurcation graft, by fashioning intrathoracic side branches from a tube graft, to prevent superior mediastinal compression phenomena when the sternotomy is wired closed.

CONCLUSIONS

For management of traumatic lesions of the great vessels of the aortic arch, there is no alternative to transthoracic exposure and repair. Management of atherosclerotic lesions of the aortic arch vessels, however, has undergone significant evolution over the past 30 years. In the 1950s, transthoracic operations were associated with a 20 to 40% mortality rate. Now, employing better patient selection and improved operative techniques, contemporary mortality rates approximate 5% for elective transthoracic arterial reconstruction.[3,7,8,12] Furthermore, durability of transthoracic reconstruction is superior to extrathoracic repair.[3,7] Consequently, a less than perfect result should not be compromised by inappropriate use of extrathoracic extraanatomic arterial reconstruction, recognizing that lesions requiring transthoracic arterial reconstruction are rarely encountered.

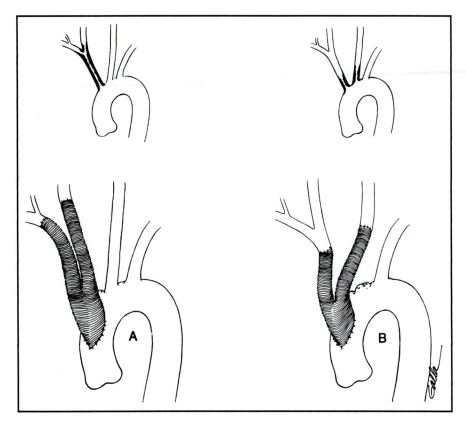

Figure 16-7. A. Aortosubclavian and right common carotid bifurcation graft bypass. **B.** Aortoinnominate and left common carotid bifurcation graft bypass. A minimally diseased segment of intrapericardial aortic arch is used for proximal anastomosis. (*From Brewster DC, Moncure AC, et al.: J Vasc Surg 2:99, 1985.*)

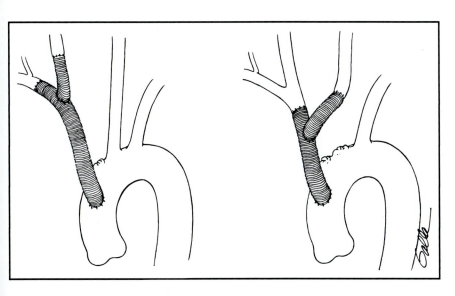

Figure 16-8. A. Aortosubclavian bypass graft with side arm to right common carotid artery. **B.** Aortoinnominate bypass graft with side arm to left common carotid artery. These bypass graft configurations may be required to decrease the bulk of prosthetic material occupying anterior superior mediastinum in order to prevent compression phenomena. A minimally diseased segment of intrapericardial aortic arch is used for the proximal anastomosis. (*From Brewster DC, Moncure AC, et al.: Vasc Surg 2:99, 1985.*)

REFERENCES

1. Crawford ES, DeBakey ME, et al.: Surgical treatment of the occlusion of innominate, common carotid, and subclavian arteries: A ten years' experience. Surgery 65:17, 1969.
2. Whitehouse WM Jr., Zelenock GB, et al.: Arterial bypass grafts for upper extremity ischemia. J Vasc Surg 3:569, 1986.
3. Crawford ES, Strowe CL, Powers RW: Occlusion of the innominate, common carotid, and subclavian arteries: Long-term results of surgical treatment. Surgery 94:781, 1983.
4. Halsted W: Ligation of the first portion of the left subclavian artery and excision of a subclavian artery aneurysm. Bull Johns Hopkins Hosp 3:93, 1892.
5. Schaff HV, Brawley RK: Operative management of penetrating vascular injuries of the thoracic outlet. Surgery 82:182, 1977.
6. Ernst CB: Exposure of inaccessible arteries. I: Carotid and arm exposure. Surg Rounds 8:21, 1985.
7. Vogt DP, Hertzer NR, et al.: Brachiocephalic arterial reconstruction. Ann Surg 196:541, 1982.
8. Zelenock GB, Cronenwett JL, et al.: Brachiocephalic arterial occlusions and stenoses: Manifestations and management of complex lesions. Arch Surg 120:370, 1985.
9. Brewster DC, Moncure AC, et al.: Innominate artery lesions: Problems encountered and lessons learned. J Vasc Surg 2:99, 1985.
10. Steenburg RW, Ravitch MM: Cervicothoracic approach for subclavian vessel injury from compound fracture of the clavicle. Ann Surg 157:839, 1963.
11. Mattox KL: Aortic arch and proximal brachiocephalic penetrating injury, in Ernst CB, Stanley JC (eds): Current Therapy in Vascular Surgery. Philadelphia, BC Decker, 1987, p 262.
12. Carlson RE, Ehrenfeld WK, et al.: Innominate endarterectomy: A 16-year experience. Arch Surg 112:1389, 1977.
13. Hewitt RL, Brewer PL, Drapanas T: Aortic arch anomalies. J Thorac Cardiovasc Surg 60:746, 1970.
14. DeBakey ME, Morris GC, et al.: Segmental thrombobliterative disease of branches of aortic arch. JAMA 166:988, 1958.

CHAPTER 17
Transperitoneal Exposure of Abdominal Aorta and Iliac Arteries

Henry Haimovici

ANATOMIC REVIEW

The abdominal aorta extends from the aortic hiatus of the diaphragm, in front of the lower border of the twelfth thoracic vertebra, and ends on the body of the fourth lumbar vertebra by dividing into the two common iliac arteries. The projection of the bifurcation of the aorta to the anterior abdominal wall corresponds to the midpoint of a line joining the two iliac crests. Generally, this point is situated at about 2 to 3 cm below the umbilicus (Fig. 17-1). The length of the abdominal aorta is about 13 cm, and its diameter, variable according to pathologic conditions, ranges between 25 and 40 mm under normal conditions.

The abdominal aorta is situated in the retroperitoneal space, and because of its relations with a large number of viscera and vascular structures, its surgical access may be difficult. From a surgical point of view, the abdominal aorta may be conveniently divided into infrarenal and suprarenal segments.

Anteriorly, the abdominal aorta is covered by the lesser omentum and stomach, behind which are the branches of the celiac artery and the celiac plexus. Below these structures, the aorta is covered by the splenic vein, the pancreas, the left renal vein, the inferior part of the duodenum, the mesentery, and the aortic plexus. Posteriorly, it is separated from the lumbar vertebrae and intervertebral fibrocartilages by the anterior longitudinal ligament and left lumbar veins. On the right side, above, it is in relation with the azygos veins, cisterna chyli, thoracic duct, and right crus of the diaphragm, the latter separating it from the upper part of the inferior vena cava and from the right celiac ganglion; below, the inferior vena cava is in closer contact with the aorta. On the left side are the left crus of the diaphragm, the celiac ganglion, the ascending part of the duodenum, and some coils of the small intestine. The aorta gives off a large number of visceral and parietal branches.

The visceral branches comprise the celiac, superior and inferior mesenteric, renal, spermatic, and ovarian arteries. The relation between point of origin of the visceral branches of the abdominal aorta and the vertebrae is highly variable.

The parietal branches are the paired inferior phrenic and lumbar arteries. The latter are arranged in four pairs. At the medial border of the psoas muscle, each lumbar artery divides into dorsal branches, which supply the muscles of the spine, and ventral branches, which supply the muscles of the abdominal wall.

Of the vascular structures in close contact with the aorta, the inferior vena cava and its tributaries have a significant surgical relationship. The inferior vena caval system receives the veins of the lower extremities and those from the abdominal and pelvic cavities, except the veins of the

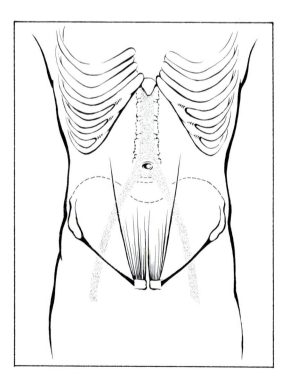

Figure 17-1. Diagram of the topography of the abdominal aorta and iliac arteries.

portal system. At the level of the fifth lumbar vertebra, from its origin with the two common iliac veins, the inferior vena cava increases in size from below upward, with the accession of the various tributaries, and becomes the largest of the body veins. It maintains a close relationship with the abdominal aorta through the major part of its course. Laterally, it lies in contact with the right psoas major muscle and is related closely to the descending duodenum, the head of the pancreas, and the medial margin of the right kidney.

Variations in the caval patterns, although infrequent, may be striking and have important surgical implications. Figure 17-2A is an example of doubling of the inferior vena cava, the two vessels being of approximately the same caliber. Figure 17-2B shows a left-sided inferior vena cava, which on occasion can be even larger than the right normal vein. Figure 17-2C indicates a doubling of the inferior vena cava, the left renal vein being retroaortic. Figure 17-2D indicates that, although the inferior vena cava is in its normal position, the iliac veins are preaortic. Figure 17-2E indicates that the left renal vein is double and appears as a circumaortic venous collar.

These vena caval anomalies, as well as others, and their surgical management will be reviewed in more detail in Chapter 47 on abdominal aneurysms.

Lymphatic structures are situated in the retroperitoneal space and form a chain extending from the inguinal ligaments to the diaphragm. The lumboaortic nodes are remarkable for their large number. They lie in superficial and deep grooves about the aorta and inferior vena cava and receive the efferents of the intestines and their mesenteries.

The lumbar sympathetic ganglia lie in the retroperito-

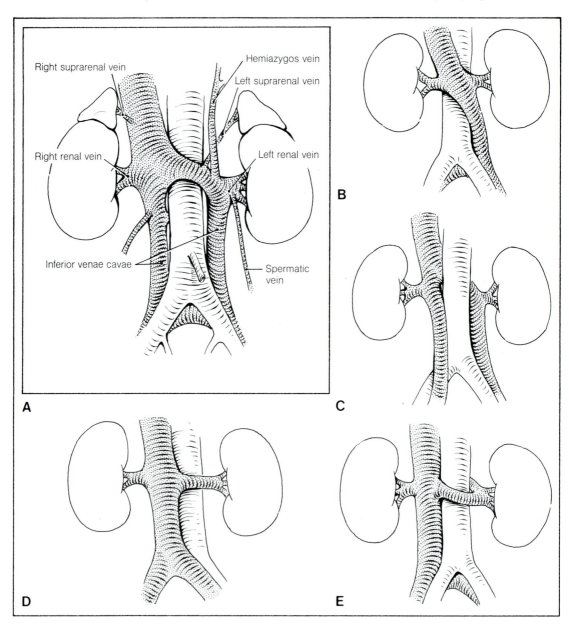

Figure 17-2. Inferior vena cava anomalies (see text).

neal space, anterior to the lumbar vertebrae and medial to the psoas major muscle. The left lumbar chain is concealed partially by the aorta, the right by the vena cava.

Anomalies of the abdominal aorta and of its major branches, although infrequent, may assume important surgical significance. Its bifurcation, instead of being at the level of the fourth lumbar vertebra, may be more proximal. The more frequent anomalies are found among its branches, especially of the renal arteries. (See Chapter 57 on renal arterial surgery.)

TRANSPERITONEAL INFRARENAL AORTIC EXPOSURE

Exposure of the infrarenal abdominal aorta is best achieved by a transperitoneal approach. An extraperitoneal exposure as an alternative may be indicated in some instances. The transperitoneal approach may be median or paramedian.

The *median xiphopubic celiotomy* is the incision of choice (Fig. 17-3A). It is carried out from the xiphoid process to the pubic symphysis and goes through the subcutaneous tissue down to and including the linea alba. The rectus muscles form bulging bands on each side of the linea alba. As depicted in Figure 17-3A, the incision starts from the upper end and is carried straight down, except that the umbilicus is skirted in an elliptical fashion. The linea alba is first opened above the umbilicus where it is broadest. Below, because the rectus muscles approach the midline, the inadvertent opening of their sheaths is occasionally unavoidable, as the incision is carried toward the pubis. The properitoneal fat is separated to expose the peritoneum, and the two layers are then opened with scissors.

Although the midline incision may be made more rapidly, the *left paramedian incision* (Fig. 17-3B) is considered to offer a more secure closure, since there are two layers of fascia with an intervening layer of muscle. In addition, the nerve supply to the rectus muscle is preserved, since the muscle is mobilized from medial to lateral.

As shown in Figure 17-3B, the skin incision starts from the lateral border of the xiphoid process and is extended laterally to the midline by about 2 to 4 cm and then downward to the pubic symphysis. The incision is deepened to the anterior rectus sheath, which is opened in line with that of the skin. The rectus muscle is reflected from medial to lateral, and the posterior rectus sheath and peritoneum are opened in line with the previous incision.

The anatomic structures of the posterior sheath are different in its upper two thirds from those below. The rectus is closed in a sheath formed by the aponeuroses of the three lateral muscles, which are arranged in such a way that, from midway between the umbilicus and the symphysis pubis, the posterior wall of the sheath contains no aponeurosis of the three muscles, since they all pass in front of the rectus. As a result, the posterior sheath ends in a thin curved margin, the linea semicircularis, the concavity of which is directed downward. The rectus, in the situation where its sheath is deficient below, is separated from the peritoneum by the transversalis fascia. Figure 17-3C depicts a cross-section of the abdominal wall: (1)

above the umbilicus it indicates the anterior and posterior sheath, and (2) below, there is only the anterior sheath, whereas posteriorly there are the fascia transversalis and peritoneum.

Immediately upon entering the peritoneal cavity, before exposing the aorta, it is mandatory to explore and verify the conditions of all the intraabdominal viscera (stomach, gallbladder, liver, pancreas, colon, and small bowel). In addition, the major visceral branches of the aorta should be explored for the possibility of associated vascular lesions by determining the presence of a thrill or diminished pulsation.

Next, the small bowel is eviscerated and placed in a sac or on the upper right side of the abdomen and protected with wet towels.

The posterior parietal peritoneum overlying the abdominal aorta is then incised (Fig. 17-4A). The peritoneal layer is lifted up with forceps lateral to the duodenojejunal angle. The first jejunal loop is put under slight tension to facilitate the section of the ligament of Treitz. The peritoneal incision is extended toward the lower part of the abdominal aorta into the pelvic area. In the process, the third and fourth portions of the duodenum are separated from the aortic surface toward the right. The preaortic sheath is then incised, care being taken at this point to carry out hemostasis of the small vessels found at this level.

Dissection of the peritoneum is continued toward the pelvic cavity, staying to the right of the mesosigmoid. The preaortic sheath is then opened in the same direction. Exposure of the left renal vein is carried out after completing the incision of the preaortic sheath. Avoidance of excision of the preaortic autonomic plexus may help prevent postoperative sexual dysfunction.

The left border of the aorta is dissected after identifying the inferior mesenteric artery and vein, the latter near the angle of Treitz.

The inferior mesenteric artery, in cases of an abdominal aortic aneurysm, must be ligated and divided (Fig. 17-5A,B). Care must be taken to ligate it close to its origin from the abdominal aorta. Before doing so, it is essential to identify its bifurcation and to determine the presence or absence of a pulsation in its distal and proximal segments. If necessary, the inferior mesenteric vein may be ligated and divided above the left renal vein as it crosses this vessel proximally (Fig. 17-5C).

In isolating and mobilizing the left renal vein, the spermatic or ovarian veins should be identified and their origin and course be ascertained.

To expose the renal arteries, the left renal vein must be retracted proximally by passing a rubber vessel loop about it (Fig. 17-5D).

Mobilization and freeing of the posterior wall of the aorta is a more tedious step, requiring greater care than for the anterior surface. On the right, its separation from the adjacent inferior vena cava may be more hazardous and must be done with extreme care.

The proximal mobilization of the aorta below the renal vessels should be carried out after identifying the retroaortic vessels, namely, the lumbar veins, in order to avoid their injury.

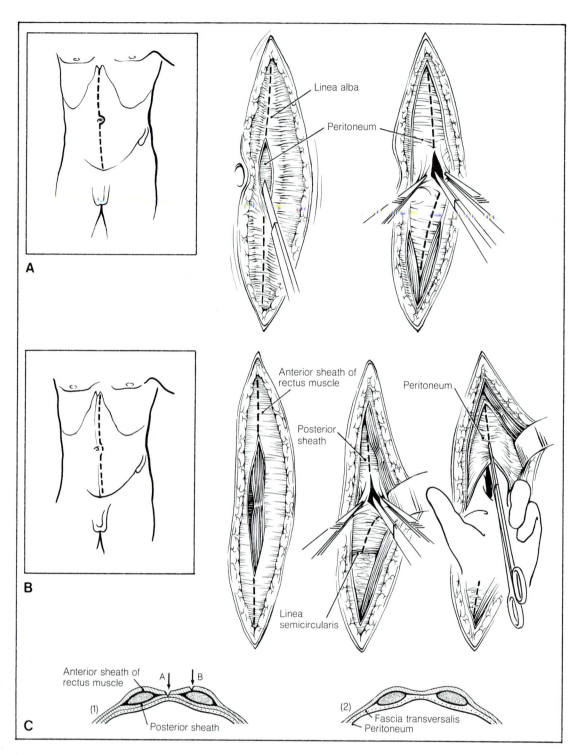

Figure 17-3. A. Xiphopubic midline incision. **B.** Xiphopubic left paramedian incision. **C.** (1) Cross-section of the abdominal wall proximal to the umbilicus. (2) Cross-section of the abdominal wall midway between the umbilicus and pubic symphysis (below the linea semicircularis).

Mobilization of the bifurcation of the aorta is best carried out distal to it, around the common iliac arteries close to the latter's division into internal and external iliac vessels. The reason for this maneuver stems from the fact that the normal confluence of the two iliac veins behind the bifurca-

tion of the aorta renders its dissection at this level more difficult and dangerous. In mobilizing the bifurcation of the common iliac, it is necessary to identify the ureter to avoid its injury. Other pitfalls to be avoided, as already mentioned above, are (1) injuries to the lumbar veins and

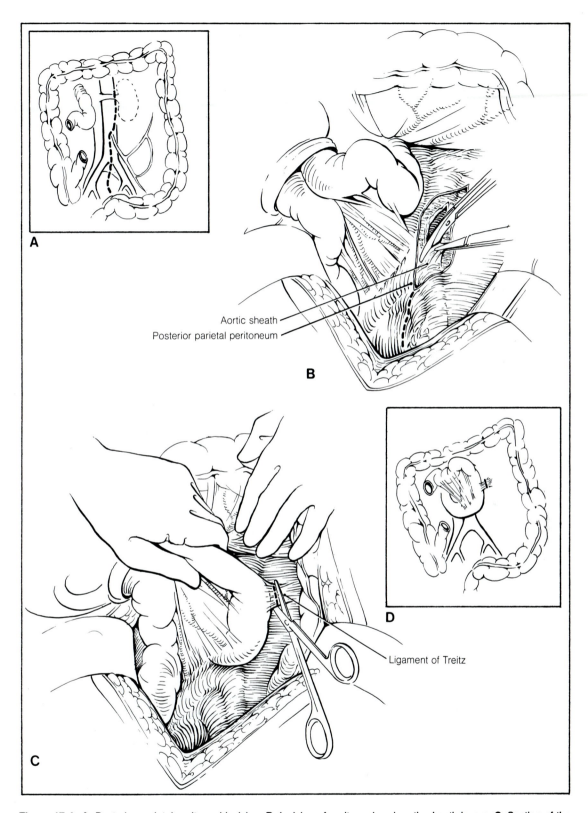

A

B

Aortic sheath
Posterior parietal peritoneum

C

D

Ligament of Treitz

Figure 17-4. A. Posterior parietal peritoneal incision. **B.** Incision of peritoneal and aortic sheath layers. **C.** Section of the ligament of Treitz at the duodenojejunal angle. **D.** Inset indicating the relative positions of the abdominal structures during aortic exposure.

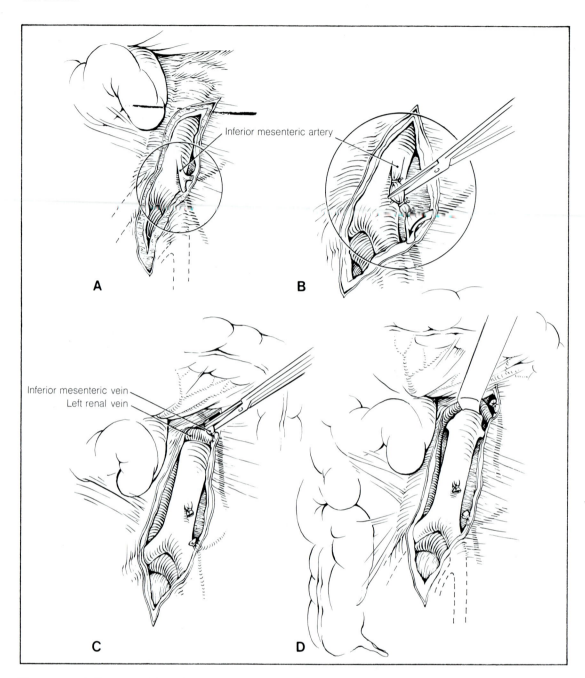

Figure 17-5. A. Exposure of the inferior mesenteric artery. **B.** Ligation and section of the inferior mesenteric artery. **C.** Ligation and section of the inferior mesenteric vein, proximally to the left renal vein. **D.** Exposure of renal arteries by proximal retraction of the left renal vein.

(2) difficulties that may arise in the presence of a left-sided or retroaortic inferior vena cava, (3) a horseshoe kidney, or (4) a lower-pole renal artery.

This approach to the infrarenal abdominal aorta has the advantage of affording distal extension for exploring the iliac or femoral arteries. Proximal extension of the exposure may be more difficult and would afford reaching the superior mesenteric artery only by retracting the left renal vein and exposing the suprarenal viscera.

Exposure of the suprarenal abdominal aorta through the lesser omentum is somewhat more difficult, especially

in heavy-set individuals. In these instances, a thoracoabdominal approach is the method of choice (see Chapter 18).

PHYSIOPATHOLOGIC CONSIDERATIONS IN AORTIC SURGERY

Clamping of the infrarenal abdominal aorta is usually well tolerated in the majority of cases. Occasionally, however, serious ischemic manifestations of the spinal cord, intestines, and kidney may be noted. Clamping of the suprarenal abdominal aorta, by contrast, may be fraught with serious to fatal complications if necessary precautions are not undertaken during the surgical procedure. Ischemia of the spinal cord and of the colon, and renal failure are described in detail in the chapters on surgery of the thoracoabdominal aorta.

TRANSPERITONEAL EXPOSURE OF ILIAC ARTERIES

In the presence of markedly diseased or completely occluded common iliac vessels, exposure of the external iliac arteries also becomes necessary and is carried out at the level of the iliac fossa.

The decision for exposing the external iliac arteries depends on their patency as determined by prior arteriography and by the palpatory findings during this stage of surgery.

Exposure of Right External Iliac

Exposure of the right iliac fossa is achieved by retracting upward the cecum and the terminal ileum (Fig. 17-6). The posterior parietal peritoneum is incised along the iliac axis. The external iliac runs from the sacroiliac to the lateral side down to the inguinal ligament, where it becomes the femoral artery. The two branches of the external iliac, the inferior epigastric and the deep circumflex iliac, arise from its terminal segment.

After incision of the peritoneum both proximally and distally, a short segment of about 4 to 5 cm needs to be mobilized. Proximally, toward the bifurcation of the common iliac, care should be taken not to injure the ureter, which crosses the vessels at that level. After opening the vascular sheath, the artery is mobilized and tapes are placed about it.

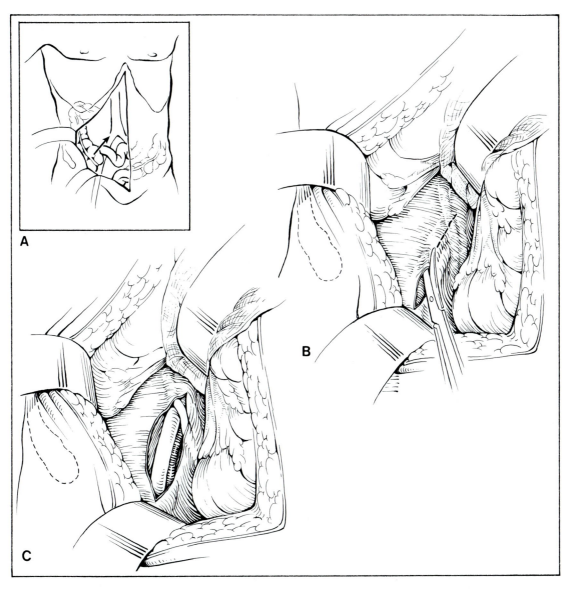

Figure 17-6. Transperitoneal exposure of the right external iliac artery (see text).

Exposure of Left External Iliac Artery

The descending colon and the sigmoid are retracted upward and medially, exposing the iliac fossa. The exposure of the left external iliac (Fig. 17-7) is carried out in a fashion similar to that on the right side.

As mentioned above, exposure of the external iliac arteries through the transperitoneal approach is usually carried out as part of an aortoiliac procedure. A retroperitoneal tunnel between the aorta and external iliac arteries on both sides is then developed. On the right, it is developed under the posterior parietal peritoneum, and on the left it is made under the mesosigmoid. In developing the retroperitoneal tunnels, it is important to bear in mind the presence of the ureter and the vessels originating from the iliac artery and the satellite veins and to avoid their injury. The ureters, once identified, should be allowed to remain in situ.

Should exposure of the external iliac prove to be inadequate for implantation of a graft or for a thromboendarterectomy, exposure of the femorals becomes mandatory. In these cases, passing of the graft is greatly facilitated through the tunnel of the iliac fossa extended to the femoral canal.

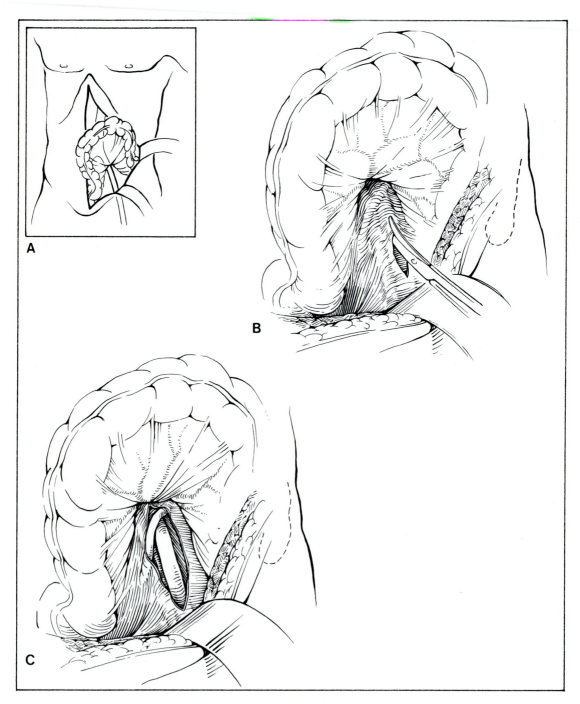

Figure 17-7. Transperitoneal exposure of the left external iliac artery (see text).

CHAPTER 18
Retroperitoneal Approach to Abdominal Aorta

Calvin B. Ernst

Since the first successful aortoiliac bypass for occlusive disease by Oudot on November 14, 1950, and the first successful abdominal aortic aneurysm repair by Dubost and his colleagues on March 21, 1951, innumerable reconstructive procedures have been performed on the abdominal aorta.[1,2] It is somewhat ironic that retroperitoneal exposure of the abdominal aorta, used by both Oudot and Dubost in their first successful aortic reconstructive procedures, has not been widely adopted. In part this relates to unfamiliarity with the retroperitoneal approach by general and vascular surgeons, who, by nature of their training and by being comfortable working in the abdomen, have continued to expose the aorta transabdominally. That the transabdominal approach is highly effective has been widely documented and, understandably, the retroperitoneal approach has few advocates. Nonetheless, under certain circumstances it is equal in effectiveness to the transabdominal approach and is preferred in some circumstances.

It has been suggested that retroperitoneal aortic reconstruction is less stressful for the patient with less postoperative ileus, less third-space fluid shifts, and fewer pulmonary complications than transperitoneal aortic reconstruction.[3–5] Consequently, retroperitoneal aortic reconstruction has been recommended for elderly high-risk patients. However, until randomized prospective data are available comparing standard transperitoneal approaches with the retroperitoneal approach, no definite conclusions can be drawn favoring either approach.

Indications for retroperitoneal aortic exposure include small infrarenal aneurysms localized to the aorta, suprarenal or juxtarenal aneurysms, aortic reconstruction requiring left renal arterial or mesenteric revascularization, patients with horseshoe kidneys, patients with right-sided ostomies, and some morbidly obese individuals. The retroperitoneal approach is also indicated for patients who have a hostile abdomen resulting from extensive intraabdominal adhesions, radiation therapy, or inflammatory processes, and those undergoing secondary aortic reconstruction.

Contraindications to use of the retroperitoneal approach include the need for right renal arterial reconstruction, need to assess intraabdominal organs, and extensive aneurysmal involvement of the right iliac system. A relative contraindication is needed to expose the right groin vessels.

To the uninitiated, several pitfalls exist when performing retroperitoneal aortic reconstruction. All may be avoided; when one anticipates such problems, alternative approaches are available including variations on the transabdominal approach. One of these is the transperitoneal-retroperitoneal approach that offers the advantages of retroperitoneal exposure, particularly to the visceral vessels.[6]

RETROPERITONEAL INFRARENAL AORTIC EXPOSURE

Several authors have provided detailed descriptions of retroperitoneal infrarenal aortic exposure utilizing transverse,[7] midline,[8] or perimedian incisions.[9] Clearly, a variety of incisions are available, all providing access to the aorta and proximal common iliac arteries.

Proper positioning of the patient is important. The left thorax should be elevated 45 to 60 degrees. To provide access to the right groin, the hips should lie as flat as possible. Flexing the table and maintaining the patient's position with an air-vacuum styrofoam bean bag causes the wound to spiral open (Fig. 18-1). The midpoint between the right costal margin and the right iliac crest is centered over the table flexion point. With the surgeon standing on the left, the table may be rotated away (during dissection of the aorta) or toward him (if groin incisions are required). During closure of the incision, the table is flattened, bringing the wound edges into apposition.

A transverse skin incision is made from the edge of the rectus sheath, midway between the umbilicus and symphysis pubis, 8 to 10 cm into the eleventh intercostal space (Fig. 18-1). The abdominal wall and intercostal muscles are divided in the line of the incision, taking care not to injure the eleventh and twelfth dorsal neurovascular bundles. Damage to these nerves denervates the abdominal wall

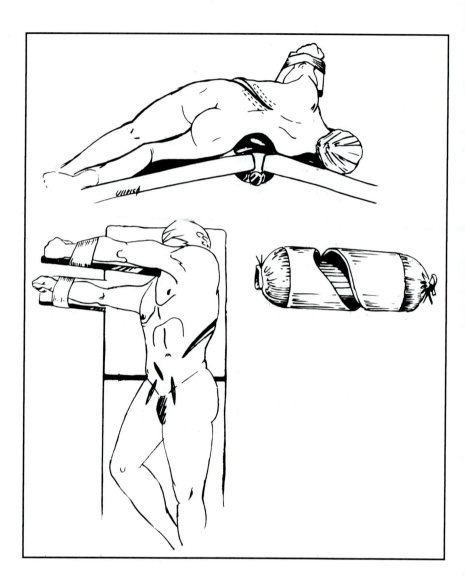

Figure 18-1. Patient position for retroperitoneal aortic exposure. Flexing the operating table causes the incision to spiral open. (*From Shepard AD, Scott GR, et al.: Arch Surg 121:444, 1986.*)

musculature, leading to muscle weakness manifest by an asymmetric abdominal contour with unsightly bulging. Excising a short segment of the twelfth rib facilitates wound closure.

The retroperitoneal space is entered at the tip of the twelfth rib. With blunt dissection the peritoneum is stripped from the underlying iliac fossa and psoas muscle. Peritoneum is also stripped from the undersurface of the abdominal wall, taking care as the linea semilunaris is approached to avoid tearing the peritoneum, which thins out and is adherent to the transversalis fascia as the midline is approached. Posterolaterally, the peritoneum is stripped from the flank, psoas muscles, and inferior surface of the diaphragm. The peritoneum and its contents are swept and retracted anteromedially. A dissection plane is developed along the lumbodorsal fascia behind the left kidney and ureter, which are further mobilized and retracted anteriorally (Figs. 18-2 and 18-3). Alternatively, dissection may proceed anterior to the left kidney and ureter, but a major advantage of the retroperitoneal approach is partially lost: by leaving the kidney in situ, the left renal vein obscures the juxtarenal aorta.

With the kidney and ureter retracted anteromedially, the aorta is exposed from the level of the left renal artery to the aortic bifurcation. Any self-retaining retractor firmly attached to the operating table simplifies and maintains fixed exposure and is the key to maintaining such exposure. By exposing the aorta from its bifurcation to the level of the left renal vein, the left renal artery is identified at the level of the lumbar branch of the left renal vein. The lumbar branch of the left renal vein is a fairly constant structure and serves as a marker to the origin of the left renal artery (Fig. 18-3). After the lumbar branch of the left renal vein is ligated and divided, the infrarenal aorta comes into complete view.

Retroperitoneal aortic exposure for occlusive disease requires limited infrarenal dissection, preserving the inferior mesenteric artery (IMA). When managing a large aneurysm, however, sometimes the IMA must be ligated and divided flush with the aneurysm to gain access to the right common iliac vessels. For aneurysms confined to the aorta, the IMA is kept intact and distal dissection proceeds posterior to the IMA origin. Dissection of the aortic bifurcation from the underlying vena cava and iliac vein confluens must

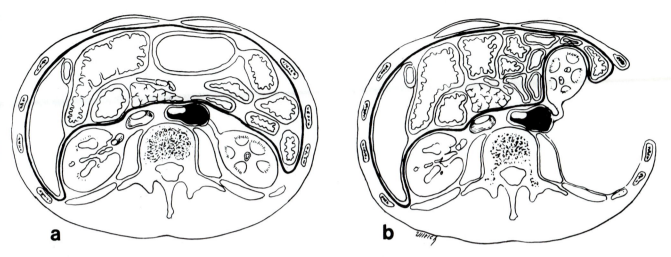

Figure 18-2. Transverse section at the level of left renal artery. Peritoneum depicted by bold line, **a.** Dissection plane is developed along the lumbodorsal fascia behind the left kidney, which is mobilized anteromedially and to the right, **b.** (*From Shepard AD, Scott GR, et al.: Arch Surg 121:444, 1986.*)

proceed with caution lest venous injury occur. Venous repair, particularly on the right of the aorta at this level and through the retroperitoneal approach, is difficult if not impossible. Distal arterial control is facilitated by dissecting the common iliac arteries individually, thus avoiding the hazardous aortic bifurcation caval area. Large aneurysms requiring extensive right iliac dissection are a relative contraindication to the retroperitoneal approach. Required dis-

section of the right common iliac bifurcation is challenging because of marginal exposure. Dissection and mobilization of the right iliac arterial system under such circumstances is hazardous and should be avoided. Distal control and occlusion of the right iliac artery during aneurysm repair should be obtained by a balloon occlusion catheter threaded through the opened aneurysm (Fig. 18-4). Some authors recommend extending the abdominal incision across the

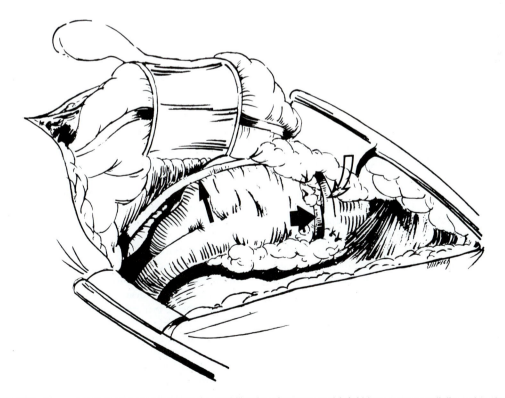

Figure 18-3. Aneurysm exposed by retracting the mobilized peritoneum and left kidney anteromedially and to the right. Lumbar branch of left renal vein (*arrowhead*) serves as a marker to the left renal artery (*open arrow*). Ureter (*arrow*) is swept anteromedially. (*From Shepard AD, Scott GR, et al.: Arch Surg 121:444, 1986.*)

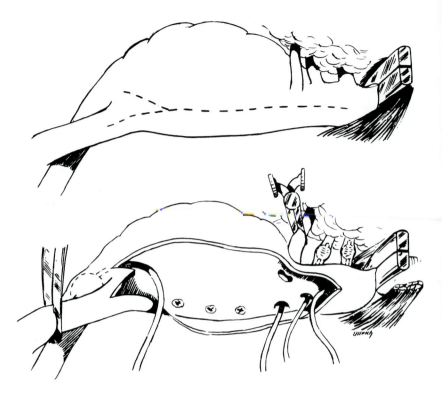

Figure 18-4. Proximal aortic occlusive clamp placed just cephalad to celiac trunk. Line of incision into aneurysmal sac is posterolateral to visceral vessels (*top*). Occlusion balloon catheter passed through opened aneurysm controls backbleeding from celiac trunk, superior mesenteric artery, and right renal artery (only orifice shown with catheter). Left renal artery and left common iliac artery occluded with vascular clamps. Right common iliac artery backbleeding controlled with intraluminal occlusion balloon catheter (*bottom*). (*From Shepard AD, Scott GR, et al.: Arch Surg 121:444, 1986.*)

midline to the right lower quadrant to facilitate right iliac arterial exposure.[4] Dissection of the left common iliac artery, however, is easy because this vessel, with its branches, is apparent throughout its entire length.

Whether one is managing aneurysmal or occlusive disease, circumaortic dissection is unnecessary for proximal aortic clamping. Only small tunnels anterior and posterior to the infrarenal aorta are required, just sufficient to accommodate the blades of a vascular clamp. Caval injury is not a concern at this level because it is not immediately adjacent to the aorta as it is at the aortic bifurcation.

RETROPERITONEAL APPROACH FOR JUXTARENAL AND SUPRARENAL AORTIC EXPOSURE

The retroperitoneal approach is ideal for juxtarenal or suprarenal aortic exposure because the obscuring left renal vein and body of the pancreas are not limiting factors, as they are with the transperitoneal approach. Occasionally, however, a combined transperitoneal-retroperitoneal approach may be required, particularly for large juxtarenal aortic aneurysms with extensive iliac arterial involvement.[6] The transperitoneal component of the exposure facilitates iliac dissection, and the retroperitoneal component facilitates suprarenal aortic exposure.

As with dissection of the infrarenal aorta, positioning the patient is the key to ease of exposure. Positioning is the same as for exposing the infrarenal aorta, with the exception that left chest elevation must be closer to 75 than 60 degrees.

A transverse skin incision begins at the lateral border of the rectus sheath, starting between the umbilicus and symphysis pubis, and extends 15 to 20 cm into the tenth intercostal space. Through such an incision, the supramesenteric aorta may be adequately exposed. Exposure of the celiac segment of the aorta requires an incision into the eighth intercostal space and a formal thoracoabdominal incision (Fig. 18-5) (see Chapter 46).

The abdominal wall and intercostal muscles are divided in the line of the incision. The retroperitoneal space is entered near the tip of the tenth rib, and with blunt dissection the peritoneum is stripped from the underlying iliac fossa and psoas muscle, developing a plane along the lumbodorsal fascia behind the left kidney and ureter, which are mobilized and retracted anteromedially. By sweeping the retroperitoneum cephalad and medially, the undersurface of the diaphragm is exposed. The lateral extent of the incision is deepened into the left thorax, and a short length of diaphragm is incised radially, which facilitates proximal exposure.

After placement of appropriate packs, the peritoneal sac and wound edges are retracted by any self-retaining retractor firmly attached to the operating table.

Dissection proceeds like the infrarenal exposure described above but with further cephalad exposure of the suprarenal aorta obtained by dividing the diaphragmatic crus enveloping the aorta. Suture ligation of an areolar tissue surrounding the origin of the superior mesenteric artery (SMA) prevents or minimizes lymphatic leaks.

After dividing the diaphragmatic crus, further sharp dissection exposes the SMA 1 to 2 cm proximal to the left renal artery. Circumferential aortic dissection is not required

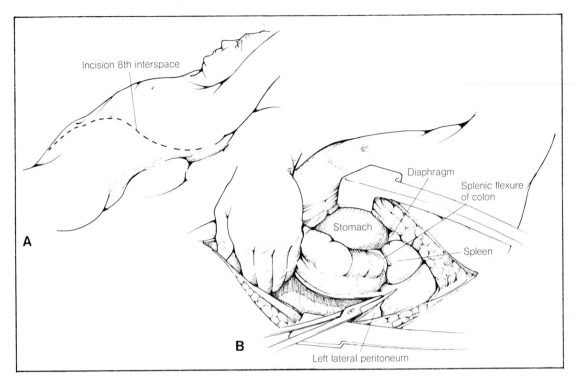

Figure 18-5. Incision for retroperitoneal suprarenal aortic exposure. **A.** An eighth interspace incision is required to adequately expose the aorta proximal to the celiac trunk. **B.** Transperitoneal-extraperitoneal approach mobilizes descending colon, spleen, stomach, and pancreas anteromedially to the right. (*Courtesy of H. Haimovici.*)

for suprarenal or supramesenteric aortic occlusion. Only narrow tunnels anterior and posterior to the aorta are made, just sufficient to accommodate the blades of a vascular clamp.

After the aneurysm is opened, backbleeding from individual vessel orifices may be controlled by threading intraluminal balloon occlusion catheters into the respective ostea or by small bulldog clamps placed individually on the SMA and left renal arteries (Fig. 18-4). Because the right renal artery is obscure, clamping is not possible. Therefore, an occlusion balloon catheter may be used, or alternatively the operative field may be kept dry by cell-saver suction and reinfusion of blood lost from the right renal orifice. During the time required for construction of the aortic anastomosis, only a small amount of blood is lost from the right renal artery. In addition, no longer than 30 minutes are usually required for suprarenal occlusion and resulting renal ischemia. Consequently, no special precautions are taken to cool the kidneys or infuse solutions into the renal arteries. Anticipating prolonged suprarenal occlusion, however, demands renal protection by infusion of 200 to 300 ml of iced Ringer's lactate solution (containing mannitol and sodium bicarbonate) into each renal artery.

Closure of incisions for both infrarenal and suprarenal aortic exposure is straightforward and facilitated by flattening the table. If the left chest has been entered, a 20 French catheter is placed during closure and removed after evacuating air from the chest.

PITFALLS OF RETROPERITONEAL AORTIC RECONSTRUCTION

Certain pitfalls of retroperitoneal aortic reconstruction deserve comment. These include injury to the vena cava, which is difficult to manage through the retroperitoneal approach. Vigorous retraction in the upper aspects of the operative field may lead to unrecognized splenic trauma. This should be minimized by using self-retaining retractors. The lumbar branch of the left renal vein must be identified because it serves as a marker to the left renal artery and to avoid injuring it as well. Similarly, a retroaortic left renal vein or circumaortic left renal vein can cause problems if not identified, although this is rare. During mobilization of the retroperitoneum, it is important to identify the left gonadal vein so that it is not avulsed from the left renal vein during the course of sweeping the retroperitoneum anteriorly. A left pneumothorax may occur and be unrecognized, particularly if the left eleventh intercostal space incision is not made carefully.

Both the IMA and the left renal artery are swept anteriorly when retrorenal dissection is performed and must be identified to prevent injury. To preserve continuity of the IMA, it is important to incise the aneurysm posterior to its origin. The left ureter must be identified and swept anteriorly with the kidney and retroperitoneal structures to avoid injury. The left ureter is particularly vulnerable to traction injury during secondary aortic procedures when it may be tethered in the pelvis and is not as mobile as it might be in a virgin retroperitoneum.

Postoperative problems following retroperitoneal aortic reconstruction include the potential for development of an aortoenteric fistula, if the aneurysm sac is not imbricated over the prostheses or if the duodenum lies on the graft following aortic reconstruction for occlusive disease.

Excessive blunt retroperitoneal dissection may cause tearing of small veins and subsequent oozing with postoperative retroperitoneal hematoma formation. Precise dissection and careful hemostasis prevent this complication. Closed suction drainage for 24 hours has been suggested by some to minimize retroperitoneal hematoma formation.[3,10] However, I have an aversion to placing drains near a fresh aortic graft. A left flank hernia may develop if precise multiple-layer closure of the wound is not performed.

REFERENCES

1. Oudot J: La greffe vasculaire dans les thromboses du carrefour aortique. Presse Med 59:234, 1951.
2. Dubost C, Allary M, Oeconomos N: Resection of an aneurysm of the abdominal aorta: Reestablishment of the continuity by a preserved human arterial graft, with result after five months. Arch Surg 64:405, 1952.
3. Shepard AD, Scott GR, et al.: Retroperitoneal approach to high-risk abdominal aortic aneurysms. Arch Surg 121:444, 1986.
4. Sicard GA, Freeman MB, et al.: Comparison between the trans-abdominal and retroperitoneal approach for reconstruction of the infrarenal abdominal aorta. J Vasc Surg 5:19, 1987.
5. Williams GM, Ricotta J, et al.: The extended retroperitoneal approach for treatment of extensive atherosclerosis of the aorta and renal vessels. Surgery 88:846, 1980.
6. Ernst CB: Exposure of inaccessible arteries. Part II: Abdomen and leg exposure. Surg Rounds 8:26, 1985.
7. Rob C: Extraperitoneal approach to the abdominal aorta. Surgery 53:87, 1963.
8. Shumacker HB: Midline exposure of the abdominal aorta and iliac arteries. Surg Gynecol Obstet 135:791, 1972.
9. Taheri SA, Sawronski S, Smith D: Paramedian approach to the abdominal aorta. J Cardiovasc Surg 24:529, 1983.
10. O'Mara CS, Williams GM: Extended retroperitoneal approach for abdominal aortic aneurysm repair, in: Bergan JJ, Yao JST (eds): Aneurysms: Diagnosis and Treatment. New York, Grune & Stratton, Inc, 1982, pp 327–343.

CHAPTER 19
Retroperitoneal Approach to Iliac Arteries

Henry Haimovici

ANATOMIC REVIEW

Access to the iliac arteries by the retroperitoneal approach is obtained through incisions made through the anterolateral abdominal wall. The skin of the abdomen at this level is attached loosely to the subjacent structures except at the umbilicus, where it adheres firmly. The superficial fascia of the lower abdomen is divided into two layers: the superficial, called Camper's fascia, which lies in the bulk of the subcutaneous fat, and the deep layer, called Scarpa's fascia, which is denser and is applied more closely to the abdominal muscles.

The flat muscles of the abdomen and the recti are the main structures of the abdominal wall protecting its contents (Fig. 19-1). The most superficial of the flat muscles is the *external oblique,* which lies on the lateral and anterior parts of the abdomen. It is broad, thin, and irregularly quadrilateral, its muscular portion occupying the side and its aponeurosis occupying the anterior wall of the abdomen. The fleshy fibers of this muscle proceed in various directions, some of which are inserted into the anterior half of the outer lip of the iliac crest, with others ending in an aponeurosis. The aponeurosis of this muscle is a thin but strong membranous structure, the fibers of which are directed downward and medialward. The portion of the aponeurosis that extends between the anterior superior iliac spine and the pubic tubercle is a thick band, folded inward, that continues below with the fascia lata. It is called the inguinal ligament, or Poupart's ligament.

The second flat muscle is the *internal oblique,* which is thinner and smaller than the external, beneath which it lies. It is an irregularly quadrilateral form and is situated at the lateral and anterior part of the abdomen. It arises by fleshy fibers from the lateral half of the grooved upper surface of the inguinal ligament, from the anterior two thirds of the middle of the iliac crest, and from the posterior lamella of the lumbodorsal fascia. From its origin, the fibers diverge. Those from the inguinal ligament, few in number and paler in color than the rest, arch downward and medialward across the spermatic cord or the round ligament of the

uterus. The fibers from the anterior third of the iliac origin are horizontal in their direction and, becoming tendinous along the lower fourth of the linea semilunaris, pass in front of the rectus abdominis to be inserted into the linea alba. The fibers arising from the middle third of the origin run obliquely upward and medialward and end in an aponeurosis.

The *transversus muscle,* so-called from the direction of its fibers, is the most internal of the flat muscles of the abdomen, being placed immediately beneath the internal oblique muscle. The muscle ends in front of a broad aponeurosis. It passes horizontally to the middle line and is inserted into the linea alba. Its upper three fourths lies behind the rectus and blends with the posterior lamella of the aponeurosis of the internal oblique. Its lower fourth is in front of the rectus.

The *rectus abdominis* is a long, flat muscle that extends along the whole length of the front of the abdomen and is separated from its fellow of the opposite side by the linea alba. The rectus is enclosed in a sheath formed by the aponeuroses of the two oblique and transversus muscles. This arrangement of the aponeurosis originates from the costal margin, extending to midway between the umbilicus and the symphysis pubis, where the posterior wall of the sheath ends in a thin, curved margin, the linea semicircularis, the concavity of which is directed downward. Below this level, all three muscles pass in front of the rectus.

The *transversalis fascia* is a thin aponeurotic membrane that lies between the inner surface of the transversalis muscle and the extraperitoneal fat. It forms part of the general layer of fascia lining the abdominal wall and is directly continuous with the iliac and pelvic fasciae.

Iliac Arteries

The abdominal aorta, as stated above, divides on the left side of the body of the fourth lumbar vertebra into the two common iliac arteries, each about 5 cm in length.

The *right common iliac artery* is usually somewhat longer

251

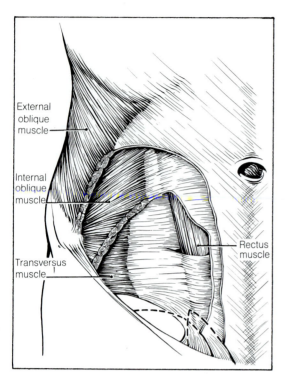

Figure 19-1. Diagram of the anterolateral muscles of the abdomen.

than the left and passes more obliquely across the body of the last lumbar vertebra. In front of it are the peritoneum, the small intestines, branches of the sympathetic nerves, and, at its point of division, the ureter. Behind, it is separated from the body of the fourth and fifth lumbar vertebrae and the intervening fibrocartilage by the terminations of the two common iliac veins and the commencement of the inferior vena cava. Laterally, it is in relation, above, with the inferior vena cava and the right common iliac vein and, below, with the psoas major. Medial to it, above, is the left iliac vein.

The *left common iliac artery* is in relation, in front, with the peritoneum, the small intestines, branches of the sympathetic nerves, and the superior hemorrhoidal artery. At this point it is crossed by the ureter. The left common iliac vein lies partly medial to and partly behind the artery. Laterally, the artery is in relation with the psoas major.

The *external iliac artery*, a continuation of the common iliac, passes obliquely downward and lateralward along the medial border of the psoas major, midway between the anterior superior spine of the ilium and the symphysis pubis, where it enters the thigh and becomes the femoral artery. Its relations, in front and medially, are with the peritoneum, subperitoneal areolar tissue, the termination of the ileum, and, frequently, the vermiform process on the right side; on the left side, the external iliac artery is in relation to the sigmoid colon and a thin layer of fascia, derived from the iliac fossa, that surrounds the artery and vein. Behind, it is in relation with the medial border of the psoas major. Laterally, it rests against this muscle, from which it is separated by the iliac fascia. Numerous lymphatic vessels and lymph glands lie on the front and on the medial

side of the vessel. Besides several small branches, the external iliac artery gives off two collaterals of considerable size: the inferior epigastric artery and the deep iliac circumflex artery. Both of these branches arise from the external iliac immediately above the inguinal ligament.

The *hypogastric artery* (internal iliac artery) arises at the bifurcation of the common iliac artery, opposite the lumbosacral articulation, and divides into two large trunks, an anterior and a posterior. This artery supplies the walls and viscera of the pelvis, the buttock, the generative organs, and the medial side of the thigh. It is a short, thick vessel, smaller than the external iliac, of about 4 cm in length.

EXPOSURE OF EXTERNAL ILIAC ARTERY

The patient is placed in the supine position (Fig. 19-2). A rolled sheet or a small sandbag is placed under the buttocks to elevate this area by about 10 to 15 degrees. A skin incision is made parallel with and about 1 cm above the inguinal ligament, the incision being in the middle third of a line extending from the anterior superior iliac spine to the pubic symphysis and slightly curved proximally (Fig. 19-2A). After hemostasis of subcutaneous vessels is carried out, the aponeuroses of the external oblique, internal oblique, and transversus muscles are incised, always parallel to the inguinal ligament. These three structures are then reflected upward and medialward, the transversalis fascia is opened, the properitoneal adipose tissue is retracted gently in the same direction as the muscles, and the retroperitoneal space is entered. The external iliac artery is exposed, its sheath opened, and a tape placed about it. On its anterior surface one finds two small, fragile venules that are branches of the satellite veins. This anatomic feature indicates the necessity for dissection of the external iliac artery above this point, where it presents no other than the external iliac vein as the only important anatomic relationship.

Extraperitoneal Exposure of Iliac Axis

There are several approaches to the iliac axis. Our personal preference is indicated in Figure 19-3, which illustrates the exposure of the right iliac vessels.

The patient is placed in the supine position, with a hard pillow under the right thoracolumbar region, thus elevating the body by about 10 to 15 degrees. Figure 19-3A shows the skin incision, which begins at the level of the anterior axillary line at the midpoint between the subcostal margin and the iliac crest. From there, it continues in an S-shaped line, the first part being directed toward the umbilicus and the second portion parallel to the inguinal ligament and about 3 cm above it. The skin incision exceeds slightly the lateral border of the rectus abdominis.

The incision is then carried down to the external oblique (Fig. 19-3B). The lateral edge of the skin flap is retracted laterally and downward. Incision of the external oblique is done closer to the inguinal ligament than to the lateral border of the rectus abdominis. The aponeurotic portion of the muscle is incised along its fibers. Then the muscular portion is elevated and separated from the underlying struc-

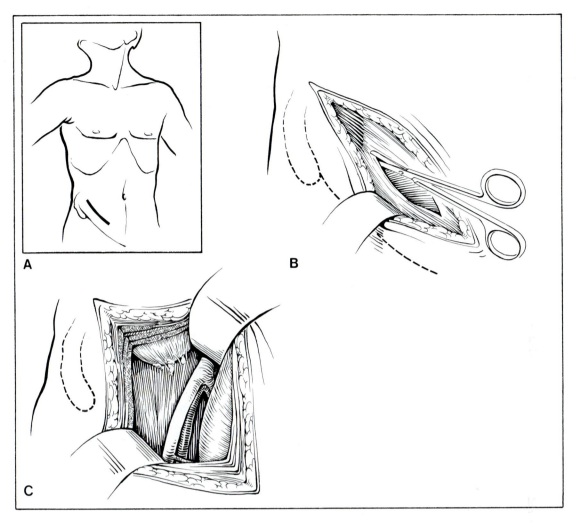

Figure 19-2. Extraperitoneal exposure of the right external iliac artery.

tures, and the incision is extended proximally along its fibers.

Figure 19-3C and D indicates the section of the internal oblique and the transversus. Transection of these two muscles may require sacrificing two or three minor neurovascular bundles encountered during the cutting of these structures.

Proximal and medial retraction of the three sectioned muscles, as well as retraction of the lateral edges of the same structures, exposes the properitoneal adipose tissue (Fig. 19-3E). Detachment of the abdominal contents, starting toward the lower angle of the exposure, facilitates the separation of the peritoneum from the psoas muscle. One should avoid separating the abdominal contents by entering the retroperitoneal space at the upper angle of the incision, which may lead to the quadratus lumborum muscle. After the abdominal contents are retracted and protected with moist laparotomy sheets, the iliac vessels are ready to be exposed (Fig. 19-3F). Two wide retractors of the Deaver type are adequate for retraction and exposure of the entire iliac axis. The ureter must be identified and protected from any undue injury in the course of retraction. Injury to the lymph nodes and lymphatics should be avoided. If they

are injured, ligation should be done routinely to prevent lymphorrhea, which may be troublesome.

Retraction of the upper angle may be difficult, especially in an obese patient, if the aorta is also to be exposed. If necessary, section of the lateral border of the rectus abdominis may facilitate the retraction.

The advantage of this approach is in its easy and clear exposure not only of the iliac axis but also of the bifurcation of the aorta. Pitfalls to be avoided during the mobilization of the iliac artery are injuries to the inferior vena cava or the satellite iliac veins. Another pitfall may be related to the inadvertent sacrifice of the nerves of the internal oblique and transversus muscles.

Closure of the abdominal wall should be meticulous, although hernias after this procedure occur extremely rarely.

Exposure of the left iliac axis is illustrated in Figure 19-4. The approach to the left iliac vessels is similar, if not identical, to the approach to those on the right side. The only difference in exposure is that the aortic bifurcation is more accessible and much easier to mobilize on the left side.

In both right and left exposures, a concomitant lumbar

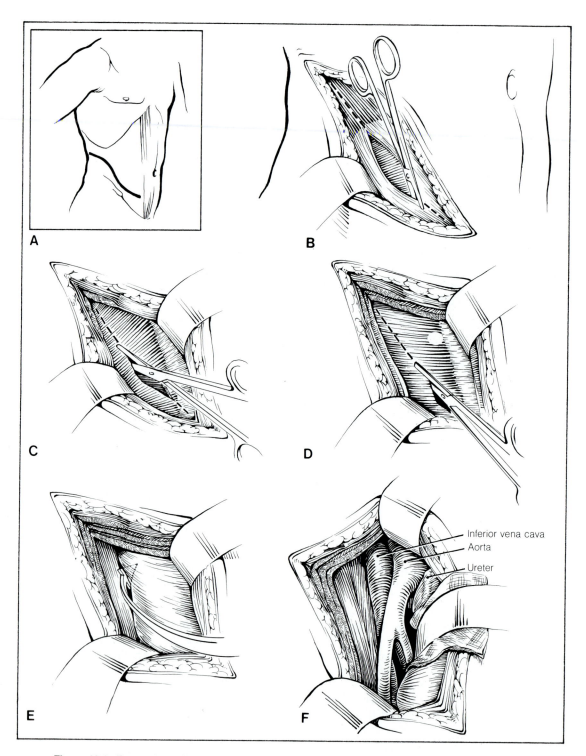

Figure 19-3. Extraperitoneal exposure of the right iliac vessels, including the terminal abdominal aorta.

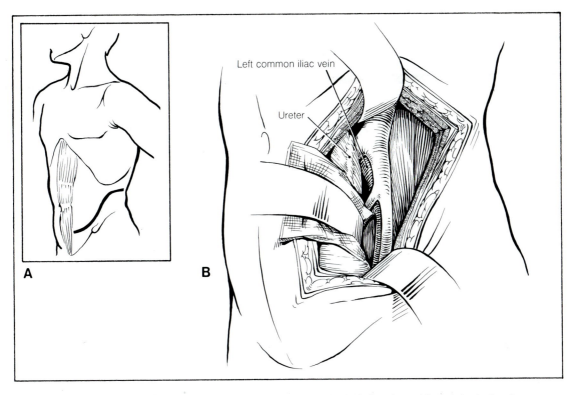

Figure 19-4. Extraperitoneal exposure of the left iliac vessels, including the terminal abdominal aorta.

sympathectomy can be achieved through these extraperitoneal approaches.

COMBINED ILIAC AND FEMORAL EXPOSURES

The iliac and femoral vessels can be approached either by two separate incisions or by a combined abdominal-thigh incision.

Separate Abdominal and Thigh Incisions

If separate incisions are to be made (Fig. 19-6), the two separate approaches to the femoral and iliac vessels are carried out as previously described. Since this combined exposure is normally intended to revascularize the lower extremity through the femoral artery, it is wise to start first by exposing the latter. (See the section Femoral Artery, in Chapter 20.) The iliac exposure is carried out after the quality of the femoral vessels is ascertained.

In this combined procedure, a tunnel between the iliac and femoral regions must be developed for passage of a graft. Proper dilation of the femoral canal is important in preventing a possible constriction at this level.

Combined Abdominal and Thigh Incision

If a combined abdominal-thigh incision is to be used, the skin incision is as indicated in Figure 19-5A. It starts at the anterior axillary line and is directed toward the angle between the lateral border of the rectus abdominis and the inguinal ligament. At this point, it is redirected distally and curved slightly, with its convexity lateral along the femoral vessels. The thigh incision is slightly lateral to the femoral as it is extended along the medial border of the sartorius.

The abdominal incision is first completed in a fashion similar to the extraperitoneal exposure of the iliac vessels (Fig. 19-5B). The external oblique is divided along its fibers. The internal oblique and transversus muscles are transected parallel to the inguinal ligament, and the retroperitoneal space is entered after the abdominal contents are retracted superiorly and medially.

The inguinal ligament is transected about 1 cm lateral to the femoral artery (Fig. 19-5C). It is important to identify the anatomic planes: the aponeurosis of the external oblique, the inguinal ligament, and the iliopubic ramus.

In dividing the inguinal ligament, one should avoid injuring the inferior epigastric and the circumflex iliac arteries found behind this structure. A few smaller arterioles, supplying the adjacent lymph nodes, and a few small venules can be sacrificed without any adverse effect.

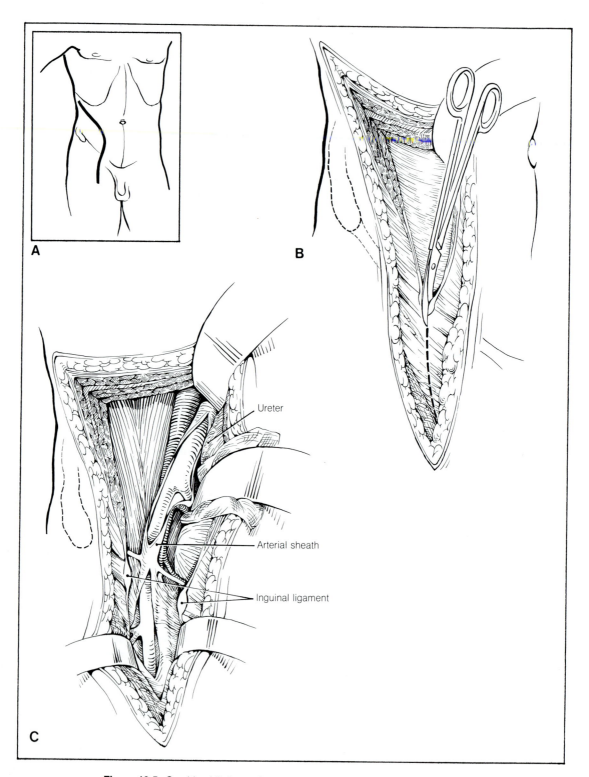

Figure 19-5. Combined iliofemoral exposure with division of the inguinal ligament.

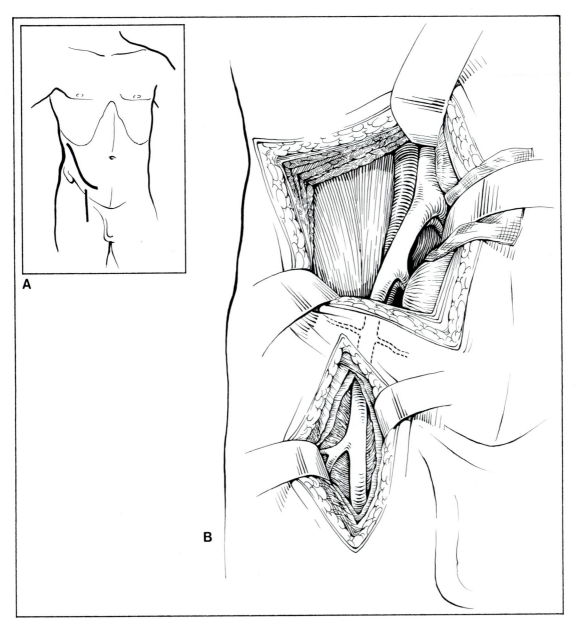

Figure 19-6. Combined iliac and femoral exposures, with separate approaches used.

In dissecting the distal end of the external iliac artery, one may encounter enlarged lymph nodes because of chronically infected ischemic lesions of the foot. Undue trauma to these lymph nodes should be avoided for obvious reasons (lymphorrhea).

In the course of this combined approach to the iliofemoral arteries, extraperitoneal exposure of the terminal abdominal aorta is also possible, being much easier to achieve on the left side. By contrast, on the right side, this approach offers better control of the origin of the inferior vena cava, whereas that of the bifurcation of the aorta is less adequate.

Exposure of the femoral vessels is carried out in similar fashion, as previously described (Fig. 19-5).

One of the critical steps in this combined iliofemoral exposure may be at the time of closure of the inguinal ligament. The anatomic reconstitution must be meticulous and must avoid any stricture of the femoral canal.

The advantages of this combined iliofemoral exposure are obvious. First, all these vessels can be handled under direct vision. Second, should it be necessary to expose the superficial femoral or popliteal artery, further extension of the previous incision can be easily achieved.

NOTE: See the Bibliography at end of Chapter 20.

CHAPTER 20
The Lower Extremity

Henry Haimovici

FEMORAL ARTERY

Anatomic Review

The femoral artery (Fig. 20-1), a direct continuation of the external iliac artery, enters the thigh behind the inguinal ligament (Poupart's ligament) midway between the anterior superior iliac spine and the pubic tubercle. From this point, the artery follows an almost straight course, gradually inclining from the anterior to the posteromedial aspect of the thigh. As a result of this direction, the femoral artery is comparatively superficial in its initial segment but be-

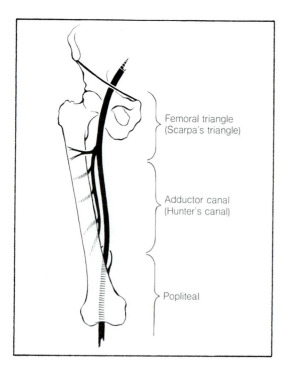

Figure 20-1. Diagram of the femoral artery and its divisions (Scarpa's triangle, Hunter's canal).

comes deeply located at its terminal portion. In its proximal part, it is located in what is known anatomically as the femoral triangle or the triangle of Scarpa. In its distal portion, it is located in an anatomic area known as the adductor or Hunter's canal.

The anatomic landmarks of *Scarpa's triangle* include the soft parts of the root of the thigh. This region is bounded proximally by the inguinal ligament, laterally by the sartorius muscle, and medially by the pectineus and adductor muscles. Distally, the apex of the triangle is formed by the overlapping of these muscles. The roof of this area consists of the fascia lata, which completely covers the space anteriorly. The floor is made up of two inclined planes, which form a well-marked medium groove at their junction. The laterally inclined plane consists of the iliopsoas muscle invested by a thin layer of fascia. In this compartment are included the femoral vessels and nerve and their large branches. Among the latter structures are the termination of the great saphenous vein and the deep subinguinal lymph vessels and glands embedded in a quantity of loose fat tissue. This space communicates with the abdomen through the lacuna vasorum.

Exposure of Femoral Artery in Triangle of Scarpa

The patient is placed in the supine position, with the thigh in abduction and slight external rotation. A curved skin incision is made, extending from above the inguinal ligament and with a concavity medialward, along the medial border of the sartorius (Fig. 20-2A). The incision is carried through the subcutaneous tissue at the site of retraction of the lateral edge of the skin, to avoid injuring the lymphatic vessels or the lymph nodes. Should some of the lymphatics or lymph nodes be divided, their ligation or cauterization should be carried out to avoid any lymphorrhea in the postoperative period. The incision of the deep fascia is then carried out medial to the medial border of the sartorius (Fig. 20-2B). This incision is extended upward toward Poupart's ligament and distal to the apex of the region.

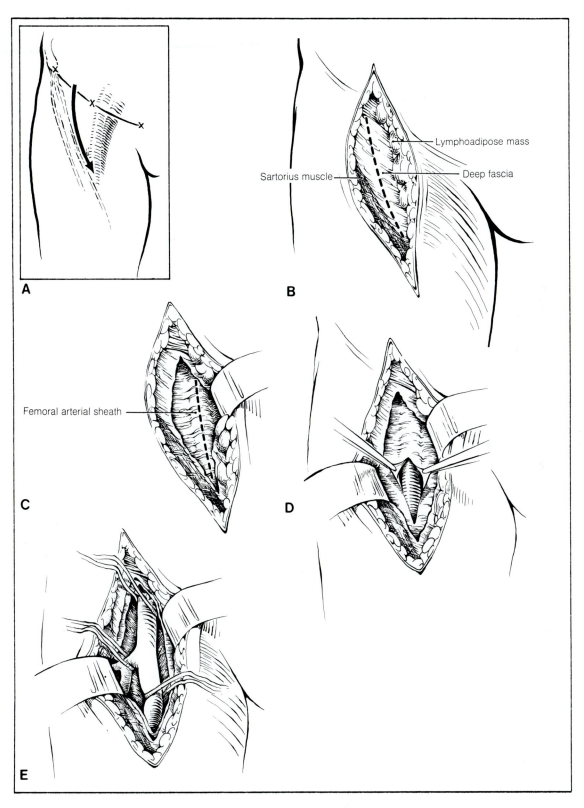

Figure 20-2. Exposure of the femoral artery in Scarpa's triangle.

The arterial sheath is then opened along its entire length, thus enabling the artery to be mobilized (Fig. 20-2C,D). This sheath, a sleevelike prolongation of the fascial envelopment of the abdomen, passes downward into the thigh behind the inguinal ligament. It extends downward as far as the origin of the profunda femoris artery, where it fuses with the outer coat of the femoral vessels. Two septa divide the sheath into arterial, venous, and lymphatic compartments. In the mobilization of the common femoral artery proximally, care should be taken to avoid injuring the epigastric and the deep circumflex iliac arteries, the latter two branches being at the junction between the femoral and the external iliac arteries under Poupart's ligament. After the common femoral is mobilized, umbilical or rubber vessel loops are placed about it (Fig. 20-2E). Next, the superficial femoral artery is mobilized just 1 to 2 cm below the origin of the profunda, and a tape is placed about it in a similar fashion. Slight traction on these two tapes will facilitate the location of the origin of the profunda femoris artery, which is then mobilized by further opening of the sheath that extends around its origin. The profunda emerges posteriorly and usually courses laterally to the main trunk. Anterior to the origin of the profunda there is a fibrous band that has to be incised in order to mobilize it. In so doing, care must be taken not to injure the branches of the profunda femoris vein, which pass in front of the artery. These may be clamped, divided, and ligated. A tape is placed about the origin of the profunda and around some of its major branches.

In addition to the common, superficial, and profunda vessels, the epigastric, circumflex iliac, and a few other branches that may come off the common or superficial femoral also have to be controlled before the surgery of the vessel is undertaken.

In retracting these structures after the exposure of the vessels, it is important that the lymphoadipose tissue situated between Scarpa's fascia and the deep fascia be retracted medially out of the operative field. Through the same incision, if the saphenous vein is to be used as a bypass graft, the procedure shifts to the medial aspect, and the dissection of the vein starts at that level.

Exposure of Superficial Femoral Artery in Hunter's Canal

Brief Anatomic Review

The superficial femoral artery is contained in the adductor or Hunter's canal, which extends from the apex of the femoral triangle to the tendinous hiatus of the adductor magnus muscle. This canal is an intermuscular space on the medial aspect of the middle third of the thigh. Its main structures are the femoral vessels and the saphenous nerve. The boundaries of this canal include the lateral wall formed by the vastus medialis muscle and the posterior wall formed by the adductor longus muscle proximally and the adductor magnus muscle distally. The roof of the canal is a layer of deep fascia running from the adductor longus and magnus muscles to the vastus medialis. The sartorius muscle covers the space.

The femoral artery is bound closely by connective tissue to the femoral vein, which at first lies posterior to and then slightly to the lateral side of the artery. The superior genicular artery (anastomotica magna) branches off from the femoral near its termination. Distal to it, when the artery goes through the adductor hiatus, the artery becomes the popliteal. The saphenous nerve crosses anterior to the femoral artery, and from the tendinous hiatus it passes downward under the sartorius muscle to the distribution over the medial aspect of the leg and ankle.

Exposure of Superficial Femoral Artery

For exposure of the superficial femoral artery (Fig. 20-3), the patient should be in the supine position, with the lower extremity placed in external rotation and the knee flexed (Fig. 20-3A).

The skin incision is made along a line extending from the apex of the femoral triangle to the adductor tubercle. The incision is deepened through the superficial fascia overlying the sartorius (Fig. 20-3B). The saphenous vein is retracted medially. The muscle is then mobilized from its fascial investment, and the roof of the canal is exposed (Fig. 20-3C). The strong fascia is opened, and the femoral vessels are exposed, with the saphenous nerve lying on its anterior surface (Fig. 20-3D). The saphenous nerve is then protected by placing a tape around it and retracting it medially without too much tension. The artery is surrounded by a network of venules that may hamper its dissection and mobilization at this level (Fig. 20-3D). Several muscle branches emerge from the superficial femoral artery at this point, and they may have to be spared. Especially important is the highest genicular artery, located at the lower angle (Fig. 20-3E). Distal to it is the adductor hiatus, which may have to be opened for greater access to the junction between the superficial femoral and popliteal arteries. Usually, at this level there are marked arteriosclerotic changes of the artery.

Variants of these exposures depend on the extent of the pathologic findings in the vessels proximally or distally. If the external iliac artery is also involved, and if it is necessary to expose it, an extraperitoneal approach is indicated. (See the section on Exposure of External Iliac Artery, in Chapter 19.)

Should it be necessary to expose the entire femoral artery, the incision is made from the groin down to the adductor tubercle, with the two incisions combined as described.

POPLITEAL ARTERY

Anatomic Review

The popliteal artery is situated behind the structures of the knee joint and constitutes the longitudinal axis of the region. The popliteal fossa is a lozenge-shaped space consisting of an upper, or femoral, and a lower, or tibial, triangle.

The popliteal artery, a continuation of the superficial femoral artery, enters the superior and medial part of the popliteal space through the tendinous part of the adductor magnus muscle (adductor magnus hiatus). As it passes

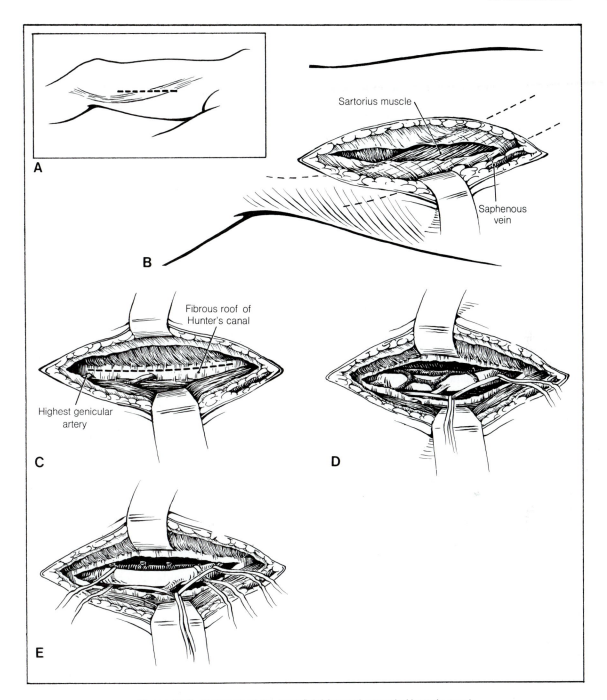

Figure 20-3. Exposure of the superficial femoral artery in Hunter's canal.

through the popliteal space, it inclines laterally along the outer border of the semitendinosus muscle until it reaches the middle of the limb. It then descends vertically to the distal border of the popliteus muscle and terminates by dividing into the anterior and posterior tibial arteries. The popliteal artery throughout its course is placed deeply and lies in direct contact with the posterior ligaments of the knee joint.

Three pairs of branches are given off by the popliteal artery at three different levels and are distributed mainly about the bony part of the knee. The superior genicular

arteries, lateral and medial, originate at the level of the femoral condyles. The middle genicular artery pierces the oblique popliteal ligament and supplies the ligaments and synovial membrane in the interior of the articulation. The inferior genicular arteries, lateral and medial, wind around the front of the knee and anastomose with each other deep to the patellar ligament.

The popliteal vein, formed by the junction of the anterior and posterior tibial veins, lies superficial to the artery, medial to it distally, and lateral to it proximally. The short saphenous vein, which pierces the deep fascia in the lower part of the popliteal space, divides into two branches, one entering the popliteal vein and the other the great saphenous. The popliteal vein and artery are bound wall to wall in a resistant connective tissue sheath, a relationship that explains their simultaneous injury and the formation of an arteriovenous fistula.

The sciatic nerve, with its two branches (tibial and common peroneal), is found at the upper angle of the popliteal space. The two branches continue in their known direction, the tibial along the popliteal vessels and the peroneal leaving the popliteal space at its lower end.

From a surgical point of view, the popliteal artery is divided into proximal and distal segments. Each of these segments can be exposed alone, or it may be necessary sometimes to expose the vessel in its entirety.

Exposure of Popliteal Artery

There are three different approaches to exposure of the popliteal artery: (1) medial, (2) posterior, and (3) mixed posteromedial. The medial exposure may be used for the proximal or distal or the entire popliteal artery.

Medial Exposure of Proximal Popliteal Artery

The patient is placed in the supine position, with the lower extremity in slight external rotation and the knee in 30-degree flexion and supported by a rolled sheet (Fig. 20-4A). The skin incision is made in the lower third of the thigh along the anterior border of the sartorius muscle and is carried through to the superficial fascia (Fig. 20-4B), care being taken not to injure the long saphenous vein, which is located slightly posterior outside the sartorius. After the deep fascia is opened, the sartorius muscle is retracted medially. The dissection is continued from the angle of the upper incision, which is bordered by the vastus medialis laterally and the sartorius medially and posteriorly. By retracting these two muscles, one encounters the tendon of the adductor magnus (Fig. 20-4C,D), which hides the most proximal portion of the popliteal artery at its emergence from the adductor canal. The highest genicular artery pierces the deep fascia; it should be identified and preserved (Fig. 20-4E). The tendon of the adductor magnus at its insertion on the femur is divided to facilitate exposure of the popliteal vessels. A thin fascial structure covering a layer of adipose tissue surrounds the vascular bundle. The vascular sheath is opened longitudinally. The two satellite popliteal veins are located lateral and posterior to the artery. Often, communicating venous tributaries between the medial and lateral popliteal veins cross the artery, necessitating their division and ligation (Fig. 20-4C). The popliteal artery is then freed in its segment chosen for the selected surgical procedure. Usually a 3- to 4-cm length is suitable for its control (Fig. 20-4F). In exposing the popliteal vessels, it is essential to identify the saphenous nerve and retract it out of the field.

The thick adipose tissue layer must be disassociated from the vascular bundle, which is relatively deep and is situated behind the lower portion of the femur shaft. The adipose layer is covered by a thin aponeurotic sheath, which has to be opened before the blood vessels are reached.

The vascular sheath is common to the artery and vein.

The vein has a thick wall and may be confused at times with the artery, to which it is intimately attached by a dense perivascular tissue. Because of this tissue, the separation of the two vessels may sometimes be difficult. The artery is usually surrounded by the venous plexus formed by collateral veins between the two medial and lateral popliteal veins.

The advantages of medial exposure stem from the fact that the supine position of the patient affords easy access also to the femoral artery and to the saphenous vein without any difficulty and with relatively little trauma.

Exposure of Entire Popliteal Artery

As in the previous exposure, the patient is placed in the supine position, with the extremity in slight external rotation and the knee in a 30-degree flexion, supported with a rolled sheet placed under it. A curved skin incision is made along the anterior border of the sartorius muscle in the lower one third of the thigh and extended across the knee joint along the posteromedial edge of the tibia (Fig. 20-5A). The deep fascia is incised anteriorly to the sartorius muscle, and the popliteal space is entered below the adductor magnus tendon, in the lower angle of which four muscles are identified and mobilized at their lower insertions. The sartorius, semimembranosus, gracilis, and semitendinosus muscles are inserted in that order and are transected near the tibia (Fig. 20-5B). Next, the origin of the medial head of the gastrocnemius muscle is divided near the medial femoral condyle through its musculotendinous portion.

After division of these muscle insertions, the exposure of the popliteal vessels from the proximal end through their division into anterior and posterior tibial arteries becomes easy. As in the previously described procedure, the adipose tissue layer and its thin fascia are displaced until the vascular bundle is exposed. The artery lies medial to it, and the veins are posterior and lateral to it. A venous plexus is usually present around the artery after the sheath has been opened. These communicating vessels between the two popliteal veins have to be dissected away from the arterial wall for free access to the artery (Fig. 20-5C).

The distal portion of the popliteal may not be entirely accessible, in which instance the soleus muscle may have to be split open to expose the bifurcation of the artery.

After the vascular procedure is completed, the tendons and muscular structures are reconstituted, with interrupted mattress sutures used for the approximation of the divided ends. Of these, the reconstitution of the medial head of the gastrocnemius is most important. Because catgut ligatures may not hold, it is important that the sutures be of nonabsorbable material. With this type of repair, there is no weakness or difficulty of the knee joint postoperatively. Although the operative time is prolonged because of the reconstitution of the divided musculotendinous structures, the technical requirements for good exposure of the popliteal artery at this level justify the extra effort put into it.

Exposure of Distal Popliteal Artery

For exposure of the distal popliteal artery (Fig. 20-6), the patient is placed in the supine position, with the knee flexed about 30 degrees and supported by a rolled sheet under it. A medial exposure is used, as for the previous two approaches to the popliteal artery.

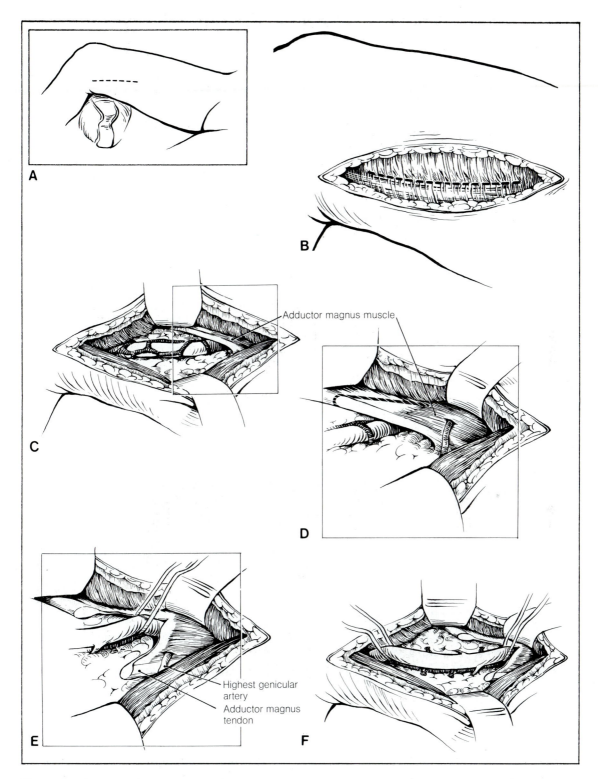

Figure 20-4. Medial exposure of the proximal popliteal artery. **A.** Position of the lower extremity, knee flexed and supported by a bolster. **B.** Deep fascia incision, anterior to the sartorius muscle. **C.** Exposure of the proximal popliteal artery and adductor magnus tendon. **D.** Close-up view of the adductor magnus covering the proximal end of the artery. **E.** Division of the adductor magnus tendon for better exposure of the vessel. **F.** Popliteal artery freed of the venous plexus and mobilized between two tapes.

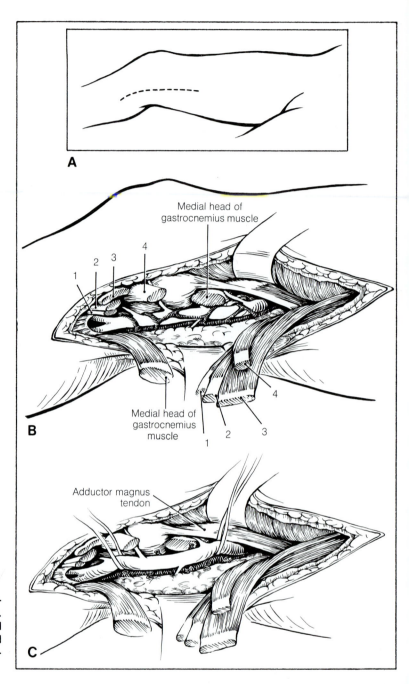

Figure 20-5. Medial exposure of the entire popliteal artery. **A.** Position of the extremity and the line of incision. **B.** Identification of divided muscles covering the popliteal artery: (1) semitendinosus, (2) gracilis, (3) sartorius, and (4) semimembranosus muscles. **C.** Popliteal artery exposed, freed, and mobilized between two tapes.

The skin incision starts about 1 cm below the posterior border of the medial condyle of the femur and is extended parallel to the posteromedial border of the tibia and about 1 cm behind it (Fig. 20-6A). The length of the incision is about 8 to 10 cm. In carrying out the skin incision, one should take care to avoid injury to the saphenous vein except for its branches, which are divided and ligated.

The crural fascia is exposed and incised below the tendons of the semitendinosus and gracilis. After the deep fascia is incised from end to end, the medial head of the gastrocnemius is retracted posteriorly and medially, thus exposing the soleus muscle and the neurovascular bundle (Fig. 20-6D). The latter is usually situated deep against the bony surface, which is covered by the popliteus.

The vascular sheath is opened, and the first structures in the bundle to appear are usually two popliteal veins, one posteromedial and the other anterolateral. As in the previous segments of the popliteal, a number of communicating veins between the two popliteals are present, necessitating their division and ligation to expose the artery. Its distal dissection and mobilization may have to be achieved by division of the arcade of the soleus muscle, which covers the bifurcation of the popliteal at this level. The tibial nerve, which lies medial and posterior to the vessels, should be protected against any possible injury during the retraction of the artery. Tapes are placed about the popliteal artery (Fig. 20-6E). By a combined motion of slight elevation and medial traction, the artery comes into view.

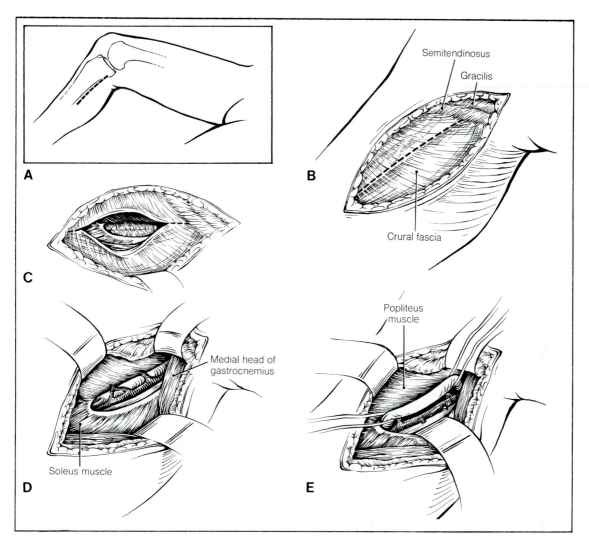

Figure 20-6. Medial exposure of the distal popliteal artery. **A.** Position of the limb, knee flexed, and the line of skin incision. **B.** Exposure of the crural fascia and the line of incision. **C.** Fascia incised, exposing the vascular bundle. **D.** Exposure of the distal popliteal vessels and the arcade of the soleus muscle. **E.** Popliteal freed and mobilized.

Advantages of exposing the distal popliteal artery are that at this level there are usually no significant collateral vessels arising from either popliteal or from the posterior tibial and anterior tibial arteries below. Although this segment is smaller than the proximal popliteal, the infragenual segment is of sufficient caliber for easy graft attachment. Of particular significance has been the finding that this segment tends to be better preserved and is usually free of atheromatous degenerative changes in comparison with the proximal popliteal.

Should the exposure just described be insufficient, a proximal extension of the incision with division of the tendons may be necessary, as described previously for the exposure of the entire popliteal artery.

Posterior Approach to Popliteal Artery
The classic approach to the popliteal artery is the posterior approach (Fig. 20-7). The neurovascular structures appear superficial, and their exposure necessitates no muscle sec-

tions. If the vascular procedure is confined to the popliteal artery, this approach to the vessel is obviously advantageous. However, under other circumstances, there are a number of disadvantages that contraindicate its exposure through the posterior incision.

The patient is placed in a prone position, with the leg slightly flexed and supported by a small pillow under the ankle.

The length of the skin incision may depend on whether only the proximal or the entire popliteal is exposed. In the former, a median vertical incision above the popliteal fold is carried out. For the lower popliteal, the skin incision starts from the middle of the flexion fold of the knee and extends distally in a straight line in the depression between the two heads of the gastrocnemius.

Exposure of the entire popliteal artery requires an extended skin incision both above and below the knee flexion fold (Fig. 20-7A). The classic median skin incision crossing the flexion fold of the joint perpendicularly may result in

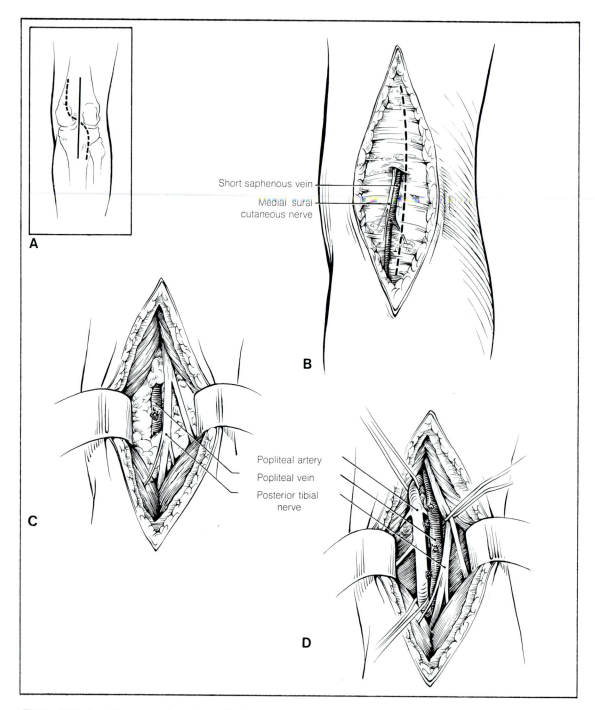

Short saphenous vein

Medial sural cutaneous nerve

A

B

Popliteal artery

Popliteal vein

Posterior tibial nerve

C

D

Figure 20-7. Posterior approach to the popliteal artery. **A.** Lines of incision. **B.** Popliteal fascia with its line of incision and short saphenous vein accompanied by the medial sural cutaneous nerve. **C, D.** Transfascial exposure of the neurovascular bundle.

a retractile scar, thus preventing a full extension of the knee joint. Because of this possibility, an S-shaped skin incision is used in most instances, as indicated in Figure 20-7A.

After the skin flaps are reflected, the deep fascia is opened longitudinally in the midline. The short saphenous vein pierces the fascia at this level, as does the posterior

cutaneous nerve of the thigh (Fig. 20-7B). After the deep fascia is opened, the tibial and peroneal nerves are identified. The sciatic nerve can also be identified at a more proximal level where the nerve usually divides into the two branches. The neural structures are the most superficial and lateral. The popliteal vein is medial to the nerve and can easily be exposed by following the short saphenous vein. The sheath surrounding the vessels is opened in the same fashion as in the exposure described above. The artery lies medially and is the deepest structure of the three in the neurovascular bundle.

The distal portion of the popliteal artery is usually surrounded by a venous plexus resulting from the communicating branches between the two popliteal veins. The two heads of the gastrocnemius must be retracted to allow access to the distal portion of the popliteal. If more distal dissection is necessary, the soleus muscle must be exposed, because the neurovascular bundle plunges under it. After incision of the latter, the bifurcation of the popliteal artery into the anterior tibial and the tibioperoneal trunk and its bifurcation into the posterior tibial and peroneal can be easily exposed.

LEG ARTERIES

Anatomic Review

The leg arteries are situated between the inferior part of the tuberosity of the tibia and the bases of the malleoli. The neurovascular bundles of the leg are situated in compartments provided by the deep crural fascia and its septa.

Figure 20-8 depicts a cross section through the upper third of the leg. As indicated in this diagram, the leg has four compartments: (1) anterior, (2) lateral, (3) superficial posterior, and (4) deep posterior.

The *anterior compartment* is bounded anteriorly by the enveloping fascia, posteriorly by the interosseous membrane and the anterior surface of the fibula, medially by the lateral surface of the tibia, and laterally by the anterior intermuscular septum. It contains the anterior tibial, extensor digitorum longus, extensor hallucis longus, and peroneus tertius muscles, the anterior tibial vessels, and the anterior tibial nerve (deep peroneal).

The *lateral compartment* is the smallest and is situated between the peroneal intermuscular septa. It contains the termination of the common peroneal nerve, the superficial peroneal nerve, and the peroneal longus and brevis muscles.

The *superficial posterior compartment* comprises the gastrocnemius, soleus, and plantaris muscles. The combined tendons of the two previous muscles are the tendo calcaneus, or Achilles tendon, which inserts into the distal half of the posterior surface of the calcaneus.

The *deep posterior compartment* is demarcated from the superficial muscles by a fascial septum that extends between the fibula and the medial border of the tibia. The posterior tibial muscle arises from the interosseous membrane and adjoining part of the tibia and fibula. In addition, the flexor digitorum longus and the flexor hallucis longus arise from the posterior surface of the tibia and the fibula, respectively. The posterior tibial and the peroneal arteries and their satellite veins, as well as the tibial nerve, are situated in the deep posterior compartment.

Exposure of Posterior Tibial Artery

Proximal Segment
For the exposure of the proximal posterior tibial artery, a 10 cm skin incision is made at mid-calf level behind the posteromedial border of the tibia (Fig. 20-9A). After incision of the deep fascia (Fig. 20-9B), the gastrocnemius muscle is retracted posteriorly. Exposure of the posterior tibial vessels can be carried out either through a transsoleus division or by detaching the latter muscle from its tibial insertion. Our preference is the former approach. The soleus is transected along its fibers, and the posterior tibial vessels are easily exposed (Fig. 20-9C). The artery is freed from its surrounding venous plexus and its two satellite veins. Care

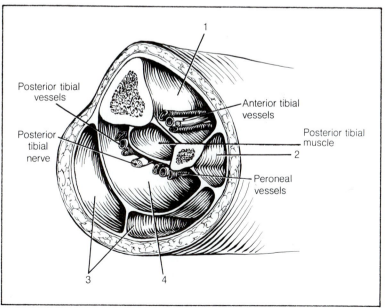

Figure 20-8. Cross section through the upper third of the leg, depicting the location of the three major neurovascular bundles and the four compartments: (1) anterior, (2) lateral, (3) superficial posterior, and (4) deep posterior.

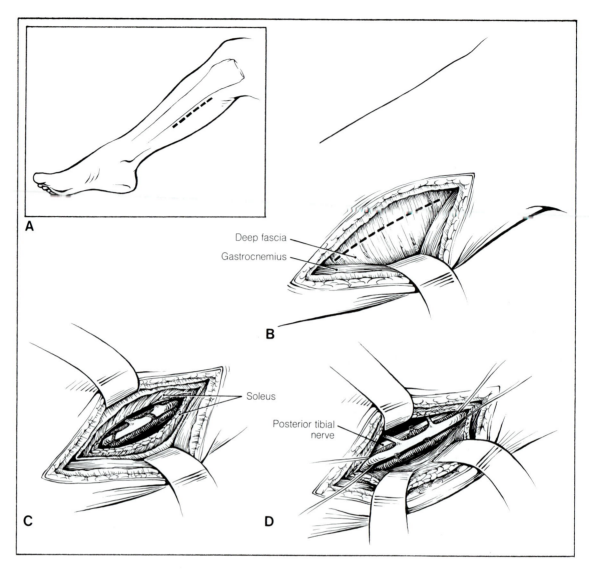

Figure 20-9. Medial exposure of the proximal posterior tibial artery. **A.** Line of skin incision. **B.** Exposure of the deep fascia and its line of incision. **C.** Transsoleus muscle exposure of the vascular bundle. **D.** Freeing and mobilization of the posterior tibial artery.

should be taken to avoid injury to the posterior tibial nerve in the process of mobilizing the vessels (Fig. 20-9D).

Distal Segment

Exposure of the distal posterior tibial artery is carried out in the lower third of the leg above the internal malleolus (Fig. 20-10A). After incision of the superficial fascia, the Achilles tendon is mobilized and retracted posteriorly. The deep fascia is then incised anteriorly, thus exposing the posterior tibial vessels (Fig. 20-10B). The flexor digitorum longus and flexor hallucis longus are situated posterior to the vessels. As in the preceding technique, the artery is freed after division of the communicating veins between the two tibial veins (Fig. 20-10C). The posterior tibial nerve in the lower third is situated posterior to the vascular bundle and should be carefully retracted to avoid any possible injury to it.

Exposure of Anterior Tibial Artery

The anterior tibial artery is composed of two distinct segments: (1) the upper third, or arched, segment, situated behind and immediately medial to the neck of the fibula and crossing the interosseous membrane, and (2) the anterior tibial trunk proper, coursing the entire length of the anterior tibial compartment.

Exposure of the arched segment of the anterior tibial artery is best carried out through the transfibular approach (see below).

Exposure of Upper Segment

The patient is placed in the supine position, with the knees slightly flexed and supported by a rolled sheet, the foot being maintained in slight internal rotation. A long skin incision of about 8 to 10 cm is made along the classic line

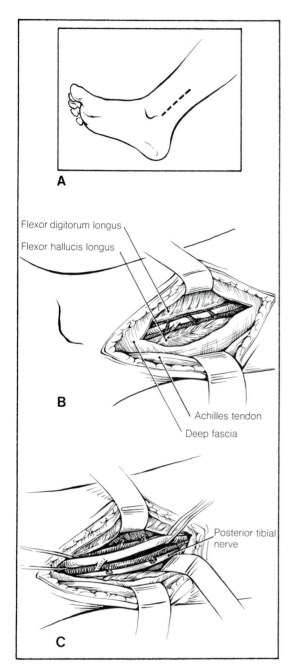

A

Flexor digitorum longus

Flexor hallucis longus

B

Achilles tendon

Deep fascia

C

Posterior tibial nerve

Figure 20-10. Medial exposure of the distal posterior tibial artery. **A.** Line of skin incision.

for the ligature of the artery (Fig. 20-11A). Proximally, this line starts medial to the head of the fibula and ends in the middle of the anterior surface of the ankle on the lateral visible edge of the tendon of the anterior tibial muscle.

The skin incision is carried down to the fascia. It is important to determine, by digital palpation, the groove between the anterior tibial and extensor digitorum longus. With the index finger, one separates the interspace of the muscles until it reaches the neurovascular bundle located on the anterior surface of the interosseous membrane. The vessels are located deep to the extensor and lie slightly lateral to the incision. By gentle retraction of the muscles,

the neurovascular bundle is exposed. The dissection of the artery from the satellite veins and anterior tibial nerve can then be achieved (Fig. 20-11). The mobilization of the various components of the neurovascular bundle may sometimes be difficult when the muscles are heavy and bulging. So that any undue pressure and trauma can be avoided, it is best to extend the incision both proximally and distally to release the pressure from the adjacent structure.

Exposure of Distal Segment
The skin incision, 6 to 8 cm long, follows the same line for the exposure of the anterior tibial artery (Fig. 20-12A), as mentioned above.

The superficial fascia is opened along the same line as the skin incision. The tendon of the anterior tibial muscle is identified, mobilized, and retracted medially, and the tendon of the extensor digitorum longus is retracted laterally (Fig. 20-12B).

The neurovascular bundle is situated lateral to the anterior tibial muscle and medial to the extensor digitorum longus. The tibial artery is situated in the background and is accompanied by its two veins. The anterior tibial nerve is located medial to it.

At this level, the artery is more superficial and is of easy access. Extension of the exposure can be carried out proximally by extending the incision and separating the muscles as indicated or, if necessary, distally toward the dorsalis pedis by dividing the annular ligament of the ankle (Fig. 20-12C).

Combined Exposure of Distal Popliteal Artery and Its Trifurcation

Exposure of the distal popliteal artery and of the posterior tibial and peroneal arteries can be achieved by the medial approach as described above. Although this approach offers easy access to the distal popliteal and posterior tibial, exposure and mobilization of the peroneal may be difficult in some instances. Under these circumstances, a lateral exposure may offer greater advantages.

Medial Exposure
The distal popliteal artery and the tibioperoneal trunk, the latter a direct continuation of the former, frequently display a combination of lesions of variable degrees, which, if inadequately repaired, may be the main cause of femoropopliteal reconstructive failures.

In *atherosclerotic lesions*, the popliteal-tibioperoneal trunk junction is often the site of stenotic or occlusive changes. This arterial segment as it enters the deep compartment of the leg is in contact with the tendinous arch of the soleus. As a result of its passage through the arch, this arterial segment undergoes chronic microtrauma that leads to mural changes, not unlike the arteriosclerotic changes in the femoral-popliteal junction in Hunter's canal. Palma coined the term "soleus syndrome" for the arterial lesion of the popliteal-tibioperoneal junction, thus identifying its initiating cause.

The technique for combined exposure of the distal popliteal and its leg branches includes the following steps: (1)

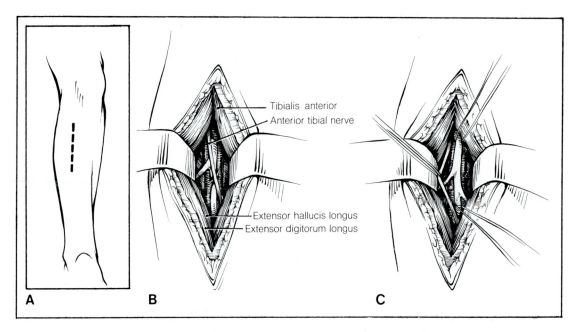

Figure 20-11. Anterolateral exposure of the proximal anterior tibial artery. **A.** Line of skin incision. **B.** Exposure of the neurovascular bundle. **C.** Mobilized anterior tibial artery and retraction of the anterior tibial nerve.

medial leg exposure of the infragenual popliteal as described under Exposure of Distal Popliteal Artery, (2) extension of the skin incision by 4 to 5 inches and exposure of the soleus muscle, (3) splitting of the arcade of the soleus and part of its muscular portion to allow adequate access to the neurovascular bundle (a variant of transecting of the soleus over the neurovascular structures is detachment of the muscle from its insertion on the tibia and retracting it laterally), (4) freeing of the tibioperoneal trunk from its satellite veins and posterior tibial nerve, and excision of the venous plexus surrounding the artery for its adequate

mobilization, and (5) identifying and mobilizing the trifurcation (Fig. 20-13).

In *popliteal artery embolism* with propagating thrombosis into the tibioperoneal trunk and beyond, complete exposure of these critical vessels will allow a thromboembolectomy under direct vision, especially if the thrombus extends into the anterior tibial artery. When the Fogarty catheter is introduced, even as close as the distal popliteal, it is often difficult, if not impossible, to direct the catheter into the anterior tibial because of its nearly right-angle takeoff. To obviate this difficulty whenever indicated, one should perform the

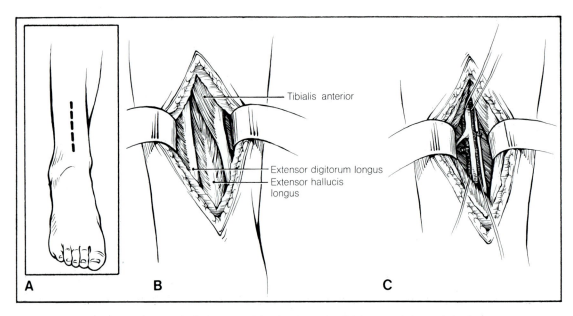

Figure 20-12. Anterolateral exposure of the distal anterior tibial artery. **A.** Line of skin incision.

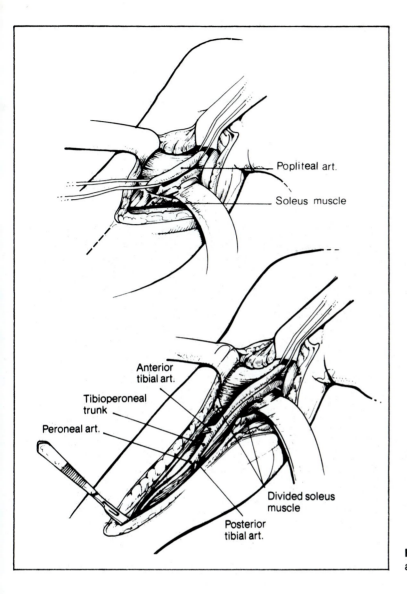

Anterior
tibial art.

Tibioperoneal
trunk

Peroneal art.

Divided soleus
muscle

Posterior
tibial art.

Popliteal art.

Soleus muscle

Figure 20-13. Combined exposure of the distal popliteal artery and its trifurcation.

arteriotomy on the tibioperoneal trunk opposite the origin of the anterior tibial.

Lateral or Transfibular Exposure

This approach offers easy access not only to the peroneal but also to the distal popliteal and the anterior and posterior tibials.

Exposure through the lateral approach by the transfibular route (Fig. 20-14) follows essentially the method described by Henry, to which a few minor modifications were introduced subsequently by others.

The patient is placed in the supine position, with the leg semiflexed and internally rotated. The skin incision begins over the lower part of the biceps tendon and is carried distally below the knee over the length of the fibula for approximately 12 to 15 cm. It begins 5 to 6 cm above the head of the fibula and continues about the same length distally (Fig. 20-14A). The landmarks for the skin incision are the cord of the biceps tendon above, the head of the fibula in the center, and the groove that separates the soleus

from the fibular head distally. This groove is the key to the plane of cleavage between the peroneal and calf muscles.

After the skin and superficial fascia are divided at the upper end of the incision, the deep fascia is opened at the medial edge of the biceps tendon. The common peroneal nerve is exposed and is placed on a rubber vessel loop for gentle traction. The division of the deep fascia is carried downward along the course of the nerve along the posterior margin of the biceps tendon. The fascial origin of the peroneus longus muscle lies directly over the groove in which the nerve passes forward across the neck of the fibula. This fascia is divided. A definite plane, the lateral intermuscular septum, between the soleus muscle posteriorly and the peroneus longus muscle anteriorly, is easily developed, and, when the muscles are separated, the lateral border of the fibula is immediately exposed (Fig. 20-14B). By the use of sharp dissection and a periosteal elevator, the periosteum can be readily stripped from the fibula and its division accomplished by means of a Gigli saw (Fig. 20-14C).

Although the fibula head can be removed without caus-

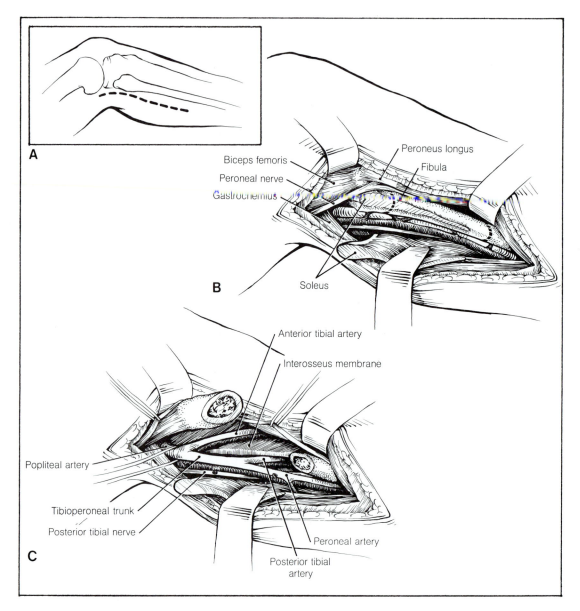

Figure 20-14. Transfibular approach to the distal popliteal artery and its three branches. **A.** Line of skin incision. **B.** Transsoleus exposure and freeing of the fibula. **C.** Resected fibula and exposure of the distal popliteal artery, anterior tibial artery, tibioperoneal trunk, and the peroneal artery.

ing any instability of the knee joint, adequate exposure of the distal popliteal artery and its three branches can be achieved without removing it. The upper third or half of the fibula is resected subperiosteally, distal to its head. The ends of the severed fibula are smoothed with rongeurs or beveled laterally to avoid any injury to the adjacent structures, especially to the peroneal nerve.

The medial aspect of the periosteum is incised. Proximal and distal dissection reveals the presence of the lower popliteal segment and its three branches.

Mobilization of the selected artery is achieved as previously described in the other techniques for the leg arteries. The entire arterial tree is now easily accessible, which thus makes possible the direct evaluation of the entire outflow tract of the leg.

Pitfalls to be avoided are injury to the peroneal nerve and the adjacent veins or arteries. Resection of the fibula per se does not result in any subsequent difficulties.

Advantages of this exposure are multiple: The arch of the anterior tibial, deeply situated, is accessible without resulting in injury to it or in subsequent hemorrhage, which may occur through another approach.

With the retraction of the soleus muscle posteriorly and the peroneus longus muscle anteriorly, the vessels are easily seen. The resected portion of the bone is not replaced.

Another advantage of this approach is that the procedures involving bypass grafts from the femoral or popliteal levels can be carried out with the patient in the supine position as indicated.

It offers the possibility of performing a local endarterectomy under direct vision with good control of the upper and lower parts of the vessel, a method that cannot be easily achieved by the medial approach.

DORSALIS PEDIS

Anatomic Review

The dorsalis pedis artery is a continuation of the anterior tibial and passes forward from the ankle joint along the medial (tibial) side of the dorsum of the foot to the proximal part of the first intermetatarsal space, where it divides into two branches, the first dorsal metatarsal and the deep plantar (Fig. 20-15).

In its course, the vessel rests on the articular capsule of the ankle joint, the talus, navicular, and second cuneiform bones. Near its termination, it is crossed by the first tendon of the extensor digitorum brevis. On the medial (tibial) side is the tendon of the extensor hallucis longus, and on its lateral (fibular) side, the first tendon of the extensor digitorum longus. The artery is accompanied by two satellite veins and is covered by the skin, fascia, and cruciate ligament; near its termination, it is crossed by the first tendon of the extensor digitorum brevis.

Branches
On its medial side, the branches are thin and usually connect with the plantar branches of the posterior tibial. On the lateral side, the branches are much larger (Fig. 20-15).

The medial tarsal arteries are two or three small branches that ramify on the medial border of the foot and join the medial malleolar network. The lateral tarsal artery passes in an arched direction laterally and supplies the extensor digitorum brevis and the joints of the tarsus.

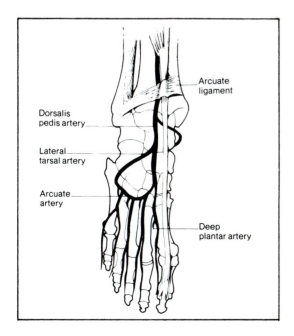

Figure 20-15. Diagram of dorsalis pedis artery and its major branches.

The arcuate artery arises a little anterior to the lateral tarsal artery and passes laterally to anastomose with the lateral tarsal and lateral plantar arteries. This vessel gives off the second, third, and fourth dorsal metatarsal arteries.

The first dorsal metatarsal artery, the termination of the dorsalis pedis, courses forward on the first interosseous space and, at the cleft between the first and second toes, divides into two branches, one of which passes beneath the tendon of the extensor hallucis longus and is distributed to the medial border of the great toe. The other bifurcates to supply the adjoining side of the great and second toes.

The deep plantar artery descends into the sole of the foot between the two heads of the first interosseous dorsalis and unites with the termination of the lateral plantar artery to complete the plantar arch. It sends a branch along the medial side of the great toe and continues forward along the first interosseous space as the first plantar metatarsal artery, which bifurcates for the supply of the adjacent side of the first and second toes.

Exposure of Dorsalis Pedis

Exposure of the dorsalis pedis is carried out close to the ankle and extends about 2 to 3 inches distally (Fig. 20-16). The incision is carried down through the skin, subcutaneous tissue, fascia, and the cruciate ligament. As mentioned, the artery is accompanied by two satellite veins and the termination of the deep peroneal (anterior tibial) nerve. In mobilizing the artery, care should be taken to avoid damaging the collaterals, which not only supply the dorsum of the foot but in the absence of a posterior tibial provide also the main inflow to the plantar arteries.

In reconstructing the leg arteries in occlusive arterial disease of the infrainguinal arteries, it is essential to determine the patency of the pedal vessels, both dorsal and plantar, and the degree of patency, an important index for achieving successful revascularization of the most distal part of the limb.

PLANTAR ARTERIES

Anatomic Review

The posterior tibial artery in its most distal parts approaches the medial side of the leg. At its bifurcation, it is situated midway between the medial malleolus and the medial process of the calcaneal tuberosity. Here it divides beneath the origin of the abductor hallucis into the medial and lateral plantar arteries.

The *medial plantar artery*, much smaller than the lateral, passes forward along the medial side of the foot. At the base of the first metatarsal, it passes along the medial border of the first toe, anastomosing with the first dorsal metatarsal artery (Fig. 20-17). Small superficial digital branches accompany digital branches of the medial plantar nerve and join the plantar metatarsal arteries of the first three spaces.

The *lateral plantar artery*, much larger than the medial, passes laterally and forward to the base of the fifth metatarsal bone. It unites with the deep plantar branch of the

Image labels: Arcuate ligament, Dorsalis pedis artery, Lateral tarsal artery, Arcuate artery, Deep plantar artery

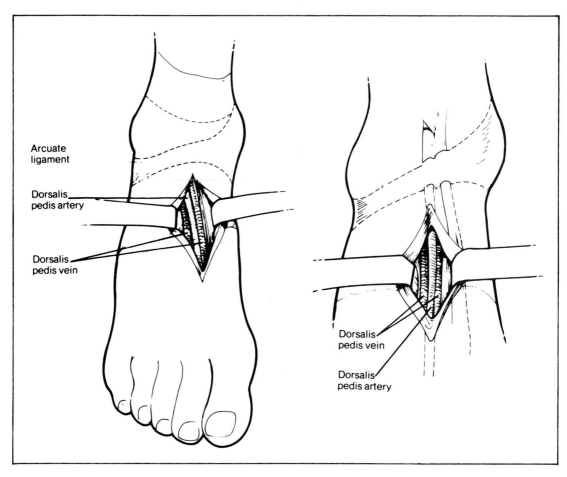

Figure 20-16. Exposure of the dorsalis pedis (see text for details).

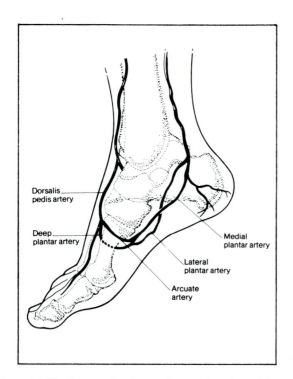

Figure 20-17. Diagram of major arteries and branches of the foot seen in the lateral position.

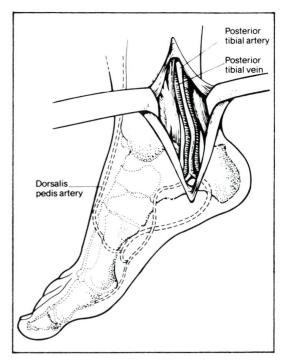

Figure 20-18. Exposure of posterior tibial artery and its bifurcation (see text for details).

dorsalis pedis artery, thus completing the plantar arch. The arch is deeply situated and extends from the base of the fifth metatarsal bone to the proximal part of the first interosseous space to complete the plantar arch. It is convexed forward and lies below the base of the second, third, and fourth metatarsal bones and the corresponding interossei muscles. The plantar arch, besides distributing numerous branches to the muscles, skin, fasciae, and the sole, gives off the perforating and plantar metatarsal branches.

Exposure of Terminal Posterior Tibial Artery and Origin of Plantar Arteries

Revascularization of the plantar structures via the plantar branches can be achieved by implanting the graft behind the medial malleolus (Fig. 20-18). By division of the laciniate ligament, which covers the tendons, the blood vessels and the nerve are exposed at the junction between the heel and the plantar surface. In the presence of complete occlusion of the posterior tibial, indirect revascularization of the plantar flap can best be achieved by revascularizing the dorsalis pedis, provided the collaterals of the lateral plantar artery anastomose with the plantar branches. Repair of plantar arteries may be indicated in traumatic lesions and may require microvascular technique, these branches being otherwise too small for reanastomosis.

BIBLIOGRAPHY

Anson BJ, McVay CB: Surgical Anatomy, 5th ed. Philadelphia, Saunders, 1971, p 1241.

Arnulf G, Benichoux R: Découverte large de la fémoropoplitée (tiers inférieur de la fémorale et totalité de la poplitée). Lyon Chir 44:203, 1949.

Cormier JM, Sautot J, et al.: Nouveau traité de technique chirurgicale. Artères Veines, Lymphatiques 5:628, 1970.

DeBakey ME, Creech O Jr, Morris GC: Aneurysm of thoracoabdominal aorta involving the celiac, superior mesenteric and renal arteries. Ann Surg 144:549, 1956.

Elkin DC: Exposure of blood vessels. JAMA 132:421, 1946.

Elkins RC, DeMeester TR, Brawley RK: Surgical exposure of the upper abdominal aorta and its branches. Surgery 70:622, 1971.

Feller I, Woodburne RT: Surgical anatomy of the abdominal aorta. Ann Surg [Suppl] 154:239, 1961.

Fiolle J, Delmas J: Découverte des Vaisseaux Profonds par des Voies d'Accès Larges. Paris, Masson et Cie, 1940.

Haimovici H: Arterial circulation of the extremities, in Schwartz CJ, Werthessen NT, Wolf A (eds): Structure and Function of the Circulation. New York, Plenum Press, 1980, vol 1, pp 425–485.

Haimovici H, Steinman C, et al.: Excision of a saccular aneurysm of the upper abdominal aorta involving the major branches, iliac-visceral revascularization via bypass graft. Ann Surg 159:368, 1964.

Henry AK: Extensile Exposure, 2d ed. Baltimore, Williams & Wilkins, 1957, p 320.

Lacombe M: Voies d'abord des artères des membres, in Techniques Chirurgicales. Chirurgie vasculaire 43010, 43020, Encyclopédie Médico-Chirurgicale, Paris.

Palma EC: The soleus syndrome: Hemodynamic arteriosclerosis of the posterior tibial artery and its two branches treatment. J Cardiovasc Surg 19:615, 1978.

Rob C: Extraperitoneal approach to the abdominal aorta. Surgery 53:87, 1963.

Shumacker HB Jr: Midline extraperitoneal exposure of the abdominal aorta and iliac arteries. Surg Gynecol Obstet 135:791, 1972.

PART III
Basic Arterial Techniques

CHAPTER 21
Vascular Sutures and Anastomoses

Henry Haimovici and Frank J. Veith

The history of vascular sutures and anastomoses is that of the beginning of blood vessel surgery itself (Chapter 1). It was not until 1889 that a successful repair of arteries was achieved by Jassinowsky.[1] He used fine curved needles and fine silk and made interrupted stitches placed close together but avoided penetrating the intima. In 1899, Dörfler[2] published the essential features of his method, which consisted of continuous sutures embracing all the coats of the vessel. He was the first to point out that the penetration of the intima did not lead to any changes or interfere with the patency of the lumen. In 1901, Clermont[3] reunited successfully the ends of a divided inferior vena cava by means of a continuous fine silk suture.

In 1900, Carrel[4] began his pioneering studies of vascular anastomoses. In the beginning, his method differed from Dörfler's in that he avoided penetrating the intima. Later, together with Guthrie, he discontinued avoiding the intima and instead included it in suturing the vessel. Carrel and Guthrie[5] added other modifications to this technique until it was well adapted for arterioarterial, venovenous, or arteriovenous anastomoses.

The list of surgeons who contributed before and after the basic principles were evolved by Carrel is a long one. Suffice it to mention only that, since the advent of the contemporary vascular era, a number of further improvements were made to meet the needs of newer and more complex vascular techniques.

EXPOSURE AND MOBILIZATION OF ARTERIES

After the various anatomic layers covering the vessels have been divided and the involved vascular bundle has been exposed, attention is directed to the actual dissection and mobilization of the artery or vein or both.

If the vessels are surrounded by a vascular sheath, as most are, the latter can be lifted off and opened. A vascular sheath is a tubular structure investing both the artery and its adjacent vein. Its structural characteristics are variable and depend on the location and the specific segment of the vessel. Usually a thin layer of cellular tissue separates the sheath from the vascular wall.

The ease of exposing and mobilizing an artery or vein depends largely on whether the vessel is normal or diseased.

A *normal artery* can be easily mobilized by identifying and opening its sheath (Fig. 21-1A,B). Often this procedure can be facilitated by ligating and dividing small crossing veins that course between larger accompanying veins, particularly those which parallel arteries peripheral to the groin. After incision of the sheath along its axis, the artery is freed on each side by means of the blunt tip of curved scissors (Fig. 21-1C). In dissecting its posterior wall, great care is necessary to avoid injuring a possible invisible branch. This is achieved by using the tip of a Mixter clamp, which facilitates the dissection from one side of the artery to the other until the clamp passes behind the artery without difficulty. Then an umbilical or silicon rubber tape is passed around the artery (Fig. 21-1D). By lifting the artery with the tape, the dissection can proceed proximally and distally under direct vision.

Exposure of a major artery with a significant branch is made by first mobilizing the main trunk above and below the branch, and then freeing the latter (Fig. 21-2A,B).

A similar procedure is used in mobilizing a bifurcation (Fig. 21-2C). In doing so, care must be taken to avoid injuring the collateral vessels as well as the adjacent vein and its tributaries (Fig. 21-2D).

A *diseased artery* is often more difficult to mobilize because of loss of identity of its sheath as a result of perivascular fibrosis. Injection of a few milliliters of saline solution or procaine under the superficial layer of the sheath may help in lifting it from the underlying artery. After a cleavage plane is developed with the tip of blunt scissors or a fine clamp, the sheath is opened longitudinally. Mobilization of the diseased artery, however, may be more laborious and difficult than for a normal one because of extensive

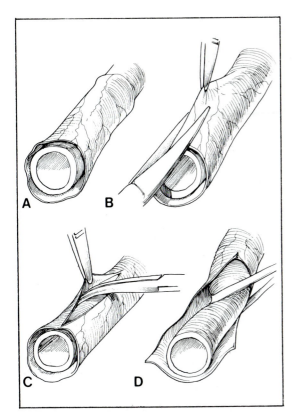

Figure 21-1. Diagram of an artery and its sheath. (*Redrawn from Cormier JM: Techniques générales de chirurgie artëielle, in Nouveau Traité de Technique Chirurgicale. Paris, Masson & Cie, 1970.*)

and dense perivascular fibrosis and hypervascularization of the sheath. Because the same process extends to the collateral branches from the main trunk, great care must be exercised in freeing not only the main trunk but its branches as well.

CLAMPING OF AN ARTERY

Temporary control of arteries can be achieved either by occluding tapes or by cross or lateral clamping (Fig. 21-3). The latter results in only a partial occlusion of the lumen, usually useful in operations, perhaps in procedures involving the thoracic aorta. Before clamping is done, digitial palpation of the arterial wall may disclose the extent of calcified plaques and soft areas. The best way to assess the degree of mural involvement is to compress the artery between the index finger and the thumb, after temporary occlusion is obtained with tapes placed tightly around the vessel.

Arterial clamps are of several designs. They are devised to prevent damage to the vessel, notably to the intima and its atherosclerotic plaques. Unfortunately, few of the current arterial clamps are entirely atraumatic, and they must be used with extreme care and minimal force if injury is to be minimized. For a medium-sized artery, such as the femoral, popliteal, axillary, or brachial, it is best to use double-looped silicon rubber vessel loops. For the aorta or iliac, arterial clamps are most suitable.

Although cross-clamping is most commonly used for temporary control, lateral clamping may be indicated in some cases, except in the ascending or descending thoracic aorta. One of the possible complications of lateral clamping, especially of the abdominal aorta, is fracture or a calcific plaque, usually located on its posterior wall. If the latter is noted beforehand, it may contraindicate lateral clamping for fear of intimal damage with subsequent thrombosis.

Tolerance of tissues to temporary arterial clamping varies with the area involved. The brain and the kidney, as is well known, are extremely sensitive to anoxia due to clamping of the respective artery. Similarly, cross-clamping of the thoracic aorta cannot usually be tolerated for more than 30 to 45 minutes because of the ensuing paraplegia unless preexisting collaterals are present. Prolonged cross-clamping of the infrarenal abdominal aorta is another such

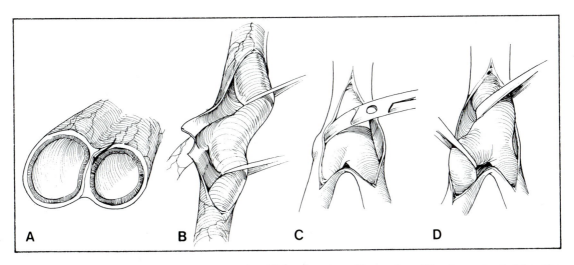

Figure 21-2. Freeing from sheath of an artery and mobilizing the artery with a major collateral vessel or its bifurcation. (*Redrawn from Cormier JM: Techniques générales de chirurgie artérielle, in Nouveau Traité de Technique Chirurgicale. Paris, Masson & Cie, 1970.*)

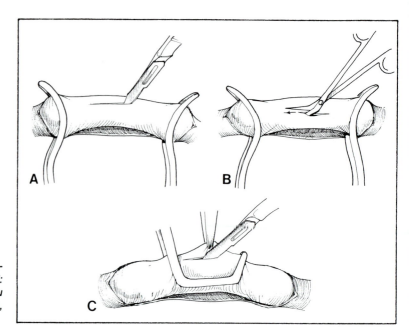

Figure 21-3. Clamping of an artery. **A, B.** Cross-clamping. **C.** Lateral clamping. (*Redrawn from Cormier JM: Techniques générales de chirurgie artérielle, in Nouveau Traité de Technique Chirurgicale. Paris, Masson & Cie, 1970.*)

example, albeit of a lesser intolerance. Thus striated muscle ischemia may induce a serious metabolic syndrome, which may lead to myoglobinuria, renal shutdown, and possible gangrene of the extremities. It behooves the surgeon, therefore, to minimize the duration of clamping of a major artery or to use methods to minimize ischemia.

ARTERIAL LIGATION

Arterial ligations are rarely indicated today, except as a temporary measure for hemorrhage control or in cases where the vessels cannot be repaired because of the extent of the lesions, presence of infection, or poor general condition of the injured individual. Although arterial ligations were practiced mostly for battle casualties, they may also be indicated in civilian injuries, but to a lesser extent. Since the Korean War, the introduction of arterial repairs has superseded arterial ligation whenever possible.

Unlike the practice in the past, ligations are rarely used today as a definitive treatment in certain instances of arterial aneurysms or arteriovenous fistulas.

Technique of Ligation

In the presence of vascular injury, the first step is control of the hemorrhage. Indeed, preliminary hemostasis is absolutely necessary before a formal ligation of the traumatized vessel can be achieved. This may be accomplished by the use of a tourniquet around the root of the extremity proximal to the traumatized vessel. An alternative method is digital compression or application of vascular clamps on the injured vessels, both proximal and distal to the injury whenever possible.

Wide exposure of the vessels is essential for good access to an adequate segment both above and below the laceration of the vessels. In doing so, every effort must be made to

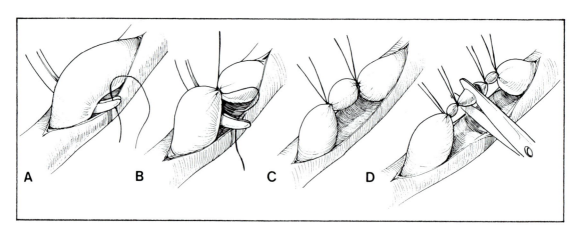

Figure 21-4. Types of arterial ligations. (*Redrawn from Cormier JM: Techniques générales de chirurgie artérielle, in Nouveau Traité de Technique Chirurgicale. Paris, Masson & Cie, 1970.*)

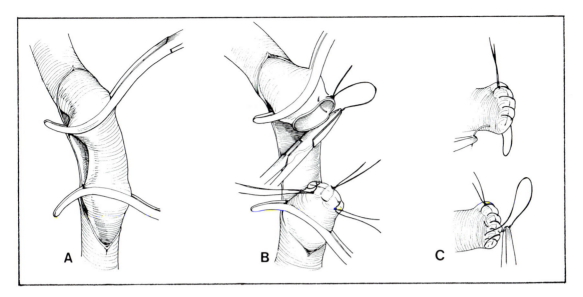

Figure 21-5. Division and suturing of arterial ends. (*Redrawn from Cormier JM: Techniques générales de chirurgie artérielle, in Nouveau Traité de Technique Chirurgicale. Paris, Masson & Cie, 1970.*)

preserve the collaterals, especially the muscular branches.

Once hemostasis and exposure have been achieved, mobilization of the involved artery is carried out according to the principles described above.

The material used for ligation of the arteries depends on the size of the vessel. For small vessels, a simple or double ligature of the fine catgut or silk or synthetic fibers may suffice. For arteries of medium-sized diameter, the vessel may have to be divided and double ligatures placed on each end (Fig. 21-4). The first ligature is a simple one. The second is a suture ligature placed distal to the previous one. For larger arteries, in addition to ligation of the vessel, oversewing of the stump with one or two rows of a continuous suture is a safety measure, and it is particularly important if the available length of vessel is limited or the surgeon is dealing with a diseased artery (Fig. 21-5). Release of the clamp after completion of the ligation should be slow and progressive.

Ligation of a medium-sized collateral should be done by dividing the vessel, double-ligating the distal end, and closing its origin with a lateral over-and-over suture (Fig. 21-6A), care being taken to avoid narrowing the main artery. The alternative to a lateral suture is ligating the divided stump close to its origin. The pitfall of this maneuver may be a blowout of the stump or, if the stump is too long, subsequent thrombus formation and potential embolization. It should therefore be avoided (Fig. 21-6B).

Results of arterial ligations for injuries or any other cause depend on the arterial segment involved. If the ligation is below a major branch that may assume the role of collateral supply, the effects of the ligation may be minimal. Certain arterial segments are more vulnerable than others. The common iliac, common femoral, and, particularly, popliteal arteries are critical anatomic locations. Their ligation may lead to a high rate of gangrene. By contrast, the external iliac, superficial femoral, and tibial arteries are less critical and usually tolerate ligations with few ischemic changes.

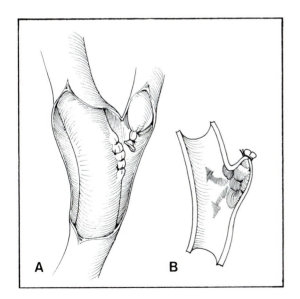

Figure 21-6. Division of a major collateral, and lateral closure of its origin on the parent vessel. **A.** Correct procedure. **B.** Incorrect ligation of collateral. (*Redrawn from Cormier JM: Techniques générales de chirurgie artérielle, in Nouveau Traité de Technique Chirurgicale. Paris, Masson & Cie, 1970.*)

ARTERIOTOMY

The chosen segment for arteriotomy is exposed, mobilized, and isolated. Occlusion of the vessels is not carried out until everything is ready for the arteriotomy, thus minimizing the occlusion time. The arteriotomy for most purposes should be longitudinal. The opening of the artery is done with the cutting-blade edge of the scalpel, not with its point.

The *longitudinal arteriotomy* is initiated first with a short opening of the lumen, which is signaled by the extrusion

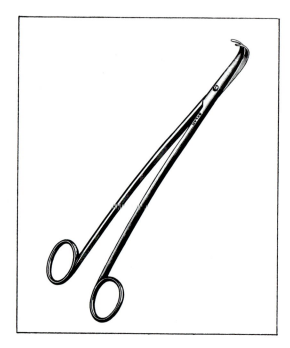

Figure 21-7. Arteriotomy scissors.

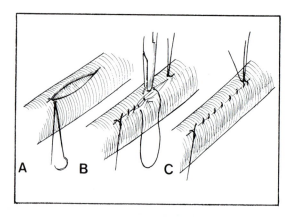

Figure 21-9. Closure of a longitudinal arteriotomy, with a continuous over-and-over suture.

of a few drops of blood. The arteriotomy is then completed by introducing a Potts-angled scissors in the lumen. Alternatively, the incision can be lengthened by inserting a fine clamp and continuing with a sharp new scalpel blade. This method is particularly useful when one is opening a diseased artery in preparation for anastomosis with a bypass graft. The length of the arteriotomy depends on the type of procedure contemplated. For an embolectomy or a thrombectomy, it should not exceed 0.75 to 1 cm; if it is intended for an anastomotic area, it may be somewhat longer.

A *transverse arteriotomy* is usually semicircular and is carried out in the same technical fashion as the longitudinal one. Care should be taken to avoid using the point of the scalpel blade and thus possibly entering too far into the artery and injuring its posterior wall.

Control of large (aorta, iliac) vessels may be gained occasionally, either by cross or lateral clamping. The latter

is carried out by means of a Satinsky clamp of suitable size, thus obviating complete arrest of arterial flow. In this instance, the arteriotomy is longitudinal and is used for anastomosing a graft.

In contrast to the type of arteriotomy that is easy to make in a soft, normal arterial wall, this procedure in an arteriosclerotic artery may result in dissection of an atherosclerotic plaque from the outer layer of the arterial wall. Calcification of an artery may render the arteriotomy and subsequent procedure more difficult. If the linear incision of the artery is changed into an elliptical opening, excision of the edges with ordinary scissors most often results in a jagged arteriotomy with loose intima.

The factors responsible for these technical difficulties are accounted for by the arteriosclerotic changes of the arterial tissue. Indeed, the increased thickness of the artery, the existence of a cleavage plane between the intima and media, and the presence of uneven calcific plaques make it difficult to obtain clean-cut arteriotomy edges. Scissors with a powerful shearing action and the capability of providing sharply delineated edges (Fig. 21-7) were specifically designed for this purpose by the author.[6] Recently, another technique was described. It consists of an intraoperative fracture technique used to overcome the rigidity of the arterial wall in calcified arteries. This technique, described by Ascer et al.,[7] did not prevent the implantation of the grafts, which resulted in patency and limb salvage.

The steps are simple and consist, first, of a longitudinal linear arteriotomy and then, with the arteriotomy scissors, excision of its edges one at a time. This results in a minor ellipsis-shaped arteriotomy (Fig. 21-8). These scissors[*] are available in two sizes, a large one for the aorta and iliac and a smaller one for the femoral and popliteal vessels. The resulting clean-cut arteriotomy greatly facilitates an end-to-side graft anastomosis in arteries with marked arteriosclerotic and calcific changes.

Closure of a longitudinal linear arteriotomy may be done with a continuous over-and-over suture or interrupted stitches (Fig. 21-9). One of the pitfalls of closing a longitudinal arteriotomy, especially in a medium-sized or small ar-

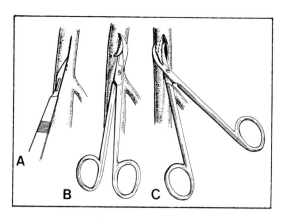

Figure 21-8. Arteriotomy: three steps using the arteriotomy scissors. (*From Haimovici H: Surgery 54:745, 1963.*)

---

*Manufactured by J. Sklar Manufacturing Co.

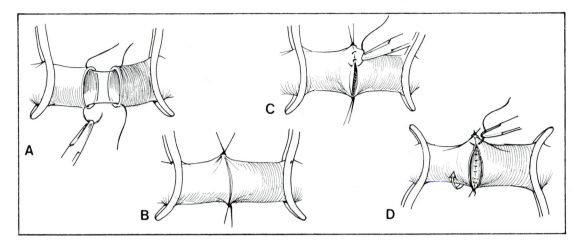

Figure 21-10. End-to-end anastomosis by means of two guy stitches (**A, B**). **C.** Anterior wall anastomosis. **D.** Posterior wall anastomosis after 180-degree rotation of the two vessels.

tery, may be its narrowing by the suture. In such cases, use of a patch graft is indicated (see Chapter 22.)

Closure of a transverse arteriotomy is best carried out by interrupted stitches. One should start with the placement of guy stitches at each angle and then proceed with the others between these two points taking care to include the entire thickness of the arterial wall and to have intima-to-intima coaptation.

VASCULAR ANASTOMOSES

End-to-End Anastomosis

Various types of techniques are available for anastomoses of blood vessels. They can be accomplished by an over-and-over suture or by a continuous everting mattress suture.

Approximation of the two ends of the divided vessels can be accomplished by several methods: (1) two stitches placed on the posterior wall close to each other, (2) equidistant stitches placed at each angle, (3) three stitches placed at equal distance (triangulation of Carre[4]), or (4) placement of four equidistant stitches (quadrangulation of Frouin[8]).

Figure 21-10 depicts the anastomosis of two vessels by means of two guy stitches and a continuous over-and-over stitch. First, the anterior wall is approximated by this suture technique. The vessels are then rotated by 180 degrees, and the anastomosis is completed on the posterior wall, in an anterior position.

Figure 21-11 shows an end-to-end anastomosis performed by suturing the posterior wall through the lumen of the vessel. After intraluminal closure on the posterior wall, the anterior row is completed in the usual fashion, by the extraluminal technique.

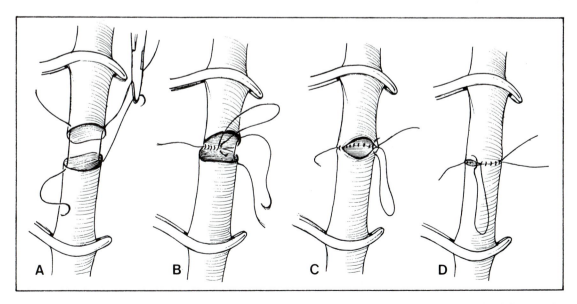

Figure 21-11. End-to-end anastomosis, performed by means of the intraluminal technique anastomosis of the posterior wall (**B**).

End-to-Side Anastomosis

Figure 21-12 depicts an end-to-end anastomosis, which is applicable to both large and small vessels. The arteriotomy indicated in Figure 21-12A and B can be used as an ellipsis-shaped opening for medium-sized arteries or as a rectangular-shaped opening for small vessels, although recently we have found that even with tiny arteries in the foot, anastomoses can be fashioned effectively to an elliptical anastomosis (Veith). Figure 21-12C demonstrates the direction of the sutures, starting from one end and proceeding by a continuous over-and-over stitch. The graft is then flipped over to provide direct vision for the anastomosis of the opposite edges, as indicated in Figure 21-12D and E. Alternatives to this are a four-stay suture technique for the end-to-side anastomosis, as described previously,[9] (Fig. 21-13) or a technique with heel-and-toe suture run down each side and tied at the midpoints of the anastomosis.

Figure 21-14 depicts an end-to-side anastomosis, similar to the previous one, except that the posterior wall of the vessels is anastomosed by the intraluminal technique. The anterior row is sutured by the usual extraluminal method.

Side-to-Side Anastomosis

Figure 21-15 depicts a side-to-side anastomosis of two vessels. Two guy sutures are placed at each angle, and the anterior edges of the vessels are retracted by means of stay sutures placed in their center. The needle of the upper angle is passed back through the vessel into the lumen, and the anastomosis of the posterior wall is carried out by an intraluminal technique as indicated in Figure 21-15C. After the intraluminal anastomosis is completed, the two sutures are tied together, and the distal needle is then used for the anastomosis of the anterior wall by an extraluminal technique, as indicated in Figure 21-15D and E.

Everting Suture Technique

Use of the everting technique for intraluminal vascular suturing was introduced by Blalock and Taussig[10] for the shunt procedure in the treatment of the tetralogy of Fallot. The technique consisted of placing a continuous everting mat-

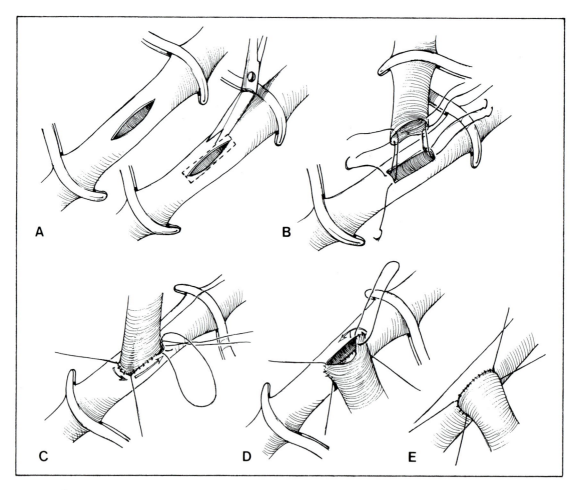

Figure 21-12. End-to-side anastomosis, with four guy sutures and a continuous over-and-over stitch.

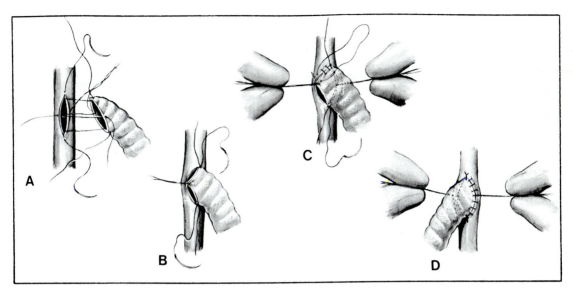

Figure 21-13. End-to-side anastomosis, with the four-stay suture technique. (*From Haimovici H: Surgery 47:266, 1960.*)

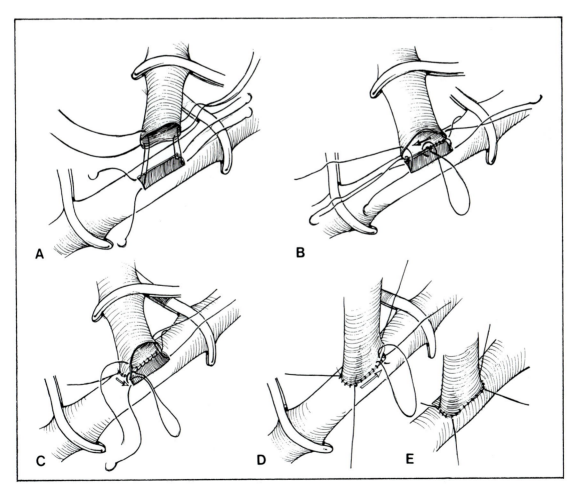

Figure 21-14. End-to-side anastomosis in which the posterior wall of the vessels is anastomosed by the intraluminal technique.

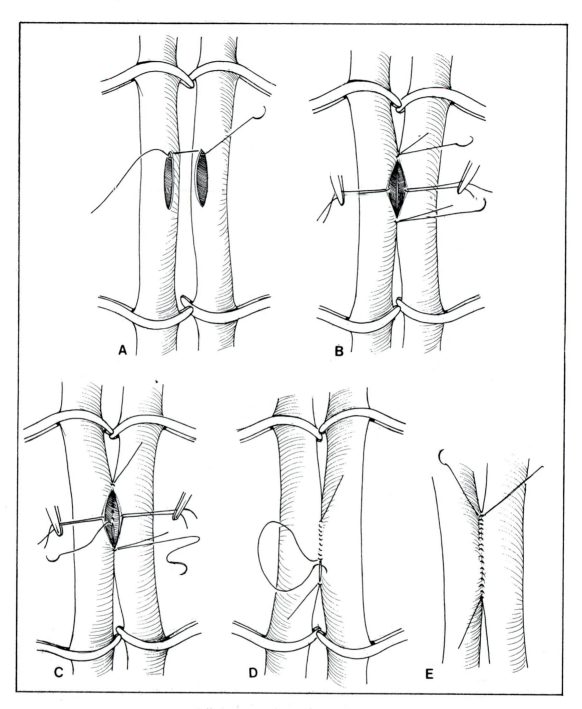

Figure 21-15. Side-to-side anastomosis.

tress suture along the posterior half of the circumference of the anastomosis before approximating the vessels and drawing the suture taut. This procedure has proved useful in areas where there are short cuffs or other limitations of exposure, necessitating suturing of the back walls from within the lumina.[11]

Use of this type of vascular suturing is applicable to end-to-end anastomoses as well as to end-to-side anastomoses, as depicted in Figures 21-16 and 21-17. The parachute technique can be used with continuous and everting techniques and is facilitated by monofilament polypropylene sutures.

Specific techniques for some graft implantations will be found in subsequent chapters.

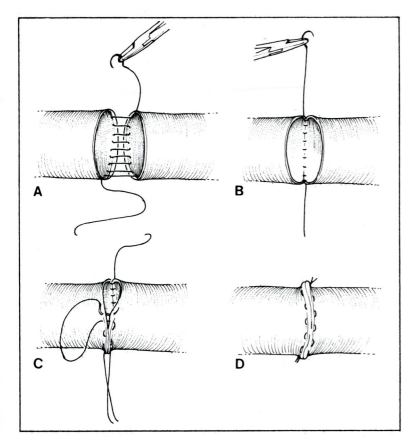

Figure 21-16. End-to-end anastomosis, with an eversion technique and intraluminal vascular suturing.

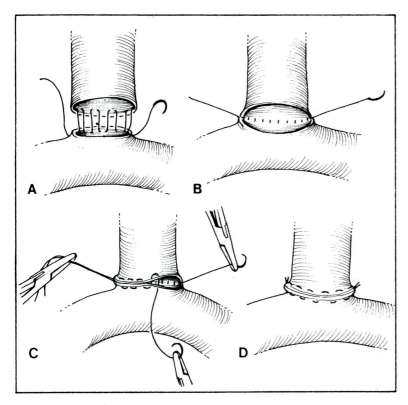

Figure 21-17. End-to-side anastomosis, with an eversion technique and intraluminal vascular suturing.

REFERENCES

1. Jassinowsky A: Die Arteriennaht: Eine experimentelle Studie. Inaug Diss Dorpat, 1889.
2. Dörfler J: Über Arteriennaht. Beitr Klin Chir 25:781, 1899.
3. Clermont G: Suture latérale et circulaire des veines. Presse Med 1:229, 1901.
4. Carrel A: La technique opératoire des anastomoses vasculaires et la transplantation des viscères. Lyon Med 98:859, 1902.
5. Carrel A, Guthrie CC: Uniterminal and biterminal venous transplantation. Surg Gynecol Obstet 2:266, 1906.
6. Haimovici H: Arteriotomy scissors. Surgery 54:745, 1963.
7. Ascer E, Veith FJ, Flores SAW: Infrapopliteal bypasses to heavily calcified rock-like arteries: Management and results. Am J Surg 152:220, 1986.
8. Frouin A: Sur la suture des vaisseaux. Presse Med 16:233, 1908.
9. Haimovici H: A four-stay suture technique for end-to-side arterial anastomoses. Surgery 47:266, 1960.
10. Blalock A, Taussig HR: Surgical treatment of malformations of the heart in which there is pulmonary stenosis or atresia. JAMA 128:189, 1945.
11. Shumacker HB Jr, Muhm HY: Arterial suture techniques and grafts: Past, present, and future. Surgery 66:419, 1969.

CHAPTER 22
Patch Graft Angioplasty

Henry Haimovici

HISTORICAL DATA

One of the important limiting factors in the reconstruction of vessels, especially of medium and small arteries, is the constriction of the lumen resulting from closure of a longitudinal arteriotomy. Prevention of this luminal constriction can easily be achieved by use of a patch graft. This principle of arterial repair, widely used today, was demonstrated experimentally by Carrel and Guthrie[1,2] as early as 1906.

They defined this procedure as follows: "The patching consists of closing an opening in the wall of a vessel by fitting and sewing to its edges a flap taken from another vessel or from some other structure such as the peritoneum." In describing anastomosis of blood vessels by the patching method and transplantation of the kidney, they further stated: "The anastomosis by the patching method consists of extirpating a vessel together with an area or patch from the vessel of origin, the patch being so cut that the mouth of the extirpated vessel is situated in the center of the patch. The edges of the patch are then fixed to the edges of a suitable opening made in the wall of another vessel" (Fig. 22-1).

Although Carrel and Guthrie[1,2] long ago demonstrated the feasibility of this surgical technique, it is only since the advent of the current reconstructive arterial surgical era that this procedure has assumed a significant place among corrective vascular methods. In 1959, Crawford et al.[3] and Senning[4] used autogenous vein patch grafts for closure of an arteriotomy in small arteries. These experiments confirmed the concept that they widen the lumen and prevent annular constriction from a longitudinal arteriotomy or even a circular suture line. In 1962, DeBakey et al.[5] reported extensive clinical use of patch graft angioplasty in the treatment of all types of occlusive arterial diseases and aneurysms. Subsequently, several investigators evaluated different types of patch material for the closure of arteriotomy of small arteries.[6-12] Reinforced by these recent laboratory and clinical experiences, patch graft arterial repair is now a well-establised procedure.

INDICATIONS

Indications for patch graft angioplasty are determined by three main factors: (1) size of arteries, (2) longitudinal arteriotomy, and (3) nature and extent of the mural lesion necessitating partial excision of the wall. In brief, any closure of an arteriotomy of a longitudinal wound that consumes the arterial circumference represents a major indication for this procedure. Its principal aim is to prevent stenosis and thrombosis at the site of the arteriotomy, especially since the patch graft is used in arteriosclerotic lesions and embolic occlusion of medium and small arteries (Fig. 22-2).

PATCH GRAFT MATERIAL

Carrel and Guthrie,[1,2] in their original experiments, used autogenous arterial, venous, and peritoneal patches. Clinically, both tissue and prosthetic materials are used for that purpose. Autogenous vein patches, favored by most surgeons, are indicated mostly for medium-sized and small arteries. Synthetic material is more suitable in larger vessels, such as the aorta and iliac arteries.

The histologic changes that take place in different patch graft materials over long periods of observation have been the subject of several investigations.[6-12]

Healing of grafts in the large vessels occurs almost uniformly, irrespective of the type of patch material. Its critical test, however, is in the smaller arteries. There is general agreement that both autogenous vein patches and autogenous arterial patches are usually less susceptible to local complications than are the synthetic grafts.

Vein Patch Grafts

The autogenous vein patch graft is soon incorporated into the host artery. Arteriographic studies and gross examination cannot readily identify them unless there is some stric-

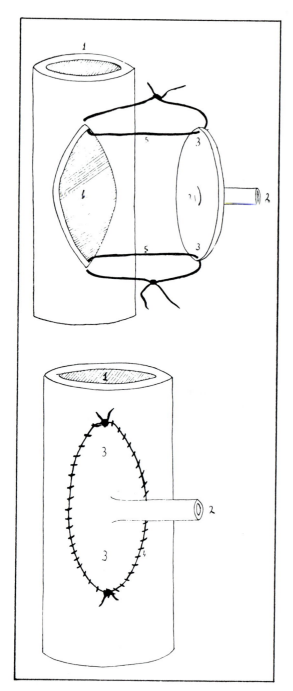

Figure 22-1. Diagrams of transplantation of a renal artery, together with a segment of the aortic wall implanted as a patch graft. (*From Carrel A, Guthrie CC: JAMA 47:1648, 1906.*)

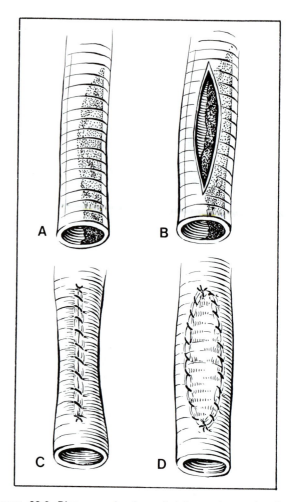

Figure 22-2. Diagrams showing arteriotomy closure by direct method and patch graft. **A.** Artery containing a mural lesion. **B.** Longitudinal arteriotomy over the lesion. **C.** Direct closure of arteriotomy, resulting in constriction of lumen. **D.** Patch graft closure illustrating prevention of constriction.

ture at the suture line. In such cases, the arteriogram displays a slight narrowing at that level. Localized dilation may be present if the patch graft is too large. Macroscopically, most of these grafts display a smooth intimal lining.

Histologic studies of vein patches have shown progressive alterations within a few weeks after implantation. Although in some of the grafts there is a partial preservation of normal venous architecture, consisting of elastic fibers with recognizable layers of the vein wall, smooth muscle disappears and is replaced by extensive fibrosis. The en-dothelial surface appears to remain intact without any accumulation of fibrin. Although the histologic vein structure is lost completely in many instances and replaced by fibrous tissue, it still functions properly without evidence of dilation or narrowing of the host artery.[7,10]

Arterial Patch Grafts

Autogenous arterial patches have significantly fewer degenerative changes and seem to be preferred over vein patches whenever possible.[6,8] Although the arterial patch retains some of its histologic characteristics, unlike the veins, arteries are not readily available or expandable and are therefore rarely used as patch grafts.

Prosthetic Patch Grafts

The healing patterns of Dacron patch grafts are similar to those reported by investigators of synthetic tubular grafts. Within 2 or 3 weeks, the patch acquires an inner lining, which in the beginning is loosely attached. A marked fibrotic reaction is usually found surrounding the graft.[9,10] This increases gradually and forms a thick layer by the end of 6 weeks.

Dacron velour displays less thrombosis and fibrotic reaction than the conventional Dacron material.[12] The histologic appearance indicates a good incorporation of this fabric into the host artery, with only minimal thickening of the neo-intima.

PTFE (Gore-Tex) vascular patch material, available in sheet form, almost immediately develops a layer of proteinaceous material on the luminal surface, while the outer wall is surrounded by wound tissue and blood clot. Within 2 weeks, the clot is absorbed, a healed connective tissue capsule is being formed, and collagen penetration into the wall is noted. The healing reaction is more an incorporation than a simple encapsulation (see Chapter 10).

METHODS AND TECHNIQUE OF PATCHING

Patch graft angioplasty is most suitable for short arteriotomy closures, rather than for long segments. Its use for the latter, especially if they exceed 8 cm, may lead to poor long-term results. This procedure may be used as an isolated modality, but more often it is combined with other reconstructive surgical techniques, such as thromboendarterectomy, excision with graft replacement, or bypass graft. Need for a patch graft may be anticipated from the arteriographic findings, or it may become necessary in the course of a surgical reconstructive procedure.

If one anticipates the use of a vein graft, preoperative preparation of the area supplying the vein should be carried out. If it is in the area of the femoral or popliteal artery, the saphenous vein is easily accessible. Otherwise, one should prepare the skin if the patch is to be secured from another area.

The segment of the saphenous vein is opened longitudinally and reserved. Its length is tailored to the arteriotomy to be closed. The resulting patch is rectangular in shape. Two methods may be used for its implantation: (1) The retangular shape is maintained, and the graft is attached to the edges of the arteriotomy by four stay stitches placed through the four corners (Fig. 22-3). (2) The alternative is to excise the corners of the rectangle so as to obtain an oval shape at each end of the patch graft (Fig. 22-4).

The graft is attached at each end of the arteriotomy with double-arm No. 5-0 fine synthetic suture material. Silk, because of its eventual loss of tensile strength, is to be avoided. A continuous everting stitch is used between the stay sutures. The patch must be under tension to allow good approximation between the graft and the edges of the host artery. Aneurysmal dilation is avoided by limiting the width of the patch graft. To achieve a patch without redundancy, the surgeon must use stay sutures at each end and at the midpoint of each edge of the arteriotomy (Fig. 22-4). The direction of the stitch, as in any other implant, goes from the graft to the host artery.

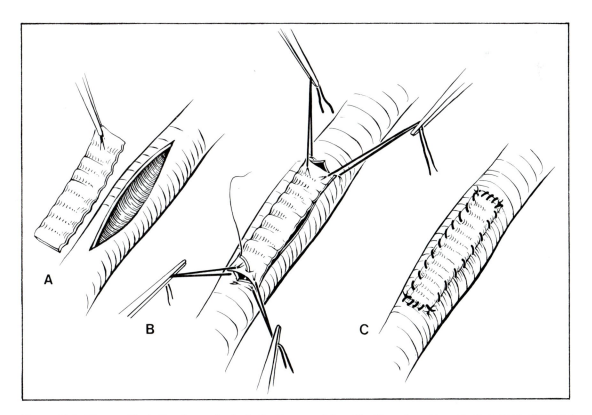

Figure 22-3. Diagram illustrating the method of attaching a patch graft with rectangular ends to a longitudinal oval arteriotomy. **A.** Rectangular piece of graft and arteriotomy. **B.** Placement of the stay sutures in the four angles and anchoring of the patch to the edges of the arteriotomy. **C.** Continuous everting stitch, resulting in a rectangular patch with prevention of narrowing of the lumen.

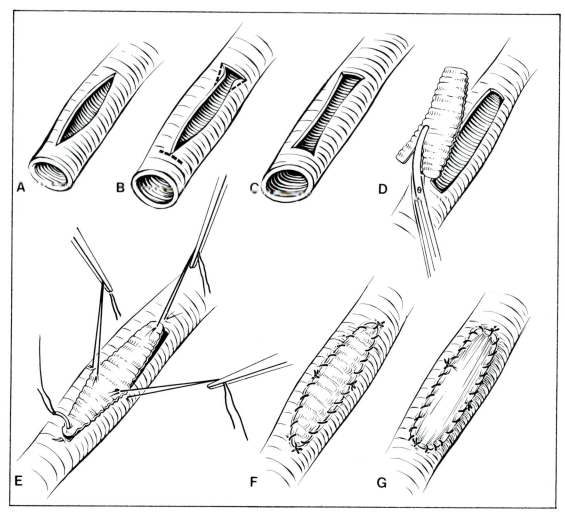

Figure 22-4. Diagrams illustrating oval patch grafts. **A.** Longitudinal arteriotomy. **B.** Excision of the angles of the arteriotomy. **C.** Rectangular arteriotomy. **D.** Tailoring of a patch graft to match the arteriotomy. **E.** Use of the four-stay suture technique for graft implantation. **F.** Prosthetic patch graft completed. **G.** Vein patch graft completed.

Before the patch is completed, it is essential to check the proximal and distal arterial tree for possible thrombosis. Once the patency has been checked, the suturing of the graft is completed.

Patching at Different Arterial Sites

Although the technique of patching varies somewhat with the location and extent of the arterial lesion, the principle is essentially the same for all areas. The best results obtained are in short segmental occlusions.

Localized segmental lesions occurring in the common iliac, common femoral, internal carotid, vertebral, renal, popliteal, and axillary arteries are the most suitable indications for patch graft angioplasty. The incision of the artery extends from the uninvolved proximal segment through the region of the obstruction into the uninvolved distal

segment. After the endarterectomy is completed, the patch is attached in the manner described above. In the arteries below the inguinal ligament or those in the neck, vein patch grafts are most suitable, whereas in the aorta or the iliac artery, Dacron or another synthetic material can be used to advantage.

When a patch graft is used at the level of a relatively large vessel that divides into two branches, such as the common femoral, which bifurcates into a superficial and a profunda vessel, the patch graft can be placed in three different manners.[*]

1. *Patch attached to the common and superficial femoral.* It is usually exceptional to stop the patch graft in the common

---

[*]These modalities are applicable to all arteries of similar anatomic configurations (e.g., carotid, iliac, aorta).

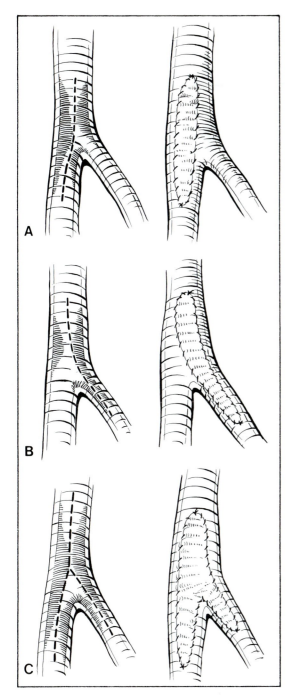

Figure 22-5. Diagram of a patch graft at a femoral arterial bifurcation. **A.** Patch to the common and superficial femoral. **B.** Patch to the common femoral and profunda. **C.** Y-shaped patch to the common femoral and its two branches.

2. *Patch attached to the common femoral and to the profunda.* The patch is tailored in such a way as to extend from the common to the profunda beyond its origin, usually to the level of the bifurcation of the latter vessel (Fig. 22-5B).

3. *Patch attached to the common femoral and both branches.* In some instances where both the superficial and profunda femoral vessels are involved by the arteriosclerotic process, a Y-shaped patch is necessary for closing of the arteriotomy of these three vessels (Fig. 22-5C).

Combination Graft Procedures

Patch graft angioplasty may be associated with bypass grafts. Three main combination procedures may be used:

1. A patch graft attached to the main artery may provide an area for the anastomosis of a tubular graft. The necessity for this modality is the presence of a small, narrowed artery or the loss of the anterior wall because of severe arteriosclerotic changes with calcification (Fig. 22-6A).

2. At a bifurcation of a major artery, a patch graft may be combined with a tubular graft implanted proximal to the patch (Fig. 22-6B).

3. A combination of tubular graft with extended patch may be used in certain cases if the distal end of a graft has to be attached to an area of extensive involvement of the arterial wall. Then the beveling of the graft is fashioned with a long flap that offers this combination (Fig. 22-6C).

A number of other combinations of these various techniques may be necessitated by pathologic findings involving both occlusive and eurysmal disease.

Complications and Pitfalls

Complications of patching of arteries may result from technical errors or from the type of patch graft material. Early thrombosis or hemorrhage may occur as a result of a technical error. Late thrombosis or hemorrhage may be due to the disruption of the anastomosis or to the progression of the degenerative changes of the arterial wall. Local infection is a potential hazard to which one should always be alert.

Pitfalls to be avoided are excessive length or width of the graft, which may lead to aneurysmal formation at the site of the graft.

SUMMARY

Patch graft angioplasty has proved to be useful in performing the various reconstructive surgical procedures. The main advantages are prevention of stenosis at the site of the closure of an arteriotomy, especially in a small vessel. The long-term results obtained with this procedure are gratifying.

femoral, since the superficial, at least at its initial segment, is also involved by the atherosclerotic process. Therefore, the patch should always extend beyond the origin of the superficial femoral by about 3 to 5 cm (Fig. 22-5A).

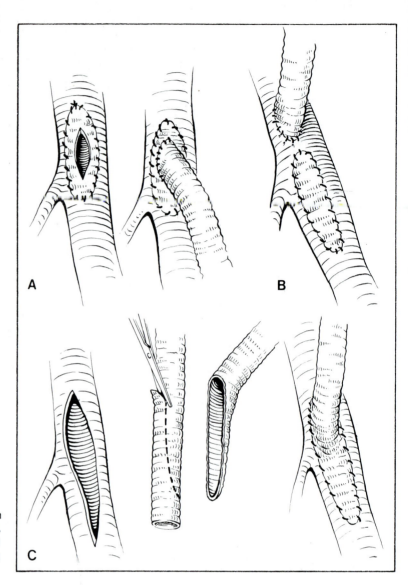

Figure 22-6. Diagram of patch grafts combined with tubular grafts. **A.** Tubular graft attached to a patch. **B.** Tubular graft attached proximal to a patch. **C.** Long bevel of a tubular graft with an additional patch for closing an extensive arteriotomy.

REFERENCES

1. Carrel A, Guthrie CC: Résultats du patching des artères. C R Soc Biol (Paris) 60:1009, 1906.
2. Carrel A, Guthrie CC: Anastomosis of blood vessels by the patching method and transplantation of the kidney. JAMA 47:1648, 1906.
3. Crawford ES, Beall AC, et al.: A technic permitting operation upon small arteries. Surg Forum 10:671, 1959.
4. Senning A: Strip-graft technique. Acta Chir Scand 118:81, 1959.
5. DeBakey ME, Crawford ES, et al.: Patch graft angioplasty in vascular surgery. J Cardiovasc Surg 3:106, 1962.
6. Chatarjee KN, Warren R, Gore I: Long-term functional and histologic fate of arteriotomy patches of autogenous arterial and venous tissue: Observations on arterialization. J Surg Res 4:106, 1964.
7. Norton LW, Spencer FC: Long-term comparison of vein patch with direct suture. Technique of anastomosis of small arteries. Arch Surg 89:1083, 1964.
8. Rossi NP, Koepke JA, Spencer FC: Histologic changes in long-term arterial patch grafts in coronary arteries. Surgery 57:335, 1965.
9. Dale WA, Lewis MR: Experimental arterial patch grafts. J Cardiovasc Surg 6:24, 1965.
10. Pena LI, Husni EA: A comparative study of autogenous vein and Dacron patch grafts in the dog. Arch Surg 96:369, 1968.
11. Wagner M, Ruel G, et al.: The use of Spandex as a vascular patch graft material. Surg Gynecol Obstet 127:805, 1968.
12. Menon SMR, Talwar JR, et al.: Comparison of Dacron velour and venous patch grafts for arterial reconstruction. Surgery 73:423, 1973.

CHAPTER 23
Endarterectomy

Henry Haimovici

HISTORICAL BACKGROUND

Endarterectomy, first performed by J. Cid dos Santos in 1946, was originally designed for simple removal of thrombi but turned out to be more than a simple thrombectomy.[1,2] Attempts at disobstruction of occluded arteries by simple thrombectomy were not new. Severeanu in 1880,[3] Jianu in 1909,[4] and Delbet in 1906 and again in 1911[5] are credited with attempting arterial thrombectomy.

These early trials were all unsuccessful. The procedure was thus relegated to oblivion until 1946, when dos Santos decided to do this operation with the patient under the cover of heparin. The first patient on whom he tested this concept was a 66-year-old man with a left ischemic limb due to an iliofemoral occlusion. The procedure resulted in patency of the vessels lasting three days, at which time the patient died of advanced uremia. The arteriograms taken after the procedure and at postmortem confirmed the patency of the iliofemoral vessels. Histopathologic examination of the removed specimen showed not only the thrombus but also the whole intima and part of the media. In spite of this histopathologic finding, there was no rethrombosis.

Encouraged by these findings, dos Santos next used this procedure on a 35-year-old woman with a subclavian-axillary arterial thrombosis associated with a cervical rib. The histopathologic findings were similar to those in the first case. The clinical recovery with patency of the subclavian-axillary artery persisted for 29 years, as of the date of his publication in 1976.[6]

The data provided by these two cases were quite revealing, and dos Santos stated: "I really had performed a different operation from the one I originally intended to do; and I could conclude that, under heparin action, blood could flow against muscle without giving place to thrombosis."[2] He thus felt that the integrity of the intima as a requirement for a successful surgical procedure is no longer always mandatory. This new procedure, later called thromboendarterectomy, represented a wholly new concept in arterial surgery. It appeared as a revolutionary idea be-

cause it seemed to negate the prevailing concept according to which an injured intima leads inevitably to vascular thrombosis. Indeed, unlike embolectomy, in which only the thrombus is removed, in thromboendarterectomy both the thrombus and the endartery (intima and part of the inner media) are excised.

The accidental finding that arterial thrombosis does not necessarily occur after removal of the intimal lining and a portion of the media is a typical example of serendipity. As a result of these findings, a new chapter emerged in the field of vascular surgery.

Dos Santos's pioneering efforts were soon confirmed and expanded by Bazy, et al.,[7] Leriche and Kunlin,[8] Wylie,[9,10] Cannon and Barker,[11] and a few others.

Although sporadic reports started to appear shortly thereafter, greater acceptance of this new operation had to await further technical refinements and improvements in instrumentation, since, as stated by dos Santos, "At the beginning failure was the usual, success the occasional." This procedure, even after 37 years, is still not entirely without some controversies.

Terminology

Originally dos Santos named this operation "arterial disobstruction" or "disobliteration." Later Bazy and Reboul[12] coined the term *endarterectomy*, but Leriche[8] preferred the more comprehensive term *thromboendarterectomy*.* These two terms, often used interchangeably, are designed to indicate removal not only of the intima and thrombus but also of the media. Consequently, since "endartery" and "intima" are used as synonyms, the term *endarterectomy* appears to convey an incomplete meaning of the procedure. Sanctioned by long-time usage, however, these terms are widely accepted, notwithstanding the above semantic limitations.

---

*These terms are also spelled endarter*i*ectomy or thromboendarter*i*ectomy.

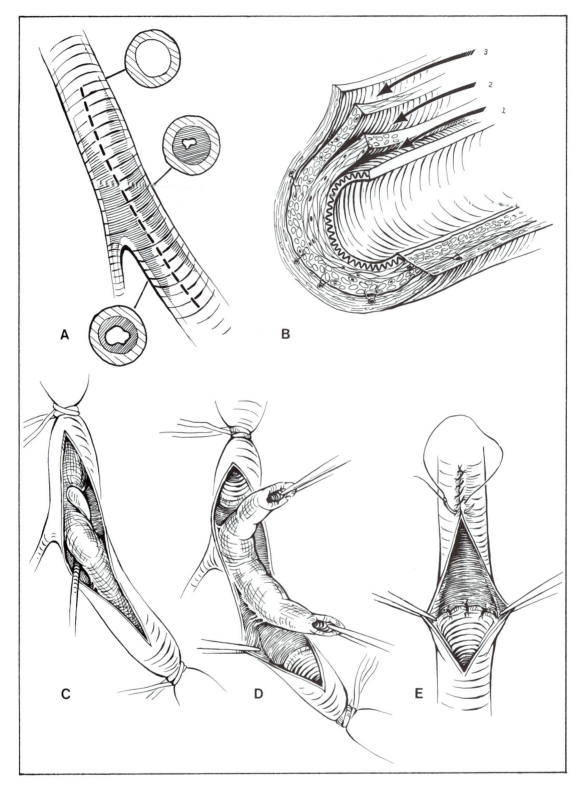

Figure 23-1. Principles of endarterectomy. **A.** Longitudinal arteriotomy extending beyond the occluding core and three cross sections at different levels of the arterial lesions. **B.** Planes of cleavage *1,* subintimal, *2,* transmedial, *3,* subadventital. Note the two muscular fiber layers of the media, the circular (internal) and longitudinal (external). **C.** Dissection and mobilization of an atherothrombotic occluding core. **D.** Excision of the core. **E.** Distal intimal edge reattached to the arterial wall with interrupted stitches.

PRINCIPLES OF ENDARTERECTOMY

Early arteriosclerotic lesions involve mostly the intima and, to a lesser extent, the media. At a later stage, the internal elastic membrane is usually fragmented, and the atheromatous changes invade the medial coat. When the lumen is partially or completely occluded, a fibrosclerotic core is present with or without an organized thrombus.

Cleavage Plane

A cleavage plane, usually present in the outer portion of the arterial wall, represents the mural pathologic component that is the key to the performance of an endarterectomy. The cleavage plane varies with the size, location, and pathology of the particular artery. In arteries of the muscular type, such as the superficial femoral, the media includes circular fibers in its inner three quarters and longitudinal ones in its external quarter. The latter layer also has elastic fibers, which increase in number and thickness in the vicinity of the external elastic membrane. As a consequence of this anatomic characteristic, the cleavage plane in such an artery is situated between the inner three quarters and the outer quarter of the media, as determined by the different orientation of the two layers of muscular fibers (Fig. 23-1).

The cleavage planes are not all situated at the same level.[13] As a rule, normal planes of cleavage are close to either the internal or external elastic membrane. Based on the extent and location of the mural lesions, the following three cleavage planes are found most commonly: subintimal, transmedial, and subadventitial (Fig. 23-1B).

Subintimal
The subintimal cleavage plane is located between the intima and the media along the outside of the internal elastic membrane.

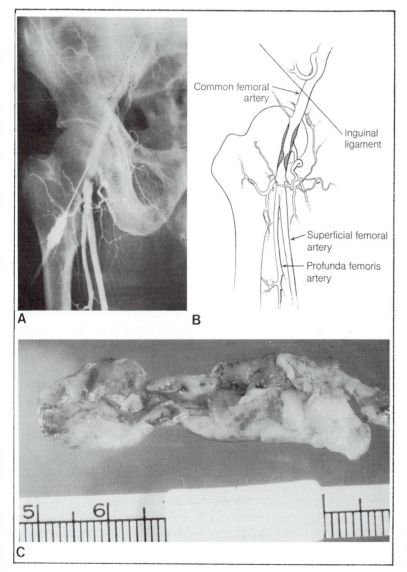

A.

B. Common femoral artery — Inguinal ligament — Superficial femoral artery — Profunda femoris artery

C.

Figure 23.2. A. Femoral arteriogram indicating marked stenosis of the common femoral artery proximal to its bifurcation. **B.** Artist's reproduction of the arteriogram. **C.** Endarterectomy specimen.

Transmedial

The transmedial plane lies between the involved and intact layer of the media, usually between the inner three quarters and the outer quarter.

Subadventitial

The subadventitial plane is situated between the media and the adventitia along the inner surface of the external elastic membrane.

Since it is not possible to know preoperatively which cleavage plane is available, great care should be exercised to determine its exact location in each individual case. As a rule, the best planes to use are either subadventitial or transmedial. Use of the subintimal plane may lead to thrombosis and should be avoided.

Pathology of Lesions

Endarterectomized Specimen

Such a specimen has the appearance of an irregular, flattened plaque of grayish white tissue, speckled with yellow streaks (Fig. 23-2). Often, segments of thrombotic material are encrusted in the folds of the intima. Some of the plaques are ulcerated and are covered with thrombi. Histologically, the endothelial layer is difficult or impossible to identify, the internal elastic membrane is usually fragmented or absent, and lipid infiltration with cholesterol crystal clefts and fibrotic lesions are present in the subintimal region

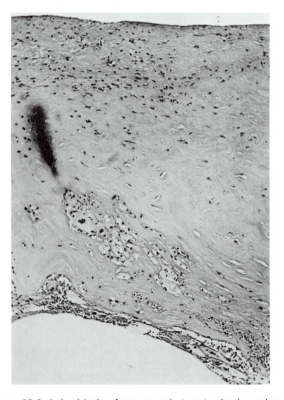

Figure 23-3. Intimal lesion from an endarterectomized specimen.

and media, with frequent calcific degenerative changes in the latter (Fig. 23-3).

Thromboendarterectomized Specimen

This specimen consists of a tubular structure resembling the arterial wall on the outside, with the lumen totally occluded by a thrombus that is firmly attached to the wall (Fig. 23-4). Histologically, the arterial wall shows thickening, hyalinization, cholesterol deposition, and calcification, with a well-organized thrombus. In some areas, the organization is represented by early fibroblastic infiltration and minimal iron pigment deposition.

Residual Arterial Wall

The residual arterial wall is usually glistening without any evidence of atheromatous tissue. If the cleavage plane is close to the external elastic membrane, all the circular fibers should have been removed. If shreds of this layer are still present, they should be carefully stripped away. Microscopically, the residual arterial wall includes in variable amounts medial fibers, the external elastic membrane, and the adventitia.

Within minutes after completion of the surgical procedure, the inner surface of the residual wall becomes covered with a fibrin layer. Subsequently, an inner fibrous coat is formed, which may lead occasionally to reduction of the arterial lumen. For this reason, as mentioned previously, the most external cleavage plane should be used to avoid possible subsequent stenosis.

The existence of a neo-intima in the endarterectomized artery is still a moot question. Neointimal hyperplasia, especially in anastomotic areas, is a frequent complication. Periarterial fibrotic reaction to the endarterectomy is often noted, although its degree varies from case to case.

Hemodynamic Factors

Endarterectomy is designed to reconstruct the arterial lumen with at least part of its original characteristics, namely, with a diameter that allows near-adequate capacity and a geometrical shape that ensures normal flow. This ideal aim, however, cannot always be achieved, since it is nearly impossible to restore the arterial wall once it has lost its original tissue characteristics and its normal physical properties. Nevertheless, it may be feasible to obtain a reasonably uniform cross section of the lumen in all its involved segments. This may be achieved either by direct suturing of the arterial wall or by means of a patch graft angioplasty, which is partiularly advisable in the vicinity of bifurcations.[14]

Arteries after endarterectomy become obviously thin-walled and soft. In spite of these morphologic changes, the endarterectomized vessel is able to withstand arterial pressures and to maintain the suture line. The endarterectomized segments appear to contain less smooth muscle but more nonprotein material, as compared with normal arteries, and owe their high elastic stiffness primarily to the collagen fibers concentrated in the outer layers of the wall.[15]

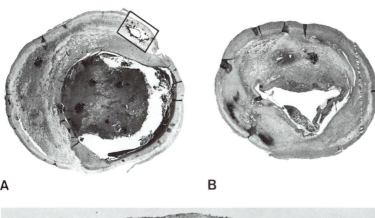

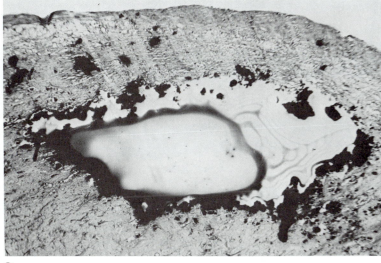

Figure 23-4. Cross section of a thromboendarterectomy specimen at two different levels. **A.** Lumen filled by recent thrombus. **B.** Lumen is filled by fibrosclerotic mass. **C.** Enlargement of the calcified area as seen in the medial coat of **A.**

The conventional technique of endarterectomy can be performed through the semiclosed or the open method.

SEMICLOSED ENDARTERECTOMY

Exposure and Mobilization of the Vessel

Wide exposure is essential for proximal and distal control not only of the main artery but also of all collaterals. Exposure of the artery is usually made by means of two or three skin incisions, not exceeding 8 to 10 cm, along the involved vessel (Fig. 23-5A).

A longitudinal arteriotomy is carried out at each end of the involved vessel.

After the cleavage plane is developed, a lateral dissector separates the lesion circumferentially. Then the distal end of the lesion is transected sharply.

Dissection of the lesion (Fig. 23-5B) is carried out by using a combination of lateral and ring dissectors. The entire occluding core is mobilized and then extruded through either the lower or upper incision (Fig. 23-5C). Great care must be exercised in handling the distal intimal flap, reat-

taching it, if necessary, to the rest of the arterial wall with interrupted stitches across its edge (Fig. 23-1E).

Closure

The arteriotomies are closed by a simple arteriorrhaphy or by a patch graft angioplasty.

Overpass

Dos Santos in 1963 described this technical detail, not only for securing the distal edge of the endartery better but also for allowing direct visualization of the outflow area (Fig. 23-5F). A vein patch is implanted at this level for additional safety.[16]

Pitfalls

Pitfalls of the semiclosed method, especially for long segments, may be quite serious and consist of (1) incomplete removal of the lesion, leaving residual strands of media that could lead to rethrombosis, (2) rupture of the arterial wall with subsequent troublesome hemorrhage, and (3)

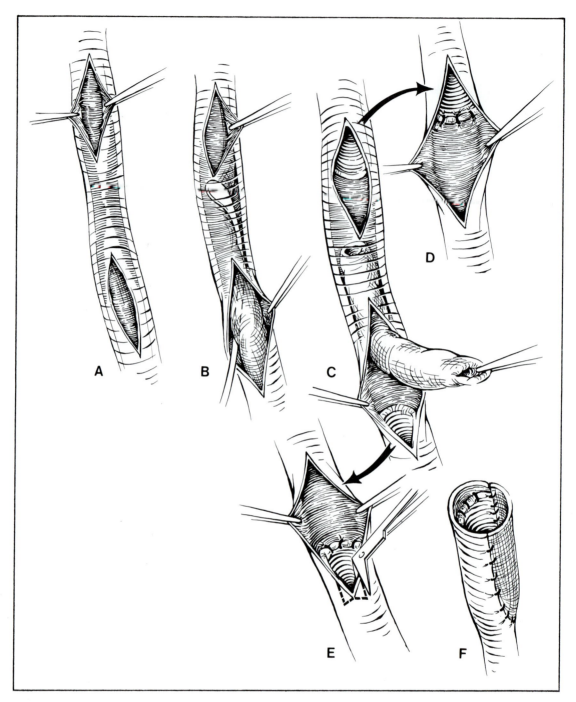

Figure 23-5. Semiclosed endarterectomy. **A.** Two small separate arteriotomies carried through the subadventitial cleavage plane. **B.** Dissection and mobilization of an atherothrombotic core with a lateral dissector. **C.** Removal of the occluding core after sharp transection at both ends. **D.** Proximal intimal edge fixed to the arterial wall with interrupted stitches. **E.** Distal intimal edge fixed in a similar fashion. **F.** Overpass (see text).

retrograde bleeding during the procedure due to inadequate control of collaterals.

OPEN ENDARTERECTOMY

Open endarterectomy is unquestionably more adequate and safer than the semiclosed method.

Exposure

The vessel is exposed along its entire length and is mobilized from end to end together with all its collaterals.

A longitudinal arteriotomy is carried out slightly proximal from the uninvolved area through the lesion and distally beyond the obliterating core.

Cleavage Plane

The dissection of the lesion is started by a limited arteriotomy through the adventitia and the external layer of the media, for the purpose of developing a cleavage plane. The initial limited arteriotomy is then extended both proximally and distally along the cleavage plane. Once the core is mobilized, the two ends are transected sharply. Sometimes the hypertrophied intima tapers off at the distal end. The occluding mass is then removed.

Reattachment

It is not mandatory to reattach the proximal end of the intimal flap, although in some instances it may be necessary to do so. The distal end is treated in a fashion similar to the semiclosed method. A patch may be attached to this area, especially if the artery is of small caliber. In such a case, it may be necessary to consider changing the acute angle of the distal arteriotomy into a broader end. This can be accomplished in two ways, as described in Chapter 22, Patch Graft Angioplasty (see Figs. 23-5F and 23-6C).

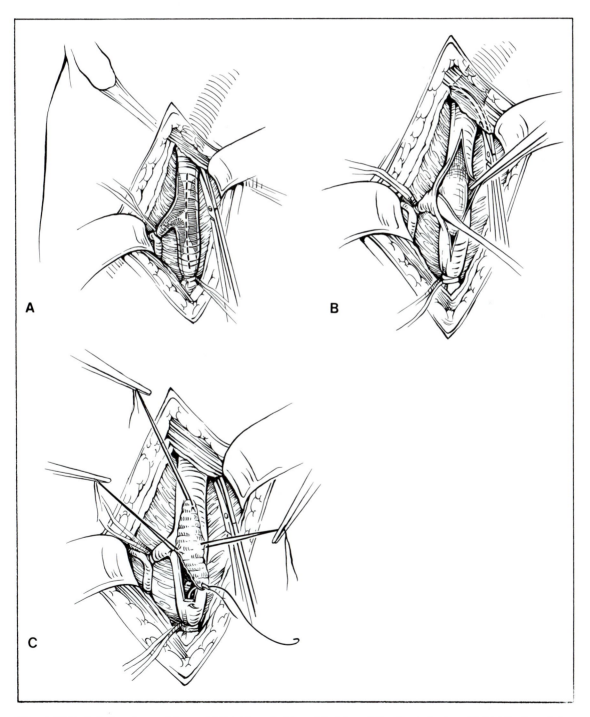

Figure 23-6. Endarterectomy of femoral bifurcation. **A.** Line of incision of the femoral artery. **B.** Mobilization of the occluding core. **C.** Closure of the arteriotomy with a patch graft.

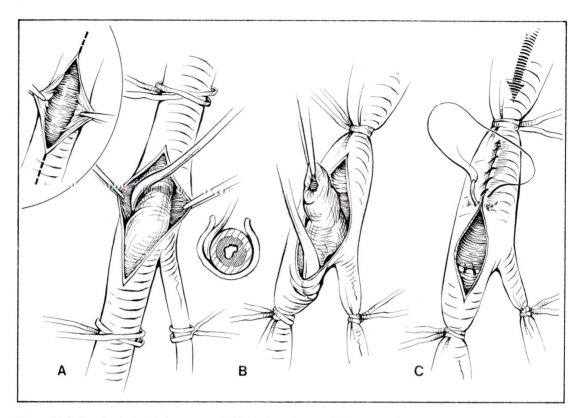

Figure 23-7. Extraluminal endarterectomy. **A.** Dissection of an occluding core after arteriotomy performed through a subadventitial cleavage plane. The arteries proximal and distal to the procedure remain intact at this phase. **B.** Excision of the occluding core. Occlusion of proximal and distal segments is necessary at this phase. **C.** Closure of arteriotomy.

Dissection

Whenever possible, an extraluminal dissection of the occluding core is desirable. This may offer a twofold advantage: it facilitates the dissection of the lesion, and it may shorten the period of total arterial occlusion. This may be of great value in visceral arterial endarterectomy (Figs. 23-7 and 23-8).

The indication for open vs. semiclosed endarterectomy may be determined by the extent of the lesion or by the preference of the individual surgeon. The author prefers the open technique.

Heparin

A combination of systemic and local heparinization offers the best method for preventing thrombosis during these usually long procedures. Postoperative heparinization has been abandoned because the possible troublesome complications outweigh its effectiveness in preventing thrombosis at this stage.

COMBINED PROCEDURES

Endarterectomy is often necessary prior to the distal implantation of a graft because of severe stenosis or occlusion at that level. Such cases may be encountered in any arterial segments but are more common in aortofemoral or femoropopliteal bypass procedures.

In arterial embolism, it is not uncommon to find the embolus impacted into a bifurcation involved with severe atherosclerotic changes. It is then essential to perform, in conjunction with the balloon catheterization, a meticulous endarterectomy before completing the embolectomy.

COMMENTS: ENDARTERECTOMY VS. PERCUTANEOUS BALLOON CATHETERIZATION

With the advent of the percutaneous balloon catheter or laser angioplasty for management of arterial stenosis or occlusion, the indications for endarterectomy have been reassessed. The interventional radiologic procedures are often helpful either as a definitive treatment or as an adjunct to arterial surgery.

Endarterectomy still represents the most widely used operation for well-defined arterial lesions for which the radiologic interventions appear unsuitable. Of these, carotid endarterectomy as mentioned above is a most widely used operation. In order of decreasing incidence, other indications are atherosclerotic lesions, stenosis or occlusion of the abdominal aorta, and as an adjunct in grafting limb arteries in which the balloon catheter is unsuitable anatomically.[17]

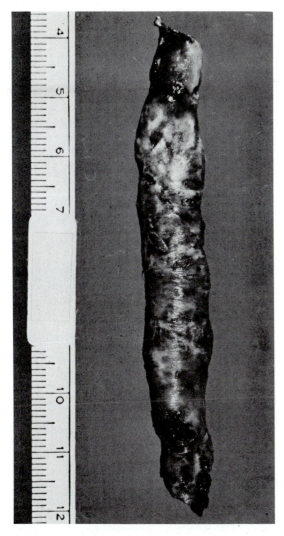

Figure 23-8. Specimen removed from the right common femoral artery extraluminal dissection of the occluded core.

Knowledge of the basic principles of endarterectomy, of the anatomopathology of the lesions, and of the healing of the arterial wall is essential for understanding the scope and extent of the surgical procedure. This knowledge also provides a better comparison with the results of the mural response following the angioplasty techniques.

Notwithstanding the fact that nonsurgical methods have superseded endarterectomy in some cases, the useful-ness of the latter nevertheless remains widely applicable in well-defined arterial lesions.

REFERENCES

1. Dos Santos JC: Sur la désobstruction des thromboses arté-rielles anciennes. Mem Acad Chir 73:409, 1947.
2. Dos Santos JC: Introduction to a Round Table on Endarterec-tomy. J Cardiovasc Surg (Special Issue for the 15th International Congress of the European Society of Cardiovascular Surgery), p 223, 1966.
3. Severaneau: Quoted in reference 4.
4. Jinau I: Thrombectomia arteriala pentru un caz de gangrene uscata a piciorului. Soc Chir (Bucarest) 27:11, 1912.
5. Delbet P: Chirurgie arterielle et veineuse, in Les Modernes Acquisitions. Paris, Bailliere, 1906, p 104.
6. Dos Santos JC: From embolectomy to endarterectomy, or the fall of a myth. J Cardiovasc Surg 17:113, 1976.
7. Bazy L, Huguier J, et al.: Désobliteration d'une thrombose ancienne segmentaire, de 17 cm long, dans une artère fémorale superficielle, atteinte d'artérite pariétale calcifée. Mem Acad Chir 73:602, 1947.
8. Leriche R, Kunlin J: Essais de désobstruction des artères throm-bosés suivant la technique de Jean Cid Dos Santos, Lyon Chir 42:475, 1947.
9. Wylie EJ, Kerr E, Davis O: Experimental and clinical experiences with the use of fascia lata applied as a graft about major arteries after thromboendarterectomy and aneurysmorrhaphy. Surg Gynecol Obstet 92:257, 1951.
10. Wylie EJ: Thromboendarterectomy for arteriosclerotic thrombo-sis of major arteries. Surgery 23:275, 1952.
11. Cannon J, Barker W: Successful management of obstructive femoral arteriosclerosis by endarterectomy. Surgery 38:48, 1955.
12. Bazy L, Reboul H: Technique de l'endartériectomie désobliter-ante. J Int Chir 65:196, 1950.
13. Malan E, Botta JC: Normal and pathologic planes of cleavage. J Cardiovasc Surg (Special Issue for the 15th International Con-gress of the European Society of Cardiovascular Surgery), p 261, 1966.
14. Malan E, Longo T: Hemodynamic factors in endarterectomy. J Cardiovasc Surg (Special Issue for the 15th International Con-gress of the European Society of Cardiovascular Surgery), p 265, 1966.
15. Sumner DS, Hokanson DE, Strandness DE: Arterial walls be-fore and after endarterectomy. Stress-strain characteristics and collagen-elastin content. Arch Surg 99:606, 1969.
16. Dos Santos JC: Late results of reconstructive arterial surgery (restoration, disobliteration, replacement with the establish-ment of some operative principles). J Cardiovasc Surg 5:445, 1964.
17. Inahara T: Endarterectomy for segmental occlusive disease of the superficial femoral artery. Arch Surg 116:1547, 1981.

CHAPTER 24
Percutaneous Transluminal Angioplasty in Peripheral Vascular Disease

Barry T. Katzen

HISTORICAL BACKGROUND

Percutaneous transluminal angioplasty (PTA) was first described by Dotter and Judkins in 1964 in a landmark publication describing its use in the treatment of atherosclerotic peripheral vascular disease.[1] This technique evolved from the observation that inadvertent passage of guide wires through occlusions occurred occasionally during angiography and led to an original system developed by Dotter, which used a stiff 8 French Teflon catheter inserted over a guide wire and followed by a 12 French catheter, which coaxially dilated the artery. Although this technique was successful, it was greeted with little enthusiasm in the United States, with many vascular surgeons believing that it was dangerous, because it introduced the possibility of showering of atherosclerotic debris, and that in all likelihood it would not be effective in most patients. Nonetheless, the technique was exported to Europe, where it was refined and widely used by Zeitler et al.,[2] van Andel,[3] Porstmann,[4] and Gruntzig[5] with considerable success.

The application of the Dotter catheter system was limited by many technical factors, including the stiffness of the catheters, the size of the arterial puncture wound, the difficulty in obtaining hemostasis around the various components of the coaxial system, and the potential for vascular trauma created by forward shearing forces.

This latter limitation was addressed by a series of graduated, tapered catheters developed by van Andel[3] to reduce the risk of distal embolus formation and to increase the success in progressive dilatation. These devices remained limited by the fact that they could effect dilatation only to the size of the puncture site and therefore required extremely large arterial holes, particularly when treating large vessels. Initial attempts to develop a balloon dilatation system were described by Porstmann[4] and involved the use of a latex balloon that was "caged" inside a Teflon catheter to provide overdilatation. Although this device was effective, it too had many technical limitations, which led to the development in 1974 by Gruntzig of a revolutionary system that used a flexible double-lumen catheter and a so-called "rigid" balloon. Applying plastics technology, Gruntzig[6] developed a polyvinyl balloon catheter that would not inflate more than 1 to 3 mm beyond the designated size.

The Gruntzig balloon catheter revolutionized PTA from a technical point of view, making it simpler, less traumatic, and more effective, thus leading to higher success rates. Continued evolution of this design concept has produced high-pressure balloons, balloons with lower profiles, and extremely small balloons, in the 4 to 5 French size, and has greatly reduced the puncture site trauma by producing dilatation of large caliber, with catheters of a size similar to those used today for outpatient angiography.

PATHOPHYSIOLOGY OF VASCULAR DILATATION

Initially, Dotter and Judkins[1] postulated that compression of the atheromatous material was the primary mechanism of transluminal angioplasty, and it was believed that the volume of the plaque was reduced by releasing fluids and some of the lipid content from the lesion.[7] Although somewhat difficult to accept, this concept was widely believed until more recent experimental studies[8–13] helped clarify the mechanism of angioplasty. Transluminal angioplasty is in effect a traumatic process and is a complex injury including some desquamation of the endothelium, stretching of the vessel wall, and an actual split and disruption of the plaque, which may be associated with fissures of the intima and media. After transluminal angioplasty, healing of the disrupted layers forms a neointima similar to that formed after a surgical endarterectomy. The process may be summarized as one of "controlled injury," produced by the dilatation itself, and a healing process that forms a smooth-walled lumen.

INDICATIONS FOR TRANSLUMINAL ANGIOPLASTY IN THE LOWER EXTREMITIES

As in all methods of treatment of vascular disease, indications for the use of transluminal angioplasty are based on both clinical and morphologic criteria. Transluminal angioplasty is indicated for symptomatic patients; however, the degree of symptoms may be less than those necessary for surgical intervention because of the reduced morbidity associated with the procedure. Although serious complications that may require surgical intervention occur rarely, PTA should not be attempted without considerable deliberation in patients who could not withstand surgery in the event a complication occurred.

Although some exceptions may be made, clinical indications for balloon angioplasty are similar to those for surgical intervention:

- Intermittent claudication affecting life-style
- Rest pain
- Ischemic ulceration or poor wound healing with vascular compromise
- Limb salvage

ANATOMIC INDICATIONS

As in all technical procedures, patient selection is extremely critical in assuring high success rates with low complication rates. More than 15 years of experience have led to some general principles for defining lesions that are ideal and some lesions that are less ideal or contraindicated.

Ideal anatomic lesions include the following:

- Short stenosis of the abdominal aorta
- Short stenosis involving the aortic bifurcation, including the common iliac artery origins
- Short iliac artery stenosis and some short iliac occlusions
- Short solitary or multiple isolated stenoses of the superficial femoral artery and occlusions less than 15 cm
- Short stenoses of the popliteal arteries and some occlusions, with better results occurring in shorter lesions

Some types of lesions may also be treated with high degrees of success but with somewhat lower success rates than the more ideal lesions:

- Long-segment stenoses in the iliac arteries
- Branches of the popliteal artery below the knee, including short stenoses.

In general, stenoses that occur in extremely long segments and in particular, in arteries such as long-segment stenoses in the external iliac arteries and long-segment irregularity in the abdominal aorta, are less ideal for angioplasty and are best treated initially by surgery. Nonetheless, the lesions may be treated for symptomatic relief if the patient is not considered a good surgical candidate for a variety of reasons. The initial and long-term success rates, however, may be somewhat reduced. By reviewing the clinical findings and the anatomic indications and considering the risk-benefit ratio of competitive therapies, the best possible initial and long-term success rates and lowest complication rates will be achieved.

Contraindications to PTA may exist based on anatomic features; however, they are generally relative and must be assessed in light of risk-benefit ratios of PTA, as well as alternative procedures. For instance, certain lesions that might ordinarily be thought not technically possible might be attempted and even completed successfully in the event of limb salvage. The following situations may be associated with both reduced success rates and high complication rates:

- Patients with long-segment iliac occlusions in tortuous vessels
- Patients in whom occlusions are present and in whom thrombus is suspected clinically or angiographically
- Patients who may have aneurysms in direct apposition with a stenotic segment, particularly in the renal and iliac vessels

Recent experience with thrombolysis has demonstrated that some types of occlusions may be converted into stenotic lesions with catheter-directed lytic therapy.[14] Therefore lytic therapy of the thrombotic component of any occlusion must be considered before angioplasty.

Traditionally the presence of calcium at the site of stenosis has been believed an indication of nondilatable lesions. Recent developments in balloon technology, particularly with the development of higher pressure balloons and other devices, now make treatment of these types of lesions technically possible. Similar experience has been gained with eccentric lesions. In patients with "blue-toe" syndrome and isolated stenosis, transluminal angioplasty can generally be performed easily; however, the angiographer should be alert for the presence of thrombus. More recent experience has led to the use of percutaneous atherectomy, a new procedure for treatment of these types of lesions percutaneously.

Clinical experience has now demonstrated that certain lesions are more ideal than others for PTA, and technical improvements have led to the ability to treat certain types of lesions that previously were nontreatable by PTA. Patient selection should depend on a cooperative approach between the vascular surgeon and interventional radiologist to choose the appropriate therapy and to tailor the use of various modalities in the best interest of patient care.

In some clinical settings angioplasty may be of value in conjunction with surgical procedures, that is, by limiting the degree of surgical intervention necessary or by making surgery possible in otherwise inoperable patients:

- Treatment of iliac stenosis before femoropopliteal bypass or other distal procedures
- Treatment of postoperative strictures
- Treatment of native inflow or outflow vessels in the presence of a bypass graft in which continued patency may be threatened

Angioplasty may be a useful alternative to surgical intervention or an adjunct to surgical intervention or may be used after surgical intervention in selected patients.

TECHNICAL PRINCIPLES OF BALLOON ANGIOPLASTY

Techniques vary in various parts of the circulatory system, and rapid improvement in balloon catheter and guide wire technology is continually being made. Nonetheless, certain principles of angioplasty are generally applied. The steps of angioplasty might be simplified as follows:

1. Percutaneous access
2. Initial detailed evaluation of the lesion and detailed circulation in multiple oblique projections
3. Careful passage through the lesion or recanalization
4. Exchange for appropriately sized balloon catheter
5. Balloon inflation to 5 to 6 atmospheres of pressure across entire segment of the lesion
6. Withdrawal of catheter over the guide wire
7. Injection of contrast over the guide wire from a point proximal to the dilatation site
8. Removal of the catheter, and puncture site compression

In the past, passage of the guide wire through a stenotic lesion represented the most likely area in which technical problems might be encountered and complications could occur. Recently, the development of steerable, or torque, guide wires have made this a much less traumatic procedure and have given the angiographer greater control over the process.

During balloon inflation, the patient should experience mild discomfort, which is a sign of adventitial stretching. In an alert, cooperative patient, the lack of significant discomfort during balloon inflation is a reliable sign of under dilatation, whereas severe pain may be an early warning sign of rupture and, when present, should result in some reduction in inflation pressure. Part of the art of angioplasty is in selection of correct balloon size; too little dilatation may lead to early restenosis, whereas too much dilatation may lead to excessive trauma and possible arterial rupture.

ADJUNCTIVE PHARMACOLOGY

The use of anticoagulation during angioplasty varies among angiographers, as well as among anatomic sites. The risk of thrombosis during PTA is dependent on several factors, including the degree of vascular trauma, the presence of arterial spasm, the degree of flow present in the angioplasty environment, and the anatomic location. It is generally not necessary to provide anticoagulation in larger vessels such as the iliac arteries, whereas in smaller vessels such as the tibioperoneal vessels, anticoagulation is more useful. When heparin is used, it is generally in boluses of 2,000 to 7,000 U, with the goal of immediate systemic anticoagulation. Generally, anticoagulation is used primarily after tibial angioplasty.

The use of antispasmodic agents, particularly through an intraarterial bolus, may be of value. They are usually administered prophylactically before and after several key parts of the angioplasty procedure, including before guide wire passage, after passage of the guide wire, before dilatation, and after dilatation. The most frequently used agent is nitroglycerin, given in 100 μg increments (in a volume of 1 ml), which may be of particular value in the treatment of spasm demonstrated angiographically. Frequent administration is well tolerated because of the low dose and short half-life of the agent. This method of administration is of little value in larger vessels such as in the iliac circulation, but in the renal arteries and vessels below the knee, administration of nitroglycerin may be of particular value.

Systemic vasodilators may also be used, including nitroglycerin patches, nitroglycerin tablets administered sublingually, and nifedipine or other calcium channel blockers. Nifedipine is generally administered sublingually, giving the contents of a broken capsule sublingually 20 minutes before the procedure.

PATIENT CARE

Percutaneous transluminal angioplasty requires only local anesthesia and mild sedation, with medication administered before the procedure as necessary. If the diagnostic evaluation has been completed on an outpatient basis, the procedure is performed the day of admission. The patient is maintained on bed rest overnight, and early ambulation the next morning is encouraged. If no complications or adverse reactions have occurred, discharge the day after the procedure is the rule. Noninvasive evaluation is performed before the procedure and immediately after the procedure to assess the hemodynamic effects of PTA. Patients are generally examined at 2- and 6-month intervals for confirmation of patency. As in all forms of treatment of vascular disease, risk factors such as diet, smoking, and exercise are addressed in both the preprocedure and postprocedure periods.

RESULTS

As with any interventional procedure, the results of PTA vary, depending on a number of factors, including extent of the disease, location of the lesion, underlying risk factors, and the degree of initial success. Experience during the past 10 years has adequately documented the efficacy of PTA, and results are predictable. In general, initial and long-term results of PTA are better in larger vessels than in smaller vessels.

In the iliac arteries, success rates from 75 to 100% have been reported.[15–28] Initial success rates greater than 90% can be anticipated in the treatment of iliac artery stenoses (Fig. 24-1). Long-term results vary from 61 to 100%, with variations in the methods of reporting; however, most of these studies were reported before the advent of more effective balloon catheters. In 1983 I reported an initial success rate of 95% and a 3-year patency of 93%.[27]

Reports indicate an initial success rate in the superficial femoral and proximal popliteal arteries ranging from 76 to 90%.[18,20,24,29–36] Perhaps in these arteries more than in any other anatomic area, specifics of morphology such as the presence of calcium, length of disease, presence of occlusion, and status of distal runoff, play an important role. Additionally, the experience of the angiographer may have a direct bearing on the initial success rate, as indicated by Krepel et al.,[36] who had an initial success rate in the first

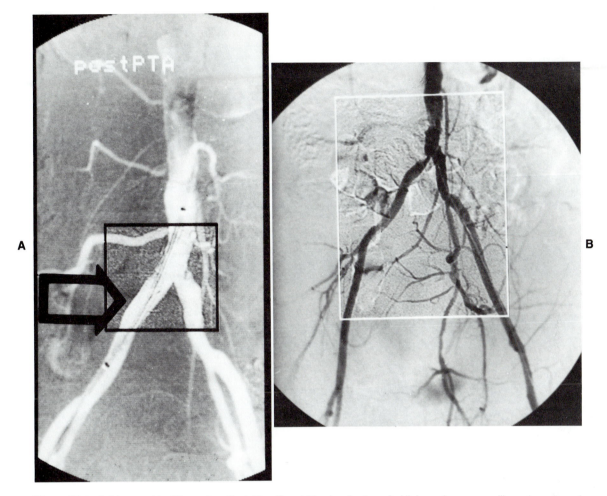

Figure 24-1. A 64-year-old white male with right calf and hip claudication. **A.** High-grade common iliac artery stenosis with 40 mm Hg pressure grading. **B.** After transluminal angioplasty with 8 mm outer diameter balloon, obliteration of underlying pressure grading and morphologic improvement.

77 procedures of 77% and an initial success rate in the next 87 procedures of 91%.

These reports also indicate that the long-term success rate of femoral and popliteal angioplasty for stenoses averages approximately 70% at 3 years (Fig. 24-2). The long-term success rates for occlusions, however, are lower, varying from 57 to 70% in most series, with the length of the occlusion having a direct bearing on long-term success rates (Fig. 24-3).

Despite the fact that results of PTA are poor in long occlusions, in patients with long occlusions who may not be candidates for surgery, successful PTA can be performed, particularly when the measurable clinical result is limb salvage.

The results of successful angioplasty are immediately apparent—improvement in pulses, capillary filling, and other measures of perfusion. The problems of restenosis are currently being widely investigated, with some authors believing that the placement of intravascular stents will ultimately prevent or retard restenosis.[37] These investigational devices are currently in their early stages of evalua-

tion, and it is too early to draw conclusions about their efficacy.

DISTAL POPLITEAL AND TIBIOPERONEAL ANGIOPLASTY

One of the areas of significant advance in PTA is in the treatment of distal popliteal artery and branch lesions. Previous experience had been associated with relatively poor results due to the small vessel size, the lack of available tools, and the associated vasospasm that accompanied the treatment of these vessels. With the development of new, miniaturized balloons and guide wires and the better understanding of the pharmacologic control of the angioplasty environment, treatment of these lesions has become much more successful.[38] The technical approach is more careful and controlled, using sheaths, systemic anticoagulation, and a variety of possible small guide wires and balloons. Initial success rates of 90% and higher have been reported, with associated clinical success rates.[38]

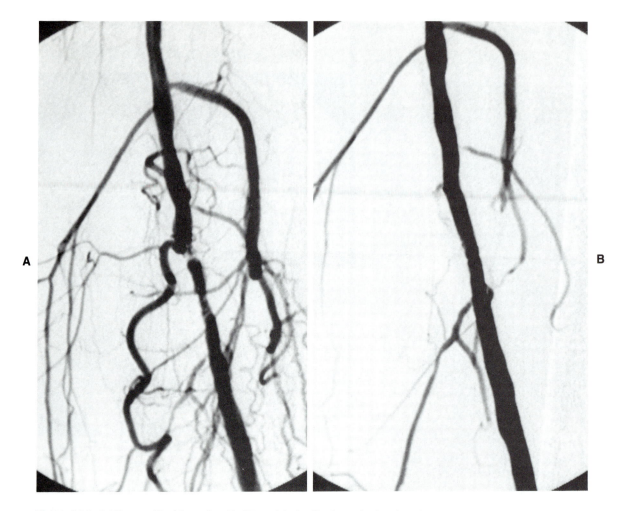

Figure 24-2. A 70-year-old white male with 50 yards' claudication, who is otherwise active. **A.** High-grade superficial femoral artery stenosis over short segment with abundant collateralization. **B.** After transluminal angioplasty with 6 mm outer diameter balloon, marked morphologic improvement with reduction in collateral flow.

RENAL ANGIOPLASTY

One of the significant benefits of the development of a flexible balloon catheter by Gruntzig was the application of transluminal angioplasty to renal artery lesions.

The diagnosis of renovascular hypertension is extremely difficult. Even its definition is not universally agreed on. In general, patients who have underlying hypertension, demonstrable renal artery lesions, and elevated renal vein renin levels are considered candidates for transluminal angioplasty. Angiographers widely believe that, given the reduced risk, expense, hospital stay, and general benefits of transluminal angioplasty, indications for treatment may be less stringent than those applied for surgical revascularization of the renal arteries.[39] In my clinical experience the increasing use of beta blockers for the treatment of coronary vascular disease has frequently masked the presence of renovascular hypertension, and while blood pressures have remained normal, renal function and size gradually have deteriorated.

Renal angioplasty is technically more complicated than other types of peripheral angioplasty and is best performed by experienced interventionists in an environment in which a capable and cooperative surgical team is present.

RESULTS OF RENAL PTA

Because of the complex nature of renovascular hypertension and the presence of both anatomic and physiologic disorders, evaluation of the results is somewhat complex. Initial success rates based on morphology and physiologic response are 75 to 94% (Fig. 24-4). Results are better in patients with fibromuscular dysphasia, in whom initial success rates are greater than 90% and long-term success rates greater than 90% are anticipated.[40-43] Similarly, skilled interventionists have reported successful recanalization and dilatation of occluded renal arteries in patients with renal vascular hypertension by employing fibrinolytic agents and angioplasty.[14]

It is generally agreed that in patients with the appropri-

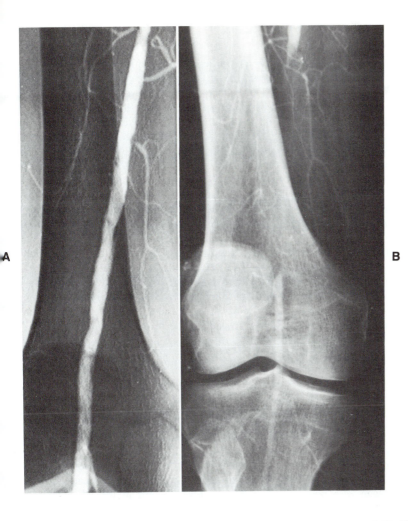

A

B

Figure 24-3. A 60-year-old male with limiting claudication, night cramps. **A.** A 10 cm distal superficial femoral artery occlusion. **B.** After recanalization in transluminal dilatation, abundant antegrade flow through the occluded segment.

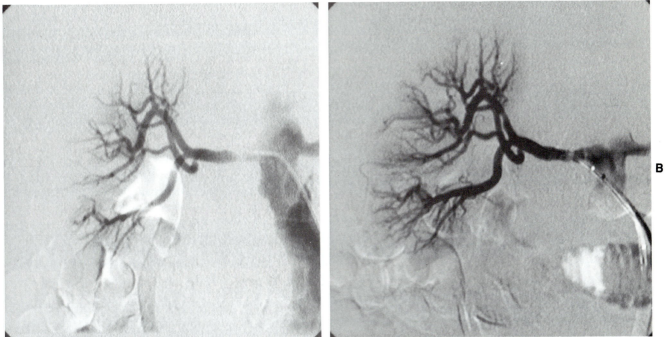

A

B

Figure 24-4. A 75-year-white male with peripheral vascular disease, who has severe hypertension requiring three antihypertensive medications. **A.** High-grade stenosis of the right renal artery distal to the catheter tip; some reduction in renal size is demonstrated. **B.** After angioplasty a widely patent lumen with accrued filling of all distal branches.

ate clinical and anatomic setting, angioplasty of the renal artery should be attempted before surgical intervention.

ANGIOPLASTY OF BYPASS GRAFTS

PTA is an effective method of treating postoperative strictures that occur at the site of the surgical anastomosis, particularly because repeat surgery is more difficult than the original procedure. The stenoses generally occur at anastomoses of the grafts and are due to intimal proliferation and fibrotic scar formation. Technical approaches include direct puncture of the graft proximal to the lesion or distal to the lesion in a retrograde fashion, such as in a saphenous vein bypass graft in the thigh; however, direct puncture of saphenous vein grafts is generally discouraged. Once synthetic grafts are punctured, the puncture site should be dilated, and sheaths are generally used to reduce the degree of trauma associated with multiple catheter exchanges. Data on treatment of bypass grafts is not widely available; however, in general practice they are treated by transluminal angioplasty, before surgical revision, when stenoses are present.

COMPLICATIONS OF TRANSLUMINAL ANGIOPLASTY

Complications may be associated with almost any aspect of the transluminal angioplasty procedure and have been reported with a frequency of 2 to 18.8%.[30,44–46] In general, the incidence of complications requiring surgical intervention or prolonging hospital stay occur approximately 2 to 3% of the time.

Complications may be associated with the percutaneous access, attempts to traverse the lesion, dilatation itself, and contrast agents used during the course of the procedure. These possible complications should be discussed in detail with the patient before the procedure.

Complications occurring at the puncture site and associated with percutaneous access may include bleeding, thrombosis, development of false aneurysm, and, rarely, neurologic deficit. At the angioplasty site, dissection by a guide wire traversing a lesion may lead to a complete occlusion; in addition, a large intimal defect may lead to spasmodic thrombosis. On rare occasions, arterial rupture may occur at the puncture site as well. Rarely, distal embolus formation can occur, most often associated with the treatment of occlusions, and may be treated by fibrinolytic agents, although direct surgical intervention distal to the angioplasty site is generally performed.

Renal failure, hypotension due to bleeding, and adverse contrast reactions may also occur.

It is extremely unusual for a complication to occur more than 24 hours after the angioplasty procedure, although in the case of false aneurysms, diagnosis may be delayed.

Technical advances in imaging such as sophisticated fluoroscopy and digital subtraction angiography, smaller balloon catheters, and improved guide wires, as well as new contrast agents, continue to improve the safety of angioplasty.

CONCLUSIONS

PTA has become an accepted method of treatment for patients with peripheral vascular disease, based on a worldwide experience since the procedure was conceived and developed by Charles Dotter and refined and popularized by Andreas Gruntzig.[1,8] Wider application of angioplasty is now being evaluated, including the application to brachiocephalic vessels to small vessels in the distal calf and foot, as well as postoperative applications. Recently, considerable interest has been shown by both the medical and lay communities in the associated use of lasers, mechanical recanalization devices, and devices to perform percutaneous atherectomy. Nonetheless, it is the procedure of PTA against which these new devices must be compared, as well as against the long-standing results of surgical intervention.

It is imperative that all physicians who treat peripheral vascular disease be familiar with alternative methods of therapy and their associated benefits, risks, and disadvantages so that proper application, patient education, and the best clinical results can be provided.

EXPERIENCE WITH A NEW DIGITAL SUBTRACTION ANGIOGRAPHIC SYSTEM DESIGNED FOR INTERVENTIONAL RADIOLOGY

Since the initial development of digital subtraction angiography, varying degrees of acceptance have been obtained because of limiting factors present in the production of high quality images. Among the variables are the image intensification system, as well as the entire computerized angiographic components. Although limitations exist, when all components are optimal, the benefits of digital subtraction angiography, including reduced contrast, reduced catheter size, reduced time of the examination, and production of instantaneous data, are of great benefit to patient care.

Experience using a digital subtraction angiographic unit designed specifically for applications in interventional vascular radiology reveals advantages, including total operation of the important aspects of the device at the tabletop by the interventional radiologist, operation of the entire device as a "spot-filming" device, using a foot petal, and the ability to store selected images on-line in an electronic view box. Additionally, instantaneous real-time subtraction, or "road mapping," has been of particular value. Application of the inherent digital system has also been used to produce "digital spot films" in nonvascular cases such as biliary, genitourinary, and biopsy procedures. The advantages of electronic contrast enhancement of both the fluoroscopic and radiographic images have been of significant benefit.

In conclusion, the production of a system specifically designed for use in interventional radiology has led to significant patient benefit by reducing procedure time, providing better quality and more rapid diagnostic information on-line, facilitating decision making during the procedure, and producing image quality comparable to film screen imaging.

REFERENCES

1. Dotter CT, Judkins MP: Transluminal treatment of arteriosclerotic obstruction: Description of a new technic and a preliminary report of its application. Circulation 30:654, 1964.
2. Zeitler E, Gruntzig A, Schoop W (eds): Percutaneous Vascular Recanalization: Technique, Application, Clinical Results, Berlin, Springer-Verlag, 1978.
3. van Andel GJ: Percutaneous Transluminal Angioplasty: The Dotter Procedure. Amsterdam, Excerpta Medica, 1976.
4. Porstmann W: Ein neuer Korsett-ballonkatheter zur transluminalen Rekanalisation nach Dotter unter besonderer Berucksichtigung von Obliterationen an den Bechenarterien. Radiol Diagn (Berl) 14:239, 1973.
5. Gruntzig A: Die Perkutane Transluminale Rekanalisation Chronischer Arterienverschlusse mit Einer Neuen Dilatationstechnik. Baden-Baden, Verlag Gerhard Witzstrock, 1977.
6. Gruntzig A, Hopff H: Perkutane Rekanalisation chronischer arterieller Verschlusse mit einem neuen Dilatationskatheter: Modifikation der Dotter-Technik. Dtsch Med Wochenschr 99:2502, 1974.
7. Dotter CT, Judkins MP, Rosch J: Nonoperative treatment of arterial occlusive disease: A radiologically facilitated technique. Radiol Clin North Am 5:531, 1967.
8. Castaneda-Zuniga WR, Formanek A, et al.: The mechanism of balloon angioplasty. Radiology 135:565, 1980.
9. Block PC, Baughman KL, et al.: Transluminal angioplasty: Correlation of morphologic and angiographic findings in an experimental model. Circulation 61:778, 1980.
10. Block PC, Fallon JT, Elmer D: Experimental angioplasty: Lessons from the laboratory. AJR 135:907, 1980.
11. Pasternak RC, Baughman KL, et al.: Scanning electron microscopy after coronary transluminal angioplasty of normal canine coronary arteries. Am J Cardiol 45:591, 1980.
12. Kinney TB, Chin Ak, et al.: Transluminal angioplasty: A mechanical-pathophysiological correlation of its physical mechanisms. Radiology 153:85, 1984.
13. Zollikofer CL, Chain J, et al.: Percutaneous transluminal angioplasty of the aorta. Radiology 151:355, 1984.
14. Katzen BT, van Breda A: The current status of catheter directed fibrinolysis in the treatment of arterial and graft occlusions, in Arterial Surgery: New Diagnostic and Operative Techniques. New York, Grune & Stratton, Inc, 1988, p 119.
15. Colapinto RF, Harries-Jones EP, Johnston KW: Percutaneous transluminal recanalization of complete iliac artery occlusions. Arch Surg 116:277, 1981.
16. Dotter CT, Rosch J, et al.: Transluminal iliac artery dilatation: Nonsurgical catheter treatment of atheromatous narrowing. JAMA 230:117, 1974.
17. Schoop W, Levy H, et al.: Early and late results of PTA in iliac stenosis, in Zeitler E, Gruntzig A, Schoop W (eds): Percutaneous Vascular Recanalization. New York, Springer-Verlag New York, Inc, 1978.
18. Gruntzig A, Kumpe DA: Technique of percutaneous transluminal angioplasty with the Gruntzig balloon catheter. AJR 132:547, 1979.
19. Alpert JR, Ring EJ, et al.: Treatment of stenosis of the iliac artery by balloon catheter dilatation. Surg Gynecol Obstet 150:481, 1980.
20. Colapinto RF, Harries-Jones EP, Johnston KW: Percutaneous transluminal angioplasty of peripheral vascular disease: A 2-year experience. Cardiovasc Intervent Radiol 3:213, 1980.
21. Dotter CJ: Transluminal angioplasty: A long view. Radiology 135:561, 1980.
22. Motarjeme A, Keifer JW, Zuska AJ: Percutaneous transluminal angioplasty of the iliac arteries: 66 experiences. AJR 135:937, 1980.
23. Waltman AC: Percutaneous transluminal angioplasty: Iliac and deep femoral arteries. AJR 135:921, 1980.
24. Zeitler E: Percutaneous dilatation and recanalization of iliac and femoral arteries. Cardiovasc Intervent Radiol 3:207, 1980.
25. Neiman HL, Bergan JJ, et al.: Hemodynamic assessment of transluminal angioplasty for lower extremity ischemia. Radiology 143:639, 1982.
26. Kadir S, White RI Jr, et al.: Long-term results of aortoiliac angioplasty. Surgery 94:10, 1983.
27. Katzen BT: Transluminal angioplasty in ischemic peripheral vascular disease, in Castaneda-Zuniga W (ed): Transluminal Angioplasty. New York, Thieme-Stratton, Inc, 1983.
28. van Andel GJ, van Erp WFM, et al.: Percutaneous transluminal dilatation of the iliac artery: Long-term results. Radiology 156:321, 1985.
29. Katzen BT, Chang J: Percutaneous transluminal angioplasty with the Gruntzig balloon catheter. Radiology 130:623, 1979.
30. Greenfield AJ: Femoral, popliteal, and tibial arteries: Percutaneous transluminal angioplasty. AJR 135:927, 1980.
31. Martin EC, Fankuchen EI, et al.: Angioplasty for femoral artery occlusion: Comparison with surgery. AJR 137:915, 1981.
32. Spence RK, Freiman DB, et al.: Long-term results of transluminal angioplasty of the iliac and femoral arteries. Arch Surg 116:1377, 1981.
33. Tamura S, Sniderman KW, et al.: Percutaneous transluminal angioplasty of the popliteal artery and its branches. Radiology 143:645, 1982.
34. Lu CT, Zarins CK, et al.: Long-segment arterial occlusion: Percutaneous transluminal angioplasty. AJR 138:119, 1982.
35. Probst P, Cerny P, et al.: Patency after femoral angioplasty: Correlation of angiographic appearance with clinical findings. AJR 140:1227, 1983.
36. Krepel VM, van Andel GJ, et al.: Percutaneous transluminal angioplasty of the femoropopliteal artery: Initial and long-term results. Radiology 156:325, 1985.
37. Rousseau H, Puel J, et al.: Self-expanding endovascular prosthesis: An experimental study. Radiology 164:709, Sept 1987.
38. Schwarten, D.
39. Tegtmeyer CJ: Percutaneous Transluminal Angioplasty. Current Problems in Diagnostic Radiology 1987. Chicago, Year Book Medical Publishers, Inc., 1987.
40. Tegtmeyer CJ, Elson J, et al.: Percutaneous transluminal angioplasty: The treatment of choice for renovascular hypertension due to fibromuscular dysplasia. Radiology 143:631, 1982.
41. Tegtmeyer CJ, Tegtmeyer VL, et al.: Percutaneous transluminal angioplasty: The treatment of choice for vascular lesions caused by fibromuscular dysplasia. Semin Intervent Radiol 1:289, 1984.
42. Tegtmeyer CJ, Kellum CD, Ayers C: Percutaneous transluminal angioplasty of the renal artery: Results and long-term follow-up. Radiology 153:77, 1984.
43. Geyskes GG, Puijlaert CBAJ, et al.: Follow-up study of 70 patients with renal artery stenosis treated by percutaneous transluminal dilatation. Br Med J (Clin Res) 287:333, 1983.
44. Gruntzig A: Die Perkutane Transluminale Rekanalisation Chronischer Arterienverschlusse mit Einer Neuen Dilatationstechnik. Baden-Baden, Verlag Gerhard Witzstrock, 1977.
45. Zeitler E: Complications in and after PTR, in Zeitler E, Gruntzig A, Schoop W (eds): Percutaneous Vascular Recanalization. Heidelberg, Springer-Verlag, 1978, p 120.
46. Gardiner GA Jr, Meverovitz MF, et al.: Complications of transluminal angioplasty. Radiology 159:201, 1986.

CHAPTER 25
The Current Status of Catheter-Directed Fibrinolysis in the Treatment of Arterial and Graft Occlusions

Barry T. Katzen

Since the discovery of thrombolytic agents, there has been interest in applying the benefits of lysis to patients with peripheral vascular occlusive disease in which thrombosis is an integral part of the pathophysiologic process. Enthusiasm has varied widely, and development has been limited by the relatively recent availability of thrombolytic agents for general use. The development of interventional vascular radiology in the past 10 to 15 years has been accompanied by increasing investigation of the applicability of these agents to peripheral vascular disease. Local thrombolysis is a technique that has evolved more recently and has continued to improve in safety and efficacy. It should be familiar to all angiographers, particularly those performing transluminal angioplasty and other percutaneous interventions. Thrombolysis has become significant as an adjunct to angioplasty in two major areas: the treatment of thrombotic complications and the treatment of atherosclerotic occlusions associated with both thrombotic and atherosclerotic components. Additionally, catheter-directed lysis can be extremely valuable in the management of bypass graft occlusions. The following discussion reviews the current status of thrombolysis in the management of vascular disease.

PHARMACOLOGY OF FIBRINOLYSIS

The body's natural fibrinolytic and hemostatic systems are in equilibrium to preserve vascular integrity and patency. The fibrinolytic system can be activated by endogenous factors in the blood, vascular endothelium, and other tissues or by thrombolytic agents (exogenous activators). Activation occurs through conversion of the inactive precursor plasminogen, present in circulating blood or bound to fibrin in clot, to the active proteolytic enzyme plasmin, which hydrolyzes a solid clot into peptide fragments called fibrin degradation products. Plasminogen is synthesized rapidly and, if depleted during thrombolytic activity, returns to normal within 24 hours of cessation of therapy. Plasmin has a short half-life because of its nearly immediate inactivation in the blood by antiplasmin, a specific inhibitor. In a

thrombus, the presence of fibrin prevents plasmin inactivation, allowing plasmin activity and fibrin breakdown. Activation of the fibrinolytic mechanism is normally controlled by specific inhibitors at various steps to maintain hemostasis and prevent fibrinolysis except in areas of high fibrin concentration such as a thrombus.

To activate the fibrinolytic mechanism, endogenous activators must be released, or exogenous activators must be administered. Agents such as nicotine are known to induce release of endogenous activators, but they are not clinically useful. Therefore exogenous activators are necessary to produce controlled therapeutic thrombolysis.

Streptokinase

The agent most frequently used for fibrinolytic therapy is streptokinase (SK), a nonenzymatic protein derived from β-hemolytic streptococci that activates fibrinolysis by combining in a 1:1 molar ratio with plasminogen to form an activator complex. The SK-plasminogen is effective in converting free plasminogen into plasmin. The effectiveness of SK is therefore dependent on a sufficient quantity of plasminogen to form the activator complex and to act as a substrate for the conversion to plasmin.

SK is antigenic, and prior streptococcal infection induces a variety of antibodies, including a specific SK antibody that directly inactivates the agent by forming an irreversible complex in a 1:1 ratio. Therefore all the antibody sites must be saturated by an initial loading dose of SK before subsequent doses can act systemically. Antibody titers can vary greatly from individual to individual. Calculation of the loading dose requirements formerly was performed during initial clinical trials and was based on antibodies in a large patient sample population. Currently, a standardized loading dose of 250,000 U is used, because this dose will neutralize antibodies in 90% of the American population.[1] Although the importance of antibodies in systemic fibrinolytic therapy is obvious, the role of antibodies during direct infusion of SK into clot is not known. The antigenicity of SK can cause occasional pyretic reactions (in 5 to 10% of patients) and cases of serum sickness.[2,3] Anaphylaxis has been reported, but it is extremely rare[14] and may have occurred only in earlier preparations.

The half-life of SK is short; however, altered coagulation may persist for hours because of the depletion of fibrinogen and other clotting factors, as well as the presence of fibrin split products, which may produce an anticoagulant effect.[5]

Urokinase

The other agent frequently used for fibrinolysis, urokinase (UK), differs from SK in several significant aspects. As opposed to SK, UK is nonantigenic, being derived from human fetal renal-cell cultures. Since there are no antibodies to cause inactivation, no loading dose is necessary. Biochemically, UK is a direct plasminogen activator and does not form an intermediate activator complex. All molecules of plasminogen are converted to plasmin in a 1:1 ratio. Because of these characteristics, UK should have a more direct and predictable thrombolytic effect. To date, there has been much greater clinical experience with SK because of its greater availability and reduced cost, but further evaluation of these agents should clarify these differences.

The half-life of UK is short; however, as with SK, prolonged abnormalities after systemic use can result from depleted clotting factors.

Tissue Plasminogen Activator

Currently a new thrombolytic agent is being evaluated—tissue plasminogen activator (tPA).[6] This agent is an endogenous activator of plasminogen that was originally prepared from human uterine tissue and is now manufactured by biogenetic engineering techniques. It is normally present in a variety of tissues and is a more specific agent in that it will only activate plasminogen in the presence of fibrin, theoretically limiting its effect to areas of thrombus and avoiding depletion of fibrinogen systemically. Initial results have demonstrated that systemic fibrinogen levels can be significantly reduced, indicating further evaluation and understanding of the mechanism of action is necessary. It is hoped that tPA will provide more specific activity and a more predictable response and may obviate the need for local infusions.[7-9]

ANGIOGRAPHIC APPLICATIONS OF FIBRINOLYTIC THERAPY

Patient Selection After Angioplasty or Angiographic Complications

Acute thrombosis may complicate angioplasty in 2 to 3% of patients.[10] Because of the presence of a fresh thrombus, these situations represent ideal applications of catheter-directed therapy, and it should be used before surgical intervention if the clinical setting permits. Factors that make these occlusions so amenable to thrombolysis include the acute nature of the thrombus, the knowledge of vascular anatomy afforded by the preceding angiography, and the fact that an angiographic catheter is generally in place after the angioplasty. Thrombolysis is generally rapid in these patients, often within a few hours, and the success rates are high.[11,12]

These occlusions are often associated with significant spasm, most likely related to the trauma of angioplasty or the abnormal flap that may have occurred, and vigorous use of intra-arterial vasodilators should accompany therapy, particularly in the acute phase while waiting for initiation of the infusion. As in all patients with acute arterial occlusions, the degree of ischemia should be carefully assessed, and if neurologic deficit or motor abnormalities are present, immediate surgical intervention should be considered. However, these patients commonly have sufficient collateralization due to their underlying disease so that tolerance of the occlusion may allow time for thrombolytic infusion.

Occlusions that occur after diagnostic angiographic procedures are generally the result of underlying pathology such as diffuse atherosclerotic disease or arterial spasm. Low-dose infusions into areas including the puncture site have been performed with safety, although careful observation of the infusion site is necessary. The use of vasodilators may also be of value and is recommended.

Embolization after transluminal angioplasty should be approached with caution since the nature of the embolic material is uncertain and may be atheromatous or thrombotic. Careful clinical assessment is made, and if thrombolytic therapy is used, rapid reperfusion should occur, or surgical therapy should follow expeditiously. Because of the distal location of occlusion in these patients, clinical status may not allow time for infusion.

Occlusions of Native Vessels

The nature of an atherosclerotic occlusion is difficult to assess angiographically and may be purely atherosclerotic or a combination of atheromatous plaque and superimposed thrombus. Most occlusions probably consist of both elements. Although recanalization of total occlusions is possible and can be associated with successful angioplasty, total occlusions may be associated with a higher risk of emboli, particularly in the iliac artery.[10]

It has been my experience that the thrombotic component of many occlusions can be lysed with thrombolytic therapy.[13] The likelihood of successful lysis is partially dependent on the age of the thrombus, but this may be difficult to evaluate angiographically and is difficult to assess clinically since there may be little hemodynamic difference between a high-grade stenosis and total occlusion. Data show that success of thrombolysis in relatively acute occlusions of native vessels is high, with total success rates of 82 to 90%, but overall success rates of 75 to 80% were noted in occlusions of more than 3 weeks' duration.[13]

The angiographic appearance of occlusions can suggest a recent event even in the presence of chronic symptoms. An irregular proximal or distal end of an occlusion, the lack of well-developed collateral circulation, and an occlusion that does not begin or end at a collateral branch are all suggestive findings, especially in an appropriate clinical setting.

Because of the uncertainties described above, after review of the clinical and angiographic findings by all medical specialists involved, a trial of thrombolytic therapy is frequently used in native vessel occlusions. If lysis is successful, angioplasty or another intervention will follow; and if it is not, surgical therapy is used. Approximately 70% of native vessel occlusions treated electively have been successfully lysed.[13]

Thrombolysis of Occluded Bypass Grafts

Treatment of occluded arterial bypass grafts is another important application of catheter-directed thrombolysis. As with all forms of occlusions, a thrombus is a manifestation of underlying pathology, and this method of therapy offers both diagnostic and therapeutic benefits. Stenoses at graft anastomoses can occur at both the proximal and distal sites and can be difficult to document intraoperatively. In the case of saphenous vein bypass grafts, therapy and transluminal angioplasty may save the saphenous vein and obviate the need for revision and replacement with synthetic material. There may be prognostic significance in the success of thrombolytic therapy; in two series, when poor runoff was the cause of graft occlusion, repeated occlusions occurred unless some other runoff was established surgically.[14,15] Patients with occluded bypass grafts who are initially seen with other medical abnormalities are poor surgical candidates. Thrombolysis may also allow operation to be delayed in patients who are poor operative risks.[15]

General principles of patient selection are similar to those described previously. Acute occlusions of grafts that are less than 6 weeks old are generally the result of technical problems and are better treated surgically.[16] This approach also avoids the potential problems of infusing a recent operative site. The clinical situation should be taken into account, and if operation is not feasible and there is a potential for limb loss, thrombolysis should be attempted.

There have been reports of extravasation of contrast during thrombolytic therapy performed in Dacron grafts because of leakage through interstices of the graft.[17] Most of them have been asymptomatic or nonsignificant, but significant bleeding can occur.[15] In my experience this has not been noted with the use of urokinase. In the extremities, sites of infusion can be observed clinically, but bleeding from intra-abdominal sites can go unrecognized for a time, and this potentially severe complication should be borne in mind.

Dosage and Selection of Fibrinolytic Agents

Since the initial description of catheter-directed fibrinolysis, several regimens for administration have been described using both streptokinase and urokinase. My therapeutic objective is to achieve successful clot lysis in the most expeditious fashion, with the least complications and with little or no systemic effect. Because of indwelling arterial catheters and frequently the presence of medical conditions associated with higher risks of bleeding from systemic lysis and because catheter directed therapy requires lower doses of the active agent, the technique of "low dose" catheter-directed therapy has evolved. By delivering the fibrinolytic agent directly into the thrombus, it is possible to activate plasminogen bound to fibrin without activating circulating plasminogen. This important principle leads to greater efficacy when compared to the use of systemic doses to treat arterial occlusions and provides the basis for achieving no significant systemic effect. This concept was first demonstrated by Dotter[18] who achieved successful lysis with doses as low as one twentieth of systemic doses.

Most subsequent series have reported use of SK in low doses (5000 to 10,000 U/h) because of its low cost and ready availability.[12,14,15,18–22]

Hess et al.[23] described a more rapid, higher dose SK infusion technique in which 1,000 to 3,000 U boluses were injected directly into the thrombus.[23] After several minutes and under fluoroscopic observation, thrombus and lytic products were vigorously aspirated, and the catheter was advanced. This process was then repeated. The duration of these infusions ranged from 1 to 5 hours, with the patient remaining on the angiographic table throughout the procedure. Overall success rates were similar to those reported with low-dose, slower infusions, but this technique has not been widely used in the United States, probably, in part, because of the time constraints in most angiography departments. Bleeding complications are reportedly lower, possibly because of the smaller total SK dose.

Higher rates of intra-arterial SK infusion have rarely been used for peripheral vascular occlusions, although they are commonly used in the treatment of acute coronary occlusions. The necessity for rapid revascularization in patients with coronary occlusions to prevent myocardial necrosis does not apply to most peripheral arterial occlusions. Limited experience with higher doses of SK fails to demonstrate any significant improvement in success rates or lysis time in the peripheral circulation.

More recently, investigators have been evaluating the use of UK for catheter-directed thrombolysis, and significant clinical differences apparently exist, leading to UK's becoming the preferred agent. It is not neutralized by circulating antibodies, as is SK, and this may result in increased success rates.[24] Additionally, it appears to have little or no systemic effect. I generally infuse 40,000 to 80,000 U/h in a manner similar to that described for SK. Another protocol described by McNamara[25] described improve results using initially higher doses of UK followed by lower hourly dose rates. Infusions were started at 4,000 U/min for 2 hours followed by 1,000 U/min, and included the use of concomitant heparin administration. A recent series of 122 patients by van Breda and Katzen[13] confirmed the higher success rates and reduced complication rates of infusions of UK. Additionally, little significant difference was noted between doses of 50,000 U/h and doses exceeding 100,000 U/h. McNamara uses an initial regimen of 4,000 U/min for 2 hours, followed by longer infusion of 1,000 U/min (60,000 U/h). With this regimen, too, a higher success rate and lower incidence of bleeding were noted. Despite its increased cost, the increased safety and efficacy of UK make it the agent of choice for catheter-directed thrombolytic therapy.

Patient Care

Once fibrinolytic infusions are initiated, patients are placed in an intensive care unit for monitoring of the puncture site, bleeding parameters, and clinical status of the affected extremity. This monitoring includes frequent Doppler examinations and close observation for bleeding.

Periodic angiographic monitoring is performed by returning the patient to the angiographic suite and advancing the catheter, if necessary, as lysis progresses. Care is taken to minimize manipulation at the puncture site. The coaxial system described under technique allows advancement of the small infusion guide wire or catheter without manipulation at the puncture site. Contamination of the puncture site during repeat manipulations probably occurs but has not been clinically significant. Nonetheless, because of the potentially devastating complications from the use of vascular prostheses, these patients are given broad-spectrum antibiotics.

If no progress is noted during the first 6 to 12 hours, the infusion is terminated. During this time some evidence of lysis generally is noted, possibly associated with clinical improvement; if no further progress is noted in the subsequent 12- to 24-hour period, the infusion is stopped. All decisions are made in the context of the clinical status of the patient and the therapeutic alternatives.

At the completion of thrombolytic therapy, angiography is again performed to outline any underlying stenosis or other cause of occlusion, which may then be treated immediately by angioplasty, if feasible, or surgery if necessary. In patients in whom complete lysis is achieved and no underlying cause is found, consideration should be given to long-term anticoagulation therapy. Patients who are treated with angioplasty after lysis do not generally receive anticoagulation therapy.

Hematologic Monitoring

Many attempts to avoid or minimize systemic effects during locally administered fibrinolysis have been made, a task made more difficult by the lack of a single laboratory parameter that accurately predicts the likelihood of bleeding. Thrombin time is the single most useful parameter,[5] but significant bleeding can occur with a normal thrombin time. In addition, the thrombin time is altered in the presence of heparin, which some have used concomitantly during fibrinolytic infusions. Fibrinogen depletion occurs during systemic fibrinolysis but should be reduced during lower-dose infusions, and depletion has been associated with an increased incidence of bleeding complications.[12]

Recommendations for laboratory monitoring, based on my clinical experience, include a baseline coagulation profile of thrombin time, fibrinogen, partial thromboplastin time, and prothrombin time at the start of therapy, primarily to screen for unsuspected underlying abnormalities. Thrombin time and fibrinogen are repeated at 4 hours to identify patients with an abnormally rapid onset of systemic effect, which has occurred clinically only in patients being infused with SK. If this rapid onset occurs, the hourly dose is reduced or discontinued, and laboratory work is repeated in 4 hours. If no significant alteration is noted, the thrombin time and fibrinolytic are repeated at 12 hours or immediately before the next angiographic check. If the fibrinogen level falls below 100 mg/dl the infusion is slowed or discontinued, and cryoprecipitate or fresh frozen plasm is administered to restore fibrinogen levels. In clinical experience this has

not been necessary during infusions of UK, where significant reduction in fibrinogen has been observed only rarely.

Some authors recommend concommitant anticoagulation to reduce the risk of pericatheter thrombosis; however, this has been unnecessary in my experience when a small coaxial infusion technique is used and the placement of catheters through areas of reduced flow is avoided.

Tissue plasminogen activator is currently under evaluation for use in peripheral arterial occlusions at lower doses than those used for myocardial infarction and with techniques similar to those described above. At this time there is insufficient data to make conclusions as to its efficacy or safety compared to urokinase.

Results

Positive results of catheter-directed fibrinolytic infusions have varied as questions regarding agents of choice, technique, and dose have been evaluated in the literature ranging from 40 to 90%, with an average of approximately 75%. Comparisons of success rates in various studies are difficult because of the many factors that may influence success. First, as is true with systemic thrombolysis, acute occlusions respond better than chronic ones. For example, angioplasty-induced thromboses respond quite well, with complete or significant lysis noted in most patients.[13] In my experience with 18 postangioplasty thromboses, successful lysis was achieved in 17, with the single failure due to extensive atheromatous disease with poor runoff.

A second general observation is that short occlusions tend to lyse more successfully than longer ones. Success rates with bypass grafts are similar to those with native vessel occlusions, with the same mechanical factors affecting success.

Urokinase produces higher success rates with reduced morbidity and is currently the agent of choice. Further studies by other investigators may confirm further improvement in results.

Complications: Recognition and Treatment

Although in my experience the safety of fibrinolytic therapy has improved significantly, treatment is complex and technical, and complications can occur. They may result from the angiographic aspects of the procedure such as puncture site thrombosis or may be specific to the thrombolytic therapy such as hemorrhage, distal embolization, or pericatheter thrombosis. Additionally, adverse reaction to some agents can occur.

Pericatheter Thrombosis
Development of thrombus along the angiographic catheter in spite of successful lysis at the distal end has been reported in as many as 35% of infusions[22,25,26] and was noted by me occasionally in earlier experience. Several factors may contribute to this phenomenon, but poor flow in the presence of distal occlusion, coupled with the almost universal presence of diffuse vascular disease along the path of the catheter, is the primary reason for thrombosis, and the presence of an angiographic catheter further compromises

flow and is probably the precipitating factor in thrombus formation. In addition there may be an increased thrombogenic milieu in some patients with ongoing thrombosis. My observation is that thrombosis can occur in the presence of adequate systemic anticoagulation if flow is reduced severely.

For this reason, the smallest possible infusion device should be used, particularly in the more distal vessels, and the intravascular course of the infusion catheter should be kept to a minimum (i.e., using antegrade puncture and access to the superficial femoral artery rather than approaching from the contralateral femoral artery). Use of coaxial systems employing a 5 French catheter maintained in a proximal position and of an open-ended guide wire positioned in the occlusion is the most ideal arrangement and is used most frequently. In cases of infusions of the superficial femoral artery, the 5 French catheter may be used for distal manipulation, but once the open-ended guide wire is in place, the catheter is withdrawn to the approximate level of the lesser trochanter. Contrast should be injected proximally in the artery before the initial distal manipulation to assist in assessing the degree of flow around the catheter.

In cases of common iliac occlusion, open-ended guide wires and coaxial devices are not generally used, but they are used in occlusions of the more distal external iliac artery or in cases of long-segment graft occlusions.

Hemorrhage

The most significant potential problem with low-dose thrombolysis, as with systemic infusions, is hemorrhage, although the objective of low-dose infusions is to reduce this risk to negligible levels. The rate of bleeding in reported series varies from 4 to 25%[14,15,18–20,22,25] and is worse with SK than with UK in my most recent experience. Most bleeding occurs at the arterial puncture site, but bleeding at remote sites has been noted, including intracranial bleeding with SK. Concomitant heparinization adds to the risk of bleeding and may create confusion as to the cause of bleeding when it occurs. Local bleeding can generally be controlled by manual compression and by terminating the infusion. Patients with known intracranial pathology are at higher risk for bleeding if systemic effects occur but can probably be treated more safely with low dose UK. Similarly, patients with known gastrointestinal bleeding or other bleeding problems would not be treated. Because of potentially life-threatening risks, thrombolytic therapy should not be undertaken without due consideration of the risk-benefit ratio and treatment alternatives. However, in my experience, low-dose UK has been used safely in patients with many underlying risk factors, including use in intraoperative settings.

Laboratory monitoring of thrombolytic infusions does not accurately predict the likelihood of bleeding or of successful lysis. The risk of bleeding does seem to increase with length of infusion, and I therefore attempt to limit the length of infusion to 24 hours. Maintaining fibrinogen levels above 100 mg/dl may help prevent bleeding complications, and infusion of cryoprecipitate should be considered if fibrinogen falls below this level. Additionally, thrombolysis of synthetic prosthetic grafts, especially those made of Dacron, carries the risk of extravasation through the graft interstices, which could possibly cause life-threatening hemorrhage, although this has not been noted in my clinical experience.

Embolization

Some patients experience dramatic worsening of ischemia during thrombolytic therapy; this is usually due to distal embolus formation from thrombotic material as lysis progresses. Careful angiographic evaluation after therapy may demonstrate some evidence of distal emboli,[15,19,23,27] but most often the clinical status improves within 1 hour as lysis progresses. Documented distal embolus formation, in most reports, has responded to continued thrombolytic therapy. If significant clinical deterioration persists longer than 1 hour, angiography should be repeated, and surgical intervention performed if necessary; but, in general, continued thrombolytic therapy will result in clinical improvement.

Fatal bilateral renal embolism and mesenteric artery embolism have been reported during attempted lysis of aortic occlusions.[28] Lysis of abdominal aortic occlusions is not recommended, unless no therapeutic options are present, because of the amount of thrombus present, reducing the likelihood of success and increasing the likelihood of complications.

Embolization of thrombus due to contrast injection at the origin of an occlusion can occur if injection is made too forcefully. These injections should be made carefully when occlusions are at the origin of a vessel, such as in the superficial femoral artery, where thrombus could reflux into the profunda femoral artery. If reflux of thrombus should occur, initial thrombolytic therapy should be directed at this site, but surgery may be necessary if significant clinical deterioration occurs.

In general, all catheter manipulations during thrombolysis should be performed with caution, since the clot softens before total lysis.

Allergic Reactions

Early preparations of SK were associated with a high incidence of allergic reactions, including pyrexia, musculoskeletal pain, and even anaphylaxis. Allergic reactions to UK are extremely rare and generally are not clinically significant. Pretreatment with corticosteroids is not recommended. Anti-pyretics and symptomatic treatment are generally sufficient. If SK is being used, conversion to UK during infusion will avoid allergic manifestations.

CONCLUSIONS

Intraarterial thrombolytic infusion has a definite role in today's management of peripheral vascular disease and is an important part of the interventional radiologist's armamentarium. In addition to its therapeutic benefits, it has contributed significantly to our understanding of the nature of atherosclerotic occlusion and has raised many questions, including the age at which a thrombus in the occluded vessel can still be lysed.

An intraarterial thrombolytic infusion is useful in patients with occlusions related to vascular intervention such as transluminal angioplasty or catheterization procedures and also plays a significant role in the treatment of occlusions of native vessels and grafts. Careful clinical assessment of patients and consideration of therapeutic alternatives are necessary to minimize the risk and maximize the benefits. The pharmacology and physiology of thrombolysis should be familiar to practicing angiographers and others interested in this field.

BIBLIOGRAPHY

Tillet WS, Garner RL: The fibrinolytic activity of hemolytic streptococci. J Exp Med 58:485, 1933.

MacFarlane RG, Pilling J: Observations on fibrinolysis: Plasminogen plasmin and antiplasmin content of human blood. Lancet 2:562, 1946.

Tillett WS, Johnson AJ, McCarthy WF: The intravenous infusion of the streptococcal fibrinolytic principle (streptokinase) into patients. J Clin Invest 34:169, 1955.

Guril NJ, Callahan W, Hufnagel HV: High dose short term local urokinase for clearing femoral thrombi by vasodilation and thrombolysis. J Surg Res 20:381, 1976.

Freeman AH, Bang NV, et al.: Factors affecting the formation and dissolution of experimental thrombi. Am J Cardiol 6:426, 1960.

Boyles, PW, Meyer WH, Graff J: Comparative effectiveness of intravenous and intra-arterial fibrinolysin therapy. Am J Cardiol 6:439, 1960.

Biggs JC: Thrombolytic therapy in arterial and venous thrombosis. Aust Ann Med 19(suppl):19, 1970.

Weimar W, Stibbe J, et al.: Specific lysis of an iliofemoral thrombus by administration of extrinsic (tissue-type) plasminogen activator. Lancet 2:1018, 1981.

Rosner NH, Doris PE: Contrast extravasation through a Gore-Tex graft: A sequela of low dose streptokinase therapy. AJR 143:633, 1984.

Graor RA, Risius B, et al.: Low dose streptokinase for selective thrombolysis: Systemic effects and complications. Radiology 152:35, 1984.

Katzen BT, Edwards KC, et al.: Low dose fibrinolysis in peripheral vascular disease. J Vasc Dis 1:718, 1984.

Mori KW, Bookstein JJ, et al.: Selective streptokinase infusion: Clinical and laboratory correlates. Radiology 148:667, 1983.

Hargrove WC, Barker CF, et al.: Treatment of acute arterial and graft thromboses with low dose streptokinase. Surgery 92:981, 1982.

REFERENCES

1. Sharma GVRK, Cella G, et al.: Thrombolytic therapy. N Engl J Med 306:1268, 1982.
2. Totty WG, Romano T, et al.: Serum sickness following streptokinase therapy. AJR 138:143, 1982.
3. Weatherbee TC, Esterbrooks DJ, et al.: Serum sickness following selective intracoronary streptokinase. Curr Therapeut Res 35:433, 1984.
4. Baumgartner TG, Davis RG: Streptokinase induced anaphylactic reaction. Clin Pharmacol Ther 1:470, 1982.
5. Bell WR, Meek AG: Guidelines for the use of thrombolytic agents. N Engl J Med 301:1266, 1979.
6. Collen D: On the regulation and control of fibrinolysis. Haemostasis 43:77, 1980.
7. Collen D, Rijken DC, et al.: Purification of human tissue-type plasminogen activator. Thromb Haemost 48:294, 1982.
8. Van de Werf F, Ludbrook PA, Bergmann SR: Coronary thrombolysis with tissue-type plasminogen activator in patients with evolving myocardial infarction. N Engl J Med 310:609, 1984.
9. Collen D, Verstack M: Systemic thrombolytic therapy of acute myocardial infarction. Circulation 68:462, 1983.
10. Katzen BT: Percutaneous transluminal angioplasty for arterial disease of the lower extremities. AJR 142:23, 1984.
11. Van Breda A, Waltman AC: Low dose thrombolysis for arterial disease of the lower extremities. Int Angiol 2:75, 1983.
12. Totty WG, Gilula LA, et al.: Low dose intravascular thrombolytic therapy. Radiology 143:59, 1982.
13. Van Breda A, Katzen BT, et al.: Results of catheter directed urokinase infusion in 122 patients. Paper presented at the 72nd annual meeting and scientific assembly of the Radiologic Society of North America, Nov 1986.
14. Risius B, Zelch M, et al.: Catheter-directed low dose streptokinase infusion: A preliminary experience. Radiology 150:349, 1984.
15. Van Breda A, Robison JC, et al.: Local thrombolysis in the treatment of graft occlusions. J Vasc Surg 1:103, 1984.
16. Whittemore AD, Clowes AW, et al.: Secondary femoropopliteal reconstruction. Ann Surg 193:35, 1981.
17. Rabe FE, Becker GJ, et al.: Contrast extravasation through Dacron grafts: A sequela of low dose streptokinase therapy. AJR 138:917, 1982.
18. Dotter CT, Rosch J, Seamen AJ: Selective clot lysis with low dose streptokinase. Radiology 111:31, 1974.
19. Katzen BT, van Breda A: Low dose streptokinase in the treatment of arterial occlusions. AJR 136:1171, 1981.
20. Bernie GA, Dandyk DF, et al.: Streptokinase treatment of acute arterial occlusions. Ann Surg 198:185, 1983.
21. Hargrove WC, Berkowitz HD, et al.: Recanalization of totally occluded femoropopliteal vein grafts with low dose streptokinase infusion. Surgery 92:890, 1982.
22. Becker GJ, Rabe FE, et al.: Low dose fibrinolytic therapy. Radiology 148:668, 1983.
23. Hess H, Inguish H, et al.: Local low dose fibrinolytic infusions of peripheral arterial occlusions. N Engl J Med 307:1627, 1982.
24. Van Breda A, Katzen BT: Streptokinase vs. urokinase in local thrombolytic infusions. (In press.)
25. McNamara TO, Fischer R: Thrombolysis of peripheral arterial and graft occlusions: Improved results using high dose urokinase. AJR 144:769, 1985.
26. Eskridge JM, Becker GJ, et al.: Catheter related thrombosis and fibrinolytic therapy. Radiology 149:429, 1983.
27. Wolfson RH, Kumpfe DA, Lutherford RB: Role of intra-arterial streptokinase in treatment of arterial thromboembolism. Arch Surg 119:697, 1984.
28. Wook WA, Tisnado J, Cho SR: Visceral embolization during low dose fibrinolysis of aortic graft occlusion. AJR 141:1055, 1983.

CHAPTER 26
Intraoperative Transluminal Angioplasty

Thomas J. Fogarty and Albert K. Chin

HISTORICAL DEVELOPMENT

Intraluminal balloon catheter treatment of occlusive vascular disease originated in the radiology suite. In 1964, Dotter successfully dilated an iliac artery stenosis with a standard Fogarty balloon embolectomy catheter.[1] In general, though, he found the compliant embolectomy balloon unsuitable for dilating atherosclerotic plaque. He realized catheters of a constant shape and size were needed for successful arterial dilatation. In an attempt to answer this need, he and Judkins developed a system of concentric tapered catheters that were passed over one another to dilate the stenosis. Using similar technology, van Andel[2] subsequently treated arterial lesions using separate tapered dilators. Portsmann,[3] on the other hand, attempted to adapt the balloon catheter to the purpose: he used latex balloons caged by an external meshwork to control the balloon shape.

None of these designs proved satisfactory for transluminal angioplasty. The coaxial tapered catheters and the caged balloon catheters resulted in a high rate of embolic complications, and early thrombosis occurred following their use.

Transluminal angioplasty did not develop into an effective procedure until Gruntzig designed a constant volume balloon catheter constructed of a nondistensible plastic material. This catheter employed techniques commonly applied in diagnostic angiography.[4] The initial passage of a spring guidewire through the stenosis was followed by the coaxial passage of the balloon angioplasty catheter over the guidewire (Fig. 26-1). If the lesion proved too tight to allow the passage of the Gruntzig balloon catheter, a tapered van Andel catheter was initially used to enlarge the lumen.

The guidewire and coaxial balloon dilatation catheter system has also been applied in the surgical suite as an intraoperative procedure. Concern over the possibility of guidewire and catheter dissection and perforation in severely stenotic lesions led Fogarty and Chin to introduce the linear extrusion catheter[5] (Fig. 26-2). This catheter does not require prior guidewire placement, and the balloon does not need to be accurately centered within the stenosis

for effective dilatation. Consequently, elaborate radiographic control is not required to perform the intraoperative angioplasty.

PHYSICAL PRINCIPLES

Successful application of transluminal angioplasty relies on an understanding of several underlying physical principles.

Mechanism of Dilatation

Transluminal angioplasty involves the development of fracture planes through the plaque and the intimal surface. These fractures allow the diseased vessel to distend under physiologic pressure, with a resultant increase in lumen diameter (Fig. 26-3). This mechanism of transluminal angioplasty has been documented using histopathologic studies, as well as quantitative materials analysis.[6-8] These studies

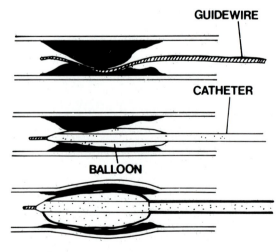

Figure 26-1. Coaxial balloon angioplasty catheter concept.

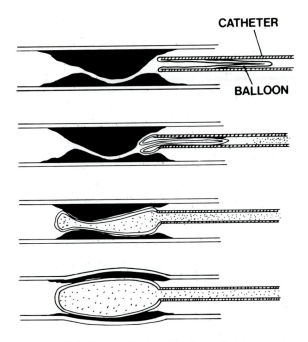

Figure 26-2. Linear extrusion dilatation catheter concept.

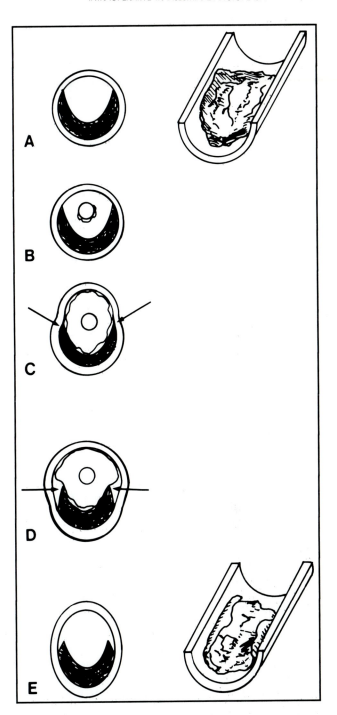

Figure 26-3. Mechanism of balloon dilatation. **A.** Cross section of a diseased artery. **B.** Placement of an uninflated balloon dilatation catheter. **C.** Stress exerted at the plaque–normal artery junction during balloon inflation. **D.** Plaque separation and fracture during continued balloon inflation. **E.** Resultant cross-sectional appearance of the artery after dilatation.

demonstrate that minimal plaque compresssion occurs during balloon dilatation. From our observations, plaque fractures occur more frequently along the longitudinal direction. This may account for the relative scarcity of intimal flap formation following transluminal angioplasty, because the blood flow is less apt to lift the leading edge of a longitudinal tear.

Balloon Sizing

Angioplasty balloons are constructed of a nonelastomeric material. A constant balloon shape, regardless of inflation pressure, is necessary to prevent overdistension and vessel rupture during dilatation. Arterial dilatation should never be attempted with an embolectomy balloon. The elastomeric embolectomy balloon bulges out on either side of a stenosis, exerting a greater stress on the normal than on the diseased portions of the vessel.

The angioplasty balloon's diameter should not exceed the native vessel's diameter adjacent to the stenosis. The largest appropriate balloon size should be used to achieve the maximal dilating force, as illustrated in Figure 26-4, which depicts a cross section of an angioplasty balloon inside a stenotic artery. The inflation pressure stretches the balloon surface against the raised plaque, exerting tension and leading to dilatation. This tension, also known as hoop stress, is directly proportional to the inflation pressure multiplied by the radius of the balloon (Laplace's law). Thus for a given inflation pressure, a larger balloon diameter leads to a greater dilatation force.

Transluminal dilatation is effective because of the resultant increase in the lumen's cross-sectional area. It is important to realize that a small percentage of reduction in the degree of stenosis may result in a large percentage of improvement in the amount of blood flow. This result occurs because arterial flow is related to the fourth power of the lumen diameter (Poiseuille's law).[9] For example, an 8 mm iliac artery with a 95% stenosis and a 60 mm Hg gradient is partially dilated to an 80% stenosis and a 20 mm Hg gradient. A 100% improvement in flow rate would result

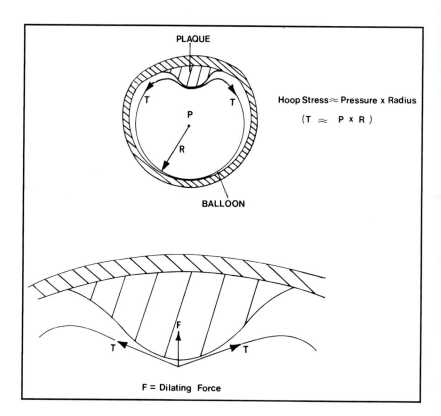

Figure 26-4. Inflation pressure and its relationship to dilating force.

from this mild decrease in the degree of stenosis. Thus dilatation to the full native diameter may not be necessary— or advisable. In lesions with concentric calcification, for instance, dilatation to the native diameter may cause arterial rupture.

Shear Force

Shear force is another physical principle of importance in transluminal angioplasty. Shear force is the frictional force exerted between two surfaces in contact, moving with respect to one another. In tight stenoses, centering a coaxial balloon dilatation catheter within the lesion may apply significant shear force to the plaque surface. This shear force may cause plaque dislodgment or vessel dissection.

The linear extrusion catheter minimizes shear force by unrolling a balloon through the stenosis. The force exerted by the balloon remains perpendicular to the contours of the plaque. There is no axial movement of the balloon with respect to the artery, decreasing the possibility of plaque dislodgment. Previous measurements in models of high-grade stenoses have shown that linear extrusion catheter use may decrease shear force up to a magnitude of 40 times when compared with coaxial balloon angioplasty catheter passage[10] (Fig. 26-5).

Balloon Inflation

Once properly situated, coaxial angioplasty balloons are inflated to 4 to 5 atm (approximately 60 to 75 psi) for several minutes to achieve adequate dilatation. Under fluoroscopy,

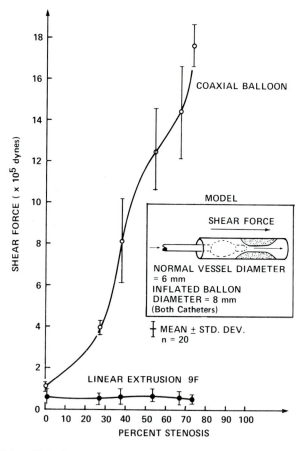

Figure 26-5. Decreased shear force with the use of the linear extrusion balloon in tight lesions.

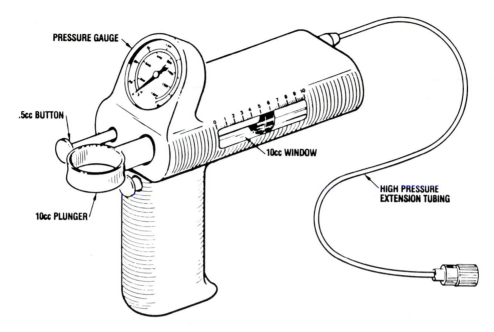

Figure 26-6. Specialized inflation device to control balloon eversion.

the balloon may have an initial hourglass shape that converts to a cylindrical outline, indicating that dilatation has
occurred.

Linear extrusion balloon eversion requires a high initial
inflation pressure to overcome the internal balloon friction
present in the fully inverted balloon. Once the balloon has
begun to evert, much less inflation pressure is required
to unroll the balloon. The inflation pressure rises again as
a stenosis is reached. When a single syringe is used for
inflation, the high initial inflation pressure followed by the
lower pressure requirement causes sudden eversion of the
linear extrusion balloon. The use of a specialized inflation
device allowing repeated high-pressure injections of a 0.5
ml volume helps control the eversion process (Fig. 26-6).

PATIENT SELECTION

Intraoperative balloon angioplasty is performed in three
modes of application: (1) as a primary procedure, (2) as
an adjunct to scheduled vascular reconstructions, and (3)
as a staged procedure following percutaneous transluminal
angioplasty.

Primary Balloon Angioplasty

Primary intraoperative balloon angioplasty is used in situations in which percutaneous transluminal angioplasty is
potentially unsafe because of, for example, patient obesity
or calcification at the site of dilatation. Introduction of the
balloon dilatation catheter into an open vessel in an operative setting decreases the chance of complications in these
circumstances.

In some situations, increased vessel control during
transluminal angioplasty is necessary. For example, balloon

angioplasty of carotid fibromuscular lesions should be performed intraoperatively. This allows the surgeon to obtain
adequate proximal and distal control, and to backflush the
vessel after dilatation. Primary operative transluminal angioplasty is also useful for treating limiting claudication
caused by an isolated lesion in the iliac or superficial femoral
artery. When applied in this situation, transluminal angioplasty is a low-risk procedure and may be of benefit to
debilitated patients in whom formal reconstruction would
be difficult.

Adjunctive Balloon Angioplasty

Adjunctive intraoperative balloon angioplasty is used to
decrease the magnitude of a surgical procedure. Thus dilatation of inflow iliac lesions during the course of a femoropopliteal bypass graft may serve to avert an aortobifemoral
reconstruction. Similarly, outflow stenoses in the femoral
or popliteal arteries may be dilated in conjunction with
the placement of an aortobifemoral bypass graft. This may
spare the patient a staged femoropopliteal bypass procedure. In addition, this procedure may relieve the claudication that would ordinarily be present postoperatively if the
aortofemoral reconstruction alone were performed in a patient with concomitant proximal and distal disease.

Adjunctive balloon dilatation may also allow the placement of an extraanatomic bypass graft in otherwise unfavorable situations. For example, a patient may have bilateral
iliac disease with an occlusion on one side and a localized
stenosis on the other. Balloon dilatation of the localized
lesion may allow that side to be used as the donor limb
for a femorofemoral graft (Fig. 26-7).

Transluminal angioplasty, when used as an adjunct
to a scheduled vascular reconstructive procedure, may enhance flow through a newly placed graft. Correction of

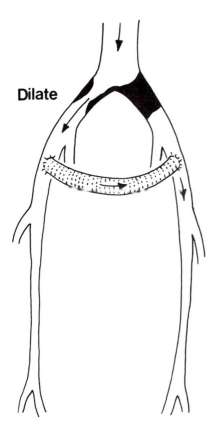

Dilate

Figure 26-7. Intraoperative dilatation to permit placement of a femorofemoral bypass graft. The right iliac artery is dilated and used as the donor limb of the graft.

inflow or outflow lesions is accomplished with little additional operative time.

In cases of acute thrombosis due to the presence of a significant arterial stenosis, adjunctive balloon angioplasty may give the patient maximal benefit with the application of a minimal procedure. Intraoperative balloon dilatation is performed after balloon catheter embolectomy. The dilatation procedure protects the patient from rethrombosis due to underlying occlusive disease. It may be used as the primary mode of correction or as a temporary maneuver in the acute stage of sudden arterial occlusion. Combined embolectomy and balloon angioplasty buys the surgeon precious time, which may be used to stabilize the patient and to plan the best tactic for future revascularization.

Staged Balloon Angioplasty

Staged transluminal angioplasty may be useful in certain situations. A percutaneous transluminal angioplasty may be performed on an inflow lesion, days or weeks before a scheduled vascular reconstruction. During surgery the dilated lesion is reevaluated, with intraoperative balloon dilatation of the lesion repeated if necessary. In this case, the primary purpose of staged balloon angioplasty is to allow the success of the inflow dilatation to be determined before one embarks on a possibly complex distal procedure.

In general, staged percutaneous dilatation is useful for complex lesions, including total occlusions or severe stenoses greater than 5 cm in length. On the other hand, lesions that appear circumscribed on the arteriogram can usually be managed with adjunctive intraoperative dilatation.

CONTRAINDICATIONS

The same conditions that preclude the use of percutaneous transluminal angioplasty also contraindicate intraoperative balloon dilatation. These contraindications include severe stenoses greater than 10 cm in length, lesions located at critical bifurcations, and ulcerative or thrombosed lesions. Lesions greater than 10 cm in length represent a relative contraindication. These lesions have a low probability of successful improvement after transluminal dilatation. When applying the balloon dilatation to bifurcations, one must exercise caution. Balloon angioplasty of one branch at a bifurcation may result in occlusion of the other branch. Ulcerated or thrombotic lesions have significant embolic potential when subjected to transluminal angioplasty. However, an acute thrombosis may be treated with a combination of balloon embolectomy and balloon angioplasty as discussed previously.

TECHNIQUE

Coaxial Balloon Dilatation Catheter

A spring guidewire is introduced through the arteriotomy and is passed across the stenosis. A floppy, or J-tipped, guidewire is used to decrease the possibility of perforation during guidewire passage. After successful negotiation of the guidewire through the lesion, the coaxial balloon dilatation catheter is threaded over the guidewire and under fluroscopy is centered within the stenosis. The balloon is inflated to its rated pressure for several minutes. When viewed on X-ray film, the dilatation balloon may initially assume an hourglass configuration and then resolve into a normal cylindrical conformation, suggesting that successful dilatation has occurred.

In tight lesions or tortuous vessels, initial guidewire passage may be difficult or impossible. In other cases, successful guidewire passage may be followed by unsuccessful placement of a coaxial balloon angioplasty catheter within the stenosis. In both of these situations, the linear extrusion catheter has been useful in crossing the lesion without causing arterial dissection.

Linear Extrusion Catheter

The linear extrusion catheter is introduced through an arteriotomy. In adjunctive intraoperative dilatation, this may be the arteriotomy used for the proximal or distal graft anastamosis.

Before dilatation catheter insertion, the distance between the arteriotomy and the stenosis site is determined, as well as the diameter of the native vessel immediately proximal to the stenosis. These measurements are made using a Fogarty balloon calibrator. The calibrator is inserted into the arteriotomy, and the balloon is partially inflated with saline. The calibrator is advanced until the balloon meets the leading edge of the stenosis (Fig. 26-8). This distance is measured using length markers on the calibrator body. The calibrator balloon is then inflated until it contacts the wall of the artery proximal to the stenosis. The volume of saline required for this inflation is noted. The balloon is deflated, and the calibrator removed from the artery. Reinflation of the balloon is conducted with the measured volume of saline, and the diameter of the balloon is determined using a circle template. This method yields an accurate measurement of the native vessel diameter.

Selection is made of a Fogarty-Chin linear extrusion catheter whose inflation diameter most closely approximates, but does not exceed, the calibrated arterial diameter. The linear extrusion catheter is purged of air and is connected to a high-pressure inflation device. The dilatation catheter is inserted into the arteriotomy and is advanced 2 cm short of the calibrated distance to the stenosis (Fig. 26-9). The movable silicone marker on the catheter body is advanced to the arteriotomy site and is grasped with a pair of forceps or a clamp. This prevents the catheter from backing out of the vessel during balloon extrusion.

Initial inflation of the linear extrusion catheter requires a high pressure to overcome the internal friction of the fully inverted balloon. This pressure typically exceeds the maximum rated balloon pressure at full inflation. This excess should not cause alarm—balloon rupture will not occur during this initial pressurization. Once the balloon begins to evert, an immediate drop in pressure is noted. As a stenosis is approached, a moderate pressure rise again occurs. When the balloon has been fully extruded, the catheter is pressurized to the recommended value and left in place for several minutes to achieve full dilatation. During adjunctive dilatation procedures, we keep the linear extrusion balloon inflated while the graft anastomosis is being completed. The dilatation balloon is used as an occlusion device during the reconstructive procedure, with arterial flow restored immediately after dilatation catheter removal. Immediate restoration of arterial flow in the newly dilated vessel prevents collapse of disrupted vessel wall segments and possible early arterial occlusion. After linear extrusion catheter removal, a completion arteriogram is performed without repeated balloon calibration.

PHARMACOLOGIC THERAPY

No additional anticoagulation is used with intraoperative transluminal angioplasty, aside from the regimen normally applied in routine reconstructive procedures. Postoperative heparin use is indicated for patients who are initially seen with preoperative embolism or acute thrombosis.

Antiplatelet agents are used for all reconstructions below the inguinal ligament. We commonly prescribe a half tablet (2.5 grains) of aspirin per day postoperatively, to be continued on a long-term basis. Dipyridamole (Persantine) may also be added, although we do not routinely do so.

Thrombolytic agents such as streptokinase, urokinase, and tissue plasminogen activator have been applied in conjunction with balloon angioplasty for the treatment of acute thrombosis and embolism.[11,12] We do not use these agents. Rather, we find the most expedient method of treating acute arterial occlusion involves balloon embolectomy followed by adjunctive transluminal angioplasty as needed for underlying atherosclerotic disease.

RESULTS

In general, the results achieved with intraoperative balloon dilatation parallel those experienced with percutaneous transluminal angioplasty. After transluminal dilatation, lesions in larger diameter vessels have a better patency rate than lesions in smaller diameter vessels. An isolated iliac stenosis is the most favorable lesion to dilate.[13,14] In comparison with aortofemoral bypass grafts, isolated iliac artery dilatations have slightly lower long-term patency rates. Femoral and popliteal lesions are also amenable to balloon dilatation. Long-term patency rates are superior with reversed saphenous vein grafts in the femoropopliteal region. However, when prosthetic graft material is used, translumi-

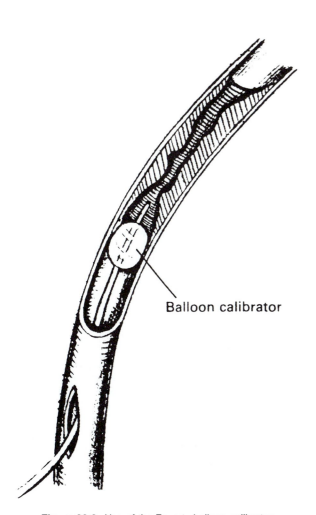

Figure 26-8. Use of the Fogarty balloon calibrator.

Balloon calibrator

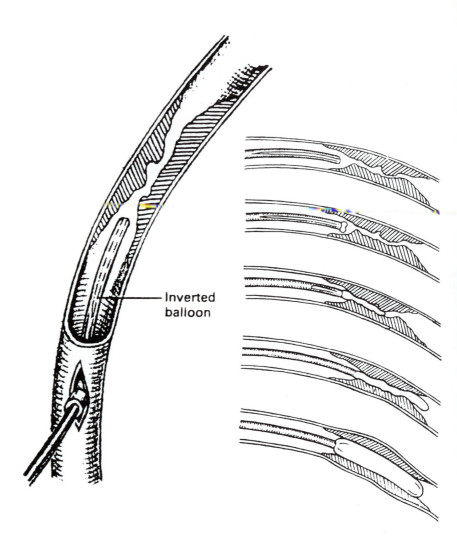

Figure 26-9. Advancement of the linear extrusion catheter and adjustment of the silicone ring marker before balloon eversion.

nal dilatation yields better results than femoropopliteal bypass grafting[15–20] (Table 26-1).

The following are the results of a recent long-term follow-up of 77 patients who underwent intraoperative transluminal dilatation of 96 sites. The mean follow-up for this series was 17.5 months. Lesions dilated in this study ranged from 1 to 9 cm in length. The superficial femoral artery was dilated in more than one half of the cases, with the next largest group comprising iliac artery dilatations. Lesser numbers of popliteal and profunda femoral dilata-

tions are performed, and one each was performed in the tibioperoneal trunk, renal, carotid, and subclavian arteries. An initial success rate of 98.7% decreased to an 82% patency rate and to a 53% patency rate by the end of the first and the fifth years, respectively.

Twenty total occlusions were dilated in this series, with 60% remaining patent during the course of the study. The only initial failure involved the inability of the balloon to pass through a totally occluded superficial femoral lesion. Two other dilatations of total occlusions resulted in early closure, one at 1 day and another at 1 week after the dilatations.

Only one complication occurred—a rupture of a calcified superficial femoral artery. This rupture required a bypass graft placement with no additional adverse effects. No surgical deaths occurred. Eighteen percent of the patients died during the follow-up period; most of these deaths were due to concomitant cardiac disease.

COMPLICATIONS

Complications that may occur with the use of coaxial or linear extrusion balloon dilatation catheters include vessel rupture, thrombosis, or embolism.[21–23] Because vessel rupture may result from the use of an oversized dilatation

TABLE 26-1. COMPARISON OF LONG-TERM PATENCY RATES AFTER SURGERY VS. PERCUTANEOUS TRANSLUMINAL ANGIOPLASTY (PTA)

	Patency (%)		
Procedure	1 Yr	3 Yr	5 Yr
Aortobifemoral bypass	98.7	94.9	91.2
Iliac artery PTA	86	84	83
Femoropopliteal bypass			
Saphenous vein	83	77	73
Prosthetic graft	64	48	35
Femoral artery PTA	79	67	64

balloon, careful balloon sizing is important in preventing overdistention. Thrombosis may occur after dilatation, particularly if a good flow rate is not established immediately after balloon removal. Also, embolism may occur during and after balloon angioplasty. Therefore lesions containing thrombus should not be dilated.

Other complications are more prone to occur with one catheter system vs. the other. The coaxial balloon dilatation catheter requires prior guidewire placement. The possibility of guidewire- or dilatation-catheter–related arterial dissection and perforation increases in severely stenotic lesions. After guidewire placement, the force required to center the coaxial balloon within the lesion may cause plaque dislodgment and distal embolization. Attempts to thread a guidewire through tortuous or stenotic vessels may lead to the creation of false passages. Use of the linear extrusion catheter is preferable in these situations.

The balloon in the linear extrusion catheter unrolls through the straightest pathway. Therefore selective cannulation is needed for the dilatation of a lesion in a branch that angles away from the main trunk. In the linear extrusion catheter system, the balloon length may also be critical. A rapidly tapering vessel may be ruptured by a long balloon, even though the balloon diameter has been correctly sized for the intended lesion.

FUTURE DIRECTIONS

Catheter treatment of intravascular disorders has just begun. The use of balloon catheters, first for embolectomy and now for dilatation, has initiated the trend towards less invasive vascular surgical procedures.

Future developments in intravascular catheter technology include the use of lasers, heated probes, and extruding sheaths to recanalize occlusions. These systems will be complemented by the use of advanced means for vascular imaging. Flexible fiberoptic angioscopes are currently available in diameters less than 1 mm. More sophisticated ultrasonic and radiographic imaging devices will soon be added. This extended visualization capability will facilitate the use of instruments that dilate or remove vascular occlusions.

It is important that vascular surgeons, who best appreciate the pathophysiology of arterial occlusive disease, become familiar with the proper use of these new developments in surgical technique. Only then will the interest of the vascular patient be best served.

REFERENCES

1. Dotter CT, Judkins MP: Transluminal treatment of arteriosclerotic obstruction: Description of a new technique and a preliminary report of its application. Circulation 30:654, 1964.
2. van Andel GJ: Percutaneous transluminal angioplasty: The Dotter procedure. Amsterdam, Excerpta Medica, 1976, p. 92.
3. Portsmann W: Ein neur Korsett-balloonkatheter zur tranluminalen Rekanalisation nach Dotter unter besonderer Berucksichtigung von Obliterationen an den Beckenarterien. Radiol Diagn (Berl) 14:239, 1973.
4. Gruntzig AR, Kumpe DA: Technique of percutaneous transluminal angioplasty with the Gruntzig balloon catheter. AJR 132:547, 1979.
5. Fogarty TH, Chin A, et al.: Adjunctive intraoperative arterial dilatation: Simplified instrumentation technique. Arch Surg 116:1391, 1981.
6. Block PC, Myler RK, et al.: Morphology after transluminal angioplasty in human beings. N Engl J Med 307:382, 1981.
7. Chin AK, Kinney TB, et al.: A physical measurement of the mechanisms of transluminal angioplasty. Surgery 95(2):196, 1983.
8. Zarins CK, Lu CT, et al.: Arterial disruption and remodeling following balloon dilatation. Surgery 92(6):1086, 1982.
9. Strandness DE Jr, Sumner DS: Hemodynamics for surgeons. New York, Grune & Stratton Inc, 1975.
10. Kinney TB, Fan M, et al.: Shear force in angioplasty: Its relation to catheter design and function. AJR 144:115, 1985.
11. Murray PD, Garnic JD, Bettmann MA: Pharmacology of angioplasty and intravascular thrombolysis. AJR 139:795, 1982.
12. Graor RA, Risins, B, et al.: Low-dose streptokinase for selective thrombolysis: Systemic effects and complications. Radiology 152:35, 1984.
13. Kadir S: Percutaneous transluminal angioplasty of the iliac and common femoral arteries and their accessory vessels, in Jang GD (ed): Angioplasty. New York, McGraw-Hill Book Co, 1986, p. 36.
14. Kadir S, White RI Jr, et al.: Long term results of aortoiliac angioplasty. Surgery 94:10, 1983.
15. Gallino A, Mahler F, et al.: Percutaneous transluminal angioplasty of the arteries of the lower limbs: A 5 year follow-up. Circulation 70(4):619, 1984.
16. Simonetti G, Urigo F, et al.: Iliac artery lesions: A comparison between percutaneous transluminal angioplasty and surgery. Ann Radiol 29(2):127, 1986.
17. Hewes RC, White RI Jr, et al.: Long-term results of superficial femoral artery angioplasty. AJR 146:1025, 1986.
18. Roberts B, McLean GK: Role of percutaneous angioplasty in the treatment of peripheral arterial disease. Adv Surg 19:329, 1986.
19. Brewster DC, Darling RC: Optimal methods of aortoiliac reconstruction. Surgery 84:739, 1978.
20. Brewster D, LaSalle AJ, et al.: Factors affecting patency of femoropopliteal bypass grafts. Surg Gynecol Obstet 157:437, 1983.
21. Connolly JR, Kwaan JHM, McCart PM: Complications after percutaneous transluminal angioplasty. Am J Surg 142:60, 1981.
22. Ring EJ, Freiman DB, et al.: Percutaneous recanalization of common iliac artery occlusions: An unacceptable complication rate? AJR 139:587, 1982.
23. Katzen BT, Chang J: Percutaneous transluminal angioplasty with the Gruntzig balloon catheter. Radiology 130:623, 1979.

CHAPTER 27
Angioscopy and Laser Angioplasty

Warren S. Grundfest and Frank Litvack

We have played an active role in developing two new technologies which may have a significant impact on the practice of vascular surgery. Angioscopy allows the vascular surgeon to inspect the intimal surface and observe luminal details of blood vessels at points distant from the operative site. Angioplasty, with lasers and mechanical and electrical devices, remodels the vessel lumen with partial removal of atherosclerotic lesions. These new tools allow either percutaneous or intraoperative restoration of blood flow in obstructed coronary and peripheral vessels. This chapter presents an overview of these two new fields. These technologies are rapidly developing, and further significant improvements are likely.

ANGIOSCOPY

Methodology

Early attempts at intravascular observation were hampered by the lack of appropriate devices. Until recently, the fiberoptic imaging bundle could not be miniaturized, and the

The authors would like to express their appreciation to the surgeons who participated in this research and helped to collect much of the angioscopic data: vascular surgeons Robert Foran, M.D.; Lewis Cohen, M.D.; Philip Levin, M.D.; David Cossman, M.D.; Richard Treiman, M.D.; and Robert Carroll, M.D.; and cardiovascular surgeons Myles Lee, M.D.; Aurelio Chaux, M.D.; Jack Matloff, M.D.; Carlos Blanche, M.D.; and Robert Kass, M.D.

The authors gratefully acknowledge the contributions of Tsvi Goldenberg, Ph.D., James Laudenslager, Ph.D., Tom Pacala, Ph.D., and Thannasis Papaioannou, M.S., of the Cedars-Sinai Laser Research Center.

This work is supported in part by the Imperial Grand Sweepstakes, the Grand Sweepstakes, and the Medallions Fund of Cedars-Sinai Medical Center. These generous contributions are gratefully acknowledged.

This work is supported in part by the Specialized Centers of Research in Ischemic Heart Disease of the National Heart, Lung, and Blood Institute, award #HL-17651.

Drs. Grundfest and Litvack are recipients of NHLBI Clinical Investigator Awards #1KOHL-01522 and #KO8HL-01381-01, respectively.

smallest endoscopes were not practical for intravascular use. Attempts at rigid endoscopy were hampered by the limited scope of application. In 1983, Spears et al.[1] published a report outlining the use of a small prototype flexible endoscope to view the coronary ostium via a guide catheter. This report heralded a new era in fiberoptics: the development of miniaturized endoscopes.

Our group at Cedars-Sinai then developed miniaturized devices for vascular endoscopy.[2,3] Commercially available angioscopes range in size from 2.8 to 0.5 mm in outer diameter. To view larger diameter vessels (greater than 3 mm), we employ angioscopes that are 1.0 to 2.8 mm in diameter (Olympus, Rye, N.Y., and American Edwards, Santa Ana, Calif.). For smaller vessels, we have used angioscopes as small as 0.5 mm in diameter. This new technology pioneered by our colleague Dr. Tsvi Goldenberg (Advanced Interventional Systems, Costa Mesa, Calif.) permits percutaneous insertion and imaging in coronary and distal tibial vessels. In these small endoscopes, an imaging bundle of 3,000 to 8,000 imaging fibers is surrounded by a concentric ring of illumination fibers. The optical system is then packaged in a plastic catheter. The stiffness of the imaging bundle and the catheter material determines the flexibility of the endoscope. At present, only the devices larger than 2.5 mm are steerable. Illumination is delivered through a side port on the endoscope to a concentric ring of illumination fibers. We employ a 1,000-watt xenon light source (Storz Corp., Los Angeles); although in most situations, a 500-watt source is acceptable.

The optical image presented at the proximal end of a miniaturized bundle is too small for useful direct visual observation. We therefore interface the endoscope to a video camera via a specially designed video endoscope coupler. These couplers have varying degrees of magnification. Several coupler models are commercially available, but as yet, none are optimal for our use. A variety of video cameras are also available for endoscopy. When we want high quality permanent video records, we employ a low-noise, high-gain (Sharp XC801RP), three-tube camera. This camera is cumbersome, and when we want adequate clinical informa-

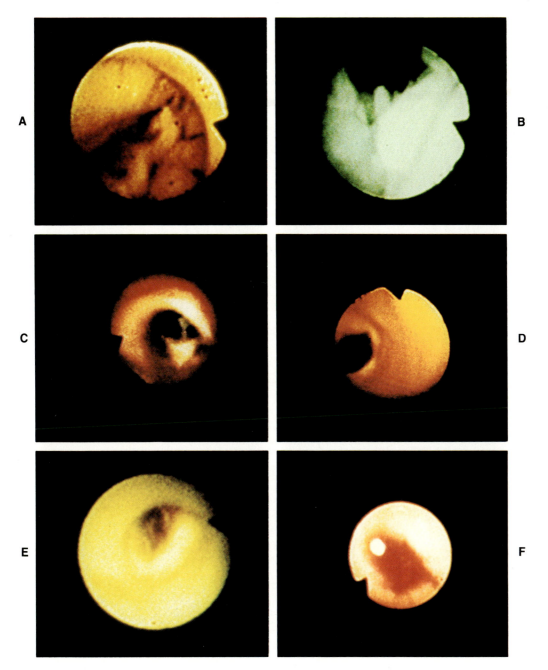

Figure 27-1. A. Distal half of a distal anastomosis of a Gortex supergeniculate femoropopliteal bypass graft. A large intimal flap stretching from the center of the field to the 6:30 position obstructs the outflow track. Based on this angioscopic image, this anastomosis was revised. **B.** Angioscopic image obtained after completion of an in situ infrageniculate femoro-popliteal bypass graft. While the distal lumen of the anastomosis was widely patent, a few small and probably insignificant flaps were seen. These flaps were left in place and did not appear to accumulate thrombus. **C.** Angioscopic image obtained from a 73-year-old man undergoing embolectomy and thrombectomy of a vein graft. After multiple attempts, thrombectomy angioscopy was used to inspect the proximal portion of the vein. Upon inspection, this large flap, seen between the 3 and 5 o'clock positions, was noted, as well as considerable residual thrombus. Under direct visualization, a Fogarty embolectomy balloon was passed, and after three additional tries, good results were achieved. **D.** The middle third of a left interior descending coronary artery in a 71-year-old patient with chronic stable angina. A lesion is seen encroaching on the lumen. The intimal surface is smooth, yellow-white, and without intimal ulcerations. **E.** Intimal surface of a patient with 2 weeks of accelerated angina. In the upper portion of the field the discolored irregular surface is an ulcerated plaque with subintimal hemorrhage. **F.** Angioscopic view taken from the left anterior descending coronary artery of a patient undergoing urgent bypass for acute recurrent ischemia shows the thrombotic nature of this coronary occlusion. The light of the angioscope can be seen reflecting off the thrombus in the upper left corner at approximately the 10 o'clock position. Despite vigorous irrigation, this thrombus could not be dislodged.

tion only, we use small "chip" cameras weighing only a few ounces. Because of the lower resolution and contrast specifications, images obtained with these solid state cameras are not as clear as those obtained with the three-tube professional cameras. However, the advantages of small size, low weight, and ease of use of the chip cameras makes these devices generally preferable for angioscopic applications. Images are always viewed on a high-resolution color monitor. The videotape recorder also significantly affects the resolution of the stored images. We employ a $\frac{3}{4}$ in. Sony tape deck.

Current endoscopes tend to be fragile; imaging bundles or illumination fibers break easily. After 20 to 30 uses, the image quality degrades because of mechanical fracture of the fibers. The development of disposable low-cost endoscopes is in progress, but they are not yet commercially available. We keep detailed records on the quality of the imaging bundles as they are delivered from the factory. All endoscopes are tested for minimum focus, spatial resolution, and flaws in the jacketing. Devices with minimum focal lengths greater than 5 mm are not applicable in intravascular imaging. The spatial resolution of currently available endoscopes exceeds 200 μm at 5 mm. Therefore, it is possible to obtain high-resolution images with these devices.

The most common cause for poor images is the inability to remove blood from the imaging field. At present, no adequate commerical irrigation systems are available. We employ a variety of systems depending on the surgical site. In peripheral vascular applications, a pressurized crystalloid solution is delivered through either a concentric or coaxial irrigating catheter. This irrigating system usually consists of an 8 or 9 in. introducer catheter with a side port, or a 16- or 18- gauge, 5 in. long intravenous catheter.

In the coronary system, angioscopy is performed during bypass surgery. Crystalloid cardioplegia is infused, either through the aortic root or via an 18- or 20-gauge, 2 in. intravenous catheter. We are starting to perform percutaneous coronary angioscopy using crystalloid irrigation at body temperature delivered via the guide catheter.

At surgery, the angioscope is inserted through an arteriotomy. Both proximal and distal lumens are inspected. After completion of a distal graft anastomosis, the angioscope is inserted through the proximal limb of the graft to view the anastomosis.

In peripheral vascular bypass surgery, the angioscope can be inserted through vein graft or synthetic graft as the operator desires. However, it is essential to have vascular control prior to angioscope insertion, because blood causes failure to obtain an image. When retrograde visualization is planned, a Fogarty balloon embolectomy catheter can be advanced proximally and the vessel irrigated prior to inspection. This works particularly well in the inspection of occluded limbs of aortobifemoral grafts. At present, all angioscopes lack distance markers, which would be helpful in determining lesion locations. We guide these first-generation angioscopes by gentle manipulation of the vessel and rotation of the angioscope while it is being advanced. In many instances, better images are obtained on withdrawal of the angioscope than on insertion. To date, we have performed more than 130 coronary and 85 peripheral vascular

angioscopies, obtaining more than 250 angioscopic images. We have a 15% failure rate, primarily due to inability to deliver sufficient volume of fluid to clear the imaging field.

Results of Angioscopic Investigation

Peripheral Vascular Angioscopy

We have detected a variety of unsuspected technical errors that occur during vascular surgery. Of the 37 peripheral anastomoses angioscoped, five (13%) were revised based on angioscopic images[4] (our rate of revision has fallen from about 25% in our earliest experience,[5] suggesting the procedure has a learning value even for the experienced surgeon). Three of the revisions occurred in femoropopliteal bypass grafts, one in an axillary bypass graft, and one in the distal limb of an aortobifemoral bypass graft. Revisions were for redundancy of graft material, intraluminal flaps, or misplaced sutures that caused significant obstruction of flow. Figure 27-1A shows a typical example of a large, filamentous flap obstructing the distal outflow in a femoropopliteal bypass graft.[*] The novice angioscoper must learn that to the inexperienced observer, a small flap can appear enormous when it is close to the distal tip of the angioscope. Whenever possible, lesions should be compared to the size of the distal or proximal orifice or adjacent suture material to estimate relative sizes. Of the 32 anastomoses which were felt to be technically successful by traditional surgical criteria, angioscopic inspection often revealed small intimal fragments which did not compromise flow. Figure 27-1B is an angioscopic photograph taken from an infrageniculate in situ femoropopliteal bypass graft. Several small flaps were seen angioscopically, the largest of which is in the center of this photograph. The lumen which occupies the upper quarter of the frame appears adequate, and this anastomosis was left intact.

Although we have only anecdotal information about the prognostic value of angioscopy, it seems likely that the information we obtain is both unique and important. In three cases, we have performed angioscopic inspection. After completion, arteriography showed a normal anastomosis and outflow tract. Angioscopy showed obstructing vascular webs or thrombosis in all three. In two cases, no action was taken, and the vessels occluded 1 to 2 days postoperatively. In the third case, the thrombus was removed and an intimal flap was secured, with an uneventful follow-up.

We have angioscoped 68 patients during femoropopliteal bypass surgery. Various techniques were used to create the bypass graft. Of these, 15 employed reverse saphenous vein, 17 used in situ saphenous veins, and 36 used Gortex. Of the 17 in situ procedures, eight veins had intact valves at angioscopy, which led to repeat valve disruption. Angioscopy often revealed sclerotic vein segments in both in situ and reverse saphenous vein grafts. Usually dilatation or removal of overlying connective tissue was sufficient to achieve appropriate luminal diameter (<3 mm). However, in 3 of 28 veins, angioscopic findings of localized sclerosis

---

[*] Figure 27-1 is a color plate inserted between pp 324 and 325.

led to excision of the segment. In the eight thrombectomies we examined by angioscopy, seven revealed residual thrombus, intimal flaps, or disrupted plaque. Figure 27-1C demonstrates the lumen of a Gortex graft after an apparently successful attempt at embolectomy. On angioscopic inspection, a significant portion of the lumen was still occupied by thrombus and neointimal debris, as shown in this figure. Repeat thrombectomy under angioscopic guidance resulted in a debris-free lumen in all cases.

Coronary Angioscopy

Angioscopy during coronary artery bypass surgery has revealed a smaller number of technical errors. In newly created anastomoses, 3 of 36 were found to have either misplaced sutures or intimal flaps. In three other cases, angioscopy led to revision of an old graft or placement of an additional graft.

Angioscopy has given us new insights into the nature of coronary ischemic syndromes. In patients with chronic stable angina, the intimal surface typically was smooth, yellow-white, and glistening, without evidence of disruption, as illustrated in Figure 27-1D.[6] In contrast, most patients with acute ischemic syndromes were observed to have intimal ulcerations and thrombus.[7] In patients with accelerated angina (defined as increasing frequency of angina without rest pain), we observed intimal ulcers and associated platelet aggregates. Figure 27-1E is an angioscopic view from a left anterior descending coronary artery in a patient with a 2-week history of accelerated angina. The posterior intimal surface in the center of the image is ulcerated and irregular, with subintimal hemorrhage. In 18 patients with unstable angina at rest, the "offending" artery (by ECG criteria) revealed thrombus and ulceration.[8] Figure 27-1F shows a typical obstructive thrombus taken from a patient with impending infarction. Of arteries observed after infarction, some showed a variable combination of thrombus, ulceration, and intimal strands. Angioscopy provided information not seen at angiography. In most cases, the endothelial ulcer and the partially occlusive thrombus were not detected by angiography. In six additional patients who had acute percutaneous transluminal coronary angioplasty (PTCA) failure, intimal flaps and thrombus were seen in all but were seen angiographically in only two.[9]

In peripheral vascular disease, correlation with the clinical syndromes is intrinsically less certain because the syndromes are not as rigidly defined. In five patients with acute onset of leg pain at rest, we have observed ulcerative and thrombotic lesions in four.[10] Additionally, we have seen ulcerated and thrombotic lesions proximal to total obstructions in the superficial femoral artery. These observations suggest that endothelial ulceration often leads to thrombosis or distal embolization, that is, that the ulcerative lesion with its subsequent sequela is the primary cause of acute vascular syndromes.

Complications

Initial designs of angioscopes were primitive. The early devices (some of which are still available) had sharp distal ends which could cause endothelial abrasion and relatively stiff, unyielding, shafts which made them difficult to manipulate in the vascular tree. A new generation of angioscopes has largely overcome these problems. Nevertheless, forceful manipulation, particularly when there is no image, is dangerous. One should also avoid using a large angioscope in a small vessel, because forced dilatation can lead to intimal disruption over a long segment. In the peripheral vascular circulation, we usually employ no more than 200 to 300 ml of crystalloid solution per angioscopic inspection. In coronary applications, we have found that irrigation through the aortic root can lead to excessive infusion of cardioplegia, and therefore the preferred route of irrigant delivery is by coaxial catheter. We have had no complications from fluid overload. To date, using first-generation devices, we have observed four intimal flaps, which may have resulted from angioscopy. In one case, a flap at a newly created distal anastamosis was thought to be secondary to vigorous angioscopic inspection. This anastomosis required revision. In the other three cases, small flaps were identified and were thought to be due to the sharp angioscopic tip. In these three cases, no clinical sequelae were observed.

Technical Limitations

Present commercially available angioscopes lack intrinsic steering and irrigating systems. Another limitation is the time required to assemble the system. However, new prototype systems with improved instrumentation may overcome some limitations. Disposable angioscopes and angioscopes with in situ valve cutters which can be operated under direct vision are currently in development. Construction of more flexible devices, with further miniaturization of the optics is also in progress, with the goals of developing a more user-friendly system and percutaneous coronary angioscopy.

LASER ANGIOPLASTY

Balloon angioplasty has demonstrated that mechanical dilatation of discreet atherosclerotic lesions can remodel the vessel lumen, with resulting increase in blood. However, balloon angioplasty is ineffective in vessels with diffuse disease, multiple lesions, or total chronic obstructions. The limitations of balloon techniques have initiated a search for alternative percutaneous and intraoperative methodology, including laser angioplasty. Because of a lack of understanding of the interaction of laser light with a biologic tissue, initial attempts at laser angioplasty were unsuccessful.[11,12] The use of sharp optical fibers, rigid, high-profile catheters, and excessive amounts of laser energy resulted in an unacceptably high perforation rate. In the rest of this chapter, we will describe the various types of lasers, the energy they produce, and the effects of that energy on biologic tissue. We conclude the chapter with a brief discussion of the present status of clinical laser angioplasty and mechanical devices.

Lasers convert electrical or chemical energy into a unidirectional, coherent, monochromatic beam of light. This energy conversion is achieved by exciting the molecules or atoms called the "active medium" of the laser. The active medium is contained within a chamber with mirrors at each end. The active medium of a laser can be solid, liquid, or gas. When sufficient energy is delivered into the cavity, the molecules of the active medium become excited. In returning to their stable, unexcited state, the activated molecules release this absorbed energy as photons of light. The photons strike other excited molecules causing additional release of photons, "amplifying" the original process. Thus, when one photon strikes an already excited molecule, two photons are emitted. As long as the population of excited molecules is maintained by pumping energy into the system, the amplification process continues. As the photons are reflected back and forth between the mirrors, the photon intensity within the optical chamber builds by many orders of magnitude. The mirror at one end of the optical chamber is only partially reflective, allowing a portion of the light to escape the chamber as a high-intensity unidirectional beam of one color.[13] The energy conversion process is an inefficient one. Energy that is not emitted as light is converted to heat. Thus, most lasers have significant cooling requirements.

Delivery of light to the intravascular target is usually accomplished by fiberoptic waveguide. The waveguide typically is composed of a core of highly transparent quartz fibers. Each fiber is surrounded by "cladding" that has a different index of refraction. Thus light that enters a fiber is internally reflected along the fiber axis and does not escape into the cladding. In addition to the core and cladding, most fiberoptic systems are surrounded by a plastic jacket. The combination of fiber stiffness and plastic tends to make fiberoptics inappropriately rigid for vascular use.

Laser-Tissue Interaction

The major advantage of the laser is the capacity to deliver spatially and temporally confined energy to a remote location. This allows the surgeon to deliver very high levels of light energy to a small area of tissue without open surgical exposure of the area being treated. The interaction of the tissue with light and subsequent healing response determines the medical results. Reflected light produces no biologic effect. If the light is absorbed and then re-emitted at a longer wavelength, fluorescence occurs. When the light energy is absorbed and converted to heat, a range of processes from protein coagulation to tissue ablation and pyrolysis occurs.[14] In contrast, direct electronic excitation of chemical bonds can be induced by use of the appropriate wavelength and parameters.[15] High-energy ultraviolet photons (greater than 3.6 eV) can produce electronic bond breaking with subsequent ejection of molecular fragments. This process is called photochemical desorption and can result in tissue ablation with only minimal generation of heat.[16] Since only the irradiated tissue is subject to bond breaking and ablation, the process is precise.

The *carbon dioxide* laser can be operated in the continuous wave or pulsed wave mode depending upon its excitation source. This laser emits light in the far infrared region of the spectrum at 10,600 μm. This wavelength is not transmissible through quartz or glass fiberoptics and must be delivered by articulated arms or metal tubes, which limits its use in the cardiovascular setting. This wavelength is absorbed primarily by the water molecules in tissue. The absorbed energy is converted to heat, and the water within tissue boils when temperature exceeds 100° C.[17]

Three lasers have found applications in surgical procedures. The *argon ion* laser uses a high-voltage electrical discharge to excite argon gas, which emits blue-green light at 488 and 514 nm. This wavelength is readily transmitted through quartz or glass fiberoptics and is strongly absorbed by chromophores such as hemoglobin and porphyrins. The primary effect of the argon laser energy is to generate heat at the site of chromophore absorption, which subsequently leads to water vaporization and tissue ablation.[18]

The *Nd:YAG* laser employs a garnet crystal doped with neodymium and yttrium (two rare earth elements) as the active medium. A flashlamp is used for the outside energy source. To produce laser light at 1,060 nm the Nd:YAG laser can be operated in either the continuous wave or pulsed mode. Through the technique of Q-switching, intense 10 ns pulses or less can be obtained. When operating in the continuous wave mode, this laser emits light that is easily transmitted through standard silica fiberoptic waveguides. However, in the pulsed mode, fiberoptic transmission is difficult.[19]

The absorption of this wavelength energy is primarily by tissue protein. This wavelength tends to penetrate deeply, unless very dark pigments are present. The wide breadth and depth of penetration produces volume heating, and therefore this laser is used to induce coagulation necrosis.[20]

By changing the doping element from neodymium to erbium or lanthanum, different wavelengths can be created. These lasers emit light in the 3,000 μm range, which is strongly absorbed by water. These new lasers are in experimental development, as are the zirconium fluoride fibers necessary for transmission of this wavelength. The advantage of these new lasers is the intense water absorption (similar to the CO_2 laser) combined with the potential for fiberoptic transmission.[21] It is uncertain, however, that these devices will ever reach clinical application.

The *excimer* lasers are a class of gas lasers that employ a noble gas such as xenon, krypton, or argon with a halogen compound such as hydrogen fluoride or hydrogen chloride. Until recently, these devices were purely experimental. They emit brief nanosecond pulses of light in the ultraviolet portion of the spectrum, and the wavelength of the emitted light is dependent upon the gas mixture employed. The xenon fluoride excimer laser emits light at 351 nm, the xenon chloride excimer laser emits light at 308 nm, and argon fluoride excimer emits light at 193 nm. Of all the possible combinations, only the longer ultraviolet wavelengths of 351 and 308 nm are suitable for fiberoptic transmission. Fiberoptic transmission of this intense ultraviolet light is achieved through "long pulses," which permit delivery of sufficient energies to ablate even hard, calcified lesions.[22] At a given wavelength, tissue effects appear to vary little as the pulse duration is increased from 7 to 300 ns. The advantage of this shorter wavelength laser light is that it produces precise incisions without adjacent thermal injury. The ablation itself is also much more controllable by the operator. Such precision and control is ideal for recanalization of small blood vessels. In both in vitro and in vivo experiments, ablation of vascular tissue by 308 nm irradiation proceeded at temperatures below 60° C.[23] In a separate set of experiments, completely obstructed canine femoral arteries were recanalized by 308 nm excimer laser energy transmitted through fiberoptics.[23] Our group has recently received FDA approval to conduct clinical trials of 308 nm excimer laser angioplasty in peripheral vessels, and the first clinical trials are now in progress.

Laser Angioplasty in Man

Experience with laser angioplasty in man is limited. Initial studies using bare fibers to conduct argon or YAG laser energy met with little success. These attempts produced small channels, charred the arterial surface, and had a high early reocclusion rate. These early clinical failures led to the development of multiple new devices. No one technique has yet emerged as clearly superior. The first of these devices to undergo clinical trials is the "hot tip" device.[24]

The hot tip is a bullet-shaped, metal cap mechanically attached to the end of a fiberoptic waveguide. Argon laser irradiation is used to heat the cap. Since the metal conducts heat quickly, the entire cap is heated uniformly to 300 to 400° C. The cap rapidly destroys soft intravascular obstructions. By April 1987, more than 300 patients with peripheral vascular disease had been treated, always followed by balloon angioplasty. In the first 219 patients reported, 51 (23%) had vascular lesions classified as "impossible" to cross with balloons; an additional 45 were classified as "difficult." Seventy-four percent of the total occlusions and 88% of the difficult lesions were recanalized. In the remaining patients, the procedure was successful in all. One-year clinical follow up in 74 patients showed a long-term patency rate of 65%, using only clinical criteria.[25,26] No follow-up angiograms have been reported. Based on this experience, it now appears that the hot tip technology may have a role in recanalization of large, completely obstructed vessels. However, the results in both coronary and distal peripheral vessels have been less encouraging. Anecdotal reports of 14 coronary procedures show six successful recanalizations, four failures to pass the lesion, one perforation, and three coronary occlusions within hours of the procedure.[27,28]

Several groups, including our own, have developed alternative methods to generate heat at the tip of the catheter. These new devices, which are based on radio frequency energy, are far less complex and more reliable than the current laser generators. Like the laser hot tip, these devices open total occlusion in the canine femoral artery.[29] The ease of fabrication of electrically based hot tips permits improved tip temperature control and more effective distribution of the thermal energy through better tip design.[30] These electrical thermal angioplasty devices can be powered by relatively small, inexpensive power supplies. The simplicity of the procedure and equipment and the initial success of the hot tip methodology suggest that percutaneous therapy for femoral popliteal occlusive disease will become a reality. However, evaluation of this technology will be complete only when long-term studies compare patency and limb salvage rates over a 5-year period.

A second strategy actively being explored is the use of mechanical recanalization devices. Simpson et al. have developed a catheter that entraps an atheroma within a shielded housing.[31] A rotating blade is advanced within the housing, and the atheroma is shaved off and captured in the distal lumen of the catheter. Three problems have been encountered with its use: the size of the housing has precluded its use in small vessels, it cannot be used in total occlusions, and multiple lesions require a significant amount of operator time. In addition, preliminary reports suggest a relatively high restenosis rate of 30% or greater. Despite these disadvantages, the catheter has been successfully employed to remove subtotal occlusions in the superficial femoral artery in 120 of 124 cases.

A second device is a sophisticated catheter developed by Kinsey.[32] At the catheter tip is a cam rotating at >90,000 rpm. Behind the cam, a continuous jet of saline is propelled laterally against the arterial wall. The combination of the saline jet and the mechanical cam emulsifies the atheroma and expands the vessel. The high velocity fluid debrides the lateral wall while the cam moves forward along the long axis of the vessel. In 53 patients, a success rate of 85% immediately after surgery has been reported. There are no long-term follow-up studies, and perforation may be a problem.

Hansen et al. have developed a drill bit studded with 30 μm diameter diamond chips.[33] This bit is rotated at more than 100,000 rmp, and debris is cleared by a continuous flow of saline irrigation. Remarkably, distal embolization using these mechanical devices has not been a recognizable problem in preliminary human trials or animal experimentation.

These new techniques are all at the earliest investigational stage. Thus, it is not possible for us to predict which devices will have long-term clinical utility. Nevertheless, with the great impetus provided by balloon angioplasty and the early success of these newer technologies, it seems likely that the future vascular surgeon will use both intraoperative and percutaneous methods of recanalization.

REFERENCES

1. Spears JR, Marais HJ, Serur J.: In vivo coronary angioscopy. J Am Coll Cardiol 51:1311, 1983.
2. Litvack F, Grundfest WS, et al.: Angioscopic visualization of blood vessel interior in animals and humans. Clin Cardiol 8:65, 1985.
3. Grundfest WS, Litvack F, Sherman CT: Delineation of peripheral and coronary detail by intraoperative angioscopy. Ann Surg 202:394, 1984.
4. Glick D, Grundfest WS, et al. Intraoperative decisions based on angioscopy. Circulation 78(suppl 1, no. 3):13, 1988.
5. Grundfest WS, Litvack F, et al.: The current status of angioscopy and laser angioplasty. J Vasc Surg 5(4):667, 1987.
6. Chaux A, Lee M, et al.: Intraoperative coronary angioscopy: Technique and results in the initial 58 patients. J Thorac Cardiovasc Surg 92:972, 1986.
7. Forrester JS, Litvack F, et al.: A perspective of coronary disease as seen through the arteries of living man. Circulation 75(3):50, 1987.
8. Grundfest WS, Litvack F, et al.: Definition of new pathophysiologic mechanisms and altered decisions: An outcome of intravascular angioscopy. J Am Coll Cardiol 2:153a, 1986.

9. Hickey A, Litvack F, et al.: In vivo angioscopy following balloon angioplasty. Circulation 74(suppl. 2) 1986.
10. Glick DG, Grundfest WS, et al.: Intraoperative decisions based on angioscopy in peripheral vascular surgery. Society for Clinical Vascular Surgery, 15th Symposium. March 1987, p 44.
11. Choy DSJ, Stertzer SH, et al.: Human coronary laser recanalization. Clin Cardiol 7:377, 1984.
12. Ginsberg R, Kim DS, et al.: Salvage of an ischemic limb by laser angioplasty: Description of a new technique. Clin Cardiol 7:54, 1984.
13. Laudenslager J: Laser fundamentals, in White R, Grundfest WS (eds): Lasers in Cardiovascular Disease. Chicago, Year Book Medical Publishers, 1987, pp 7–26.
14. Grundfest WS, Litvack F, et al.: Laser tissue interactions: Considerations for cardiovascular applications, in White R, Grundfest WS (eds): Lasers in Cardiovascular Disease, Chicago, Year Book Medical Publishers, 1987, pp. 32-37.
15. Srinivasan R: Ablation of polymers and biological tissue by ultraviolet lasers. Science 234:559, 1986.
16. Grundfest WS, Litvack F, et al.: Effect of excimer laser irradiation on human atherosclerotic aorta: Amelioration of laser induced thermal damage. Technical Digest of Conference on Lasers and Electro-optics. June, 1984.
17. Grundfest W, Litvack F, et al.: Comparison of in vitro and in vivo thermal effects of argon and excimer lasers for laser angioplasty. Circulation 74(suppl 11):813A, 1986.
18. Laudenslager J: Laser fundamentals, in White R, Grundfest WS (eds): Lasers in Cardiovascular Disease. Chicago, Year Book Medical Publishers, 1987, pp 26–31.
19. Grundfest WS, Litvack F, et al.: Pulsed ultraviolet lasers and the potential for safe laser angioplasty. Am J Surg 150:220, 1985.
20. Grundfest WS, Litvack F, et al.: Laser tissue interactions: Considerations for cardiovascular applications, in White R, Grundfest WS (eds): Lasers in Cardiovascular Disease. Chicago, Year Book Medical Publishers, 1987, pp 32–43.
21. Leon M, Smith P, Bonner R.: Laser angioplasty delivery systems: Design considerations, in White R, Grundfest WS (eds): Lasers in Cardiovascular Disease. Chicago, Year Book Medical Publishers, 1987, pp 44–62.
22. Litvack F, Grundfest WS, et al.: Laser angioplasty: Status and prospects. Semin Intervent Radiol 3(1):75, 1986.
23. Litvack F, Grundfest WS, et al.: In vivo excimer laser angioplasty and a new, flexible, blunt tipped delivery system. Circulation 76(4), 1987.
24. Sanborn T: Laser thermal angioplasty, in White R, Grundfest WS (eds): Lasers in Cardiovascular Disease. Chicago, Year Book Medical Publishers, 1987, pp 75–90.
25. Cumberland D: Peripheral and coronary percutaneous laser assisted balloon angioplasty: Clinical results. Third European Laser Assoc. Amsterdam, Lasers in Medicine, 1986.
26. Sanborn TA, Cumberland DC, et al.: Six months follow-up of laserprobe assisted balloon angioplasty. Circulation 74(suppl 11):1819A, 1976.
27. Cumberland D, Oakley GDG, et al.: Percutaneous laser assisted coronary angioplasty (letter). Lancet 2(8500):214, 1986.
28. Crea F, Davies G, et al.: Percutaneous laser recanalization of coronary arteries (letter). Lancet 2(8500):214, 1986.
29. Doyle L, Litvack F, et al.: An in vivo model for testing laser angioplasty systems (abstract). Circulation 74(4)(suppl 2):1440a:361, 1986.
30. Litvack F, Grundfest WS, et al.: Hot tip angioplasty by a novel radiofrequency catheter. J Am Coll Cardiol 2(2):108A, 1988.
31. Simpson JB, Zimmerman JJ, et al.: Transluminal atherectomy: Initial clinical results in 27 patients (abstract). Circulation 74(suppl 2):203, 1986.
32. Kinsey K. Personal communication. June 1987.
33. Hansen D, Auth D, et al.: Rotating mechanical angioplasty in atherosclerotic iliac arteries in rabbits. J Am Coll Cardiol 7:213A, 1986.

PART IV
Occlusive Arterial Diseases

CHAPTER 28
Arterial Embolism of the Extremities and Technique of Embolectomy

Henry Haimovici

Arterial embolectomy, designed to restore patency of an acutely occluded vessel by a thromboembolus, is one of the earliest known reconstructive arterial procedures. Although attempted since 1895 by several surgeons, it was not until 1911 that the first successful embolectomy was performed by Georges Labey and reported by Mosny and Dumont.[1] In their comments on this case, it is of interest to note the authors' clear perception of what the ideal indications ought to be for a successful procedure. They stated that to be acceptable, it is important that "the operation should be undertaken without delay, that the embolus be aseptic and easily accessible, that the patient be young and his arteries healthy." Obviously, these principles were then and still are today most applicable to ideal situations. However, the wide spectrum of clinical forms deals with less favorable conditions, as has been illustrated abundantly since 1911.

Shortly after this first success, the procedure was extended to include patients of all ages and different clinical and pathologic circumstances. Because of the pioneering efforts of Einar Key of Sweden, this procedure gained increasing acceptance.[2] The publications in the ensuing 3 to 4 decades pointed out, among other factors, the necessity of early operative intervention to avoid irreversible intimal damage and secondary thrombosis distal to the embolic occlusion.[3,4] It is very likely that incomplete removal of the secondary or propagated thrombi often contributed to its poor results. Among the attempts to overcome this technical difficulty was the introduction of retrograde arterial flushing with saline for the removal of the propagated thrombi.[5–7] This technique, however, often failed to achieve its goal.

A more significant advance in the management of arterial embolism was the introduction in 1940 of anticoagulant agents, especially heparin, used during and after surgery.[8,9]

However, it was not until 1963 that a most notable advance in the performance of arterial embolectomy was achieved by the introduction of the balloon catheter by Fogarty et al.[10] This simple instrument represents an important landmark in the history and management of arterial embolism, as well as in vascular surgery in general. Concurrently, further progress has been accomplished by better understanding of the hemodynamics of embolic occlusion, by greater awareness of the possibility of metabolic complications associated with severe ischemia of skeletal muscle,[11–13] and by wider use of open heart surgery for cardiovalvular repair.

At present, in spite of all these advances responsible for the current higher rate of limb salvage and reduced mortality in some groups of patients previously considered high-risk surgical groups, the concept of arterial embolism and its management is still undergoing changes.[14–16] It seems that while progress was being achieved in one area, a few old challenges continued to persist and new ones emerged. Thus, despite the fact that the balloon catheter has greatly improved the technique of embolectomy, limb loss and mortality rates still remain high in a certain group of patients.[17] The cardiac nature of the emboligenic factors and the extent of the ischemic impact on the involved tissues (especially the skeletal muscles) with the metabolic repercussions are among the determinant features responsible for the persistent severity of an arterial embolism. Its etiology and the clinical, metabolic, and operative aspects will be reviewed here to provide some of the answers to the persisting, challenging problems engendered by arterial embolism.

CLINICAL AND PATHOLOGIC DATA

Arterial embolism is a complication of a severe cardiopathy. The heart is the source of embolism in 90 to 96% of the published cases.[18–20] The relative incidence of the types of the cardiopathy has changed in recent years. Rheumatic valvular disease is no longer as preponderant as before,[16] in contrast to a greater etiologic role played by arteriosclerotic heart disease and myocardial infarction. Although atrial fibrillation is common in both the rheumatic and arteriosclerotic heart diseases, its relative incidence in the latter

TABLE 28-1. NATURE OF CARDIOPATHY IN ARTERIAL EMBOLISM

	Percentage	
Etiology	Before 1960 (228 Patients)*	After 1963 (83 Patients)†
RHD	40.4	7.7
ASHD	50.8	84.0
ASHD/RHD	1.25	10.5

* Data from Haimovici H: Angiology 1:20, 1950.
† Data from Haimovici H, et al.: Surgery 78:409, 1975.

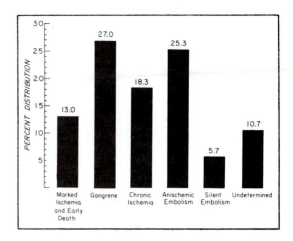

Figure 28-1. Natural course of 300 cases of surgically untreated arterial embolism of the extremities. (*Based on data from Haimovici H: Angiology, 1:20, 1950.*)

group has increased in the decades since 1950 (Table 28-1).

Mural thrombi associated with myocardial infarction, occurring about 11% of the time, may sometimes embolize long before clinical and electrocardiographic evidence of their origin becomes available. In such cases of silent myocardial infarction, the differential diagnosis of embolism from arterial thrombosis may be difficult or even impossible.[20]

Arterial embolism may occur at any age, although the peak incidence is in the fifth, sixth, and seventh decades. The sex incidence varies with the cardiopathy. In a group with rheumatic heart disease, 78.3% were females, whereas in a group with myocardial infarction, 73.6% were males.[20]

The natural clinical course of a peripheral arterial embolism (Fig. 28-1) depends upon the location of the occlusion, the degree of completeness of the luminal obliteration, the extent of secondary thrombosis and the degree of spontaneous restoration of the collateral circulation. Among these, secondary thrombosis is one of the most important local factors. Indeed, by its occurrence, from an initial short segmental obstruction induced by the embolus, the secondary thrombus extends the occlusion distally to the main arterial trunk and its collaterals (Fig. 28-2). Thus, the latter, by involving a long segment, is a lesion far more dangerous to the viability of the limb than is the original relatively small embolus.

Multiple emboli are known to occur either in the same extremity or at different arterial sites. It is usually assumed that they are the result of a shower of emboli and occur at about the same time (Fig. 28-3). The possibility of multiple embolic occlusions in the same extremity or at different

locations including the visceral arteries, although well known, is not always appreciated (Fig. 28-4). Failure to do so may be responsible for the unsuccessful results in some cases of embolectomy.[20–24]

Recurrent emboli may occur in different locations or in the same vessel. In the latter case, one may suspect the possibility of in situ thrombosis, a differential diagnosis that should be kept in mind. The interval of recurrence may take a few days to several months. The possibility of recurrent embolization emphasizes the necessity for eradicating its source, whether it be valvular disease, atrial thrombosis, or some other cause of vascular or nonvascular origin.

Atheroembolism, arterial embolism of atheromatous material, has been reported in recent years with increasing frequency.[25–29] They may occur (1) as microemboli following release of cholesterol crystals or other atheromatous debris from an ulcerated plaque and (2) as macroemboli resulting from major atheromatous plaques mixed with thrombi and cholesterol crystals that lodge in major systemic arteries.

These atheroemboli may originate in an abdominal aneurysm or a nonaneurysmal lesion of the aorta or may follow surgical manipulation of the latter. Their differential diagnosis from a cardiogenic embolism is usually helped by the absence of any emboligenic heart condition.

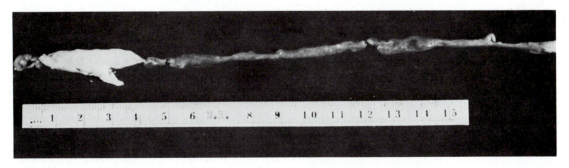

Figure 28-2. Note the small size of a femoral embolus (light color) involving the bifurcation and the long secondary thrombus (dark color) removed from the superficial femoral and popliteal arteries.

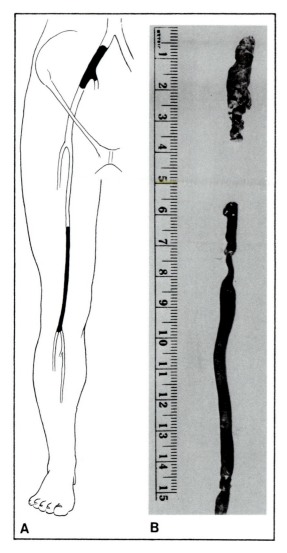

Figure 28-3. A. Diagram of right iliac and popliteal emboli. **B.** Photographs of specimens of emboli removed during the same surgical procedure.

The clinical picture varies with the location of the involved arterial segment. The atheroemboli may go unrecognized or unsuspected, especially in the group of microemboli. Greater awareness of the source of atheroembolism is basic for recognition of this entity.[29] (See Chapter 30 on Atheroembolism.)

TOPOGRAPHIC DIAGNOSIS

The site of an embolic occlusion is generally easily identifiable (Fig. 28-5). The clinical criteria are (1) the site of the initial pain, (2) the level where the normal pulsation disappears, (3) the noninvasive diagnostic modalities, (4) the extent of the circulatory disturbances, and (5) knowledge that emboli usually lodge at bifurcations. Unfortunately, in a certain number of cases, especially in those with preexisting occlusive disease, the exact localization of the embolus

may be difficult to determine without arteriography. Indeed, presence of an atherosclerotic stenosis, either proximally or distally away from bifurcations, may represent a potential site of entrapment of the embolus. Because of this possible unconventional location of an embolus, it is essential that preoperative arteriography be carried out in cases suspected of associated preexisting arterial lesions.

DIFFERENTIAL DIAGNOSIS

The recognition of a peripheral arterial embolism is usually simple. Although a sudden onset is quite characteristic, occurring in 81% of cases,[20] in 1 of 5 cases, there may be a progressive onset. Lack of routine evaluation of the extremities in patients with advanced heart disease may sometimes be responsible for the failure of prompt recognition of an arterial embolism. Conditions that may otherwise be confused with peripheral embolism are phlegmasia cerulea dolens, acute arterial thrombosis, acute thrombosis of a popliteal aneurysm, acute thrombosis of a nonarteriosclerotic artery, low-flow syndrome due to circulatory failure, dissecting aortic aneurysm, and arterial spasm. Awareness of these entities is essential in the differential diagnosis.

Associated Visceral Arterial Embolism

Visceral emboli, isolated or associated with peripheral emboli, occur with greater frequency than is generally recognized (Fig. 28-6). It is well known that there is a considerable discrepancy between their clinical diagnosis and autopsy findings. Clinically, visceral emboli, if small, are often undetectable or remain unsuspected, whereas major embolic occlusions display significant and often rapidly irreversible and lethal changes when occurring in cerebral, mesenteric, renal, or coronary vessels. (See Chapters 55 to 57 for their descriptions.)

INDICATIONS FOR EMBOLECTOMY

It is hardly necessary to point out that conservative measures (heparin, vasodilator drugs, fibrinolytic agents) are only adjuncts to, not substitutes for, arterial embolectomy, which is the method of choice and is applicable in almost all cases.*

Early embolectomy, 8 to 12 hours after onset—considered the optimal time for this procedure since the first successful case performed in 1911—is still a valid principle today. However, in late cases, the physiologic state of the limb rather than the elapsed time from the onset of the occlusion will determine operability.

Late arterial embolectomy thus may still be indicated and is often successful if the limb still exhibits signs of viable tissues. Analysis of the clinical and pathologic data of late

---

*Percutaneous aspiration thromboembolectomy has been described recently as an alternative in cases below the femoral bifurcation (Turnspeed WD, et al,: J Vasc Surg 3:437, 1986).

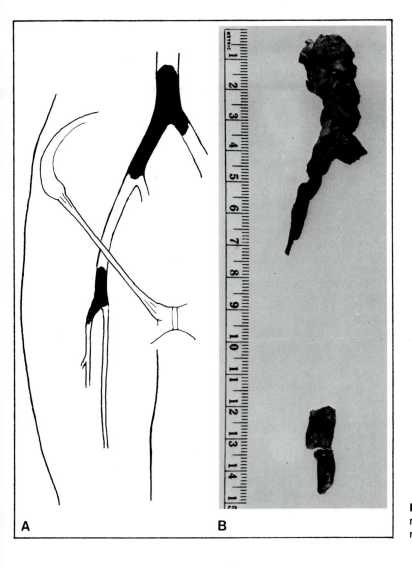

Figure 28-4. A. Diagram of saddle aortic and right common femoral emboli. **B.** Photograph of specimens removed during surgery.

arterial embolectomies suggests that four factors govern their successful outcome: (1) a relatively damage-free arterial intima, (2) nonadherence of the embolus and secondary thrombus to the intima, (3) a patent distal arterial tree prior to embolization, and (4) pretreatment with anticoagulants. These factors facilitate a more complete extraction of the secondary thrombi so essential for achieving adequate revascularization of the limb. Contraindication to a late arterial embolectomy is frank gangrene involving part of the extremity.[30]

Grading of Embolic Ischemia of Lower Extremity

In its simplest form, an arterial embolus by itself occludes only a short segment of an artery, and in the absence of spasm or secondary thrombosis, the restoration of the distal circulation may be effected through collateral channels. However, a peripheral arterial embolism usually occurs in a more complex clinicopathologic setting.

On the basis of our previous study concerning the degree of spontaneous restoration of the circulation in a series of untreated cases,[20] the grading of arterial embolism is as follows:

Grade I *Moderate* ischemia with early pulse return: an ischemic embolism (29.5%)

Grade II *Advanced* ischemia with only partial late recovery: chronic postembolic ischemia (22.2%)

Grade III *Severe* ischemia leading to variable degrees of gangrene, often with metabolic complications (28%)

Grade IV *Very severe* ischemia with early fatal outcome, mainly the result of advanced heart failure or associated visceral emboli (11.3%)

PREOPERATIVE EVALUATION

Evaluation of an embolic occlusion and its ischemic manifestations is based on examination of the pulses, skin temperature and color changes, motion and sensory deficits, and the degree of contracture of the calf or forearm. Paralysis and anesthesia of the distal or entire limb are ominous signs. Embolectomy may still be attempted but not without

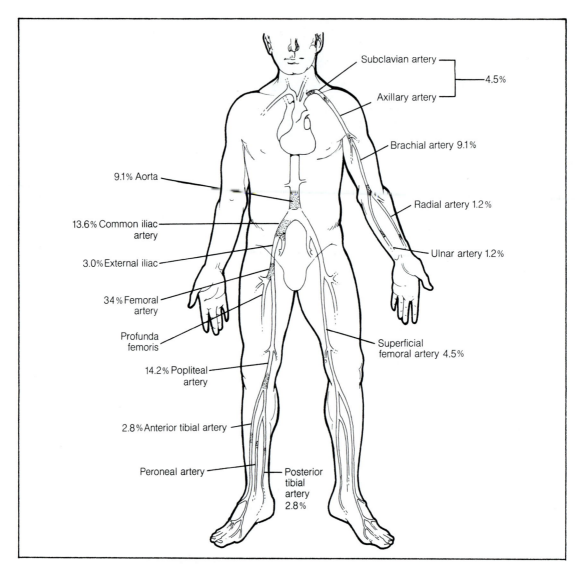

Figure 28-5. Incidence of location of peripheral emboli in a series of 330 cases.[20]

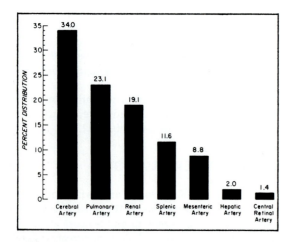

Figure 28-6. Sites and incidence of visceral emboli in 96 cases out of 228 patients.[20]

some reservation, especially if limb rigidity is present. If the location of the embolus and the preembolic status of the distal arterial tree are in doubt, and if Doppler evaluation is equivocal, arteriography appears essential (Fig. 28-7).

Assessment of the underlying heart disease, source of the embolism, and its correction should be undertaken without delay. The cardiac condition may determine, to some extent, how aggressively one should treat the arterial complication. In the presence of myocardial infarction, heart failure, or shock, a vigorous treatment should be instituted prior to embolectomy. During the few hours necessary to correct to an acceptable degree the cardiac function, heparin should be administered intravenously. Fibrinolysins, if available, may be injected directly into the involved artery. Their value, however, is still not well established.

Routine blood chemistries, a hematologic profile, and examination of urine for myoglobin may be of value in cases with early rigidity of calf or forearm muscles.

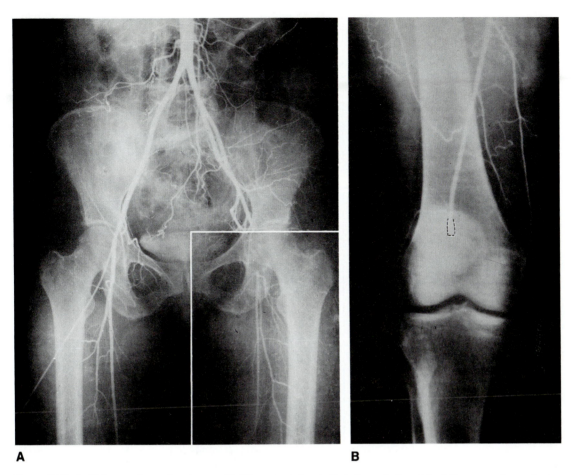

A   B

Figure 28-7. A. Right transfemoral aortogram (Seldinger technique). Embolic occlusion of the left common femoral artery in a 58-year-old woman who had mitral stenosis and auricular fibrillation. Note the smooth outline of the arterial tree. **B.** The same arteriographic study disclosed an embolic occlusion of the right popliteal artery.

ANESTHESIA AND MONITORING OF PATIENT DURING SURGERY

In the majority of cases, local anesthesia can be used to great advantage. Since the introduction of the balloon catheter, this method is applicable in almost all cases of embolectomy. However, a light general anesthesia or additional sedation can be used if the patient is apprehensive. Epidural or spinal anesthesia may be advisable if the procedure entails exposure not only of the groin vessels but also of the popliteal and leg arteries.

Monitoring of the patient's electrocardiogram, blood pressure, and blood gases of the involved limb may be helpful, mostly in late cases of embolectomy with possible involvement of skeletal muscles.

OPERATIVE TECHNIQUES

Since the introduction of the balloon catheter, the technique of embolectomy has been simplified and the approach to the various vessels has been reduced to a few critical areas. Although in most instances the latter provide access to any occluded vessel, direct exposure of the involved arteries

may nevertheless be necessary in some cases (Fig. 28-8). The technique of embolectomy will be described for (1) femoral, (2) aortic bifurcation, (3) iliac, (4) popliteal, and (5) upper limb arteries.

Femoral Embolectomy

Preparation of Limb
Although the procedure may be confined to the groin at the level of Scarpa's triangle, it is essential to prepare also the abdomen and the entire lower extremity.

Exposure of Femoral Vessels
Exposure should be adequate to afford easy access to the common, superficial, and deep femoral vessels. A longitudinal incision is carried out over the course of the femoral artery and is extended slightly superiorly above Poupart's ligament and inferiorly by approximately 3 to 4 inches.

The femoral artery occluded by an embolus appears fusiformly dilated and slightly bluish. Proximally, there is a vigorous pulsation, whereas distally, pulsation is usually completely absent. However, a transmitted pulsation may be perceived occasionally by palpation. This should not

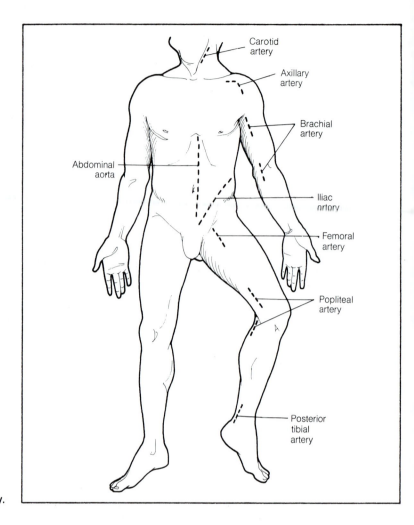

Figure 28-8. Sites of embolectomy.

mislead into the belief that the occlusion is more distal. Gentle palpation of the vessels may identify the exact extent of the embolic or thrombotic occlusion, except for a recent soft thrombus that may be difficult to feel.

After the femoral sheath is opened, the vessels are easily mobilized. Double-looped nontraumatic occluding clamps with Silastic pads (Vesseloops, Med General) are placed around the superficial, profunda, and common femoral vessels. To prevent migration or breaking off of the embolus and propagated thrombus through the profunda or superficial femoral artery, the double-looped tapes are not or are only moderately tightened without occluding the vessel completely (Fig. 28-9A,B).

Arteriotomy
A longitudinal incision about 1.0 to 1.5 cm long is carried out in the common femoral artery down to the origin of the profunda. This type of incision is preferable, especially if the artery is arteriosclerotic. A transverse arteriotomy may be indicated if the artery seems devoid of mural lesions.

Extraction of Embolus and Secondary Thrombus
Upon completion of the arteriotomy, the embolus tends to extrude by itself. A balloon catheter of an appropriate

size (5F) is then introduced into the superficial femoral artery. In the absence of preexisting arteriosclerotic occlusion, the passage of the catheter usually reaches easily the tibial vessels. After achieving patency of the main arterial axis, a 4F catheter is introduced into the profunda femoris. Each of its primary branches is catheterized until all suspected thrombi are removed. A 6F catheter is then passed proximally toward the iliac artery or aorta for removal of a possible unsuspected thrombus. The balloon catheters may have to be passed more than once in all vessels to obtain a normal flow. Upon completion of the embolectomy or, rather, thromboembolectomy, the arteries are copiously irrigated with a 5% heparin-saline solution. The femoral vessels are reclamped and the arteriotomy is closed (Fig. 28-10).

Closure of Arteriotomy
Closure can be carried out either by a continuous running stitch, using No. 5 or No. 6 synthetic (polypropylene) suture material, or by interrupted stitches, especially in a transverse arteriotomy. Irrespective of the type of closure, it is essential to prevent stenosis of the artery by careful approximation of the arteriotomy edges or by vein patch angioplasty, if indicated.

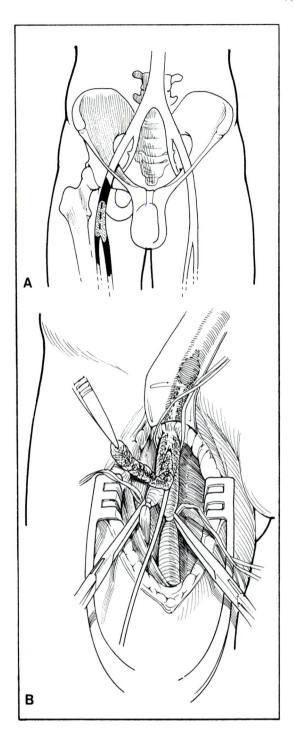

Figure 28-9. Femoral embolectomy. **A.** Diagram depicting a right common femoral embolus (stippled area) with secondary thrombosis both proximal and distal to it. **B.** Balloon catheter being withdrawn from the external iliac artery and pushing out the embolus and thrombus.

Checking Reestablishment of Patency

The proximal patency is usually easily ascertained by the presence of a vigorous pulsation. The more difficult evaluation of patency is confined to the distal pulses. Their return in the profunda and superficial femoral arteries, indicative

though the pulses may be, does not, however, guarantee the patency of the popliteal and tibial arteries. Although back bleeding during the procedure may be considered a significant sign of distal patency, it does not necessarily indicate absence of residual thrombi. It should be pointed out that the retrograde bleeding may originate from a proximal major collateral.

Because of these considerations, it is important, before leaving the operating room, to ascertain the presence of the popliteal and pedal pulses. Their restoration can be anticipated only in those patients in whom the arterial tree was patent in the preembolic episode. However, if there is a history of preexisting arteriosclerotic occlusive disease, unless there is a return of distal pulses, the nature of the restoration of the arterial tree cannot be ascertained on clinical grounds alone. If in doubt, arteriography may then allow identification of the distal arterial lesion. This is particularly true in a late arterial embolectomy (see below).

Closure of Incision

This procedure is carried out in layers in the usual fashion. A correct closure of the incision is obviously important to prevent any possible collection of serum, blood, or lymph, all of which may lead to infection.

Heparinization

During the procedure, the patient is heparinized either systemically by the intravenous route or directly through the involved arterial tree. In addition to the heparinized solution used during the procedure, 3,000 to 5,000 units of heparin is also injected prior to the closure of the incision.

Postoperative Clinical Evaluation

Immediately after arterial restoration, the pain disappears, together with return of motor and sensory functions and of normal color and warmth of the skin. In patients with incomplete restoration of arterial circulation, it may be several hours before partial or complete return of these signs and symptoms can be expected.

The cardiac condition responsible for the peripheral embolism dominates to a large extent, in most cases, the postoperative care. It is essential to monitor the cardiopathy, restore cardiac rhythm, and use heparin postoperatively as prophylaxis against further embolization.

Aortic Bifurcation Embolectomy

Embolic occlusion of the aortic bifurcation results in a dramatic clinical picture and usually occurs in a critically ill patient. Its incidence is about 10% of all emboli of the extremities. The prognosis for both limb and life before the present era was extremely poor, whether with or without surgery. Use of the retrograde technique has improved substantially the overall outcome.

Diagnosis of an aortic saddle embolism is relatively simple. The presence of a cardiopathy with the suddenness of bilateral ischemia with paraplegia leaves little doubt about the diagnosis. A dissecting aortic aneurysm, rather rarely encountered, may mimic an embolic syndrome and should be suspected in the presence of an atypical clinical picture.[31]

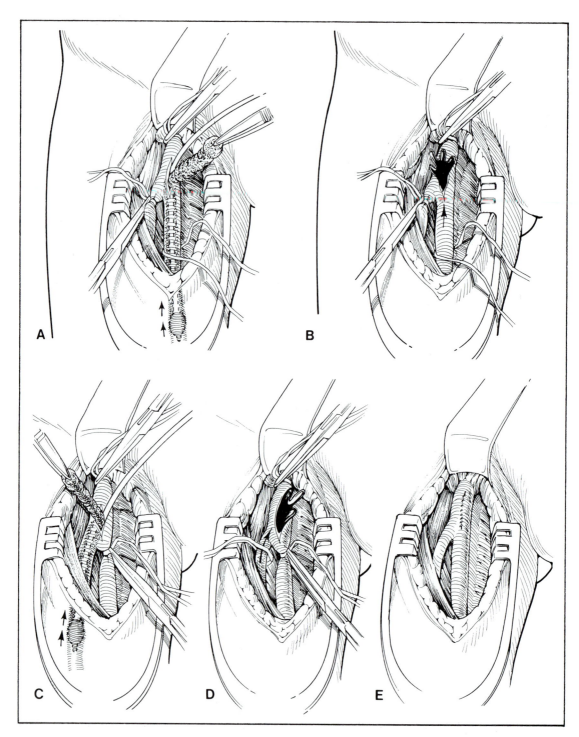

Figure 28-10. Extraction of embolus and secondary thrombus. **A.** Balloon catheter in the superficial femoral artery being withdrawn through the arteriotomy and achieving extrusion of secondary thrombus. **B.** Back bleeding from the superficial femoral after thrombectomy. **C.** Balloon catheter being withdrawn from the profunda femoris together with the secondary thrombus. **D.** Back bleeding from the profunda femoris after thrombectomy. **E.** Closed arteriotomy.

At the other end of the diagnostic spectrum, an incomplete aortic occlusion may be mistaken for a more distal embolism (Fig. 28-11). A translumbar or intravenous aortogram, usually optional, may be helpful in such cases in settling the diagnosis.

Several technical approaches are available for aortic embolectomy: (1) transfemoral or retrograde, the most com- monly used, (2) transperitoneal, and (3) retroperitoneal, the last two being rarely indicated nowadays.

Retrograde or Transfemoral Embolectomy
Since the introduction of the Fogarty balloon catheter (Fig. 28-12), the results of disobstruction of the aortic bifurcation have improved considerably because of a more complete

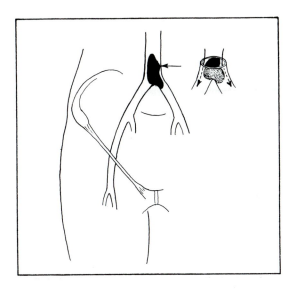

Figure 28-11. Diagram of a riding aortic embolus, incompletely occluding the aortic bifurcation.

and easier retrieval of the embolus and the propagated thrombi.

Advantages. The advantages of the retrograde technique are (1) simple groin exposure of the femorals under local anesthesia, (2) direct evaluation of distal propagated

thrombi and of preexisting femoral arteriosclerotic lesions, (3) lack of operative shock, and (4) usually uncomplicated postoperative course.

Disadvantages. Being a blind procedure, a successful embolectomy may sometimes be difficult to achieve in cases of (1) severe atherosclerotic lesions of the aortoiliac segment, (2) marked iliac tortuosity, (3) coexistence of visceral emboli, especially of the mesenteric artery, (4) emboli of the hypogastric vessels, the latter being missed through this approach, and (5) an undetected, acutely thrombosed, small aortic aneurysm. These conditions are fortunately not common. The advantages of the retrograde approach outweigh by far the occasional pitfalls, which may be avoided if one bears in mind such possibilities.

Technique. Although the technique consists of a bilateral transfemoral approach, it is essential to prepare also the abdominal region and both lower extremities. This wide operative field preparation may be necessary if a different or additional arterial exposure is required.

Both femoral arteries in the groin are exposed through the standard longitudinal incision. Local anesthesia and monitoring of the patient are similar to those previously described for a simple femoral embolectomy.

The common, superficial, and profunda femoris vessels are mobilized, and tapes are placed about them. After care-

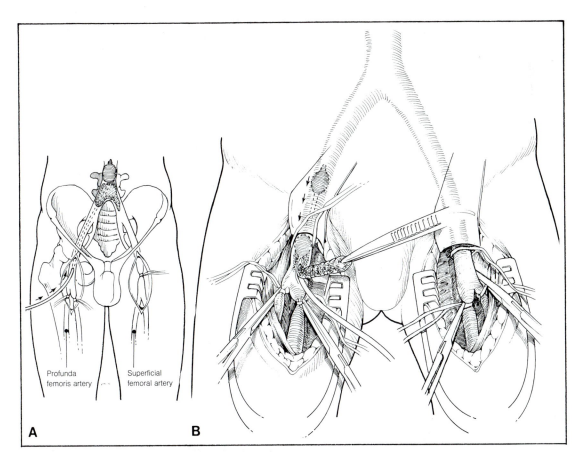

Figure 28-12. Aortic embolectomy. **A.** Balloon catheter maximally distended in the abdominal aorta above the embolus. **B.** Catheter being withdrawn through the right femoral arteriotomy together with the aortic embolus.

ful palpation of the vessel for determining the presence of either arteriosclerotic lesions or thrombotic material, the distal branches may not be clamped or only partially closed by incompletely tightening the tapes.

The best and most expeditious way for handling the two groins is by two surgical teams.

Arteriotomy is carried out in one common femoral artery, preferably on the side where the ischemia is most pronounced. On the opposite side, the superficial and profunda femoris vessels are occluded by atraumatic tapes.

Disobliteration of the distal vessels is carried out first, by means of a Fogarty catheter of an appropriate caliber (4F or 5F), starting with the superficial femoral artery and then checking the profunda femoris. After obtaining a good or acceptable backflow, the two vessels are irrigated with heparinized solution.

Proximal disobliteration is carried out with a large-caliber catheter (6F) which is introduced up to the renal vessels. The balloon is then inflated until an elastic resistance is perceived. At this point, the catheter is withdrawn through the arteriotomy. As the balloon catheter passes from the

aortic level to the iliac, the balloon must be slightly deflated in order to readjust it to the diameter of the iliac. This maneuver may have to be repeated until one obtains a vigorous systolic flow.

After a good pulsation is obtained above the arteriotomy, the attention is shifted to the opposite side. A good pulsation should be obtained on the contralateral femoral as determined by palpation. Should there be the slightest suspicion of a thrombus at this level, exploration of the femoral is mandatory. A similar set of maneuvers is then carried out, first in the superficial and profunda femoral vessels, and then proximally in the iliac artery and aorta. When patency of both sides is achieved, the arteriotomy of both femoral arteries is closed in the usual fashion (Fig. 28-13).

Distal Arterial Patency. Immediately after the arteriotomies are closed, the distal pulses must be ascertained. Their appearance, in addition to return of the normal color of the skin and filling of the superficial veins, is indicative of good flow. Intraoperative use of Doppler pulse determi-

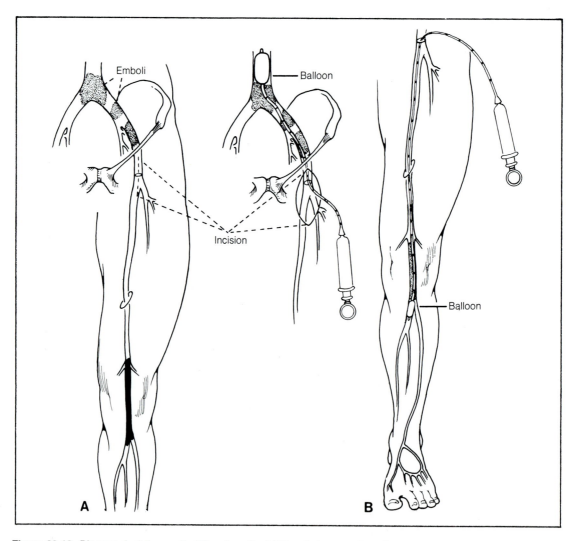

Figure 23-13. Diagram depicting aortic (**A**) and popliteal (**B**) embolectomy through a common femoral arteriotomy. Note the inflated balloon in the aorta (**A**) and the posterior tibial trunk (**B**).

nation of the peripheral vessels may be quite helpful. If unsatisfactory, intraoperative arteriography should be used. Any doubt about the quality of patency of the distal arterial tree in one or both lower extremities makes mandatory reexploration of one or both.

Immediately postoperatively, examination of the abdomen should also be carried out clinically and, if necessary, radiologically in order to determine whether there is any involvement of the mesenteric vessels.

Pitfalls. The preceding technique is simple and easy to carry out in the presence of normal arteries or arteries at least devoid of any major arteriosclerotic changes. However, in the presence of severe mural lesions or of secondary thrombosis involving the distal arterial tree, it becomes necessary to explore the superficial femoral or the popliteal artery (Fig. 28-13B).

Transperitoneal Aortic Embolectomy

Indications for this approach are rare nowadays. However, in the presence of an incomplete disobliteration through the femoral arteries, it is necessary to expose the aortic bifurcation directly. The reason for this difficulty resides primarily in the associated stenotic arteriosclerotic changes of the bifurcation.

Advantages of such an exposure are obvious, since the lesions of the aortic bifurcation and of the iliac arteries can be properly evaluated and dealt with. *Disadvantages*, however, include a more extensive surgical exposure, necessitating general or spinal anesthesia. The operative risk is obviously much greater than in the previous approach.

Technique. The technique consists of a median or left paramedian incision extending from the pubis to above the umbilicus and, if necessary, up to the xiphoid process. The small bowel is eviscerated, and the posterior parietal peritoneum is incised along the aortic pulsation down to the pelvis. The abdominal aorta is mobilized below the inferior mesenteric artery. The two common iliac arteries are mobilized, and tapes are placed about them. An arteriotomy is carried out, preferably in one of the common iliac arteries, through which the embolus and the thrombus are extruded, including the one from the opposite side, if present. The distal arterial tree is cleared through the arteriotomy by means of a Fogarty catheter. Should any suspicion exist about the opposite side, its patency should be ascertained through a separate arteriotomy. After the arteriotomies are closed and the arterial flow is reestablished, the abdominal closure is carried out in the usual fashion.

Retroperitoneal Aortic Embolectomy

The aorta and its bifurcation may be exposed through a left retroperitoneal approach, using the technique described in Chapter 18.

Advantages of this exposure, especially in a thin individual, are obvious. The operative risk is certainly less than with the transperitoneal approach. *Disadvantages*, especially in an obese individual, may be due to inadequate exposure of the right iliac artery. However, incision of the left rectus abdominis may facilitate the exposure, and an arteriotomy can be done without too much difficulty.

Technique. The embolectomy is carried out through an arteriotomy in the left common iliac artery, as previously described. The patency of the distal arterial tree on this side is easily evaluated by means of an appropriate balloon catheter. On the opposite side, if necessary, a catheter can be introduced through a separate arteriotomy in the contralateral common iliac.

Should there be any need, this exposure also offers easy access for a lumbar sympathectomy. This may be particularly indicated if there is a history of preexisting arteriosclerotic lesions of the distal arterial tree.

Postoperative Care

Special attention must immediately be directed toward both the cardiopulmonary function and the lower extremities. The patient is transferred to the intensive care unit, where cardiac monitoring and pulmonary function are closely supervised.

Anticoagulation may be deferred for 12 to 24 hours to avoid hematomas because of the extensive abdominal or retroperitoneal dissections. After this period, intravenous heparin is administered in order to prevent any further embolization and possibly distal rethrombosis. Aspirin and dipyridamole are administered as soon as feasible postoperatively. Oral anticoagulation should be instituted and maintained for life.

The lower extremities are checked carefully for pulses or for any sign of recurrence of ischemia. Doppler ultrasonic technique is most helpful, short of arteriography, for ascertaining patency and arterial flow.

Revascularization complications should be watched for very closely (see below).

Iliac Embolectomy

The embolus usually blocks the common iliac artery and extends into the external and internal iliac arteries. The clinical picture is that of major sudden ischemia of one lower extremity. Bilateral iliac embolism is indistinguishable from the clinical picture of a saddle embolus of the aorta.

The technical approaches available for an iliac embolectomy are (1) transfemoral or retrograde, the most commonly used, and (2) retroperitoneal.

Retrograde or Transfemoral Embolectomy

Despite the fact that this is a unilateral procedure through the groin, it is important to bear in mind two possibilities: (1) difficulty of complete removal of the embolus and propagated thrombus or (2) inadvertent proximal dislocation of the thrombotic material into the aorta and the opposite iliac artery. Consequently, a wide preoperative preparation of the abdomen and of both thighs is mandatory should it become necessary to expose directly the iliac or the opposite femoral artery.

Local anesthesia and the various steps of the techniques are identical with those described for aortic embolectomy.

Retroperitoneal Embolectomy

Although a local anesthesia can be used, because of discomfort it is most often desirable to use a spinal or epidural or even a general anesthesia. A wide retroperitoneal exposure of the iliac vessels as well as of the aortic bifurcation is necessary for an adequate procedure. The arteriotomy, whether longitudinal or transverse, is best carried out in the common iliac artery just above its division into the internal and external branches. This affords easy access to the latter for thrombectomy, if indicated. A possible difficulty may result from the thrombus propagated into the femoral artery, especially into its superficial and profunda vessels. Exposure of the latter may then become necessary.

Popliteal Embolectomy

A popliteal embolism may carry a more serious prognosis than that of a femoral artery. This is especially true in older patients with preexisting arteriosclerotic lesions of the tibial arteries, primarily in diabetic patients in whom the leg arteries are much more severely involved than in nondiabetics. Early embolectomy appears mandatory, therefore, to avoid secondary thrombosis in the most distal branches and thereby help salvage the limb.

A preoperative femoral arteriogram, with special emphasis on visualizing the popliteal and leg arteries, is essential. The popliteal embolus may be approached indirectly through the femoral artery in the groin or directly through a medial exposure of the lower third of the thigh above the knee (Fig. 28-14). While these conventional approaches may be suitable in some cases, in most instances it is best to expose the infragenual popliteal artery for its direct access together with the origin of the tibial arteries (anterior tibial and tibioperoneal trunk with its two branches).

One of the advantages of exposing the distal popliteal artery is the absence of significant collaterals arising from it or its branches. Although this segment is smaller than the proximal popliteal, the infragenual segment is of sufficient caliber for easy graft attachment. In addition, this segment tends to be better preserved and is usually free of artheromatous degenerative changes, in contrast to the proximal popliteal.

Exposure of the distal popliteal is achieved through a medial paratibial route. The anatomic details of this exposure are described in Chapter 20. Essentially, the steps

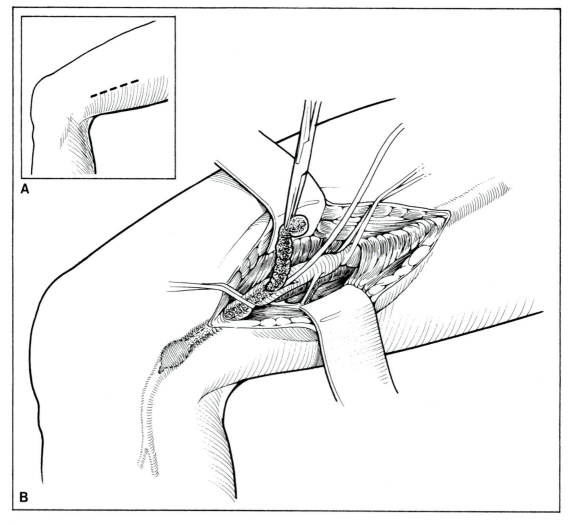

Figure 28-14. Popliteal embolectomy. **A.** Skin incision (dotted line) for the lower third medial-thigh approach to the popliteal artery. **B.** Balloon catheter embolectomy performed through a longitudinal arteriotomy.

for this exposure consist of a skin incision 8 to 10 cm long parallel to the posterior medial border of the tibia, opening of the crural fascia below the tendons of the semitendinosus and gracilis, exposure of the neurovascular bundle, which is usually situated quite deep against the bone surface covered by the popliteus muscle, opening of the vascular sheath surrounding the vessels, freeing of the popliteal artery from its satellite veins, section and ligation of the network of venules surrounding the artery, and division of the soleus muscle for exposure of the distal segment of the popliteal with its branches.

The arteriotomy of the popliteal is carried out in its distal segment facing the origin of the anterior tibial and extended down to the tibioperoneal trunk (Fig. 28-15). This arteriotomy facilitates the insertion of the Fogarty catheter into the anterior tibial artery through direct vision of its ostium, as well as the introduction of the catheter into the posterior tibial and peroneal arteries. (See Chapter 20.) Should the thromboembolic material not be retrieved com-

pletely, a retrograde irrigation of these vessels through the retromalleolar incision of the posterior tibial artery may be attempted, although this procedure has given very few positive results.

In a popliteal embolectomy, perhaps more than in any other, caution should be exercised in inflating the balloon catheter. Overdistention may cause damage to the intima or even its avulsion, especially in diabetic patients with arteriosclerotic lesions of the tibial arteries. Removal of the catheter should be done with great gentleness, with neither overdistention nor underdistention.

Results of Embolectomy of Lower Extremity

The many factors that may determine the outcome of an embolectomy are not always uniformly interpreted in the published reports.[22,32] The relative significance of the individual factors may vary substantially. In a recent review

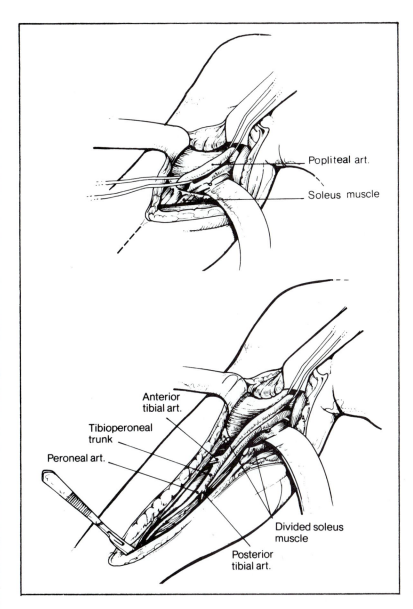

Poplicial art.

Soleus muscle

Anterior tibial art.

Tibioperoneal trunk

Peroneal art.

Divided soleus muscle

Posterior tibial art.

Figure 28-15. Medial leg exposure of below-knee popliteal artery and its trifurcation branches. (See text for embolectomy procedure at this level.)

TABLE 28-2. DISTRIBUTION OF EMBOLI OF UPPER EXTREMITY

Author	Subclavian	Axillary	Brachial	Radial	Ulnar
Haimovici[39]	—	15	30	4	4
Daley et al.[23]	—	3	36	—	—
Baird & Lajos[33]	10	22	64	4	4
Darling et al.[21]	4	20	44	—	—
McGowan & Mooneeram[35]	2	3	17	2	—
Raithel[36]	4	5	15	—	—
Savelyev et al.[38]	47	66	143	3	1
Totals	67	134	349	13	9
Percent	11.7%	23.4%	61.0%	2.3%	1.6%

of 35 collected series, Blaisdell et al.[18] found 14 reports with mortality rates ranging from 15 to 24%, 11 reports with rates between 30 and 48%, and a median group of 10 series reporting mortality rates of 25 to 29%. The same wide range holds true for limb salvage, with rates between 40 and 81%. The entire series included 3,330 embolectomies, with an average limb salvage rate of 63% and an average mortality rate of 28%.

The highest mortality rate is due to congestive heart failure and acute myocardial infarction, with pulmonary embolism being the second major cause. The other factors are strokes, mesenteric infarction, hepatic coma, and miscellaneous etiologies. In reporting causes of mortality, the literature rarely mentions that metabolic and renal complications may be due to ischemic rhabdomyolysis and the revascularization syndrome. (See Chapter 32.)

In the assessment of rates of limb salvage, amputation, and mortality, it appears that the published criteria are far from standardized. Hence, these reports contain a number of built-in statistical errors inherent in the method of estimating the various postoperative findings.

In evaluating the results of embolectomy, it is essential to properly identify gradations of the severity of ischemia along with the systemic factors. Finally, in reporting limb salvage, it is important to indicate whether rates are calculated for the survivors or for the entire series, a fact not always mentioned. As useful as they may be, statistical compilations may not provide an accurate and meaningful picture of the underlying factors that govern results of an arterial embolectomy.

Therapeutic guidelines derived from such widely diverse statistics are nevertheless compelling. Treatment without delay remains the mandatory principle. Early arterial embolectomy and heparinization, either alone or combined, along with management of the patient's cardiopulmonary and metabolic problems, are the best means at our disposal for improving limb salvage and patient survival rates.

Arterial Embolectomy for Upper Limb Embolism

The relative *incidence* of upper limb emboli as related to the total number of peripheral emboli is variably reported and ranges between 16 and 32.6%. These percentages indicate that this embolic location is less infrequent than had been reported earlier.[20,33–39]

The *nature* of the cardiopathy, which is the source of emboli, has changed radically during the past 3 decades, as indicated earlier in this chapter.

Distribution of emboli assumes a rather constant pattern. Their relative distribution is shown in Table 28-2. These data are based on the compilation of seven statistical studies. As can be seen, the greater incidence in the brachial artery

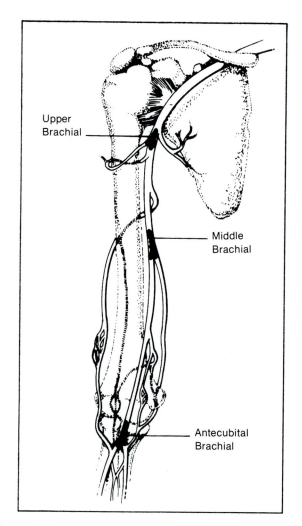

Figure 28-16. Diagram indicating the three major locations of brachial emboli (upper, middle, and antecubital brachial).

suggests that the majority of upper limb emboli are of small size.

Symptomatology varies according to the arterial level involved. In a *subclavian-axillary* artery embolism, the proximal pulsation is usually found in the supraclavicular fossa, with ischemic manifestations detectable to midarm level. In a *brachial* artery embolism, the occlusion may occur either in the upper third of the arm, just above the profunda brachii, in the midarm at the origin of the superior ulnar collateral artery, or at the bifurcation of the brachial artery in the antecubital fossa. Therefore, the brachial pulse may be felt either at the distal axillary or at midarm or above the antecubital fossa. In these cases, the ischemic manifestations involve the hand and forearm up to or below the elbow (Fig. 28-16).

In an embolic occlusion of the *radial* or *ulnar* arteries,

clinical manifestations are usually less pronounced and remain localized to the distal forearm and hand.

Evaluation of the degree of viability of the hand or forearm may be determined by the color, temperature of skin, motion of fingers or wrist, sensory perception, degree of muscle edema, or rigidity. Noninvasive procedures, such as pulse volume recording (PVR) and Doppler pulse recording, may be helpful in assessing the level of arterial blockage. However, arteriography is the decisive diagnostic means, especially when clinical and noninvasive evaluation cannot identify the presumptive locations and extent of the occlusive process (Fig. 28-17). An intraoperative arteriogram often may be necessary for assessing the result of the embolectomy. When properly performed, arteriography carries few risks as measured against the valuable information it may provide.

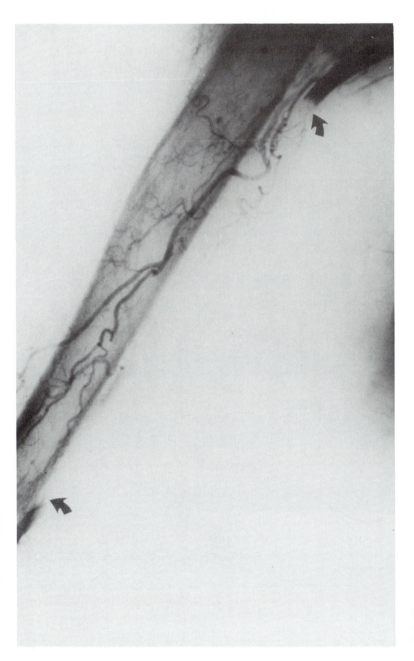

Figure 28-17. Brachial arteriogram indicating a massive occlusion between the distal axillary and antecubital fossa.

Prognosis

Although the potential hazards to the viability of the upper limb are thought to be less than those of an embolism of the lower limb, morbidity and mortality rates in these cases are far from negligible (Table 28-3). Thus, in an earlier reported series of untreated surgical patients, 11 of 46, or 24%, died either with gangrene or before development of necrosis of the hand. In addition, gangrene occurred in 7% of the survivors, requiring a major amputation either of the hand or arm, thus raising the total percentage of gangrene to 31%. Furthermore, a number of patients developed functional impairment of the limb associated with occasional gangrene or one of several fingers. Several recent publications and our own experience clearly show that in unoperated patients, either persistent postembolic ischemic changes or frank gangrene of fingers or hand may occur in a rather substantial percentage of patients.

Indications

The indications for embolectomy, which is usually performed under local anesthesia, are widely applicable, while contraindications are minimal and practically confined to a few seriously ill patients.

Technique of embolectomy needs no elaboration except for reemphasis of its preferential use in certain anatomic areas of the arterial tree (Figs. 28-18 and 28-19).

Subclavian-axillary embolectomy can be performed

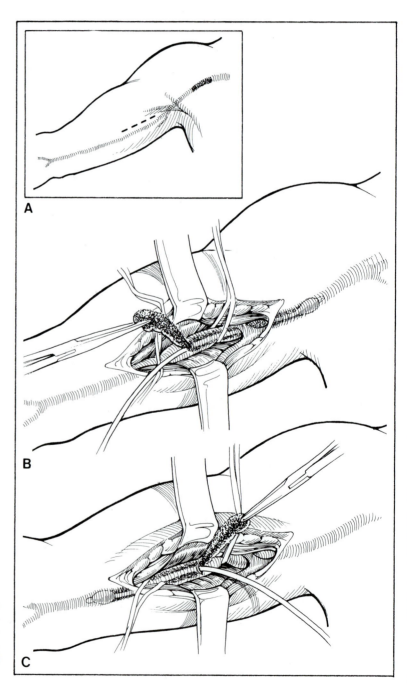

Figure 28-18. Subclavian-axillary embolectomy. **A.** Skin incision (dotted line) for the upper third medial-arm approach of the brachial artery. **B.** Subclavian-axillary passage of a balloon catheter for removal of an embolus. **C.** Distal brachial passage of the catheter for removal of secondary thrombi.

TABLE 28.3. NATURAL COURSE OF NONSURGICALLY TREATED ARTERIAL EMBOLISM OF UPPER EXTREMITY BASED ON LOCATION

	Cases		Gangrene and Early Death		Gangrene and Amputation		Recovery	
	No.	%	No.	%	No.	%	No.	%
Axillary	13	28.3	4	30.8	1	7.7	8	61.5
Brachial	25	54.3	4	16.0	1	4.0	20	80.0
Radial-Ulnar	8	17.4	0	0	1	12.5	7	87.5

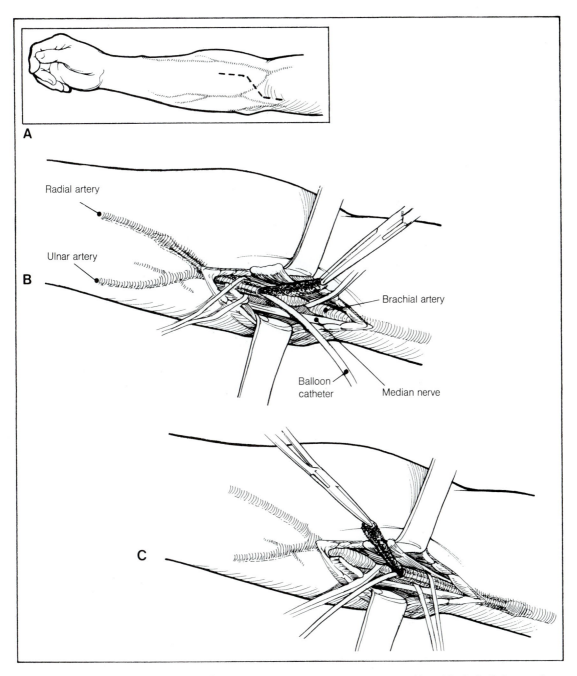

Figure 28-19. Brachial artery embolectomy at the antecubital level. **A.** Skin incision (dotted line). **B.** Balloon catheter being withdrawn from the radial artery together with an embolus and secondary thrombus. **C.** Catheter being withdrawn from proximal arteries (brachial and axillary) together with a thrombus.

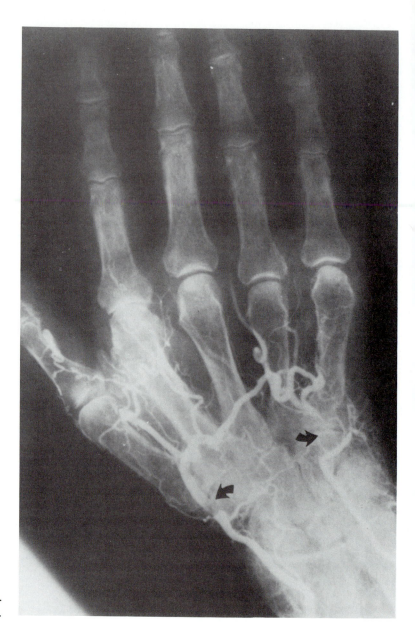

Figure 28-20. Proximal hand and wrist arteriograms indicating emboli of the radial and ulnar arteries of left hand.

through a skin incision of the upper third of the arm using a medial approach to the brachial artery. The balloon catheter is first passed proximally until a forceful systolic jet is obtained behind the removal of the embolus. The catheter is then passed distally for retrieval of secondary thrombi. However, for anatomic reasons, the catheter may not reach the distal thromboembolic material through a midbrachial artery exposure. The procedure is then carried out through a distal brachial arteriotomy.

Removal of emboli through the distal brachial artery is best achieved by its exposure in the antecubital fossa and is the most adequate approach not only for this location but for the axillary-subclavian embolectomy as well. It provides also a better access to the peripheral arterial tree in the event that other thromboemboli occurred distally.

The antecubital fossa is exposed in the usual fashion, and the artery is mobilized with its bifurcation of the radial and ulnar. Fogarty catheters 2F and 3F can be introduced under direct vision into the two branches and thus help

retrieve most of the peripheral thromboembolic material. Embolectomy of the *proximal palmar arch* may be attempted in certain instances when the hand remains partially symptomatic in spite of the presence of wrist pulses (Fig. 28-20).

Fasciotomy may be indicated in a small number of cases only if the edema of the muscles is severe enough to produce tension in the forearm. In general, the edema of the forearm in patients with restoration of arterial flow subsides within a few days.

Results of arterial embolectomy for upper limb embolism are indicated in Table 28-4, which reviews 322 instances compiled from six reports. Briefly, successful embolectomies were divided into those with return of wrist pulses and complete circulatory restoration (55%) and those with salvage of the limb without return of wrist pulses (23.9%), making a combined limb salvage rate of 78.9%. Gangrene occurred in 9.3% and mortality in 11.8%. In general, mortality following embolectomy was primarily related to the grav-

TABLE 28-4. RESULTS OF ARTERIAL EMBOLECTOMY OF THE UPPER EXTREMITY

Author/Year	No. of Cases	Salvage with Pulses	Salvage without Pulses	Gangrene	Operative Mortality
Champion & Gill[34]	7	4	3	0	0
Baird & Lajos[33]	17	15	1	1	0
McGowan & Mooneeram[35]	20	10	10	0	0
Darling et al.[21]	52	26	15	4	7
Savelyev et al.[38]	101	28	42	19	12
Sachatello et al.[37]	20	14	3	3	0
Savelyev et al.[38]	105	80	3	3	19
Totals	322	177(55%)	77(23.9%)	30(9.3%)	38(11.8%)
		78.9%			

ity of the cardiopathy and least related to the surgical procedure per se.

SPECIAL PROBLEMS IN ARTERIAL EMBOLISM

Associated Atherosclerosis of the Arterial Tree

Preexisting arteriosclerotic occlusion of the superficial femoral artery is not an unusual finding in patients with arteriosclerotic heart disease. The latter is more prevalent today as a cause of peripheral emboli than in the past, and it is,

therefore, not surprising that these patients may have associated arteriosclerotic lesions of the peripheral arterial tree. Many of these patients may have past histories of intermittent claudication, clearly suggesting the coexistence of this associated occlusive disease. Furthermore, asymptomatic arteriosclerosis due to mild or moderate stenosis is often found in such patients. In these cases, the results of embolectomy can be adversely affected by such lesions, especially in diabetic patients. In a specific example in which an occlusion of the superficial femoral artery is present but not detected preoperatively, an awareness of an embolus to the common femoral bifurcation may result in more dramatic ischemic and neurologic changes than in an uninvolved peripheral arterial tree (Fig. 28-21). Because of the simultaneous embolic blockage of the profunda femoris,

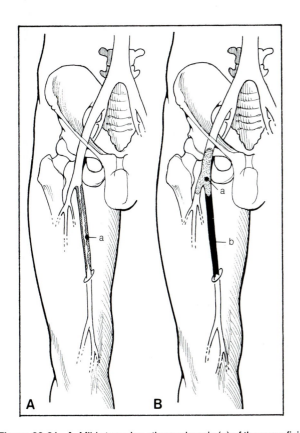

Figure 28-21. A. Mild stenosing atherosclerosis (*a*) of the superficial femoral artery. **B.** Embolic occlusion of the common femoral and its bifurcation (*a*), and thrombotic occlusion of the superficial femoral (*b*).

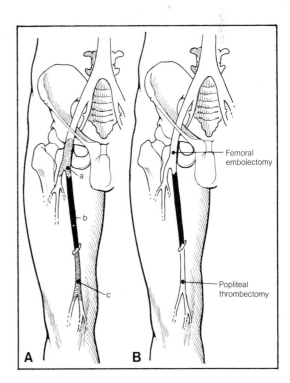

Figure 28-22. A. Secondary thrombosis of the popliteal artery (*c*). **B.** Reestablishment of patency of the common femoral by embolectomy and of the popliteal by thrombectomy.

thrombosis of the popliteal artery may occur distal to the existing arteriosclerotic occlusion of the superficial femoral (Fig. 28-22). In such instances, if the femoral embolectomy is unable to restore the collateral supply to the leg and foot, it is necessary to explore the popliteal artery, either by means of an arteriogram or by direct exploration of the popliteal artery through a medial approach in the lower third of the thigh. Often, a soft thrombus may be found in it, the removal of which may be crucial for a successful outcome of the femoral embolectomy. It should be reemphasized that intraoperative arteriography is essential to properly manage the situation.

Results of Late Arterial Embolectomy

Reported results of late arterial embolectomy, i.e., beyond 10 hours after onset, indicate that even if the operation is performed one or several days beyond the accepted optimal time, complete or adequate restoration of arterial flow to the limb may be achieved, although morbidity and mortality are usually increased. Thus, in my series of 28 cases of embolectomy performed after a delay ranging from 22 hours to 21 days after onset,[30] revascularization was achieved in 18 cases, or 64.3%. Limb salvage reported by others ranged between 55.5 and 77%.[40–42] While early embolectomy remains the best treatment, indications for late arterial embolectomy should be based primarily on the physiologic state of the limb and to a lesser extent on the chronologic factor.

The absolute percentages of limb salvage and mortality reported for late arterial embolectomy series may not be entirely dependable, since patients with such conditions may have survived arterial embolic occlusions that threatened only moderately the viability of their limb. With a less select group, it is possible that limb loss and mortality rates could be much higher than in the isolated published reports, especially if they are not considered in the context of the total group of embolic cases.

COMPLICATIONS

Complications associated with arterial embolectomy may be related to (1) venous thromboembolism, (2) technical pitfalls, and (3) metabolic effects.

Venous Thromboembolism

Venous thrombosis of the extremity involved with arterial embolism is perhaps more frequent than the literature would indicate, this being especially true in cases with late or prolonged occlusions. In an early study,[20] this condition was noted in 7% of our cases. Fogarty et al.[10] reported a 27% incidence of active venous thrombosis in their series. After a successful embolectomy, the limb may not be salvageable if there is an associated massive venous thrombosis. Routine inspection of the adjacent vein for presence of thrombosis is recommended. If such a lesion is suspected, a venotomy should be carried out and the venous tree explored with a venous Fogarty catheter introduced both proximally and distally to ascertain its patency. Venous

aspiration, if required, should be accompanied by heparinization of the limb on the operating table. This maneuver may avert pulmonary embolism.[43,44]

Technical Pitfalls

Clamping

Clamping of an arteriosclerotic and calcific artery may result in damage to the wall, which may necessitate an endarterectomy to prevent local thrombus formation. Before clamping the artery, therefore, it is recommended to avoid areas of mural calcification and to attempt to place the clamps in soft areas or use Vesseloops or nontraumatic clamps with Silastic pads.

Complications Associated with Embolectomy Balloon Catheters

These have been noticed ever since the introduction of balloon catheters in the management of occlusive arterial disease. Though the great advantages of the balloon catheter are well recognized, its use is indeed not always free of some potential hazards.[45–48] Several possible complications associated with its use are (1) perforation of the arterial wall, followed by extravasation of blood in varying degrees, (2) intimal dissection, which may result in ulceration with secondary thrombosis, (3) avulsion of atherosclerotic plaques, (4) breakage of a catheter, with its retention in the arterial lumen, (5) impaction of an embolus or thrombus into the distal arterial tree or shifting of the thrombus from one branch to another, which may lead to severe ischemia, and (6) arteriovenous fistulas. Although some of these complications may not always jeopardize the viability of the limb, their repair in most instances is mandatory as soon as they are recognized.

Prevention

Knowledge of the nature of the vascular pathology, especially the association of thromboembolism with arteriosclerosis, and a clear understanding of the function and limitations of the balloon catheter are essential for avoiding some of the more common hazards.

Gentle manipulation of the catheter is the key to avoiding pitfalls and complications. After the uninflated catheter is introduced as far as is necessary, the balloon is slowly inflated until the feeling of complete occlusion of the lumen is deemed to be sufficient. At that point, withdrawal of the balloon is started (Fig.28-23), and its volume is adjusted in accordance with the diameter of the artery either from the proximal to the distal or from the distal to the proximal area of its introduction. For instance, in passing the catheter into the aortoiliac segment, the balloon is inflated until complete obliteration of the lumen is achieved. Then, as the catheter is being withdrawn toward the femoral artery, the tension in the balloon must be progressively reduced. Conversely, if the catheter is first introduced distally into the tibial vessels, the volume of the balloon has to be gently and cautiously increased as it travels from the ankle toward the popliteal and into the femoral artery. The initial withdrawal of the catheter should be effected with extreme caution and gentleness, with progressive inflation for complete removal of the distal thrombus and embolus. While the

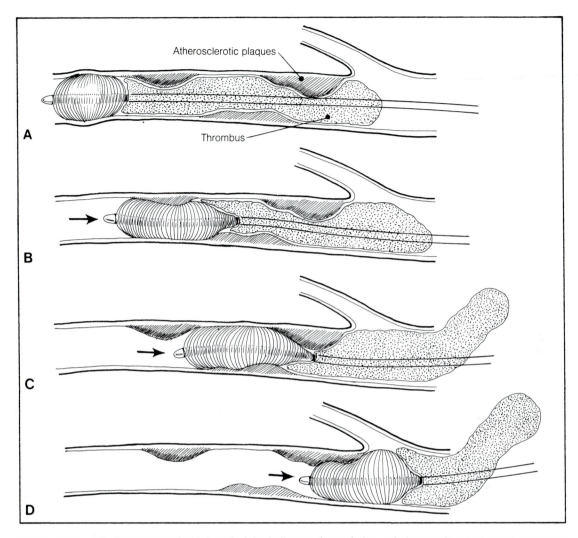

Figure 28-23. A-D. Progression of withdrawal of the balloon catheter during embolectomy in an atherosclerotic artery. Note the changes in the degree of balloon inflation matching the luminal diameters.

passage is usually smooth in the presence of a free and normal distal or proximal arterial tree, associated stenotic arteriosclerotic arterial changes may present serious hazards. Most complications occur in this type of arterial setting. Progression of the withdrawal of the balloon catheter during embolectomy in an atherosclerotic artery should, therefore, proceed with greater caution to adjust periodically the distension of the balloon to the luminal diameters. This can be effected only by manual appraisal of the pressure of the balloon through the ease with which it passes from one area to another in its withdrawal. To achieve this goal, it is essential that the surgeon control the degree of balloon distension and deflation throughout the withdrawal of the catheter.

Metabolic Complications Associated with Severe Embolic Ischemia

While reestablishment of arterial flow to an extremity following an acute embolic occlusion results in morphologic and functional recovery in a large percentage of patients, in a small number of instances (7.5 to 15%), however, even if arterial patency is achieved, a complex myopathic-nephro-pathic-metabolic syndrome may be observed, leading often to loss of limb and life.[11–13,49]

The manifestations of this syndrome are divided into three stages: (1) the ischemic or devascularization phase, (2) the revascularization phase, and (3) the reperfusion of the ischemic muscles. In the first phase, the clinical and metabolic findings are quite characteristic. The clinical imprint of four outstanding findings characterizes the ischemic or devascularization phase: excruciating pain, pronounced ischemia of tissues, rigidity of the limb, and massive edema. Besides the degree of pain, the most striking of these signs is the rigidity (rigor mortis) of the extremity. This sign, which I consider the most important alarm signal, is always present many hours before other clinical and laboratory findings, and is highly suggestive of the nature of the underlying pathologic condition. Within 10 to 12 hours after the onset of the acute arterial occlusion, the patient displays oliguria, azotemia, and myoglobinuria together with variable degrees of metabolic acidosis.

During the revascularization phase, the clinical picture

and the metabolic changes, even if unnoticed during the acute phase, appear extremely severe. Shortly after blood flow reestablishment, massive edema and huge blisters of the limb occur, together with rewarming of the skin, although distal gangrene and necrosis of the calf appear. Often, even after a successful embolectomy, the muscles remain edematous. Because of the unyielding fascial compression around the calf muscles, the latter many turn into frank gangrene in such cases. It is then imperative to perform one or several fasciotomies in order to relieve the tension and release the edema from the muscles. This may be a limb-saving procedure.

During the reperfusion of the ischemic muscles, metabolic studies indicate a decreased blood pH, an effluent low venous oxygen tension (Po_2), an effluent high venous carbon dioxide tension (Pco_2), elevation of serum potassium and creatine phosphokinase (CPK) concentrations, and alterations of other enzymes related to the striated muscle, such as lactic dehydrogenase (LDH) and serum glutamic oxaloacetic transaminase (SGOT).

Because of the sequence of the clinicopathologic events, I have proposed the term myonephropathic-metabolic syndrome for this condition.[11–13,49] (See Chapter 32.)

Management of these metabolic complications depends essentially on their immediate recognition. It is imperative to reestablish the electrolyte balance, especially to reduce serum potassium to normal levels by oral or rectal administration of exchange resins and, if necessary, by hemodialysis. Alkalinization of the patient to combat acidosis should be carried out without delay. This treatment is all the more mandatory if myoglobinuria is present or suspected, since myoglobin precipitates readily in the renal tubules in an acid milieu. Use of bicarbonates is essential in the prevention of the renal complication. In the presence of renal failure, hemodialysis should be used until kidney function is restored. Fasciotomies should be carried out in the presence of muscle edema as mentioned above. The CPK serum level is usually high. Its degree is an index of the extent of muscle necrosis. Mannitol and tromethamine (THAM) are to be used without delay, to avoid further metabolite release. Amputation, so often necessary because of massive gangrene, may be indicated even in the presence of ischemic lesions without frank gangrene as a prophylactic measure to remove the source of the metabolites from the necrosed skeletal muscles.

REFERENCES

1. Mosny E, Dumont J: Embolie femorale au cours d'un restrecissement mitral pur. Arteriotomie. Guerison. Bull Acad Med (Paris) 66:358, 1911.
2. Key E: Embolectomy in the treatment of circulatory disturbances in the extremities. Surg Gynecol Obstet 36:309, 1923.
3. Key E: Embolectomy of the vessels of the extremities. Br J Surg 24:350, 1936.
4. Haimovici H: Les Embolies Arterielles des Membres. Paris, Masson et Cie, 1937, 337 pp.
5. Lerman J, Miller FR, Lund CC: Arterial embolism and embolectomy, JAMA 94:1128, 1930.
6. Crawford ES, DeBakey ME: The retrograde flush procedure in embolectomy and thrombectomy. Surgery 40:737, 1956.
7. Kartchner MM: Retrograde arterial embolectomy for limb salvage. Arch Surg 104:532, 1972.
8. Murray DWG, Best CH: The use of heparin in thrombosis. Ann Surg 108:163, 1938.
9. Murray DWG: Heparin in thrombosis and embolism. Br J Surg 27:567, 1940.
10. Fogarty TJ, Cranley JJ, et al.: A method for extraction of arterial emboli and thrombi. Surg Gynecol Obstet 116:241, 1963.
11. Haimovici H: Arterial embolism with acute massive ischemic myopathy and myoglobinuria: Evaluation of a hitherto unreported syndrome with report of two cases. Surgery 47:739, 1960.
12. Haimovici H: Arterial embolism, myoglobinuria and renal tubular necrosis, Arch Surg 100:639, 1970.
13. Haimovici H: Muscular, renal and metabolic complications of acute arterial occlusions: Myonephropathic-metabolic syndrome. Surgery 85:461, 1979.
14. Freund U, Romanoff H, Floman Y: Mortality rate following lower limb arterial embolectomy: Causative factors. Surgery 77:201, 1975.
15. Green RM, DeWeese JA, Rob CG: Arterial embolectomy before and after the Fogarty catheter. Surgery 77:24, 1975.
16. Haimovici H, Moss CM, Veith FJ: Arterial embolectomy revisited (editorial). Surgery 78:209, 1975.
17. Haimovici H: Unpublished data.
18. Blaisdell FW, Steele M, Allen RE: Management of acute lower extremity arterial ischemia due to embolism and thrombosis. Surgery 84:822, 1978.
19. Warren R, Linton RR: The treatment of arterial embolism. N Engl J Med 238:421, 1948.
20. Haimovici H: Peripheral arterial embolism. A study of 330 unselected cases of embolism of the extremities. Angiology 1:20, 1950.
21. Darling RC, Austen WG, Linton RR: Arterial embolism. Surg Gynecol Obstet 124:106, 1967.
22. Haimovici H: Arterial embolism: Peripheral and visceral, in Haimovici H (ed): The Surgical Management of Vascular Diseases. Philadelphia, Lippincott, 1970, p 71.
23. Daley R, Mattingly TW, et al.: Systemic arterial embolism in rheumatic heart disease. Am Heart J 42:566, 1951.
24. Hara M, Williams GO: Multiple arterial emboli. Surgery 60:804, 1966.
25. Gore I, Collins DP: Spontaneous atheromatous embolization: Review of the literature and a report of 16 additional cases. Am J Clin Pathol 33:415, 1960.
26. Wagner RB, Martin AS: Peripheral atheroembolism: Confirmation of a clinical concept, with a case report and review of the literature. Surgery 73:353, 1973.
27. Kwaan JHM, Connolly JE: Peripheral atheroembolism. Arch Surg 112:987, 1977.
28. Kempczinski RF: Lower extremity arterial emboli from ulcerating atherosclerotic plaques. JAMA 241:807, 1979.
29. Haimovici H: Atheroembolism, in Haimovici H (ed): Vascular Emergencies. New York, Appleton-Century-Crofts, 1982, Chap 12, p 205.
30. Haimovici H: Late arterial embolectomy. Surgery 46:775, 1959.
31. Amer NC, Schaefer HC, et al.: Aortic dissection presenting as iliac arterial occlusion: Aid to early diagnosis. N Engl J Med 266:1040, 1962.
32. Eriksson I, Holmberg JT: Analysis of factors affecting limb salvage and mortality after embolectomy. Acta Chir Scand 143:237, 1977.
33. Baird RJ, Lajos TZ: Emboli to the arm. Ann Surg 160:905, 1964.
34. Champion HR, Gill W: Arterial embolus to the upper limb. Br J Surg 60:505, 1973.
35. MacGowan WAL, Mooneeram R: A review of 174 patients with arterial embolism. Br J Surg 60:11, 1973.

36. Raithel D: Surgical treatment of acute embolization and acute arterial thrombosis: A review of 342 cases. J Cardiovasc Surg 61, 1973.
37. Sachatello CR, Ernst CB, Griffen WO: The acutely ischemic upper extremity: Selective management. Surgery 76:1002, 1974.
38. Savelyev VS, Zatevakhin II, Stepanov NV: Artery embolism of the upper limbs. Surgery 81:367, 1977.
39. Haimovici H: Cardiogenic embolism of the upper extremity. J Cardiovasc Surg 23:3, 1982.
40. Ammann J, Seiler H, Vogt B: Delayed arterial embolectomy: A plea for a more active surgical approach. Br J Surg 63:73, 1976.
41. Robbs JV, Baker LW: Late revascularization of the lower limb following acute arterial occlusion. Br J Surg 66:129, 1979.
42. Jarrett F, Dacumos GC, et al.: Late appearance of arterial emboli: Diagnosis and management. Surgery 86:898, 1979.
43. Jackson BB: Venous aspiration as an adjunct in the management of late arterial embolectomy. Surgery 57:358, 1965.
44. Blaisdell FW, Lim RC Jr, et al.: Pulmonary microembolism: A cause of morbidity and death after major vascular surgery. Arch Surg 93:776, 1966.
45. Foster JH, Carter JW, et al.: Arterial injuries secondary to the use of the Fogarty catheter. Ann Surg 171:971, 1970.
46. Rob C, Battle S: Arteriovenous fistula after Fogarty catheter thrombectomy. Arch Surg 105:90, 1972.
47. Dainko EA: Complications of the use of the Fogarty balloon catheter. Arch Surg 105:79, 1972.
48. Byrnes G, MacGowan WAL: The injury potential of Fogarty balloon catheters. J Cardiovasc Surg (Torino) 16:590, 1975.
49. Haimovici H: Metabolic syndrome secondary to acute arterial occlusions, in Haimovici H (ed): Vascular Emergencies. New York, Appleton-Century-Crofts, 1982, Chap 18, p 267.

CHAPTER 29
Acute Arterial Thrombosis

Henry Haimovici

Recognition of acute arterial thrombosis of the extremities, as distinct from arterial embolism, is often difficult, if not impossible. It is then not surprising that it is frequently misdiagnosed, yet its clinical-pathologic background, natural history, and surgical management are essentially different from those of arterial embolism. It is, therefore, important that these lesions be dealt with separately from embolism.

Acute arterial thrombosis may occur as a result of a great number of local arterial factors or as a consequence of systemic diseases.

The major categories of acute arterial thrombosis are:

1. Acute atherosclerotic thrombosis
2. Acute iatrogenic thrombosis
3. Acute thrombosis of small arteries

ACUTE ATHEROSCLEROTIC THROMBOSIS

Atherosclerosis is the most common predisposing cause of acute thrombosis. It may occur either as a *primary* thrombosis in an asymptomatic ulcerated atherosclerotic plaque or as a *secondary* thrombosis superimposed on a known preexisting arteriosclerotic stenotic or occlusive process with a long-standing history of arterial insufficiency.

Incidence

The relative incidence of acute thrombosis vs. arterial embolism is not always easy to establish, especially in elderly patients with combined cardiopathy and peripheral arteriosclerosis.[1] As a result, all episodes of acute arterial obstruction, regardless of origin and etiology, are often classified as "acute arterial occlusions."[2,3] One of the reasons for the lack of clarity in this classification is the fact that the diagnosis of the nature of an acute arterial occlusion is often based more on a clinical suspicion than on a documentation by means of arteriography, operative findings, and pathologic data.[1,3] However, the distinction between the two entities is not merely a problem of semantics or nomenclature. Most often, is has therapeutic and prognostic significance. In a compilation of seven statistical studies recently published, of a total 1576 cases, there were 892 embolic and 684 thrombotic arterial occlusions.[4] The incidence of arterial embolism ranged from 37 to 70%, with an average of 56.6%. Similarly, the incidence of acute throm-

TABLE 29-1. RELATIVE INCIDENCE OF ARTERIAL EMBOLISM AND ACUTE THROMBOSIS

Authors	Total Number of Arterial Occlusions	Embolism		Thrombosis	
		No.	%	No.	%
Horton et al.[5]	216	89	40	127	60
Pietri et al.[6]	127	79	82	48	38
Dale[7]	79	42	53	37	47
Planell[8]	400	220	55	180	45
Enjalbert et al.[9]	204	76	37	128	63
Koch and Kraft-Kinz[10]	208	146	70	62	30
Raithel[11]	342	240	70	102	30
Totals	1,576	892	56.6	684	43.4

bosis ranged from 50 to 63%, with an average of 43.4%. While the ratios of embolism to thrombosis vary widely in these seven reports, statistically the overall ratio indicates that embolic occlusions are more prevalent than are those of acute thrombosis (Table 29-1).

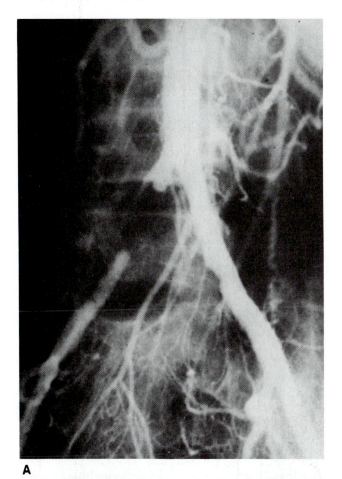

A

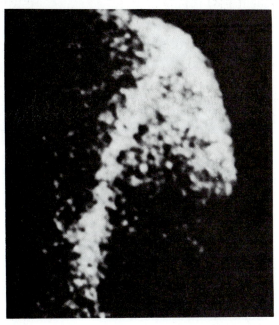

B

The incidence of the various levels of arterial occlusion is also somewhat different in the two conditions. In embolism, the level of occlusion depends essentially on the size of the embolus and the local arterial response to its sudden impact. In acute thrombosis, the level of occlusion depends on pre-existing arterial lesions and their preponderance in certain areas of greater susceptibility to atherosclerosis.

The relative incidence of acute thrombosis in patients with known arteriosclerosis has been variably estimated. The occurrence of this complication varies with the location in the arterial tree and with the type of primary or secondary acute occlusion. The primary occlusions are those occurring on the basis of an ulcerated plaque, while secondary acute thrombosis is the type that occurs as a superimposed thrombosis in an already stenotic lesion of the artery. The greatest incidence of both primary and secondary acute thrombosis occurs in the femoral-popliteal segment and to a lesser degree in the aortoiliac location. Finally, the incidence of acute thrombosis in the popliteal-tibial vessels of diabetics is somewhat greater than in nondiabetic patients.

Clinical Manifestations

The majority of cases of acute arterial thrombosis occur in the lower extremity, and only a small percentage occur in the upper limb. This is somewhat different from arterial embolism, in which a larger percentage of arterial emboli occur in the upper extremity. The type of clinical manifestations and their degree of ischemia are determined by two major factors: (1) the location and extent of the thrombosis and (2) whether the thrombosis is in a nonocclusive atherosclerotic artery (primary) or in a previously chronically occluded arterial tree (secondary).

Primary acute occlusions are not unlike those occurring in an arterial embolism (Fig. 29-1). The onset is sudden and characterized by severe pain, paresthesias, and numbness in the toes and foot.

Secondary acute arterial thrombosis, which is slightly more frequent (68 vs. 42%) is characterized by a less sudden or dramatic onset than in those with primary acute occlusions.[12]

Figure 29-1. A. Transfemoral aortogram showing a segmental occlusion of the right common iliac artery in a 52-year-old woman with a history of sudden pain in the right lower extremity. The patient had had an aortic valve replacement 5 years prior to this arterial episode and was taking warfarin (Coumadin) up to 5 weeks before. Shortly after stopping the anticoagulant because of gum bleeding, she developed sudden pain in the right leg. A right transfemoral balloon catheter failed to retrieve the embolus originally diagnosed. It was felt that the occlusion was due to thrombosis. A transluminal dilatation with the balloon catheter succeeded in restoring the iliac patency. **B.** This radioisotope angiogram performed 3 months postoperatively by Dr. A Rudavsky shows complete patency of the iliac artery. One year after this angiogram, all pulses were easily palpable. (*From Haimovici H: Vascular Emergencies. New York, Appleton-Century-Crofts, 1982, p 219.*)

TABLE 29-2. RELATIVE INCIDENCE OF ARTERIAL OCCLUSION BY LOCATION IN EMBOLISM AND ACUTE THROMBOSIS

	Aorta (%)	Iliac (%)	Femoral (%)	Popliteal (%)	Tibials (%)
Embolism					
Horton et al.[5]	17	21	46	10	4
Dale[7]	7.1	7.1	50	28.6	7.2
Raithel[11]	16	17.7	52	14.3	—
Enjalbert et al.[9]	19.6	29.6	50.8	—	—
Average Incidence	14.9	18.8	51.9	17.6	5.6
Acute Thrombosis					
Horton et al.	10	14	55	18	1
Dale[7]	—	25	32.1	28.6	14.3
Raithel[11]	10	35.9	42.9	11.2	—
Enjalbert et al.[9]	2.5	33.6	60.6	3.3	—
Average Incidence	7.5	27.1	47.7	15.3	7.6

Clinicopathologic Forms According to the Location of Arterial Occlusion (Table 29-2)

Acute Aortic Thrombosis

Acute infrarenal aortic thrombosis is infrequent in contrast to the common entity of chronic aortoiliac occlusive disease (Leriche syndrome). Its sudden occurrence has the earmarks of a catastrophic event, not unlike a massive saddle embolism, which it mimics in all its clinical aspects. The pathophysiology and hemodynamics are quite different in chronic from those in acute thrombotic occlusions. In the former, the increments of the atherosclerotic lesions of the aortic wall proceed slowly over many years until the reduction of the lumen reaches a critical stenosis (80% of the cross-sectional area).[13] If acute thrombosis occurs at this stage, it may be well tolerated. However, when the terminal aortic thrombosis occurs in a lumen still below the critical stenosis or in a nearly normal lumen, the ischemic effects are sudden and severe, with pain in both legs followed by paresis or paraplegia (primary thrombosis).

The physical findings are similar to those in an aortic bifurcation embolism: absent pulses below the umbilicus, coldness, mottled cyanosis of the skin distal to the midabdomen and buttocks, and numbness and loss of motion in both lower extremities.

The medical background of this group of patients shows frequently associated disease due to generalized arteriosclerosis, involving the legs, the kidneys, the cerebral circulation, and the heart. Although these patients may display cardiac decompensation, they usually do not have an emboligenic cardiopathy.

Differential Diagnosis. The differential diagnosis is obviously focused first on the presence or absence of an emboligenic cardiopathy (atrial fibrillation) without a prior history of intermittent claudication. The differentiation is not always easy. A dissecting aneurysm may mimic an acute occlusion, especially if it involves the abdominal aorta and iliac arteries. Chest and abdominal pain, together with an enlarged mediastinum and double lumen on the aortogram, will help establish the correct diagnosis.

Aortography, if used cautiously and if not contraindicated by the general condition of the patient, may be useful not only for possible differentiation from a saddle embolus but also for determining the quality of the runoff and the collaterals.

Prognosis. The prognosis for an acute aortic thrombosis usually carries extremely serious risks, not only for the lower extremities but also for survival of the patient. This is in contrast to the prognosis of this entity below the inguinal ligament.[14]

Management. If in doubt of the thrombotic nature of the aortic occlusion, one may attempt a thromboembolectomy through the transfemoral approach. With few exceptions, however, this will fail to achieve a forceful and sustained arterial flow, which should indicate the nonembolic nature of the occlusion. Nonoperative treatment leads to a fatal outcome, although heparin should be used as a first step in all instances. Thromboendartectomy is not recommended as a safe procedure, since rethrombosis occurs often. Aortofemoral bypass and axillary-bifemoral bypass (preferably the latter) are the best available means of correcting this condition. Mortality rates of surgery range from 25 to 33%. Since the natural course of these cases is ominous, aggressive efforts may be rewarded by salvage of some of these gravely at-risk patients.

Acute Thrombosis of Aortic and Iliac Aneurysms

While rupture is more common in aneurysms of the abdominal aorta, sudden complete thrombosis of the aneurysmal sac is rarely reported. A few recent publications have disclosed that such a complication is associated with severe clinical manifestations and high mortality rates. The clinical picture is that of an acute Leriche syndrome. Most of the aneurysms appear to be rather small (around 4 to 5 cm), but they are associated with severe arteriosclerotic disease distal to the aneurysm. One of the clinical manifestations is the mottling noted to the level of the iliac crest or even to the umbilicus. The symptoms and findings are those of sudden ischemia, including severe pain, paresthesias, absence of pulses, and paraplegia.[15–18]

Management of this catastrophic event presents a major surgical emergency. The operative procedure may consist of aneurysmectomy with graft replacement or, if that is contraindicated because of the general condition, an axillobifemoral graft. The metabolic complications should be anticipated, and the patient should be managed with hydration and intravenous bicarbonate to combat prophylactically the metabolic acidosis and prevent possible precipitation of myoglobin in the renal tubules.

Acute Graft Thrombosis

Acute thrombosis complicating previously implanted arterial grafts for aneurysmal or occlusive disease is not an uncommon event. Both after the graft occlusion and following a restoration of the circulation, one may occasionally observe massive muscle ischemia, with metabolic and renal repercussions. Recently, in a personal report on a group of over 200 cases of acute arterial occlusions, the author noted this syndrome in 10 patients with embolism and in 5 with acute graft thrombosis. Of the latter, 2 involved bypass grafts of the abdominal aorta, 1 of the common iliac artery, and 2 of the femoropopliteal artery. These five patients had seven involved limbs, and all were severely ischemic. Their clinical and metabolic complications were similar to those described in arterial embolism. However, whereas in arterial embolism management consists essentially of thromboembolectomy, that of a failed graft appears more elaborate and complex. A brief account of one such case may best illustrate its clinical and management aspects.

A 66-year-old man developed a sudden occlusion of his graft 6 years after an aortoiliac Dacron bypass. Operative finding 8 hours after clinical onset revealed thrombosis of the graft and disruption of its aortic anastomosis. Because of technical problems, reimplantation of a new graft was impossible. Instead, an axillofemoral bypass to the right leg, the more severely ischemic limb, helped to restore the circulation. The left limb appeared viable. In spite of adequate alkalinization, fasciotomies of the right calf, hemodialysis, and restoration of acid-base balance, the patient developed a very severe metabolic and renal syndrome, myoglobinuria, progressive azotoemia, massive levels of CPK, and other findings (Table 29-3). The patient died on the fifteenth postoperative day. Acute tubular necrosis and rhabdomyolysis were confirmed histologically.

The course of femoral popliteal graft thrombosis is much more easily controlled than that of aortoiliac graft failures, and most of the metabolic complications are reversible. To my knowledge, the literature on acute graft failures rarely if ever mentions these metabolic repercussions in cases of limb amputations or mortality. It is likely that awareness of such complications may help in detecting them early and in preventing their disastrous consequences.[19]

TABLE 29-3. LABORATORY FINDINGS IN A PATIENT WITH A FAILED GRAFT

	Day 1	Day 9	Day 14
BUN (mg/dl)	20	171	264
Creatinine (mg/dl)	1.3	10.5	17.1
Uric acid (mg/dl)	8.2	19.8	30.6
Calcium (mg/dl)	10.3	6.4	5.3
Phosphate (mg/dl)	1.9	6.9	8.7
LDH (IU/L)	210	2,745	1,485
SGOT (IU/L)	50	1.980	1,593
CPK (IU/L)	210	10,800	17,910

BUN, blood urea nitrogen; LDH, lactic dehydrogenase; SGOT, serum glutamic oxaloacetic transaminase; CPK, creatine phosphokinase.

Acute Femoropopliteal Thrombosis

Incidence. The absolute frequency of isolated acute superficial femoral or popliteal thrombosis is difficult to assess unless supported by correlative anatomic, arteriographic, and pathologic criteria. By contrast, combined femoropopliteal thrombosis is more common than that of the isolated segments. Our studies of the patterns of arteriosclerotic lesions of the lower extremities support this view on the basis of arteriographic visualization of the entire proximal and distal arterial tree associated with the femoropopliteal segment.[8,10,20]

Involvement of the femoropopliteal area consists of lesions initiated on each side of the foramen of the adductor magnus, at the junction between Hunter's canal and the origin of the popliteal. Their combination with either proximal or distal lesions is the most common arterial pattern of the lower extremity.

Primary acute thrombosis may occur in an atherosclerotic femoral or popliteal segment not previously occluded. The atherosclerotic changes are primarily of the intimal type, located essentially in the lower half of the superficial femoral and proximal popliteal arteries. The clinical picture in these instances is not unlike the one seen in arterial embolism of the femoral or popliteal artery. The onset may be sudden, but the symptoms and signs may be less severe. The arteriogram of an acute thrombosis fails to disclose the characteristic radiologic picture of an embolic occlusion, which is that of a sharp, dome-shaped line. Furthermore, in incomplete embolic occlusions, some contrast medium may seep between the embolus and the arterial wall, which does not occur in acute thrombosis.

Secondary acute thrombosis of the femoropopliteal artery occurs as a superimposed lesion of a preexisting stenosis or blockage of the distal portion of Hunter's canal. The symptomatology in this type of acute thrombosis is perhaps less pronounced than in the primary cases. However, there is a distinctive deterioration or worsening of the preexisting intermittent claudication, with sudden ischemic changes of the skin temperature, impairment, or loss of motion and sensation in the distal leg and foot.

Evaluation of the arterial occlusion and its extent should include both the noninvasive modalities, e.g., pulse volume recording (PVR), Doppler, and skin temperature, and arteriography. The latter is essential for delineating the exact location and extent of the lesion.

Prognosis. The prognosis of an acute thrombotic occlusion of the femoral or popliteal artery alone or associated with the tibial-peroneal segments depends on whether a distal runoff is present or whether there is a diffuse blockage of the distal arterial tree. In the former instance, a reconstructive procedure is possible, but in the latter instance, a thrombectomy alone is totally insufficient for salvage of the limb. Local prognosis may be as severe in the femoropopliteal artery and especially in tibial occlusions as in the aortoiliac lesions.

Management. Conservative management is only an adjunct to a surgical procedure in most instances. Intravenous heparin (1,000 to 2,000 units per hour) should be instituted immediately if the diagnosis of acute occlusion is suspected.

A loading dose of 4,000 to 5,000 units may be used in the very severe type of ischemia. Heparinization of the patient should in no way interfere with the arteriogram, since its action can be readily reversed with protamine sulfate should the need arise. After adequate arteriographic evaluation of the arterial tree, a decision can be made as to whether revascularization is feasible. Exploration of the vessels at the level of the occlusion should be facilitated by these findings. As an alternative, intraarterial streptokinase should be considered.

A thrombectomy is rarely, if ever, useful in these acute arterial occlusions. A bypass graft is necessary in the majority of cases, provided a runoff is delineated by an adequate arteriogram. Nevertheless, thrombectomy alone was reported to provide good results in 53% of cases by Planell and 65% of cases by Enjalbert et al.[8,9] On the other hand, thromboendarterectomy in segmental occlusions resulted in arterial patency in 93% of cases, as reported by Koch and Kraft-Kinz.[10] In contrast to the above, Raither found that thrombectomy alone is only a palliative procedure. The Fogarty catheter is not helpful in such cases, as passage through the arteriosclerotic occlusion is often impossible. Raithel, in using a ring-stripper together with a Fogarty catheter, was able to facilitate the pullout of the occluding thrombus with the involved arterial intima.[20] However, in later arterial thrombotic lesions with organized thrombus percutaneous angioplasty may be attempted more successfully with less operative risk. Our personal approach in selected cases favors bypass grafts, which may offer a much better outlook against rethrombosis. The overall results of emergency procedures in these cases of acute arterial thrombosis are less encouraging than are those in embolectomy.

IATROGENIC ACUTE ARTERIAL THROMBOSIS

Acute thrombosis secondary to injuries of peripheral arteries following their catheterization may result in such complications as reported in increasing numbers in recent decades. With the widespread use of these catheterization procedures, thrombotic complications, while infrequent, may pose serious threats to limb or life. These complications occur either after angiography or blood-gas monitoring or catheterization for therapeutic purposes. They may follow retrograde catheterization of the brachial and radial arteries or transcutaneous catheterization of the femoral artery either for angiography or for placement of intraaortic balloon pumping.

Recognition of these potential hazards and complications is essential for adequate and immediate treatment of the thrombotic lesion. Delay in their management may lead to irreversible changes, with either gangrene of digits or of skin, but rarely the loss of an entire extremity.

In the presence of a *brachial postcatheterization* arterial thrombosis, the type of procedure used for repair of these arterial lesions will depend on the type of operative findings.[21,22] In the acute cases, a simple thrombectomy, if performed within 12 to 48 hours, may restore the arterial circulation. Thrombectomy at a later stage may not be as successful as in the earlier phase. Resection and reanastomosis of the involved arterial segment may be necessary either directly or with interposition of a saphenous vein or by the use of a bypass. It is likely that, when performed early, thrombectomy is an appropriate treatment for this iatrogenic complication in normal arterial tissues, although in an atherosclerotic artery, resection and end-to-end anastomosis or interposition of a graft may be necessary.

In the presence of *radial thrombosis* following catherization associated with ischemic manifestations present in the fingers or hand, intravenous low-molecular-weight dextran and heparin associated with possible cervicodorsal sympathetic blocks may be used in the hope of improving palmar circulation. Thrombectomy should obviously be reserved when thrombosis is demonstrated in the presence of critical ischemia.[23]

Following *femoral percutaneous angiography*, the complication in the majority of cases is due to thrombi found at the puncture site. Exploration of the femoral artery under local infiltration anesthesia should be carried out when evidence of occlusion and ischemic manifestations is noted. A Fogarty embolectomy catheter is employed to extract proximally and distally all the propagated thrombi. Full restoration of the arterial circulation can be achieved in almost all cases, especially if the arterial insufficiency is recognized early and the repair is carried out within 24 hours. In patients seen after an interval of several days, either because of an error in diagnosis or because of delayed manifestations of ischemia, salvage may still be possible, particularly in younger individuals. Only minor necrosis of the skin and soft tissue in the toes occasionally occurs, for which conservative management may suffice.[24]

In the presence of acute arterial thrombosis complicating *intraaortic balloon pumping*, surgical correction should be undertaken without delay. Thrombectomy alone may suffice in some instances, but, more often than not, thrombectomy combined with a femoral crossover graft may be indicated, which can be carried out while the patient is on the pump. Crossover grafting is preferable to transfer of the balloon to the opposite side and to ipsilateral replacement. Massive thrombosis of the aorta has rarely been reported, although it is a serious potential complication. Femoral endarterectomy or transluminal angioplasty may be necessary at the time of the insertion of the balloon, as may catheter thrombectomy during an intraaortic balloon pumping. In rare instances, acute gangrene has occurred during the intraaortic balloon pumping, requiring major leg amputation. One of the frequent complications noted during or after the removal of the pump is acute compartment syndrome, requiring not only arterial reconstruction but also adequate and appropriate fasciotomies. While it is unquestionable that intraaortic balloon counterpulsation is an important treatment for acute left ventricular failure, it should be emphasized that it also carries serious morbidity and mortality rates. Awareness of this and improved technique with routine evaluation of the arterial status of the lower extremity preoperatively, intraoperatively, and postoperatively, and the use of heparin as soon as the balloon is inserted may represent significant prophylactic measures.[25,26]

ACUTE THROMBOSIS OF SMALL ARTERIES

Acute thrombosis of small arteries may occur in a wide and varied spectrum of entities. The most common etiologic factors are organic arterial diseases, posttraumatic occupational vasospastic syndromes, frostbite, collagen diseases, and hematologic disorders.[27,28]

Of the organic arterial diseases, the most common are those associated with thromboangiitis obliterans, idiopathic acute thrombosis, and acute ischemia secondary to a low-flow syndrome.[29,30]

Posttraumatic Raynaud's phenomenon may be associated with acute thrombosis of small arteries, primarily of the hand. Workers using vibrating tools, machinists, laborers, and farmers whose hands are subjected to repeated blunt trauma may complain of pain, coldness, and color changes typical of Raynaud's phenomenon. The arterial occlusive process may specifically involve the ulnar artery as a result of occupational use of the hypothenar portion of the hand.

Frostbite, at the acute stage, (Fig 29-2) is the result of vasoconstriction, which, if unrelieved, may lead to severe ischemia as a result of superimposed acute thrombosis of smaller arteries. On the basis of recent experience, rapid thawing is preferable to slow rewarming. Vasodilator procedures and the use of heparin have been advocated by some and have been found to be of no value by others. In the presence of tissue damage and gangrene, amputation should be delayed as long as possible, since the lesions may be superficial. Conservative therapy and local debridgment may result in healing without major loss of tissue.

Of the hematologic conditions, polycythemia vera is known to result in a certain percentage of cases with vascular complications, involving arteries as well as veins. The nature of these complications is generally thrombotic and only occasionally embolic. The latter may occur as a result of arterioarterial embolism. It is important that active treatment of polycythemia be undertaken concurrently with treatment of the vascular lesions. Besides peripheral manifestations, awareness of the multiplicity of visceral involvement should evoke the possibility of these lesions in every patient with polycythemia vera. Once the diagnosis is established, management with appropriate therapy should in most cases give a satisfactory response.[31–34]

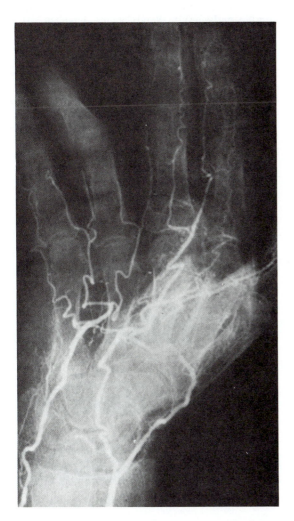

Figure 29-2. Arteriogram of the left hand of a 70-year-old man with an acute syndrome of sudden pain, cyanosis, and coldness of the fourth and fifth fingers. Note the occlusion of the distal half of the digital arterioles in the two fingers, which led eventually to distal gangrene and partial digital amputation. (*From Haimovici H: Vascular Emergencies. New York, Appleton-Century-Crofts, 1982, p 234.*)

REFERENCES

1. Wessler S, Sheps SG, et al: Studies in peripheral arterial occlusive disease, III: Acute arterial occlusion. Circulation 17:512, 1958.
2. Cambria RP, Abbott WM: Acute arterial thrombosis of the lower extremity. Its natural history contrasted with arterial embolism. Arch Surg 119:784, 1984.
3. Blaisdell GS, Steele M, Allen RE: Management of acute lower extremity arterial ischemia due to embolism and thrombosis. Surgery 84:822, 1978.
4. Haimovici H: Acute atherosclerotic thrombosis, in Haimovici H (ed): Vascular Emergencies. New York, Appleton-Century-Crofts, 1982, pp 213–223.
5. Horton VH, Bernatz PE, Fairbairn JF II: Acute arterial occlusion, in Fairbairn, Juergens, Spitell (eds): Peripheral Vascular Disease. Philadelphia, Saunders, 1972.
6. Pietri G, Alagni R, et al: Isquemias agudas de las arterias pifericas. Angiology 29:161, 1975.
7. Dale WA: Differential management of acute ischemia of the lower extremity. J Cardiovasc Surg (Special Issue: 11th World Congress, International Cardiovascular Society, Barcelona, Sept. 1973).
8. Planell ES: Emergency thrombectomy in the treatment of acute arterial thrombosis. J Cardiovasc Surg (Special Issue: 11th World Congress International Cardiovascular Society, Barcelona, Sept. 1973).
9. Enjalbert A, Gedeon A, Puel P, et al: Emergency thrombectomy in acute arterial obliterations: Experience with 204 operated cases. J Cardiovasc Surg (Special Issue: 11th World Congress, International Cardiovascular Society, Barcelona, Sept. 1973).
10. Koch G, Kraft-Kinz J: Treatment of arterial thrombosis and arterial embolism. J Cardiovasc Surg (Special Issue: 11th World Congress, International Cardiovascular Society, Barcelona, Sept. 1973).

11. Raithel D: Surgical treatment of acute embolization and acute arterial thrombosis. J Cardiovasc Surg (Special Issue: 11th World Congress, International Cardiovascular Society, Barcelona, Sept. 1973).

12. Humphries AW, deWolfe VG, et al.: Evaluation of the natural history and the results of treatment in occlusive arteriosclerosis involving the lower extremities, in Wesolowski SA, Dennis C (eds): Fundamentals of Vascular Grafting. New York, McGraw-Hill Book Co., 1963, p 423.

13. Haimovici H, Escher DJW: Aorto-iliac stenosis: Diagnostic significance of vascular hemodynamics. Arch Surg 72:107, 1956.

14. Danto LA, Fry WJ, Kraft RI: Acute aortic thrombosis. Arch Surg 106:66, 1971.

15. Johnson JM, Gaspar MR, et al.: Sudden complete thrombosis of aortic and iliac aneurysms. Arch Surg 108, 1974.

16. Subram AN, Duncan JM: Acute limb ischemia from sudden thrombosis of an abdominal aortic aneurysm: A case report. Tex Heart Inst J 9:1, 1982.

17. Criado FJ: Acute thrombosis of abdominal aortic aneurysm. Tex Heart Inst J 9:367, 1982.

18. Bridges KG, Donnelly JC Jr: Acute occlusion of an abdominal aortic aneurysm complicated by bilateral lower extremity venous thrombosis: A case report. Cardiovasc Dis 8:1, 1981.

19. Haimovici H: Metabolic syndrome secondary to acute arterial occlusions, in Haimovici H (ed): Vascular Emergencies. New York, Appleton-Century-Crofts, 1982, pp 267–289.

20. Raithel E: Ein neuartiger Katheter-Stripper zue Behandlung der akuten Gliemassenischaemie. Chirug 44:434, 1973.

21. Brener BJ, Couch NP: Peripheral arterial complications of left heart catheterization and their management. Am J Surg 125:521, 1973.

22. Nicholas GG, DeMuth WE: Long-term results of brachial thrombectomy following cardiac catheterization. Ann Surg 183:436, 1976.

23. Baker RJ, Chunprapaph B, Nyhus LM: Severe ischemia of the hand following radial artery catheterization. Surgery 80:449, 1976.

24. Yellin AE, Shore EH: Surgical management of arterial occlusion following percutaneous femoral angiography. Surgery 73:772, 1973.

25. Alpert J, Goldenkramz RJ, et al.: Limb ischemia during intra-aortic balloon pumping: Indication for femorofemoral crossover graft? Ann Thorac Cardiovasc Surg 79:729, 1980.

26. Pace PD, Tilney NL, et al.: Peripheral arterial complications of intraaortic balloon counterpulsation. Arch Surg 111:1070, 1976.

27. Baur GM, Porter JM, et al.: Rapid onset of hand ischemia of unknown etiology. Ann Surg 186:184, 1977.

28. McNamara MF, Takkaki HS, et al.: A systematic approach to severe hand ischemia. Surgery 83:1, 1978.

29. McKusick VA, Harris WS, et al.: Buerger's disease: A distinct clinical and pathologic entity. JAMA 181:5, 1962.

30. Veith RJ, Sprayregen S, et al.: Asymmetrical nonocclusive ischemia of the extremity mimicking arterial embolus. J Cardiovasc Surg (Special Issue: 11th World Congress, International Cardiovascular Society, Barcelona, Sept. 1973, p 83.)

31. Hardy JD, Conn JH, Fain WR: Nonatherosclerotic occlusive lesions of small arteries. Surgery 57:1, 1965.

32. Brown GE, Griffin HZ: Peripheral arterial disease in polycythemia vera. Arch Intern Med 46:705, 1930.

33. Barabas AP, Offen DN, Meinhard EA: The arterial complications of polycythemia vera. Br J Surg 60;183, 1973.

34. Haimovici H: Disease of small arteries of the extremities, in Hardy JD (ed): Rhoads Textbook of Surgery: Principles and Practice. Philadelphia, J.B. Lippincott, 1977, p 1827.

CHAPTER 30
Atheroembolism

Richard F. Kempczinski

The term *atheroembolism* is a misnomer to the degree that it suggests that such emboli invariably originate from atherosclerotic lesions. In fact, they have also been seen following traumatic arterial injury,[1,2] thoracic outlet compression,[3] and arterial fibromuscular dysplasia.[4] A more accurate, albeit more cumbersome, designation might be "arterio-arterial" emboli. However, "atheroembolism" has become so entrenched in the medical literature that we will continue to use it despite its recognized limitations.

The concept of atheroembolism originated with Panum's description in 1862 of a fatal coronary artery occlusion due to an atheromatous plaque.[5] However, it was not until 1945 when Flory observed cholesterol containing "thrombi" in the visceral and muscular arterioles of elderly patients with advanced aortic atherosclerosis that the pathophysiology became clear. He correlated the frequency of the cholesterol emboli with the severity of the proximal aortic atherosclerosis and concluded that such lesions were, in fact, emboli of atherosclerotic debris. He tested this hypothesis by scraping some of the atheromatous material from the aorta of his human subjects and injecting it into the ear vein of rabbits. Subsequent postmortem examination identified typical atheroembolic lesions in the pulmonary arteries of his experimental animals.[6]

The first documentation of a lower extremity embolus composed of atherosclerotic plaque was reported by Venet in 1952.[7] Seven years later, cholesterol embolization causing peripheral gangrene, the "blue toe syndrome," was reported.[8] Thurlbeck and Castleman drew attention to the frequency of atheroembolism following aortic surgery,[9] and in 1960, livedo reticularis of the extremities resulting from disseminated atheromatous emboli was described.[10] Thus, the pathophysiology and clinical features of atheroembolism have been well described for more than 25 years.

PATHOPHYSIOLOGY

Atheroemboli can originate from any artery in line with and proximal to the point of impact. As the name implies, atherosclerosis and the changes it produces in the luminal surface of arteries are usually the underlying cause. However, any pathologic process that creates irregularity or ulceration of the arterial intima is potentially capable of giving rise to "atheroemboli."

There are two pathologically distinct types of atheroemboli[11]:

Macroscopic emboli generally originate on ulcerative, irregular aortic plaques or within arterial aneurysms and usually consist of large clumps of white thrombus. They may also contain fragments of the atherosclerotic plaque itself.[12,13] Typically, such emboli lodge at major arterial bifurcations and produce symptoms and signs indistinguishable from emboli of cardiac origin.

Microscopic atheroemboli consist of fibrinoplatelet aggregates or cholesterol crystals. Such emboli are generally much smaller and, therefore, lodge in more peripheral vessels ranging in size from 150 to 1,100 μm in diameter (average, 460 μm).[14] Because such vessels are typically muscular or dermal arterioles, peripheral pulses are generally intact, but the patients complain of the sudden onset of painful cyanosis at the tip of one or more digits, the blue toe syndrome. Rarely, release of atheromatous material from within the plaque may be an isolated event and the proximal arterial lesion may actually undergo "healing." In such cases, the peripheral lesions generally resolve, although the affected digits frequently remain sensitive to cold and the patients may complain of persistent dysesthesias. Often, the true cause of the patient's symptoms goes unrecognized, and their complaints are attributed to "vasospasm or vasculitis."

The lower limbs, which are a major site for impaction of atheroemboli, can accommodate a significant amount of atheromatous material before symptoms are recognized. This is due in part to the capacity for extensive collateral formation in the lower limbs and to the small size of the vessels typically occluded by microscopic atheroemboli. However, in an experimental model, Warren and Lytton confirmed that there was a "critical atheromatous load" for each arterial bed beyond which progressive, ascending thrombosis of major vessels resulted in gangrene or death of the animal or both.[15] This experimental observation helps

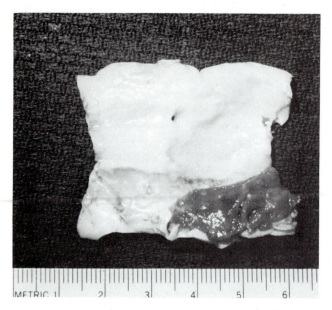

Figure 30-1. Aortic endarterectomy specimen from a patient with a macroscopic embolus to his leg. There is an ulcerative atheroma with a large, loosely adherent, fresh thrombus. (From Kempczinski RF: Lower-extremity arterial emboli from ulcerating atherosclerotic plaques. JAMA 241:807, 1979. Copyright 1979 American Medical Association.)

explain the clinical syndrome of gradually progressive obliteration of the distal arterial bed in the absence of discrete, major embolic events. It appears to result from multiple subclinical emboli that gradually occlude the distal small vessels until the runoff is so compromised that major proximal arterial thrombosis occurs, culminating in severe arterial insufficiency and potential limb loss. It is most commonly seen in the upper extremity as a complication of subclavian arterial aneurysms or thoracic outlet compression[3] and in the lower extremities distal to popliteal aneurysms. It is a particularly frustrating type of arterial occlusion to treat, since the reconstructed arterial segment frequently reoccludes, despite successful removal of the proximal thrombus. Lesions predisposing to this complication must be promptly recognized and corrected prior to arterial thrombosis, since treatment of the established condition is gener-

ally unsatisfactory and usually results in amputation. Although they have not been widely used for the treatment of atheroemboli, intraarterial infusion of thrombolytic drugs[16] may be used to clear the distal runoff bed, and the creation of a small, distal arteriovenous fistula[17] may theoretically provide additional runoff, thus helping to maintain patency of the major proximal arteries and providing an opportunity for recanalization of the distal thrombi.

Although abdominal aortic aneurysms are a well-recognized source of macroscopic peripheral emboli,[18] the incidence of this complication remains controversial. It ranges from 0.6 to 10% of all major arterial emboli, whereas microscopic embolization has been reported in more than 30% of unresected aortic aneurysms when it is searched for carefully.[9,18,19] Peripheral aneurysms can also be the source of distal embolus. In fact, this is one of the more common complications of such lesions. In the upper extremity, atheroemboli have been reported from subclavian or axillary aneurysms as well as from the poststenotic dilation that occurs secondary to thoracic outlet compression.[3] In the lower extremity, femoral and popliteal aneurysms are commonly responsible for this complication.

Mural thrombus forming on ulcerative aortic plaque (Fig. 30-1) is an important, frequently neglected cause of large peripheral emboli that is being reported with increasing frequency.[20,21] Based on the necropsy studies first reported by Flory, the frequency of atheroembolism varies in proportion to the severity of the underlying atherosclerosis.[6] He found cholesterol emboli in the visceral organs in 12 to 16% of patients with severe erosive aortic atherosclerosis. Since muscle samples from their lower extremities were not examined, the incidence of embolization may in fact be much higher. Although the aortic disease was quite diffuse in these patients, it may on occasion be surprisingly localized.

Although no single experience with atheroembolization is sufficiently large to accurately reveal the usual origin of atheroemboli, most reported cases have arisen in the infrarenal aorta or iliac arteries (Table 30-1). However, in at least one large series, 75% of digital microemboli originated in the femoral or popliteal arteries.[22]

Regardless of their source, the local effects of atheroemboli are similar. If large thrombi occlude major arterial bifurcations, patients will typically experience the sudden onset

TABLE 30-1. PROXIMAL SOURCE OF ATHEROEMBOLI

Author	No. of Patients	Aortoiliac	Femoropopliteal
Karmody et al.[22]	31	8	23
Kealy[14]	16	16	0
Kempczinski[23]	21	18	3
Kwann & Connolly[24]	15	15	0
Lee et al.[26]	10	9	1
Mehigan and Stoney[25]	12	5	7
Perdue and Smith[28]	13	11	2
Wingo et al.[27]	52*	24	28
Totals	170	106 (62%)	64 (38%)

* Some of their 40 patients had lesions in both locations and were double counted.

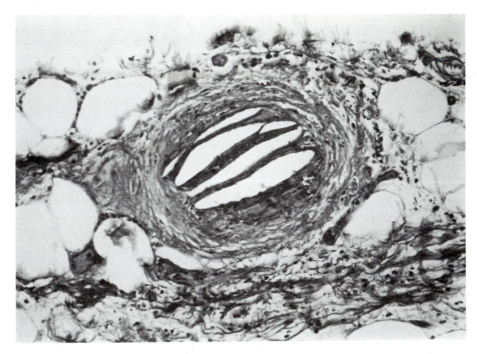

Figure 30-2. Small, subdermal artery occluded by recent thrombus containing cholesterol crystals. Such lesions are typically found in areas of cutaneous gangrene or livedo reticularis.

of pain, pallor, paralysis, and parasthesias in the affected extremity with loss of pulses distal to the point of impaction.

Cholesterol emboli, however, evoke some unique reactions in the vessels where they impact.[29,30,31] Initially, the vessel becomes occluded by the atheromatous material and the thrombus it induces (Fig. 30-2). If the wall remains viable, there is partial reabsorption of the thrombus and some of the amorphous, atheromatous debris within 24 to 48 hours, leaving behind the cholesterol crystals, which in turn are engulfed by macrophages and foreign body giant cells. This phase is followed by endothelial cell and fibroblast proliferation with a variable lymphocytic perivascular infiltration. The precise sequence of events following impaction appears to depend on the content and the nature of the cholesterol crystals. Penetration of such crystals through the vessel wall with fibrin deposition has also been occasionally observed. The end stage of this process is an obliterative endarteritis that is impossible to distinguish from chronic atherosclerotic arterial thrombosis.

INCIDENCE

Because the manifestations of atheroembolism are so protean, they are frequently confused with other pathologic conditions and the true incidence of this problem is difficult to determine. However, several authors have emphasized that it is almost certainly more frequent than presently suspected.[13,20,23] In a series of more than 2,000 consecutive necropsies, Kealy found evidence of microscopic atheroembolism in 0.8% of the patients.[14] In a more recent report, Wingo et al. indicated that the "blue toe syndrome" had prompted 1.4% of 3,417 noninvasive, arterial examinations performed in their Vascular Diagnostic Laboratory over a

6-year period.[27] In another postmortem study, multiple random biopsies of the skin and lower extremity musculature were obtained on 100 consecutive adult autopsies. Atheroemboli were identified in 4% of these patients.[32]

The incidence of macroscopic atheroemboli is even more difficult to determine, because they are so often misattributed to a cardiac source. However, during a recent 5-year period, careful radiologic examination of the abdominal aorta demonstrated the presence of large, luminal filling defects in 20 of 39 patients with sudden occlusion of a distal artery.[20] Machleder et al. found 48 cases of nonaneurysmal aortic mural thrombus in 10,671 consecutive autopsies (0.45% incidence). Eight of these patients (17%) had evidence of distal embolization and three (6%) had major thromboembolic occlusions that were considered the proximate cause of death.[21] In most large series of arterial embolization, the proximate source of the embolus is "undetermined" in 6 to 10% of cases.[13,19] It would not be unreasonable to suggest that the majority of these thrombi had originated from an unrecognized proximal aortic source.

CLINICAL FEATURES

Atheroembolism has been rightly called "The Great Masquerader."[33] Depending on the size and distribution of the emboli, atheroembolism can mimic a variety of systemic and extremity clinical syndromes (Table 30-2).

As previously described, macroemboli consist largely of clumps of white thrombus but on occasion may also contain portions of the atheromatous plaque from which they originated. Macroscopic emboli occlude major arterial bifurcations and present with a clinical syndrome indistin-

TABLE 30-2. POSSIBLE CLINICAL MANIFESTATIONS OF ATHEROEMBOLISM

Large, peripheral emboli occluding major arteries
Digital cyanosis and palpable pulses (blue toe syndrome)
Livedo reticularis
Polyarteritis nodosa–like syndrome
Myalgias and muscle tenderness
Progressive obliteration of distal arterial runoff

guishable from that of arterial emboli of cardiac origin. Only the absence of a legitimate cardiac source, a high index of suspicion, and aggressive biplanar angiography will uncover the true responsible lesion in such patients.[20]

Microscopic cholesterol emboli present an even more challenging problem. Although we will not discuss atheroembolism to visceral arteries in detail, they are quite common, especially to the renal and pancreatic vessels.[34,35] Patients with diffuse microembolization may present with low-grade fever, eosinophilia, and elevated erythrocyte sedimentation rate (ESR). Such patients are frequently misdiagnosed as collagen vascular disease, polyarteritis nodosa, systemic bacterial endocarditis, vasculitis, polymyositis, and a variety of gastrointestinal complaints.[34,36]

The spectrum of cutaneous lesions is equally diverse. The characteristic "blue toe" occurs in only a small percentage of patients suffering dermal microemboli. A typical lesion occurs suddenly, is characteristically localized to the tip of the finger or toe, is quite painful, cyanotic, and surrounded by erythema or mottling of the skin (Fig. 30-3). Adjacent digits on the ipsilateral or contralateral extremity may demonstrate evidence of previous embolization or show signs of less complete digital vascular occlusion. Characteristically, peripheral pulses are intact, and if embolization does not recur, such lesions may regress. In addition to these characteristic, well described lesions, similar changes may occur on the skin on the medial aspect of the heel, the prepatellar skin, and the scrotum.[37] Livedo reticularis, which appears as a fixed, reticulated cyanosis, typically involving the skin of the lower extremities (Fig. 30-4) and torso, may also result from disseminated microscopic atheroembolism.[10,38,39] Deschamps et al. described a patient with livedo reticularis and skin nodules resembling polyarteritis nodosa that were shown to be due to emboli of cholesterol crystals.[39] Although the association with cutaneous nodules was most unusual, they felt that livedo reticularis was the most common cutaneous manifestation of atheroembolism.

Perdue and Smith described yet another variant of atheroembolism in patients with peripheral gangrene that was

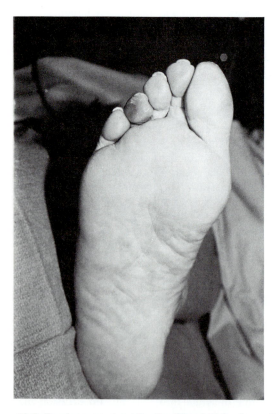

Figure 30-3. Tender cyanosis at the tip of the right fourth toe (the blue toe syndrome) is characteristically seen in patients with microscopic atheroemboli.

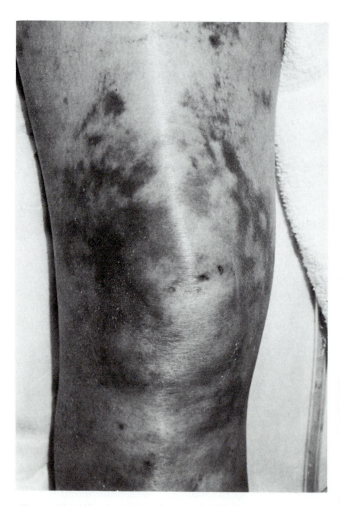

Figure 30-4. Fixed, reticulated cyanosis (livedo reticularis) of the prepatellar skin of the right leg in a patient who sustained intraoperative atheroembolization.

disproportionate to the degree of arterial insufficiency present, did not involve pressure points, and was occasionally accompanied by tender areas of lividity.[28] Peripheral pulses were generally present, and many of the patients complained of myalgia, muscle tenderness, and an unusual distribution of livedo reticularis or gangrene. Arteriography revealed unsuspected aortic aneurysms in four patients, femoral arterial aneurysms in two, and severe, ulcerative aortic atherosclerosis in the remaining seven patients.

Although most cases of atheroembolism appear to occur spontaneously, it may be precipitated by blunt abdominal trauma,[1,2] aortic surgery,[9,40] arteriography,[41] cardiac catheterization,[42] tenesmus,[43] and possibly by the use of anticoagulants.[36,44]

The problem of intraoperative atheromatous embolization is a particularly distressing event because it often involves the extremity in which preexisting arterial occlusive disease was minimal; once it occurs, the development of gangrene ultimately requiring amputation may be inevitable (Fig. 30-5). Several authors have described modifications in their operative technique during aortic reconstruction to minimize this complication.[45,46]

In a recent report, Flinn et al. identified 15 patients in whom vascular graft failure was caused by an atheroembolic event.[47] There was an almost even distribution between immediate postoperative graft failures and delayed occlusions. The authors concluded that distal bypass graft failure in the absence of an identifiable technical problem or significant outflow disease may frequently be due to atheroembolism from a proximal, nonocclusive atheromatous lesion. Although we have described the various visceral and peripheral manifestations of atheroembolism as separate and distinct clinical entities, they often overlap; individuals may exhibit one or more syndromes at the same time.

DIAGNOSIS

A high index of suspicion is essential for the early recognition of atheroemboli. This is especially true of macroembolization in which the signs and symptoms may be indistinguishable from emboli of cardiac origin. The diagnosis should be especially considered in patients in whom no good cardiac source of emboli can be uncovered, in cases in which embolization has recurred despite adequate anticoagulation, and, finally, in patients with multiple distal emboli and severe symptomatic proximal aortic atherosclerosis or aneurysm.

Patients with cutaneous or visceral microembolization present a particularly challenging differential diagnosis. The presence of systemic complaints, such as fever, eosinophilia, and elevated ESR in conjunction with visceral complaints will often suggest some form of collagen vascular disease, such as polyarteritis or vasculitis. It is only when more typical cutaneous lesions appear that the diagnosis may be suspected. The presence of painful, digital cyanosis and palpable proximal pulses is highly suggestive of atheroembolism. However, additional conditions such as vasospasm, thromboangiitis obliterans, and digital artery thrombosis must be considered. In those situations in which the diagnosis appears unclear, additional tests may prove helpful.

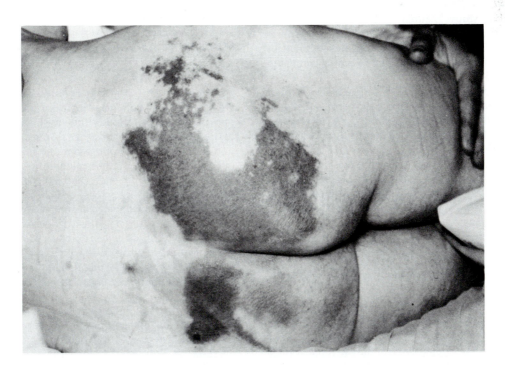

Figure 30-5. Infarction of the skin of both buttocks due to intraoperative atheroembolism. The central area of each lesion became necrotic and required surgical excision. Pathologic examination confirmed cholesterol emboli occluding many of the dermal and subdermal arterioles.

Noninvasive Vascular Testing

Patients with macroemboli occluding the bifurcation of major arteries present with acute extremity ischemia and absent peripheral pulses. Although noninvasive testing may confirm the clinical impression in such situations and may help identify the site of occlusion, it is by no means essential. However, in patients with the blue toe syndrome, it may be useful in identifying clinically occult proximal stenoses and certainly will help in focusing subsequent angiography. In a recent publication the hemodynamic findings in 67 lower extremities of patients with the blue toe syndrome were reported.[77] Segmental limb pressures and arm-ankle pressure indexes were normal in 53% of the limbs examined. However, an abnormal toe-ankle pressure index was present in 43% of these. The noninvasive diagnostic tests were helpful in documenting the relative contribution of proximal arterial obstruction and distal pedal or digital artery occlusions in these patients. When angiography was subsequently performed, there was good correlation with the noninvasive tests, with an overall sensitivity of 84% and a specificity of 100%. However, the negative predictive value of 68% emphasized the importance of proceeding to angiography even in patients with apparently "normal" noninvasive studies.

Histologic Diagnosis

Biopsy of suspicious cutaneous lesions may be helpful in establishing the diagnosis when the clinical presentation is otherwise confusing.[29] Furthermore, muscle biopsies from the lower extremities have also been used to confirm the diagnosis of atheroembolism.[48] Based on the results of their necropsy study, Maurizi et al. concluded that the lower extremities are a major impaction site for distal atheromatous emboli. They also observed that muscle biopsies were positive for emboli in all patients with documented atheromatous emboli to the kidneys.[32]

When macroscopic emboli are recovered, they should be carefully inspected by the operating surgeon, and suspicious areas should be separately submitted for microscopic examination. In those cases in which there is a strong clinical suspicion of atheroembolism, but no atheroma grossly visible within the embolus, serial sectioning of the specimen is imperative. Although atheromatous fragments are only rarely identified,[12,13] the finding is pathognomonic when present.

Careful pathologic examination of amputated gangrenous digits is rarely diagnostic, since such amputations are usually performed distal to the point at which the emboli impact; the digital arteries are found to contain only propagated thrombus.[22]

Arteriography

High quality, biplanar arteriography of the proximal arterial tree remains the cornerstone of diagnosis for this condition (Fig. 30-6). The extent and precise location of the radiologic examination will be, in part, guided by the location of the

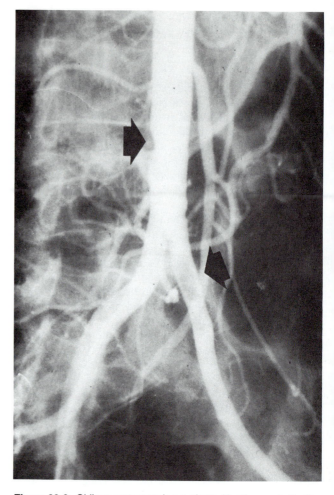

Figure 30-6. Oblique aortogram in a patient with atheroembolization to both lower extremities. Note ulcerative atheroma in the aorta immediately above the bifurcation (*top arrow*) and large intraluminal filling defect in the left common iliac artery (*lower arrow*).

emboli and by the previous noninvasive vascular studies. Occasionally, in patients with diffuse bilateral emboli, it may be necessary to study the entire aorta from the heart to the bifurcation to discover the responsible lesion. In addition to the usual anteroposterior and lateral views, special oblique projections may be required to demonstrate small ulcerative lesions. In such cases, the traditional views of the aorta may be surprisingly normal in appearance.

Patients with extensive ulcerative atherosclerosis of the aorta are at increased risk of iatrogenic emboli during arteriography unless great care is exercised and excessive manipulation with rigid catheters is avoided.[41] In such cases, translumbar aortography, despite its limited versatility, may be safer than the more common transfemoral Seldinger technique.

In general, to implicate a proximal lesion as the source of distal emboli, an open main channel must be demonstrable from the lesion to the point of impaction. Although microscopic cholesterol emboli can theoretically traverse the intervening collateral network around an arterial occlusion and impact in the terminal arterial bed, this situation is thought to occur only rarely. Thus, lesions proximal to complete arterial occlusions are rarely the source of distal emboli.

PROGNOSIS

Despite the deceptively benign appearance of an isolated "blue toe" in a patient with palpable peripheral pulses, microscopic atheroembolism is characterized by its tendency to recur with increasing likelihood of tissue loss.[22,23] In the largest series of patients with atheromatous embolism followed for a period long enough to give reliable information on prognosis, only 44% of the affected extremities had a benign course.[27;] 38% showed initial or subsequent tissue loss, and 14% manifested evidence of recurrent atheroembolism. Twenty-two percent of patients ultimately suffered amputation. The cumulative amputation rate was 32% during 7 years of follow-up in these patients. Twenty percent of the patients died, with a cumulative mortality rate of 52%. Although spontaneous healing without recurrence is theoretically possible, this is distinctly uncommon in most reported series.

TREATMENT

Medical Alternatives

When atheromatous macroembolization occurs, systemic anticoagulation should be initiated as soon as the diagnosis is made to prevent extension of the thrombus. The use of anticoagulation during the early stages of microembolization, although logical in similar grounds, is less clearly established. Chronic anticoagulation has been generally unsuccessful in preventing recurrent atheroemboli. In fact, it may actually favor repetitive embolization by preventing the formation of a "protective" thrombus over the eroded ulcerative plaque.[36,44]

Although antiplatelet drugs such as aspirin and dipyridamole have been used successfully to reduce the frequency of transient cerebral ischemic attacks, data regarding their use in lower extremity atheroembolism is insufficient to recommend their use.

Surgical Management

The principles of surgical treatment of atheroembolism include removal of the embolic source and restoration of arterial continuity. The type of operation used to accomplish this purpose will, of course, vary with the underlying disease. If a localized lesion appears to be the embolic source, thromboendarterectomy with or without patch angioplasty may be adequate in preventing recurrent embolization.[11] This form of therapy is best exemplified by endarterectomy of the carotid bifurcation but may be equally suitable for localized aortoiliac or femoropopliteal disease.

When multiple tandem lesions are present on the affected side, precise localization may be impossible. Under such circumstances, several principles might be useful in determining appropriate therapy:

1. If stenotic lesions are of unequal severity, the most severe lesion should be treated first.
2. If lesions are of equal severity, the more proximal lesion should be treated.
3. If an arterial aneurysm is identified, it should be promptly replaced because of the potential for rupture or thrombosis.

When treating arterial aneurysms or more diffuse atherosclerotic disease that is not amenable to localized throm-

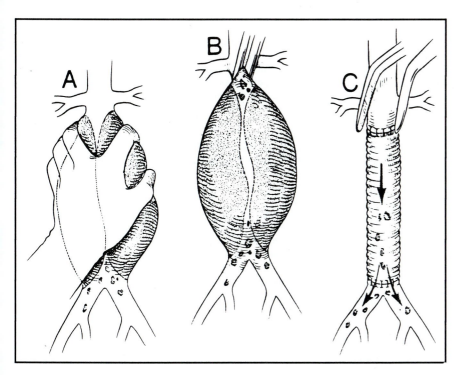

Figure 30-7. Mechanism of distal embolization during resection of abdominal aortic aneurysm. Embolism may occur during manipulation of the aorta before clamping **(A)**, during application of proximal aortic clamp **(B)**, or when the clamps are released following reconstruction **(C)**. (From Starr DS, Lawrie GM, Morris GC Jr: Prevention of distal embolism during arterial reconstruction. Am J Surg 138:764, 1979.)

boendarterectomy, complete arterial replacement with a prosthetic graft is essential. Bypass grafts with end-to-side anastomoses without exclusion of the native vessels will not remove the embolic source and may permit recurrent embolization.[23]

The potential for intraoperative atheroembolism is especially acute in these patients because the arterial segment being replaced is frequently filled with loose, friable material that may be dislodged by the surgeon during dissection of the vessels. Starr et al. have emphasized that this event may occur at several stages during the operation.[46] Care should be taken during the dissection lest manipulation of the vessels liberate debris. In addition, vascular clamps should be applied distally first to prevent showering the circulation with atheroma if the vessel wall is friable. Finally, once the arterial reconstruction is complete but before release of the vascular clamps, the graft should be carefully flushed and aspirated to prevent material proximal to the vascular clamp from being embolized distally (Fig. 30-7). Intraoperative atheromatous embolization during aortic or iliac reconstruction may result not only in distal extremity ischemia, but has also been reported as responsible for spinal cord ischemia[40,49] as well as renal infarction.[9] Once diffuse intraoperative microembolization has occurred, no effective form of medical or surgical therapy presently exists, and amputation may be inevitable. This point reemphasizes the necessity for careful intraoperative technique to prevent embolization.

When embolization has resulted in chronic cutaneous ischemia that will not be improved by proximal macrovascular bypass, adjunctive lumbar sympathectomy has been advocated as a means of increasing skin blood flow and reducing tissue loss.[26]

SUMMARY

Any lesion that results in disruption or ulceration of an artery's luminal surface may become the focus for fibrino-platelet aggregates that could dislodge and embolize to a more distal site. Because atherosclerosis is most frequently responsible for this form of arterioarterial embolization, the term *atheroembolism* is commonly used to describe this syndrome. It is characterized by two distinct forms.

1. Embolization of large aggregates of fibrin or white thrombus that are capable of occluding major arterial bifurcations and that present with a clinical picture indistinguishable from emboli of cardiac origin.
2. Diffuse embolization of small, microscopic aggregates of platelets or cholesterol debris that typically cause distal cutaneous cyanosis or gangrene, often with intact proximal pulses. This so-called blue toe syndrome is the most commonly recognized form of atheromatous embolization.

Regardless of the form atheromatous embolization takes, it is characterized by a tendency to recur with increasing risk of tissue loss and ultimately amputation. The use of chronic, long-term anticoagulation has not successfully prevented recurrence and is generally inadequate for treating this condition. Surgical therapy is based on the principles of removing the embolic source and restoring arterial continuity. With localized lesions, simple thromboendarterectomy and closure may be adequate. For more diffuse forms of disease, graft replacement is essential. The diseased segment must be excluded from the circulation to prevent recurrent embolization. With appropriate therapy, recurrent embolization and tissue loss are uncommon and long-term patency is generally satisfactory.

REFERENCES

1. Roon AJ, Sauvage LR: Blue toe syndrome—A warning sign of unsuspected vascular injury. Surgery 93:722, 1983.
2. Hertzer NR: Peripheral atheromatous embolization following blunt abdominal trauma. Surgery 82:244, 1977.
3. Banis JC Jr., Rich N, Whelan TJ Jr.: Ischemia of the upper extremity due to noncardiac emboli. Am J Surg 134:131, 1977.
4. Mehigan JT, Stoney RJ: Arterial microemboli and fibromuscular dysplasia of the external iliac arteries. Surgery 81:484, 1977.
5. Panum PL: Experimentalle beitrage zur lahre von der embolie. Virchows Arch [A] 25:308, 1862.
6. Flory CM: Arterial occlusions produced by emboli from eroded aortic atheromatous plaques. Am J Pathol 21:549, 1945.
7. Venet L, Friedfeld L: Avulsion and embolization of a calcific arterial plaque: Femoral embolectomy. Surgery 32:119, 1952.
8. Hoye SJ, Teitelbaum S, et al.: Atheromatous embolization: A factor in peripheral gangrene. N Engl J Med 261:128, 1959.
9. Thurlbeck WM, Castleman B: Atheromatous emboli to the kidneys after aortic surgery. N Engl J Med 257:442, 1957.
10. Fisher ER, Hellstrom HR, Myers JD: Disseminated atheromatous emboli. Am J Med 29:176, 1960.
11. Brenowitz JB, Edwards WS: The management of atheromatous emboli to the lower extremities. Surg Gynecol Obstet 143:941, 1976.
12. Edwards EA, Tilney N, Lindquist RR: Causes of peripheral embolism and their significance. JAMA 196:119, 1966.
13. Wagner RB, Martin AS: Peripheral atheroembolism: Confirmation of a clinical concept, with a case report and review of the literature. Surgery 73:353, 1973.
14. Kealy WF: Atheroembolism. J Clin Pathol 31:984, 1978.
15. Warren BA, Lytton DG: The effects and morphology of atheroembolism in limb arteries: An experimental study. Pathology 8:231, 1976.
16. Lawhorne TW Jr., Sanders RA: Ulnar artery aneurysm complicated by distal embolization: Management with regional thrombolysis and resection. J Vasc Surg 3:663, 1986.
17. Ibrahim IM, Sussman B, Dardik I, et al.: Adjunctive arteriovenous fistula with tibial and peroneal reconstruction for limb salvage. Am J Surg 140:246, 1980.
18. Lord JW, Rossi G, Daliana M, et al.: Unsuspected abdominal aortic aneurysms as the cause of peripheral arterial occlusive disease. Ann Surg 177:767, 1973.
19. Heiskell CA, Conn J Jr.: Aortoarterial emboli. Am J Surg 132:4, 1976.
20. Williams GM, Harrington D, et al.: Mural thrombus of the aorta. An important, frequently neglected cause of large peripheral emboli. Ann Surg 194:737, 1981.
21. Machleder HI, Takiff H, et al.: Aortic mural thrombus: An occult source of arterial thromboembolism. J Vasc Surg 4:473, 1986.
22. Karmody AM, Powers SR, et al.: "Blue toe" syndrome. An indication for limb salvage surgery. Arch Surg 111:1263, 1976.
23. Kempczinski RF: Lower-extremity arterial emboli from ulcerating atherosclerotic plaques. JAMA 241:807, 1979.
24. Kwaan JHM, Connolly JE: Peripheral atheroembolism. An enigma. Arch Surg 112:987, 1977.

25. Mehigan JT, Stoney RJ: Lower extremity atheromatous embolization. Am J Surg 132:163, 1976.

26. Lee BY, Brancato RF, et al.: Blue digit syndrome: Urgent indication for digital salvage. Am J Surg 147:418, 1984.

27. Wingo JP, Nix ML, et al.: The blue toe syndrome: Hemodynamics and therapeutic correlates of outcome. J Vasc Surg 3:475, 1986.

28. Perdue GD, Smith RB: Atheromatous microemboli. Ann Surg 169:954, 1969.

29. Snyder HE, Shapiro JL: A correlative study of atheromatous embolism in human beings and experimental animals. Surgery 49:195, 1961.

30. Warren BA, Vales O: Electron microscopy of the sequence of events in the atheroembolic occlusion of cerebral arteries in an animal model. Br J Exp Path 56:205, 1975.

31. Warren BA, Vales O: The ultrastructure of the reaction of arterial walls to cholesterol crystals in atheroembolism. Br J Exp Path 57:67–77, 1976.

32. Maurizi CP, Barker AE, Trueheart RE: Atheromatous emboli. A postmortem study with special reference to the lower extremities. Arch Pathol 86:528, 1968.

33. Darsee JR: Cholesterol embolism: The great masquerader. South Med J 72:174–180, 1979.

34. Retan JW, Miller RE: Microembolic complications of atherosclerosis. Literature review and report of a patient. Arch Intern Med 118:534, 1966.

35. Kassirer JP: Atheroembolic renal disease. N Engl J Med 280:812, 1969.

36. Moldveen-Geronimus M, Merriam JC Jr.: Cholesterol embolization. From pathological curiosity to clinical entity. Circulation 35:946, 1967.

37. Rosansky SJ: Multiple cholesterol emboli syndrome. South Med J 75:677, 1982.

38. Kazmier FJ, Sheps SG, et al.: Livedo reticularis and digital infarcts: A syndrome due to cholesterol emboli arising from atheromatous abdominal aortic aneurysms. Vasc Dis 3:12, 1966.

39. Deschamps P, Leroy D, et al.: Livedo reticularis and nodules due to cholesterol embolism in the lower extremities. Br J Dermatol 97:93, 1977.

40. Perry MO: Spinal cord injury following aortorenal bypass. J Cardiovasc Surg 20:261–264, 1979.

41. Harrington JT, Sommers SC, Kassirer JP: Atheromatous emboli with progressive renal failure. Renal arteriography as the probable inciting factor. Ann Intern Med 68:152, 1968.

42. Judkins MP: Percutaneous transfemoral selective coronary arteriography. Radiol Clin North Am 6:467, 1968.

43. Eliot RS, Kanjuh VI, Edwards JE: Atheromatous embolism. Circulation 30:611, 1964.

44. Roberts B, Rosato FE, Rosato EF: Heparin—a cause of arterial emboli? Surgery 55:803, 1964.

45. Robicsek F: Prevention of cholesterol embolism (trash foot) during aortoiliac reconstruction using a blood filtering device. J Cardiovasc Surg 27:63, 1986.

46. Starr DS, Lawrie GM, Morris GC Jr.: Prevention of distal embolism during arterial reconstruction. Am J Surg 138:764, 1979.

47. Flinn WR, Harris JP, et al.: Atheroembolism as cause of graft failure in femoral distal reconstruction. Surgery 90:698, 1981.

48. Anderson WR, Richards AMacD: Evaluation of lower extremity muscle biopsies in the diagnosis of atheroembolism. Arch Pathol 86:535–541, 1968.

49. Slavin RE, Gonzalex-Vitale JC, Marin OSM: Atheromatous emboli to the lumbosacral spinal cord. Stroke 6:411–416, 1975.

CHAPTER 31
Vascular Trauma

Kenneth L. Mattox

Surgery for vascular trauma differs from other vascular surgery in many important ways. The trauma patient presents with marked physiologic derangements, is frequently hypothermic, hypovolemic, hypoxemic, acidotic, and perhaps even hyperkalemic. The vascular trauma surgeon interfaces with paramedics, emergency room physicians, and trauma nurse coordinators. Because vascular injury frequently occurs outside routine working hours, radiologic evaluation is often unobtainable or incomplete. Available blood must be typed and crossed on an urgent basis, and the patient history is often incomplete or incorrect.

The decision-making process used in the management of peripheral vascular trauma and the techniques of vascular reconstruction for specific peripheral vascular injuries are the subjects of this chapter.

HISTORICAL PERSPECTIVE

Although vascular trauma frequently has been ascribed to the war zone, treatment of such injuries is now quite common in civilian practice.[1,2,3] Although extensive reviews of vascular injuries were undertaken during the first and second World Wars, it was not until the Korean Conflict and Vietnamese War that a deliberate program for vascular reconstructive procedures was initiated.[4-9] Early military reports focused on amputation associated with specific injuries. Current military and civilian reports relate to issues of evaluation, choice of vascular prostheses, methods of exposure, and adjuvant techniques such as autotransfusion. Ninety-five percent of military vascular injuries occur in the extremities; approximately 60 to 65% of civilian vascular injuries are in the extremities.

PREHOSPITAL AND EMERGENCY ROOM ISSUES

The patient with potential vascular injury should always be transported to a designated regional trauma center.[10] If injury occurs in an urban setting and within 30 minutes of a major trauma center, paramedics should transport the patient as quickly as possible without wasting valuable time to insert intravenous lines, summon air ambulance transportation, or apply antishock garments.[11-14] A patient with a systolic blood pressure between 80 and 90 mm Hg is bleeding at a rate of 60 to 200 ml/min. It requires an average of 10 minutes for a paramedic to insert an intravenous line. The average prehospital time (response-scene-transport) is 20 to 30 minutes, and the average volume of fluid infused before the patient reaches the hospital is 700 to 1,000 ml. Therefore, for a transport time of less than 35 minutes, the patient is bleeding faster than fluids can be reinfused.[12] Although the data are sparse, it appears, especially in urban areas, that the time required to reach a hospital by air ambulance exceeds the time required by ground ambulance.[13] A recent prospective, randomized controlled study demonstrated the pneumatic antishock garment to be ineffectual with regard to improved survival or reduction of length of hospital stay when the garment is applied in the prehospital phase to patients with vascular injury who are in shock.[14]

When alerted that a patient with potential vascular injury is arriving, or as soon as a patient with multisystem trauma and the potential for vascular injury arrives, the emergency room physician should immediately summon a vascular trauma surgeon. Decisions for evaluative tests, timing, and type of arteriography and operation should be made by the surgeon who will carry out these procedures rather than the emergency room physician.

SIGNS AND SYMPTOMS OF VASCULAR INJURY

History, physical examination, and suggestive radiologic signs prompt the trauma surgeon to suspect a vascular injury. Indicative clues obtained from the patient's history include the following:

1. Posterior dislocation of the knee
2. Bright red arterial bleeding from a puncture site

3. Prehospital hypotension in conjunction with a trauma score less than 12
4. Extensive blood loss at accident site or in transport
5. Accident involving a head-on collision
6. Marked deformity of the automobile passenger compartment
7. Marked energy transfer (such as a fall from a significant height)

Physical findings suggestive of vascular injury may be divided into general findings, "hard signs," and "soft signs" (Table 31-1).[15,16] Although some truncal vascular injuries and some peripheral vascular injuries may not yield hard or soft signs, one must be able to recognize symptoms that are present.

General signs include hypotension, tachycardia, pale sweaty skin, decreased capillary refill, trauma score of less than 12, hemothorax, tamponade, and distended abdomen with or without positive peritoneal lavage.

There are several hard signs to look for in the patient with possible vascular injury (Table 31-1). Except for vascular injuries in zones one and three of the neck or thoracic outlet, patients with hard signs of vascular injury do not require arteriography and should be taken directly to the operating room for reconstructive procedures.

Several soft signs of arterial injury have been noted (Table 31-1). For patients with only soft signs of arterial injury, arteriography is necessary before the decision to perform surgery can be made. The location and type of arteriography depend on logistics and the availability of interventional radiologic procedures. For most peripheral vascular injuries of the upper and lower extremities, single-shot arteriography performed in the emergency center by the trauma surgeon is extremely useful and cost effective, with essentially no false positive or false negative results.[17–19] Confirmation of suspected blunt injury to the ascending aorta, innominate artery, or descending thoracic aorta is best accomplished in a special radiology suite.[20–23]

Several roentgenologic findings are suggestive of vascular injury in the chest:

1. Widening of the mediastinum, either at the thoracic outlet or aortic isthmus

2. Loss of the aortic knob contour
3. Hematoma in the left apical hemithorax
4. Deviation of the trachea, nasogastric tube, or esophagus to the right
5. Depression of the left mainstem bronchus[24–25]

In the abdomen, roentgenologic findings suggestive of major vascular injury include the following:

1. Widening of the space between the kidneys and ureters
2. Anterior displacement of the intestines
3. Displacement of contrast medium within the bladder

In an extremity, proximity of a missile to a vessel should prompt the physician to perform a confirmatory arteriogram. Arteriograms may reveal complete disruption, thrombosis, intimal defect, traumatic aneurysm, traumatic arteriovenous fistula, or spasm. Because spasm may be the harbinger of an underlying injury, the arteriogram should be repeated or additional consultation should be obtained to rule out an injury.

SPECIAL IMAGING TECHNIQUES

Magnetic resonance imaging and computed tomography scanning have little place in the evaluation of vascular trauma, but digital subtraction angiography, especially digital arterial subtraction angiography, may be helpful.[26–27] Interventional radiologists may be helpful in embolizing material into a bleeding vessel to encourage clotting.[28] This procedure is especially helpful in blunt injury to the pelvis. At other times, special coils and materials may be used to close a small arteriovenous fistula in the neck, lung, or distal vasculature of the upper and lower extremity. Balloon occlusion may control bleeding or an arteriovenous fistula in inaccessible areas.

SPECIAL PHARMACOLOGIC AGENTS

Except for cardiopulmonary bypass, heparin should not be used systemically. However, a small dose (10 to 30 ml) of local heparin solution (100 U/ml) are useful for distal vascular injuries. No more than a total of 5,000 units should be given, because a greater amount of heparinization results in total body heparinization. If heparin is used in the extracorporeal circuit of the autotransfusion device, the excess fluid should be centrifuged off the red cells and the red cells washed with saline solution to prevent total body heparinization. Obtaining intraoperative activated clotting times will determine whether or not excessive heparinization has occurred. This simple technique may prevent a major complication by signifying the need for heparin reversal with protamine.[29]

For small grafts (<8 mm), arterial reconstructive procedures below the popliteal artery, and for venous reconstruction, the postoperative use of aspirin, dipyridamole (Persantine), nonsteroidal antiinflammatory agents, and other such drugs may help to maintain short-term patency. Long-term drug use has not been shown beneficial for maintaining long-term patency. Prostaglandin, prostaglandin inhibitors, tissue plasminogen activators, urokinase, and streptokinase

TABLE 31-1. "HARD" AND "SOFT" SIGNS OF VASCULAR TRAUMA

Hard Signs	Soft Signs
Absent distal pulse	Proximity of injury to artery
Obvious arterial bleeding	History of arterial bleeding at scene of accident
Expanding or pulsatile hematoma	Diminished distal pulse
Bruit or thrill at injury site	Small nonpulsatile hematoma
Nerve deficit distal to injury	Questionable neurologic deficit
Six "Ps" of vascular injury	
Pulselessness	
Pallor	
Pain	
Poikilothermia	
Paresthesia	
Paralysis	

to dissolve thrombi associated with vascular trauma are not widely used.

Venography has been performed infrequently after repair of a venous injury. In a limited number of cases in which venography has been performed, the thrombosis rate may be as high as 70 to 80%.[30,31] In the majority of cases, even those patients with venous thrombosis are asymptomatic. Despite the high thrombosis rate, a venous reconstruction during the acute phase of trauma is important because the acute swelling may discourage venous collateralization. Even vena cava and iliac vein reconstructions have a high thrombosis rate. Venous thrombosis and lower extremity swelling are decreased in vena cava or lower extremity reconstruction when the lower extremity is elevated for several days after surgery. For major iliac and femoral vein reconstructions or ligations, one should consider long-term use of a fitted, graded pressure stocking to minimize long-term edema.

TECHNIQUES OF RECONSTRUCTION

Application of Vascular Clamps

A bloodless "dry" vascular field is achieved by the application of vascular occluding clamps, which are of a special noncrushing design. A clamp of an appropriate size and angle is chosen and applied with only enough pressure to stop bleeding in the operative field. Clamping with too much pressure damages the intima and results in spasm (demonstrated on postoperative arteriogram). Also, the objective is to apply the clamp only once. Multiple applications in the same area or to multiple sites create damage and spasm. The clamp handle is placed so that it does not interfere with vision or technical maneuvering. In some locations, inflated intraluminal occluding Fogarty balloons may

be used instead of vascular clamps to afford the same "dry" operative field. Doubly looped, heavy silk suture may be tightened around a collateral vessel to achieve hemostasis. After reconstruction, this encircling loop is removed to allow flow to return.

Fogarty Thrombectomy and Application of Local Heparin

Surgeons must assume the presence of thrombus distal to the injury, and choose an appropriately sized Fogarty catheter. At times a proximal Fogarty thrombectomy also will be required. The surgeon should visualize good forward pulsatile flow and usually, good distal vessel flow. Following the Fogarty thrombectomy, a small amount of heparinized solution is instilled locally, both proximally and distally. Because locally instilled heparin rapidly becomes incorporated into the systemic circulation and can result in total body heparinization, no more than a total of 5,000 units should be administered during the operative procedure.

Completion arteriography is performed after vascular reconstruction and is accomplished by inserting a small needle proximal to the reconstruction. The area of clamp application, the anastomosis, and the distal circulation are visualized for spasm, narrowing, presence of thrombus, and adequacy of distal circulation.

Suture Material

In general, synthetic monofilament suture material, usually polypropylene, is used. For reconstruction of smaller arteries, from the femoral artery and brachial artery distally, 5–0 or 6–0 monofilament suture is used. For very small vessel reconstruction, an interrupted suture technique may

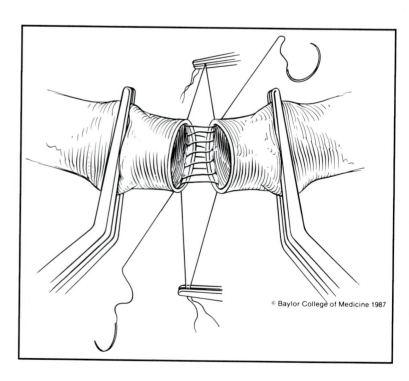

Figure 31-1. Technique of open running anastomosis. Note that stay sutures keep ends oriented, and occluding clamps are placed to avoid tension on the suture line.

© Baylor College of Medicine 1987

be indicated. For reconstruction of the thoracic and abdominal aorta and the vena cava, 3–0 or 4–0 polypropylene is the suture of choice. The suture for the larger vessels is applied in a running manner, usually with an open anastomosis (Fig. 31-1).

Substitute Conduits

To bridge a gap when a vessel has been so traumatized that end-to-end anastomosis without tension cannot be accomplished, a variety of substitute conduits may be utilized. These include transposed autologous artery, transposed autologous vein, homologous artery or vein, expanded polytetrafluoroethylene (PTFE), woven or knitted Dacron, homologous umbilical vein, and commercially available bovine artery. Currently, the most popular substitute conduits are Dacron tube grafts for replacement of the thoracic and abdominal aorta, PTFE for renal artery reconstruction, PTFE or Dacron for arterial reconstruction of vessels greater than 6 to 8 mm in diameter, and autogenous saphenous vein for artery or venous reconstruction of less than 5 mm in diameter. The transposed autologous vein or artery, as well as homologous and xenograft vascular material, are in essence collagen tubes subject to dissolution by collagenase activity of bacteria if the conduit becomes infected. Numerous studies have indicated the superiority of synthetic material (nylon, Dacron, PTFE) if infection occurs around the substitute conduit.[32–42] The primary complications after insertion of a synthetic prosthesis are thrombosis and inability to maintain long-term patency, especially in vessels less than 5 mm in diameter. For the patient with multisystem trauma who is in shock and who requires an expedient vascular reconstruction, substitute conduits of PTFE and Dacron in sizes greater than 6 mm are acceptable and have been used extensively in numerous trauma centers with large volumes of vascular trauma cases.[43–46]

Antibiotics

Antibiotics should be administered at least 48 hours after injury to patients with vascular trauma. Broad-spectrum antibiotics are indicated, especially to cover gram-negative organisms if abdominal penetration has occurred and *Staphylococcus epidermidis* and *S. aureus* are present. In patients with continued fever, leukocytosis, and signs of sepsis, antibiotics should be continued based on cultures taken at the time of surgery, on subsequent culture results taken from the surgical area, or on blood cultures.

Autotransfusion

A variety of autotransfusion devices have been developed for the emergency room, operating room, and intensive care unit. In the emergency room and intensive care unit, the Sorenson Trauma Autotransfuser (Abbott Laboratories, Hospital Products Division, Abbott Park, Ill. 60064) can collect hemothorax or mediastinal blood and reinfuse it directly without processing. Intraoperative blood may be collected, concentrated, washed, and reinfused using a variety of devices, that is, the Baylor Rapid Autotransfuser (BRAT) (Cardiovascular Systems Inc., 2408 Timberloch, Site B-11, The Woodlands, Tex. 77380), Haemonetics Cell Saver (Haemonetics Corporation, 400 Wood Road, Braintree, Mass. 02184), and the Didacto (Electromedics, 7337 Revere Parkway, Englewood, Colorado 80112). If enteric contamination occurs, scavenged blood should not be reinfused unless compatible blood is unavailable.

SURGICAL APPROACH TO SPECIFIC INJURIES

Carotid Artery

Carotid artery injuries account for approximately 5% of vascular injuries. Penetrating trauma is responsible for approximately 80% of these, and blunt injury accounts for the remainder.[47,48] If left untreated, carotid artery injuries result in large traumatic false aneurysms, airway obstruction, and carotid occlusion. Because a large hematoma in the neck is frequently present when the patient arrives, early awake nasotracheal intubation in the emergency center is strongly recommended. When a carotid injury at the base of the neck (zone 1) or higher than the angle of the jaw (zone 3) is suspected, preoperative angiography is required to plan proper operative management.

Carotid injuries at the thoracic outlet (zone 1) are best managed via a median sternotomy and ipsilateral anterior neck incision. Most carotid injuries are exposed via an incision anterior to the sternocleidomastoid muscle. Exposure for injuries at the base of the skull can be enhanced by deliberate dislocation of the temporomandibular joint and movement of the jaw forward.

Revascularization may be achieved via lateral arteriorrhaphy or ligation for injuries of the external carotid artery. A lateral or end-to-end arteriorrhaphy is possible for most common and internal carotid artery lesions. Graft interposition may be used for more extensive injuries of the common or internal carotid arteries. For vessels requiring a graft smaller than 5 mm in diameter, autogenous saphenous vein graft is the conduit of choice. A small amount of locally instilled heparin may be infused into the distal carotid, with care being taken not to inject any air or clot debris. Blunt injuries involving intimal tear and dissection of the internal carotid artery are managed with ligation and division. For penetrating injuries with loss of substance of the internal carotid artery, mobilizing the branches of the external carotid and moving the external carotid artery laterally to serve as the conduit to the more distal internal carotid artery may be safely accomplished (Fig. 31-2). Rarely, balloon occlusion of a very high carotid artery injury may be necessary; this has been accomplished both intraoperatively and in the angiography suite.

The controversial issues focus on the patient with a carotid artery injury and fixed neurologic deficit with no retrograde flow from the open end of the carotid. Ligation is probably preferable in these patients. In all other cases, especially if the surgery occurs within 4 hours of injury, revascularization is strongly recommended.[48] With concomitant tracheal or esophageal lesions, the arterial repair

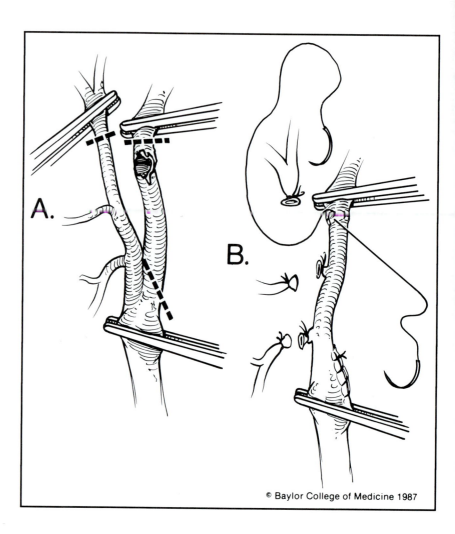

Figure 31-2. Technique of mobilizing noninjured external carotid artery to provide autogenous conduit for injured internal carotid artery.

© Baylor College of Medicine 1987

should be covered with a flap of muscle (i.e., sternocleidomastoid), to protect against repair blowout if infection in the region occurs.

Thoracic Outlet

Thoracic outlet vascular injury accounts for less than 3% of vascular trauma cases.[49] Vessels at risk in the thoracic outlet include the innominate artery, proximal carotid arteries, subclavian arteries, arch of the aorta, innominate vein, superior vena cava, and azygos vein. Blunt injury to the upper sternum may produce injury to the proximal innominate artery. Blunt injury fractures of the clavicle may produce subclavian vascular injury. Most other injuries to the thoracic outlet vessels are secondary to penetrating trauma. On occasion, iatrogenic injuries occur when tracheostomy tubes or percutaneous catheters for intravenous access or long-term medical therapy are inserted. If left untreated, such injuries may result in disabling arteriovenous fistulas, aneurysm, or compression of vital adjacent structures (such as the trachea, brachial plexus, and other extremity venous return). Injuries of the innominate artery and vein and the aortic arch are managed via a median sternotomy, with liberal extension into the proximal neck on the ipsilateral side of the injury.[50]

Because of the rich collateral circulation, injuries of the innominate artery, common carotid arteries, and subclavian arteries can be reconstructed without hypothermia, complex shunts, cardiopulmonary bypass, or heparinization (Fig. 31-3). After sternotomy, the ascending aorta is exposed intrapericardially, and an 8 to 12 mm knitted Dacron graft is affixed using a partially occluding clamp. The distal innominate (or distal common carotid artery) is exposed, taking care to enter the injury hematoma just as the occluding clamps are applied. The previously "flushed" graft is sutured end-to-end into the distal artery, taking care to "flush" and "back flush" any clot or debris before completing the suture line. The injury is then oversewn with a running suture. An injured innominate vein may be ligated with impunity (Fig. 31-4).

The incision for subclavian vascular injury must be individualized. It may be as simple as a single supraclavicular incision. On occasion, injury in this location may be extremely complex and require an en block supraclavicular partial sternotomy with an anterior third interspace extension (book or trap door incision). There is a high association of brachial plexus injury with subclavian vascular injury, and the subclavian artery is, in general, friable.[51] Because of the numerous adjacent structures and difficulty in exposure, graft interposition is preferable to extensive mobilization and end-to-end anastomosis if lateral arteriorrhaphy

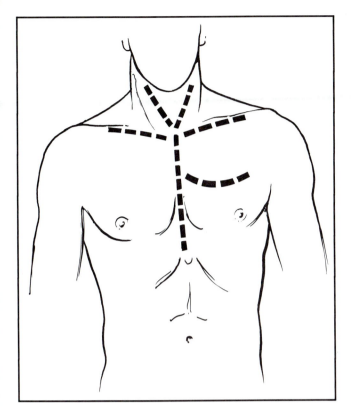

Figure 31-3. Incisions available for thoracic outlet injuries. The "trap door" incision is used only for repair of left subclavian artery injuries.

or venorrhaphy cannot be accomplished. The mortality rate associated with subclavian artery injuries is approximately 6% and is primarily secondary to associated injuries or exsanguinating hemorrhage before arrival at a hospital. Special considerations concerning exposure and proximal and distal control of subclavian vascular injuries are important. For the surgeon who may only occasionally operate on this type of injury, at times a very extensive, seemingly radical incision is the most logical. Extensive intraoperative blood loss and iatrogenic injury may occur if the incision is too small or is made at or distal to the site of the injury. Preoperative arteriogram can be helpful in planning the incision.

Descending Thoracic Aorta

Each year more than 8,000 persons in the United States sustain injury to the descending thoracic aorta as a result of decelerative trauma. Only 15% of these patients arrive at an emergency facility alive.[52] If the injury is untreated, most of these patients will have rupture of the contained hematoma within the first week of injury. Fifty percent of patients with this injury will have no external signs of trauma. The diagnosis is suspected when a history of deceleration injury is related, when external signs of significant thoracic deceleration are present, and when radiologic clues suggestive of mediastinal hematomas are evident and confirmed with arteriography (Table 31-2).[53,54] Computed to-

TABLE 31-2. RADIOLOGIC CLUES SUGGESTIVE OF THORACIC GREAT VESSEL INJURY

On Anteroposterior or Erect Posteroanterior Chest X-Ray
  Widening of mediastinum >8 mm
  Depression of left mainstem bronchus >140 degrees
  Lateral deviation of trachea
  Lateral deviation of nasogastric tube in esophagus
  Left apical hematoma
  Obliteration of aortic knob contour
  Fracture of first or second ribs
  Multiple left rib fractures
  Massive left hemothorax
  Obvious aortic double shadow with or without calcium layering
  Fracture of sternum or scapula
On Lateral Chest X-ray
  Loss of aortopulmonary window
  Anterior displacement of trachea
  Fracture dislocation of thoracic spine
  Fracture of sternum

mography scans and magnetic resonance imaging are misleading and should not replace arteriography as the confirming diagnostic test.[26,27]

After the diagnosis is confirmed, the patient is taken to the operating room where proximal and distal control of the injury is achieved via a left fourth interspace posterolateral incision. Several intraoperative management techniques are available to the surgeon. Although total cardiopulmonary bypass with total body heparinization and use of heparin-bonded shunts were popular during the 1960s and 1970s, recent successes with clamp-repair techniques are extremely gratifying.[22–26,55–60] Approximately 15% of the patients undergoing operation can have primary repair, but the majority will require graft interposition. The mortality rate for those reaching a hospital alive is approximately 15%, and the paraplegia rate is approximately 7%, regardless of the intraoperative management technique. Paraplegia is secondary to multiple factors (Table 31-3). The use of centrifugal pump shunts and sophisticated monitoring of sensory evoked potentials have not decreased the dread complication of paraplegia. The current litigious atmosphere makes it imperative that the patient and family have a clear understanding of the potential for this complication.

TABLE 31-3. FACTORS CONTRIBUTING TO PARAPLEGIA

Paralysis on admission
Pseudocoarctation syndrome
Spinal cord contusion or laceration
Spinal canal compartment syndrome
Perioperative hypotension
Number of intercostals injured or sacrificed
Questionable Factors
? Length of cross-clamp time
? Blood alcohol level
? Thrombus or debris embolization
? Intercostal arteriography
? Pharmacologic spinal circulation alteration

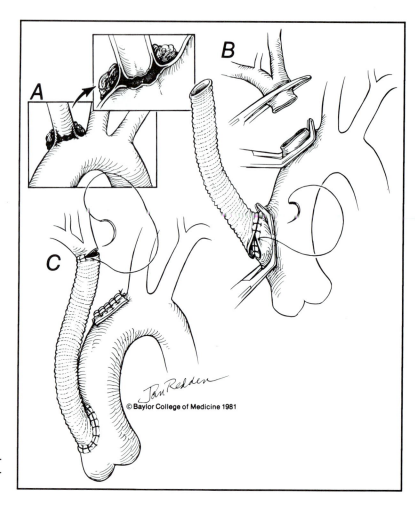

Figure 31-4. Technique of innominate artery revascularization. Knitted Dacron or PTFE grafts are preferred.

Abdominal Vascular Injury

Patients with abdominal vascular injury account for 15 to 30% of all vascular injuries encountered in civilian practice. Except for blunt injuries to the retrohepatic vena cava and venous and arterial bleeding from pelvic fractures, almost all such injuries are secondary to penetrating trauma. Many patients with abdominal injuries arrive in the emergency room hypotensive, hypovolemic, acidotic, and hypothermic and will die from continued exsanguinating hemorrhage if the injury goes untreated. A few untreated patients will develop chronic aneurysm or arteriovenous fistula. All abdominal vascular injuries are approached through a long midline incision. Exposure of the suprarenal abdominal aorta is facilitated by medial rotation of the left upper quadrant abdominal viscera, taking care to stay behind the kidney in this acute injury (Figs. 31-5 and 31-6). This maneuver, the Mattox maneuver, which has been extensively described,[3,60–62] expedites both exposure and technical control of complex injuries of the suprarenal and mesenteric arteries. Infrarenal abdominal aortic injuries and iliac artery injuries are approached through the root of the mesentery, as in an elective approach for an abdominal aortic aneurysm. The vena cava injury is approached via liberal right lateral visceral mobilization, termed a super-Kocher maneuver (Fig. 31-7). The portal vein is exposed in the portal triad,

sometimes with the aid of a Pringle maneuver and at times by deliberate division of the neck of the pancreas (Fig. 31-8).[63] The superior mesenteric artery is approached at the root of the mesentery with the transverse colon retracted superiorly.[64,65] Aortic injuries are most often repaired with lateral aortorrhaphy; however, for the suprarenal position, interposition grafting with Dacron material can be used successfully. For patients with exsanguinating hemorrhage, ligation of iliac artery, iliac vein, and celiac axis has been successfully achieved with revascularization of the lower extremity using secondary femoral-femoral bypass if necessary.[66,67] For the nonexsanguinating hypothermic patient, reconstruction of the iliac artery with end-to-end anastomosis or Dacron or PTFE interposition can be used with success. Vena cavorrhaphy is accomplished by lateral venorrhaphy in most instances, although graft interposition has been successfully used.[62,68–70] At times, enlarging the anterior hole in the cava may be necessary to repair a posterior hole before anterior venorrhaphy. On rare occasion, injury to the suprarenal retrohepatic vena cava may be treated with observation if there is no free bleeding into the peritoneal cavity.[71,72] If free bleeding from the retrohepatic injury is noted, early cannulation from the right heart to the inferior vena cava, developing a bypass shunt, may be lifesaving in some instances.[73] In recent experience, a 30% survival rate has been achieved with this shunt.[74] The occurrence

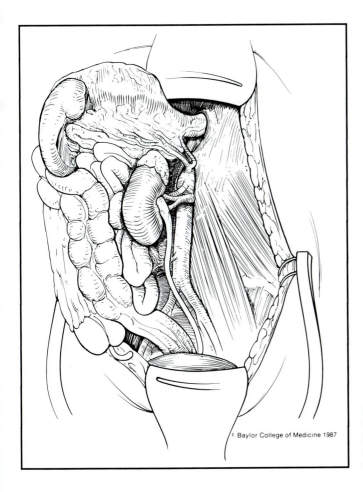

Figure 31-5. Ventral view demonstrating Mattox maneuver, a technique of medial mobilization of left abdominal viscera behind the kidney for exposure of suprarenal aortic injuries. CAUTION: Mobilization anterior to the kidney in acute injury results in marked blood loss and difficulty in gaining control.

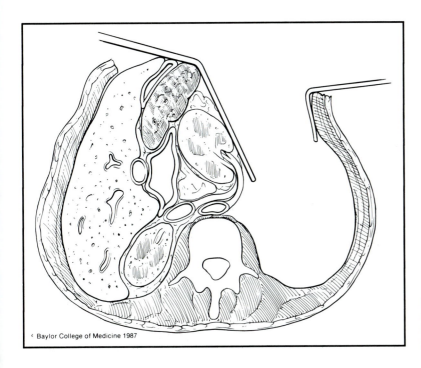

Figure 31-6. Cross-section view of the Mattox maneuver depicted in Figure 31-5. Note the mobilization plane is just anterior to the psoas muscle.

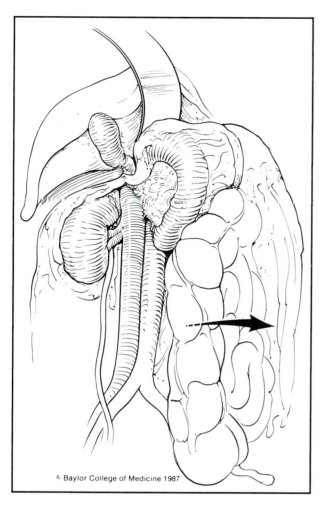

© Baylor College of Medicine 1987

Figure 31-7. Technique of a right-sided visceral mobilization (Super-Kocher maneuver) to expose injuries of the inferior vena cava, as well as the right and left common iliac arteries.

of thrombosis of the vena cava following repair is extremely high. Reconstruction of the superior mesenteric artery is perhaps best achieved with a PTFE or Dacron interposition graft from the aorta or iliac artery to the portion of superior mesenteric artery just distal to the takeoff of the middle colic artery. Renal artery revascularization is recommended if one encounters a blunt or penetrating injury to the renal artery that has been occluded for less than 4 hours. Unfortunately, many renal artery repairs occur late, or concomitant renal hilar injury necessitates a nephrectomy.[75,76]

Mortality from abdominal aortic injury approaches 60 to 80%, whereas the mortality for vena cava injuries is 30 to 50%; the mortality rate for iliac artery injuries may approach 30 to 40%.

Axillary, Brachial, Radial, and Ulnar Arterial Injury

Although fracture of an adjacent bone may cause blunt injury to the brachial artery, most upper extremity vascular injuries are secondary to penetrating trauma. Iatrogenic injury to the brachial artery may occur during diagnostic

and therapeutic procedures. If the injury goes untreated, thrombosis or false aneurysm formation can occur. Upper extremity claudication is not uncommon with thrombosis. For penetrating injuries with hard signs of vascular injury, a liberal incision is made proximal and distal to the site of injury to achieve adequate exposure. In the area of the antecubital fossa, a sigmoid shape incision may prevent scar contracture deformity. Care is taken to identify concomitant venous or nerve injury. This procedure should be carefully documented in the dictated operative record. Lateral arteriorrhaphy can be accomplished in the majority of upper extremity vascular injuries, although in the axillary or brachial artery, use of PTFE or Dacron (5 mm or greater) is possible. For injuries of smaller vessels that cannot be repaired by arteriorrhaphy, an autogenous saphenous vein interposition is preferred. Extraanatomic routing is recommended for infected and potentially infected areas. Upper extremity amputation secondary to vascular injury is rare. Such amputations are usually necessary when the injury is a shotgun blast to the antecubital fossa or to the forearm.

Femoral Vascular Injury

Injury to the common, superficial, and profunda femoral arteries and to the femoral veins accounts for more than 20% of all vascular injuries seen in civilian practice and an even higher percentage of military vascular trauma.[77] Although fracture of the femur may produce superficial femoral artery tears, most injuries to the femoral vessels are caused by penetrating trauma, including penetration from diagnostic and therapeutic catheters.[78,79]

Most femoral vascular wounds can be exposed through an extensive groin incision, although some distal superficial artery injuries may require an incision extended almost to midthigh. Lateral and end-to-end arteriorrhaphy may be accomplished in most cases and may require some mobilization of the superficial femoral artery. One should not hesitate to use patch graft angioplasty of Dacron or PTFE. Interposition grafting using PTFE or Dacron tube grafts greater than 5 mm in diameter has been extremely successful.[3,43-46] Femoral venous injuries should be repaired using appropriately sized Dacron or PTFE graft interpositions. Although the rate of thrombosis in femoral venous injury repair is high, a venous graft interposition that remains patent for several days until the leg edema has resolved may result in a functional extremity. Patients with femoral and iliac venous repairs should have elevation of the lower extremity and be given medications that alter platelet function (such as aspirin or dipyridamole). For patients with a large blast cavity and injury to the femoral vessels, either extraanatomic routing or synthetic prosthetic material and muscle flap coverage has been used successfully. If the substitute conduit cannot be adequately covered with viable tissue and extraanatomic routing is not possible, the use of synthetic conduits is strongly recommended. The conduits should be covered daily with commercial pig skin until enough granulation tissue has formed to allow for swinging of a muscle flap for adequate autogenous coverage.[80] Mortality from femoral vascular injury is rare, and amputations from such injuries currently occur only

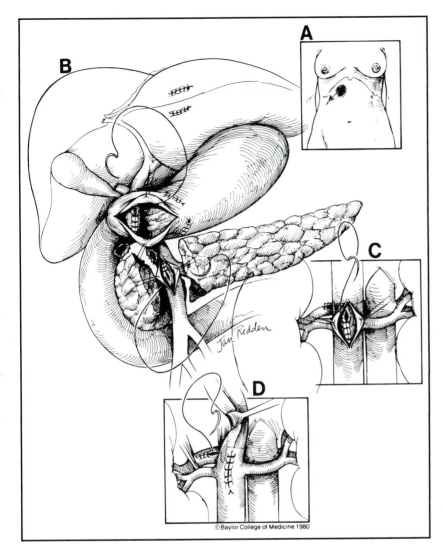

Figure 31-8. Technique of deliberate division of the neck of the pancreas to expose a portal vein injury. Note the complex injury to the vena cava, duodenum, and pancreas is treated with a pyloric exclusion procedure to decrease the potential for postrepair vascular complication.

©Baylor College of Medicine 1980

with extensive combined venous, arterial, and neurologic injury at the groin.

Popliteal and Tibial Vascular Injury

Popliteal and tibial injuries account for less than 10% of all civilian vascular trauma. These injuries may be caused by automobile or motorcycle crush injuries, penetrating trauma, or iatrogenic injury occurring during orthopedic procedures in and about the knee. In addition, popliteal and tibial vascular injuries may be caused by blast or high-velocity missile wounds; this last cause usually occurs in military situations.

With extensive soft tissue injury either from blunt trauma or high-velocity wounds, untreated popliteal vascular injury results in an amputation rate in excess of 50%. For civilian injuries caused by penetrating trauma, the amputation rate is less than 10%.

Preoperative arteriography assists in the decision for medial thigh vs. medial calf incision. If possible, repair of both popliteal vein and artery injuries is currently recom-mended. If a substitute conduit is required for repair of popliteal venous or arterial injury, the contralateral saphenous vein is the conduit of choice. If autogenous saphenous vein is not adequate for use as a conduit, externally supported PTFE or Dacron 5 mm or larger in diameter should be used. Following tibial or popliteal venous repair or ligation, the leg should be elevated and the patient placed on aspirin or dipyridamole. If extensive injury to the popliteal nerve, artery, and vein is present, as well as to the tibia and soft tissue of the knee, primary amputation should be considered and discussed preoperatively with the patient and family.

OTHER CONSIDERATIONS

Vascular reconstruction following trauma was uncommon prior to the Korean Conflict. Until the 1950s, primary arterial or venous ligation was the treatment of choice for vascular wounds. Secondary amputation was described as a measure of outcome for most vascular trauma reports before the Vietnamese War. Today, primary and secondary amputa-

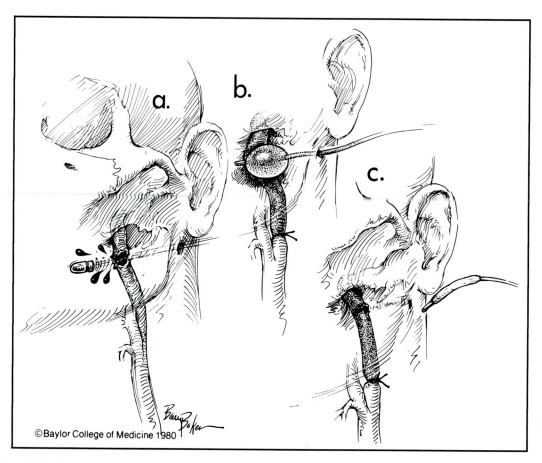

Figure 31-9. Technique of *extra*vascular balloon occlusion of uncontrolled bleeding from a high neck gunshot wound. Balloon was deflated and removed without incident on postoperative day 3.

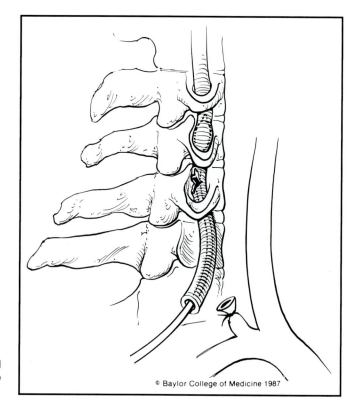

Figure 31-10. Technique of *intra*vascular occlusion of an injured vertebral artery within the foramen transversarum. Balloon may be removed on day 3.

tion is rarely even considered, much less performed. Primary amputation should be considered only in the patient with extensive soft tissue injury with concomitant injury to bone, nerves, arteries, veins, and soft tissue. Although replantation of digits, hands, and other appendices have been achieved using microvascular techniques, candidates for replantation should be carefully chosen. A patient's acceptance of extremity amputation is better if amputation is performed early, rather than in a delayed setting.

Balloons/Shunts

A variety of balloons and shunts is available to the vascular surgeon. Balloons may be intravascular occluding, extravascular occluding, or may be used to remove a clot.[81,82] Occluding balloons may achieve vascular control when injury exposure is impossible (i.e., injuries at the base of the skull, deep within the neck, or to the vertebral or hypogastric arteries) (Figs. 31-9 and 31-10).

Heparin-bonded shunts have been used from the heart or ascending aorta to the distal thoracic aorta or the femoral artery for lesions of the descending thoracic aorta.[56] Temporary shunts have been placed in femoral and popliteal arteries and veins during orthopedic repair procedures with vascular reconstruction following orthopedic stabilization.[83–86] In a few instances when the medical situation precluded vascular reconstruction and ligation was not possible, shunts have been left in place for several days until the patient is stable and elective reconstruction is possible.[87]

Medical Legal Considerations

Law suits after vascular trauma reconstruction are quite common. These suits involve cases of surgery on the descending thoracic aorta with postoperative paraplegia, vascular trauma requiring amputation, soft tissue or graft infection, concomitant nerve injury, and compartment syndromes. These manifestations may be related more to the severity of the initial injury than to a complication of the surgical reconstructive technique and therefore may be totally beyond the surgeon's control. The preoperative notes should clearly reflect that real and potential complications were specifically discussed with the patient and family, and that they understood the proposed procedures as well as possible complications.[88]

Technique of Fasciotomy

Although occasionally necessary in the upper extremity, fasciotomy is most often required for compartment syndromes in the calf. These compartment syndromes may be secondary to prolonged ischemia, direct injury, venous outflow occlusion, or to a combination of factors.[80,90]

The need for fasciotomy can be determined either by physical examination, measured pedal venous pressure, or measured compartment pressures.[91,92] Compartment and pedal pressures in excess of 40 cm H_2O may suggest

the need for fasciotomy. Despite sophisticated instrumentation, the clinical evaluation is still perhaps the most reliable.

Numerous techniques of performing fasciotomy have been described, including medial and lateral with long incisions, four-compartment, and fibulectomy fasciotomy.[93,94] Medial and lateral fasciotomy also has been described using small skin incisions and long scissors to divide the deep fascia. Fasciotomy of the tight compartments is perhaps most practically achieved through long medial and lateral incisions, care being taken not to injure the perineal nerve and the lateral aspects of the calf just below the knee (Fig. 31-11). All four compartments of the leg can be decompressed through these incisions. Skin grafting or primary closure may be accomplished several days later. Currently, small incisions in the skin with long incisions in the encircling muscle fascia are not recommended because the skin then becomes the limiting constriction.

Traumatic Aneurysm

Traumatic aneurysm may result from a delay in diagnosis, breakdown of the suture line, or infection. A false aneurysm may cause pain or may become increasingly larger, compressing adjacent structures. On rare occasions, an enlarging false aneurysm may rupture into a body cavity with exsanguinating hemorrhage.[95] Such aneurysms are uncommon with the current practice of primary adequate repair of vascular trauma.

Arteriovenous Fistula

Arteriovenous fistulas were commonly described many years ago after delayed recognition and repair of vascular injuries. Currently, primary arteriovenous fistulas are discovered at the time of primary repair and are rarely seen in a delayed setting. Should recognition of an arteriovenous fistula be delayed, adequate arterial and venous reconstruction requires proximal and distal control with appropriate separation after reconstruction.[96,97] This may be accomplished using prosthetic grafts or muscle interposition between the repairs.

Primary Ligation

Vascular reconstruction is always preferred in the stable patient. Primary ligation may be considered because of hypothermia, hypotension, acidosis, or extensive injury. In the unstable patient, primary ligation of the intrathoracic left subclavian artery, celiac axis, internal mammary artery, intercostal artery, or iliac arteries is possible and has been reportedly accomplished with success.[3,5,51] Primary ligation of the internal jugular vein, innominate vein, subclavian vein, or the iliac vein is well tolerated. Success following primary ligation of the portal vein, femoral veins, popliteal veins, superior vena cava, and inferior vena cava is less substantially documented. If primary ligation is performed

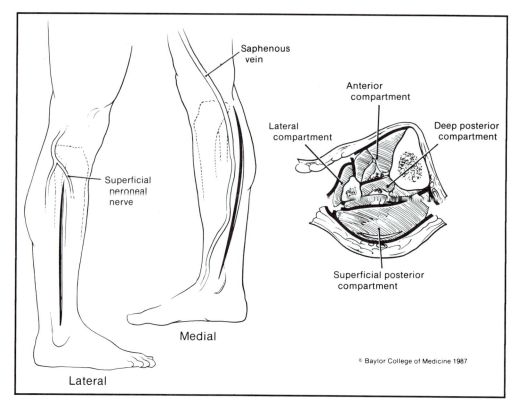

Figure 31-11. Technique of lower leg fasciotomy via *two* incisions. Note that all four fascial compartments are decompressed.

as a desperate measure in the moribund patient, reoperation within 24 hours for a second look should be considered. Secondary extraanatomic routing, such as femoral-femoral, axillary-femoral bypass will accomplish vascular reconstruction under such complex circumstances.

Sympathectomy

Although occasionally discussed as a means of maintaining patency of distal vascular reconstructions, sympathectomy in patients with vascular trauma who do not have concomitant arteriosclerosis has little value. Currently, sympathectomy in trauma is indicated for causalgia and not as a part of vascular trauma reconstruction.

Muscle Flaps

Muscle flaps are helpful in covering soft tissue defects or in isolating a vascular reconstruction when secondary contamination is considered a possibility. Muscle flaps are especially useful in the neck when concomitant carotid and tracheal or esophageal injury are present. With thoracic aortic and esophageal trauma, a muscle flap from the latissimus dorsi or intercostal muscle will be used to separate the repairs. Muscle flaps are also useful after femoral artery or vein reconstruction. Muscle flaps are developed primarily; however, with secondary reconstruction, free muscle flaps using microvascular techniques may be indicated.

Potentially Contaminated Wounds/Prostheses

Primary end-to-end anastomosis or lateral arteriorrhaphy is the procedure of choice when managing vascular wounds in contaminated or potentially contaminated areas. Ligation or extraanatomic routing outside the area of infection also may be considered in such cases, but is impossible to perform in some locations. Considerable debate exists in the literature concerning the appropriate conduit to use for vascular injuries in areas of infection or potential infection. Extensive laboratory research and clinical experience have shown that the complication rates associated with insertion of synthetic prosthetic material are identical to the complication rates seen with insertion of autogenous material. The specific complications encountered, however, are very different.

At the time of its transposition, the autogenous saphenous vein is not living tissue. It is a collagen tube deprived of its vasculature and is subject to all the complications of other foreign bodies, infection being the complication of primary concern. Infection around a transposed saphenous vein or autogenous artery results in dissolution of that vessel through the collagenase activity of the bacteria.

Complications associated with a synthetic prosthetic graft are graft infection, thrombosis, and suture line aneurysm, all of which are easier to manage than are the complications associated with use of transposed saphenous vein. Extensive clinical and laboratory research now indicates that adequately sized synthetic prostheses (5 mm or larger in diameter) are the conduits of choice for vascular wounds in contaminated and potentially contaminated areas.[32–42]

TABLE 31-4. RADIOLOGIC "CLUES" SUGGESTIVE OF THE PRESENCE OF A MIGRATORY MISSILE

Bullet out of focus superimposed over cardiac silhouette

Confusing "course" of bullet

Stable patient when "course" of bullet suggests devastating injuries

"Missing" or "moving" bullet on serial X-ray films

Bullet in intravascular location with a distant entry site

Missile Embolism

Intravascular migratory foreign bodies (usually missiles) create both diagnostic and therapeutic dilemmas[98,99] (Table 31-4). Missiles migrate via veins to the right ventricle and pulmonary arteries as well as from central arteries (and the heart) to peripheral arteries. Once the diagnosis is suspected, arteriography is unnecessary to confirm the diagnosis. Because of the risk of exsanguinating hemorrhage or pericardial tamponade, the entry site (usually easily deduced) is controlled first.[100] Migratory missiles frequently have passed through the bowel before entering the blood stream; therefore, they should be considered nonsterile. Complications of embolized missiles include infection, valve malfunction, erosion, occlusion of a major artery with peripheral ischemia, and psychogenic fears for the informed patient. Except for small pellet-sized missiles, migratory bullets are removed. Cardiac missile emboli usually require cardiopulmonary bypass for removal via the right atrium.

ACKNOWLEDGMENT

I wish to acknowledge the patient and diligent technical assistance of Ms. Mary Katherine Allen, without which this chapter would not have gone to press.

REFERENCES

1. Drapanas T, Hewitt RL, et al.: Civilian vascular injuries: A critical appraisal of three decades of management. Ann Surg 172:351, 1970.
2. Morris GC Jr, Beall AC Jr, et al.: Surgical experience with 220 acute arterial injuries in civilian practice. Am J Surg 99:775, 1960.
3. Feliciano DV, Bitondo CG, et al.: Civilian trauma in the 1980s: A 1-year experience with 456 vascular and cardiac injuries. Ann Surg 199:717, 1984.
4. Makins GH: On the vascular lesions produced by gunshot injuries and their results. Br J Surg 3:353, 1916.
5. DeBakey ME, Simeone FA: Battle injuries of the arteries in World War II. Ann Surg 123:534, 1946.
6. Hughes CW: Arterial repair during the Korean War. Ann Surg 147:555, 1958.
7. Hughes CW: Acute vascular trauma in Korean War casualties: An analysis of 180 cases. Surg Gynecol Obstet 99:91, 1970.
8. Rich NM, Baugh JH, Hughes CW: Acute arterial injuries in Vietnam: 1000 cases. J Trauma 10:359, 1970.
9. Chandler JG, Knapp RW: Early definitive treatment of vascular injuries in the Vietnam Conflict. JAMA 202:136, 1967.
10. American College of Surgeons Committee on Trauma: Hospital and prehospital resources for optimal care of the injured patient. Chicago, American College of Surgeons, 1987.
11. Border JR, Lewis FR, et al.: Panel: Prehospital care—Stabilize or scoop and run. J Trauma 23:708, 1983.
12. Lewis FR: Prehospital intravenous fluid therapy: Physiologic computer modeling. J Trauma 26:804, 1986.
13. Baxt WG, Moody P: The impact of rotorcraft aeromedical emergency care service on trauma mortality. JAMA 249:3047, 1983.
14. Mattox KL, Bickell WH, et al.: Prospective randomized evaluation of antishock MAST in posttraumatic hypotension. J Trauma 26:779, 1986.
15. Yao J, Plant J, Wilson RF: Peripheral vascular injuries, in Walt A, Wilson R (eds): Management of Trauma. Pitfalls and Practice. Philadelphia, Lea & Febiger, 1975, p 403.
16. Snyder WH, Thal ER, et al.: The validity of normal arteriography in penetrating trauma. Arch Surg 113:424, 1978.
17. O'Gorman RB, Feliciano DV, et al.: Emergency center arteriography in the evaluation of suspected peripheral vascular injuries. Arch Surg 119:568, 1984.
18. McCorkell SJ, Harley JD, et al.: Indications for angiography in extremity trauma. Am J Radiol 145:1245, 1985.
19. Lim RC, Glickman MG, Hunt TK: Angiography in patients with blunt trauma to the chest and abdomen. Surg Clin North Am 52:551, 1972.
20. Kirsh MM, Crane JD, et al.: Roentgenographic evaluation of traumatic rupture of the aorta. Surg Gynecol Obstet 131:900, 1970.
21. Mattox KL: Aortic arch and proximal brachiocephalic penetrating injury, in Ernst CB, Stanley JC (eds): Current Therapy in Vascular Surgery. Philadelphia, BC Decker, 1987, pp 262–265.
22. DeWeese JA, Mattox KL, et al.: Symposium on traumatic thoracic aortic rupture. Contemp Surg 24:109, 1984.
23. Mattox KL: Evolving concepts in the management of decelerative injury to the thoracic aorta, in Najarian JS, Delaney JP (eds): Trauma and Critical Care Surgery. Chicago Year Book Medical Publishers, 1987, p 81.
24. Akins CW, Buckley MJ, et al.: Acute traumatic disruption of the thoracic aorta: A ten-year experience. Ann Thorac Surg 31:305, 1980.
25. Mattox KL: Decelerating aortic injuries, in Bergan JJ, Yao JST (eds): Vascular Surgery Emergencies. New York, Grune & Stratton, 1986, p 341.
26. Egan TJ, Neiman HL, et al.: Computed tomography in the diagnosis of aortic aneurysm dissection of traumatic injury. Radiology 136:141, 1980.
27. Heiberg E, Wolverson MK, et al.: CT in aortic trauma. AJR 140:1119, 1983.
28. Tadavarthy S, Knight L, et al.: Therapeutic transcatheter arterial embolization. Radiology 112:13, 1974.
29. Mattox KL, Guinn GA, et al.: Use of activated coagulation time in the intraoperative heparin reversal for cardiopulmonary surgery. Ann Thorac Surg 19:634, 1975.
30. Phifer TJ, Gerlock AJ, Rich NM: Long-term patency of venous repairs demonstrated by venography. J Trauma 25:342, 1985.
31. Timberlake GA, O'Connell RC, Kerstein MD: Venous injury: To repair or ligate, the dilemma. J Vasc Surg 4:553, 1986.
32. Bricker DL, Beall AC Jr, DeBakey ME: The differential response to infection of autogenous vein versus Dacron arterial prosthesis. Chest 58:566, 1970.
33. Martin TD, Mattox KL: Synthetic materials in vascular trauma, in Kerstein MD (ed): Management of Vascular Trauma. Baltimore, University Park Press, 1984, pp 52–62.
34. Harrison JH: Influence of infection on homografts and synthetic (Teflon) grafts. Arch Surg 76:67, 1958.
35. Schramel RJ, Creech O Jr: Effects of infection and exposure on synthetic arterial prostheses. Arch Surg 78:271, 1959.

36. Foster JH, Berzins T, Scott HW Jr: An experimental study of arterial replacement in the presence of bacterial infection. Surg Gynecol Obstet 108:141, 1959.
37. Brown RB, Hoofer WD, et al.: Vascular replacement in grossly contaminated wounds: An experimental study comparing formalin preserved homografts and plastic prosthesis. J Trauma 1:322, 1961.
38. Weiss JP, Lorenzo FV, et al.: The behavior of infected arterial prostheses of expanded polytetrafluoroethylene (Gore-Tex). J Thorac Cardiovasc Surg 73:630, 1977.
39. Knott LH, Crawford FA Jr, Grogan JB: Comparison of autogenous vein, Dacron and Gore-Tex in infected wounds. J Surg Res 24:288, 1978.
40. Ward RE, Hudson MI, Flynn TC: Gram-negative infections of arterial substitutes. J Surg Res 33:510, 1982.
41. Stone KS, Walshaw R, et al.: Polytetrafluoroethylene versus autogenous vein grafts for vascular reconstruction in contaminated wounds. Am J Surg 147:692, 1984.
42. Richardson RL, Pate JW, et al.: The outcome of antibiotic-soaked arterial grafts in guinea pig wounds contaminated with E. coli or S. aureus. J Thorac Cardiovasc Surg 59:635, 1970.
43. Lau JM, Mattox KL, et al.: Use of substitute conduits in traumatic vascular injury. J Trauma 17:541, 1977.
44. Shah DM, Leather RP, et al.: Polytetrafluoroethylene grafts in the rapid reconstruction of acute contaminated peripheral vascular injuries. Am J Surg 148:229, 1984.
45. Vaughan GD, Mattox KL, et al.: Surgical experience with expanded polytetrafluoroethylene (PTFE) as a replacement graft for traumatized vessels. J Trauma 19:403, 1979.
46. Shah PM, Ito K, et al.: Expanded microporous polytetrafluoroethylene (PTFE) grafts in contaminated wounds: experimental and clinical study. J Trauma 23:1030, 1983.
47. Rubio RA, Reul GJ Jr, et al.: Acute carotid artery injury: 25 years experience. J Trauma 14:967, 1974.
48. Brown MF, Graham JM, et al.: Carotid artery injuries. Am J Surg 144:748, 1982.
49. Bricker DL, Noon GP, et al.: Vascular injuries of the thoracic outlet. J Trauma 10:1, 1970.
50. Graham JM, Feliciano DV, et al.: Innominate vascular injury. J Trauma 22:647, 1982.
51. Graham JM, Feliciano DV, et al.: Management of subclavian vascular injuries. J Trauma 20:537, 1980.
52. Parmley LF, Mattingly TW, et al.: Nonpenetrating traumatic injury to the aorta. Circulation 17:1086, 1958.
53. Hartford JM, Fayer RL, et al.: Transection of the thoracic aorta: Assessment of a trauma system. Am J Surg 151:224, 1986.
54. Fisher RG, Hadlock F, Ben-Menachem Y. Laceration of the thoracic and brachiocephalic arteries by blunt trauma. Radiol Clin North Am 19:91, 1981.
55. Pate JW: Traumatic rupture of the aorta: emergency operation. Ann Thorac Surg 39:531, 1985.
56. Donahoo JS, Brawley RK, Gott VL: The heparin-coated vascular shunt for thoracic aortic and great vessel procedures: A ten-year experience. Ann Thorac Surg 23:507, 1977.
57. Mattox KL, Holzman M, et al.: Clamp/repair: A safe technique for treatment of blunt injury to the descending thoracic aorta. Ann Thorac Surg 40:456, 1985.
58. Williams TE, Vasko JS, et al.: Treatment of acute and chronic traumatic rupture of the descending thoracic aorta. World J Surg 4:545, 1980.
59. Stiles QR, Cohimia GS, et al.: Management of injuries of the thoracic and abdominal aorta. Am J Surg 150:132, 1985.
60. Mattox KL, McCollum WB, et al.: Management of upper abdominal vascular trauma. Am J Surg 128:823, 1974.
61. Mattox KL, McCollum WB, et al.: Management of penetrating injuries of the suprarenal aorta. J Trauma 15:808, 1975.
62. Mattox KL, Feliciano DV: Truncal vascular trauma: Aorta, innominate vessels, vena cava, portal vein, and visceral arteries, in Wilson SE, Veith FJ, et al. (eds): Vascular Surgery Principles and Practice. New York, McGraw-Hill Book Co., 1987, p 813.
63. Graham JM, Mattox KL: The wounded soul. Texas Med 78:51, 1982.
64. Graham JM, Mattox KL, et al.: Injuries to the visceral arteries. Surgery 84:835, 1978.
65. Accola KD, Feliciano DV, et al.: Management of injuries to the superior mesenteric artery. J Trauma 26:313, 1986.
66. Mattox KL, Rea J, et al.: Penetrating injuries to the iliac arteries. Am J Surg 136:663, 1978.
67. Ryan W, Snyder W, et al.: Penetrating injuries of the iliac vessels: Early recognition and management. Am J Surg 144:642, 1982.
68. Graham JM, Mattox KL, et al.: Traumatic injuries of the inferior vena cava. Arch Surg 113:413, 1978.
69. Kudsk KA, Bongard F, Lim RC: Determinants of survival after vena caval injury. Analysis of 14-year experience. Arch Surg 119:1009, 1984.
70. Mattox KL: Abdominal venous injuries. Surgery 91:497, 1982.
71. Posner MC, Moore EE, et al.: Natural history of untreated inferior vena cava injury and assessment of venous access. J Trauma 26:698, 1986.
72. Mattox K: Discussion of Millikan JS, Moore EE, Cogbill TH et al.: Inferior vena cava injuries—A continuing challenge. J Trauma 23:211, 1983.
73. Schrock T, Blaisdell FW, Mathewson C: Management of blunt trauma to the liver and hepatic veins. Arch Surg 96:698, 1968.
74. Burch J. Personal communication, 1987.
75. Brown MF, Graham JM, et al.: Renovascular trauma. Am J Surg 140:802, 1980.
76. Guerriero WG: Management of renal trauma. Infect Surg 6(7):421, 1987.
77. Rich NM, Hobson RW II, et al.: Common femoral arterial trauma. J Trauma 1975.
78. Rich NW, Hobson RW, Fredde CW: Vascular trauma secondary to diagnostic and therapeutic procedures. Am J Surg 128:715, 1974.
79. Mills JL, Wiedeman JE, et al.: Minimizing mortality and morbidity from iatrogenic arterial injuries: The need for early recognition and prompt repair. J Vasc Surg 4:22, 1986.
80. Ledgerood AM, Lucas CE: Biologic dressings for exposed vascular grafts: A reasonable alternative. J Trauma 15:569, 1975.
81. Smiley K, Perry MO: Balloon catheter tamponade of major vascular wounds. Am J Surg 121:326, 1971.
82. Wolf RK, Berry RE: Transaxillary intra-aortic balloon tamponade in trauma. J Vasc Surg 4:95, 1986.
83. Johansen K, Bandyk K, et al.: Temporary shunts: Resolution of a management dilemma in complex vascular injuries. J Trauma 22:395, 1982.
84. Khalil IM, Livingston DH: Intravascular shunts in complex lower limb trauma. J Vasc Surg 4:582, 1986.
85. Nichols JG, Svoboda JA, Parks SN: Use of temporary intravascular shunts in selected peripheral arterial injuries. J Trauma 26:1094, 1986.
86. Majeski JA, Gauto A: Management of peripheral arterial vascular injuries with a Javid shunt. Am J Surg 138:324, 1979.
87. Khouqeer F, Mattox KL: Prolonged use of arterial shunts in vascular trauma. J Vasc Surg (submitted for publication 1988).
88. Weigel CJ: Legal Aspects of Trauma, in Mattox KL, Moore EE, Feliciano DV (eds): Trauma. Norwalk, Conn., Appleton and Lange, 1987.

89. Hye GL, Peck D, Powell DC: Compartment syndromes: Early diagnosis and a bedside operation. Ann Surg 49:563, 1983.

90. Patman RD, Poulos E, Shires GT: The management of civilian arterial injuries. Surg Gynecol Obstet 118:725, 1964.

91. Matsen F: Compartment syndrome: A unified concept. Clin Orthop 113:8, 1975.

92. Gerlock AJ: The use of the pedal venous pressure (PVP) as a guide in evaluating the patency of venous repairs. J Trauma 17:108, 1977.

93. Mubarak SJ, Owen CA: Double incision fasciotomy of the leg for decompression. J Bone Joint Surg 59:184, 1977.

94. Ernst CB, Kaufer H: Fibulectomy-fasciotomy: An important adjunct in the management of lower extremity arterial trauma. J Trauma 11:365, 1971.

95. Mattox KL: Traumatic aneurysms, in Rutherford RB (ed): Vascular Surgery. Philadelphia, W.B. Saunders Co., 1977.

96. Rich NM, Hobson RW II, Collins GJ: Traumatic arteriovenous fistulas and false aneurysms: A review of 558 lesions. Surgery 78:817, 1975.

97. Fry WJ, Kollmeyer KR, et al.: Acute and chronic traumatic arteriovenous fistula in civilians. Arch Surg 116:697, 1981.

98. Mattox KL, Beall AC, et al.: Intravascular migratory bullets. Am J Surg 37:192, 1979.

99. Graham JM, Mattox KL: Right ventricular bullet embolectomy without cardiopulmonary bypass. J Thorac Cardiovasc Surg 8:310, 1981.

100. Shannon JJ, Vo NM, et al.: Peripheral arterial missile embolization: A case report and 22-year literature review. J Vasc Surg 5:773, 1987.

CHAPTER 32

Metabolic Complications of Acute Arterial Occlusions and Related Conditions: Role of Free Radicals (Myonephropathic-Metabolic Syndrome)

Henry Haimovici

Until recently, metabolic complications secondary to acute ischemia of an extremity have received scant attention in spite of countless publications dealing with arterial thromboembolism or trauma. Although considerable progress has been achieved in the management of acute ischemic syndromes, limb salvage and mortality rates still leave much to be desired in a significant percentage of these entities. In such instances, the immediate outcome of limb and patient survival may depend on many factors, one of which may be the presence of a metabolic syndrome secondary to ischemic rhabdomyolysis, the prognosis of which may be ominous. Often, unawareness of these potential complications has been a contributing factor to the poor prognosis, as stated above.

The knowledge of the role of rhabdomyolysis in the pathogenesis of the metabolic syndrome is essential for understanding the significance of the therapeutic implications in such sudden arterial interruptions. This situation has prompted (1) a critical analysis of this problem and (2) review of a number of acute vascular and related conditions that display similar metabolic complications. A unified concept of their pathogenesis is pointed out based on their common as well as on their divergent features.

BIOLOGIC BACKGROUND: PIVOTAL ROLE OF SKELETAL MUSCLE

The skeletal muscle which represents about 42% of the entire body weight and 76% of the mass of the lower extremities, is a tissue that incorporates a multitude of biochemical substances in its structural complex. Being highly vulnerable to anoxia, the muscle may respond by releasing into the circulation some, if not most, of these biochemicals, which may be extremely harmful or even fatal to the patient. They are the major cause of the metabolic syndrome resulting from acute ischemic muscle entities.

Before one undertakes the study of the clinicopathologic aspects of this complex syndrome, the *myonephropathic-metabolic syndrome,* knowledge of the *normal* morphology and *normal* biochemistry of the skeletal muscle fiber is indispensable (Figs. 32-1 and 32-2).

It is beyond the scope of this chapter, however, to give a detailed description of all the morphologic and biochemical components of the muscle fiber. But knowledge of these components provides the basis for an understanding of the biologic repercussions of skeletal muscle iscemia and the various clinicopathologic entities resulting from them.

Morphologically, the smallest independent cellular units of the muscle are the fibers, which are multinucleate cellular structures that may vary greatly in length. These fibers contain the biochemical substances that are physiologically and pathologically of great significance for understanding both the normal functions and the metabolic complications resulting from their release into the circulation.

Physiologically, the chemical substances that determine the energetics of the muscle are the adenosinetriphosphatases (ATPases) and creatine phosphokinase (CPK). Besides participating normally in the energetics of the muscle, adenosine triphosphate (ATP) and phosphocreatine (PCr) play a significant role in the biochemical changes that occur during ischemia of muscle tissue, described below.

Of the morphologic components, the membrane of the muscle fiber plays an essential role in the physiologic and pathologic functions of the skeletal muscle. The metabolic complications resulting from ischemia of skeletal muscle are due to derangement of the transport processes across the membranes. The muscle membrane plays a fundamental role in the interchanges of the various biochemical components. Alterations in the permeability of membranes under traumatic or simple ischemic conditions may induce severe shifts in the internal space of the sarcolemmal reticulum and outside of it (Fig. 32-3).

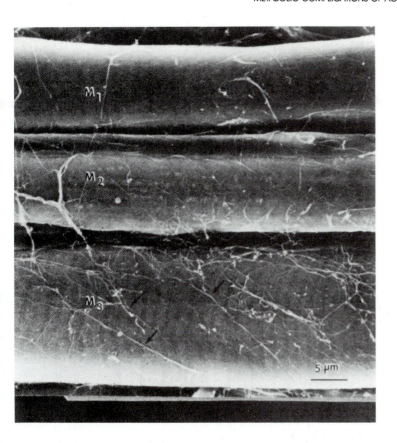

Figure 32-1. Skeletal muscle fibers appear as cylindrical units aligned in parallel bundles. Faint cross striations are visible along individual fibers. Coarse collagenous fibers of the endomysium run in various directions over and between muscle fibers (*arrows*). (*From Peachey LD, Adrian RH, Geiger SR (eds): Skeletal Muscle. Bethesda, Md., American Physiological Society, 1983, p 2.*)

The physiologic integrity of the membrane, which includes neural components, can be affected by a decrease in ATP. The ATP level is markedly reduced in ischemic muscle, resulting in abnormal membrane permeability (Fig. 32-4). In fact, the reduction in ATP level represents the underlying mechanism of the biochemical changes. These morphologic and physiologic characteristics of the membrane will be mentioned later, in the discussions of the pathogenesis of the various entities that are described in this chapter.

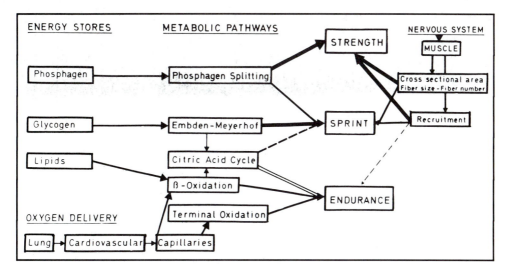

Figure 32-2. Summary of the various energy stores and metabolic pathways for performance in strength, sprint, and endurance events. The energy stores include phosphagen, glycogen, and lipids. Oxygen delivery originates in the lungs and is dispersed through the cardiovascular system down to the capillaries, which leads to the terminal oxidation of the tissues. This summary indicates not only how oxygen is delivered but also how it interacts with the nervous system and the muscles during the various performances. (*From Peachey LD, Adrian RH, Geiger SR (eds.): Skeletal Muscle. Bethesda, Md., American Physiological Society, 1983, p 566.*)

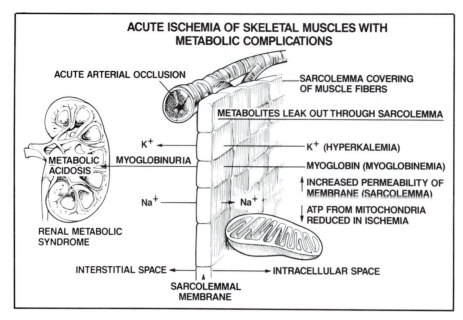

Figure 32-3. Acute ischemia of skeletal muscle associated with metabolic complications. Note the leakage through the sarcolemma of potassium and myoglobin, which leads to myoglobinuria and hyperkalemia. The mitochondria and ATP are reduced by ischemia, which leads to increased permeability of the membrane. This point will be discussed further in the pathogenesis.

CLINICAL ENTITIES

As stated earlier, the basic skeletal muscle lesion responsible for the various clinical entities is rhabdomyolysis. The generally used definition of rhabdomyolysis indicates a lesion of the skeletal muscle, resulting in morphologic damage, the nature, extent, and exact degree of which are variable.

Notwithstanding this variability, the definition of rhabdomyolysis should incorporate essentially two major parameters: (1) a muscle lesion and (2) a biologic syndrome resulting from ischemia of the muscle.

Three major etiologic types of rhabdomyolysis are being differentiated according to the nature of the factors inducing the lesions in the skeletal muscle:

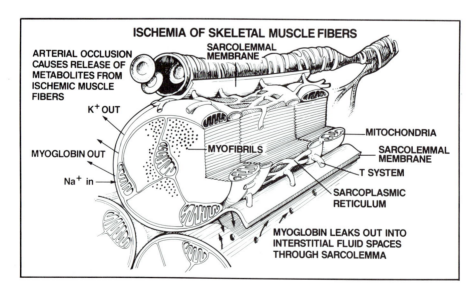

Figure 32-4. Arterial occlusion causing ischemia of skeletal muscle fibers, resulting in release of metabolites from the myofibrils. Note the sarcolemmal membrane surrounding the muscle fiber. The sarcoplasmic reticulum, mitochondria, T system, and myofibrils are seen at the cut end of the muscle fiber. Note the release of myoglobin leading out into interstitial fluid spaces through the sarcolemma (membrane). In addition, potassium leaks out while sodium enters through the sarcolemma from the interstitial fluid spaces.

1. *Acute arterial occlusions,* which may cause (a) minor or reversible muscle lesions, (b) partial limited necrosis, and (c) massive necrosis with loss of limb and often death
2. *Ischemic muscle necrosis:* the "crush syndrome," in which there is prolonged (several hours) compression of muscle tissue with or without involvement of the vessels of the traumatized region
3. *Nontraumatic injuries:* a wide spectrum of diffuse muscle cell injuries that occasionally lead to extensive muscle necrosis and that generally are due to a variety of toxins affecting the skeletal muscle fibers.

ACUTE ARTERIAL OCCLUSIONS

The causes of acute arterial occlusions most commonly associated with the metabolic syndrome secondary to rhabdomyolysis include (1) arterial embolism, (2) acute thrombosis, (3) acute arterial graft thrombosis, (4) cross-clamping of major arteries during reconstructive surgery, (5) arterial cannulation during cardiopulmonary bypass, and (6) arterial trauma.

Arterial Embolism

Since 1960, when two cases of arterial embolism with massive ischemic myopathy, myoglobinuria, hyperkalemia, and metabolic acidosis were reported, an increasing number of publications have confirmed the fact that a certain percentage of such cases may be associated with a syndrome of severe and often fatal metabolic complications.

The *incidence* of this group of cases, as it relates to the overall experience with arterial embolism, is still difficult to assess because reports on the importance of potential metabolic repercussions are rare. The paucity of these reports may be due to an unawareness of such complications or to a clinical picture obscured by cardiovascular manifestations, which are often present. The persistent high rates of morbidity, amputation, and mortality are then attributed to a cardiac origin, rather than to the true rhabdomyolytic cause.

Based on a collective series of 2,447 patients with acute arterial occlusions, the incidence of this syndrome ranged between 7.0 and 37.5%, with an average of 13.7% representing a total of 178 patients. It should be pointed out that the data which served as a basis for including the 2,447 patients were rather selective and were based on those that have been published in recent years. The exact incidence, however, is still not known. For example, in a 1979 personal study of over 200 acute arterial occlusions, the overall incidence of both fatal and recovered cases associated with this syndrome was 7.5%.

Clinical Manifestations

The most striking clinical feature of arterial embolism is the unusual and extreme severity of both local and systemic manifestations. These manifestations may be observed (1) initially during the acute ischemic or devascularization phase, (2) after the revascularization of the extremity, and (3) after the reperfusion of the distal ischemic tissues. The clinical and metabolic manifestations differ in degree and extent in the three phases. Recognition of the early phase is of paramount significance, as was pointed out previously.

Ischemic (Devascularization) Phase. The clinical picture in this phase is characteristic and dramatic, inasmuch as it differs greatly from the usual form. In all instances the clinical onset is ushered in by *excruciating pain.* Any attempt at mobilizing or examining the extremity is accompanied by exacerbation of pain. The profound ischemia of the tissues is characterized by coldness, waxy pallor mixed with cyanotic mottling, and sensory anesthesia. The severity of the ischemia is due to massive obstruction of the main arterial axis and its collateral network, which is translated into extensive rhabdomyolysis. The most striking and characteristic feature of this clinical syndrome is the *rigidity of the extremity,* or *rigor mortis.* Muscle contracture and stiffness of the joints appear so pronounced that their presence, together with an acute embolism or thrombosis, should evoke the possibility of ischemic myopathy associated with myoglobinuria. Indeed, limb rigidity was found in all cases and may be considered an "alarm signal" heralding the metabolic syndrome. The joints, especially the distal ones such as the ankle or knee, appear "frozen" (Fig. 32-5).

Edema of the extremity is nonpitting, unlike that of a venous thrombosis. Massive swelling occurs within 12 to 24 hours and usually involves the entire extremity, although the swelling of the thigh may be more pronounced than that of the leg. The swollen limb is usually tender, tense, of woody consistency, and nonpitting. The edema is mostly in the muscles. The association of coldness and cyanosis may lead to confusion with phlegmasia cerulea dolens. However, unlike its distribution in venous thrombosis, the edema is most pronounced in the muscles and less pronounced in the subcutaneous tissue. This is obvious if one considers the biologic changes that take place in the muscles during the ischemic period.

Because of the pain and the metabolic disturbances, the patient often appears to be agitated, confused, and disoriented. The so-called neuropsychiatric manifestations are probably the result of the combination of azotemia and the effects of other metabolites on the brain function as well.

During this ischemic phase, variable degrees of metabolic acidosis, together with incipient azotemia and hyperkalemia, are already present, all of which, if uncorrected, may lead to serious complications or even the death of the patient. The significance of recognizing this early phase cannot be overemphasized.

Revascularization Phase. Restoration of arterial flow to the previously acutely and severely ischemic extremity has been reported sporadically in the past to result in a syndrome of pain, edema, and tenderness of the muscles. However, the metabolic complications in these cases were rarely noted or fully appreciated. At present, a fairly large body of experimental and clinical information on the revascularization phase and its metabolic repercussions is available.

The clinical picture varies according to the degree of ischemia. In severe cases the pain may increase in intensity,

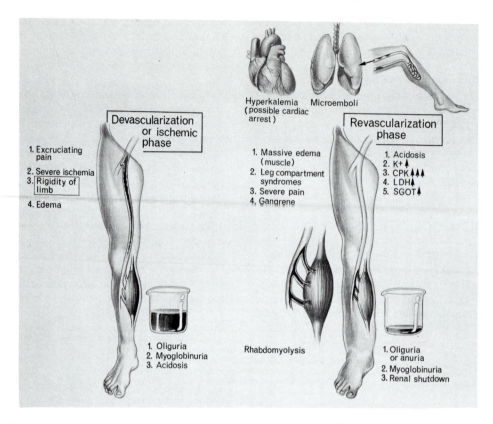

Figure 32-5. The two clinical phases with the corresponding major muscle, renal, biochemical, and morphologic alterations. During the acute *devascularization* phase the dominating features are (a) severe ischemia and ridigity of the limb (muscle contracture) and (b) oliguria, incipient myoglobinuria, and acidosis. During the immediate *postrevascularization* phase the dominating features are (a) edema and leg compartment syndromes, (b) rhabdomyolysis, and (c) renal shutdown. The *reperfusion* phase, not depicted here, is associated with muscle ischemia due to free radicals and superimposed necrosis.

despite revascularization, because of incomplete reperfusion of the distal tissues. The reason for this incompleteness may be that the intramuscular branches of the arterial tree are occluded more severely than the major branches. Edema of the limb becomes more pronounced than it was before the operation, whereas the muscular contracture and rigidity may subside. *Leg or forearm compartment syndromes are almost always present.* Although the overall tissue perfusion may become adequate, ischemia may remain severe in the distal portion of the limb. The prognosis in this phase depends essentially on the extent of the muscle mass involved and its degree of necrosis.

After revascularization, microemboli containing platelets and fibrin may invade the pulmonary circulation as a result of embolectomy, thrombectomy, or the declamping of the aorta.

Metabolic Syndrome
Most patients display metabolic manifestations, which may be transient or prolonged, shortly after onset of arterial occlusion and especially after limb revascularization.

Metabolic Acidosis. Metabolic acidosis may be of variable degree, *but it is always present.* It is the response to the accumulation of acid metabolites. Tissue hypoxia or anoxia leads to a decrease in aerobic oxidation through the Krebs

cycle, followed by an increase in anaerobic glycolysis of the Embden-Meyerhof pathway, resulting in lactic acid and pyruvic acid. Levels of both lactate and pyruvate increase initially, and lactate levels later increase more than pyruvate levels, producing an increased lactate-pyruvate ratio.

The blood pH and CO_2 content fall. There is a decrease in bicarbonates, and the numbers of cations and anions increase considerably. Before revascularization of the limb, the pH of the venous efflux of the involved extremity varies with the degree of metabolic acidosis already present. If the initial pH is less than or equal to 7.2, the prognosis appears to be poor, especially if the subsequent pH falls even farther. Treatment requires a considerable amount of buffer substances (sodium bicarbonate or tromethamine) to neutralize the fresh appearance of the hydrogen ions after revascularization.

Electrolytic Changes. The serum sodium level appears to be within normal limits in the majority of cases. This is in contrast to the serum potassium level, which in the beginning may be normal in the venous blood from both the ischemic limb and systemic circulation; after release of the clamp, however, there is an increase in serum potassium levels. Although, in milder cases, hyperkalemia can be controlled without difficulty, in severe cases, noted in the venous efflux from the ischemic limb, it must be treated vigorously to prevent a dangerous effect on the heart function. It represents a poor prognostic factor that may translate into muscle cytolysis, and sudden release of the clamping may lead to cardiac arrest.

The venous Po_2 concentration in the ischemic limb is significantly lower than in the systemic venous blood. The venous Po_2 of concentration in the ischemic limb is higher than in the systemic blood. After restoration of the arterial circulation, venous Po_2 and Pco_2 concentrations may return to normal within a variable period of time, depending on the degree and duration of ischemia.

Enzymatic Changes. The serum creatine phosphokinase (CPK) concentration is usually slightly elevated in the systemic blood before revascularization. However, it is far higher in the venous blood from the ischemic limb. After restoration of the arterial flow by removal of the arterial clamp, the average CPK volume rises even farther in most cases. Elevation of this enzyme concentration is direct evidence of damaged striated muscle. High values of the enzyme usually reflect advanced muscle necrosis. Preservation of intact skin in such cases may be misleading, because it is not always an index of viability of the underlying muscles. In mild cases the serum level of CPK may decrease within several hours or within 1 or 2 days after revascularization. From experimental studies, the CPK disappears much more slowly than do other metabolites such as myoglobin. In moderately severe cases it may increase over a period of several days to 1,000 or 2,000 units and then return progressively to a normal level within 10 to 12 days. However, in severe and fatal cases, as the CPK level keeps increasing progressively, it may reach 20,000 units or even higher.

Lactate dehydrogenase (LDH) and serum glutamic-oxaloacetic transaminase (SGOT) levels are also elevated in all forms of acute arterial occlusions displaying this syndrome. The levels of the transaminases (SGOT, serum glutamic-pyruvic transaminase [SGPT]) are increased in proportion to the degree of ischemia. In patients with very severe muscle damage, persistence of high levels of transaminase indicates irreversible changes of the tissue.

In recent years, determination of total LDH and total CPK activities has been made in a wide spectrum of diseases, of which myocardial infarction is the most frequent entity. Because patients with severe occlusive disease may also have myocardial damage, it is essential to identify the specific LDH and CPK isoenzymes in the blood. Thus, two of the five isoenzymes of LDH—LDH_1 and LDH_2—usually have significantly increased levels in myocardial infarction, whereas LDH_4 and LDH_5 are more specific for striated muscle damage. Likewise, of the isoenzymes of CPK, fraction 2, or the MB fraction, is indicative of myocardial necrosis, whereas CPK-MM is found predominantly in skeletal muscle. A decrease or a return to normal blood levels of these enzymes may reflect resolution of muscle damage. Interpretation of these serum enzyme values carries a number of pitfalls because of the wide spectrum of diseases in which the enzymes are positively identified.

Myoglobinuria. Within a few hours after the onset of arterial occlusion, the urinary output is usually decreased and the urine displays a dark cherry-red or burgundy-red color, because of the presence of myoglobin. *Myoglobinuria* may reach a peak within 48 hours that may last several days, depending on the extent and severity of the rhabdomyolysis. Occasionally myoglobinuria may escape detection because of either laboratory mishap or delay in testing the urine. The presence of myoglobin can be determined as a guaiac- or benzidine-positive or an orthotolidine-positive pigment in the urine containing no red blood cells, especially if the serum is clear. The most common mistaken diagnosis in myoglobinuria is hemoglobinuria. Berman (1977) suggested that a naked-eye look at the plasma may suffice to arouse suspicion of myoglobin by application of this rule: Red plasma plus red urine equals hemoglobin; clear plasma plus red urine equals myoglobin. Of course, the specific chemical tests available for detecting these pigments in the urine (described later) provide the final accurate diagnosis. The methods available for estimating myoglobin are chemical, spectrophotometric, and immunologic.

Most of these tests are primarily qualitative in nature. Recent methods have been described for quantitative investigation of myoglobin in the urine, thus making possible the earlier and more accurate detection of myoglobin in both the serum and urine.

Myoglobinemia. Among the possible pitfalls of detecting myoglobin in the urine are the delay in myoglobin clearance through the kidney and the small amounts that may be cleared. Therefore it is difficult to demonstrate myoglobinuria. However, testing for myoglobin in the serum or plasma, that is, myoglobinema, can and should be done because myoglobin may be easier to identify in the blood before it reaches the urine through the kidney clearance. Therefore, because a number of cases of myoglobinuria have been missed, one must think in terms of myoglobinemia, especially in those patients in whom rhabdomyolysis due to ischemia is highly suspected.

Hypocalcemia and Hypercalcemia. *Hypocalcemia* with concurrent hyperphosphatemia and oliguria has been noted in more than half of the patients. Conversely, *hypercalcemia* has been reported in 22 to 25% of the patients with nontraumatic rhabdomyolysis during the diuretic phase. The mechanism of alteration of the calcium-phosphorus ratio in the oliguric phase is attributed to the overall changes in sarcolemmal (membrane) permeability. Thus in normal muscle the calcium ion concentration is three to four times lower than in the extracellular fluid. If the calcium ion concentration in the muscle sarcoplasm reaches equilibrium with the extracellular space, contraction of the muscle will be increased, which may explain the rigidity. On the other hand, the presence of hypocalcemia in acute renal failure may account for the twitching and seizures noted in some patients.

Rhabdomyolysis: Acute Muscle Devascularization

The degree of ischemic damage to the skeletal muscle is of central significance, because it determines the viability of the limb and, to a great extent, whether the metabolic syndrome will result. Surprisingly, scant attention has been paid to the pathologic change that take place in the acutely devascularized muscle in arterial occlusions. In an effort to acquire some missing information concerning this phase of rhabdomyolysis, a number of experimental investigations have produced a substantial body of data. These data have been based on the effects of acute ligations or tourniquet ischemia in animals and therefore bear only limited resemblance to the findings in human subjects. The significance of the data, however, derives from the chronologic evaluation of damaged muscle fibers, which indicates the various stages of the histopathologic changes, as related to the duration and extent of the ischemia.

During surgery performed within hours of an acute arterial occlusion pallor and swelling of moderate intensity have been observed in human muscle (Fig. 32-6). These changes become more pronounced within 24 hours, when the swollen, pallid muscles take on an appearance described as that of "fish flesh." After 24 hours the muscles appear grossly congested, purple, and hard. On fascial incision, if the muscles are still viable, they turn pink and herniate through the opening of the fasciotomy. If unrelieved by decompression of the involved area, edema usually increases further after additional revascularization of the limb. Beyond this stage, the muscle may also display variable degrees of necrosis, ranging from focal to extensive areas.

Microscopically, some fibers show initially well-preserved outlines. In some areas the absence of nuclei is noted and the cytoplasm is slightly coagulated and granular. Such findings are characteristic of early anoxic changes. Within 24 hours, individual fibers display swelling and hyalinization. At a later phase (48 to 72 hours), the lesions consist of foci of loss of striation and sarcolemmal nuclei of muscular fibers. Specimens from amputated limbs may show regeneration of muscle fibers ranging from slight to moderate to degenerative changes, to actual necrosis (Fig. 32-7). The muscle cell changes are translated into biochemical alterations and metabolic complications (Fig. 32-8). It is well known that the sarcoplasm contains a large number of chemical substances and enzymes, including myocin and actin. The normal relationship among myoglobin, myocin, and actin is disrupted by loss of ATP and the muscle enzymes, all of which is attributable to altered permeability of the muscle cell membrane.

Acute Renal Failure

Acute renal impairment usually varies with the degree of muscle ischemia, acidosis, and myoglobinuria. In mild or moderately severe cases, renal function is only temporarily impaired and is completely reversible. Urinary output may be decreased during the devascularization phase and may be further impaired after revascularization. Most patients display either oliguria or anuria. Their blood urea nitrogen and creatinine concentrations rapidly rise to very high levels after renal impairment is detected clinically. In patients with severe complications, prolonged myoglobinuria in the presence of acidosis, if not treated promptly with vigorous peritoneal dialysis or preferably with hemodialysis, leads to irreversible renal shutdown and usually to the death of the patient.

Histologically the renal tubules contain casts of myoglobin, with reactive epithelial cells occasionally indicating their regeneration (Fig. 32-9). The evidence for acute tubular necrotic lesions depends on tubular clogging by myoglobin and possibly, to some degree, by hemoglobin. The pathologic picture presented above is commonly referred to as myoglobinuric nephrosis or nephropathy. Sometimes the

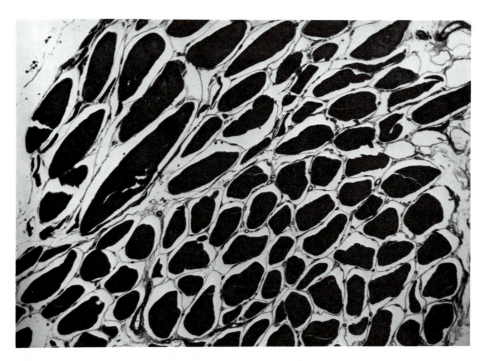

Figure 32-6. Swelling of individual muscle fibers and their hyalinization. (H & E; ×250.). (*From Haimovici H: J Cardiovasc Surg 14:589, 1973.*)

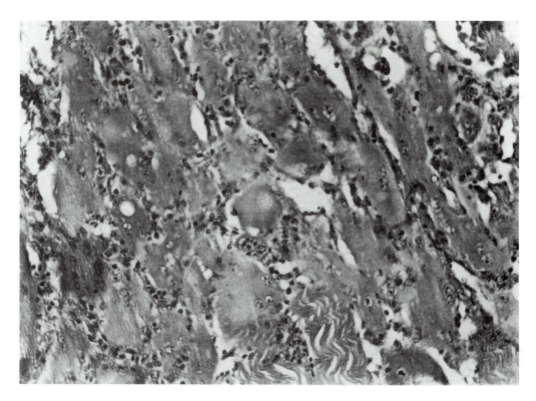

Figure 32-7. Photomicrograph showing sarcolemmal proliferation and regeneration of muscle fibers. (H & E; ×400.) (*From Haimovici H: J Cardiovasc Surg 14:589, 1973.*)

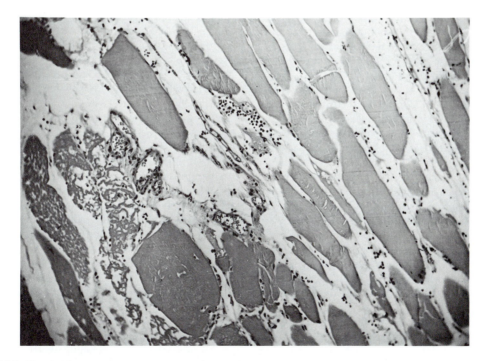

Figure 32-8. Muscle biopsy specimen during fasciotomy from anterior leg compartment of an ischemic lesion after acute arterial embolic occlusion indicates the loss of sarcolemmal nuclei, homogeneous appearance of cytoplasm with loss of striations, interstitial edema, and infiltration of polymorphonuclear and mononuclear leukocytes. (×440.)

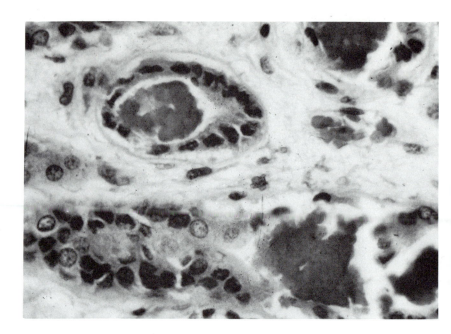

Figure 32-9. Renal tubules containing casts of myoglobin and showing reactive epithelium cells indicating regeneration. (×440.) (*From Haimovici H: Arch Surg 100:639, 1970.*)

latter findings are mixed with preexisting nephrosclerotic lesions, which are apt to aggravate the prognosis.

The pathogenesis of acute renal failure associated with the syndrome of myoglobinuria has brought to light some unsolved problems. On the basis of the histologic data reported above, obtained from both human autopsy material and experimental animal models, the presence of myoglobin casts in the renal tubules seems to strongly suggest a causal relationship between tubular mechanical blockage by the myoglobin casts and acute renal shutdown. The suggested theory that myoglobin has a direct toxic effect on the tubules has been debated because experimental infusion of this pigment has failed to induce acute renal failure.

Skeletal Muscle Reperfusion Phase

The initial ischemia in skeletal muscle results in rhabdomyolysis and during the reperfusion phase is further complicated by free radical–induced ischemia leading to an additional superimposed necrosis. In the past few years, a large body of evidence regarding this complication has been accumulated, mostly in connection with ischemic myocardium, caused by primary occlusion of the coronary arteries or secondary to coronary artery bypass surgery. By analogy, it was assumed and subsequently demonstrated that with reflow or reperfusion into a region of hypoxic or ischemic skeletal muscle, paradoxical results, consisting of a marked increase of ischemic damage, may be observed. A number of experimental studies have shown that obstruction of blood flow to skeletal muscle for from 30 minutes to several hours may result in edema formation after release of the occlusion.

Thus Korthuis et al. and Harris et al. showed that prolonged ischemia followed by reperfusion produces morphologic alterations in skeletal muscle similar to those seen after reperfusion of ischemic myocardium, intestine, brain, and kidney. In skeletal muscle studies, Korthuis et al. showed that the role of oxygen-derived free radicals in the genesis of increased vascular permeability could prevent the production of active oxygen species when the patient is subjected to pretreatment with specific oxygen radical scavengers. According to their studies, ATP is converted to adenosine monophosphate (AMP) during ischemia. When AMP levels are elevated, AMP is catabolized by hypoxanthine, a substrate for xanthine oxidase. These particular biochemical conversions have been shown to be present in various organs, such as the heart, brain, and intestine. Thus xanthine oxidase, which normally exists in the cell as $NAD+$-reducing dehydrogenase, is formed by the action of a protease in response to the low oxygen tension produced by ischemia. These investigators noted that most of the damage to skeletal muscle occurred, not during the ischemic period, but after reoxygenation has been restored (Fig. 32-10).

Harris et al. also showed that changes in the intramuscular metabolites vary with the duration of ischemia. At two hours, minimal ultrastructural damage occurred, followed by complete regeneration of intramuscular phophagens and glycogen on reperfusion, with complete normalization of lipid oxidation products. In contrast, one 7-hour ischemic insult resulted in profound injury at the ultrastructural level, with inability to restore intramuscular phosphagens and glycogen on reperfusion. Their results pointed out that there was "prolonged glycolytic activity of skeletal muscle during global ischemia which could be documented by increased production of oxygen–free radical–mediated lipid oxidation products in irreversibly injured muscle."

Role of Scavenging Agents. Ischemia-induced injury of skeletal muscle, regardless of the cause, results in vascular permeability at the microvascular level. The mechanism underlying the increase in permeability is not entirely elucidated. Reperfusion of ischemic skeletal muscle results in a more dramatic increase in microvascular permeability, leading to additional tissue necrosis.

Recent investigation of a few substances, called scavenging agents, indicates that these agents have the

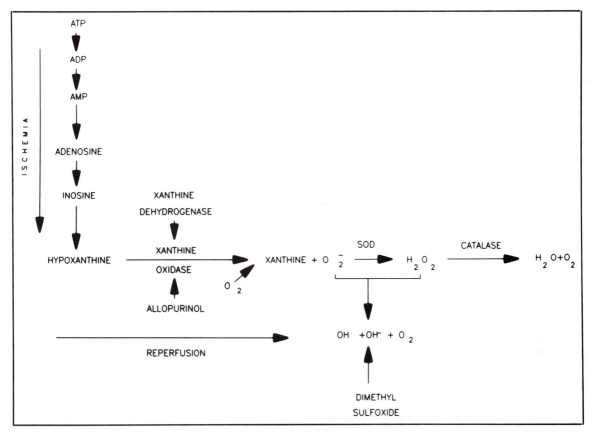

Figure 32-10. Biochemical mechanisms of reperfusion of ischemic muscle. This phase of the ischemic skeletal muscle is produced by oxygen radicals as a result of conversion of ATP to ADP followed by adenosine monophosphate (AMP). The elevated AMP is catabolized to hypoxanthine, a substrate for xanthine oxidase. For the production of oxygen radicals, molecular oxygen is required before hypoxanthine and xanthine oxidase can react to form superoxide anion. O_2 represents the hydroxyl radical. Most of the damage to skeletal muscle occurs after reoxygenation is restored, essentially because of xanthine oxidase, which appears as the source of oxygen radicals in ischemic skeletal muscle. (*Modified from Korthuis et al.*[73])

ability to alter the permeability increase. The main agents used, mostly experimentally and to some extent clinically, are superoxide dismutase, allopurinol, catalase, and mannitol. α-Tocopherol (vitamin E) has been used recently as a scavenging agent and is being added to this group of antidotes. All these agents have the ability, in various degrees, to prevent ischemic injury to skeletal muscle, hyperosmotic mannitol is known to reduce ischemic cell swelling and to minimize both myocardial necrosis and muscle ischemia. For some time, the physiologic and therapeutic properties of mannitol have been clearly established, and its use preceded that of free radicals in postischemic reperfusion lesions. Its administration before, during, and especially after emergency vascular reconstruction may be of great therapeutic significance. On the basis of current research, it is anticipated that besides the above-mentioned scavengers, including mannitol, new substances are potentially displaying similar properties. The field is in the midst of expansion, and no definitive statements are as yet available.

Clinical Course: Prognosis

The clinical course of this syndrome of myonephropathic-metabolic changes varies with the severity and duration

of the complications, which in turn depend on the extent and degree of tissue damage. In mild or moderate cases of ischemia, the metabolic alterations—including hyperkalemia, myoglobinuria, and elevation of CPK levels—may last only a short time and are completely reversible. In severe cases of ischemia, the metabolic and structural repercussions are often largely irreversible (Fig. 32-11). Although some of these metabolic changes can be easily corrected, hyperkalemia and myoglobinuria may reach dangerous levels because of massive muscle necrosis.

Clinical course may be affected by several factors, of which the most important are

1. The number, extent, and level of arterial occlusions
2. The duration of the occlusions
3. The extent of the involvement of intramuscular arterioles and venules
4. The awareness and early recognition of this syndrome
5. The immediate aggressive treatment of the ischemia and of its early metabolic manifestations, including those occurring as a result of the free radicals' effect.

Limb loss due to gangrene is high, ranging between 30 and 50%. In our experience, gangrene was present in

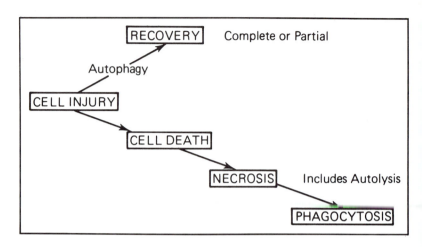

Figure 32-11. Five types of disruption of the normal structure of muscle and the types of myofiber breakdown. Essentially, the alternative histopathologic events after cellular injury are listed. At the bottom, following cell injury, the events would lead to cell death, which ends in necrosis and finally includes autolysis. On the other hand, if the disease should progress from autophagy of damaged cells through a scavenging process, a complete or partial recovery would result. (*From Cullen MJ, et al.: Ann NY Acad Sci 317:440, 1979.*)

25% of the survivors and in 36% of the fatal cases. The more proximal the acute occlusion (e.g., in the aortoiliac artery), the more massive the rhabdomyolysis (Fig. 32-12). This leads to higher amputation rates and lower survival rates than are found in patients with femoropopliteal occlusions. Although late or delayed thromboembolectomy may represent a negative prognostic factor, it is primarily the degree of ischemia, and not the chronology, that is the determining factor in these cases.

The reported mortality rates range from 30 to 80%. Sarrazin and Cassar, each studying his own group of 23 patients, reported a mortality rate of only 30%, whereas Gutierrez Carreno and Sanchez Fabela noted a mortality rate of 44.4% in a group of nine patients. In our series, 7 of 15 patients, or 47%, died. On the other hand, Cormier and Devin reported a mortality rate in 25 cases of 80%. The high rate of fatality is usually attributed to hyperkalemia, uncontrolled acidosis, and acute renal shutdown, with its inherent complications.

Pathogenesis

It is apparent from the preceding data that the cases of arterial embolism that result in the above-reported metabolic complications exhibit different features from those of the common clinical form. Among the several underlying factors differentiating these severe forms from the common clinical form are the following:

1. A massive obliterating process that leads to an "absolute" ischemia, not necessarily related to its duration because the clinical metabolic sydrome often assumes an "explosive" onset
2. A poor or ineffective collateral network, as a corollary of the massive occlusion of the main arterial tree (Fig. 32-13)
3. Widespread irreversible ischemic lesions of the skeletal muscles
4. Combined severe hemodynamic and metabolic phenomena

In cases of mild and transient hemodynamic and metabolic effects, by contrast, the severe myonephropathic-metabolic syndrome appears to be less frequent.

The pathogenic mechanism of the metabolic events appear to be a successive series of biochemical alterations.

The common denominator of most of the changes is the initiating severe ischemia of the skeletal muscle, as mentioned previously. The onset of these alterations is sometimes difficult to assess clinically. If muscle tenderness and rigidity are considered as an index, the muscle involvement must be present at a very early stage and is probably the first sign in the chain of events leading to the biochemical and metabolic changes. Among these, CPK and myoglobin are the most important chemical indicators of ischemia. In some of my cases in which the patient was operated on within 4 to 6 hours, the muscles appeared edematous and pale. It is of interest to note that Carlstrom, a veterinarian, described an equine paroxysmal myoglobinuria syndrome in which the iliopsoas and the quadriceps femoris muscles appeared edematous and pale, a condition apparently caused by thrombosis of the abdominal aorta.

Microscopically, there is a great variety of morphologic changes of the muscle fibers, ranging from slight to moderate degenerative changes to actual necrosis. As a result of these morphologic alterations, chemical changes occur at the cellular level where substances such as myoglobin, potassium, and CPK are released into the blood and lymph streams. *The basic morphologic derangement resides in the increased permability of the membrane, which is due to decreased ATP levels resulting from ischemia of the membrane.*

Since most of these patients display metabolic acidosis from the beginning of the syndrome in the ischemic phase, the acidosis will result in a predisposition to the precipitation of myoglobin in the tubules. The therapeutic implication is clear and indicates the need for therapeutic alkalinization to prevent or counteract the acidosis, as already emphasized on several occasions.

Elevated CPK levels, which will vary according to the degree of muscle damage, and hyperkalemia, which may result in variable degrees from the membrane disturbance and from the potassium in the muscle fibers, constitute two major markers of ischemia. The awareness of this and the other biochemical complications resulting from muscle ischemia should evoke appropriate therapeutic measures for the prevention of a serious outcome.

Therapeutic Orientation

The management of the metabolic complications associated with the syndrome of rhabdomyolysis must be oriented concomitantly to local and systemic manifestations. Aware-

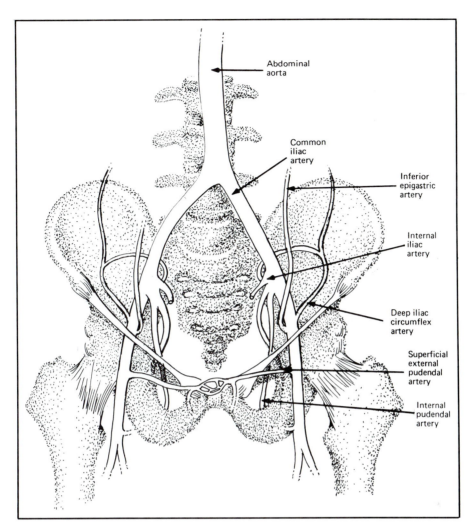

Figure 32-12. The aortoiliac-femoral arterial tree. These segments provide the arterial supply to large masses of skeletal muscles. As a result, the myonephropathic-metabolic syndrome is more prone to occur in these areas. As indicated in this diagram, this syndrome occurred in 36.7% of the cases in the abdominal aorta, in the common iliac in 9.5%, and in the femoral in 6.3%. These percentages seem to correlate with a muscle mass irrigated by the various segments.

ness of potential complications represents the key to prevention, diagnosis, and immediate and specific treatment.

Two major signs must be first ascertained: (1) the presence of dark red urine containing myoglobin, as detected by the tests previously described, and (2) rigidity of the calf muscles, including edema of the extremity due to severe muscle ischemia. First, the essential biochemical parameters from both the systemic circulation and the involved limb, such as the pH, myoglobin, CPK, P_{CO_2}, P_{O_2}, and blood volume, are to be ascertained. Under these circumstances, arterial and venous infusion should be established without delay.

Initial Management. Without going into the details of the various principles of treatment, it is essential to point out that fluid replacement and restoration of electrolyte balance is a first step for appropriate management of blood loss, with fluids and electrolytes used in immediate management.

Whether the color of the urine is dark red and myoglobin is detectable or not, sodium bicarbonate must be used to correct the possible or definite presence of acidosis.

If there is evidence of rigidity of the skeletal muscle in the calf or higher, fasciotomy is mandatory, even before arterial repair. The fasciotomy of the leg may involve one or three compartments, or all four, depending on the extent of the edema of the muscles and the viability of the tissue observed.

Operative Procedures. After these measures, thromboembolectomy or any other necessary reconstructive arterial procedure should be undertaken at that point without delay.

In the *postrevascularization stage*, after the early reestablishment of blood flow of the acutely ischemic extremity, prevention of muscle damage by the use of mannitol and by alkalinization of the patient should be continued during and after the operation, until the blood pH, especially in the involved limb, has been restored to a normal level. This treatment is even more essential if myoglobin is present or suspected, because it precipitates readily in the acid milieu of the renal tubules. Concurrently, reestablishment of electrolyte balance, including especially reducing serum potassium to normal levels, is essential. In the presence of

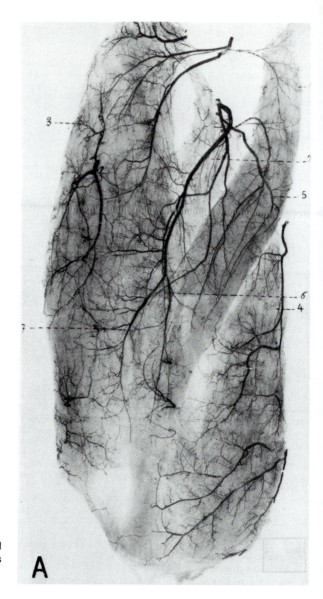

Figure 32-13. A. The intramuscular arterial supply to the rectus femoris and the vastus muscles.

A

severe renal dysfunction—oliguria or anuria—hemodialysis, rather than peritoneal dialysis, should be started until renal function can be restored. This may sometimes take several days to several weeks.

In the presence of suspected free radical damage to the skeletal muscle after reperfusion, mannitol, as already mentioned, plus superoxide dismutase, allopurinol, or catalase, depending on which of the antioxidants are available, should be used without delay to prevent further damage to skeletal muscle.

Amputation, which is necessary in the presence of frank gangrene, is sometimes indicated even in the absence of frank necrosis as a prophylactic measure to eliminate the source of metabolites from the ischemic skeletal muscles, more particularly if severe and extensive rhabdomyolysis is present.

During *fasciotomy*, which may be performed before revascularization of the limb, the nonviable skeletal muscle, especially in delayed procedures, should be excised, with only the viable tissue left attached to the limb, if feasible. Occasionally one may excise a large mass of muscle down

to the interosseous membrane. Healing by secondary intention may be achieved, and the limb may be salvaged if revascularization is effective.

Prognosis of these revascularization cases depends on a number of factors, which were indicated above.

The brief description of the therapeutic orientation in arterial embolism may serve as a prototype for other cases of acute arterial occlusion, descriptions of which will follow in the next few sections of this chapter.

Nonembolic Acute Arterial Occlusions

As mentioned earlier, the most common causes of acute arterial occlusion, besides arterial embolism, that may be associated with the metabolic syndrome due to rhabdomyolysis include the following:

1. Acute thrombosis of the nonaneurysmal abdominal aorta
2. Acute thrombosis of the abdominal aortic aneurysm
3. Cross-clamping of major arteries during reconstructive surgery

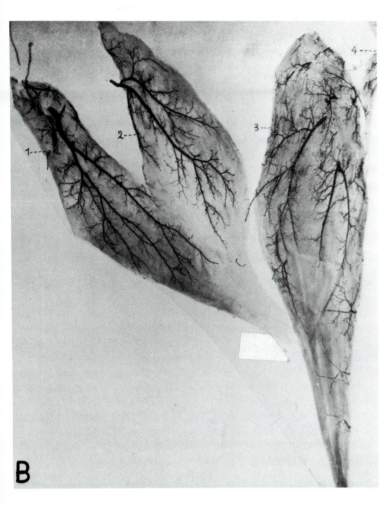

Fig. 32-13 cont. B. The intramuscular arterial supply to the gastrocnemius, soleus, and plantares. Involvement of these intramuscular branches from whatever cause—thrombotic, embolic, or traumatic—results in overwhelming pathologic changes and is directly responsible for the degree of severity of the rhabdomyolytic process. (*From Salmon M and Dor J: Publ. Masson & Cie, Paris, 1933. From Haimovici H: Arterial circulation of the extremities, in Structure and Function of the Circulation, vol. 1, Plenum Press, New York, 1980, p 425.*)

4. Arterial cannulation during cardiopulmonary bypass
5. Arterial trauma
6. Ischemic muscle necrosis (the "crush syndrome")
7. Nontraumatic and nonocclusive arterial rhabdomyolysis with acute renal failure, which includes a wide spectrum of entities in which diffuse muscle cell injuries predominate but in which extensive muscular necrosis may occasionally occur with the metabolic syndrome. These entities, described in other sections of this textbook, will be mentioned here only insofar as their metabolic complications are concerned.

Acute Abdominal Aortic Occlusions

Acute occlusion of the terminal abdominal aorta and its bifurcation displays clinical manifestations that most often are of a catastrophic nature. Two major etiologic factors are generally responsible for this condition: (1) saddle embolus of the aortic bifurcation and (2) acute arterial thrombosis.

In a previously published review compiled of a total of 1,576 cases of acute arterial occlusion of the lower extremities, 892 (56.6%) were due to embolism and 684 (43.4%) were due to acute thrombosis. Of these, the relative incidence of acute occlusion of the aorta due to embolism and that due to acute thrombosis also differed. The former occurred in 14.9% and the latter in 7.5%. It therefore appears that the nature of acute aortic occlusion is predominantly embolic.

Acute infrarenal aortic thrombosis is less frequent than embolic occlusion and is also infrequent in contrast to the common entity of chronic aortoiliac occlusive disease (Leriche syndrome). Its sudden occurrence has the earmarks of a catastrophic event, not unlike a massive saddle embolism, which it mimics in all its clinical manifestations. The physical findings are similar to those encountered in aortic saddle embolism: absent pulses below the umbilicus, coldness, mottled cyanosis of the skin distal to the midportion of the abdomen and of the buttocks, and numbness and loss of motion of both lower extremities.

A suspected diagnosis of either embolic or thrombotic occlusion of the abdominal aorta mandates the immediate use of intravenously administered heparin, as well as fluids, including Ringer's lactate solution and sodium bicarbonate, given in large amounts in an attempt to overcome potential metabolic acidosis, which is frequently encountered but rarely mentioned in published discussions of this subject. This treatment approach has a double advantage. First, it provides the necessary fluids for the patient, who is often hypovolemic. Second and more important, it provides the necessary antidote to the metabolic acidosis and prevents the myoglobin from precipitating into the tubules, thus preventing renal failure. Although myoglobin is one of the important metabolites released by the ischemic muscle, other biochemical factors, released by the same muscles through the damaged myofibrillar membranes, are rarely mentioned. Levels of CPK, potassium, calcium, LDH, and SGOT, for example, are significant from diagnostic and prognostic points of view. All these biochemical factors will determine not only the viability of the limb but also the survival of the patient.

Time Interval to Revascularization. Early or immediate recognition of the acute condition is essential for the successful management of acute embolic or thrombotic occlusions of the abdominal aorta. Recognition of the diagnosis in acute thrombosis appears to be somewhat delayed in comparison with that in acute embolic occlusion. Thus the time from the onset of symptoms until revascularization of the extremity averaged 10.3 hours in embolic cases, in contrast to 26.1 hours in cases of acute thrombosis (Littooy and Baker). The delay between the onset of the symptoms and the revascularization of the extremities results, in many cases, in metabolic complications due to acute rhabdomyolysis, as reported by these authors. Thus renal failure and mortality rates are much higher in cases of acute thrombosis that is recognized late than in cases of acute embolic occlusion that are seen earlier. Renal failure occurred in 11 patients reported by Littooy and Baker. Death occurred in 8 of 11 patients, probably because of acute myoglobinuria with acute tubular necrosis. Although these findings were not mentioned specifically in this article, it was inferred that "as a result of muscle cell ischemia and cell death, these would lead to the release of myoglobin, potassium and lactic acid." Myoglobin develops and peaks about 3 hours after reperfusion, which may lead to precipitation into the renal tubules if the urine is concentrated and acidic.

If preliminary findings suggest embolism, one may attempt a thromboembolectomy through a transfemoral approach. With few exceptions, however, in acute thrombotic lesions this will fail to achieve a forceful and sustained arterial flow, indicating the nonembolic nature of the occlusion. Nonoperative treatment of acute aortic embolic or thrombotic occlusion leads to a fatal outcome in approximately 75% of cases.

Because of the potential for metabolic complications and because of the risks involved, the *prognosis* is extremely serious, not only for the salvage of the lower extremity but also for the survival of the patient. This is in contrast to the prognosis in arterial occlusion below the inguinal ligament, even when etiologic factors are similar. This fact is consistent with the well-documented prognostic rule regarding the size of the occluded vessel: the larger the acutely occluded artery, the greater the potential for loss of limb and for the death of the patient as a result of metabolic complications.

Acute Thrombosis of Abdominal Aortic Aneurysms

In contrast to the well-known tendency to rupture, sudden, complete occlusion of an abdominal aneurysm sac is a somewhat less frequent event, but it is no less dangerous. A few recent publications have disclosed such complications associated with severe clinical and metabolic manifestations and high mortality rates. Since 1974, when Johnson et al. collected 10 cases from the literature and added seven of

their own, cases of this nature have been reported in the literature, especially from 1981 to the present. It is somewhat surprising that with the recently increasing incidence of aortic aneurysms, acute thrombosis of the terminal abdominal aorta is not being reported more frequently.

Clinical manifestations are those of sudden paraplegia, with mottling noted to the level of the umbilicus or the iliac crests. In addition to the symptoms and findings of severe ischemia and paraplegia, a significant number of these cases result in death related to renal complications. The immediate cause of death was irreversible shock, myocardial infarction, cerebral vascular accidents, and, as mentioned, renal failure. Myoglobinuria due to severe ischemia of the muscles most likely played an important part in renal tubular dysfunction, as noted by Johnson et al. in a few other, more recent reports.

The differential diagnosis in these cases is with saddle embolus, acute atherosclerotic thrombosis of the terminal abdominal aorta, acute aortic dissection, and acute thrombosis of an abdominal aortic aneurysm. The prognosis of acute thrombosis of an abdominal aneurysm appears to be catastrophic, and the condition presents a major surgical emergency. The chosen procedure may depend on the nature of the lesions and the condition of the patient.

Because of the metabolic complications, which are among the more serious events and therefore should be anticipated, surgery consisting of direct aneurysmectomy is not the wisest option. A bilateral axillofemoral bypass and vigorous treatment of the metabolic complications are the important therapeutic gestures to undertake. In the event that renal thrombosis is also diagnosed, dysobstruction is lifesaving when the thrombotic process extends to a critical level involving the origin of renal vessels. Presumption of this condition is based on the presence of oliguria that is unresponsive to fluid challenge, prompting the performance of preoperative aortography.

It is important to point out, without going into details presented elsewhere, that acute, complete thrombosis of abdominal aortic aneurysms is, first, a rare but catastrophic event with a frequently dramatic presentation similar to that of an acute Leriche syndrome. Ultrasound examination should be used to delineate the existence and size of the aneurysm, and management should be an emergent procedure consisting of not only systemic heparinization but also rapid restoration of fluids, correction of metabolic acidosis, and assessment of the renal response to intravascular fluid replenishment. Axillobifemoral grafting, instead of aneurysm replacement, should be considered in most instances where an operative risk is too great to enter the abdomen.

Arterial Clamping During Reconstructive Vascular Surgery

Declamping of a major artery (aorta, iliac, femoral) after temporary occlusion may result in mild to severe hypotension, often associated with variable degrees of metabolic change. The sudden decrease in blood pressure, known as the "declamping phenomenon" or "declamping shock," has been studied extensively both in laboratory animals and to some extent in conjunction with human reconstructive arterial surgery.

Experimental Data
The results of declamping after experimentally induced occlusion of the abdominal aorta are dependent essentially on the method and extent of the associated arterial occlusions.

Isolated Aortic Clamping. In temporary aortic cross-clamping the hemodynamic and metabolic changes are usually mild and transient. Occluding the infrarenal aorta in dogs for 1 hour, Strandness et al. found, at declamping, a 23% decrease of the average mean aortic pressure and a 21% decrease of the average cardiac output. Associated with those findings was a decreased hind leg volume after clamping and an increased volume within 60 seconds after declamping, returning later to normal values. However, Baue and McClerkin, also using 1-hour cross-clamping, found no evidence for a change in myocardial function, as measured by ventricular contractile force. After release of the clamp, both arterial and venous pH fell—from 7.38 to 7.28 and from 7.31 to 7.16, respectively. This acidosis lasted 5 to 15 minutes. The acute drop in blood pressure was attributed to a translocation or to transient pooling of blood into a temporarily hypovolemic vascular bed. The magnitude of pressure drop was unrelated to the length of time of clamping, which ranged from a few seconds to 2 to 3 minutes. The declamping phenomenon in these studies was shown to be prevented or completely eliminated by the use of a vasopressor distal to the clamp immediately before its removal.

Combined Aortic Clamping with Multiple Ligations of Major Branches. To obtain an experimental setting approaching clinical situations, investigators designed experiments to exclude not only the aorta but also multiple branches between the renal arteries and the aortic bifurcation with its distal branches. The results thus obtained differed significantly. Thus Engler, using a combination technique consisting of cross-clamping with multiple-branch ligation, obtained sustained hypotension associated with hypoxia and acidosis. These changes were prevented by using a small shunt from the aorta above the point of occlusion to the aorta below. These experiments strongly suggested that the changes were due to inadequate arterial pressure perfusion of the muscles distal to the clamped aorta. Lim et al., Perry, and Provan et al. essentially confirmed these findings.

The experiments discussed above induced only temporary and transient changes; a more profound degree of ischemia appeared necessary to achieve results that would parallel those in human subjects. Thus a greater number of branches must be excluded from the vascular system. Winninger, when excluding, in addition, all major branches below the femoral artery, was able to reproduce hemodynamic and metabolic changes similar to those observed in acute occlusions in human subjects. The declamping hypotension reached the level of 35 to 41% of the preclamping level, and the arterial pH was markedly decreased, together with a severe systemic acidosis. Stipa et al., using an even more extensive arterial exclusion technique, showed that during the declamping of the femoral arteries after a 10-hour ischemia, there was progressive acidosis and at least a 50% increase in limb volume associated with shock and rapid death.

In summary, to reproduce experimentally the hemodynamic and metabolic changes seen in clinical situations, one must obtain a wider interruption of the arterial supply than is obtained with the simple cross-clamping of a major artery.

Human Data
The human data obtained with arterial clamping in vascular surgery reflect the above findings to some extent. Although metabolic alterations may be noted after the declamping of most major arteries, serious hemodynamic changes usually occur only after replacement of an aortic aneurysm.

Muscle hypoxia due to chronic occlusive disease in patients with only claudicating limbs is associated with a decrease in pH and an increase in blood lactate and pyruvate levels. During reconstructive vascular surgery for such patients, arterial clamping has been shown to accentuate the oxygen deficit of the tissues distal to the clamp. The extent to which such cross-clamping of the aortoiliac and femoropopliteal segments produces significant metabolic changes during reconstructive arterial surgery is not widely known, because it has been seldom reported.

Recently, O'Donnell et al. published a study on metabolic evaluation of 35 patients with chronic occlusive arterial disease, based primarily on muscle surface measurements of pH using the medial belly of the gastrocnemius. Their observations on pH appeared to correlate well with the clinical degree of ischemia. Thus tissue metabolism of lactate, glucose, and oxygen showed no difference between control cases and the claudication group. By contrast, a lower pH value, with a significant increase in lactate release and in glucose and oxygen extraction, was observed in the groups with rest pain and ischemic gangrene. After aortofemoral or femoropopliteal arterial reconstruction, muscle surface pH values were comparable with those of the control group (7.42 ± 0.05). Although these pH determinations are indirect measurements of tissue perfusion, O'Donnell considers them to be a sensitive index and a useful clinical approach to metabolic evaluation in muscle ischemia.

Sorlie et al., in a study of metabolic changes during *prolonged clamping of the common femoral artery* for femoropopliteal reconstruction, also reported significant changes. Regardless of the degree of preexisting chronic occlusive disease, femoral cross-clamping for 80 to 180 minutes represents an important superimposed acute ischemia. A battery of biochemical determinations was carried out before, during, and after the release of the femoral clamp. The pH, P_{CO_2}, and P_{O_2} values, the O_2 saturation, and the lactate, LDH, and CPK levels were studied in the popliteal venous effluent and the systemic blood of eight patients. Marked acidosis with a rise in lactate, phosphate, and creatinine levels was found in all patients. The pH value decreased to a mean value of 7.18, and the P_{CO_2} value increased from

45 to 62 mm Hg. There was no statistically significant correlation between the occlusion time and the degree of hypoxia. Of the electrolytes, the potassium concentration increased by 20% in the venous effluent, in comparison with the preocclusion level. Of the muscle enzymes, only the CPK activity increased, gradually reaching its peak after 8 to 15 hours (mean value 700 U/L) and returning to normal values in 5 days. As a rule, the maximum CPK level correlated well with the femoral occlusion time. The significance of these metabolic changes, as judged by the CPK activity in the eight patients, was moderate, and no clinical repercussions were apparent.

Cross-clamping of the infrarenal abdominal aorta, which induces ischemia of a larger muscle mass than does cross-clamping of the common femoral artery, was reported by Andersson and Eklof and their associates. As in femoral artery clamping during reconstructive aortic surgery, the necessary cross-clamping of the aorta will temporarily lower the distal blood flow still further. The hemodynamic and metabolic changes thus induced decrease further and more severely in those patients having aortic aneurysm repair than in those operated on for occlusive aortic disease. These studies, carried out over a period of several years, were performed to determine disturbances in the energy-rich phosphagen metabolites in skeletal muscle of the ischemic limb and in the efferent venous blood. The hemodynamic and metabolic changes were reported to occur on aortic reconstructive surgery in 14 patients, 12 having occlusive aortic disease and two undergoing surgery for aortic aneurysm repair. Occlusion time of the investigated leg lasted for 69 to 150 minutes (mean 107). Before cross-clamping, and before and 30 minutes after aortic declamping, muscle biopsy specimens were obtained from the lateral vastus muscle of the ischemic leg. Glycogen, lactate, PCr, creatine (Cr), ATP, adenosine diphosphate (ADP), and AMP were measured by means of enzymatic fluorometric techniques. The results of the cross-clamping and declamping showed that lactate content increased fourfold and glycogen levels decreased. Although the PCr content fell, the muscle ATP concentration could not be maintained. However, the muscle creatinine level did not significantly decline. Thirty minutes after aortic declamping, the metabolic changes were more dramatic. However, in spite of recirculation of the limb, the lactate level was still high. Levels of both ATP and ADP decreased significantly, together with PCr and creatine content. Except for one patient with an abdominal aneurysm, no declamping hypotension was noted in these cases. There was a significant postclamping increase in mean lactate levels, as already mentioned, and in the pyruvate concentration in the iliac venous blood over the values noted before aortic clamping. The values for lactate and pyruvate ranged from 1.49 to 2.80 and from 0.08 to 0.19, respectively, 60 minutes after declamping. The metabolite concentration and the muscle samples 20 minutes after aortic declamping disclosed several significant alterations. The glucose, lactate, and pyruvate levels and the lactate/pyruvate ratio had all increased, whereas PCr, ATP, ADP, and AMP levels showed a significant decline to 80% of the preclamping values. These investigators postulated that their findings "might indicate damage in the mitochondria and the cellular membranes in skeletal muscle after temporary arterial occlusion," which is in accordance with the conclusions of other investigators.

The plasma concentrations of CPK, creatine, and hypoxanthine in efferent venous blood from the investigated limb showed that although hypoxanthine arteriovenous differences are small, the plasma creatine content was found to increase throughout the procedure. On the other hand, the PCr level did not change significantly. The hypoxanthine concentration rose during ischemia and the initial reperfusion but returned to basal level after 10 minutes of recirculation. The hypoxanthine arteriovenous differences indicate a sharp outflow of this substance on the release of the clamp and during the first 5 to 10 minutes of reoxygenation. In brief, in patients undergoing aortic repair, the mean muscle blood flow is decreased by 50 to 90% during cross-clamping, depending on the size of persistent blood flow through the developed collateral vessels. Thus a limited supply of oxygen and exogenous substrate is still possible. As mentioned, there are several changes in the phosphagen components, but all metabolites return to basal level within 5 minutes of recirculation except for the lactate content. As shown by these investigators and others, the cellular transmembrane potential seems to lag behind in restoration and is not normalized until an hour later. The cross-clamping in the latest study induced only minor changes. One of the important conclusions from the latest study is that a significant rise in the creatine level in efferent venous blood occurs during reperfusion, which, in the opinion of the investigators, strongly supports the concept of leakage through disrupted muscle cellular membranes.

Current observations confirm the possibility of injury to the muscles in the presence of an oxygen-dependent autolytic degradation of the tissue resulting from the low remaining perfusion. The formation of oxygen radicals appears to be a contributing factor, as pointed out elsewhere in this monograph.

In accordance with recent concepts pertaining to free radicals, these authors adapted their own thinking to this new understanding to the reperfusion syndrome. It appears, therefore, that it is not sufficient simply to restore effective perfusion of previously ischemic tissue; it is also necessary to protect membrane function at the time of reperfusion. Without mentioning the solutions to these problems, however, they mention that the multipharmacologic approach seems to be necessary. Probably severely ischemic limbs should be specifically treated before and during revascularization to avoid the adverse results of reoxygenation.

Abdominal Aortic Aneurysm: Ruptured Lesions and Metabolic Complications. Unlike the hemodynamic and metabolic responses to clamping and declamping of the aorta for aortoiliac occlusive disease, those observed in aortic aneurysms appear more complex by far. Ever since the early days of this surgery, cross-clamping of the infrarenal aorta has received greater attention because of potential metabolic and renal complications. A great variety of opinions have been expressed concerning the mechanism of "declamping shock," including redistribution of blood volume below the clamp, a fall in cardiac output, and liberation of a vasodilator substance from the hypoxic tissues during aortic occlusion. It is likely that more than one of these factors, and perhaps others, are responsible for these complications, the most recently incriminated being prostaglandin E.

Mansberger et al., studying the metabolic responses in 15 patients undergoing *elective resection* of abdominal aortic aneurysms, consistently found a "washout acidosis" after aortic declamping. This was evidenced by a significant fall in pH, elevation of lactate and pyruvate levels in their absolute values, and by excess lactate during occlusion. The venous P_{O_2} value and its saturation were profoundly decreased.

In *ruptured* aortic aneurysms, metabolic and renal repercussions are manifold, especially in patients with severe shock or prolonged cross-clamping or in those undergoing massive transfusion. Of these complications, renal failure represents the single most important cause of death, with the mortality rate ranging from 50 to 90%. Several mechanisms have been postulated to account for the renal complications: aortorenal reflexes with renovascular spasm, renal atheromatous embolization, and hypovolemic shock associated with multisystem failures. Although some of the mechanisms, such as the aortorenal vasoconstrictor stimuli, were not corroborated, hypovolemic shock is recognized as playing an important etiologic role in prerenal failure. The sudden decrease in renal perfusion associated with myoglobinuria provides the intrinsic tubular factor ultimately responsible for acute renal failure. The incidence of the latter factor, rarely mentioned in the current literature, is difficult to ascertain. Admittedly, a large number of other factors contribute to renal complications, of which rhabdomyolysis and myoglobinuria may play a significant role in a number of cases as yet undetermined. McCombs and Roberts reported 17 cases of acute renal failure in a series of 398 cases of abdominal aortic aneurysms, nine of which were resected electively and eight after rupture. The overall incidence was 2.5% after elective operations and 21% after rupture. Of the 17 patients, nine had peripheral embolization, with known myonecrosis in four. Other factors, however, such as prolonged cross-clamping and preoperative-intraoperative hypotension in 11 other patients, were likely to have contributed to the renal problem. The surgeon's ability to deal with the multiple factors leading to renal complications is often limited, but renal protective measures during aortic cross-clamping must be vigorously applied against such complications as acidosis, myoglobinuria, and hyperkalemia. In some cases, extracorporeal shunting during aneurysmal repair may be considered, as advocated recently.

Arterial Cannulation During Cardiopulmonary Bypass

Although cannulation of a common femoral artery for extracorporeal circulation is less frequent than in the past, it may result in metabolic acidosis and more severe metabolic complications because of prolonged ischemia of the lower extremity. Although such cases have been reported only rarely, one should remain aware of a potential complication during cardiac surgery.

This complication of open-heart surgery is due primarily to prolonged femoral artery occlusion. Several reports have appeared in the literature pointing out catastrophic complications that may lead not only to loss of a limb but also to loss of the patient's life. Because of this possibility, systematic search for myoglobinuria after cardiac surgery, especially in prolonged procedures, may help detect more instances than are presently suspected.

Kagen, in 1977, reported six cases of myoglobinuria in a group of 16 patients after open-heart surgery for valvular replacement. Kugimiya and associates reported similar cases of cardiopulmonary bypass complicated by ischemia of the lower extremity after femoral artery cannulation. Massive ischemic myopathy with myoglobinuria occurred in eight patients, or 1.9% of his 420 patients. Most of Kugimiya's patients were an average age of 10 years, ranging from 4 to 17 years. They had congenital heart disease, and cardiopulmonary bypass surgery ranged from 52 minutes to 2 hours 42 minutes. Kugimiya reported that in the last 444 cases of cardiopulmonary bypass with femoral artery cannulation or direct aortic cannulation, the cooling of the extremity was helpful in preventing the appearance of the myonephropathic-metabolic syndrome.

Although such complications as those reported in connection with cardiopulmonary bypass and femoral artery cannulation are encountered infrequently, because of awareness of them and because of much better handling of the ischemic metabolites, these cases are becoming less common.

In connection with arterial cannulation during cardiopulmonary bypass, it may be mentioned that certain reports in the literature raise serious questions about the validity of the diagnosis and management. Thus it is known that a number of renal complications occur as a result of these open heart procedures. Whether renal dysfunction after a cardiac surgical procedure is due to myoglobinuria in these cases remains a problem open to question in the absence of specific biochemical documentation. One may only speculate on the possible contribution of myoglobinuria to a number of renal complications reported in connection with open heart surgery. Abel et al., for instance, in reviewing the records of 507 survivors of open heart surgery, found that 198 patients (39%) had serious renal complications, some with acute tubular necrosis, the mortality rate was 30.3%. Except for blood urea nitrogen and creatinine levels, no other biochemical determinations, including myoglobin, were mentioned. Awareness of this muscle metabolite, which may cause some cases of renal failure in open heart surgery, may help to prevent such a complication if it is treated vigorously before irreversible damage occurs.

Vascular Trauma

Arterial injuries, whether they are penetrating or blunt, may often induce a syndrome of acute arterial occlusion. As in cases of acute thromboembolism, traumatic arterial interruption may still be amenable to surgical correction many hours after the event, provided that adequate collateral supply is still available by maintaining viability. Unfortunately, an arterial injury may often become aggravated by a number of associated features induced by the original trauma.

It is not within the scope of this section to delve into these associated lesions, which are clearly described in Chapter 31. Suffice it to mention that in the present context, the concomitant evaluation of these lesions is essential because they may contribute significantly to the myonecrosis-renal-metabolic syndrome. The main subject of this section, therefore, deals only briefly with the events relevant to the syndrome of complications that are mentioned above.

The clinical picture of arterial trauma varies greatly because of a large number of factors. Rhabdomyolysis and its biochemical complications seem to occur infrequently in simple arterial injuries, in contrast to those associated with other lesions. Indeed, development of the metabolic-renal syndrome due to arterial trauma is usually the result of the following:

1. Delayed repair
2. Multiple traumatic lesions
3. Fractures and dislocations
4. Soft tissue trauma
5. Venous injuries
6. Nerve lesions
7. Traumatic shock.

The two most significant determinants of the outcome are extensive soft tissue trauma, involving primarily the skeletal muscles, and delayed vascular repair. The resulting clinical picture is not unlike that of a crush syndrome. It is important to point out, without going into detail, that few publications on major arterial trauma deal with metabolic complications resulting from these skeletal muscle lesions. Thus Robbs and Baker, for example, reported arterial reconstruction in 14 cases, resulting in eight salvage and six major amputations, but failed to mention the metabolic components of the clinical picture of these patients, even though clinically it appeared that these complications were undoubtedly associated with biochemical changes due to skeletal muscle injury occurring concomitantly with the arterial injuries.

However, a few publications, especially in the European literature, have pointed out the significance of these metabolic complications and acute renal failure. Unawareness of the metabolic complications resulting from skeletal muscle injury is responsible for the lack of reports on this subject. Of course, it is possible that such complications do not occur when patients' lesions are treated without delay, as they were, for example, during the Vietnam war, when there were no reports of any of the biochemical or renal complications. This is only a presumption, however, and it is not based on any statistical studies that would provide the necessary data to support such a contention.

The basic principles for management of acute arterial occlusions and of the crush syndrome are obviously applicable in vascular trauma with metabolic complications. The use of hypertonic mannitol, in addition to other fluids, is important for replacement of blood and electrolytes. Revascularization of the limb will depend, of course, on the general condition of the patient and the extent of the arterial lesions. The viability of the extremity and the absence of advanced rigor of the muscles are clear indications that arterial surgery should be performed without delay. Furthermore, swelling of the limbs is most often due to the compartment syndrome and requires wide fasciotomies.

Even in the presence of rigor, revascularization of the limb should be undertaken without delay. Primary amputation may be avoided if the muscles and bones can be handled without sacrificing the limb before an attempt at these conservative measures. However, in the presence of frank myonecrosis involving large muscle mass, primary amputation may be unavoidable. By contrast, in the presence of focal myonecrosis, excision of the lesion may not represent a major contraindication to revascularization.

It is important to restate that prevention of reperfusion side effects must be kept in mind. Mannitol, or superoxide dismutase, allopurinol, or catalase, whichever is available and indicated, must be administered before vascular repair and concurrently with all the other procedures designed to combat the biochemical-induced metabolic complications.

ISCHEMIC MUSCLE NECROSIS: THE CRUSH SYNDROME

The crush syndrome, due to a compression of a limb beneath debris for several hours, occur during war or in civilian accidents (e.g., automobile accidents or debris falling from a demolished house). The original impression from these cases, observed especially during the blitz of Great Britain during World War II, was that the patient was suffering from an entity akin to "shock." Shortly afterward, it was found that the clinical syndrome of shock was only one of several complications.

At the level of the injury of the limb, edema increases either spontaneously or after intravenous infusion of fluid. Occasionally, fasciotomy was carried out along the course of the artery, with much serous fluid seeping from the wound and pale, necrotic muscle bulging out. Of great significance, however, from a pathologic and prognostic point of view, is the renal dysfunction in these patients. On admission to an emergency department, such a patient's urine pH is as low as 4.6 and displays dark brown sediment consisting of acid hematin granules. After the urine is centrifuged, the pigment shows a benzidine-positive reaction, as demonstrated by experimental studies published by Duncan and Blalock.

From a pathologic point of view, it was stressed by Bywaters and subsequent observers that the essential lesion of crushing injury in the muscle leads to necrosis. This may be due to ischemia caused by direct compression of the muscle, or it may be due to ischemia from interference with the main arterial supply, by sudden spasm, thrombosis, or rupture or obstruction of the vessels.

The treatment of these cases was similar to what is being done today to treat shock or the so-called crush syndrome. It consists of the administration of fluids and an alkali such as sodium bicarbonate (the treatment of shock consisting of hydration and alkalinization, as mentioned above), to overcome "oligemic shock." Shock is found in spite of the blood pressure reading, which remains normal for a time because of vasoconstriction. One of the most important complications is renal failure, the treatment of which consisted of infusion with insulin and dextrose. This proved to be of some value, but the most important procedure is present-day hemodialysis.

Bywaters and his comtemporary British colleagues have been credited with providing evidence of the biochemical changes that result from skeletal muscle damage. As stated earlier, the evidence of "traumatization" that Cannon and Bayliss obtained in their experiments, in which they produced shock, is to some extent similar to that of Bywaters and the British team, who observed injuries to the skeletal muscles during the battle of Britain. It is difficult to differentiate biologically what was meant by traumatic shock, as described by Cannon in the initial stage of this process, from that of the crush syndrome, seen also in the initial symptoms and signs that were seen subsequently during the blitz of London and other parts of Great Britain. The biochemical findings in this syndrome have been of great impetus in the study of traumatic shock and other conditions that had been observed in civilian patients, such as acute arterial occlusions or vascular trauma, as well as other nontraumatic lesions in which the rhabdomyolytic process dominated as the initiating cause of these changes. The pathogenesis of myoglobinuria and of other biochemical changes that occur as a result of traumatic lesions of the muscles remains to be analyzed and explained. The next few contributions will attempt to answer these questions.

These biochemical changes were actually demonstrated by laboratory experiments in which skeletal muscle injuries were produced by several methods. Montagnani and Simeone have reported experiments in 1953 and described in detail the time relationships regarding the appearance of myoglobin in body fluids after release of limb ischemia produced by tourniquets placed across the thigh and hip.

Other types of experiments were carried out by American (Thompson and Campbell) and, more recently, by a few Japanese investigators. All of them have demonstrated the role of injury to the skeletal muscle that results in a biochemical response leading to a metabolic syndrome, as already described in this chapter.

All these experimental studies have essentially reproduced the crush syndrome, consisting of declamping hypotension, hyperkalemia, and acute tubular degeneration of the kidneys. In addition, the earlier expeiiments showed that "washing out," or perfusion, of the ischemic limbs before release of the damaged muscle could decrease significantly the degree of myoglobinemia, myoglobinuria, and hemoglobinuria. More recent studies have also shown that renal function is altered in proportion to the severity of induced ischemia after revascularization in dogs, in which ischemia was induced by a tourniquet applied around the groin and hind limbs.

All these experiments confirm the clinical observations that have been alluded to in the earlier part of this section.

NONTRAUMATIC AND NONOCCLUSIVE ARTERIAL RHABDOMYOLYSIS WITH ACUTE RENAL FAILURE

Nontraumatic muscle injuries, although they have no connection with acute arterial occlusions, have great clinical significance because of the rhabdomyolysis and acute renal failure associated with them. Originally, these cases were observed in such medical subspecialties as nephrology, neurology, and biochemistry. These patients were seen because of skeletal muscle complaints associated with urinary changes, including the presence of myoglobin. Recently in medical subspecialties an increasing number of patients have been noted to display the above-mentioned syndrome of myoglobinemia and myoglobinuria in association with rhabdomyolytic processes. At the present time, it appears that such cases are more frequent than was originally suspected.

The presence of rhabdomyolysis in nontraumatic and nonarterial occlusive disease is of great significance because of the serious potential complications of the skeletal muscle injury and the renal failure.

The specific case studies demonstrating the presence of myoglobinuria and rhabdomyolysis reported evidence of myoglobin in the urine, with an estimation of the serum CPK and aldolase levels and a report of increased serum levels of potassium, uric acid, and calcium. A few of the important references concerning these entities are herein included for readers who are interested in this group of so-called medical conditions with these metabolic complications.

A great variety of medical conditions are responsible for nontraumatic rhabdomyolysis, including, for example, a large number of myopathies, grand mal seizures, prolonged coma (the latter related especially to drug abuse and its associated toxic effects or to muscle injury due to compression during immobility in the course of the comatose stage), infections (either bacterial or viral), burns, epilepsy, and poisoning with various metals.

Although rhabdomyolysis is common in all these entities, myoglobinuric renal failure has not always been demonstrable or demonstrated, probably because of the method of testing the urine or the blood for the presence of myoglobin. Some of these methods are probably not as sensitive as others, one factor being the competence of the laboratory. It appears, however, that the renal failure noted in all these cases may have been mostly myoglobinuric or nonmyoglobinuric associated with rhabdomyolysis.

Among these conditions, which are mostly nonmedical, inflammatory myopathies and myoglobinurias have been reported in association with a great variety of etiologic factors. It is not the intent of this chapter to review or incorporate all the varieties of cases that have been published in the past few years. One cause, however, is to be mentioned because of the current reports on acute myoglobinuria associated with drug abuse, which has been the subject of several articles in recent years. Whether heroin or cocaine is directly responsible for kidney and muscle damage remains to be interpreted in each case, depending on the superimposed factors that lead to the crushing of the muscles during the comatose state of these patients.

In brief, the increasing reports on the various factors responsible for skeletal muscle ischemia have made the medical profession aware of the frequency with which muscle damage is responsible for a great variety of other types of organ damage in the body. Knowledge of such damage has helped our understanding of the closure of major arteries by direct pressure on the muscle or by the effect of a large variety of toxins that may attack the muscle directly through the bloodstream. As a result of the greater number of reports on this subject, the role of acute ischemia of the skeletal muscle, leading to a profound metabolic compromise of the homeostatic mechanisms of the human body, has became a well-accepted concept.

CONCLUDING COMMENTS

The great variety of entities described in this chapter, ranging from acute arterial occlusions and traumatic lesions to a host of lesions caused by endogenous and exogenous toxins, have several common characteristics, including (1) acute rhabdomyolytic changes involving mostly the muscles of the extremities and (2) metabolic complications that often lead to renal failure and a fatal outcome. Among the biochemical factors common to most, if not all, of these entities are myoglobinuria and muscular enzymatic alterations, such as a change in CPK levels. Myoglobin and CPK are the two major biochemical markers responsible for the metabolic characteristics of these entities, for which I coined the term "myonephropathic-metabolic syndrome." Knowledge of their clinicopathologic features and aggressive treatment of the metabolic complications are the key to salvage in most of these cases.

BIBLIOGRAPHY

Abel RM, Wick J, Beck CH Jr: Renal dysfunction following open heart operations. Arch Surg 108:175, 1974.

Andersson J, Eklof B, et al.: Metabolic changes in blood and skeletal muscle in reconstructive aortic surgery. Ann Surg 283, 1979.

Baker WH, Munns Jr: Aneurysmectomy in the aged. Arch Surg 110:531, 1975.

Barry KG, Cohen A: Mannitolization, I: Prevention and therapy of oliguria associated with cross-clamping of the abdominal aorta. Surgery 50:335, 1961.

Baue AE, McClerkin WW: A study of shock: Acidosis and the declamping phenomenon. Ann Surg 161:40, 1965.

Bell JW: Acute thrombosis of the subrenal abdominal aorta. Arch Surg 95:681, 1967.

Benichoux R: Metabolic acidosis following regional circulatory arrest: Treatment by T.H.A.M., hyperventilation and hyperbaric oxygen. J Cardiovasc Surg 15:573, 1973.

Berman LB: When the urine is red. JAMA 237:2752, 1977.

Biörk G: On myoglobin and its occurrence in man. Acta Med Scand (Suppl) 226:1, 1949.

Bizet LMO, Lopez FF, et al.: Clampeo aortico infrarenal: Cambios metabolicos y su repercusion sobre la funcion renal. Angiologia 34:21, 1982.

Blaisdell FW: Traumatic shock: The search for a toxic factor. Am Coll Bull 68:2, 1983.

Blaisdell GS, Steele M, Allen RE: Management of acute lower ex-

tremity arterial ischemia due to embolism and thrombosis. Surgery 84:822, 1978.

Bridges KG, Donnelly JC Jr: Acute occlusion of an abdominal aortic aneurysm complicated by bilateral lower extremity venous thrombosis: A case report. Cardiovasc Dis Bull Texas Heart Inst 8:93, 1981.

Bruner JM: Time, pressure and temperature factors in the safe use of the tourniquet. The Hand 3:39, 1970.

Buchbinder D, Karmody AM, et al.: Hypertonic mannitol, its use in the prevention of revascularization syndrome after acute arterial ischemia. Arch Surg 116:414, 1981.

Bulkley GB, Morris JB: Role of oxygen-derived free radicals as mediators of post-ischemic injury: A clinically oriented overview, in Rotilio G (ed): Superoxide and Superoxide Dismutase in Chemistry, Biology and Medicine. Amsterdam, Elsevier, 1986, pp 565–570.

Burton KP, McCord JM, Ghai G: Myocardial alterations due to free radical generation. Am J Physiol 246:H776, 1984.

Busuttil RW, Keehn G, et al.: Aortic saddle embolus: A twenty-year experience. Ann Surg 197:698, 1983.

Bywaters EGL: Ischemic muscle necrosis, crushing injury, traumatic edema, the crush syndrome, traumatic anuria, compression syndrome: A type of injury seen in air raid casualties following burial beneath debris. JAMA 124:1103, 1944.

Cannon WB: Traumatic Shock. New York, Appleton, 1923, pp 142–159.

Carlson BM, Faulkner JA: The regeneration of skeletal muscle fibers following injury: A review. Med Sci Sports Exerc 15:187, 1983.

Carlström B: Uber die Atiologie und Pathogenese der Kreulahme des Pferdes. Skand Arch Physiol 61:161, 1931.

Cassar JP: Contribution a l'etude des troubles metaboliques lies a l'ischemie aigue des membres: Leurs variations au cours des gestes therapeutiques. These, Universite Scientifigue et Medicale de Grenoble, 1974.

Chawla SK, Najafi H, et al: Acute renal failure complicating ruptured abdominal aortic aneurysm. Arch Surg 110:521, 1976.

Chiu D, Wang HH, Blumenthal MR: Creatine phosphokinase release as a measure of tourniquet effect on skeletal muscle. Arch Surg 111:71, 1976.

Chugh KS, Nath IVS, et al.: Acute renal failure due to nontraumatic rhabdomyolysis. Postgrad Med J 55:386, 1979.

Colmers (von): Arch Klin Chir 90:701, 1909.

Corcoran AC, Page IH: Renal damage from ferroheme pigments myoglobin, hemoglobin and hematin. Texas Rep Biol Med 3:528, 1945.

Cormier JM, Devin R: Traitement des obliterations artirielles aigues des membres: Consequences generales de l'ischemie aigue. 7enu Congres Francais de Chirurgie, 1969.

Criado FJ: Acute thrombosis of abdominal aortic aneurysm. Texas Heart Inst J 9:367, 1982.

Cullen MJ, Appleyard ST, Bindoff L: Morphologic aspects of muscle breakdown and lysosomal activation. Ann NY Acad Sci 371:440, 1979.

Dahlback L: Effects of tourniquet ischemia on striated muscle fibers and motor end-plates. Scand J Plast Reconst Surg (Suppl) 7:7, 1970.

Danto LA, Fry WJ, Kraft RO: Acute aortic thrombosis. Arch Surg 104:569, 1972.

Del Maestro RF: An approach to free radicals in medicine and biology. Acta Physiol Scand (Suppl) 492:744, 1980.

Dunant J, Nosbaum J, Waibel P: Metabolic changes during induced ischemia of the leg. J Cardiovasc Surg 14:586, 1973.

Duncan GW, Blalock A: The uniform production of experimental shock by crush injury: Possible relationship to clinical crush syndrome. Ann Surg 115:684, 1942.

Eiken O, Nabseth DC, et al.: Limb replantation, II: The pathophysiological effects. Arch Surg 88:54, 1964.

Eklof B, Neglen P, Thomson D: Temporary incomplete ischemia of the legs induced by aortic clamping in man. Ann Surg 89, Jan 1981.

Elliott JP, Hageman JH, et al.: Arterial embolization: Problems of source, multiplicity, recurrence and delayed treatments. Surgery 88:333, 1980.

Engler HS, Ellison LT, et al.: Shock following release of aortic cross-clamping. Arch Surg 86:791, 1963.

Esato K, Nakano H, et al.: Methods of suppression of myonephropathic metabolic syndrome. J Cardiovasc Surg 26:473, 1985.

Famos M, Radu EW, Harder F: Rhabdomyolysis and the compartment syndrome in heroin addiction. Helv Chir Acta 50:745, 1984.

Fisher RD, Fogarty TJ, Morrow AG: Clinical and biochemical observations of the effect of transient femoral artery occlusion in man. Surgery 68:323, 1970.

Fleischman AH: Ischemic necrosis of tibialis anticus muscle with renal syndrome. Bull Hosp Joint Dis 22:146, 1961.

Francisco J Jr, Miranda F Jr, et al.: The Haimovici-LeGrain-Cormier Syndrome in Arterial Embolectomy: The Myonephropathic-Metabolic Syndrome. Personal communication, to be published.

Gardner TJ, Stewart JR, et al.: Reduction of myocardial ischemic injury with oxygen-derived free radical scavengers. Surg 94:423, 1983.

Gilmour JR: Myoglobinuria and the crush syndrome. Lancet 1:524, 1941.

Green RM, deWeese JA, Rob CG: Arterial enbolectomy before and after the Fogarty catheter. Surgery 77:24, 1975.

Griffiths DL: Volkmann's ischaemic contracture. Br J Surg 28:239, 1940–1941.

Grossman RA, Hamilton RW, Morse BM: Nontraumatic rhabdomyolysis and acute renal failure. N Engl J Med 291:807, 1974.

Gutierrez Carreno R, Sanchez Fabela C: Sindrome miopatico metabolico renal post revascularizacion de los miembros inferiores. Rev Mex Angiol 4:5, 1977.

Haimovici H: Acute atherosclerotic thrombosis, in Haimovici H (ed): Vascular Emergencies. New York, Appleton-Century-Crofts, 1982, pp 213–223.

Haimovici H: Arterial circulation of the extremities, in Structure and Function of the Circulation, vol 1. New York, Plenum Press, 1980, p 425.

Haimovici H: Arterial embolism, myoglobinuria and renal tubular necrosis. Arch Surg 100:639, 1970.

Haimovici H: Ischemic Forms of Venous Thrombosis: Phlegmasia Cerulea Dolens, Venous Gangrene. Springfield, Ill., Thomas, 1971.

Haimovici H: Metabolic complications of acute arterial occlusions. J Cardiovasc Surg 20:349, 1979.

Haimovici H: Metabolic syndrome secondary to acute arterial lesions, in Haimovici H (ed): Vascular Emergencies. New York, Appleton-Century-Crofts, 1982, pp 267–289.

Haimovici H: Muscular, renal and metabolic complications of acute arterial occlusions: Myonephropathic-metabolic syndrome. Surgery 85:451, 1979.

Haimovici H: Myonephropathic-metabolic syndrome. Key address to the XVII Japanese Cardiovascular Surgery Congress, Tokyo, May 1–2, 1987.

Haljamae H, Enger E: Human skeletal muscle energy metabolism during and after complete tourniquet ischemia. Ann Surg 182:9, 1975.

Harman JW: The significance of local vascular phenomena in production of ischemic necrosis in skeletal muscle. Am J Pathol 24:625, 1948.

Harris K, Walker PM, et al.: Metabolic response of skeletal muscle to ischemia. Am J Physiol 250:H213, 1986.

Humphries AW, DeWolfe VG, Young JR: Evaluation of the natural history and the results of treatment in occlusive arteriosclerosis involving the lower extremities in 1850 patients, in Wesolowski

SA, Dennis C (eds): Fundamentals of Vascular Grafting. New York, McGraw-Hill, 1963, p 423.

Husfeldt E, Bjering T: Renal lesion from traumatic shock. Acta Med Scand 91:279, 1937.

Jacobs AL: Arterial Embolism in the Limbs. Edinburgh, Livingston, 1959, p 60.

Janetta PJ, Roberts B: Sudden complete thrombosis of an aneurysm of the abdominal aorta. N Engl J Med 264:434, 1961.

Jepson P: Ischaemic contracture: Experimental study. Ann Surg 84:785, 1926.

Johnson JM, Gaspar MR, et al.: Sudden complete thrombosis of aortic and iliac aneurysms. Arch Surg 108:792, 1974.

Kagen LJ: Myoglobin: Biochemical, Physiological, and Clinical Aspects. New York,. Columbia University Press, 1973, pp 1–451.

Kagen LJ: Myoglobinemia in inflammatory myopathies. JAMA 237:1448, 1977.

Keaveny TV, O'Boyle A, Fitzgerald PA: Effect of surgical procedure on muscle ATP. J Cardiovasc Surg 14:601, 1973.

Knochel JP: Exertional rhabdomyolysis. N Engl J Med 287:927, 1972.

Koffler A, Friedler RM, Massry SG: Acute renal failure due to nontraumatic rhabdomyolysis. Ann Intern Med 85:23, 1976.

Kornmesser TW, Trippel OH, Haid SP: Acute occlusion of the abdominal aorta, in Bergan JJ, Yao JST (ed): Surgery of the Aorta and Its Body Branches. New York, Grune & Stratton, 1979.

Korthuis RJ, Granger DN, et al.: The role of oxygen-derived free radicals in ischemia-induced increases in canine skeletal muscle vascular permeability. Circ Res 57:599, 1985.

Kreitzer SM, Ehrenpreis M, Migue E: Acute myoglobinuric renal failure in polymyositis. NY State J Med 78:295, 1978.

Kugimiya T, Shirabe J, et al.: Myonephropathic-metabolic syndrome as a complication of cardiopulmonary bypass. Jpn J Surg 13:431, 1983.

Lang EK: Streptokinase therapy: Complications of intra-arterial use. Radiology 154:75, 1985.

LaPorta MA, Linde HW, et al: Elevation of creatine phosphokinase in young men after recreational exercise. JAMA 239: 1978.

Letac R, Letac S, Chassaigne JP: Syndrome de Bywaters apparu a la suite d'une plaie de l'artere femorale commune sans traumatisme musculaire. Ann Chir Thorac Cardiol 2:469, 1963.

Lie JT, Sun SC: Ultrastructure of ischemic contracture of the left ventricle ("stone heart"). Mayo Clinic Proc 51:785, 1976.

Lim RC, Bergentz SE, Lewis DH: Metabolic and tissue blood flow changes resulting from aortic cross-clamping. Surgery 65:304, 1969.

Little JM, Ferguson DA: The incidence of hypothenar hammer syndrome. Arch Surg 105:684, 1972.

Littooy FN, Baker WH: Acute aortic occlusion: A multifaceted catastrophe. J Vasc Surg 4:211, 1986.

Malan E, Haimovici H: Round table on acute ischemia of the limbs and revascularization syndrome: XXI Congress of the European Society of Cardiovascular Surgery. J Cardiovasc Surg 14:573, 1973.

Mansberger AR Jr, Cox EF, et al.: "Washout" acidosis following resection of aortic aneurysms: Clinical metabolic study of reactive hyperemia and effect of dextran on excess lactate and pH. Ann Surg 163(5):778, 1966.

Markowitz H, Wobig GH: Quantitative method for estimating myoglobin in urine. Clin Chem 23:1689, 1977.

Matolo NM, Cheung L, et al.: Acute occlusion of the infrarenal aorta. Am J Surg 126:788, 1973.

McCombs R, Roberts B: Acute renal failure following resection of abdominal aortic aneurysm. Surg Gynecol Obstet 148:175, 1979.

McCord JM: Oxygen-derived free radicals in postischemic tissue injury. N Engl J Med 312:159, 1985.

Mehl RR, Paul HA, Beattie EJ Jr: Successful treatment of shock after experimental replantation of extremities severed for long periods. Lancet 1:1419, 1964.

Millikan GA: Muscle hemoglobin. Physiol Rev 19:503, 1939.

Moloney WC, Stovall SL, Sprong DH Jr: Renal damage due to ischemic muscle necrosis. JAMA 131:1419, 1946.

Montagnani CA, Simeone FA: Observations on the liberation and elimination of myohemoglobin and of muscle ischemia. Surgery 34:169, 1953.

Morton JH, Southgate WA, DeWeese JA: Arterial injuries of the extremities. Surg Gynecol Obstet, 1966.

Mullick S: The tourniquet in operations upon the extremities. Surg Gynecol Obstet 146:821, 1978.

Natali J, Lacombe M, et al.: Les traumatismes arteriels vus tardivement conduite a tenir en leur presence. Presse Med 39:2273, 1964.

Nolan B, McQuillan WM: A study of acute traumatic limb ischaemia. Br J Surg 52:559, 1965.

O'Donnell TF Jr, Clowes GHA Jr, et al.: A metabolic approach to the evaluation of peripheral vascular disease. Surg Gynecol Obstet 144:51, 1977.

Peachey LD, Adrian RH, Geiger SR: Skeletal muscle. Bethesda, Md., American Physiological Society, 1983, p 1–688.

Peachey LD, Armstrong CF: Structure and function of membrane systems of skeletal muscle cells, in Peachey LD, Adrian RH, Geiger SR (eds): Skeletal Muscle. Bethesda, Md., American Physiological Society, 1983, pp 23–71.

Perdue GD: Thrombosis of aneurysms of the abdominal aorta. J Med Assoc Ga 52:201, 1963.

Perry MO: The hemodynamics of temporary abdominal aortic occlusion. Ann Surg 168:193, 1968.

Pirovino M, Neff MS, Sharon E: Myoglobinuria and acute renal failure with acute polymyositis. NY State J Med 79:764, 1979.

Planell ES: Emergency thrombectomy in the treatment of acute arterial thrombosis. J Cardiovasc Surg (Special Issue), XI World Congress, International Cadiovascular Society, Barcelona, Spain, 1973.

Powell WJ, DiBona DR, et al.: The protective effect of hyperosmotic mannitol in myocardial ischemia and necrosis. Circulation 54:603, 1976.

Powers SR, Boba A, Stein A: The mechanism and prevention of distal tubular necrosis following aneurysmectomy. Surgery 142:146, 1957.

Provan JL, Fraenkel GJ, Austen WG: Metabolic and hemodynamic changes after temporary aortic occlusion in dogs. Surg Gynecol Obstet p 544, 1966.

Rich NM, Spencer FC: Vascular Trauma, Philadelphia, WB Saunders, 1978, pp 1–610.

Robbs JV, Baker LW: Major arterial trauma: Review of experience with 267 injuries. Br J Surg 65:532, 1978.

Rowland LP, Fahn S, et al.: Myoglobinuria. Arch Neurol 10:537, 1964.

Sapir DG, Dandy WE Jr, et al.: Acute renal failure following ruptured abdominal aneurysms: An improved clinical prognosis. Crit Care Med 7:59, 1979.

Saranchak HJ, Bernstein SH: A new diagnostic test for acute myocardial infarction: The detection of myoglobinuria by radioimmunodiffusion assay. JAMA 228:1251, 1974.

Sarrazin R: Metabolic troubles in limb ischemia and their variations during surgical therapy. J Cardiovasc Surg 14:627, 1973.

Savalyev VS, Zatevakhin II, Stepanow NV: Artery embolism of the upper limb. Surgery 81:367, 1977.

Schaff HV, Flaherty JT, et al.: Hyperosmolar reperfusion following ischemic cardiac arrest: Critical importance of timing of mannitol administration on myocardial structure and function. Surgery 89:141, 1981.

Scully RE, Hughes CW: The pathology of ischemia of skeletal muscle in man: A description of early changes in muscles of the extremities following damage to major peripheral arteries on the battlefield. Am J Pathol 32:805, 1956.

Seddon H: Volkmann's ischaemia. Br Med J 1:1587, 1964.

Seidenberg B, Stern J, Hurwitt ES: Thrombotic occlusion of abdominal aortic aneurysm following distal embolization. Circulation 25:995, 1962.

Shumacker H: Surgical treatment of aortic aneurysms. Postgrad Med 25:535, 1959.

Siegel AJ, Silverman LM, Evans WJ: Elevated skeletal muscle creatine kinase MB isoenzyme levels in marathon runners. JAMA 250:2835, 1983.

Snyder DD, Campbell GS: Humoral effects of experimental crush syndrome. Surgery 47:2, 1960.

Sorlie D, Huseby NE, Kluge T: Ischaemia during arterial reconstructive surgery: Biochemical changes as reflected in popliteal vein samples. Scand J Thorac Cardiovasc Surg 11:151, 1977.

Stallone RJ, Blaisdell FW, Cafferata HT: Analysis of morbidity and mortality from arterial embolectomy. Surgery 1:207, 1969.

Stipa S, Cavallaro A, Privitera L: Treatment of shock following prolonged ischemia of the limbs. J Cardiovasc Surg 8:529, 1967.

Strandness DE Jr, Parrish DG, Bell JW: Mechanism of declamping shock in operations on the abdominal aorta. Surgery 50:488, 1961.

Subram AN, Duncan JM: Acute limb ischemia from sudden thrombosis of an abdominal aortic aneurysm: A case report. Texas Heart Inst J 9:97, 1982.

Thompson WW, Campbell GS: Studies on myoglobin and hemoglobin in experimental crush syndrome in dogs. Ann Surg 149:235, 1959.

Weeks SR: The crush syndrome. Surg Gynecol Obstet p 369, 1968.

Whelton A: Post-traumatic acute renal failure. Bull NY Acad Med 55:151, 1979.

Willerson J, Powell WJ Jr, Guney TE: Improvement in myocardial function and coronary blood flow in ischemic myocardium after mannitol. J Clin Invest 51:2989, 1972.

Winninger A: Biopathological disturbances in the revascularization stage of ischemic limbs. J Cardiovasc Surg 14:640, 1973.

Zuber WF, Gaspar MR, Rothchild PD: Anterior spinal artery syndrome: A complication of abdominal aortic surgery. Ann Surg 172:909, 1970.

NOTE: For more detailed references for this chapter see Haimovici H: Metabolic Complications of Acute Arterial Occlusions and Related Conditions (Myonephropathic-Metabolic Syndrome). Mount Kisco, N.Y., Futura Publishing Co., 1988.

CHAPTER 33
Arteriographic Patterns of Atherosclerotic Occlusive Disease of the Lower Extremity

Henry Haimovici

It is well recognized that the pathologic features of atherosclerosis are variable from individual to individual and from one arterial segment to another. As a result, the patterns emerging from the innumerable combinations of lesions are varied and complex. However, in terms of location and extent of the atherosclerotic process, it is possible to identify a certain number of broad patterns. Thus the arteriographic findings may lend themselves to an overall classification of three major groups (Fig. 33-1):

1. Aortoiliac
2. Femoropopliteal
3. Tibioperoneal

METHODS OF STUDY

Computerized technology has been used recently for visualization of the entire vascular system.[1] Achieved by intravenous injection of standard contrast agents, this method can be carried out as an outpatient procedure and in general does not entail the hazards of the conventional intraarterial injections. The results of this new technique, while helpful as a screening method, do not yield as yet the same qualitative details as standard arteriography for the lower extremities, especially when excellent information about the arterial lesions is needed. (See Chapter 5 for the correlation of the two methods.) Duplex ultrasonography, the newest modality for arterial imaging, may enable better evaluation of arterial patterns (Chapter 7).

The data to be described herein were obtained with the standard conventional arteriography and are the basis for the classifications of the arteriosclerotic patterns.

Whether one deals with any one of the three patterns, it is essential that evaluation of these arterial lesions include the entire vascular tree from its origin to its final ramifications. A comprehensive assessment must therefore be based on the study of the inflow and outflow tracts of the arterial lesions from the infrarenal abdominal aorta to the pedal arterial network.[2]

Serial angiography is a prerequisite for proper evaluation of the arterial lesions (Fig. 33-2). Principles of angiography will not be reviewed here, since they are fully described in Chapter 5. Suffice it to mention only briefly that aortoarteriography of the lower extremity can be achieved either by translumbar aortography or by the transfemoral retrograde and anterograde method. The latter can be carried out either by bilateral puncture of the femoral artery, using appropriate needles, or, preferably, by means of the catheter method. General or local anesthesia, especially the latter, because the newer radiopaque substances are generally painless, may be used in nearly all cases. In any case, optimum arteriographic outlines of the vasculature are essential.

AORTOILIAC PATTERNS

The atherosclerotic process of the aortoiliac segment may begin at the bifurcation or, most frequently, in one or both common iliac arteries. The development of these lesions is slow, insidious, and progressive. From a clinicopathologic standpoint, it may be emphasized that this syndrome may go through two distinct phases: stenotic and occlusive. If the terminal abdominal aorta or its bifurcation or the two common iliac arteries become occluded, the thrombotic process progresses proximally toward the renal arteries.

The site of origin of the atherothrombotic process is not always easy to pinpoint. However, analysis of the arteriographic data strongly suggests that two major sites of origin may determine the evolution of the lesions and their subsequent patterns: (1) the aortic bifurcation and (2) the iliac arteries.

Aortic Bifurcation

Progression of the lesions that begin at the bifurcation may extend proximally up to the renal arteries, but rarely above. Consequently, one may expect to find at least three patterns of such lesions: (1) at the bifurcation itself, which includes

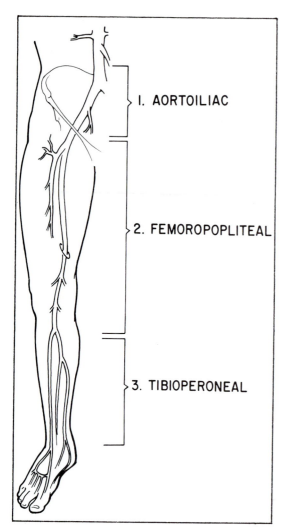

Figure 33-1. Diagram depicting the three major arteriographic patterns of the lower extremity.

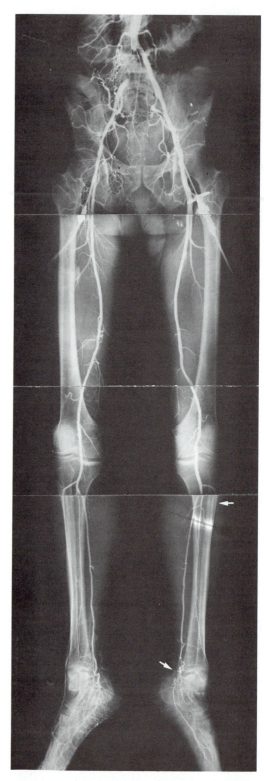

Figure 33-2. Aortography of the lower extremity by the serial angiographic technique using a bilateral transfemoral method. This procedure affords evaluation of the entire arterial tree from the abdominal aorta to the pedal vessels. Note the complete occlusion of the right common iliac artery and a few minor lesions in the left leg, as indicated by the arrows.

the terminal abdominal aorta and the origin of both iliac arteries, (2) in the distal segment, including the bifurcation and the terminal aorta up to the inferior mesenteric artery, and (3) in the entire aortic segment up to the renal arteries. The relative frequency of these three patterns is difficult to assess. The lesions range from moderate to marked stenosis (Figs. 33-3 and 33-4), to complete occlusion (Figs. 33-5, 33-6, and 33-7).

In a study of 100 aortograms, Watt[3] found the aorta to be completely occluded in 10% and the aortic bifurcation stenosed in 24%. DeBakey et al.[4] found, in a series of 448 cases, complete occlusion of the aortoiliac segment in 44% and aortoiliac stenosis in 56%. As already alluded to, the aortic occlusion is confined most often below the renal artery origin because the large flow in the latter vessels often prevents the obstruction from progressing higher. Nevertheless, stenotic atherosclerotic lesions associated with complete obstruction or stenosis of the terminal abdominal aorta are not unusual in the renal arteries.[5]

It should be pointed out that, in cases of aortoiliac

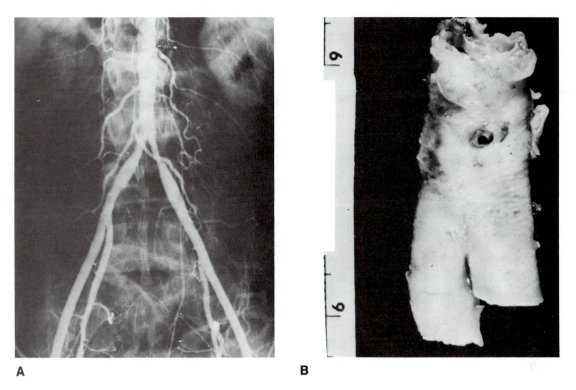

A   B

Figure 33-3. A. Aortogram indicating aortoiliac stenosis of significant hemodynamic degree necessitating an aortoiliac endarterectomy **(B).**

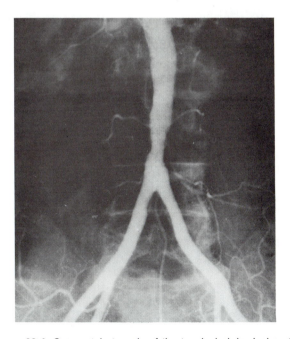

Figure 33-4. Segmental stenosis of the terminal abdominal aorta above its bifurcation.

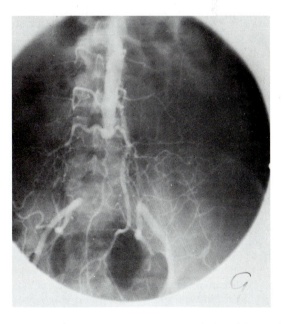

Figure 33-5. Aortogram showing complete occlusion of the terminal abdominal aorta below the inferior mesenteric artery and of both common iliac arteries.

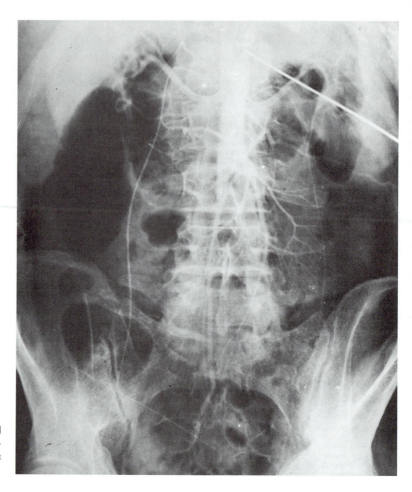

Figure 33-6. Complete abdominal aortic occlusion distal to the inferior mesenteric artery, indicating also the pathways of collateral circulation from the inferior mesenteric artery through the pelvic vessels.

stenosis, narrowing of the origin of the two iliac arteries is not always identical. For example, stenosis may either be absent or more pronounced on one side than on the other.

Iliac Arteries

The lesions of the iliac may involve either the common, the external, or the internal. In some cases, there is a combination of two or three of these occlusions.

Stenosis or occlusion of the *common iliac* artery, without aortic involvement, is the commonest form. Watt[3] found that common iliac lesions accounted for 43% of the total group of 142 lesions of the aortoiliac segment. Of these, stenosis was slightly more frequently encountered than complete occlusion. The site at which the lesion occurred was also variable: (1) near the bifurcation of the aorta (Fig. 33-8), (2) in the course of the artery itself (Figs. 33-9 and 33-10), or (3) at the level of its bifurcation (Fig. 33-11). Although it is not always easy to assess the exclusive or specific site of the iliac involvement, arteriographically one can reasonably determine the exact location and extent in most cases. It should be pointed out, however, that in the case of stenosis, the lesions found at surgery appear much more extensive than the arteriographic image would indicate. Bilateral common iliac distribution of the lesions is relatively common. Although the lesions are not always symmetric,

the rate of progression of the two sides does not appear to be synchronous.

Occlusion and stenosis are less frequent in the *external iliac artery* than in the common iliac. When the occlusion occurs, it extends distally to the origin of the inferior epigastric artery, thus leaving the common femoral patent.

Occlusion and stenosis of the *internal iliac artery* often remain asymptomatic. However, they are more commonly found in combination with the other iliac occlusions and are incidental findings in the course of the aortoiliac exploration. When an isolated lesion is present, its clinical manifestations are often not fully appreciated. The symptoms resulting from this lesion are buttock claudication and thigh and calf claudication, produced by occlusion of the main arterial channel. The latter type of claudication may overshadow the former.

Combined lesions of the common, external, and internal iliac arteries may involve two or three of these vessels. The most frequent combination of lesions is found in the common and external iliac arteries, whereas the internal iliac is often spared.

Other Associated Vascular Lesions

Aortoiliac lesions are often associated with atherosclerotic stenosis or occlusion of the femoropopliteal or tibioperoneal vessels (Fig. 33-2). DeBakey et al.[4] noted that, in a certain

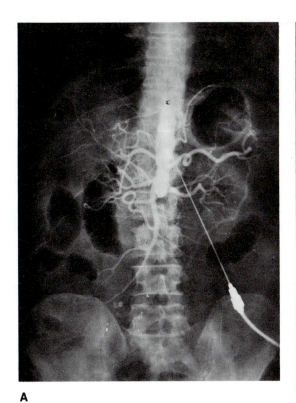

A

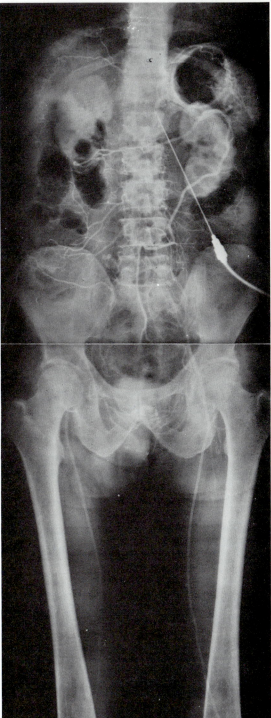

B

Figure 33-7. A. Complete abdominal aortic occlusion distal to the renal arteries. **B.** Serial aortogram, 5 and 7 seconds later, indicating reestablishment of collateral supply from the superior to the inferior mesenteric artery and from the latter to the pelvic area and thence to the external iliac, femoral, and popliteal arteries.

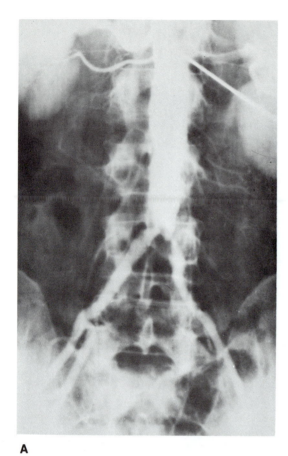

A

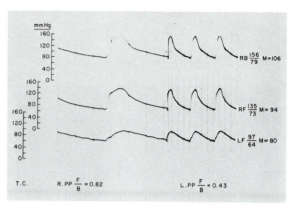

B

Figure 33-8. A. Severe aortoiliac stenosis most marked on the left side, with the patient having disabling intermittent claudication. **B.** Tracings from intrabrachial and intrafemoral arterial pressures obtained from the patient whose aortogram is shown in **A.** Upper tracing is from the right-brachial artery; middle tracing is from the right femoral artery, which shows moderate stenosis; lower tracing is from the left femoral artery, which shows marked stenosis.[8]

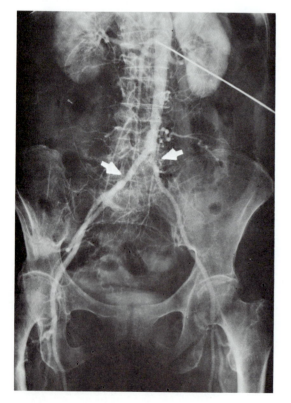

Figure 33-9. Translumbar aortogram indicating complete occlusion of the origin of the left common iliac artery and stenosis of the right midcommon iliac artery.

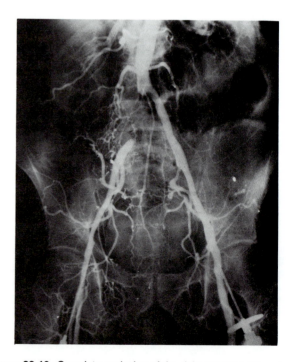

Figure 33-10. Complete occlusion of the right common iliac artery (see Fig. 33-2).

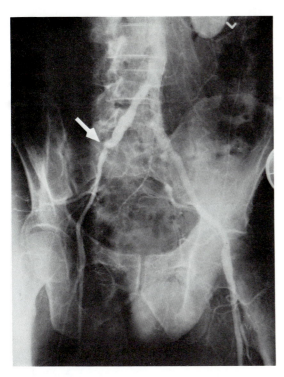

Figure 33-11. Marked stenosis of the junction between the common and external iliac arteries (*arrow*).

proportion of their cases, the aortoiliac lesions were associated with peripheral arterial occlusive disease. Thus in a series of 448 cases, 78, or 18%, had such involvement of the femoropopliteal segment. In the majority of these cases, the peripheral occlusive process was also segmental, involving primarily the superficial femoral artery with a patent lumen in the popliteal. In reviewing aortograms of 600 patients, Valdoni and Venturini[6] found 830 occlusive lesions. Of these, 24% involved the aortic bifurcation and the iliac arteries. In 50% of the aortoiliac lesions, they found the superficial femoral artery to be involved, whereas the popliteal appeared to be patent.

Collateral Circulation in Aortoiliac Occlusive Disease

When aortic obstruction occurs just below the renal arteries, the most important anastomosis occurs between the superior mesenteric by way of its middle colic branch to the left colic and thence to the inferior mesenteric artery (Fig. 33-7B). If the distal aorta is patent at and below the origin of the inferior mesenteric, it is common for it to be fed directly in this fashion. If the origin of the inferior mesenteric is occluded, the flow proceeds distally into the inferior mesenteric and superior rectal (superior hemorrhoidal) arteries, then to the anastomosing pelvic visceral and parietal branches, including the internal pudendals, lateral sacrals, vesicals, and obturators, then to the internal, common, and external iliac arteries, and then to the lower extremity (Fig. 33-7B).

The collateral vessels that provide flow to the main

vessels below the occlusion develop from existing vessels and networks. The collaterals that occur in the occlusion of the aortic bifurcation are determined by a well-known anastomotic setup known as Winslow's anastomotic system. These include, in addition to the arteries described above, the intercostals, the internal mammary, and the external iliac via the inferior epigastric artery. Riolan's arc is seen in the same type of occlusion when the marginal artery in the mesentery develops into an important link in blood supply of the lower extremity by way of the superior mesenteric artery, middle and left colic, and inferior mesenteric, and thence to the superior rectal, hypogastric, and external iliac or deep femoral arteries. Awareness of this anastomotic network becomes important when resection of the left colon has to be considered in a patient with advanced aortoiliac disease.

FEMOROPOPLITEAL PATTERNS

The extent and location of lesions in the femoropopliteal segment are extremely variable. In one study,[2] six subpatterns were identified on the basis of site and extent of occlusion (Fig. 33-12). Although almost half of the arterial lesions of the lower extremity were seen in the femoropopliteal area, they were rarely confined to this segment alone. However, isolated femoropopliteal lesions are encountered more often in nondiabetic atherosclerotic patients than in diabetic patients.

Initial lesions (Fig. 33-13) are characterized by mild to severe stenosis. One of the most common locations of such lesions is at the junction between Hunter's canal and the initial segment of the popliteal artery as well as in the distal popliteal or below the origin of the anterior tibial artery. A complete or nearly complete occlusion often occurs as an initial lesion at the level of the foramen adductor magnus area (Fig. 33-14). A short segmental lesion in the common femoral artery is not unusual (Fig. 33-15). A complete occlusion of the common femoral from its origin at the external iliac artery to the bifurcation (Fig. 33-16) and an associated occlusion of the superficial femoral are more advanced patterns (Fig. 33-17). In these cases, the collateral supply is established between the internal iliac branches and those of the profunda femoris, as shown by the arteriogram in Figure 33-17.

A complete occlusion of the superficial femoral artery may occur distally at the adductor magnus hiatus or may extend up to the bifurcation of the femoral (Figs. 33-18 and 33-19). Such lesions may often occur bilaterally, as seen in Figure 33-20. These lesions were all confined to the femoral segment. However, the incidence of isolated lesions is much smaller than that of those combined with the proximal or distal arterial tree (see below).

The popliteal lesions, like those in the femoral, are initially segmental and confined to a small area. Most often, the lesion appears either as a stenosis or complete occlusion in its midportion behind the condyles or just proximal to them (Figs. 33-21 and 33-22). A more extensive occlusion of the popliteal occurs as a result of progression of the lesion proximally, from the condyles toward Hunter's canal (Fig. 33-23). Occlusion of the entire popliteal artery, includ-

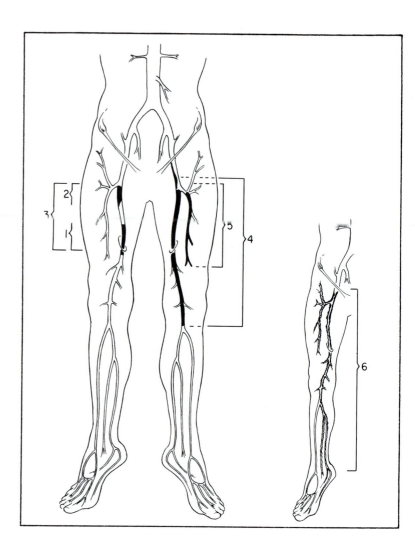

Figure 33-12. Diagram of femoropopliteal patterns showing their six divisions: (1) distal superficial femoral, (2) proximal superficial femoral, (3) entire superficial femoral, (4) entire femoral and popliteal, (5) profunda femoris, and (6) diffuse atherosclerosis with multiple stenotic areas.

ing its tibial segment, may occur in patients with diabetes or with Buerger's disease (Fig. 33-24).

In a study previously cited,[2] the incidence of a femoropopliteal segment as an isolated lesion was seen in only 10.4%, whereas the combined femoropopliteal-tibial patterns were present in 49.2% of a total of 321 cases.

Associated Aortoiliac Lesions

In the presence of a segmental femoropopliteal occlusion, it is essential to determine the condition of the outflow and inflow tracts. The concept of a segmental nature of atherosclerotic disease is an attractive one and has been propounded and propagated through the literature, but this concept may lead one to oversimplify the true features of the atherosclerotic process. By the use of the panangiographic method, we have been able to demonstrate that intimal lesions are widespread and affect certain segments with greater predilection than others. In contrast to the extent of intimal lesions, the occlusive process is usually segmental only at an early phase of the disease. As the disease progresses, the intimal lesions may increase in size and become a signficant hemodynamic lesion. In the pres-

ence of a reducing inflow, especially proximal to implantation of a graft, it is important to detect such silent lesions before undertaking the distal arterial reconstruction. An angiographic survey of the femoropopliteal segment, reported earlier, disclosed a relatively high incidence of 27% of associated aortoiliac lesions.[7]

Four basic patterns of associated lesions may be present: (1) aortoiliac stenosis, (2) iliac occlusion (unilateral), (3) aortoiliac aneurysms, and (4) tortuosity of the aortoiliac segment. These aortoiliac patterns and their respective incidence are illustrated in Figure 33-25.

Aortoiliac stenosis cannot always be accurately estimated from the arteriogram alone. Hemodynamic tests, previously described by us[8] and more recently confirmed by others,[9] may help to identify the critical stenotic lesions. Figure 33-26B indicates a severe lesion in the right iliac artery, both at its origin and above its bifurcation, in addition to the midfemoral arterial lesion indicated in Figure 33-26A.

In this study, complete iliac occlusion (unilateral) (Fig. 33-10) was found to be of low incidence, although investigation of the common iliac artery as the site of the primary lesion reveals a higher incidence of associated femoropopliteal involvement.

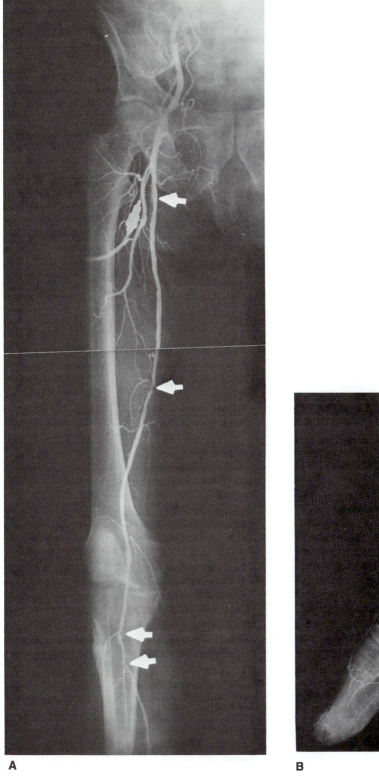

A

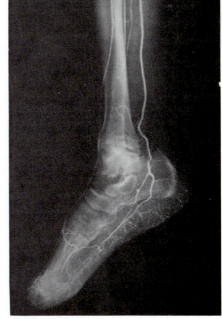

B

Figure 33-13. A. Arteriogram indicating multiple stenoses of femoral, popliteal, and tibial vessels (*site of arrows*). **B.** Note the excellent arterial supply to the leg and foot below these stenotic lesions.

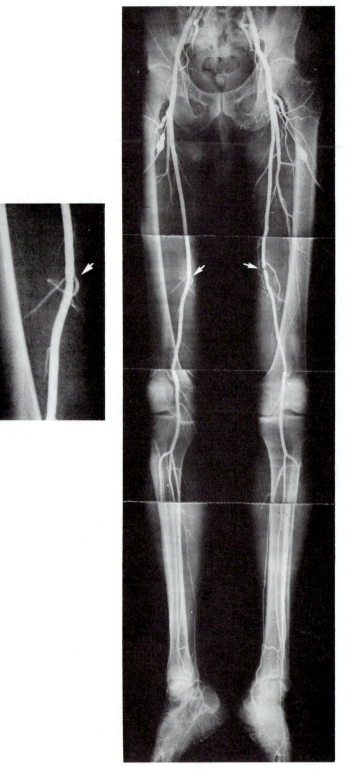
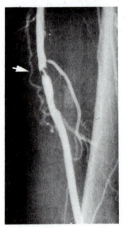

Figure 33-14. Almost complete occlusion of the superficial femoral artery at its junction with the popliteal. The arterial tree is otherwise completely normal from aorta to feet.

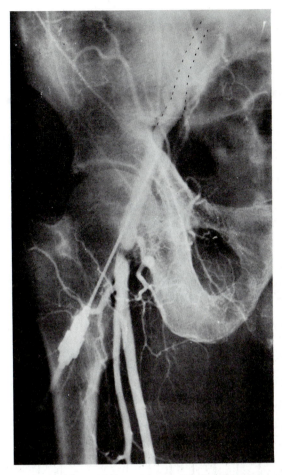

Figure 33-15. Short segmental occlusion of the common femoral artery.

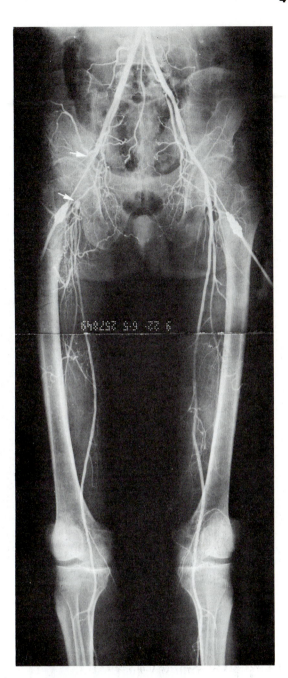

Figure 33-16. Complete occlusion of the common femoral artery from the external iliac to the profunda. Note that the superficial femoral artery, as well as the rest of the arterial tree, is completely patent.

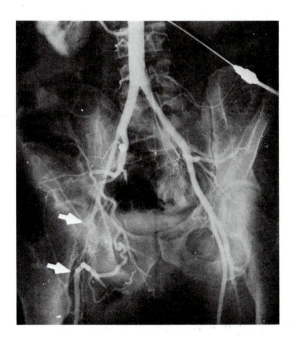

Figure 33-17. Complete occlusion of the right common femoral artery as well as the superficial. Note that the distal arterial flow of the limb is provided by the profunda femoris and the channels from the internal iliac artery, mainly through the obturator artery.

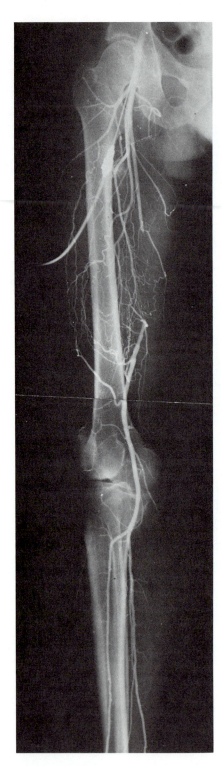

Figure 33-18. Complete occlusion of the right superficial femoral artery at its distal half. Note the patency of the popliteal and tibial vessels.

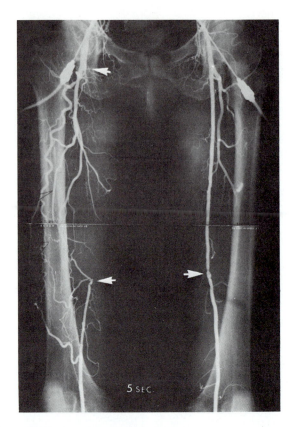

Figure 33-19. Complete occlusion of the entire superficial femoral artery from the profunda to the popliteal.

Aortoiliac aneurysms associated with the femoropopliteal segment are often not detectable clinically and are revealed only by a transfemoral aortogram. Figure 33-27 indicates a small abdominal aneurysm above its bifurcation, associated with stenosis of the iliac arteries. Figure 33-28 depicts an aortoiliac aneurysm associated with bilateral femoropopliteal occlusive disease. The associated aneurysm is usually unsuspected and is found only on arteriographic examination or aortosonography or CT scan. At surgery, these lesions are found to consist of small fusiform dilations of the aorta or iliac vessels. In some cases, only a small anterior saccular dilation is present. These aneurysms are often associated with either tortuosity or stenosis of the iliac arteries. Such combined lesions lead to further impairment of the arterial inflow to the already involved femoropopliteal segment. Figure 33-29 indicates a segmental occlusion of the distal superficial femoral associated with stenosis and tortuosity of the ipsilateral iliac vessels and with severe lesions of the internal iliac artery.

TIBIOPERONEAL PATTERNS

Occlusion of leg arteries alone occurred in 85 of 321 cases, or 26.5%, in our own study. The incidence in nondiabetic and diabetic cases was 23.9 and 29.2%, respectively. Combined occlusions of leg arteries with other arterial segments

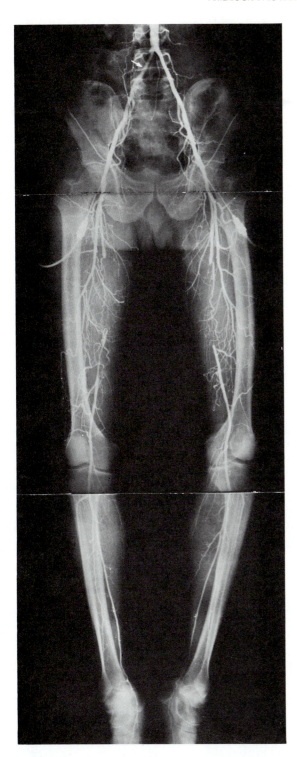

Figure 33-20. Bilateral superficial femoral occlusion with patency both proximally and distally. Right common iliac artery (*arrow*) is inadequately opacified.

occurred in all arterial patterns. Comparison of the incidence of various patterns in nondiabetic and diabetic groups shows that the atherosclerotic process is more discrete in the former and more diffuse in the latter group.

Involvement of a single artery was noted in 65% of cases of atherosclerosis and in only 31.1% of cases of atherosclerosis and diabetes (Fig. 33-30). Conversely, occlusion of two or all three leg arteries occurred in 68.9% of the cases in the latter group as compared with 35% in the nondiabetic patients (Figs. 33-31, 33-32, 33-33, and 33-34). This difference between the two groups holds true, only to a lesser degree, in the cases with combined leg and other occlusive patterns.

This difference is further demonstrated when the two groups with occlusion of the leg arteries alone are evaluated in terms of incidence of associated intimal lesions of the proximal arterial tree. These mural alterations may range from simple plaques to significant stenosing lesions. Analyzed from this angle, isolated leg arterial patterns occurred in 37.5% of cases of simple atherosclerosis and in only 4.6% of cases of atherosclerosis and diabetes. These figures indicate, therefore, that practically all diabetic patients with tibial occlusions displayed intimal lesions of the proximal arterial tree from the popliteal up to the aortoiliac area, with the highest percentage (40%) in the femoropopliteal segment (Fig. 33-35).

A further breakdown of the findings concerning the length of occlusion in the various arteries showed that in atherosclerosis the process is more segmental, in comparison with cases of atherosclerosis and diabetes, in which the process often involved the entire vessel.

It may be of some interest to note that the overall incidence of peroneal arterial occlusion is the lowest of the three arteries and that in the diabetic group, with only leg arterial involvement, the peroneal was never found occluded, although some degree of intimal change might be present. In these cases, the caliber of the peroneal appeared enlarged, obviously compensating for the absent tibials.

Finally, pedal arteries per se rarely have isolated lesions. Figure 33-36 illustrates such an example, in which the plantar arteries were involved bilaterally, together with some involvement of the dorsalis pedis.

Combined occlusions of leg arteries with those of other arterial segments occurred in all patterns, as mentioned above. Comparison of the incidence of various patterns in nondiabetic and diabetic groups shows that the atherosclerotic process is more discrete in the former but more diffuse in the latter group.

COLLATERAL CIRCULATION IN OCCLUSIVE PATTERNS OF FEMOROPOPLITEAL AND TIBIOPERONEAL SEGMENTS

The collateral pathways compensating for the various patterns of occlusion found in the femoropopliteal and tibioperoneal segments areas may be classified into five major groups[10]: (1) the profunda femoris–iliac group, (2) the profunda femoris–genicular group, (3) the genicular-tibial group, (4) the profunda femoris–genicular–tibial group, and (5) the genicular-tibial-peroneal groups.

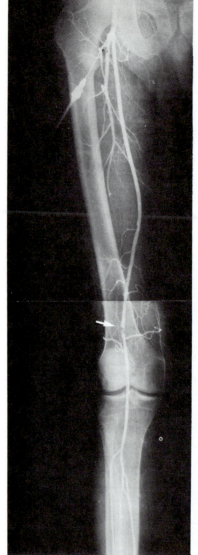

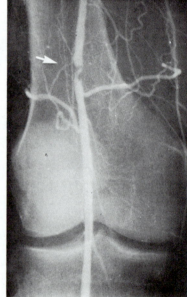

Figure 33-21. A. Segmental occlusion of the midpopliteal artery (*arrow*). **B.** Three-times magnification of the occluded segment. The arterial tree is otherwise normal proximally and distally.

A

B

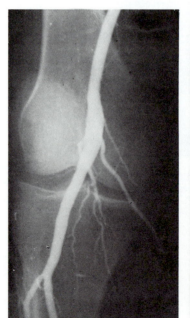

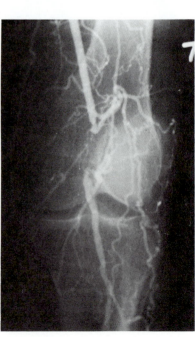

Figure 33-22. Short segmental occlusion of the left popliteal artery in the supracondylar region. Note fusiform dilation of a symmetric segment on the right side.

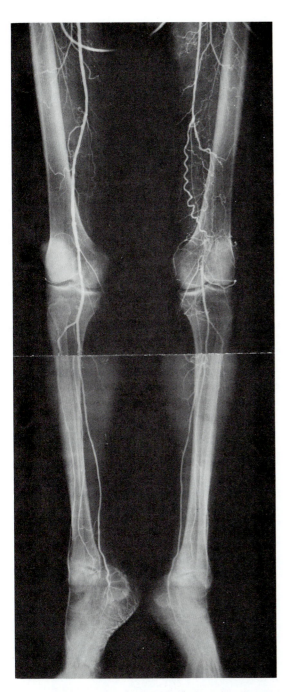

Figure 33-23. Segmental occlusion of the left popliteal artery. Note corkscrew collateral vessels compensating between the superficial femoral and distal popliteal arteries with normal leg and foot arteries.

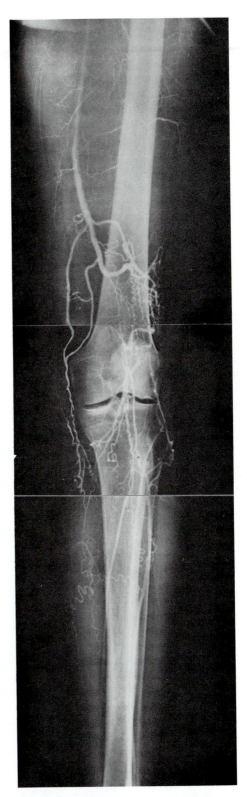

Figure 33-24. Occlusion of the proximal popliteal artery with abundant collateral vessels and a fair runoff.

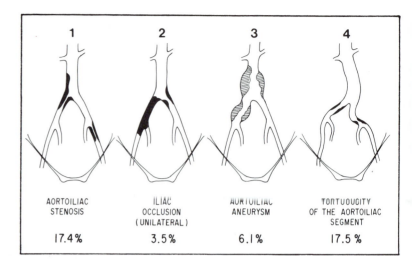

Figure 33-25. Diagrams illustrating the four aortoiliac patterns associated with femoropopliteal–tibial occlusive disease.

Profunda Femoris–Iliac Group

In occlusion of the common femoral artery, collateral vessels that bypass the arterial occlusion originate from the common, internal, and external iliac branches. Of these, the iliolumbar, the superior gluteal, the inferior gluteal, the obturator, and the deep iliac circumflex will anastomose with the branches of the profunda femoris, namely, with the lateral circumflex, the medial circumflex, and the branches of the latter.

Profunda Femoris–Genicular Group

In occlusion of the superficial femoral artery, the collateral vessels compensating for the arterial occlusion originate

from one or more branches of the profunda femoris artery and anastomose with branches of the genicular systems (Fig. 33-37). The branches of the profunda femoris most frequently assuming the role of major collaterals noted in our studies were (1) the descending branch of the lateral circumflex or the rectus femoris collateral and (2) the perforating branches, mostly the third and fourth. The branches of the genicular system most concerned in the anastomosis with the above collaterals originate from either the highest genicular or the lateral superior genicular artery. In complete occlusion of the superficial femoral artery, anastomoses between the obturator and superior gluteal arteries, along with the lateral and medial femoral circumflex arteries, supply the important link between the internal iliac and profunda femoris arteries, as in the preceding group.

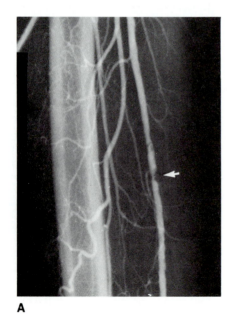

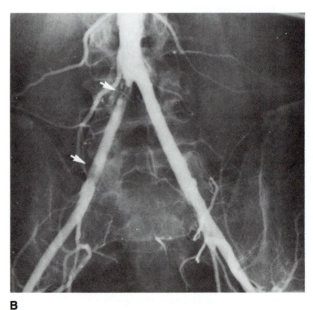

A   B

Figure 33-26. A. Segmental occlusion of the right superficial femoral artery associated with **(B)** two marked stenotic areas (*arrows*) of the right common iliac artery.

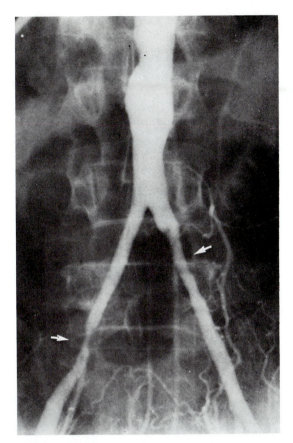

Figure 33-27. Bilateral common iliac stenosis (*arrows*) and aneurysm of the abdominal aorta proximal to its bifurcation.

Genicular–Tibial Group

In occlusion of the popliteal artery, the major collateral vessels arise from (1) the highest genicular artery, with its musculoarticular and saphenous branches, and (2) the profunda femoris artery, with its fourth perforating branch and the descending branch of the lateral femoral circumflex. These collaterals anastomose with the genicular arteries and, via this network, with the recurrent tibial arteries (Fig. 33-38). About half of our cases belong to this genicular-tibial group.[10] Although the number and size of collaterals vary with the occlusion pattern, the saphenous branch of the highest genicular, the descending branch of the lateral circumflex, and the fourth perforating branch are the most developed and constant ones.

Profunda Femoris–Genicular–Tibial Group

In combined occlusion of the superficial femoral and popliteal arteries, collateral vessels from the profunda femoris artery anastomose with branches of the genicular network, which in turn anastomose with branches of the tibial arteries (Fig. 33-39). In this group, as in the profunda femoris–genicular group, the profunda femoris receives anastomotic branches from the internal iliac artery.

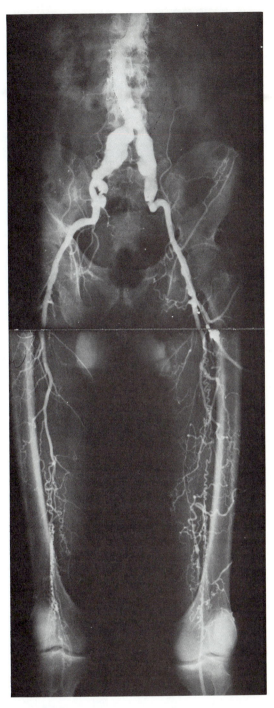

Figure 33-28. Severe occlusive arterial disease of both lower extremities with aortobiiliac aneurysm (unsuspected clinically).

Genicular–Tibial–Peroneal Group

In the group of cases of leg artery occlusions, the origin, distribution, and anastomosis of the collateral vessels are not always as well outlined as in the foregoing groups. Three sets of branches provide the anastomotic network: the genicular, the sural, and the terminal branches of the anterior and posterior tibial and peroneal arteries.

426

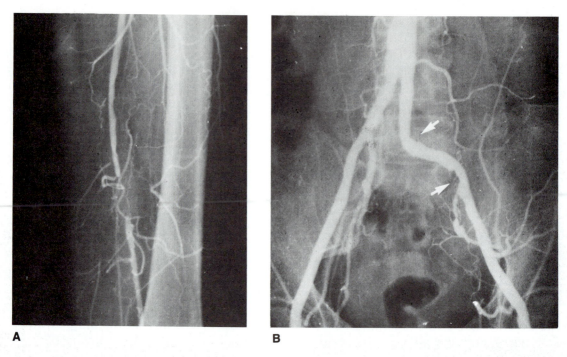

Figure 33-29. A. Segmental occlusion of the left superficial femoral. **(B)** Associated tortuosity and stenosis of the ipsilateral iliac vessels. Note the nearly complete occlusion of the internal iliac artery.

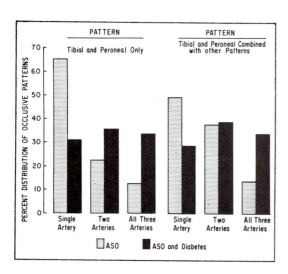

Figure 33-30. Comparative incidence of atherosclerotic lesions of the tibial and peroneal arteries alone and combined with other patterns.

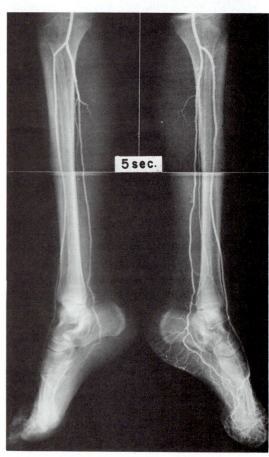

Figure 33-31. Arteriograms of leg and foot arteries, indicating the absence of the right peroneal artery, whereas all the other vessels are normal, 5 seconds after injection of radiopaque material into the femoral arteries.

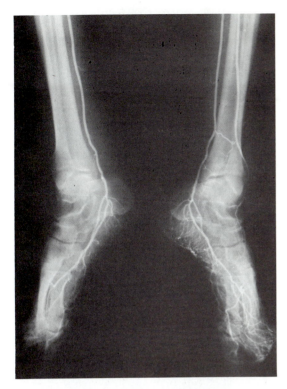

Figure 33-32. Arteriograms showing the absence of right and left anterior tibial, normal posterior tibial, and plantar vessels, a left peroneal artery giving off a small-caliber dorsalis pedis artery. The patient is nondiabetic.

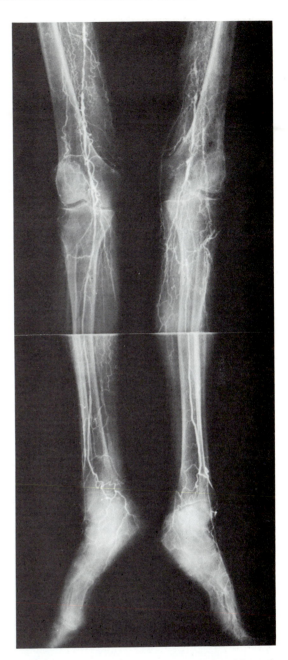

Figure 33-33. Bilateral femoral arteriogram showing diffuse atherosclerotic disease in a diabetic patient. Note patency of peroneal arteries only.

The genicular arteries form a rich but fragile network around the knee, which has connections with the collateral system from the lower third of the thigh and is linked to the anterior compartment of the leg via the anterior tibial recurrent artery. These vessels primarily supply the ligaments and the joint structures of the knee.

The sural arteries, which arise from the posterior aspect of the popliteal artery, supply the gastrocnemius muscle and have only sparse anastomoses with other muscular vessels of the leg.

The collateral vessel from the anterior tibial artery is the anterior tibial recurrent, which is a major link between the genicular system and the anterior compartment. The posterior tibial recurrent is of relatively minor importance because of its size and location.

The posterior tibial artery provides collateral vessels that occur near the ends of the vessel and do not primarily supply muscular tissue. There is a constant communicating artery that links the posterior tibial artery and the peroneal artery, usually about 2 inches above the level of the malleoli.

The peroneal artery is sometimes regarded as the termination of the popliteal, having the tibial arteries as side branches. There seems to be a reciprocal relationship between these vessels so that, at the ankle, the peroneal may replace the anterior tibial and produce the dorsalis pedis via a large perforating branch, or it may replace the lower posterior tibial artery via a communicating branch in certain cases.

The arteries of the foot (dorsalis pedis and plantar arteries) provide the pedal anastomotic networks. These two major arteries provide malleolar, tarsal, and arcuate arteries and anastomose freely with each other and with the arteries of the plantar system. The main arterial arch of the foot is completed in a dorsoplantar direction. The plantar arch of the foot gives rise to plantar metatarsal arteries in each metatarsal space. Ischemic necrosis and rest pain involving the foot must be due to more than any one of the above arteries.[11]

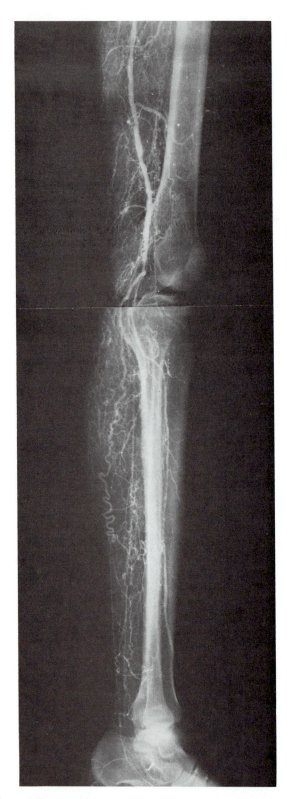

Figure 33-34. Arteriogram of a diabetic patient's leg, showing occlusion of the distal popliteal and all three leg arteries except for the distal half of the anterior tibial. Note the tenuous extensive calf collateral vessels and diffuse intimal lesions of the proximal popliteal and superficial femoral vessels.

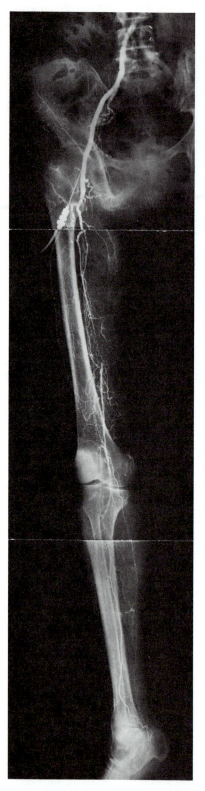

Figure 33-35. Unilateral transfemoral arteriogram of a diabetic patient. Note a nearly normal iliac and common femoral artery, complete occlusion of the superficial femoral, and diffuse disease of leg arteries, with only the peroneal artery patent.

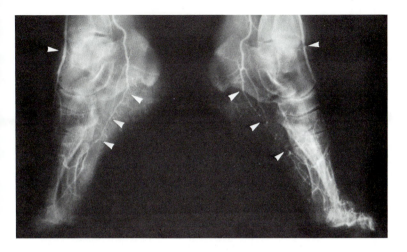

Figure 33-36. Bilateral diffuse disease of the plantar arteries, indicated by arrowheads.

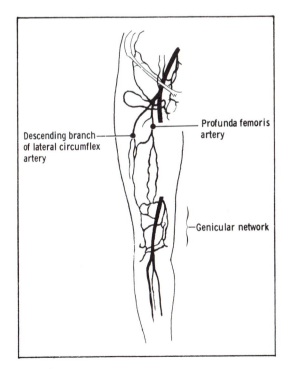

Figure 33-37. Profunda femoris–genicular group of collateral vessels.

Descending branch of lateral circumflex artery

Profunda femoris artery

Genicular network

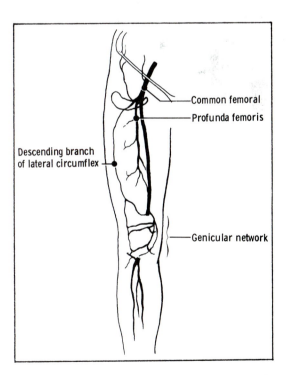

Figure 33-38. Genicular–tibial group of collateral vessels.

Common femoral

Profunda femoris

Descending branch of lateral circumflex

Genicular network

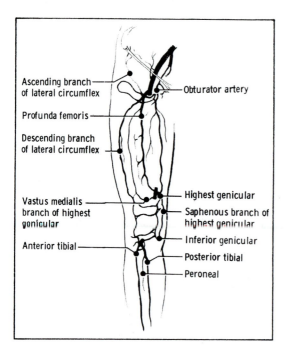

Figure 33-39. Profunda femoris–genicular–tibial group of collateral vessels.

REFERENCES

1. Turnipseed WD, Crummy AB, et al.: Computerized intravenous arteriography: A technique for visualizing the peripheral vascular system. Surgery 89:118, 1981.
2. Haimovici H: Patterns of arteriosclerotic lesions of the lower extremity. Arch Surg 95:918, 1967.
3. Watt JK: Pattern of aorto-iliac occlusion. Br Med J 2:979, 1966.
4. DeBakey ME, Crawford ES, et al.: Surgical considerations of occlusive disease of the abdominal aorta and iliac and femoral arteries: Analysis of 803 cases. Arch Surg 148:306, 1958.
5. Gomes MMR, Bernatz PE: Aorto-iliac occlusive disease: Extension cephalad to origin of renal arteries with surgical considerations and results. Arch Surg 101:161, 1970.
6. Valdoni P, Venturini A: Considerations of late results of vascular prostheses for reconstructive surgery in congenital and acquired arterial disease. J Cardiovasc Surg 5:509, 1964.
7. Haimovici H, Steinman C: Aortoiliac angiographic patterns associated with femoropopliteal occlusive disease: Significance in reconstructive arterial surgery. Surgery 65:232, 1969.
8. Haimovici H, Escher DJW: Aortoiliac stenosis, Diagnostic significance of vascular hemodynamics. Arch Surg 72:107, 1956.
9. Brener BJ, Raines JK, et al.: Measurement of systolic femoral arterial pressure during reactive hyperemia: An estimate of aortoiliac disease. Circulation [Suppl. II], 49,50:259, 1974.
10. Haimovici H, Shapiro JH, Jacobson HG: Serial femoral arteriography in occlusive disease: Clinical-roentgenologic considerations with a new classification of occlusive patterns. Am J Roentgenol Radium Ther Nucl Med 83:1042, 1960.
11. Haimovici H: Arterial circulation of the extremities, in Schwartz CJ, Werthessen NT, Wolf S (eds): Structure and Function of the Circulation. New York, Plenum Press, 1980, pp 425–485.

CHAPTER 34
Nonatherosclerotic Diseases of Small Arteries

Henry Haimovici and Yoshio Mishima

This group of diseases includes a large variety of vascular entities, many of which are still poorly understood. Their pathologic features are varied and include organic and vasospastic diseases. They may affect the vessels of both upper and lower extremities, as well as those of many vital organs.

The definition of small artery disease, in terms of vessel diameter, is often more speculative than precise. It may therefore be useful to delineate the group of arteries preferentially involved in these entities.

The small arteries are generally defined as the unnamed branches of the cognate medium-sized arteries. Included in this definition are also the arterioles and their branches, the diameters of which range from 30 to 100 μm. In the extremities, the small vessels are found distal to the medium-sized arteries of the popliteal and the brachial and represent functionally the distributive division of the arterial tree.

Although the term "diseases of small arteries" would suggest entities exclusively localized therein, it should be emphasized that the lesions may be associated in the extremities with those of the more proximal arteries, especially in the group of organic vascular diseases. Furthermore, arterioles and their smaller branches are also frequently, if not preferentially, affected in organic diseases, as well as in vasospastic and collagen diseases.

This chapter will deal only with the distinctive clinical, pathophysiologic, and therapeutic features limited to the most common entities.

The diseases causing the most common occlusive and vasospastic disorders of these vessels are listed in Table 34-1.

SMALL AND MEDIUM VESSELS

HENRY HAIMOVICI

For the sake of clarifying the complex clinicopathologic nature of the various entities, it appeared necessary to deal with them in separate sections. These will be divided into two major groups: (1) Takayasu's and Buerger's diseases and (2) the large group of the various entities indicated in Table 34-1.

The disease entities to be discussed in this chapter are distinct from those of medium and large arteries, which are due to an arteriosclerotic process. The latter represent most surgical vascular problems. Diseases of small arteries are less frequent and are rarely treated by operative procedures. Another major difference between these two groups is the pathogenesis of the small artery diseases, which is generally variable and is still poorly defined in general.

These differences are particularly relevant in connection

TABLE 34-1. NONATHEROSCLEROTIC DISEASES OF SMALL ARTERIES*

Organic diseases
  Takayasu's arteritis
  Thromboangiitis obliterans (Buerger's disease)
  Acute thrombosis of small arteries
  Arterial microemboli
  Arterial lesions of undetermined cause

Collagen diseases (immune arteritis)
  Periarteritis nodosa (Polyarteritis)
  Lupus erythematosus
  Scleroderma
  Behçet's disease

Vasospastic diseases
  Raynaud's disease or syndrome
  Acrocyanosis
  Livedo reticularis
  Frostbite

Mixed organic and vasospastic diseases
  Raynaud's phenomenon and preexisting occlusive arterial disease
  Posttraumatic occupational Raynaud's phenomenon
  Occupational trauma and secondary occlusive arterial disease of the hand

Hematologic disorders
  Polycythemia vera
  Cryoglobulinemia

*This table includes only the most common entities, usually amenable to corrective therapy.

with two diseases: Takayasu's disease and Buerger's disease. They are of the greatest interest in terms of temporal and geographic evolution characteristics of the disease process. Whereas Takayasu's disease originated in Japan and is still predominantly found in the Orient, Buerger's disease was first recognized in Western countries and until recently was predominantly found in the West. In the past two decades, for unknown reasons, Takayasu's disease is no longer exclusively seen in the Orient; by contrast, Buerger's disease is at the same time more frequent there while it is on the wane in the Western countries. Whether geographic or socioeconomic factors underlie these evolutional changes is not evident. Regardless, these two entities appeared different in the Orient and the West.

A common comprehensive review could emphasize both the similarities and the disparate features of these two diseases. The approach may appear unconventional, I believe that the Western and the Oriental experiences with these diseases could be presented independently. Thus a Japanese scholar, Professor Yoshio Mishima, will discuss the diseases from the Oriental vantage point, and I will discuss the Western experience, especially with Buerger's disease, inasmuch as I have had experience with this disease since my training days in France and later at Mt. Sinai Hospital in New York, where Leo Buerger studied and described the disease that bears his name. Consequently, two versions each of Takayasu's and Buerger's diseases, one by Mishima and the other by me, will attempt to provide an overview of the present status of these diseases in the two geographic regions.

As a result of this presentation by two different authors, there will unavoidably be repetition of some of the clinico-pathologic findings.

Takayasu's Arteritis: The Western Experience

HENRY HAIMOVICI

Initially, Takayasu's arteritis was thought to be confined mostly to the Orient, as already stated, more specifically to Japan. Subsequent reports indicated that this entity may affect all races and is worldwide in distribution.

The early reports were limited to the description of vascular lesions of the aortic arch and its branches, but later findings showed that such abnormalities may affect any segment of the aorta, with its major branches, and the pulmonary artery branches as well. Depending on the location and extent of the lesions of the branches of the aorta, Takayasu's disease is classified into four types, to be discussed in Professor Mishima's sections of this chapter.

Although atherosclerosis is recognized as the most common cause of the vascular process involving the aortic arch and its branches, Takayasu's disease was identified later as an aortitis syndrome. It was found also in the Western world as a rare but distinct possibility of a clinical and pathologic entity.

Originally, as is well known—and as stated by Mishima in his discussion—in 1908 Takayasu, a Japanese ophthalmologist, noted in younger female patients a condition of peculiar ocular manifestations consisting of capillary flush with arteriovenous anastomoses and cataracts, which could

lead to blindness. A large number of papers appeared subsequently in Japan. Among these was a paper by Shimizu and Sano in which, in addition to the above syndrome, they described the absence of pulses in the upper extremities and attributed all the manifestations to an obliterative process of the aortic arch and its main branches. They named this syndrome "pulseless disease."

The name of Takayasu attached to this syndrome remained, nevertheless, the accepted term. But besides this name, other synonyms have been used for the description of this entity: aortic arch syndrome, Martorell's syndrome, atypical coarctation, brachiocephalic arteritis, and idiopathic aortitis.

In the present chapter, the discussion of Takayasu's disease will be limited to type I. As stated earlier, most of the lesions of this type that are described in the Western literature are due to intimal atherosclerotic plaques that partially or completely obstruct the vessels. In contrast, Takayasu's arteritis has rarely been identified in the past in the Western world. On the other hand, besides Japan, even in Mexico, South America, and Africa, atherosclerosis is infrequently diagnosed in this anatomic location. Thus Kimoto in Japan found an 83% incidence of aortitis syndrome vs. a 14% incidence of arteriosclerosis, and Paramo Diaz et al. in Mexico found a similar ratio of 73% vs. 13%, respectively. In the Western world, Lande et al. and Crawford, on the basis of their personal experience, believe that most unusual lesions of the aorta and its branches, especially in young female patients, are actually due to the aortitis type, identified otherwise as Takayasu's disease.

Clinical Manifestations

Clinical manifestations progress from an early systemic phase to a late occlusive phase. Systemic manifestations include malaise, fever, leukocytosis, elevation of the erythrocyte sedimentation rate, and an increase in C-reactive protein. The incidence of these symptoms varies (35% to 53%). Recent studies incriminate immunologic factors in the development of these disease. The onset of the occlusive phase may vary from months to years after the systemic phase. Stenosis or occlusion of one or more of the aortic arch branches may produce a wide range of neurologic or ocular symptoms, including headaches, syncope, hemiplegia, hypertension, and claudication of the upper extremities.

Pathology

The nature of the disease is that of an inflammatory process of unknown origin. The arterial changes involve all layers of the arterial wall and are characterized by infiltration of giant cells in the acute phase. According to activity and duration of the inflammatory process, there may be thickening of the vessel wall, thickening of the intima, fibrosis of the media, or scarring and fibrotic reaction of the adventitia. Occlusion is associated with extension of intimal proliferation and with fibrosis of the media and adventitia.

The lesions of the aorta and its branches may progress to stenosis or occlusion and, depending on the vessel, to coarctation or aneurysm.

Stenosis or occlusion of the subclavian, carotid, and

vertebral arteries, in various combinations, is responsible for a multiplicity of cerebral and visual disturbances. The brachiocephalic lesions, with their neurologic and ophthalmologic manifestations, have been well described since Takayasu's initial observations. Depending on the affected vessels, a variety of clinical syndromes may emerge.

Arteriographic Findings

Various arteriographic patterns of the arch and its branches may be present, depending on the specific lesions. Carotid stenosis may be confined to the origin of the vessel. Not infrequently, especially in advanced cases, the stenosis may extend for a variable distance along the axis of the vessel. In these instances, it is not unusual to find a filiform narrowing extending from the aorta to the base of the skull. In general, occlusion of the brachiocephalic trunks occurs near the orifice of the artery. A flame-shaped termination of the vessel appears to be characteristic of Takayasu's arteritis. In extreme forms of brachiocephalic arteritis, all or most of its trunks are occluded. In these instances the circulation to the brain may be provided by collateral circulation, originating from a number of neck and spinal vessels.

Obstruction of the subclavian arteries may produce a subclavian steal syndrome with symptoms of cerebellar insufficiency. Some of the arteriographic characteristics should alert the clinician to the possible diagnosis of Takayasu's disease. Lande et al., among others, urge a total aortography to confirm the exact diagnosis of this disease.

Treatment

If the disease is diagnosed early, during the systemic phase, the treatment consists of the use of steroids, which may relieve symptoms in a large majority of cases. Concomitantly, arterial hypertension and heart failure are controlled by medical means, irrespective of surgical indications for the occlusive arterial lesions.

Principles and techniques of arterial reconstructive methods affecting the aortic arch branches are similar to those described earlier in this text for atherosclerotic occlusive disease (Chapter 33). Although steroids may relieve early symptoms, they do not affect the course of the established occlusive lesions.

The most applicable reconstructive methods are resection with graft interposition and bypass operations. Experience with endarterectomy has yielded poor results in most patients. The reason for the difficulties and poor outcome of endarterectomy is the lack of a cleavage plane between the thick, fibrous obstruction and the media of the wall because of the specific type of arteritis with its inflammatory lesions.

Most of the reconstructive procedures will be described in detail later in this chapter. Further descriptions of these methods may be found in Kimoto's presentation, whose experience with Takayasu's disease is extensive. Kimoto emphasizes that the best indications for reconstructive surgery are found in patients with moderate symptoms. He further states that the degree of retinal change, especially if severe, is an important guideline. In the presence of retinal changes, serious postoperative complications, such as glaucoma, retinal bleeding, or cerebral hemorrhage, could present problems.

Takayasu's Arteritis: The Japanese Experience

YOSHIO MISHIMA

In 1908, Takayasu reported the peculiar ocular manifestations seen in a young female patient with attacks of blindness and syncope. Thereafter, in 1951, Shimizu and Sano described the clinical triad of this disease, including absence of pulsation of radial arteries, arteriovenous anastomosis in the ocular fundi, and hypersensitive carotid sinus due to obliterative process of the aortic arch and its main branches. They called the syndrome "pulseless disease." Because of recent developments in clinical and laboratory studies, the concept of this disease has definitely changed, and in 1963 it was categorized as "aortitis syndrome" in Japan by Ueda et al., because the disease process involved not only the aortic arch and its branches but also the entire aorta and its branches, sometimes extended into pulmonary arteries.

Takayasu's arteritis was formerly considered almost exclusively a disease of women. In more recent years, however, there seems to have been a relative increase in the incidence of the disease among men. In our research, approximately 10% of patients with this disease are men. The number of living patients having this disease in Japan is considered to be approximately 3,000, and the annual increase of new cases is estimated to be about 100.

Pathology

From the histologic investigation of 76 autopsy cases collected over the last 16 years, Nasu (1977) classified this lesion histopathologically into three types: granulomatous inflammation type, diffuse productive inflammation type, and fibrosis type.

Granulomatous Inflammation Type (28%). Granulomas, often accompanied by Langhans' giant cells and foreign body giant cells, are formed with or without the presence of small necrotic foci and microabscesses.

Diffuse Productive Inflammation Type (14%). Diffuse infiltration of lymphocytes and plasma cells, along with proliferation of connective tissue and new growth of blood vessels, is seen in the media. A few solitary giant cells are found scattered in rare cases (Fig. 34-1).

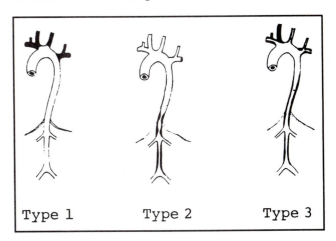

Figure 34-1. Classification.

Fibrosis Type (58%). This type was observed in a large majority of cases and was thought to be the sequela of the inflammatory changes. The severe fibrosis occurred chiefly in the media, because of scar formation after granulomatous and productive inflammation. Fibrosis of the adventitia is thought to be a protective reaction against passive distension due to diminished elasticity of the weakened media. Secondary fibrosis was also detected in the intima, and its severity depended mostly on the duration of the disease process.

In the autopsy cases, pulmonary artery involvement was detected in 45%.

Pathophysiology

Clinical pictures of Takayasu's arteritis are extremely variable because of the distribution of the arterial lesions. There has not yet been a definite classification of the disease; however, we have classified it into three types according to hemodynamic characteristics (Fig. 34-2; Table 34-2):

Type 1   A classic pulseless disease that manifests hypotension of the head and upper extremities. Dizziness, syncope, impaired vision, and claudication of the upper extremity are the commonly noted chief complaints.

Type 2   Characterized by the presence of systemic hypertension or hypertension of the upper half of the body, simulated by signs and symptoms caused by coarctation of the aorta.

Type 3   A mixed type, in which types 1 and 2 are combined, characterized by hypotension of the upper extremity and head, hypertension above the coarctated segment, and, less frequently, systemic hypertension.

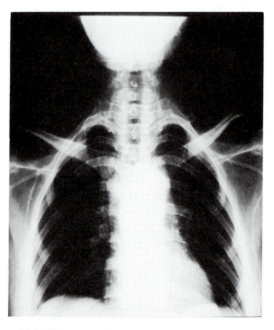

Figure 34-2. (Aortogram (a 26-year-old woman) showing occlusion of the brachiocephalic and both the carotid and subclavian arteries. Both vertebral and axillary arteries are patent through the collateral vessels.

TABLE 34-2. FREQUENCY

	Cases	Blood Pressure		
		Retinal	Ascending Aorta	Abdominal Aorta
Type 1	169	↓	Normal	Normal
Type 2	44	↑	↑	↑ ↓
Type 3	41	↓	↑	↑ ↓
Total	254			

(Inada, Ueno, Mishima)

Aortic insufficiency may be associated with Takayasu's arteritis in some cases. The pulmonary artery is also involved not uncommonly, although signs and symptoms are rarely obvious. Further, aneurysm formation can be classified as type 4 disease.

The triad pointed out by Shimizu and Sano is no longer considered to be representative of the disease. For example, the ischemic change of the ocular fundi reported by Takayasu is not so prominent as was believed, except in cases categorized as having a type 1 lesion.

The erythrocyte sedimentation rate is accelerated in the majority of cases, especially in the active stage of the disease. An increase in serum levels of α_2-globulin and γ-globulin is frequently noted. C-reactive protein is also frequently detected. These findings result from an active inflammatory process and are helpful for differentiating Takayasu's arteritis from other conditions.

The electrocardiogram frequently reveals evidence of left ventricular hypertrophy, often associated with changes in the ST segment and the T wave. They are presumably due to hypertension, or aortic insufficiency, or both, although a contribution from lesions of the coronary arteries and myocardium is not ruled out. Cardiac enlargement is a common finding on the chest x-ray film. Calcification of the aorta is also seen in some cases.

Arteriography

Aortography is the most valuable diagnostic examination and should be performed in every suspected case. Total aortography, including all brachiocephalic vessels, the entire aorta, and the renal and iliofemoral arteries, is useful for delineation of the full extent of the disease (Figs. 34-2 and 34-3).

Usually the involved arteries reveal stenosis or obstruction, but prestenotic or poststenotic dilatation may also be seen. Occasionally, aneurysm formation is recognized. In type 1 disease, as stated above, the lesions are located mostly in the aortic arch and its branches. The ascending aorta may also be affected, resulting in aortic insufficiency in some cases.

In many cases, lesions of the pulmonary arteries are detected. They are also demonstrated by pulmonary scintiscan.

Diagnosis

There are no pathognomonic symptoms of Takayasu's arteritis. Onset is often overlooked and may mimic a rheumatic or nonspecific illness with acute systemic symptoms in many cases.

General weakness and fatigability are common, espe-

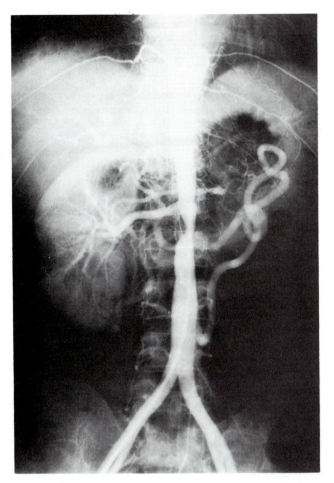

Figure 34-3. Aortogram (a 29-year-old woman) showing atypical coarctation of the aorta.

cially in the initial stage of the disease. Usually, after an asymptomatic quiescent stage of variable duration, the inflammatory lesion of the arteries becomes manifest, most commonly in the brachiocephalic vessels, with pain and tenderness of the neck, shoulders, or anterior portion of the chest. Presumably the pain is of vascular origin.

The complaints more frequently noted are due to impaired cerebral circulation, such as dizziness, headache, and visual disturbances. Ischemic symptoms of the upper extremity, such as numbness, cold sensation, and claudication, are also encountered frequently.

Clinical Course and Prognosis
The natural history of the disease is not yet fully understood. The prognosis is greatly influenced by the severity of hypertension. Aortic insufficiency is frequently associated with hypertension and is also inherent to the prognosis. Of 1,210 female patients, 664 (54.9%) have been pregnant and 622 (50.2%) have delivered a normal baby.

Treatment
Treatment currently consists of long-term steroid therapy. Subjective symptoms, together with abnormal laboratory findings, improve rapidly in most cases with administration of steroids, especially in the active stage.

Surgical intervention is mandatory in about 9% of cases.

TABLE 34-3. INDICATIONS FOR SURGICAL TREATMENT

Cerebral ischemia
Hypertension
Stenosis of the aorta
Stenosis of the renal artery
Aortic insufficiency
Aneurysm
Ischemia of upper limb

Arterial reconstructive surgery is indicated for cerebral ischemia, especially for that with progressive visual impairment, for severe hypertension, and for aneurysm with impending rupture. Aortic valve replacement may be considered in cases of severe aortic insufficiency.

From our own experience, it is desirable to perform arterial reconstructive surgery with special consideration to the hemodynamic changes caused by varying degrees of pathologic processes. Determination of arterial pressure of the various portions, such as the aorta, upper and lower extremities, and especially the retina, is the best method of further case selection for surgical treatment (Table 34-3).

Currently the most commonly used reconstruction for the cerebral ischemia is aortocarotid bypass with autologous vein graft. Earlier, we performed carotid reconstruction on both sides simultaneously. Now it is thought to be hemodynamically satisfactory to reconstruct one carotid artery on either side.

A modified technique of carotid reconstruction may also be performed. We made a first bypass between the aorta and the external carotid artery, followed by a second bypass between the graft and the internal carotid artery. Usually, a supportive maneuver such as a shunt during surgery is not necessary.

Thromboangiitis Obliterans (Buerger's Disease): The Western Experience

HENRY HAIMOVICI

As in the preceding section, there will be two versions of this discussion: one on the condition as seen at present in the United States and the remainder of the Western world and the second version on the Japanese experience with this disease.

The nature of occlusive arterial disease in young individuals has continued to be a controversial subject since 1879, when von Winiwarter first described a vascular syndrome for which he proposed the name "endarteritis obliterans." It was not until 1908, when Buerger published his classic paper, and later his book (1924), that this disease, for which he proposed the name "thromboangiitis obliterans" (TAO), became well recognized. More recently, however, the existence of this disease as an entity has been called into question, and the suggestion has been made that the cases described by Buerger were actually special examples of atherosclerosis. Subsequent critical reexamination disclosed (1) that the diagnosis of Buerger's disease was probably too frequently made in the past, (2) that the disease occurs less frequently today than it did 20 or 30 years ago, and (3) that the disease exists as a definite entity separate from atherosclerosis in a limited occurrence.

The cause of Buerger's disease is unknown. It affects primarily men (95% of the cases). Although the disease was initially thought to occur predominantly in Jews of Eastern European origin, subsequent statistical studies have shown that no race or color is known to be immune.

Heavy cigarette smoking appears to be the most important associated etiologic factor. The disease has a tendency to progress in spite of any other treatment if patients continue to smoke, whereas those who discontinue the use of cigarette smoking show improvement and seem to have no further exacerbation of the disease. A relationship between recurrence of the disease and its progression with the resumption of tobacco smoking is characteristic. Although the deleterious effects of tobacco smoking may also be encountered in arteriosclerotic occlusive disease, its almost causal relationship to the aggravation of the disease holds an unusually significant place among the diagnostic criteria for TAO.

Although the age at clinical onset of the disease is known to be between 20 and 35 years, one of the common diagnostic errors still encountered is to place patients older than 35 years who have peripheral vascular disease in the TAO category. Although occasionally this diagnosis may

be corroborated by pathologic findings in patients with clinical onset after the age of 35 or 40 years, it should be pointed out that in this age group, atherosclerosis is the most likely finding. Conversely, even in the group with an age at onset of 20 to 35 years, a number of patients may have early manifestations of atherosclerosis, as shown by findings during surgical exploration of such patients (Fig. 34-4).

Migrating thrombophlebitis is encountered in about 40% of the patients and is regarded as a characteristic component of TAO.

Involvement of all four extremities (Fig. 34-5) occurs in almost half the patients. Such distribution of the vascular lesions, although not constant, is definitely more characteristic of TAO than of any other arterial disease. Small vessels of the hand are more frequently involved by TAO than by arteriosclerosis obliterans (ASO) (Fig. 34-6).

Arteriography may reveal distinctive features of TAO, of which the most significant is a smooth outline of the arterial tree, in contrast to the intimal irregularity so characteristic of atheromatous lesions (Fig. 34-7). These arteriographic signs are important in the differential diagnosis, but it should be pointed out that they are not pathognomonic.

Histopathologic criteria deserve a critical evaluation. The disease begins in medium-sized or small arteries (poste-

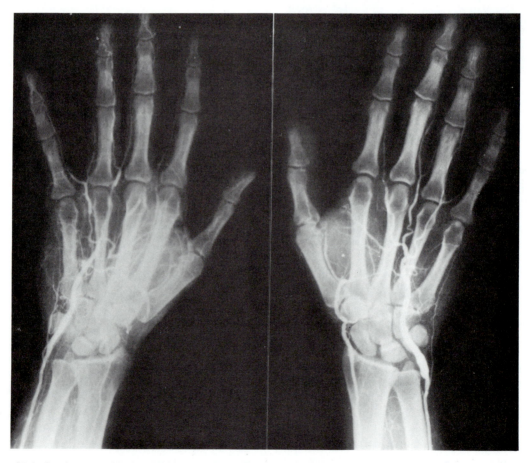

Figure 34-4. Arteriograms of both hands of a 39-year-old woman, a heavy cigarette smoker, with a 7-month history of discoloration, pain, and right index minimal fingertip ulceration. Note dilatation of ulnar artery, right more than left, occlusion of radial arteries, left more than right, and absence of opacification of most digital arterioles. Diagnosis of Buerger's disease with Raynaud's phenomenon was made. No evidence of thoracic outlet syndrome compression of vascular origin noted.

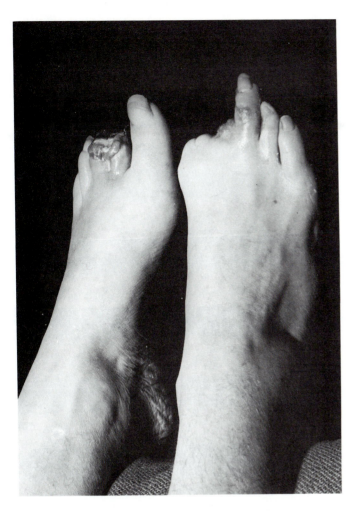

Figure 34-5. Bilateral gangrenous lesions of the toes in a woman with TAO involving all four extremities. Major peripheral arteries were patent.

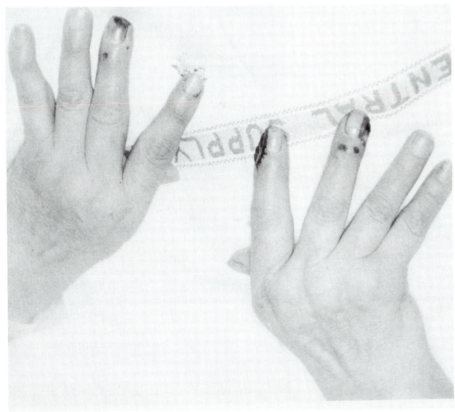

Figure 34-6. Gangrene of the fingers of both hands due to acute thrombosis of digital arterioles. Wrist pulses were normal.

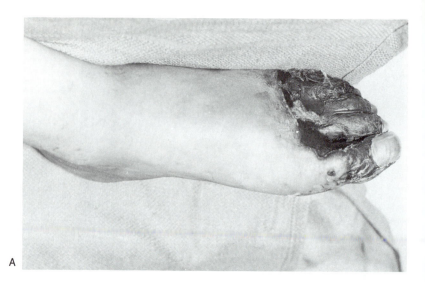

Figure 34-7. A. Gangrene of all toes of left foot in a 28-year-old man who was a heavy smoker and had involvement of all four extremities of his arteries. He underwent an above-the-knee amputation of the other lower extremity. The gangrene of the left foot developed somewhat rapidly within a matter of 2 weeks. **B.** Microscopic lesions indicate thrombosis of both artery and vein. There is a marked perivascular reaction between the artery and vein.

rior tibial, anterior tibial, radial, ulnar, plantar, palmar, or digital). The lesions are distinctly segmental and follow an episodic course. Larger arteries (popliteal, femoral, or brachial) may also be affected if the disease is severe and progressive. In the major arteries (aorta, iliac), true thromboangiitic lesions have rarely, if ever, been reported and have never been seen in our experience. This also holds true, with few exceptions, for the visceral vessels.

The histopathologic features of the vascular lesions, as described by Buerger, have perhaps been the subject of the greatest controversy. This may be due partly to the relatively wide spectrum of lesions ranging from the acute

stage to the healed thrombus. In the acute stage, Buerger described a process that consists of an acute inflammatory lesion involving all the coats of the vessel, with its lumen completely filled by a thrombus and with purulent and giant-cell foci in its periphery. These characteristic features disappear at the stage of healing (intermediate stage). The thrombus becomes organized, cellular, and recanalized. Finally, in the "healed" stage, the lumen is occluded by connective tissue representing the end product of the above-mentioned lesion, which at this time may be extremely varied in its general appearance.

Failure by some observers to demonstrate the acute

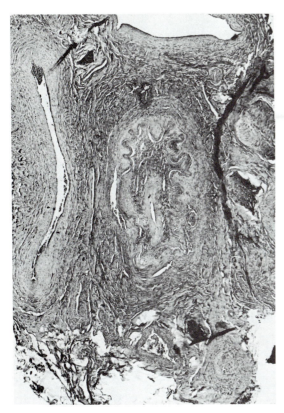
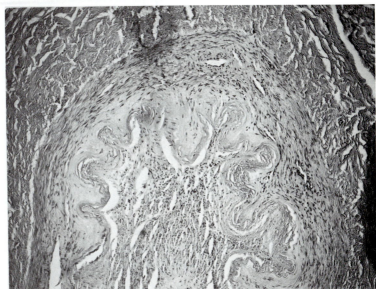

Figure 34-8. Photomicrograph of a cross section of posterior tibial vessels in a 70-year-old man who at the age of 30 years was treated for TAO. The lesions are consistent with this diagnosis. This case illustrates the possible association of Buerger's disease, which occurred at an earlier age, and arteriosclerosis of the proximal arterial tree, which developed at a later age. Most of the arteriosclerosis developed at an advanced age.

special histologic lesion is one of the sources of skepticism concerning its true significance. Recent documentary evidence has reconfirmed these characteristic lesions.

Association of TAO in the extremities with atherosclerotic changes of the aortoiliac segment or coronary or cerebral vessels is not unusual, particularly during the fifth and sixth decades of life (Fig. 34-8). Indeed, some of these patients have TAO in the medium-sized and small vessels in their young adulthood and then years later may develop atherosclerotic lesions of the major arteries or of the visceral vessels. The early peripheral vascular lesions and the late aortoiliac lesions are associated only temporally and are not related etiologically or pathogenetically. Thus it would be erroneous to attach a common label to the two vascular processes, inasmuch as a long interval separates their clinical onset (Fig. 34-9).

In relation to pathogenesis, although the description presented above clearly indicates a local reaction of a thrombus and of the arterial wall, recent studies of patients with Buerger's disease seem to have demonstrated specific cellular immunity against arterial antigens, formation of specific humoral antiarterial antibodies, and elevated levels of circulating immune complexes in many of these patients. It is necessary to point out that these studies are only of a preliminary nature and will have to be confirmed should an immunologic factor be involved in the etiology of Buerger's disease.

Diagnosis

The differential diagnosis of TAO is usually not difficult in the presence of a typical clinicopathologic picture. However, it is always necessary to keep in mind the features of ASO and idiopathic arterial thrombosis as main differential diagnoses. The main criteria for differentiating TAO from these two conditions are as outlined above. Other vascular diseases, such as vasospastic syndromes (Raynaud's disease, periarteritis nodosa, pernio, ergotism, frostbite) should not be difficult to rule out. *The histologic evidence is ultimate proof in the differential diagnosis.* In 50 patients in whom the diagnosis of TAO was made on clinical grounds, Brown et al. found only seven with clear evidence of small vessel inflammatory disease as described by Buerger.

Prognosis

The prognosis with respect to limb survival and life expectancy of patients with TAO, in comparison with those with atherosclerosis obliterans, is quite different. McPherson et al. reported a higher amputation rate in TAO in comparison with that of patients with ASO who have ischemic complications. By contrast, life expectancy appeared to be better in patients with TAO than in those with ASO.

Treatment

The treatment will vary according to the stage at which the disease presents itself. At the early stage, the arrest of progress of the disease by tobacco abstinence is absolutely

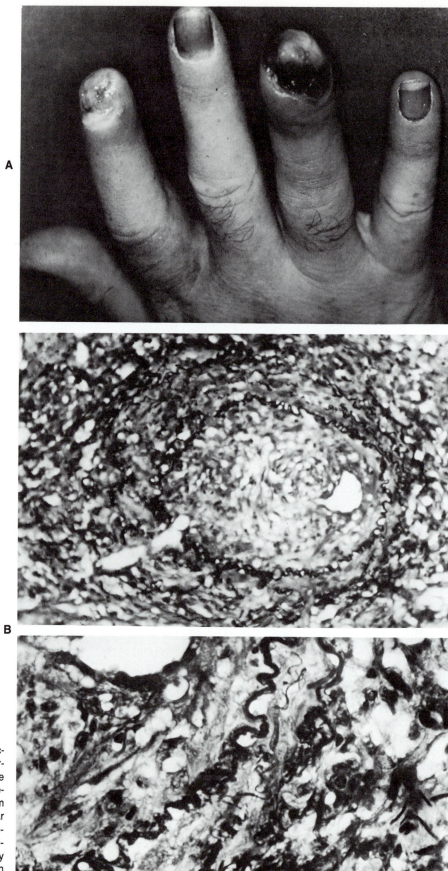

Figure 34-9. **A.** Ischemic ulcers of right second, third, and fourth fingers of a 40-year-old patient with a long history of TAO. The patient was a heavy smoker and had involvement of all four extremities. The arteriogram disclosed occlusion of the radial and ulnar arteries just proximal to the wrist and involvement of the distal portions of the digital arteries. A left upper thoracic sympathectomy was carried out, followed later by amputation of the distal phlanx of the index finger. **B.** Microscopic study of the small vessels of the digit showed lumina narrowed by proliferative endothelial lesions.

essential. Unfortunately, very few of these patients display any capability of discontinuing smoking.

The use of vasodilators may be of little effectiveness. Lumbar or upper thoracic sympathectomy may be beneficial and persistent, provided that the patient continues to abstain from smoking. In spite of a lumbar sympathectomy, it is often necessary to add destruction of a sensory nerve of the leg to achieve complete relief of pain.

Arterial reconstruction is most often not feasible in these patients. Although the posterior and anterior tibial or peroneal artery may still be patent, the multifocal lesions of the small arteries may negate the success of the bypass graft.

Amputation of toes or fingers for limited lesions is often successful, but more extensive limb loss may be unavoidable because of pain and failure to heal.

Thromboangiitis Obliterans (Buerger's Disease): The Japanese Experience

YOSHIO MISHIMA

In 1908, Leo Buerger published a paper on thromboangiitis obliterans: a study of the vascular lesions leading to presenile gangrene. As mentioned above, the description of the condition was first made by von Winiwarter. This is a segmental, inflammatory, and obliterative disease of medium-sized and small arteries affecting mainly the distal upper and lower extremities of young adult male smokers, often in association with migratory thrombophlebitis.

Although Wessler et al. recently questioned the existence of Buerger's disease as a clinical entity, many reports emphasized that there is an intense inflammatory reaction in the arteries, veins, and nerves in Buerger's disease. In Japan, many cases have been reported because Buerger's disease has been regarded with interest for a long time as spontaneous gangrene.

Etiology

The specific cause is not known. Secondary etiologic factors that have a positive effect on the disease include age, sex, race, hereditary factor (HLA antigen), autoimmune process, occupation, changes in the blood, and smoking. Smoking is the strongest secondary etiologic factor in this disease.

Pathology

Most authors agree that the inflammatory changes in all three layers of the involved vessel walls and thrombotic occlusion of the involved segments are characteristic, followed by recanalization.

In the acute stage, there may be fibroblasts and lymphocytes, and sometimes a giant cell. The occluding thrombus is very cellular and contains many nuclei of fibroblasts. Usually, the disease affects primarily the medium-sized and small arteries in segments, with relatively normal arteries between involved segments (Fig 34-10).

Migratory thrombophlebitis recurs frequently in extremities and occurs before, during, or after the onset of arterial lesions. The histologic changes in involved superficial veins are similar to those observed in the involved arteries.

In the old lesion, the involved artery is occluded by well-organized thrombi with recanalization. They are categorized as follows:

- Those with few changes in the arterial wall and involving organized thrombus and vascularization within thrombus
- Those with notable thickening of the intima
- Those with organized thrombus and with vascularization at and within the arterial wall
- Those with proliferation of elastic fibers and fragmentation of the internal elastic lamina in organized thrombus
- Those with fibroplasia, vascularization, and infiltration of round cells in arterial wall and thrombus

Therefore it is generally difficult to determine the actual cause by means of a resected specimen obtained from an old lesion.

Pathophysiology

The symptoms are those which arise from the arterial occlusion, those which depend on the inflammatory nature of the lesions, and those resulting from the breakdown of

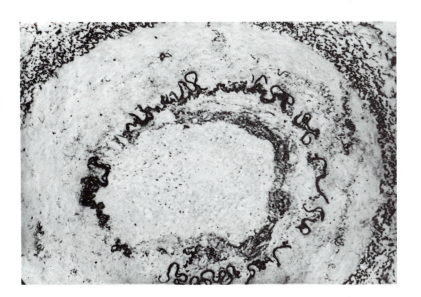

Figure 34-10. Subacute arterial lesions in the radial artery of a 32-year-old man. Proliferation of elastic fibers and fragmentations of the internal elastica in the organized thrombus are observed.

TABLE 34-4. OCCLUSIVE SITES

Upper extremities	322	22.2%
Brachial artery	25	1.7%
Radial or ulnar artery	297	20.5%
Lower extremities	1,129	77.8%
Aorto-ilio-femoral artery	25	1.7%
Popliteal artery	334	23.0%
Tibial artery	771	53.1%
	Total 1,451 limbs	

the tissue rendered ischemic by the arterial occlusion. Frequently, early symptoms include limping, caused by pain in the bottom of the foot, and gangrene, also limited to the feet. Intermittent claudication occurs but is less frequent than in arteriosclerosis obliterans, because the disease occurs mostly in the smaller vessels, such as the anterior or posterior tibial artery, often producing extensive tissue damage before claudication develops. This evidence is supported by arteriographic confirmation of the sites of arterial occlusion. In 91.9% of 322 upper extremities and in 98.7% of 1,129 lower extremities, arterial occlusion was detected distal to the cubital and popliteal bifurcations, whereas atherosclerotic occlusion developed preferably in such major channels as the iliac, femoral, and popliteal arteries (Table 34-4).

The symptoms caused by the inflammatory nature of the disease are those of ischemic neuritis, producing rest pain and the associated thrombophlebitis. Generally, the thrombophlebitis occurs in short segments and in a migratory manner. In our series, recurrent episodes of segmental superficial thombophlebitis were encountered in 29.7% of cases before, during, or after the onset of the ischemic symptoms.

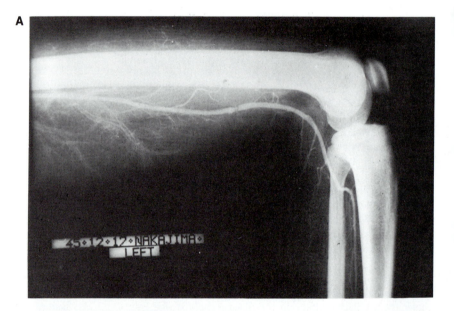

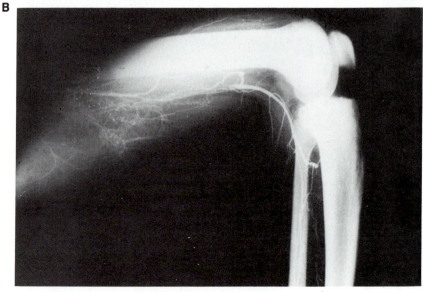

Figure 34-11. Arteriograms of a 21-year-old patient **(A)** and of the same patient at 23 years of age **(B).** In patients who clinically show acute arteritis or phlebitis, especially young patients, a small, irregular filling defect is often observed proximal to the obstructed site. This finding is considered to be the early picture of vasculitis. These lesions are often localized in small parts, but they may sometimes extend. The irregular filling defect frequently develops as an obstruction due to thrombus; especially when such lesions extend to larger parts, they easily cause acute obstruction.

The occlusive pattern and age distribution of Buerger's disease are characteristic and differ from those of arteriosclerosis obliterans. Presumably, atherosclerosis is the main cause of chronic arterial occlusion in the Western countries, whereas Buerger's disease or its related abnormality is the main cause in the Orient. Depending on the progress of the diagnostic procedures and the Europeanization of the living situation and of diet habits after World War II, the incidence of typical cases of Buerger's disease has decreased and the incidence of arteriosclerosis obliterans has increased in Japan.

Arteriography

The artery proximal to the occlusion appears smooth and of even caliber in most cases. The most characteristic occlusive patterns on the arteriogram are tapering and abrupt occlusion with tree root configuration. There are usually abundant collateral networks around the occlusion, sometimes forming a corkscrew appearance. In some cases, however, there are circumscribed stenotic lesions limited to narrow segments, followed by thrombotic occlusion in a few years.

In patients who clinically show acute arteritis or phlebitis, especially young patients, a small, irregular filling defect is often observed proximal to the obstructed site (Fig. 34-11). This finding is considered to be the early picture of vasculitis. These lesions are often localized to a small area, but they may sometimes be extensive. The irregular filling defect frequently develops as a result of obstruction by a thrombus, and especially when such lesions extend to larger parts, they can easily cause acute obstruction. Thus the arterial occlusion in Buerger's disease develops not only in an ascending fashion but also as a skip lesion. These changes may represent early stages of the disease (Fig. 34-12).

Diagnosis

The diagnostic criteria used are as follows:

- Asymmetric, abnormal coldness of the skin in the extremities
- Impairment or absence of peripheral arterial pulsations
- Exclusion of cases involving, for example, hypertension, hypercholesterolemia, albuminuria, glycosuria, calcification, abnormal electrocardiogram, or retinal atherosclerosis
- Arteriographic findings, including tapering, abrupt occlusion, and corkscrew appearance of collateral vessels
- Exclusion of cases with atheroma formation

The above-mentioned criteria are thought to be sufficient in making the clinical diagnosis, although they may include, in part, simple thrombosis or some type of nonmanifested atherosclerotic occlusions.

Clinical Course and Prognosis

From long-term observation, the cases may be classified into three groups:

Group 1 (50%)   Those with a relatively uneventful course after initial transient ischemic attacks

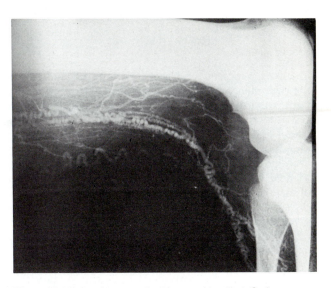

Figure 34-12. Arteriograms of a 32-year-old patient. Corkscrew appearance is due to development of collateral vessels.

Group 2 (42%)   Those with recurrence of relatively mild clinical manifestations during the follow-up period

Group 3 (8%)   Those with recurring acute episodes of severe clinical symptoms during the observation period, usually followed by major amputation

Empirically noteworthy are the cases occurring at an early age and belonging to group 3 of our classification.

In our series the patients with Buerger's disease had a practically normal survival rate, in comparison with a normal population of the same age and sex distribution. The survival curves in this series resemble those reported by McPherson et al. and both curves are distinctly better than those of the patients with arteriosclerosis obliterans.

Treatment

Suspicion of Buerger's disease is the signal for complete abstinence from smoking and the institution of a variety of other supportive measures, although none of them is specific.

To date, the vasodilating substances have been prescribed mainly for patients suffering from chronic arterial occlusive disease. In recent years, however, the rheologic study of microcirculatory disturbances in these cases has progressed both experimentally and clinically. Consequently, the agents that improve the deficient microcirculation have been noticed. In our multiclinical trials, an antiplatelet agent (Ticlopidine), an agent transforming the shape of the human red cell (Pentoxifylline), and a defibrinating agent (Batroxobin) were similarly effective for the ischemic leg ulcer caused by chronic arterial occlusion.

Surgical therapy for arterial diseases of the extremities consists of an indirect procedure for the release of vasospasm and direct arterial surgery for the reestablishment of arterial flow. In Buerger's disease, conventional arterial reconstructive surgery rarely seems to be of value.

Behçet's Disease[*]

YOSHIO MISHIMA

The main symptoms of Behçet's disease occur not only in the skin, mucosa, and eyes but also in the joints, digestive tract, vascular system, and nervous system. Its clinical course is characterized by a repeated cycle of acute exercerbation and remission in the incipient stage, and then it gradually becomes chronic. For many years, the known vascular complications in Behçet's disease have been attributed to thrombophlebitis. But a considerable number of reports have been published in recent years relating to cases with aneurysm and arterial occlusion. These vascular involvements are considered to be essential pictures of the disease process, as a part of the wide variety of clinical manifestations of this systemic disease.

Histologic changes of these arteries reveal derangements of the media, particularly of its elastic fibers (Fig. 34-13). Of the vascular changes in Behçet's disease, aneurysms develop at a relatively early age and are extremely prone to rupture. Therefore an aggressive surgical approach, initiated as soon as the diagnosis of this disease becomes definite, is mandatory for aneurysm.

At operation, the aneurysm usually adheres tightly to concomitant veins and to the perivascular tissues. It should be particularly noted that dissection from the inferior vena cava is difficult in the case of abdominal aortic aneurysm. Although all the inflammatory areas should be surgically removed, the dissection from the inferior vena cava is so difficult in the case of abdominal aortic aneurysm

EDITOR'S NOTE: Behçet's disease is largely unknown in the West. According to Behçet, it consists of a "triad of iritis, oral and scrotal ulcerations." Additional manifestations consist of vascular findings in the skin, joints, and elsewhere. This condition appears most frequently in the Middle and Far East. The most striking vascular findings are multiple central and peripheral arterial aneurysms. Bacterial infection is often associated with these vascular conditions. Their surgical repair is an extremely hazardous undertaking—*H. H.*

that complete removal of the affected areas is occasionally abandoned, and even still-active inflammation is left untouched. Because of this operative difficulty, there still remain dangers of infection of the graft and of hemorrhage from the anastomosis, which sometimes lead to the formation of a new aneurysm at the anastomotic site. So far it has also been well known that infection occurs so often in Behçet's disease that great care should be taken before, during, and after surgery.

ACUTE THROMBOSIS OF SMALL ARTERIES

HENRY HAIMOVICI

Sudden and widespread occlusion of small arteries of the hands and feet may be due to acute thrombosis in the absence of atherosclerosis. The lesions are usually limited to toes and fingers, with no previous history of intermittent claudication or impairment of the hands. The peripheral pulsations are normal in the vast number of cases. The underlying abnormality is usually an occlusive process, due to thrombosis, of the digital arterioles. Jepson described 11 cases of acute arterial thrombosis of the small arteries of the hands and feet, often in the same individual, leading in some cases to gangrene. In all these patients the acute episode was followed by a remarkable degree of recovery of the limb function, with little impairment and with Raynaud's phenomenon recurring only rarely, at a later stage. The organic occlusion of the digital arteries produced marked cyanosis of the digits and in some instances proceeded to limited gangrene. Similar cases have been described previously under the title "symmetrical digital gangrene" and have been misdiagnosed as Raynaud's disease. However, their clinicopathologic features and subsequent course do not fit the description of the latter entity.

A differential diagnosis of these acute lesions from arterial embolic or venous gangrene is usually established easily by the absence of cardinal signs of a cardiogenic source

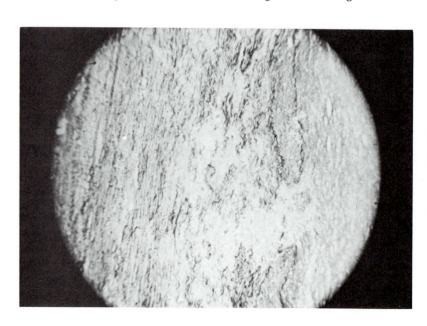

Figure 34-13. Moth-eaten appearance of the medial layer of the aorta in a patient with Behçet's disease.

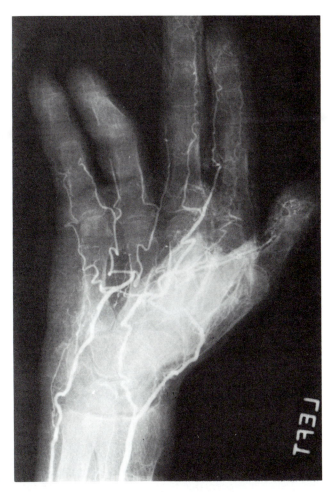

Figure 34-14. Arteriogram of left hand of a 70-year-old man with an acute syndrome of sudden pain, cyanosis, and coldness of the fourth and fifth fingers. Note occlusion of distal half of digital arterioles of these two fingers, which led eventually to gangrene and partial amputation.

for embolic lesions or by the absence of massive venous occlusion associated with gangrene (Fig. 34-14).

In the presence of severe vasospasm with incipient digital gangrene, a cervicothoracic or lumbar sympathectomy is indicated in most instances, combined, when necessary, with digital amputation.

Arterial Microemboli

Two types of microemboli may be responsible for acute occlusion of small arterial vessels: thromboembolism and atheroembolism.

Thromboembolism

Embolism resulting from a thrombus originating in a cardioarterial system (e.g., heart, aortic aneurysm) and involving the small arteries of the extremities, and even the medium-sized vessels, is rare. In a previous study of 300 cases of peripheral arterial embolism, we found 18 emboli lodged in the anterior and posterior tibial arteries and eight in the radial and ulnar arteries, a total of 26 cases representing 8.7% of the entire series. The clinical manifestations, although often minimal, may lead to severe ischemia. Such an instance is illustrated in Figure 34-15, which shows an embolus of the left radial artery and its palmar arch. Even when microthrombi occlude small arteries, localized skin lesions may result. Furthermore, occlusion of a medium-sized artery, such as the anterior tibial, may occasionally lead to ischemic gangrene of the muscles of the anterior compartment in spite of embolectomy and fasciotomy. In one instance, excision of the entire anterolateral compartment was carried out to achieve salvage of the leg.

Atheroembolism

Atheromatous emboli may arrest in multiple organs (e.g., kidney, pancreas, spleen), and in the lower extremities as well. Most such microemboli originate in the infrarenal or terminal portion of the aorta. Their size ranges from cholesterol crystals to atheromatous plaques. Embolization, primarily involving the legs, often produces a distinct clinical syndrome. Myalgia or simple muscle tenderness is frequent, and the appearance of cutaneous lesions, ranging from tender discoloration to necrosis and ulceration, is characteris-

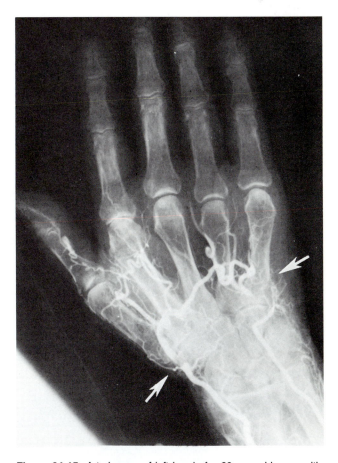

Figure 34-15. Arteriogram of left hand of a 60-year-old man, with sudden coldness, numbness, and pain of 48 hours' duration. Note embolic occlusion of the terminal segment of the radial artery extending into the palmar arch, with absence of opacification of digital arterioles. Symptoms were completely relieved after embolectomy.

tic. Peripheral pulses are usually present with microembolization, although they may be absent if preexisting occlusive disease is associated with this syndrome.

Although most atheromatous emboli may be spontaneous, some are iatrogenic in origin and occur after operation on the aorta or catheterization of the vessels. Depending on the size of the emboli, the resulting manifestations may range from a subclinical state to an obvious arterial occlusion. The diagnosis of arterial embolism in these cases may be difficult to resolve in the absence of a cardiogenic origin (atrial fibrillation, myocardial infarct) or the presence of a known abdominal aneurysm or of an aortogram indicating the presence of ulcerated lesions. Often the benign clinical manifestations are overlooked or do not receive adequate interpretation because of lack of evidence of the source of the embolism. Often, only awareness of the existence of such emboli would help one to make the correct diagnosis.

Anticoagulation may be of little value in this condition. In the presence of an ulcerated atheromatous aorta or abdominal aortic aneurysm, its resection offers the best hope to prevent further embolism.

Arterial Lesions of Undetermined Cause

As has been stated, lesions of small arteries are not always easy to identify. Frequent lack of specificity of the clinical and histopathologic features of these entities often makes it difficult to classify them with reasonable certainty. TAO is a classic example that has aroused a great deal of controversy concerning its identification and even its very existence. One of the results of this debate was reassessment and reclassification as atherosclerosis, of many cases considered earlier to be TAO.

It should be pointed out that certain pathologic features of some small vessel diseases are common to several entities, especially in the broad category of vasculitis. Thus nosologic identification of some cases is uncertain. Hardy et al. reported a typical case presenting complex thrombotic and inflammatory lesions of small arteries. The various diagnoses considered in that case range from Buerger's disease to essential polyangiitis to possible collagen disease. Such unclassified lesions are probably not unusual.

In connection with these cases of arterial lesions of undetermined cause, Inada et al., in 1974, reported on 11 patients with atypical Buerger's disease in whom the available histologic material supported an inflammatory cause more complicated than a simple reaction to thrombosis. The cases thus reported were atypical of Buerger's disease in comparison with other cases described in that article, in which 236 cases of a group of 375 were classified as Buerger's disease and only 139 cases as arteriosclerosis. This unusual type of small artery thrombosis of undetermined origin occurred in 11 of these cases of so-called Buerger's disease. There were definite inflammatory changes suggestive of the inflammatory origin of the occlusive lesion in these cases. These changes were not considered to be a reaction to simple thrombosis. The pathologic changes of Buerger's disease differed according to the stage of the disease.

Vaidya, of India, in commenting on the paper presented by Inada et al., stated that in India, Sri Lanka, and other countries of the Orient, occlusive arterial disease affecting the inferior extremity, seen predominantly in young males, frequently results in gradual vascular insufficiency, ischemia, and gangrene, similar to the cases described by Inada et al. It appears that the process of obliteration starts at the distal end and that the thrombus gradually ascends.

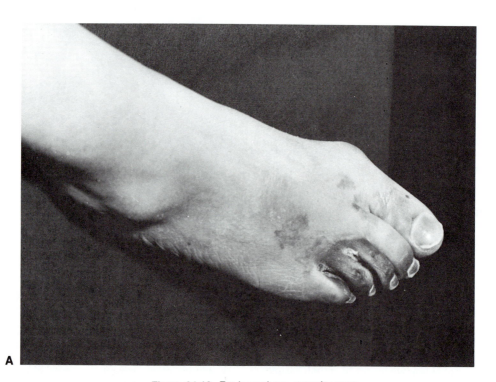

A

Figure 34-16. For legend see opposite page.

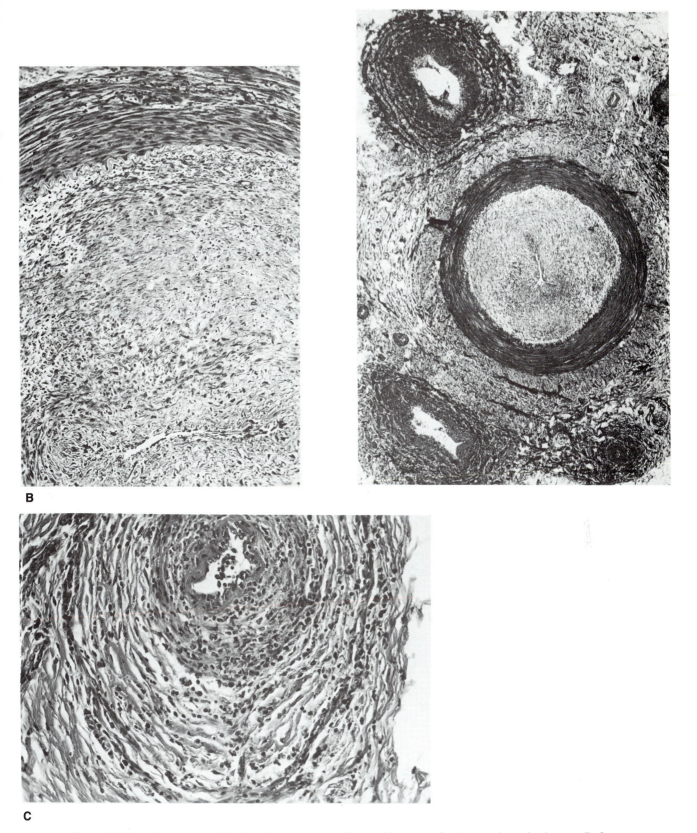

B

C

Figure 34-16. A. Gangrene of right foot of nonsmoker, a 35-year-old woman, due to an undetermined cause. **B.** Cross section (*left*) of posterior tibial artery and of venae comitantes. The microscopic lesions appear consistent with the diagnosis of thromboangiitis obliterans or arteritis of undetermined cause. (Elastica–van Gieson stain; ×30.) Magnification of a portion of the posterior tibial artery (*right*), showing greater detail of the histologic changes. (Elastica–van Gieson stain; ×60.) **C.** Photomicrograph of a section of an arteriole in the gastrocnemius muscle. Lesions are those of a panarteritis.

It may stop short at any level; in the majority of patients it stops in the popliteal artery. There are no skip lesions. It is thought that some sort of infection may be entering through the bare skin of the feet, or perhaps some kind of reaction to tubercular infection may be occurring in the arterial tree. The presence of the Langhans type of giant cells and calcification of the granulomatous inflammatory tissue surrounding the thrombus and also of the arterial wall point in this direction, although *Mycobacterium tuberculosis* has neither been seen or cultured. The lesions described by Vaidya are almost identical to those described by Inada et al., as mentioned above. Their exact nature has not yet been established. Opinions have been expressed in favor of rheumatic, tubercular, and autoimmune origin, without substantial evidence. It resembles some collagen diseases in certain characteristics as well.

I reported a case in which a 35-year-old white woman had pain in the toes of both feet and in the ankles, in association with swelling and difficulty in walking. Her condition began at the age of 14 years, and until the time of her admission to the hospital, she experienced intermittent attacks of pain and swelling of the distal portions of both lower extremities (Fig. 34-16). She finally underwent below-the-knee amputation because of spreading gangrene of the toes and severe pain. Cross section of the posterior tibial artery and of the venae comitantes showed microscopic lesions consistent with the diagnosis of TAO. However, the gangrene of the right foot due to disseminated obliterative arteritis of undetermined origin involved not only the medium-sized arteries but also their tributaries of small vessels in the muscles and skin. The lesions appeared to be typical of TAO, but in the small muscular vessels they were consistent with the diagnosis of polyarteritis nodosa. Therefore, as Hardy and Alican emphasized in their article, the histopathologic diagnosis was based on this complex clinical picture as well as on the histopathologic findings. It appears that the lesions in this particular case simply represented a combined process of two independent entities: TAO and a mixed pathologic finding of collagen disease or polyarteritis nodosa. Therefore the term "undetermined cause" must still be applied to these cases, as described by Inada et al. and Vaidya—and as indicated by my own experience in this field.

COLLAGEN DISEASES (IMMUNE ARTERITIS)

HENRY HAIMOVICI

Periarteritis Nodosa (Polyarteritis)

Periarteritis nodosa is an inflammatory disease of the medium-sized and small arteries. Since the introduction of this term in 1866 by Kussmaul and Maier, this entity has also been described by other terms; the most frequently encountered synonyms include necrotizing angiitis, polyarteritis, and panarteritis. This process may affect the arteries throughout the body. Its clinical manifestations are protean, often simulating an infectious disease with toxemia. The clinical course may be acute or chronic, with symptoms and signs referable to the organs and tissues affected. In order of decreasing frequency, the clinical features include arthralgia, skin lesions, cerebrovascular accidents, respiratory manifestations, myalgia, gastrointestinal syndromes, cardiac lesions, renal manifestations, vascular lesions involving the veins as well as the arteries, and genital complications.

The common denominator of all these clinical syndromes is the involvement of the medium-sized and small arteries, the outstanding pathologic change being a focal necrosis of the medial coat with perivascular inflammatory changes. When the process extends to the intima, the smaller vessels may become occluded. As a result, blood supply to various organs and tissues is markedly impaired, leading to necrosis, infarction, or fatty degeneration.

Because of the multiplicity of the clinical manifestations, the diagnosis of periarteritis nodosa may be extremely difficult. The disease should be suspected in any patient who has an obscure illness suggesting the presence of a diffuse systemic process with involvement of several organs and tissues, particularly joints, skin, kidneys, gastrointestinal tract, or peripheral nerves.

Laboratory findings may be helpful, if positive, but often they are nonspecific. Rapid erythrocyte sedimentation rate, leukocytosis, hypertension, and often failure of the condition to respond to conventional treatment should provide enough evidence to justify suspecting this diagnosis. Biopsy diagnosis, when positive, is the most helpful procedure, but its interpretation may be limited because of the possible inadequacy of the specimen. Histologic examination of the tissues should establish the nature of the disease. Biopsy specimens of skin or muscle may often demonstrate involvement of the small vessels or arterioles. However, biopsy specimens of the liver or kidney are rarely helpful in establishing a diagnosis—and the biopsy procedure is hazardous. In general, random biopsies should be avoided because they are of little value in establishing the nature of the vascular lesion.

Periarteritis nodosa, or polyarteritis, is seen mostly in male patients in a ratio of 2:1; the peak incidence is in the fifth decade of life. Formation of aneurysms associated with the inflammatory destruction of the media is observed relatively often. Among more frequently involved organs are the kidney, heart, lung, liver, and gastrointestinal tract, as mentioned above. Recently, in a detailed arteriographic study of 17 patients with this condition, Travers et al. reported that 10 of the patients had multiple aneurysms involving the hepatic, renal, and mesenteric vessels. Obviously, ruptured aneurysms in these locations are often unrecognized and undiagnosed before surgical exploration or postmortem examination and therefore contribute to the death of the patient. This type of aneurysm limits considerably the options of the vascular surgeon, and experience gained with these cases has been limited as a result of these clinicopathologic complications.

Therefore the prognosis for periarteritis nodosa is usually poor, although the condition is not invariably fatal. Of the criteria reflecting poor prognosis, the most significant are the visceral manifestations, especially hypertension, renal involvement, and rupture of aneurysms, as mentioned.

The use of corticosteroids has greatly improved the overall outlook. Treatment must be instituted before widespread vascular damage occurs and should be intensive and prolonged. Frohnert and Sheps, in a long-term follow-up study of periarteritis nodosa, were able to demonstrate a 5-year survival rate of 48% of patients treated with steroids. Early diagnosis is of paramount importance for adequate management of this condition, which was formerly considered fatal in most instances.

Lupus Erythematosus

The vascular manifestations associated with lupus erythematosus are varied and complex. The most common lesions involve the smaller arteries, most frequently the digital arterioles. In addition, both arterial and venous thrombosis of larger vessels is also seen. Venous thrombosis involving both superficial and deep veins and pulmonary embolism are not infrequently encountered in these patients. However, the typical vasculitis of small vessels is characteristic of lupus and is responsible for the skin infarction and the paroxysmal color changes, whereas the thrombosis of the larger arteries and veins is due to a different mechanism.

Raynaud's phenomenon is seen in about 20% of patients with systemic lupus erythematosus and seems to precede other vascular manifestations of the disease by several years. Gangrene is usually limited to the digits. Leg ulcers with systemic lupus erythematosus have been reported to be due to infarction of the skin as a result of vasculitis.

Among the laboratory findings, the LE cell phenomenon is characteristic of this syndrome. It is present in only about 75% of the patients with clinical systemic lupus erythematosus. During clinical remissions, either there is a reduction in the number of LE cells or the test result becomes negative. Acute lupus erythematosus may be fatal within a matter of a few weeks. However, in the milder forms of the disease, the clinical course is prolonged and relatively benign.

Treatment consists of large doses of corticosteroids. Continuous or intermittent steroid therapy may provide many years of remission.

Scleroderma

Patients with scleroderma often have associated Raynaud's phenomenon characterized by intermittent digital vasospasm or even persistent coldness and cyanosis. Raynaud's phenomenon is sometimes the outstanding manifestation that first brings the patient to the attention of the physician.

The pathologic skin changes in scleroderma that are associated with Raynaud's phenomenon consist of increase and swelling of collagenous connective tissue with fragmentation and swelling of the elastic fibers in the dermis. Replacement of the subcutaneous tissue by abnormal connective tissue, both within the fibrils and in the ground substance, is specific to systemic scleroderma. The epidermis may be hyperkeratotic, with melanin often accumulated in the basal cells.

The arteriolar changes in scleroderma consists of thickening of the intima, involving not only the arterioles in the skin but also those of the kidney, gastrointestinal tract, musculature, and central nervous system. The vascular manifestations seem to arise from a local fault similar to Raynaud's disease. An increase in connective tissue surrounding blood vessels has been suggested as the cause of constriction of the vessels, leading to ischemia, at least of the skin of the affected region.

Raynaud's phenomenon associated with diffuse scleroderma is seen mostly in women. The chronology of the manifestations may be variable. In some cases, Raynaud's phenomenon precedes the sclerodermal skin changes, whereas in other instances the stiffness and soreness of the joints antedate the functional organic vascular disease. As the disease progresses, the tips of the fingers or toes may become more pointed or shrunken. Occasionally, a limited gangrenous lesion of the distal phalanx of a finger or toe may be present.

The prognosis of Raynaud's phenomenon associated with diffuse scleroderma is variable. It is usually fatal in patients with renal, cardiac, and other visceral involvement.

Management of Raynaud's phenomenon associated with scleroderma includes protection against trauma or other injurious factors and use of measures to increase peripheral circulation, such as treatment with reserpine or methyldopa. Sympathectomy at the early stage of scleroderma associated with marked Raynaud's phenomenon is advocated by some but has little value in general; especially in the late stages it has no value.

VASOSPASTIC DISEASES

HENRY HAIMOVICI

Raynaud's Disease

Since the original description in 1862 by Maurice Raynaud, the disease known by his name has undergone a wide reappraisal in regard to its clinical manifestations, which has led to a reclassification of this entity. Raynaud's disease is defined as a purely vasospastic phenomenon involving mainly the digital arterioles of both hands and feet. It is characterized by a triad of intermittent color changes consisting of pallor, cyanosis, and rubor brought on by exposure to cold or by emotional stimuli. These symptoms are usually worse in the cold season and disappear or become less severe in the warm season. The onset of these manifestations is usually gradual. Originally only the tips of one or two fingers of both hands are involved, but at a later stage, involvement extends to the more proximal parts of the fingers. In the very late stages, although rarely, it may also extend to the rest of the hands. Involvement of the toes is less conspicuous but often occurs in conjunction with the vasomotor changes in the fingers and hands.

The disease is progressive, especially among women, and may become severe and disabling. Ulceration of the tips of the fingers and occasionally gangrene may cause a considerable amount of pain and discomfort. Loss of tissue in Raynaud's disease is exceptional, however, except for the distal phalanx and infected and progressively gangrenous lesions.

The exact cause of primary Raynaud's disease remains obscure. In about 80% or 90% of patients, it appears before 40 years of age. In men, it is much less severe in intensity. When Raynaud's disease occurs in the later decades, organic vascular changes are usually associated with it.

Pathology

Virtually nothing is known about pathologic changes of the digital vessels in the early stages of Raynaud's disease because biopsy specimens are not available. Lack of abnormality of the small vessels in primary Raynaud's disease is such that description of the disease does not entirely meet the definition of this chapter. Nevertheless, it is described in this chapter mainly because it may occur in association with organic or traumatic lesions. As a consequence, one has to be aware of this association to understand the more complex features of Raynaud's syndrome.

Although no biopsy or pathologic evidence exists regarding the changes in the digital arterioles, the changes may be observed in persons aged 50 years or more without Raynaud's disease, because of normal age-related changes of the arteries. At a later stage, with the advent of trophic skin lesions of the tip of the fingers, obstructive disease of the digital arteries may be present.

Diagnosis

Arteriography has been of little value in establishing the diagnosis because it has failed to demonstrate any distinctive arterial disease of the digital arterioles.

Acrocyanosis

Acrocyanosis is usually confused with Raynaud's disease. Like Raynaud's disease, it is prevalent in women and is characterized by painless and persistent coldness and cyanosis of the distal parts of the extremities. Its cause and physiopathology are obscure. Most authors tend to agree with Lewis and Landis that its disturbed physiology is reflected in the smaller vessels of the extremities. The local fault is attributed to increased vasomotor tone of the small arterioles, which leads to dilatation of the capillaries and venules even at normal environmental temperature.

Clinically, the patient notes constant coldness and bluish discoloration of the fingers and hands for many years. These signs and symptoms are more pronounced in the winter months but remain present, although to a lesser degree, in a warm environment. The color changes do not disappear on elevation of the hand. The major arteries are normal, and trophic changes do not occur in this condition.

The differentiation of acrocyanosis from Raynaud's disease should be easily determined if the triad of intermittent cold-induced color changes characteristic of the latter condition is carefully identified.

Management of acrocyanosis remains largely that of protecting the patient from cold and using vasodilator drugs, which may be of some value. In severe cases, sympathectomy, either thoracic or lumbar, offers a better prospect of a good result than that obtained in the treatment of Raynaud's disease. Prognosis is usually good in regard to viability of the limb.

Livedo Reticularis

Livedo reticularis is a vasospastic condition characterized by bluish discoloration and by blotchy reddish blue skin; it is seen mostly in women.

The basic physiologic abnormality consists of a narrowing, either organic or functional, of the arterioles, with dilatation of the capillaries and venules.

The underlying vascular abnormality is characterized primarily by thrombosis of digital arteries with absence of involvement of the larger vessels. The histopathologic changes consist of proliferation of the intima and of the isolated arterioles and small arteries. Some of these vessels are occluded completely by the proliferative process or by thrombosis, or both, with similar lesions being found in a few of the larger veins. In the presence of ulcerations of the skin due to livedo reticularis, dilated subepidermal capillaries, lymph vessels, and venules often accompany the nonspecific infiltrate of the skin.

The clinical manifestations consist of persistent bluish red mottling of the skin, not only of the lower extremities but often of the hands and arms, to a lesser degree, and occasionally of the lower part of the trunk. Coldness, numbness, dull aching, and paresthesia of the feet and legs are often present as well. Leg and foot ulcers associated with livedo reticularis are commonly recurrent during the winter months. These ulcers are usually painful and resistant to healing.

Livedo reticularis as a result of periarteritis nodosa, systemic lupus erythematosus, cryoglobulinemia, microembolism, or arteriosclerosis obliterans is a distinct possibility and should be considered in the differential diagnosis.

In mild forms of the disease, conservative management of the vasospastic condition and the ulceration may be helpful. Lumbar sympathectomy should be tried, because it may be effective in certain patients.

Frostbite

Acute frostbite is the result of vasoconstriction, which, if unrelieved, may lead to severe ischemia as a result of superimposed thrombosis of smaller arteries. Although the cause of death of the tissue is not entirely elucidated, it is well known that marked intimal changes of small arteries and arterioles may develop at a later stage. In addition, the endothelium of the terminal capillaries may also be severely damaged, affecting the permeability of the capillary wall. Stasis thrombosis then occurs in terminal arterioles and capillaries.

On the basis of the severity of tissue damage, frostbite has been classified, in a fashion similar to the classification of burns, into four degrees. However, classification into superficial and deep frostbite, as suggested more recently, appears to have more practical value.

Superficial frostbite involves the skin and superficial subcutaneous tissue, whereas deep frostbite involves—besides the skin—subcutaneous tissue, muscle, and even bone. In the mild form there is numbness, yellowing of the skin, and prickling and itching sensations. At this initial stage, rewarming of the extremity may alter the situation within a few minutes to a few hours, and recovery may be permanent.

In severe frostbite, paresthesia and stiffness are more marked than in the mild form, and there is complete loss of sensation to touch. Rewarming of the extremity is accompanied by reactive hyperemia, tenderness, burning pain, and possible formation of blisters. Necrosis or gangrene of the extremity may develop at this stage. Depending on the severity of the frostbite, the necrotic tissue may be more superficial than is suspected initially.

The diagnosis of the severe degree of frostbite is usually not difficult. In patients whose age indicates probable arteriosclerosis, it is important to determine preexisting arterial occlusive disease. Obviously, the prognosis for frostbite associated with such disease is much less favorable than that of a similar degree of frostbite with normal circulation. A history of previous intermittent claudication, cold feet, or Raynaud's phenomenon should be ascertained in each of these patients with frostbite. It may have medicolegal implications.

Frostbite should be considered as an emergency, and treatment should be instituted without delay for better salvage of the involved extremity.

In mild frostbite, restoration of natural warmth to the skin should be achieved as quickly as possible. Rubbing of the affected part should be avoided, because it may result in trauma to the skin. Likewise, overheating of the skin should be completely avoided.

In severe frostbite, avoidance of trauma and maintenance of asepsis are of great significance. On the basis of recent experience, rapid thawing is preferred to a slow rewarming. Vasodilator procedures and use of heparin have been advocated by some and found to be of no value by others. In the presence of tissue damage and gangrene, amputation should be delayed as long as possible, because the lesions may be superficial. Conservative therapy and local debridement may result in healing without major loss of tissue.

MIXED ORGANIC AND VASOSPASTIC DISEASES

HENRY HAIMOVICI

Raynaud's Phenomenon and Preexisting Occlusive Arterial Disease

Raynaud's phenomenon may occur in association with preexisting occlusive arterial disease. Vasospastic phenomena displaying the characteristics of Raynaud's triad may be encountered in Buerger's disease in about 30% of the

cases, in arteriosclerosis obliterans in about 10 to 15%, and in embolic occlusions in about 10%. This association of organic occlusive disease and Raynaud's phenomenon is generally not well recognized. It is usually precipitated by environmental coldness without emotional stimuli. It is more frequently observed in men, in contrast to Raynaud's disease, which is prevalent in women. The presence of occlusive arterial disease and the usual absence of bilaterality provide the main criteria for the differential diagnosis.

Posttraumatic Occupational Raynaud's Phenomenon

Occupational injuries of various types, such as those occurring in pianists, typists, workers using the pneumatic hammer or vibrating tools, and machinists of all types, may induce Raynaud's phenomenon. This phenomenon usually involves only one or two digits and, if severe enough, may result in occupational disability (Fig. 34-17). Protection from

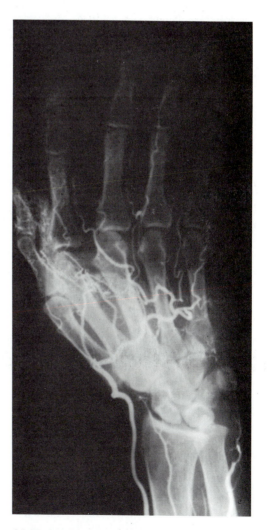

Figure 34-17. Arteriogram of right hand of 53-year-old man who injured his hand 2 years before the onset of coldness, pain, cyanosis, and ischemic ulcer of all fingertips except the tip of the thumb. Note complete occlusion of the ulnar artery just proximal to the wrist joint and lack of opacification of most digital arterioles.

exposure to cold, which is invoked as a precipitating factor, avoidance of intermittent trauma, or readjustment in the technique of a pianist or typist may be helpful. If the condition is too severe and symptoms are frequent, leading to marked disability, the temporary cessation of the occupation or permanent discontinuance may be necessary.

The use of vibrating tools has resulted in Raynaud's phenomenon after repeated percussion on the hands, a syndrome also known as pneumatic hammer disease. The phenomenon is attributed to sensitization of digital arterioles because of both rapid percussion and exposure to cold. If the occupation leads to intolerable disability, a sympathectomy may be justifiable if the occupation cannot be changed without undue hardship.

Occupational Trauma and Secondary Occlusive Arterial Disease of the Hand

Workers who use vibrating tools and machinists, laborers, and farmers, whose hands are subjected to repeated blunt trauma, may complain of pain, coldness, and color changes typical of Raynaud's phenomenon. They may have cold fingers and painful ulcers as a result of the combined arterial occlusive disease of the fingers and repeated trauma. The arterial occlusive process in these patients is usually considered a result of chronic arterial injury. Such patients may present a syndrome of ulnar occlusion due to trauma resulting from occupational use of the hypothenar portion of the hand. This latter condition is called *hypothenar traumatic syndrome*. A recent communication on 17 cases with long-term follow-up indicated the presence of thrombosis or aneurysm of the ulnar artery. Arteriography is essential for identifying the location and extent of the lesions. Local surgery may be necessary, and reconstructive vascular procedures may be feasible if involvement is confined to the proximal segment of the ulnar artery.

HEMATOLOGIC DISORDERS

Polycythemia Vera

As early as 1903, Osler recognized the frequency of vascular complications occurring in polycythemia vera. The most serious complications are thrombosis and hemorrhage. These occur in about one third to one half of the patients and are a significant cause of morbidity and death.

The thrombotic sites are most frequently seen in the peripheral, cerebral, and coronary vascular systems, with mesenteric, splenic, hepatic, and portal venous occlusions occurring less commonly. Arterial thrombosis associated with polycythemia involves primarily the smaller arteries or the digital arterioles.

The coexistence of polycythemia vera and vascular complications poses the question of their causal relationship, because some of these entities may be coincidental. On the basis of a series of 98 cases of polycythemia with 34% vascular complications, Norman and Allen concluded that a cause-and-effect relationship exists between these conditions. It is conceivable, however, that the presence of arte-

riosclerosis or TAO together with polycythemia may raise some doubts about the latter's role in the causation of vascular complications. However, it appears that the treatment of polycythemia may sometimes improve the arterial lesions, lending support in such cases to the role of the hematologic disorder in their causation. Regardless of these combined or coincidental conditions, polycythemia vera per se will induce small vessel thrombosis.

A few examples from my experience will illustrate some of the associated clinical manifestations of polycythemia vera leading to ischemic lesions.

1. A 40-year-old man developed gangrene of one toe of the right foot and cyanosis of all the other toes and the forefoot. Both pedal pulses were palpable, and an arteriogram disclosed only a short segmental stenosis of the midportion of the anterior tibial. In this case, the relationship of small vessel involvement and polycythemia appeared plausible.

2. An 80-year-old man with atherosclerosis obliterans of the distal tibial arteries developed gangrene of the great toe, requiring its subsequent amputation. Concomitant active treatment of the hematologic condition seemed to relieve the ischemic manifestations of the rest of the foot. In this case, the polycythemia appeared as an aggravating factor rather than as its initiating cause.

3. A 60-year-old man had a small ulceration of the right fifth toe, moderate arterial insufficiency, and severe burning pain due to erythromyalgia. Active treatment of the polycythemia, coupled with local management of the foot lesions, relieved the pain and helped heal the ulcer. In this case the causal relationship among polycythemia, erythromelalgia, and the arterial complications seemed questionable.

It appears, therefore, that in the presence of vascular complications associated with polycythemia, active treatment of the latter is essential. Furthermore, in addition to the peripheral manifestations, awareness of the multiplicity of visceral involvement should evoke the possibility of these lesions in every patient with polycythemia vera. Once the diagnosis is reached, management with appropriate therapy should yield a satisfactory response.

Cryoglobulinemia

Cryoglobulinemia is a result of the presence in plasma of abnormal proteins that precipitate on cooling. In 1933, Wintrobe and Buell reported such a case in a patient suffering from multiple myeloma. It was not until 1947 that Lerner and Watson suggested the name "cryoglobulins" to represent a group of proteins with a common property of precipitating from cold serum. They also noted that when the proteins are in a high concentration, they may precipitate spontaneously even at room temperature. The presence of cryoglobulins may lead to intravascular thrombosis. In addition, if cryofibrinogens are also present, both thrombosis and hemorrhage may occur. Many of the patients with this abnormal protein in the blood may have Raynaud's phenomenon, acrocyanosis, or purpura with vascular manifestations in an unusual location or of an unusual type.

In these cases, the patient should be tested for cryoglobulins, and if they are found, suspicion of the presence of multiple myeloma or similar hematologic conditions, such as leukemia, lymphoblastoma, or polycythemia vera, should be raised and the possibilities investigated. Because significant amounts of cryoglobulin may produce intravascular thrombosis, necrosis of the skin may develop, as reported by Hardy et al.

Idiopathic cryoglobulinemia is usually less amenable to treatment. In the presence of an associated underlying disease process such as myeloma, treatment of the primary disease may be partially effective. In the presence of ischemic necrosis, local treatment is obviously indicated in addition to the management of the dysproteinemia.

BIBLIOGRAPHY

Baur GM, Porter JM, et al.: Rapid onset of hand ischemia of unknown etiology. Ann Surg 186:184, 1977.

Behçet H: Uber rezidivierende apththose durch ein Virus verusachte Gerschwure Am Mund, Am Mauge und an den Genitalien. Dermatol Ubchenschr 105:1152, 1937.

Bengtsson B, Malmvall B: Giant cell arteritis. Acta Med Scand (Suppl) 658:1, 1982.

Bergan JJ, Conn J Jr, Trippel OH: Severe ischemia of the hand. Ann Surg 173:301, 1971.

Block KJ, Makin DG: Hyperviscosity syndromes associated with immunoglobulin abnormalities. Semin Hematol 10:113, 1973.

Brouet C, Clauvel J, Danon F: Biologic and clinical significance of cryoglobulins. Am J Med 57:775, 1974.

Brown H, Sellwood RA, et al.: Thromboangiitis obliterans. Br J Surg 56:59, 1969.

Buerger L: The Circulatory Disturbances of the Extremities. Philadelphia, WB Saunders, 1924.

Buerger L: The veins in thromboangiitis obliterans. JAMA 111:1320, 1909.

Buerger L: Thrombo-angiitis obliterans: A study of the vascular lesions leading to presenile spontaneous gangrene. Am J Med Sci 136:567, 1908.

Crawford ES, Crawford JL: Diseases of the Aorta. Baltimore, Williams & Wilkins, 1984, p 401.

Danaraj TJ: Primary arteritis of aorta causing renal artery stenosis and hypertension. Br Heart J 25:153, 1963.

deShazo R: The spectrum of systemic vasculitis. Postgrad Med 58:78, 1975.

Dible JH: The Pathology of Limb Ischaemia. St. Louis, Warren H. Green, 1966.

Downs AR, Gaskell P, et al.: Asessment of arterial obstruction in vessels supplying the fingers by measurement of local blood pressures and the skin temperature response test: Correlation with angiographic evidence. Surgery 77:530, 1975.

Dubois EL, Tuffanelli DL: Clinical manifestations of systemic lupus erythematosus: Computer analysis of 520 cases. JAMA 190:104, 1964.

Duncan JM, Cooley DA: Surgical considerations in aortitis with surgical emphasis on Takayasu's arteritis. Texas Heart Inst J 10:233, 1983.

Edwards EA: Postamputation radiographic evidence for small artery obstruction in arteriosclerosis. Ann Surg 150:177, 1959.

Fauci AS, Haynes BF, Katz P: The spectrum of vasculitis. Ann Intern Med 89:660, 1978.

Feldaker M, Hines EA Jr, Kierland RR: Livedo reticularis with ulcerations. Circulation 13:196, 1956.

Fitts WT, Melissinos EG: Polycythemia vera, in Sabiston DC (ed):

Textbook of Surgery, 11th ed. Philadelphia, WB Saunders, 1977, p 146.

Gulati SM, Singh KS, et al: Immunological studies in thromboangiitis obliterans (Buerger's disease). J Surg Res 27:287, 1979.

Hachiya J: Current concepts of Takayasu's arteritis. Semin Roentgenol 5:245, 1970.

Haimovici H: Aortic arch syndrome: Takayasu's arteritis, in Cirugia Vascular (Spanish edition of Vascular Surgery), Salvat, Barcelona, 1986, p 778.

Haimovici H: Arterial embolism: Peripheral and visceral, in Haimovici H (ed): The Surgical Management of Vascular Diseases. Philadelphia, JB Lippincott, 1963, Chapter 8.

Haimovici H: Diseases of small arteries of the extremities, in Hardy Rhoades' Textbook of Surgery, 5th ed. Philadelphia, JB Lippincott, 1977, p 1827.

Haimovici H: Ischemic Forms of Venous Thrombosis, Phlegmasia Cerulea Dolens, and Venous Gangrene. Springfield, Ill., Charles C Thomas, 1971.

Haimovici H: Peripheral arterial embolism: A study of 330 unselected cases of embolism of the extremities. Angiology 1:120, 1950.

Haimovici H: Thromboangiitis obliterans: A nosologic reappraisal. Editorial. J Cardiovasc Surg 4:83, 1963.

Hardy JD, Alican F: Ischemic gangrene without major organic vascular occlusion: An enlarging concept. Surgery 50:107, 1961.

Hardy JD, Conn JH, Fain WR: Nonatherosclerotic occlusive lesions of small arteries. Surgery 57:1, 1965.

Hill GL: A rational basis for management of patients with Buerger syndrome. Br J Surg 61:476, 1974.

Hill GL, Smith AH: Buerger's disease in Indonesia: Clinical course and prognostic factors. J Chronic Dis 29:205, 1974.

Hirai M, Shionoya S: Arterial obstruction of the upper limb in Buerger's disease. Br J Surg 66:124, 1979.

Hutchinson J: Acro-scleroderma following Raynaud's phenomenon. Clin J 7:240, 1896.

Hutton M, Rhodes RS, Chapman G: The lowering of postischemic compartment pressures with mannitol. J Surg Res 32:239, 1982.

Inada K, Iwashima Y, et al.: Nonatherosclerotic segmental arterial occlusion of the extremity. Arch Surg 108:663, 1974.

Inada K, Shimizu H, Yokayama T: Pulseless disease and atypical coarctation of the aorta, with special references to their genesis. Surgery 52:433, 1962.

Isaacson C: An idiopathic aortitis in young Africans. J Pathol Bacteriol, 81:69, 1961.

Ishikawa KK: Natural history and classification of occlusive thromboaortopathy (Takayasu's disease). Circulation 57:27, 1978.

Ishikawa K, Kawase S, Mishima Y: Occlusive arterial disease in extremities, with special reference to Buerger's disease. Angiology 13:399, 1962.

Jager BV: Cryofibrinogenemia. N Engl J Med 266:579, 1962.

Jenkins AM, Macpherson AS, et al: Peripheral aneurysms in Behçet's disease. Br J Surg 63:199, 1976.

Jepson RP: Widespread and sudden occlusion of the small arteries of the hands and feet. Circulation 14:1084, 1956.

Kalbfleisch JM, Bird RM: Cryofibrinogenemia. N Engl J Med 263:881, 1960.

Kimoto S: The history and present status of aortic surgery in Japan, particularly for aortitis syndrome. J Cardiovasc Surg 20:107, 1979.

Lande A, Bard R, et al.: Aortic arch syndrome (Takayasu's arteritis). J Cardiovasc Surg 19:507, 1978.

Laroche GP, Bernatz PE, et al.: Chronic arterial insufficiency of the upper extremity. Mayo Clin Proc 51:180, 1976.

Lerner AB, Watson CJ: Studies of cryoglobulins. I. Unusual purpura associated with the presence of a high concentration of cryoglobulin (cold precipitable globulin). Am J Med Sci 214:410, 1947.

Lewis T, Landis EM: Observations upon the vascular mechanism in acrocyanosis. Heart 15:229, 1930.

Liechty RD, Iob V, McMath M: Cryoproteinemia: Its relationship to peripheral vascular disease. Ann Surg 154:319, 1961.

Little AG, Zarins CK: Abdominal aortic aneurysm and Behçet's disease. Surgery 91:359, 1982.

Lupi-Herrera E, Sanchez-Torres G, et al: Takayasu's arteritis: Clinical study of 107 cases. Am Heart J 93:94, 1977.

Maekawa M, Hayase S, et al.: Obstructive aortitis with hypertension: Takayasu's disease without the eye symptoms. Jpn Circ J 27:730, 1963.

Martorell F, Fabre J: El sindrome de obliterative de los troncos supraaorticos. Med Clin (Barc) 2:26, 1944.

McKusick VA, Harris WS, et al: Buerger's disease: A distinct clinical and pathologic entity. JAMA 181:5, 1962.

McLoughlin FA, Helsby FR, et al.: Association of H1A-AI and HLA-B5 with Buerger's disease. Br Med J 2:1165, 1976.

McPherson JR, Juergens JL, Gifford RW Jr: Thromboangiitis obliterans and arteriosclerosis obliterans: Clinical and prognostic differences. Ann Intern Med 59:288, 1963.

Mozes M, Cahansky G, et al.: The association of atherosclerosis and Buerger's disease: A clinical and radiological study. J Cardiovasc Surg 2:52, 1970.

Nakao K, Ikida M, Kimata S: Takayasu's arteritis: Clinical report of eighty-four cases and immunologic studies of seven cases. Circulation 35:1141, 1967.

Norman IL, Allen EV: The vascular complications of polycythemia. Am Heart J 13:257, 1937.

O'Leary PA, Waisman M: Acrosclerosis. Arch Dermatol 47:382, 1943.

Oohashi S: Clinical, angiographical and pathological studies on Buerger's disease especially in relation to arteriosclerosis. J Jpn Surg Soc 76:491, 1975.

Paramo Diaz M, Diaz Ballesteros F, et al.: Sindrome de obliteracion de los troncos supraaorticos y enfermedad de Takayasu. Angiologia 34:111, 1982.

Perdue GD, Smith RD III: Atheromatous microemboli. Ann Surg 93:71, 1966.

Raddi HTV: Thromboangiitis obliterans and/or Buerger's disease in South India: A review of 70 cases. Int Surg 59:555, 1974.

Rivera R: Roentgenographic diagnosis of Buerger's disease. J Cardiovasc Surg 14:40, 1973.

Sanding H, Welin G: Aortic arch syndrome with special reference to rheumatoid arteritis. Acta Med Scand 170:1, 1961.

Schatz IJ: Occlusive arterial disease in the hand due to occupational trauma. N Engl J Med 268:281, 1963.

Schein CJ, Haimovici H, Young H: Arterial thrombosis associated with cervical ribs: Surgical considerations; report of a case and review of the literature. Surgery 40:428, 1956.

Sheps SG, McDuffie FC: Vasculitis, in Juergens JL, Spitell JA, Gairbairn JF (eds): Peripheral Vascular Disease, Philadelphia, WB Saunders, 1980, p 493.

Shimizu K, Sano K: Pulseless disease. J Neuropathol Exp Neurol 1:37, 1951.

Shionoya S, Ban I, et al.: Diagnosis, pathology, and treatment of Buerger's disease. Surgery 75:695, 1974.

Shionoya S, Ban I, Nakata Y: Vascular reconstruction in Buerger's disease. Br J Surg 63:841, 1976.

Swinton NW, Cook GA: Systolic hypertension and cardiac mortality of Takayasu's aortoarteritis. Angiology 27:568, 1976.

Takayasu M: Cases with unusual changes of the vessels in the retina. Acta Soc Ophthalmol Japan 12:554, 1908.

Taylor LM, Baur GM, Porter JM: Finger gangrene caused by small artery occlusive disease. Ann Surg 193:453, 1981.

Thieme WT, Strandness DE Jr, Bell JW; Buerger's disease: Further support for this entity. Northwest Med 64:264, 1965.

Travers RL, Allison DJ, et al: Polyarteritis nodosa: A clinical and angiographic analysis of 17 cases. Semin Arthritis Rheum 8:184, 1979.

Ueda H, Ito I, Okada R: Aortic arch syndrome with special reference to pulseless disease and its variants. Jpn Heart J 4:224, 1963.

von Winiwarter F: Ueber eine eigenthumliche Form von Endarteritis and Endophlebitis mit Gangran des Fusses. Arch Klin Chir 23:202, 1879.

Wessler S, Ming SC, et al.: A critical evaluation of thromboangiitis obliterans: The case against Buerger's disease. N Engl J Med 262:1149, 1960.

Wintrobe MM, and Buell MV: Hyperproteinemia associated with multiple myeloma with report of a case in which an extraordinary hyperproteinemia was associated with thrombosis of retinal veins and symptoms suggesting Raynaud's disease. Bull Johns Hopkins Hosp, 52:156, 1933.

CHAPTER 35
Aortoiliac, Aortofemoral, and Iliofemoral Arteriosclerotic Occlusive Disease

David C. Brewster

The infrarenal abdominal aorta and iliac arteries are among the most common sites of chronic obliterative atherosclerosis.[1] Indeed, atherosclerotic narrowing or occlusion of these vessels, most commonly centered around the aortic bifurcation, occurs to varying degrees in almost all patients with symptoms of arterial insufficiency of the lower extremities severe enough to require consideration for surgical revascularization.

The possibility of surgical intervention for relief of ischemic symptoms secondary to aortoiliac disease was first recognized by Leriche. Beginning in 1923, he published a series of observations of a syndrome occurring in relatively young males, consisting of bilateral intermittent claudication, diminished or absent femoral pulses, and sexual impotence. He termed this syndrome, which has subsequently come to bear his name, "aortitis terminalis" and suggested that the ideal treatment would be excision and reestablishment of vascular continuity by means of an arterial graft.[2]

Thromboendarterectomy, as introduced by Dos Santos in 1947,[3] was firmly established in the aortoiliac segment by Wylie in 1952.[4] Inspired by Gross's pioneering work with homografts,[5] resection and replacement of the diseased aorta began with arterial homografts.[6-8] With Voorhees'[9] introduction of fabric arterial grafts in 1952, the era of prosthetic graft replacement or bypass began.[10,11]

Since then, tremendous advances have occurred in this area. Currently a variety of methods exist to accurately evaluate aortoiliac occlusive disease and properly prepare the patient for arterial reconstruction. Most importantly, a variety of operative approaches and methods of revascularization are available for use in differing clinical circumstances. With proper patient selection and a carefully performed arterial reconstructive procedure, a favorable outcome and low operative morbidity and mortality may be anticipated, making surgical management of aortoiliac occlusive disease one of the most rewarding areas of vascular surgical practice today.

CLINICAL MANIFESTATIONS

The symptoms and natural history of the occlusive process is significantly influenced by its distribution and extent. Truly localized aortoiliac disease (type I), with occlusive lesions confined to the distal abdominal aorta and common iliac vessels, is seen infrequently (in 5 to 10% of patients), and, in the absence of more distally distributed disease, rarely produces limb-threatening symptoms. In such localized aortic obstruction, the potential for collateral blood flow around the aortoiliac segment is great. Collateral pathways include both visceral and parietal routes such as internal mammary to inferior epigastric, intercostal to circumflex iliac, lumbar and hypogastric to common femoral and profunda branches, and superior mesenteric to inferior mesenteric and superior hemorrhoidal pathways via the marginal artery of Drummond and arc of Riolan.

Patients with segmental disease typically present with varying degrees of claudication, most often involving the proximal musculature of the thigh, hip, or buttock areas. The symptoms may be equally severe in both limbs, although one leg usually is more severely affected than the other. More advanced ischemic complaints are absent unless distal atheroembolic complications have occurred. In males, impotence is an often-associated complaint, present in at least 30% of males with aortoiliac disease.

Patients with this segmental disease are characteristically younger, with a relatively low incidence of hypertension or diabetes, but they have a significant frequency of abnormal blood lipids, particularly type IV hyperlipoproteinemia.[12,13] In contrast to the usual male predominance in people with chronic peripheral vascular disease, almost one half of those patients with localized aortoiliac lesions are women.[14] Indeed, the frequency of aortoiliac disease in women has been increasing substantially in recent years, coincident with the increased national incidence of cigarette smoking in women. Many female patients with localized

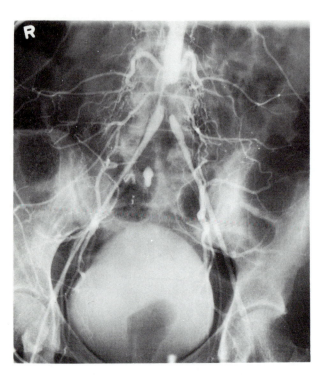

Figure 35-1. Transaxillary aortogram of patient with localized (type I) aortoiliac disease confined to the region of the aortic bifurcation and proximal iliac vessels.

aortoiliac disease constitute a characteristic clinical picture: a woman of about 50 years of age, invariably a heavy smoker, with angiographic findings of small aortic, iliac, and femoral vessels, a high aortic bifurcation, and occlusive disease often strikingly localized to the lower aorta or aortic bifurcation (Fig. 35-1).[13,15–17] Commonly, many of these patients will have had an artificial menopause induced by hysterectomy or radiation.

In more than 90% of symptomatic patients, however, the disease will be more widespread. In my experience, approximately 25% will have disease confined to the abdomen (type II), and approximately 65% will have widespread occlusive disease above and below the inguinal ligament (type III). Patients in the latter group, with "combined segment" or "multilevel" disease, are typically older, more commonly male (about 6:1 ratio), and much more likely to have diabetes, hypertension, and associated atherosclerotic disease involving cerebral, coronary, and visceral arteries. Progression of the occlusive process is also more likely in these patients as opposed to those patients with more localized aortoiliac disease.[16,18,19] For these reasons, the majority of patients with a type III pattern manifest symptoms of more advanced ischemia such as ischemic pain at rest or varying degrees of ischemic tissue necrosis and more often require revascularization for limb salvage rather than for relief of claudication alone.

DIAGNOSIS

In most instances, an accurate and detailed history and carefully performed physical examination can unequivocally establish the diagnosis of aortoiliac disease. A reliable de-

scription of claudication in one or both legs, possibly decreased sexual potency in the male, and diminished or absent femoral pulses define the characteristic triad often referred to as the Leriche syndrome. However, clinical grading of femoral pulses may sometimes be inaccurate, particularly in obese patients or in patients with groins scarred from prior operation.[20] Although proximal claudication symptoms in the distribution of thigh, hip, and buttock musculature are usually reliable indicators of clinically significant inflow disease, a significant number of patients with aortoiliac disease will nonetheless complain only of calf claudication, particularly those with multilevel disease.[21] Audible bruits may frequently be heard with a stethoscope over the lower abdomen or femoral vessels, particularly after exercise. Elevation pallor, rubor on dependency, shiny atrophic skin in the distal limbs and feet, and possible areas of ulceration or ischemic necrosis or gangrene may be noted, depending on the extent of atherosclerotic impairment.

In some instances, however, the diagnosis of aortoiliac occlusive disease may not be readily apparent, and pitfalls may exist in terms of certain complaints that may cause diagnostic confusion. In some cases, pulse evaluation and appearance of the feet may be judged entirely normal at rest, despite the presence of proximal stenoses that are physiologically significant with exercise. This is also often the case in patients presenting with distal microemboli secondary to atheroembolism, the so-called "blue toe syndrome."[22,23] In other instances, complaints of exercise-related pain in the leg, hip, buttock, or even low back may be mistaken for symptoms of degenerative hip or spine disease, nerve root irritation caused by lumbar disc herniation or spinal stenosis, diabetic neuropathy, or other neuromuscular problems. Many such patients may be distinguished from patients with true claudication by the fact that their discomfort is often relieved only by sitting or lying down, as opposed to simply stopping walking. In addition, the typical sciatic distribution of the pain and the fact that often their complaints are brought on by simply standing, as opposed to walking a certain distance, suggest nonvascular causes. However, in many such instances one or more noninvasive vascular laboratory testing modalities may be extremely valuable.[24,25]

Noninvasive studies not only improve diagnostic accuracy but also allow physiologic quantification of the severity of the disease process. This quantification may be of considerable clinical benefit, for instance in establishing the likelihood of a lesion's healing without revascularization or in differentiating neuropathic foot pain from true ischemic rest pain. Noninvasive studies may also provide a reliable and objective baseline from which to follow patients' courses and may often help in localization of the disease process. We have found use of segmental limb systolic blood pressure measurements and pulse volume recordings most useful.[26]

ARTERIOGRAPHY

If the patient's symptoms and clinical circumstances indicate sufficient disability or threat to limb survival, angiography is the next step. It should be emphasized that arteriography

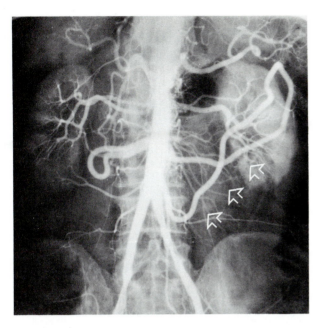

Figure 35-2. Aortogram demonstrating enlarged meandering inferior mesenteric and left colic arteries, indicators of associated occlusive disease in the superior mesenteric or celiac axis or both.

is rarely used in a truly diagnostic sense; the presence or absence of occlusive disease as a cause of the patient's symptoms can almost always be reliably established by clinical evaluation supplemented by noninvasive vascular laboratory studies performed immediately before and after exercise. Rather, angiography is employed for the anatomic information it provides the surgeon for selecting and planning an operative procedure. On occasion, the angiogram may be the final bit of data on which the decision whether to proceed with operation is based, or in other instances it may be used to determine if the occlusive disease is amenable to percutaneous transluminal balloon angioplasty. Neither of these uses is "diagnostic" in the usual sense of the word.

In addition to noting the actual anatomic distribution of occlusive disease in the aortoiliac segment and distal vessels, the surgeon should examine the films for potentially helpful or, in some instances, critical anatomic variations or associated occlusive lesions in the renal, visceral, or runoff vessels. For example, an enlarged meandering left colic artery (Fig. 35-2) may often be an indicator of associated occlusive disease in the superior mesenteric artery, which can usually be appreciated only on a lateral view. Failure to recognize this occlusion may lead to catastrophic bowel infarction if the inferior mesenteric artery is ligated at the time of aortic reconstruction.[27]

Approach

My general preference is for a retrograde transfemoral approach, which is feasible from the less involved side in most patients. In patients with severe bilateral occlusive disease or total aortic occlusion, a translumbar or transaxillary route may be employed depending on the preferences

of the angiographer or surgeon carrying out the study. A two-plane study, providing oblique or lateral views, is highly desirable and often greatly enhances the ability to determine the clinical importance of the visualized lesions.[20]

Extent of Study

For most patients, a full and complete arteriographic survey of the entire intra-abdominal aortoiliac segment and infrainguinal runoff vessels is advisable. Even if proximal operation alone is planned, knowledge of the anatomy of runoff disease is important because it helps the surgeon anticipate the probable outcome of proximal operation alone, aids in more effective management of possible technical misadventures, and is important for future planning. Only by such complete studies will unusual but highly important variations in the occlusive process, which may critically affect the conduct and outcome of the operation, be detected. It has been advocated by some that aortography is not necessary in patients with complete absence of both femoral pulses. However, most vascular surgeons currently believe angiographic study, even in these cases, is important to accurately define the exact anatomic distribution and extent of occlusive disease and to facilitate selection and the conduct of an appropriate arterial reconstruction.

In general, runoff views are obtained to at least the level of the midcalf. In selected patients with obviously advanced distal disease and threatened limbs, more distal views may be advisable, including views of the foot itself if distal infrapopliteal bypass grafting is considered likely. In these instances in which the amount of contrast reaching these distal points may be significantly impaired by multilevel occlusive lesions, supplemental use of digital subtraction angiographic techniques may enhance adequate visualization and definition of anatomy.

Hemodynamic Assessment of Multilevel Disease

Although an accurate assessment of occlusive disease is possible by traditional clinical evaluation and arteriography in most patients, difficulty may exist in some patients, particularly those with multilevel occlusive disease. Assessment of the hemodynamic distribution of occlusive disease at each segmental level is obviously of critical importance in selecting an appropriate reconstructive procedure. It is well recognized that many atherosclerotic lesions may be of only morphlologic significance on the arteriogram, with little or no actual hemodynamic importance. In such patients, proximal reconstruction alone may often fail to adequately relieve the patient's symptoms. Furthermore, if proximal disease is only modest in the presence of associated advanced distal disease, operative correction of both segmental lesions may be required in patients with advanced leg ischemia.

Despite a wide array of noninvasive vascular laboratory testing methods, none appears to accurately reflect the hemodynamic importance of aortoiliac inflow lesions, particularly in the patient with multilevel disease. All apparently are influenced by the presence of infrainguinal occlusive disease, and abnormal results may not always be reliably

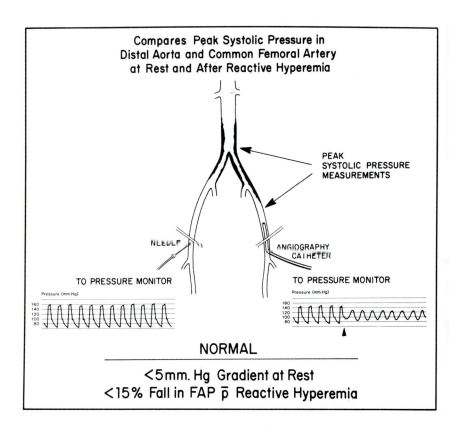

Figure 35-3. Femoral artery pressure study, an accurate means for assessing the hemodynamic importance of aortoiliac occlusive lesions. A significant fall in peak systolic femoral pressure is demonstrated on the left (*arrow*).

attributable to the proximal lesions. Deficiencies of segmental limb Doppler pressures or pulse volume recordings are well recognized in this regard. Analysis of femoral artery Doppler wave forms or calculation of a pulsatility index is also of uncertain accuracy in the presence of multisegment disease.[20,28] Reliance on the morphologic appearance of lesions on arteriograms also carries known hazards. It is now recognized that there is marked observer variability associated with the interpretation of the clinical significance of arterial lesions visualized on arteriograms.[29] In addition, although the relationship of a simple arterial stenosis and hemodynamic impairment is well documented, the multiplicity and complexity of lesions occurring in the aortoiliac system make hemodynamic assessment based on morphology alone often inaccurate.

In such instances, actual measurement of femoral artery pressure (FAP) may be of considerable value.[20,30–32] FAP measurements are usually obtainable in the arteriographic suite at the time of transfemoral catheter aortography. Separate arterial puncture by a relatively small caliber (22-gauge) needle may occasionally be required if pressure determinations are needed in the femoral artery contralateral to the angiographic catheter insertion site. As illustrated in Figure 35-3, peak systolic pressure in the femoral artery is compared to distal aortic or brachial systolic pressure. A resting systolic pressure difference greater than 5 mm Hg or a fall in FAP greater than 15% with reactive hyperemia induced pharmacologically or by inflation of an occluding thigh cuff for 3 to 5 minutes implies hemodynamically significant inflow disease. If revascularization is indicated in such patients, attention should be directed at correcting the inflow lesions. With a negative study, the surgeon may more confidently proceed directly with distal revascularization without fear of premature compromise or closure of a distal graft and without subjecting the patient to an unnecessary inflow operation.

Based on such criteria, selection of patients for an inflow procedure is greatly facilitated, and benefits are accurately predicted. In our most recent review, 96% of patients with positive results of FAP studies had satisfactory clinical improvement in ischemic symptoms with proximal arterial reconstruction alone, despite uncorrected distal disease in the majority of patients. In contrast, 57% of patients undergoing proximal operation despite a normal FAP result experienced unsatisfactory relief of symptoms and required subsequent distal procedures.[21] Similar results have been reported by other investigators using pressure determinations.[30,32]

INDICATIONS FOR OPERATION

Ischemic pain at rest or actual tissue necrosis, including ischemic ulcerations or frank gangrene, are indicative of advanced ischemia and threatened limb loss. If untreated, most such patients will deteriorate and require major amputation. Thus, all surgeons agree that these symptoms are clearcut indications for arterial reconstruction if anatomically feasible. Age is rarely an important consideration. Even elderly, frail patients or ones at high risk from multiple associated medical problems may generally be revascularized by alternative methods or balloon angioplasty if direct aortoiliac reconstruction is deemed inadvisable.

Some disagreement remains concerning the advisability of operation for claudication symptoms alone. Quite clearly, such decisions must be made on an individual basis, with consideration of the age, associated medical disease, employment requirements, and life-style preferences of each individual. In general, claudication that jeopardizes the livelihood of a patient or significantly impairs the desired life-style of an otherwise low-risk patient is considered a reasonable indication for surgical correction, assuming a favorable anatomic situation for operation exists. It is usually advisable for the surgeon to have followed such a patient conservatively for a period of time and to have thoroughly discussed the merits and possible risks of any surgical procedure. It goes without saying that the patient should have demonstrated his or her commitment to the therapeutic program by control of appropriate risk factors, most importantly elimination of cigarette smoking and appropriate weight reduction, when required, by compliance with a low-fat, low-calorie diet. In general, most surgeons are liberal in recommending operation for patients with claudication alone if symptoms can be attributed to isolated proximal inflow disease, as opposed to more distal disease in the femoropopliteal segment. This seems logical and appropriate because of the generally excellent and long-lasting results currently achieved by aortoiliac reconstruction with low risk to the patient.

Another less frequent but well-recognized indication for aortoiliac reconstruction is peripheral atheromatous emboli from proximal ulcerated atherosclerotic plaques. Clinical evidence of occlusive disease in such patients may be minimal, with little to no history of claudication. Recognition of the condition and complete angiography to investigate the presence of causative proximal lesions is important, however, to avoid repetitive episodes or even limb loss.[22,23]

No truly effective medical treatment for aortoiliac occlusive disease is currently available. Nonoperative care is aimed at limiting disease progression, encouraging development of collateral circulation, and preventing local tissue trauma or infection in the foot. With such care, spontaneous improvement may occur in a few patients, although in most instances slow progression of symptoms may be anticipated. Progression of the atheromatous process may, in some instances, be slowed by altering the patient's risk factors. Complete cessation of cigarette smoking is of paramount importance in this regard and cannot be overemphasized to the patient. Weight reduction, treatment of hypertension, correction of abnormal serum lipids, and regulation of diabetes all seem desirable and logical, although definite benefit in terms of stabilization or improvement of occlusive symptoms is less well established. A regular exercise program, often involving no more than regular walking of a specific distance on a daily basis, seems the best stimulant to collateral circulation. Good local foot care is extremely important, because trauma and digital infection are often the precipitating causes of gangrene and amputation, particularly in the diabetic patient. Although numerous vasodilator drugs exist, none are of established benefit in chronic occlusive disease.[33] None of these drugs has been shown to increase the muscle blood flow in the claudicating extremity during exercise, the critical requirement for an effective agent in the treatment of claudication. A recent multiinstitution, double-blind, placebo-controlled trial of pentoxifylline (Trental) in the treatment of patients with claudication showed a significant increase in walking distance as compared to patients receiving a placebo,[34] and the drug has been released by the U.S. Food and Drug Administration for the treatment of claudication. In my own experience, perhaps 25% of patients may find some improvement in claudication symptoms. It is often difficult to know if this is attributable to the drug, however. Although pentoxifylline may be used in patients with moderate claudication, it does not appear to change the eventual need for surgical revascularization in patients with severe claudication, resting ischemia, or more advanced symptoms.

The role of percutaneous transluminal angioplasty (PTA) is discussed more fully in Chapter 24. PTA may be a valuable treatment modality in properly selected patients with aortoiliac occlusive disease. However, patient selection is of paramount importance. To be appropriate for PTA, the lesion should be relatively localized and preferably a stenosis rather than a total occlusion. A localized stenosis of the common iliac artery less than 5 cm long is the most favorable situation for PTA, with excellent early and late patency rates.[35,36] This situation may exist in perhaps 10 to 15% of patients with aortoiliac disease who are studied arteriographically.[37] PTA is generally not recommended for patients with diffuse iliac disease, unless they are extraordinarily poor surgical candidates, or for those who have totally occluded iliac arteries because of the higher incidence of complications or recurrent occlusion.[36] Alternatives for revascularization in high-risk patients with conditions unfavorable to PTA almost always exist.

SURGICAL TREATMENT

Currently, methods of direct aortoiliac reconstruction offer the most definitive and durable means of surgical revascularization. Most often, aortofemoral bypass grafting is used, although in a limited number of cases aortoiliac endarterectomy may be feasible. Remote, or "extra-anatomic," procedures are reserved for the limited number of instances involving truly high-risk patients unable to tolerate conventional anatomic reconstruction or patients with infection or other technical problems that may hamper standard direct operation. Such procedures are discussed more fully in Chapter 39. What is evident is that a variety of inflow procedures is available to the surgeon. The proper choice of operation depends on the general condition of the patient, the extent and distribution of atherosclerotic disease, and the experience and training of the surgeon.

Preoperative Preparation

In addition to angiographic assessment, evaluation of associated cardiac, renal, and pulmonary disease is routinely performed. Any correctable deficiencies are best identified before operation and appropriately treated. For instance, patients with compromised pulmonary reserves may benefit from a period of preoperative chest physiotherapy, bronchodilator medication, and appropriate antibiotic treatment. Diminished renal function also requires evaluation, with correction of any prerenal component due to dehydration or treatment of other reversible deficiencies. Similarly, cardiac abnormalities demonstrated by clinical evaluation or ECG are evaluated and treated appropriately; in many instances consultation with a cardiologist may be quite helpful.

Without question, the most important and controversial aspect of preoperative patient evaluation is the detection and subsequent management of associated coronary artery disease. Several studies have clearly documented the existence of potentially fatal (both early and late postoperative deaths) coronary artery disease in 40% or more of patients requiring peripheral vascular reconstructive procedures.[38] However, most currently available screening methods suffer from a lack of sensitivity and specificity in predicting postoperative cardiac complications. In addition, many patients with vascular occlusive disease cannot achieve adequate exercise stress because of claudication or infirmity. Even with coronary angiography it is difficult to relate anatomic findings to surgical risk. In addition, coronary angiography is associated with its own inherent risks, and patients undergoing coronary artery bypass grafting before needed aortoiliac reconstructions are subjected to the risks and complications of both procedures.

I, as well as others, have found the use of preoperative dipyridamole-thallium 201 scintigraphy valuable in identifying the subset of preoperative vascular patients who may indeed be at high risk for perioperative myocardial ischemic events and who perhaps warrant more intensive preoperative evaluation, including coronary angiography, and perhaps coronary bypass grafting.[39-41] This process has also allowed identification of a low-risk subset of patients in whom no further evaluation or intensive intraoperative monitoring appears warranted.

DIRECT OPERATIVE PROCEDURES

Aortoiliac Endarterectomy

Aortoiliac endarterectomy may be considered for the group of approximately 5 to 10% of patients with truly localized (type I) disease. Endarterectomy offers several theoretic advantages: no prosthetic material is inserted; the infection rate is practically nonexistent; and inflow to the hypogastric arteries, potentially improving sexual potency in the male, is perhaps somewhat better than with bypass procedures. Finally, because the procedure is totally autogenous and therefore more resistant to infection, it may be used in unusual circumstances in which reoperation in a contaminated or infected field requires innovative reconstructive methods.[42]

Proper selection of patients for endarterectomy is important: disease should terminate at or just beyond the common iliac bifurcation, allowing the surgeon to achieve a satisfactory end point without extending more than 1 to 2 cm into the external iliac segment. Whether transverse or vertical arteriotomies are used is less important than ensuring a proper plane of endarterectomy at the level of the external elastic lamina and achieving a secure end point of endarterectomy, with or without the aid of tacking sutures. Primary closure or arteriotomies is generally feasible, although patch closure may occasionally be used (Fig. 35-4).

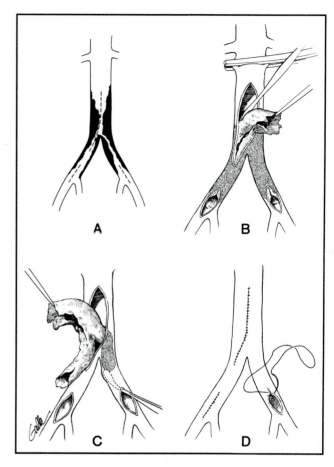

Figure 35-4. Aortoiliac endarterectomy. **A.** Occlusive disease limited to distal aorta and common iliac arteries, with location of arteriotomies indicated by dotted lines. **B.** A satisfactory endarterectomy plane is achieved, and atheromatous material is removed from the aorta from the level of the proximal clamp to the bifurcation. **C.** Satisfactory end point of the endarterectomy is achieved at the iliac bifurcation, and endarterectomy is continued proximally. Tacking sutures may be needed to secure an adequate end point. **D.** Closure of arteriotomies to complete procedure. See text for details.

Endarterectomy is definitely contraindicated in three circumstances:

1. Any evidence of aneurysmal change, which makes continued aneurysmal degeneration of the endarterectomized segment likely
2. Total occlusion of the aorta to the level of the renal arteries, which makes simple transection of the aorta several centimeters below the renal arteries with thrombectomy of the aortic cuff followed by graft insertion technically easier and far more expeditious
3. Extension of the disease process into the external iliac or distal vessels (types II and III), which is by far the most common consideration favoring bypass grafting.

Difficulties with adequate endarterectomy of the external iliac artery as a result of its smaller size, greater length, somewhat more difficult exposure, and the more muscular and adherent medial layer are well documented, with a higher incidence of both early thrombosis and late failure as a result of recurrent stenosis. For these reasons, extended aortoiliofemoral endarterectomy procedures have been generally abandoned and replaced by bypass grafting, which is simpler, faster, and associated with better late patency rates in such patients with more extensive disease.[14,43,44] In addition, aortoiliac endarterectomy is generally acknowledged as more demanding technically than bypass procedures. Therefore a bypass graft may be preferable even for localized disease if the surgeon is not adequately trained in alternative methods.

Aortofemoral Bypass Grafting

Over the past 2 decades, prosthetic graft insertion from the abdominal aorta just below the renal arteries to the femoral vessels in the groin has become the standard method of direct surgical repair for aortoiliac occlusive disease, with it used in more than 90% of such patients by most vascular surgeons. Aortofemoral grafts offer the most definitive, durable, and expeditious reconstruction currently available.[14,18,45–47]

Although the technique of aortic graft insertion has been fairly well standardized, some differences in methods do remain, and some are quite controversial. The proximal aortic anastomosis may be made either end-to-end or end-to-side. End-to-end anastomosis is clearly indicated in patients with coexisting aneurysmal disease or complete aortic occlusion extending up to the renal arteries. In addition, it is preferred by many vascular surgeons for routine use in most cases for several reasons. First, it is more sound on a hemodynamic basis, with less turbulence, better flow characteristics, and less chance of competitive flow with still-patent host iliac vessels. Such considerations have led to considerably better long-term patency of grafts done with

end-to-end proximal anastomosis in many reported series, although none have been controlled or prospective.[12,14,48,49] Second, application of partially occluding tangential clamps for construction of an end-to-side anastomosis often carries a higher risk of dislodging intra-aortic thrombus or debris that may then be irretrievably transported to the pelvic circulation or lower extremities. Finally, resection of a small segment of host aorta and use of a short body of the prosthetic bifurcation graft for end-to-end anastomosis, as shown in Fig. 35-5, allows direct placement of the prosthesis in the area of the resected aortic segment, greatly facilitating subsequent tissue coverage and reperitonealization and potentially reducing the incidence of aortoenteric fistual formation in subsequent years.

End-to-side anastomosis may be advantageous in certain anatomic patterns of disease (Fig. 35-6). For instance, if a large aberrant renal artery arises from the lower abdominal aorta or iliac arteries or if the surgeon wishes to avoid sacrifice of a large patent inferior mesenteric artery, end-to-side proximal anastomosis presumably allows preservation of these vessels. Alternatively, they may be preserved by reimplantation into the body of the graft if end-to-end insertion is preferred. Most importantly, end-to-side anastomosis is advisable if the occlusive process is located principally in the external iliac vessels. In such instances, interruption of the infrarenal aorta for end-to-end bypass to the femoral level effectively devascularizes the pelvic region, because no retrograde flow up the iliac arteries can be anticipated. This cessation of flow may potentially increase the incidence of erectile impotence in the sexually potent male.[50,51] These hemodynamic consequences may also increase the incidence of postoperative colonic ischemia, severe buttock ischemia, or even paraplegia secondary to spinal cord ischemia.[27,52] Troublesome hip claudication may also continue to plague the patient despite the presence

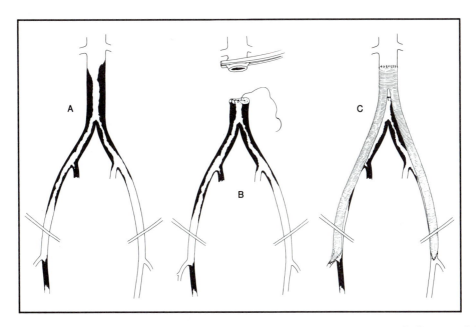

Figure 35-5. End-to-end aortofemoral graft insertion. **A.** Schematic of preoperative aortogram. **B.** Segment of diseased aorta resected and distal aortic stump oversewn. **C.** Completed procedure.

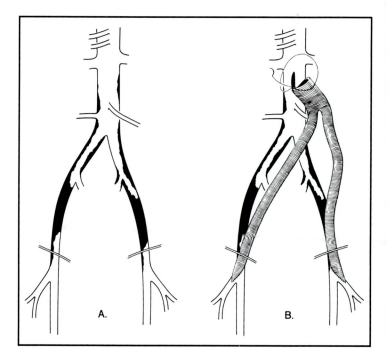

Figure 35-6. A. Anatomic circumstances or patterns of occlusive disease favoring end-to-side proximal aortic anastomosis include low-lying accessory renal arteries, an enlarged patent inferior mesenteric artery, or occlusive disease confined largely to the external iliac arteries. **B.** In these situations, the vessels may be preserved and flow maintained to the hypogastric arterial network through end-to-side graft implantation.

of excellent femoral and distal pulses. Finally, should the limb of the graft occlude in later years, the resulting limb ischemia may be particularly severe and cause difficulty with healing or even above-knee amputation should further revascularization not prove feasible. For these reasons, the surgeon may elect to use end-to-side proximal anastomosis in the anatomic circumstances described.

At present, this area is controversial, and both methods have experienced and highly skilled vascular surgeons as advocates. Regardless of the method of proximal anastomosis, the principle of placing the proximal anastomosis high in the infrarenal abdominal aorta, relatively close to the renal arteries in an area almost always less involved with the occlusive process, is of paramount importance to minimize later recurrent difficulties.

Although the distal anastomosis of the aortic graft may on occasion be accomplished at the level of the external iliac artery in the pelvis, it is almost always preferable to carry the graft to the femoral level where exposure is generally better and anastomosis easier from a technical standpoint. With adequate personnel, both femoral anastomoses may be performed simultaneously. Most importantly, anastomosis at the femoral level provides the surgeon an opportunity to ensure adequate outflow into the profunda femoris artery. Experience has demonstrated an increased late failure rate of aorto–external iliac grafts, with a higher incidence of subsequent "downstream" operations as a result of progressive disease at or just beyond the iliac anastomosis.[14,44,53] With meticulous surgical technique, proper skin preparation and draping, and a limited period of prophylactic antibiotic coverage, the anticipated higher incidence of infection if grafts were extended into the groin have not been borne out by extensive experience.[14,18,43,45–47]

Establishment of adequate graft outflow at the level of the femoral artery anastomosis, usually through the pro-

funda femoris artery in patients with disease or occlusion of the superficial femoral, has emerged as being of paramount importance in early and late graft results.[14,45,54–56] Thus, any lesion that might compromise profunda flow must be carefully evaluated and corrected at the time of distal anastomosis. Preoperative arteriography should visualize the profunda orifice, particularly when occlusion of the superficial femoral artery is demonstrated. This is usually accomplished by oblique views of the groin. At operation, the surgeon must look for possible profunda origin stenosis by palpation, gentle passage of vascular probes, or direct inspection. If any stenosis of the profunda origin exists, it should be corrected by endarterectomy or patch angioplasty techniques. My own preference is for extension of the arteriotomy down the profunda beyond the orifice stenosis, with subsequent anastomosis of the beveled tip of the graft as a patch closure (Fig. 35-7). This procedure achieves hemodynamic correction and is preferable in most instances to formal endarterectomy, which I believe may cause a higher incidence of late false aneurysm formation when the prosthetic graft is sutured to the endarterectomized segment of arterial wall. Endarterectomy of the profunda will be required if the vessel is heavily diseased, however. Other authors have preferred to use autogenous arterial or saphenous vein patches for separate profundaplasty and then anastomose the prosthesis to the common femoral artery above this. In any case, it is imperative that the surgeon use precise anastomotic technique at the end point of the profundaplasty to ensure an adequate profunda outflow tract.

Use of a graft of appropriate size is clearly important[57,58]; previously many surgeons used grafts too large in comparison to the size of outflow tract vessels, promoting sluggish flow in graft limbs and deposition of excessive laminar pseudointima in the prosthesis. This de-

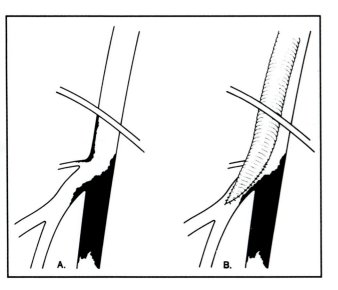

Figure 35-7. A. In patients with associated occlusion of the superficial femoral artery, graft runoff may be limited by associated occlusive disease at the profunda orifice. **B.** Extension of common femoral arteriotomy into the proximal profunda beyond significant occlusive disease with anastomosis of tapered graft tip achieves patch angioplasty of profunda orifice and enhances outflow tract and long-term patency.

posited material, in turn, often has a propensity later to fragment or dislodge, occluding one or both limbs of the graft. For treating occlusive disease, a 16 by 8 mm bifurcated graft is now most often used, although a 14 by 7 mm, or even smaller prosthesis is used without hesitation when appropriate, as is frequently the case in some female patients. The limb size of these grafts will most closely approximate the femoral arteries of patients with occlusive disease or, more particularly, the size of the profunda femoris, which often remains as the only outflow tract. In addition, many Dacron prosthetic grafts have a tendency to dilate 10 to 20% when subjected to arterial pressure. Selection of a smaller graft size helps compensate for this dilatation.

The actual type of prosthesis used does not appear to be of great importance. At present I prefer a knitted Dacron graft for aortofemoral bypass, believing that ease of handling and flexibility across the inguinal region are important. Whether internal or external velour surfaces or a combination of the two is beneficial remains unproven. Although porosity and incorporation by the host remain desirable features theoretically, the successful use of polytetrafluoroethylene (PTFE) grafts in other locations has made these considerations questionable. Woven grafts are considered inferior by many surgeons for reconstructions that must cross the inguinal ligament, but little if any factual data support such a bias. Most importantly, a product from a reputable manufacturer, with proven clinical reliability and of appropriate diameter, should be used. In many instances, any good quality prosthesis will function adequately for large vessel reconstructions, and the final decision often comes down to the preference of the individual surgeon.

CONDUCT OF THE OPERATIVE PROCEDURE

On the morning of surgery, preoperative antibiotics are administered along with other "on-call" medications before the patient is brought to the operating room. A broad-spectrum antibiotic is beneficial in instances of prosthetic vascular reconstruction.[59,60] It is routinely continued for 24 to 48 hours postoperatively. When the patient arrives in the operating room, appropriate intravenous lines and other anesthetic monitoring devices are secured. The vascular anesthetist must be fully aware of the patient's overall condition and, in particular, must know about associated vascular disease in the coronary, carotid, or renal arteries that may influence intraoperative management. Intra-arterial radial artery catheter blood pressure monitoring is virtually routine for aortic reconstruction, with pulmonary artery Swan-Ganz catheter insertion used at the discretion of the anesthesiologist in patients with potential cardiovascular instability or in other situations in which fluid shifts and blood pressure swings may present particular hazards. Liberal crystalloid intravenous fluids are administered during induction of anesthesia, guided by the available monitoring lines, to ensure adequate vascular volume and to promote good urine output.

The patient is placed supine on the operating room table, and wide preparation and draping are performed. In cases of isolated aortoiliac occlusive disease the surgical field need not extend below the upper thigh, but in most instances it is advisable to prepare both legs to the ankles in the event of unsatisfactory results or technical misadventures that may require more distal arterial exploration or reconstruction. Because of my preference for intraoperative monitoring with a segmental plethysmograph, unsterile cuffs are placed at the calf or ankle level and draped out of the operative field.[61] If more distal sterile preparation is necessary, sterile intraoperative cuffs are used for preoperative baseline recordings.

Both femoral arteries are first exposed, often simultaneously if experienced surgical assistants are available. Each common femoral artery is exposed from the inguinal ligament to 1 to 2 cm beyond its bifurcation, with separate control of both superficial femoral and deep femoral branches. At this time, the surgeon can review the preoperative arteriograms and combine this information with careful palpation of the femoral vessels, with particular attention to detecting disease at the origin or proximal portion of the deep femoral artery. This detection is particularly important, of course, in patients with preexistent superficial femoral artery occlusion in whom the profunda femoris artery must function as the principal outflow tract of the graft. The inguinal ligament is then partially divided to create space for comfortable passage of the graft. The lateral circumflex iliac vein, crossing anterior to the distal external iliac artery, is often visualized and may be divided if it will interfere with, or be traumatized, at the time of graft tunneling from the abdomen. At the conclusion of groin dissection, a moist sponge is placed in the groin wounds, and self-retaining retractors are removed.

The abdomen is then opened, generally using a midline incision from the xyphoid to within several centimeters of the symphysis pubis. The abdomen is explored, the transverse colon is elevated out of the wound, and the small bowel is gathered and covered with a moist towel. This is then retracted to the right upper quadrant, either inside or outside of the abdominal cavity. Use of apropriately designed, large, self-retaining retractors may facilitate exposure and reduce requirements for additional surgical or nursing personnel whose sole duty is to hold retractors. The importance of an adequate incision and proper exposure cannot be overemphasized.

The retroperitoneum is then opened over the midinfrarenal abdominal aorta between the duodenum and the inferior mesenteric vein. This will usually reveal the origin of the inferior mesenteric artery. Dissection is continued slightly to the right of this, along the anterior wall of the aorta until the crossing left renal vein is identified. Distally, the retroperitoneum is opened over the right side of the aorta to approximately the level of the aortic bifurcation to allow retroperitoneal tunneling to each groin incision. Dissection should be minimized in this region to spare the autonomic nerve fibers that cross the aortic bifurcation and proximal iliac vessels in this region.[51,62]

Retroperitoneal tunnels to each groin incision are then constructed by blunt finger dissection from both incisions. This is usually most easily accomplished by gaining access to the avascular plane immediately anterior and just lateral to the common iliac arteries. The surgeon must maintain this avascular plane immediately adjacent to the iliac artery to ensure passage of the prosthetic graft posterior to the ureter to minimize the chance of ureteral compression or obstruction by the graft limb or later fibrotic reaction. A long clamp is then passed from the groin to meet the surgeon's dissecting finger above and is advanced into the abdomen to complete creation of the tunnel. A Penrose drain is then grasped and drawn back through the tunnel to facilitate later passage of the graft. On the left side, the presence of the sigmoid colon and mesocolon may make tunneling more difficult, and occasionally it is safer and easier to develop the tunnel in two stages, using a retroperitoneal incision in the left iliac fossa.

If adjunctive lumbar sympathectomy is planned, it is carried out next, removing 5 to 10 cm of lumbar sympathetic chain on each side, usually encompassing the third and fourth lumbar sympathetic ganglia. If elected, this procedure is best carried out prior to systemic heparinization.

At this point, the surgeon must decide between end-to-end or end-to-side proximal anastomosis, a decision based on the criteria previously described. Final decisions in this regard are often made during the operation, however, based on finding aneurysmal change in the aorta or more advanced and calcific disease in the anterior aortic wall than had been anticipated, thus rendering end-to-side anastomosis more difficult and less desirable. Unless special circumstances indicate the advisability of preserving the inferior mesenteric artery, it is routinely divided flush with its origin from the aorta. This usually facilitates further exposure, graft insertion, and tunneling of the graft to the groins. If the inferior mesenteric artery need be preserved, this is accomplished either by end-to-side proximal anastomosis above this vessel or by preservation of a button of aortic wall around its orifice for later reimplantation into

the graft if an end-to-end proximal anastomosis is used.

Before systemic heparinization, a graft of appropriate size is selected and if necessary is preclotted with unheparinized blood. The anesthesiologist then administers 5000 to 7500 units of heparin to the patient via a reliable intravenous line. After several minutes to allow systemic circulation of the heparin, the femoral arteries are gently occluded with bulldog clamps to minimize chances of distal atheromatous embolization at the time of aortic clamp application. The proximal aortic clamp is then placed as close to the renal arteries as feasible. In general, this will be at the level of the crossing left renal vein, but occasionally the superior extent of the occlusive disease or calcification will require mobilization of the left renal vein and cephalad retraction, or even division, to allow placement of the proximal clamp immediately at the level of the renal arteries. The surgeon may or may not choose first to gain circumferential control of the aorta at the chosen level of proximal clamp application with passage of a tape or rubber catheter. My general practice is to do so unless this would be unusually difficult or hazardous because of extensive inflammatory reaction, prior surgery, or similar considerations. Distally, the aorta is occluded several centimeters above the aortic bifurcation by an angled vascular clamp.

A 2 to 3 cm segment of aorta is then removed between the clamps if end-to-end anastomosis has been elected, which is my preferred method (Fig. 35-5). Several pairs of lumbar arteries posteriorly will need to be divided and oversewn or occluded with metal clips. This segment is resected to within 1 to 2 cm of the proximal clamp. The distal cuff is then oversewn, and the distal clamp is removed.

Proximal end-to-end anastomosis is then carried out to the cuff of aorta below the proximal clamp with a running Prolene suture or an interrupted mattress suture technique if the aorta is particularly diseased, fragile, or otherwise less well-suited to a continuous suture technique (Fig. 35-8). Not infrequently, significant atheromatous disease and thickening exist in the proximal cuff, even if one is close to the renal arteries, and endarterectomy to the level of the proximal clamp is advisable to facilitate proximal anastomosis. Because the remaining aortic wall below the clamp is quite thin, I believe use of interrupted mattress sutures backed with Teflon pledgets is definitely advisable. After completion of the anastomosis, the proximal graft limbs are occluded, and the proximal clamp is released, testing the hemostatic security of the anastomosis and further preclotting the graft. The proximal clamp is reapplied, blood is evacuated from both limbs of the prosthesis, and the graft is withdrawn through the previously created retroperitoneal tunnels to each groin.

If an end-to-side aortic anastomosis is preferred, it may be performed with use of partially occluding tangential clamps or by total occlusion of the aorta by two clamps above and below the proposed level of anastomosis. I believe the latter method is usually preferable, facilitating creation of the anastomosis and, perhaps most importantly, evacuation of thrombotic material from this region.

End-to-side anastomosis is then done to each femoral artery. In the absence of significant disease in the superficial or deep femoral arteries, this is readily accomplished on each common femoral artery after creation of an arteriotomy

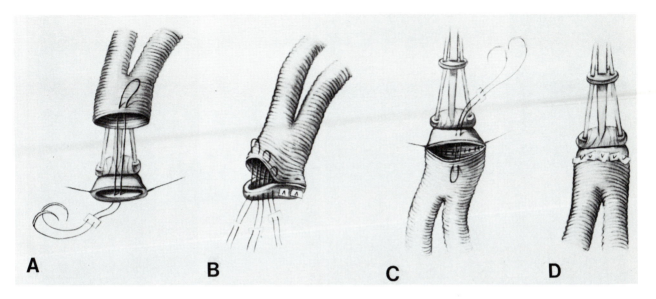

Figure 35-8. Use of interrupted mattress suture technique for proximal aortic anastomosis. **A.** Double-armed suture is passed from graft to host aorta. **B.** Posterior row of five sutures is completed and tied over pledgets of Teflon felt. **C, D.** Graft is directed toward patient's feet, and similar row of five anterior mattress sutures is tied to complete the anastomosis.

approximately 2 cm in length. If the superficial femoral artery is occluded and particularly if disease is palpated at the origin of the deep femoral artery, the arteriotomy is extended obliquely across the profunda and into the proximal aspect of this vessel, with the graft hood then sutured across it as illustrated in Figure 35-7. If more extensive profunda disease exists, a separate profundaplasty may be required rather than an excessively long anastomosis of the beveled graft tip. The surgeon should ensure that appropriate tension is placed on the graft limb before cutting it to a suitable length; excessive tension increases the likelihood of later anastomotic aneurysm formation, whereas excessive redundancy may cause kinking and subsequent occlusion of the limb.

If adequate experienced surgical assistants are available, both femoral anastomoses can be performed simultaneously. Before completion of each anastomosis, the limb is flushed in antegrade fashion, and then proximal and distal host arteries are backbled and probed. On completion of the anastomosis, distal clamps are left in place, and blood flow is restored in a retrograde fashion first. Subsequently, deep femoral and finally superficial femoral clamps are removed.

If feasible, some means of assuring adequate distal flow intraoperatively is advisable. I usually obtain pulse volume recordings at this juncture to assess this flow. Some surgeons prefer to prepare and drape the feet in transparent bags to allow visualization of their color and appearance, but this is often a more subjective and uncertain method. Alternatively, distal Doppler pressures or electromagnetic flow measurements through the opened graft limb may contribute to this judgment. Once the surgeon is assured of a satisfactory technical result on both sides, protamine is administered, and hemostasis is secured.

Closure of the retroperitoneum over the graft is performed next, ensuring complete coverage of the prosthesis

and separation from the duodenum. This is greatly facilitated if end-to-end anastomosis has been used with a short body of the prosthetic graft, allowing it to sit in the bed of the resected aorta and avoiding the forward bulge that inevitably accompanies end-to-side construction. The groin wounds are carefully closed in at least two layers. Meticulous attention to groin closure cannot be overemphasized, thus minimizing chances for poor wound healing or breakdown, with the possible dreaded complication of graft infection.

SPECIAL CONSIDERATIONS

Adjunctive Lumbar Sympathectomy

The use of a concomitant lumbar sympathectomy at the time of aortic reconstruction remains controversial. Although it is well accepted that sympathectomy does increase skin and total limb blood flow, there is little objective data to document more favorable long-term graft patency or improved limb salvage results.[63,64] Nonetheless, it is my usual policy to carry out limited (L3–4) sympathectomy at the time of aortofemoral graft insertion whenever uncorrected occlusive disease below the inguinal ligament is present. This is easily and quickly accomplished and, I believe, is beneficial to the patient with multilevel disease or limb-threatening ischemia.

The Totally Occluded Aorta

Approximately 8% of our patients undergoing operation for aortoiliac occlusive disease have a totally occluded aorta.[65] In about one half of them the occlusion has extended retrograde to the level of the renal arteries; in the remainder

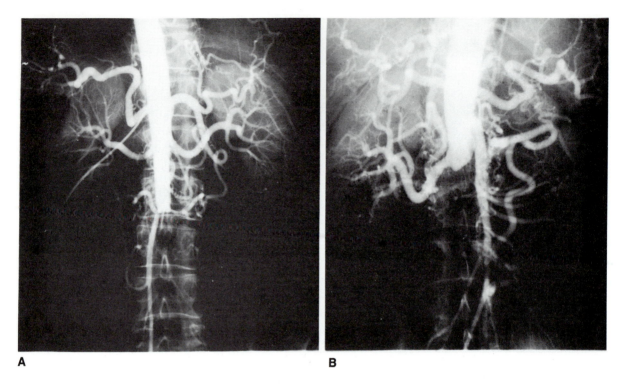

Figure 35-9. Angiographic examples of total aortic occlusion. **A.** Total occlusion extending to the midinfrarenal aorta, with patency of the proximal aorta maintained by inferior mesenteric artery and lumbar branches. **B.** Juxtarenal complete aortic occlusion, with retrograde thrombosis to the level of the renal arteries.

the occlusion has involved only the distal infrarenal aorta, with the proximal segment remaining open via runoff through a still patent inferior mesenteric artery or lumbar vessels (Fig. 35-9).

Surgical management of the latter group is straightforward and similar to standard aortic graft insertion. With extension of the occluding thrombus to a juxtarenal level, however, the operative approach is more taxing, and possible complications are more likely, particularly those complications involving disturbance of renal function. Nevertheless, surgery should be recommended for these patients, even if ischemic complaints are relatively mild and stable, because of the potential for more proximal propagation of thrombus with compromise or occlusion of neighboring renal or visceral arteries.[66]

In almost all patients with juxtarenal occlusion the bulk of the actual occlusive disease lies in the distal aorta, with the proximal occlusive material composed largely of a secondary thrombus. This proximal plug may almost always be removed by simple thrombectomy followed by routine graft insertion. Adequate dissection should be carried out to allow temporary control of the renal arteries, thus minimizing chances for renal embolization at the time of juxtarenal thrombectomy. Division of the left renal vein may facilitate exposure and is a benign procedure if carried out correctly near its insertion into the vena cava, thereby preserving collateral venous drainage. The completely occluded aorta should be opened through an arteriotomy placed several centimeters below the renal arteries. The suprarenal aorta is controlled by manual pressure or suprarenal clamp-

ing, and thrombectomy of the aortic cuff to the level of the renal arteries is carried out with a blunt clamp. This is usually terminated by aortic pressure's "blowing out" a typical organized cap of thrombus, which represents the apex of the thrombotic occlusion. The aorta is then flushed, the renal artery bulldog clamps are removed, and an appropriate vascular clamp is applied to the now patent infrarenal cuff. Graft insertion is then carried out in the routine fashion.

Formal endarterectomy should not be performed in most circumstances, because this plane may be difficult to terminate without compromise of the renal artery origins. Simple thrombectomy at this level is preferred, and it is sufficient in almost all cases.

The Calcified Aorta

Occasionally, dense calcification of the infrarenal aorta appears to preclude successful insertion of an aortic graft and causes the surgeon to consider abandoning the procedure. This is particularly true of end-to-side anastomosis with use of tangential, partially occluding clamps.

Reconstruction can always be accomplished using several possible alterations. First, a high end-to-end proximal anastomosis is preferred. By carrying dissection to or just above the left renal vein after its division or cephalad retraction, one often finds the aorta immediately below the renal arteries less involved and more manageable. Secondly, endarterectomy of a 1 to 2 cm cuff of totally transected aorta to the level of the infrarenal aortic clamp is usually possible and removes the calcification that always lies in the diseased intima and media. This procedure greatly facilitates subsequent end-to-end graft anastomosis. Although the cuff of the endarterectomized aorta, consisting of aortic adventitia and external elastic lamina, always appears fragile, it invariably proves adequate for graft anastomosis without later difficulties with bleeding, suture line disruption, or false aneurysm formation. The surgeon must use a tapered (not cutting-tip) needle, and an interrupted mattress suture technique, each suture backed with a pledget of Teflon felt as described previously (Fig. 35-8), is particularly recommended.

Clamping of calcified vessels may also be problematic. They can usually be clamped just below the renal arteries, where calcification is often less severe. Clamping in an anterior to posterior fashion, using an arterial clamp applied from a lateral direction or a Linton-Darling tourniquet clamp, may also be helpful. Finally, in truly difficult situations the aorta can be clamped above the renal arteries at the level of the diaphragm, or intraluminal balloon occlusion methods can be used.

The Small Aorta

In approximately 5% of patients the infrarenal aorta and iliac and femoral vessels are small or hypoplastic, possibly making aortic reconstruction technically difficult. Actual anatomic definition of the small aorta is obviously arbitrary. Cronenwett et al[13] have defined the syndrome as characterized by infrarenal aortas measuring less than 13.2 mm just below the renal vessels or infrarenal aortas smaller than 10.3 mm just above the aortic bifurcation. Iliac and femoral vessels are typically correspondingly small, with the common femoral vessels often only about 5 mm in size.

These patients form a unique and distinct subgroup and are frequently characterized by the "hypoplastic aorta syndrome."[15–17] Preferred surgical methods for reconstruction in patients with small vessels remain somewhat controversial; some authorities think the small size of the aorta and the iliac vessels makes endarterectomy unsuitable, whereas others favoring bypass techniques advocate the use of end-to-side proximal aortic anastomosis to avoid size discrepancies with the usual prosthetic grafts.

In our experience, because the disease in these patients is frequently localized, aortoiliac endarterectomy may often still be used. Although the small size of the vessels demands greater care and occasionally requires the use of patch closures, endarterectomy in our hands has worked well. If the disease is more diffuse, bypass grafting to the femoral vessels is preferred. Although end-to-side anastomosis is favored by many surgeons to overcome size differences between the graft and the host aorta, we nonetheless still use end-to-end techniques most often. Use of a smaller prosthesis avoids the consequences of inappropriately large grafts. In most cases, this requires the use of a 14 by 7 mm or even 12 by 6 mm bifurcation graft. The limbs of these grafts, although small, are also much more appropriate for the smaller femoral and outflow vessels of these individuals. Again, greater technical care must be exercised,

but with attention to technical detail, these grafts have not failed as a result of their small size; we much prefer the insertion of such grafts to the use of oversized prostheses. Adjunctive lumbar sympathectomy is often carried out, particularly in women.

Simultaneous Distal Grafting

A frequent practical concern in patients with multilevel occlusive disease is whether inflow operation alone will suffice. As already emphasized, diffuse combined segment disease (type III) is the most common pattern of occlusive disease, present in one half to two thirds of the patients coming to surgery.[14,43,45–47] Prior reports of patients with multilevel disease, treated in a generally accepted fashion by initial aortic reconstruction, have indicated that up to one third may fail to achieve satisfactory relief of ischemic symptoms with proximal operation alone.[19,21,45,67–69] Many patients with such unsatisfactory outcomes will require concurrent or subsequent distal bypass grafts. Identification of patients likely to have insufficient relief of ischemic symptoms with an inflow procedure alone remains difficult however.

In this regard, we reviewed a 6-year experience with 181 patients with multilevel disease who underwent aortofemoral grafting.[21] A well-performed inflow procedure will usually suffice if unequivocally severe proximal disease exists in the aortoiliac segment. Such clear-cut proximal disease is best identified by an absent or clearly reduced femoral pulse and obvious severe aortic or iliac disease on angiography, and it is confirmed, if necessary, by a positive femoral artery pressure study. Several intraoperative criteria may also be used. Restoration of an improved pulse volume recording (PVR) at the calf or ankle, as compared to preoperative tracings, can give reassurance of satisfactory improvement in distal circulation. However, improvement in PVRs or Doppler ankle pressures may not be immediately apparent in the presence of significant distal disease, especially in the cold, vasoconstricted limb. Another useful intraoperative guide in predicting a good clinical response is assessment of the anatomic size of the profunda femoris vessel itself. If the proximal profunda accepts a 4 mm probe and if a No. 3 Fogarty embolectomy catheter can be passed for a distance of 20 cm or more, it is likly that the profunda femoris artery is well developed and will function satisfactorily as an outflow tract and collateral source.

Possible benefits of simultaneous grafting include a more total correction of extremity ischemia and avoidance of the difficulties and potential complications associated with reoperation in the groin should later distal grafting prove necessary. Such advantages are usually outweighed by the greater magnitude of the synchronous two-level grafting and the fact that the majority of properly selected patients will be adequately benefited by proximal operation alone (76% in our series). Distal bypass may be carried out in the future if necessary; it was required in 17% of the patients in our series who were followed up to 6 years.[21] Such a figure is in agreement with previously reported experiences.[43,46,48,53,68]

In a small and carefully selected group of patients with

multilevel disease, synchronous proximal and distal reconstruction seems appropriate. This is a small group of patients, comprising only 4% of patients in our series, all with truly advanced limb-threatening ischemic problems in the foot. Most of these patients had only modest proximal disease, and because of the need for restoration of maximal flow to the foot because of significant distal disease, simultaneous reconstruction was elected. If the surgeon can reliably predict that a distal graft will be necessary in the future for limb salvage, we believe simultaneous grafting is preferred, offering the best chance of limb salvage and avoiding a more demanding additional operation in the groin at a later time. Certainly the use of two surgical teams can minimize the additional operation time required, and it is likely that synchronous grafting will become more common in the future.[70–73] Although success with preoperative noninvasive hemodynamic studies in selecting such patients has been claimed by some investigators,[21,71,74] others[53,67,69] have found tests of this type unreliable indicators of the need for concomitant distal bypass. Good clinical judgment remains extremely important, with reasoned and pragmatic decisions usually required.

Unilateral Iliac Disease

Not infrequently, proximal occlusive disease appears unilaterally, with fairly normal pulses and minimal to no symptoms in the contralateral extremity. Truly unilateral iliac disease is relatively infrequent, because the occlusive process is generally a more diffuse and eventually bilateral involvement. Progression of disease in the aorta or an untreated contralateral iliac artery will necessitate reoperation in a significant percentage of patients treated initially with unilateral operations for apparent one-sided disease.[44] Thus the most definitive and optimal long-term management for most patients is bilateral reconstruction with a bifurcated prosthetic graft. For these reasons, almost all vascular surgeons have abandoned use of unilateral aortofemoral grafts. In our experience, unilateral grafts were performed in 15% of patients undergoing proximal operation from 1963 to 1969, and only 4% of patients had these procedures in the 1970 to 1978 era.[14] They are virtually never performed by us today.

In patients with a well-preserved aorta and contralateral iliac artery, femorofemoral grafts have become increasingly important because of the ease of the procedure and the generally long-term results.[75–77] In certain instances, however, the surgeon may wish to avoid the contralateral side and confine reconstructive efforts to the ischemic side. For instance, the contralateral limb may be asymptomatic, but inflow in the proposed donor limb is of questionable reliability, and the patient is not a good risk for standard aortobifemoral grafting. In other instances, use of the contralateral groin may be relatively contraindicated because of heavy scarring from prior operative procedures or possible infection. In these situations, occasional direct iliofemoral grafting may be used to treat a disease that is largely unilateral at the time. A retroperitoneal approach through a separate lower quadrant incision (Fig. 35-10) usually provides

good exposure and can be performed with low patient morbidity.[78]

Associated Renal Artery or Visceral Artery Occlusive Lesions

Because of the recognized diffuse nature of atherosclerotic occlusive disease in most patients, it is not surprising that patients requiring aortic reconstruction for symptomatic lower-extremity ischemia often have associated occlusive lesions involving the renal or visceral arteries. Frequently these lesions are unsuspected and are detected only at the time of preoperative angiography. The dilemma of whether or not to attempt simultaneous correction of both abdominal aortic and visceral lesions is commonly encountered and is difficult to resolve.[79–82]

In these instances, each case must be considered individually, and no general recommendations are feasible or appropriate. Although theoretically appealing, extending aortic reconstruction to include visceral artery revascularization increases the complexity and magnitude of the operation and hence is associated almost invariably with some increased morbidity and mortality. For these reasons, truly prophylactic revascularizations should generally be avoided. The associated occlusive lesions should not be attacked simply because of their morphologic appearance on the preoperative arteriogram. However, if clinical evaluation suggests that they are symptomatic or functionally important, simultaneous correction is often appropriate.

In the asymptomatic patient with visceral artery disease, careful evaluation of the anatomic pattern of disease on the preoperative arteriogram should indicate those patients at risk for postoperative intestinal ischemia if the visceral lesions are not dealt with. As emphasized by Ernst and others, avoidance of this catastrophic postoperative problem requires preservation of an important inferior mesenteric artery in those patients with celiac or superior mesenteric artery occlusive disease or perhaps concomitant bypass grafting to the celiac or superior mesenteric artery. If associated renal artery disease is present, combined reconstruction may improve associated hypertension or overall renal function in carefully selected patients. Diminished renal function is rarely due to unilateral disease, and significant bilateral disease (either intrarenal or extrarenal) almost always must be present before overall renal function is adversely affected. The addition of a unilateral renal bypass without first proving the functional significance of the renal lesion may unnecessarily risk further compromise to excretory function in a patient who may be azotemic predominantly because of bilateral arteriolar nephrosclerosis. Therefore it seems appropriate to assess the functional significance of a unilateral renal artery lesion preoperatively and proceed with correction only when the studies are positive. If angiographically severe bilateral lesions are present and the patient has significant hypertension or diminished renal function, addition of renal revascularization to aortic reconstruction may be the best course. Such decisions require thoughtful evaluation. On occasion the surgeon may elect to stage the renal artery and aortic procedures,

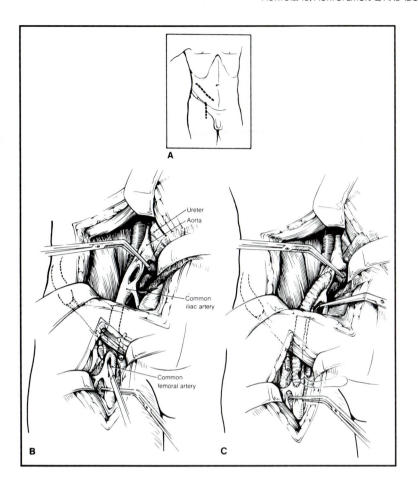

Ureter
Aorta
Common iliac artery
Common femoral artery

A
B
C

Figure 35-10. Iliofemoral bypass graft, useful for unilateral iliac occlusive disease. **A.** Lines of abdominal and groin incisions. **B.** Retroperitoneal exposure of the distal aorta and iliac vessels and exposure of right femoral vessels. **C.** Completion of iliofemoral bypass graft insertion.

in which case "extra-anatomic" means of renal artery revascularization by use of the splenic or hepatic arteries may be particularly helpful.[83,84]

RESULTS OF DIRECT AORTOILIOFEMORAL RECONSTRUCTION

Currently, generally excellent early and late results of direct aortoiliofemoral reconstructions can be anticipated and can be achieved at highly acceptable patient morbidity and mortality rates. A consensus of several large series in the modern era clearly supports this, indicating that it is reasonable to expect approximately 85 to 90% graft patency at 5 years and 70 to 75% at 10 years.[14,45–47,85] Perioperative mortality rates well below 3% are now commonplace in many centers. The mortality risk for direct reconstructions in patients with relatively localized aortoiliac disease can be expected to be extremely low, whereas those patients with multilevel disease and associated occlusive lesions in coronary, carotid, and visceral vessels will quite naturally have a somewhat greater mortality risk. In this latter group of patients, it is hoped that continued improvement of screening methods for associated disease and continued refinements in anesthetic management, intraoperative monitoring, and postoperative intensive care can further reduce the risk of serious morbidity and mortality.

Long-term survival of these patients continues to be compromised, however. The cumulative long-term survival rate for patients undergoing aortoiliac reconstruction remains 10 to 15 years less than that which might be anticipated for a normal age- and sex-matched population. Overall, approximately 25 to 30% of patients will be dead after 5 years and 50 to 60% at 10 years.[46,47,86] Not unexpectedly, most late deaths have been attributable to atherosclerotic heart disease. Patients with more localized aortoiliac disease, who have a lesser incidence of coronary artery disease, distal occlusive disease, or diabetes have a much more favorable long-term prognosis that approaches that of a normal population at risk.[85,86]

POSTOPERATIVE COMPLICATIONS

Early Complications

Early complications after aortic reconstruction are largely technical and infrequent when the procedure is carried out by an experienced surgeon and surgical team. Postoperative hemorrhage severe enough to require reoperation is seen in only 1 to 2% of patients and is usually due to failure to secure adequate hemostasis before wound closure, imprecise anastomotic techniques, inadequate reversal of intraoperative heparin, or dilutional coagulopathy associated with excessive blood loss and fluid replacement.

Acute aortofemoral graft limb occlusion may occur in 1 to 3% of patients.[87] Early graft thrombosis is similarly due to technical misadventures in most instances, most commonly at the femoral anastomosis of an aortofemoral graft. Occasionally, these problems may be attributable to twisting or kinking of the graft limb in the retroperitoneal tunnel. Thromboembolic causes of acute limb ischemia after aortic operation are more frequent than previously recognized but are usually treatable by prompt reoperation and use of embolectomy catheters.[88,89] Truly distal atheroembolic complications, often termed "trash foot," are difficult to deal with surgically and are far better prevented by minimal manipulation of the aorta, full systemic heparinization during the procedure, careful placement of gentle vascular clamps on nondiseased portions of the vascular tree, and careful flushing of the reconstruction before restoration of flow.

Acute renal failure after aortic operation is now relatively uncommon after elective surgery largely because of the recognition of the importance of administering adequate volumes of intravenous fluids during surgery, the maintenance of optimal intravascular volume and cardiac performance by careful monitoring of filling pressures, and avoidance of declamping hypotension.[90–92] Acute postoperative bowel or spinal cord ischemia is more difficult to prevent but fortunately is a relatively rare occurrence.[27,52,93–95]

Late Complications

Graft occlusion secondary to recurrent obliterative disease remains the most common late complication, reported in 5 to 10% of patients at 5 years and in 15 to 30% of patients followed 10 years of more.[87] Recurrent proximal disease extensive enough to cause failure of the entire reconstruction is unusual unless the original procedure was performed too low in the infrarenal abdominal aorta.[57] Failure of the entire reconstruction will require repeat aortofemoral grafting if the patient is an appropriate candidate[44] or extra-anatomic reconstruction for those patients believed less suitable for such extensive repeat surgery. In certain instances, the supraceliac aorta, descending thoracic aorta, or even ascending thoracic aorta may be used as an inflow source for repeat surgery if direct reoperation on the infrarenal abdominal aorta is believed ill advised or hazardous because of dense scarring, possible infection,[96–99] or other considerations. Most commonly, one limb of an aortobifemoral graft will fail, with the other limb retaining patency. In most instances, thrombectomy of the occluded graft limb can successfully restore inflow and, when combined with profundaplasty or femorodistal grafting, can maintain patency of the reoperated graft limb.[56,87,100–102] If thrombectomy is not feasible, crossover femorofemoral grafting from the uninvolved limb is the most useful alternative. Direct repeat aortic surgery for unilateral graft limb failure is rarely indicated or necessary.

Pseudoaneurysm formation may occur in 3 to 5% of patients and is most often attributable to degeneration of the host arterial wall, with subsequent dehiscence due to pulling through of the intact sutures.[47,103,104] Faulty anastomotic technique or placement of the graft limb under excessive tension is a contributing factor. Infection may be responsible and must be carefully considered in each instance of anastomotic aneurysm. The great majority of anastomotic aneurysms occur in the groin at the femoral anastomosis of an aortofemoral graft. Diagnosis in this location is readily achieved and confirmed by angiography, which is indicated to evaluate possible occult associated pseudoaneurysm formation at the proximal aortic suture line. Repeat surgery is generally easily accomplished by use of a short additional segment of graft extended to a slightly more distal anastomotic site.

Preoperative sexual dysfunction is common in patients with aortoiliac occlusive disease, but iatrogenic impotence may occur in up to one quarter of patients.[51] Although the physiology of erection and ejaculation is complex, the incidence of sexual dysfunction may be minimized by recognition of the principles of nerve-sparing dissection and graft implantation, as well as maintenance of hypogastric artery and pelvic perfusion by a variety of reconstructive techniques.[50,51,62,105,106]

Late graft infection remains a dreaded complication but is fortunately rare after elective aortoiliofemoral reconstruction. Prophylactic antibiotics in vascular reconstructions are clearly indicated and combined with meticulous sterile technique at the time of graft insertion minimize the chances of graft contamination. Once established, vascular infection usually requires removal of the prosthetic segment and revascularization through remote uncontaminated routes.[107,108]

Aortoenteric fistula formation is infrequent but carries a high likelihood of death or loss of limb. Fistula formation usually involves the proximal suture line and overlying duodenum, although the small bowel and colon may less frequently be involved. Massive gastrointestinal hemorrhage almost always occurs at some point, although frequently lesser degrees of gastrointestinal bleeding occur initially, allowing time for diagnosis and management. The diagnosis may be difficult to establish, and sometimes exploration based on a high index of suspicion is required. If present, treatment involves removal of the prosthetic graft, oversewing of the infrarenal aortic stump, closure of the gastrointestinal defect, and revascularization by extra-anatomic means.[109–112]

CONCLUSIONS

Arteriosclerotic aortoiliac occlusive disease is a common cause of lower extremity ischemic symptomatology. In the majority of patients, occlusive lesions are multifocal, involving the lower abdominal aorta, both iliac arteries, and frequently the infrainguinal arterial tree. Because of such considerations, unilateral operations are infrequently performed, and most patients are best served by aortobifemoral grafting. Before proceeding with aortic reconstructive surgery, the surgeon must document the hemodynamic significance of inflow disease. This documentation may often be accomplished by careful clinical examination and supplemented with vascular laboratory hemodynamic data and good arteriographic studies. If any doubt remains, however, direct measurement of femoral artery pressure is helpful. Because the results of surgical reconstruction in this anatomic area are so satisfactory, surgery may be considered for carefully selected patients with limiting claudication as their only symptom. More advanced limb-threatening ischemia is a clear indication for aortic reconstructions in appropriate at-risk patients. Aortoiliac endarterectomy may be used for a small group of patients, but in most instances aortofemoral grafting is the preferred procedure. The key features of aortofemoral grafting are high placement of the proximal anastomosis immediately distal to the renal arteries and careful techniques of distal anastomosis, with or without profundaplasty, to achieve adequate flow into the deep femoral artery.

Unilateral surgery is rarely indicated. Modification of surgical methods will allow successful management of associated vascular lesions or other unusual situations. Most complications can be prevented, and those that do occur may generally be successfully managed by early recognition and appropriate methods of reoperation. Highly successful long-term patency and clinical function of aortic reconstructions for occlusive disease make this one of the most rewarding areas of vascular surgery today.

REFERENCES

1. DeBakey ME, Lawrie GM, Glaeser DH: Patterns of atherosclerosis and their surgical significance. Ann Surg 201:115, 1985.
2. Leriche RR, Morel A: The syndrome of thrombotic obliteration of the aortic bifurcation. Ann Surg 127:193, 1948.
3. Dos Santos JC: Sur la desobstruction des thromboses arterielles anciennes. Mem Acad Chir 73:409, 1947.
4. Wylie EJ: Thromboendarterectomy for arteriosclerotic thrombosis of major arteries. Surgery 4:339, 1952.
5. Gross RE, Hurwitt ES, et al.: Preliminary observations on the use of human arterial grafts in the treatment of certain cardiovascular defects. N Engl J Med 239:578, 1948.
6. Oudot J: La greffe vasculaire dans les thromboses du carrefour aortique. Presse Med 59:234, 1951.
7. Julian OD, Dye WS Jr, et al.: Direct surgery of arteriosclerosis. Ann Surg 136:459, 1952.
8. DeBakey ME, Creech O Jr, Cooley DA: Occlusive disease of the aorta and its treatment by resection and homograft replacement. Ann Surg 140:290, 1954.
9. Voorhees AB Jr, Jaretzki A III, Blakemore AH: Use of tubes constructed from Vinyon "N" cloth in bridging arterial defects: Preliminary report. Ann Surg 135:332, 1952.
10. Edwards SW, Lyons C: Three years' experience with peripheral arterial grafts of crimped nylon and teflon. Surg Gynecol Obstet 107:62, 1958.
11. DeBakey ME, Cooley DA, et al.: Clinical application of a new flexible knitted Dacron arterial substitute. Am Surg 24:862, 1958.
12. Darling RC, Brewster DC, et al.: Aorto-iliac reconstruction. Surg Clin North Am 59:565, 1979.
13. Cronenwett JL, Davis JT Jr, et al.: Aortoiliac occlusive disease in women. Surgery 88:775, 1980.
14. Brewster DC, Darling RC: Optimal methods of aortoiliac reconstruction. Surgery 84:739, 1978.
15. DeLaurentis DA, Friedmann P, et al.: Atherosclerosis and the hypoplastic aortoiliac system. Surgery 83:27, 1978.
16. Staple TW: The solitary aortoiliac lesion. Surgery 64:569, 1968.
17. Greenhalgh RM: Small aorta syndrome, in Bergan JJ, Yao JST (eds): Surgery of the Aorta and Its Body Branches. New York, Grune & Stratton, 1979, p 183.
18. Moore WS, Cafferata HT, et al.: In defense of grafts across the inguinal ligament. Ann Surg 168:207, 1968.
19. Mozersky DJ, Sumner DS, Strandness DE: Long-term results of reconstructive aortoiliac surgery. Am J Surg 123:503, 1972.
20. Brewster DC, Waltman AC, et al.: Femoral artery pressure measurement during aortography. Circulation 60(suppl 1): 120, 1979.
21. Brewster DC, Perler BA, et al.: Aortofemoral graft for multilevel occlusive disease: Predictors of success and need for distal bypass. Arch Surg 117:1593, 1982.
22. Kempczinski RF: Lower extremity arterial emboli from ulcerating atherosclerotic plaques. JAMA 241:807, 1979.
23. Karmody AM, Powers FR, et al.: "Blue toe" syndrome: An indication for limb salvage surgery. Arch Surg 111:1263, 1976.
24. Kempczinski RF: Clinical application of noninvasive testing in extremity arterial insufficiency, in Kempczinski RF, Yao JST (eds): Practical Noninvasive Vascular Diagnosis. Chicago, Year Book Medical Publishers, 1982, p 343.
25. Goodreau JJ, Creasy JK, et al.: Rational approach to the differentiation of vascular and neurogenic claudication. Surgery 84:749, 1978.
26. Raines JK, Darling RC, et al.: Vascular laboratory criteria for the management of peripheral vascular disease of the lower extremities. Surgery 79:21, 1976.
27. Ernst CB: Prevention of intestinal ischemia following abdominal aortic reconstruction. Surgery 93:102, 1983.
28. Thiele BL, Bandyk DF, et al.: A systematic approach to the assessment of aortoiliac disease. Arch Surg 118:477, 1983.
29. Bruins Slot HB, Strijbosch L, Greep JM: Interobserver variability in single plane aortography. Surgery 90:497, 1981.
30. Moore WS, Hall AD: Unrecognized aortoiliac stenosis: A physiologic approach to the diagnosis. Arch Surg 103:633, 1971.
31. Brener BJ, Raines JK, et al.: Measurement of systolic femoral artery pressure during reactive hyperemia: An estimate of aortoiliac disease. Circulation 49 and 50(suppl 2):259, 1974.
32. Flanigan DP, Williams LR, et al.: Hemodynamic evaluation of the aortoiliac system based on pharmacologic vasodilatation. Surgery 93:709, 1983.
33. Coffman JD: Vasodilator drugs in peripheral vascular disease. N Engl J Med 300:713, 1979.
34. Porter JM, Cutler BS, et al.: Pentoxifylline efficacy in the treatment of intermittent claudication: Multicenter controlled double-blind trial with objective assessment of chronic occlusive arterial disease patients. Am Heart J 104:66, 1982.
35. Waltman AC, Greenfield AJ, et al.: Transluminal angioplasty of the iliac and femoropopliteal arteries: Current status. Arch Surg 117:1218, 1982.
36. Morin JF, Johnston KW, et al.: Factors that determine the long-term results of percutaneous transluminal dilatation for peripheral arterial occlusive disease. J Vasc Surg 4:68, 1986.
37. Johnston KW, Colapinto RI, Baird RJ: Transluminal dilation: An alternative? Arch Surg 117:1604, 1982.
38. Hertzer NR, Beven EG, et al.: Coronary artery disease in peripheral vascular patients: A classification of 1,000 coronary angiograms and results of surgical management. Ann Surg 199:223, 1984.
39. Brewster DC, Boucher CA, et al.: Selection of patients for preoperative coronary angiography: Use of dipyridamole-stress thallium myocardial imaging. J Vasc Surg 2:504, 1985.
40. Boucher CA, Brewster DC, et al.: Determination of cardiac risk by dipyridamole-thallium imaging before peripheral vascular surgery. N Engl J Med 312:389, 1985.
41. Cutler BS, Leppo JA: Dipyridamole-thallium 201 scintigraphy

to detect coronary artery disease before abdominal aortic surgery. J Vasc Surg 5:91, 1987.

42. Ehrenfeld WK, Wieber BC, et al.: Autogenous tissue reconstruction in the management of infected prosthetic grafts. Surgery 85:82, 1979.

43. Perdue GD, Long WD, Smith RB III: Perspective concerning aortofemoral arterial reconstruction. Ann Surg 173:940, 1971.

44. Crawford ES, Manning LG, Kelly TF: "Redo" surgery after operations for aneurysm and occlusion of the abdominal aorta. Surgery 81:41, 1977.

45. Malone JM, Moore WS, Goldstone J: The natural history of bilateral aortofemoral bypass grafts for ischemia of the lower extremities. Arch Surg 110:1300, 1975.

46. Crawford ES, Bomberger RA, et al.: Aortoiliac occlusive disease: Factors influencing survival and function following reconstructive operation over a 25 year period. Surgery 90:1555, 1981.

47. Szilagyi DE, Elliott JP Jr, et al.: A 30-year survey of the reconstructive surgical treatment of aortoiliac occlusive disease. J Vasc Surg 3:421, 1986.

48. Mulcare RJ, Royster TS, et al.: Long-term results of operative therapy for aortoiliac disease. Arch Surg 113:601, 1978.

49. Pierce GE, Turrentine M, et al.: Evaluation of end-to-side v. end-to-end proximal anastomosis in aortobifemoral bypass. Arch Surg 117:1580, 1982.

50. Queral LA, Whitehouse WM Jr, et al.: Pelvic hemodynamics after aortoiliac reconstruction. Surgery 86:799, 1979.

51. Flanigan DP, Schuler JJ, et al.: Elimination of iatrogenic impotence and improvement of sexual function after aortoiliac revascularization. Arch Surg 117:544, 1982.

52. Picone AL, Green RM, et al.: Spinal cord ischemia following operations on the abdominal aorta. J Vasc Surg 3:94, 1986.

53. Baird RJ, Feldman P, et al.: Subsequent downstream repair after aorta-iliac and aorta-femoral bypass operations. Surgery 82:785, 1977.

54. Morris GC, Edwards W, et al.: Surgical importance of profunda femoris artery: Analysis of 102 cases with combined aortoiliac and femoropopliteal occlusive disease treated by revascularization of deep femoral artery. Arch Surg 82:32, 1961.

55. Bernhard VM, Ray LI, Militello JP: The role of angioplasty of the profunda femoris artery in revascularization of the ischemic limb. Surg Gynecol Obstet 142:840, 1976.

56. Malone JM, Goldstone J, Moore WS: Autogenous profundaplasty: The key to long term patency in secondary repair of aortofemoral graft occlusion. Ann Surg 188:817, 1978.

57. Robbs JV, Wylie EJ: Factors contributing to recurrent limb ischemia following bypass surgery for aortoiliac occlusive disease, and their management. Arch Surg 193:346, 1981.

58. Sanders RJ, Kempczinski RF, et al.: The significance of graft diameter. Surgery 88:856, 1980.

59. Kaiser AB, Clayson KR, et al.: Antibiotic prophylaxis in vascular surgery. Ann Surg 188:283, 1978.

60. Pitt HA, Postier RG, et al.: Prophylactic antibiotics in vascular surgery. Ann Surg 192:356, 1980.

61. O'Hara PJ, Brewster DC, et al.: The value of intraoperative monitoring using the pulse volume recorder during peripheral vascular surgery. Surg Gynecol Obstet 152:275, 1981.

62. DePalma RG, Levine SB, Feldman S: Preservation of erectile function after aortoiliac reconstruction. Arch Surg 113:958, 1978.

63. Barnes RW, Baker WH, et al.: Value of concomitant sympathectomy in aortoiliac reconstruction. Arch Surg 112:1325, 1977.

64. Satiani B, Liapis CD, et al.: Prospective randomized study of concomitant lumbar sympathectomy in aortoiliac reconstruction. Am J Surg 143:755, 1982.

65. Corson JD, Brewster DC, Darling RC: The surgical management of infrarenal aortic occlusion. Surg Gynecol Obstet 155:369, 1982.

66. Starrett RW, Stoney RJ: Juxta-renal aortic occlusion. Surgery 76:890, 1974.

67. Sumner DS, Strandness DE Jr: Aortoiliac reconstruction in patients with combined iliac and superficial femoral arterial occlusion. Surgery 84:348, 1978.

68. Jones AF, Kempczinski RF: Aortofemoral bypass grafting: A reappraisal. Arch Surg 116:301, 1981.

69. Rutherford RB, Jones DN, et al.: Serial hemodynamic assessment of aortobifemoral bypass. J Vasc Surg 4:428, 1986.

70. Dardik H, Ibrahim IM, et al.: Synchronous aortofemoral or iliofemoral bypass with revascularization of the lower extremity. Surg Gynecol Obstet 149:676, 1979.

71. O'Donnell TF Jr, McBride KA, et al.: Management of combined segment disease. Am J Surg 141:452, 1981.

72. Baird RJ, in discussion of Brewster DC, Perler BA, et al.: Aortofemoral graft for multilevel occlusive disease. Arch Surg 117:1593, 1982.

73. Harris PL, Cave Bigley DJ, McSweeney L: Aortofemoral bypass and the role of concomitant femorodistal reconstruction. Br J Surg 72:317, 1985.

74. Garrett WV, Slaymaker EE, et al.: Intraoperative prediction of symptomatic result of aortofemoral bypass from changes in ankle pressure index. Surgery 82:504, 1977.

75. Eugene J, Goldstone J, Moore WS: Fifteen-year experience with subcutaneous bypass grafts for lower extremity ischemia. Ann Surg 186:177, 1977.

76. Brief DK, Brener BJ, et al.: Crossover femorofemoral grafts followed up 5 years or more: An analysis. Arch Surg 110:1294, 1975.

77. Dick LS, Brief DK, et al.: A 12-year experience with femorofemoral crossover grafts. Arch Surg 115:1359, 1980.

78. Couch NP, Clowes AW, et al.: The iliac-origin arterial graft: A useful alternative for iliac occlusive disease. Surgery 97:83, 1985.

79. Brewster DC, Buth J, et al.: Combined aortic and renal artery reconstruction. Am J Surg 131:457, 1976.

80. Dean RH, Keyser JE III, et al.: Aortic and renal vascular disease: Factors affecting the value of combined procedures. Ann Surg 200:336, 1984.

81. Stoney RJ, Skioldebrand CG, et al.: Juxtarenal aortic atherosclerosis: Surgical experience and functional result. Ann Surg 200:345, 1984.

82. Connolly JE, Kwaan JHM: Prophylactic revascularization of the gut. Ann Surg 190:514, 1979.

83. Brewster DC, Darling RC: Splenorenal arterial anastomosis for renovascular hypertension. Ann Surg 189:353, 1979.

84. Moncure AC, Brewster DC, et al.: Use of the splenic and hepatic arteries for renal revascularization. J Vasc Surg 3:196, 1986.

85. Martinez BD, Hertzer NR, Beven EG: Influence of distal arterial occlusive disease on prognosis following aortobifemoral bypass. Surgery 88:795, 1980.

86. Malone JM, Moore WS, Goldstone J: Life expectancy following aortofemoral arterial grafting. Surgery 81:551, 1977.

87. Brewster DC, Meier GH, et al.: Reoperation for aortofemoral graft limb occlusion: Optimal methods and long term results. J Vasc Surg 5:363, 1987.

88. Imparato AM: Abdominal aortic surgery: Prevention of lower limb ischemia. Surgery 93:112, 1983.

89. Starr DS, Lawrie GM, Morris GC Jr: Prevention of distal embolism during arterial reconstruction. Am J Surg 138:764, 1979.

90. Castronuovo JJ, Flanigan DP: Renal failure complicating vascular surgery, in Bernhard VM, Towne JB (eds): Complications

in Vascular Surgery. Orlando, Fla, Grune & Stratton, 1985, p 258.

91. Thompson JE, Vollman RW, et al.: Prevention of hypotensive and renal complications of aortic surgery using balanced salt solution: 13 year experience with 670 cases. Ann Surg 167:767, 1968.

92. Bush HL, Huse JB, et al.: Prevention of renal insufficiency after abdominal aortic aneurysm resection by optimal volume loading. Arch Surg 116:1517, 1981.

93. Ottinger LW, Darling RC, et al.: Left colon ischemia complicating aorto-iliac reconstruction. Arch Surg 105:841, 1972.

94. Szilagyi DE, Hageman, JH, et al.: Spinal cord damage in surgery of the adominal aorta. Surgery 83:38, 1978.

95. Elliott JP, Szilagyi DE, et al.: Spinal cord ischemia: Secondary to surgery of the abdominal aorta, in Bernhard VM, Towne JB (eds): Complications in Vascular Surgery. Orlando, Fla, Grune & Stratton, 1985, p 291.

96. Baird RJ, Ropchan GV, et al.: Ascending aorta to bifemoral bypass—a ventral aorta. J Vasc Surg 3:405, 1986.

97. Canepa CS, Schubart PJ, et al.: Supraceliac aortofemoral bypass. Surgery 101:323, 1987.

98. McCarthy WJ, Rubin JR, et al.: Descending thoracic aorta-to-femoral artery bypass. Arch Surg 121:681, 1986.

99. Rosenfeld JC, Savarese RP, DeLaurentis DA: Distal thoracic aorta to femoral artery bypass: A surgical alternative. J Vasc Surg 2:747, 1985.

100. Bernhard VM, Ray LI, Towne JB: The reoperation of choice for aortofemoral graft occlusion. Surgery 82:867, 1977.

101. Ernst CB, Daugherty ME: Removal of a thrombotic plug from an occluded limb of an aortofemoral graft. Arch Surg 113:301, 1978.

102. Charlesworth D: The occluded aortic and aortofemoral graft, in Bergan JJ, Yao JST (eds): Reoperative Arterial Surgery. Orlando, Fla, Grune & Stratton, 1986, p 271.

103. Satiani B: False aneurysms following arterial reconstruction: Collective review. Surg Gynecol Obstet 152:357, 1981.

104. Szilagyi DE, Smith RF, et al.: Anastomotic aneurysms after vascular reconstruction: Problems of incidence, etiology, and treatment. Surgery 78:800, 1975.

105. Flanigan DP, Sobinsky KR, et al.: Internal iliac artery revascularization in the treatment of vasculogenic impotence. Arch Surg 120:271, 1985.

106. Kempczinski RF, Birinyi LK: Impotence following aortic surgery, in Bernhard VM, Towne JB (eds): Complications in Vascular Surgery. Orlando, Fla, Grune & Stratton, 1985, p 311.

107. Qvarfordt PG, Reilly LM, et al.: Surgical management of vascular graft infections—local treatment, graft excision, and methods of revascularization, in Bernhard VM, Towne JB (eds): Complications in Vascular Surgery. Orlando, Fla, Grune & Stratton, 1985, p 499.

108. Reilly LM, Lusky RJ, et al.: Late results following surgical management of vascular graft infection. J Vasc Surg 1:36, 1984.

109. Bernhard VM: Aortoenteric fistula, in Bernhard VM, Towne JB (eds): Complications in Vascular Surgery. Orlando, Fla, Grune & Stratton, 1985, p 513.

110. Connolly JE, Kwaan JHM, et al.: Aortoenteric fistula. Ann Surg 1984:402, 1981.

111. Perdue GD Jr, Smith RB III, et al.: Impending aortoenteric hemorrhage: The effect of early recognition on improved outcome. Ann Surg 192:237, 1980.

112. Reilly LM, Ehrenfeld WK, et al.: Gastrointestinal tract involvement by prosthetic graft infection: The significance of gastrointestinal hemorrhage. Ann Surg 202:342, 1985.

CHAPTER 36
Femoropopliteal Arteriosclerotic Occlusive Disease

Henry Haimovici and Frank J. Veith

The occlusive process of the femoropopliteal segment is the most common lesion of the lower extremity, especially in patients over 60. Its preponderance, exclusive of its combination with other arterial lesions, has been documented by several statistical surveys, with its incidence ranging from 47[1] to 65.4%,[2] with an intermediate figure of 55% as shown in Figure 36-1.[3] Our studies have additionally shown that these lesions in diabetics are more prevalent in the femoropopliteal-tibial vessels than in the aortoiliac segment (75.4% vs. 24.6%).[4]

These statistical data showing an increasing incidence of femoropopliteal arterial lesions are paralleled by the widespread use of the surgical procedures for their reconstruction.

Thus, in 1972, it was estimated that of the 73,000 reconstructions of major arteries in the United States every year, more than 20,000 (over 27% of the total) are carried out in the femoropopliteal segment.[5] Furthermore, in 1982, it was reported that of a total of 339,000 major vascular procedures performed in 1978 (an increase of 117% over 1972), there were 163,000 peripheral reconstructions, thus constituting almost 50% of all vascular operations.[6] Although no specific breakdown by category of peripheral procedures was available in that report, by excluding by far the less frequent endarterectomy and aneurysmectomy procedures, it is estimated that the largest increase had occurred in the bypass grafting category.

Historically, the introduction of thromboendarterectomy by J. Cid dos Santos[7] in 1947 and the bypass graft technique by Kunlin[8] in 1948 marked the beginnings of direct revascularization methods of the lower extremity.

Of the two procedures, the bypass has gained wider acceptance and has largely superseded the former, as attested to by the vast worldwide literature on this subject.

Although functional improvement and limb salvage are being achieved in a large to a substantial degree, the results of these reconstructive procedures are the subject of an ongoing review and analysis concerning the various factors involved. These factors, which may determine the operative indications and influence their results, will be reviewed first, before describing the surgical technique.

CLINICAL BACKGROUND

Clinical, hemodynamic, and arteriographic findings provide the basis for the criteria in selecting patients with femoropopliteal occlusive disease for reconstructive surgery.

The clinical manifestations of these arterial lesions vary with their location and extent, as well as with the degree of other associated vascular lesions. They are divided into three major groups of increasing severity: (1) disabling intermittent claudication, (2) rest pain, and (3) ischemic ulcers and gangrene.

Intermittent claudication, indicating adequate arterial blood supply to contracting leg or foot muscles, varies in intensity according to the degree of arterial involvement. Mild to moderate intermittent claudication is generally not considered an indication for reconstructive surgery. By contrast, marked intermittent claudication that greatly restricts the patient's walking ability, often to the point of disability, is a major indication, especially if this symptom is a serious handicap in the life-style of a younger individual. However, an older, inactive persion whose livelihood is not threatened by this type of claudication is not considered a candidate for reconstruction, expecially if systemic manifestations of arteriosclerosis are present.

The degree of intermittent claudication is largely related to the extent and progression of the arterial disease. In the course of the evolution of the arteriosclerotic process, a superimposed acute segmental occlusion may occur, not only with a corresponding sudden aggravation of the claudication but also leading to gangrene and occasionally to foot or leg amputation. In such instances, arterial reconstruction may assume a more urgent indication than in the chronic stage.

Rest pain is a clinical picture of a more advanced arterial insufficiency. The underlying hemodynamic fact is a fall

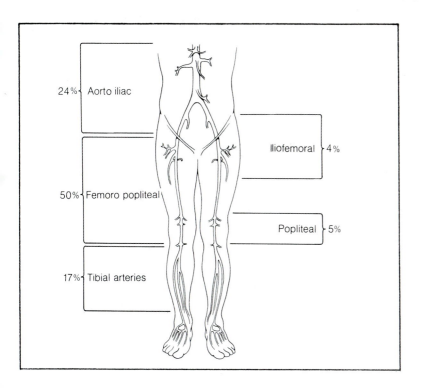

Figure 36-1. Distribution of the incidence of occlusive arteriosclerotic lesions in the lower extremities. Note the preponderance of femoropopliteal lesions. (*Based on data from Valdoni P, Venturini A: J Cardiovasc Surg 5:509, 1964.*)

in the blood flow below the level providing arterial supply to the resting limb. Clinically, rest pain involves the toes and the adjacent metatarsal area and occurs mostly at night. The patient awakes and hangs the involved limb over the side of the bed to relieve his pain. If further dependency of the limb is necessary to improve the capillary flow, the patient walks about the room before he can return to sleep. In a further advanced stage, rest pain may become continuous and be present not only during the night but also during waking hours. Associated signs of end-stage ischemia often present are a cold anesthetic or a cold edematous and discolored foot.

Ischemic ulcerative and gangrenous lesions, to be amenable to reconstructive arterial surgery, should be localized either in the toes or the heel or a combination thereof. In these cases, there may be associated infection in the interdigital web or in fissures on the heel. Meticulous local management of these lesions combined with appropriate antibiotics and avoidance of any trauma will usually limit the lesions to a small area. However, spreading gangrene may occur if local infection is not controlled, especially in diabetic patients if venous thrombosis is superimposed and if cardiac failure is present.

In attempting to establish operative criteria, it is important to take into account (1) the type of onset, (2) the age of the patient, (3) the pattern of occlusive arterial disease, and (4) the presence of diabetes.

The *mode of onset* may be insidious: sudden without prior claudication or sudden with prior claudication and a combination of associated trauma, venous occlusion, arterial embolism, and vasospastic conditions.

As to *age*, the majority of patients fall within the sixth, seventh, and eighth decades, and over 80% are males. It

is noteworthy that the relative age incidence in nondiabetic and diabetic patients varies inversely with the advancing decades. In our own study of vascular lesions in these two groups of patients, there were slightly more than 50% under age 60 in the nondiabetic group, whereas only 33% were found in the diabetic group. Conversely, after 60, the incidence in the latter group was 67% and 48.6% in the nondiabetic group.[4]

Clinical Evaluation of Arterial Disease

Before one undertakes arteriographic or other instrumental assessment, a clinical evaluation of the arterial disease is the most important part of the physical examination. The *color* of the limb, especially of the foot and toes, in the supine and dependent as well as elevated positions may provide a clue to the severity of the arterial ischemia at the microcirculatory level. The *temperature* of the skin, examined under basal conditions, may provide an indication of the degree and the location of the arterial impairment, especially if there is a difference between the two sides. Unilateral *foot coolness* or *coldness* is a manifestation of severe ischemia.

In an occlusion of the distal superficial femoral or proximal and middle popliteal, the knee on the affected side is much warmer than on the contralateral side. This finding, which we call "hyperemic knee sign," indicates an increased collateral circulation around the knee provided by the genicular system and branches of the profunda femoris artery (Fig. 36-2). The difference between the two knee temperatures may range from 2° to 5° F.[9]

Systematic palpation of all the *pulses* from the abdomi-

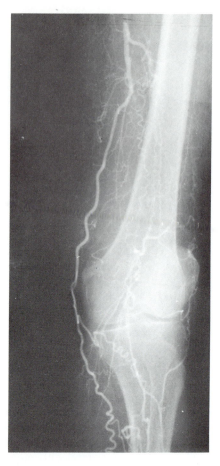

Figure 36-2. Arteriogram indicating occlusion of the superficial femoral and proximal popliteal arteries, with an enlarged saphenous branch of the highest genicular artery on the medial aspect of the knee.

nal aorta down to the pedal ones should provide a first indication about the degree and location of the arterial occlusion. *Auscultation* along the arteries from the abdominal aorta down to the popliteal artery may also indicate the presence of marked stenosis when a systolic bruit is audible.

The Doppler ultrasonic detector may provide semiquantitative information about the peripheral pulsations and their degree of amplitude. Of the noninvasive modalities, Doppler-determined segmental blood pressures and pulse volume recordings (PVRs) are generally the most useful means for evaluating lower-extremity occlusive disease. In addition, these measurements are semiquantitative and provide a permanent record of the patient's lower-extremity circulatory status at a given point in time. By comparing values at different times, the effect of interventional treatments may be assessed, and evidence of graft patency, failure, or the failing state may be obtained.[10]

Clinical Assessment of General Condition

A routine systematic evaluation of all the vital organs is essential for all patients being considered for arterial surgery and should include the following: cardiovascular status,

cerebral history with special reference to the carotid arteries, renal function, especially in diabetic patients, chest films, blood pressure determinations over a period of several days, complete blood chemistries, and lipid profile. Of these evaluations, those pertaining to cardiac function and status are the most important since perioperative myocardial infarction and other cardiac problems are the most important causes of perioperative and late morbidity and mortality.[11] In fact, aortocoronary bypass may have to be performed before the patient's peripheral lesion can be safely corrected by operation. (See Chapter 13.)

Arteriographic Patterns

A comprehensive assessment of the arterial lesions of the lower extremity, as mentioned in Chapter 33, should include the entire arterial tree from the terminal abdominal aorta to the pedal vessels (Fig. 36-3). This method is essential to provide information not only about the lesions of the femoral and popliteal arteries but also about the state of the aorta and iliac arteries (inflow tract), as well as about the tibial and pedal vessels (outflow tract). This can be achieved by serial aortoarteriography, performed preferably with local anesthesia, since new local agents are less painful. (Bilateral arteriography, should be carried out only in selected cases since in the majority of instances the arteriosclerotic process involves both lower extremities.[12])

Femoral

Our classification of the arterial disease in the *femoropopliteal* segment into six patterns is illustrated in Figure 36-4 and is based on the site and extent of the occlusion.[12] The incidence of the pattern in which the lesions are confined to the femoral and popliteal arteries is relatively low in the nondiabetic arteriosclerotic group and is even lower in patients with diabetes. Analysis of the data in the former group discloses that the lesions involved either the distal superficial femoral (about the adductor canal) or the femoropopliteal segment, with the latter extending on each side of the foramen of the adductor magnus. Occlusion of the entire superficial femoral artery is often noted. Involvement of the proximal superficial femoral artery alone is extremely rare. Diffuse stenosing atherosclerotic changes were found in approximately 20% of our series. Analysis of our arteriographic data indicate that (1) isolated femoropopliteal lesions occur primarily in nondiabetic atherosclerosis and (2) the lesions seem to be initiated at the foramen of the adductor magnus junction between Hunter's canal and the origin of the popliteal artery. The latter interpretation is in accord with the prevailing opinion of several investigators as well as with our previous findings.

Popliteal

The incidence of isolated popliteal occlusion appears to be low, especially in diabetics. The site of the occlusion process in this pattern is in the proximal half only, i.e., above the knee joint. A popliteal-tibial occlusion pattern is greater than that of the isolated popliteal lesion. In most of these cases, the site of the popliteal occlusion is in the lower half. The occlusive process appears to be in continuity

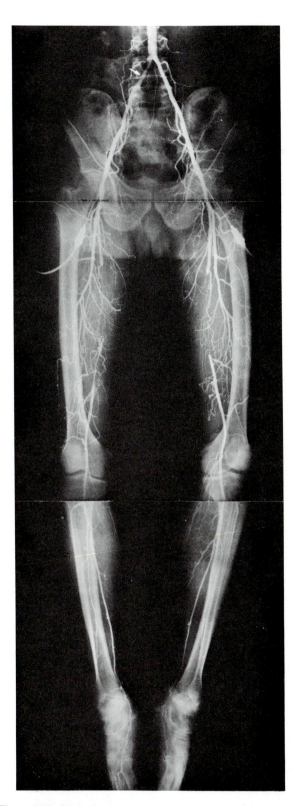

Figure 36-3. Bitransfemoral aortoarteriogram of a 62-year-old nondiabetic patient with bilateral occlusion of the superficial femoral artery. Note the right iliac displaying reduced opacification (*arrow*) due to an atherosclerotic lesion verified at surgery.

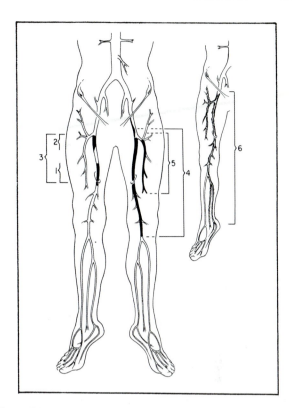

Figure 36-4. Diagram of femoropopliteal arterial patterns (see text for details): (*1*) distal superficial femoral, (*2*) proximal superficial femoral, (*3*) entire superficial femoral, (*4*) entire femoral and popliteal, (*5*) profunda femoris, (*6*) diffuse atherosclerosis with multiple stenotic areas.

with that of the leg arteries in more than half of the patients and occurs more often in diabetics than in nondiabetics.

Aortoiliac Segment (*Inflow Tract*)

Silent atherosclerotic lesions of the aortoiliac segment associated with occlusive disease of the femoropopliteal artery, as reported previously, are found in 27% of the cases.[13] Four basic patterns of this segment are present: (1) aortoiliac stenosis, (2) unilateral segmental iliac occlusion, (3) aortoiliac aneurysms, and (4) tortuosities of the aortoiliac segment. The net hemodynamic effect of all these lesions is reduction of arterial inflow of the lower extremity. Such lesions are often detected only by a panangiographic evaluation of the arterial tree, as indicated previously (see Chapter 33 for further details).

Tibial-Peroneal Segment (*Outflow Tract*)

In the presence of femoropopliteal occlusive disease, the outflow tract is rarely intact. More often than not, there are combined occlusions of leg arteries in which a single artery or two or a combination of all three arteries may be involved (Fig. 36-5). Although the incidence of combined occlusive patterns of the tibioperoneal arteries is more prevalent in diabetics, it is of some interest to note that, of the three leg vessels, the peroneal is most often patent, although some degree of intimal changes may be present, as a result of which the latter condition is often referred to as the "peroneal leg."

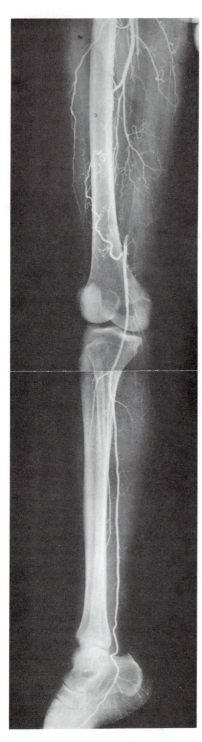

Figure 36-5. Femoral arteriogram showing occlusion of the superficial femoral, proximal popliteal, and anterior tibial arteries in a patient with moderately severe intermittent claudication.

Profunda Femoris

The profunda femoris artery, the main collateral channel of the femoropopliteal segment, may play a significant role in the overall clinicopathologic picture, since it is often involved by arteriosclerotic lesions. In the nondiabetic it is usually less involved than in the diabetic. In the majority

of instances, the arteriographic findings are those of stenosis and only rarely of complete occlusion (see Chapter 51).

Interpretation of Arteriographic Findings

From the foregoing brief description of the findings, it appears that the arterial lesions are rarely monosegmental and most often are multiple and complex. The complete occlusion of a segment is easily interpretable, but intimal lesions encroaching on the lumen are often difficult to assess in terms of their hemodynamic significance. The degree of stenosis assigned to an atheromatous lesions radiologically visible may be often misleading. Operative findings are usually more severe than the arteriographic outline would indicate. The nature of the lesions may range from a soft atheromatous to a hard fibrous or calcified plaque. The extent of the latter is rarely detectable from the angiographic image.

To avoid possibly misleading interpretations, it is essential to obtain adequate opacification of the arteriographic outline of the entire vasculature.

INDICATIONS

Based on clinical, hemodynamic, and arteriographic criteria for grading the degree of arterial insufficiency, three major indications are generally considered for femoropopliteal reconstruction:

Grade I   Severe intermittent claudication in an active person that interferes with gainful employment if the patient cannot control his condition by lifestyle modification and if he accepts the risks of operation

Grade II   Rest pain, moderate or severe, not relieved by nonsurgical conservative means

Grade III   Nonhealing ulcers or gangrene, usually limited to toes or heel or both

The indications for grade I are generally for functional improvement, if not proven otherwise. The indications for grades II and III are limb salvage.

Femoropopliteal bypass grafting and thromboendarterectomy of the femoropopliteal segment are the two major procedures commonly used for reconstructing this arterial segment.

FEMOROPOPLITEAL BYPASS GRAFT

Although Jeger[14] first described in 1913 the principle of bypass grafting for peripheral aneurysms (Fig. 36-6), it was not until 1948 that Kunlin independently introduced the procedure in the management of occlusive disease.[8] The technique described by Kunlin consists of a parallel shunt with the occluded artery, using end-to-side anastomosis both proximally and distally. The rationale for this technique is the transporting of arterial blood around an occluded segment while avoiding operative trauma and interference with collaterals or damage to concomitant veins. This technique has been widely accepted in reconstructive peripheral arterial surgery and later for aortocoronary bypass grafts.

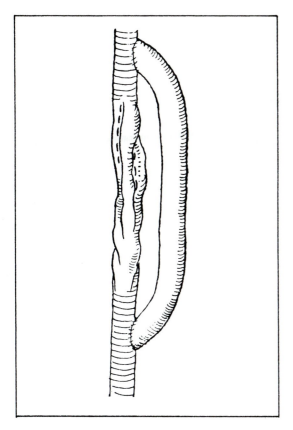

Figure 36-6. Diagram of bypass principle described by Jeger in 1913. (*From Jeger W: Die Chirurgie der Blutgefasse und des Herzens. Berlin, A. Hirschwald, 1913.*)

Graft Materials

After more than 4 decades of experience, *autogenous veins* still are the favored choice of graft material for the femoropopliteal bypass. Before the current era, at the turn of the century, there were sporadic reports of the use of autogenous veins for arterial replacements, primarily for injuries or aneurysms. Goyanes,[15] in 1906, replaced a popliteal aneurysm with the adjacent popliteal vein. Subsequently, Pringle,[16] Bernheim,[17] Lexer,[18] and others reported successful transplants of veins for replacing arterial lesions, Kunlin must be credited with the reintroduction of the autogenous vein for reconstructive occlusive arterial lesions. The autogenous saphenous vein, when available, is considered the optimal graft material. It is obtained at the time of surgery and is prepared during the procedure.

The availability of autogenous veins may be a problem in patients who have had previous surgical removal of their greater or lesser saphenous venous systems. Another problem may arise if an adequate length of saphenous vein is not available. Then, *cephalic* and *basilic veins* may be used successfully, either alone or combined with the saphenous vein.[19,20]

In the absence of autologous veins, use of fresh *homologous* veins has been reported in the past by a few surgeons. Further experience with the homologous vein grafts is necessary before their safety and feasibility are fully demon-

strated. In any event, their absolute indications appear limited. This is especially true in light of recent new graft material developments.

Newer Graft Material Developments

Among the grafts that have either gained clinical acceptance or are still being evaluated are expanded polytetrafluoroethylene, or PTFE (Gore-Tex and Impra), the glutaraldehyde-processed umbilical vein homograft (Meadox biograft), and a velour knit Dacron, which is a noncrimped and externally supported prosthesis.[23]

The detailed description of these various graft materials is found in Chapter 10, and we will mention only the highlights of each of these grafts.

The *PTFE graft* is composed of expanded Teflon arranged as nodules connected by thin fibrils. It is a remarkably inert material, provoking little perigraft inflammation, and the inner surface has a strong electronegative potential, both features of which account very likely for the graft's resistance to thrombosis. Its clinical use, particularly in limb-salvage situations, has resulted in early patency rates comparable to those achieved with saphenous veins in femoropopliteal bypasses in both above- and below-the-knee positions. However, saphenous veins have better late primary patency rates below the knee, although limb salvage rates for vein and PTFE femoropopliteal bypasses remain comparable for more than 4 years.[24]

The glutaraldehyde-stabilized *human umbilical cord vein* graft is covered with a netlike polyester mesh. The tanning agent molecule can establish crosslinks effectively and results in a stabilized graft that resists biodegradation. The umbilical vein graft is a musculocollagenous tube lined by a thromboresistant basement membrane. Although patency rates of this graft compare equally or even favorably to those of PTFE grafts in the femoropopliteal position, the high incidence of aneurysmal degeneration that has been reported with this graft seems to contraindicate its widespread use.[25,26]

New *velour Dacron* prostheses externally supported have been reported with a 78% patency rate at 4 years in the above-knee femoropopliteal site.[23] These improved results contrast with the nonsupported external velour Weft-Knit Dacron that yielded a patency rate of 56% at 4 years and 40% at 10 years for the femoropopliteal above-knee position. The results with the externally supported Dacron grafts are encouraging and represent an additional concept in the development of vascular prostheses. However, they need to be evaluated in a prospective study.

Reversed Autogenous Vein Bypass[*]

The femoropopliteal bypass graft may be carried out above or below the knee.

---

[*]Technique using the nonreversed in situ saphenous vein is described in Chapter 38, although no proof of the superiority of in situ bypasses in the femoropopliteal position has been reported.

Above-Knee Procedure

Position of Patient. The patient is placed in the supine position with the thigh externally rotated and the knee flexed approximately 30° (Fig. 36-7A). This position affords easy exposure of the femoral and popliteal arteries, as well as of the saphenous vein.

The skin of the abdomen, thigh, leg, and foot is prepared in the usual fashion. The medial aspect of the groin should be carefully draped and isolated from the adjacent perineal area by placing skin clips through the drapes and skin. The contralateral uninvolved extremity should be similarly prepared and draped in the event of need of additional saphenous vein.

Incisions. The skin incisions are made along the line of the femoral and popliteal arteries. Which artery should be exposed first depends on the arteriographic findings. If the supragenual popliteal artery appears of good caliber, the femoral is exposed first. However, should there be any question concerning the degree of involvement of the popliteal above the knee, it is best to start with its exposure.

Exposure of Femoral. A longitudinal or rather a slightly curved skin incision with the concavity facing the medial aspect is made from above the inguinal crease and extended distally for 4 to 5 inches.* The incision is made slightly later to the pulsation of the femoral to avoid the lymphatics as much as possible. Any minor bleeding or evidence of dividing lymphatics should be controlled by electrocoagulation or fine ligatures. Self-retaining retractors are placed both proximally and distally in the wound, and the lymphoadipose tissue is gently retracted medially. The deep fascia is opened along the femoral artery. The sheath of the artery is then opened along its axis. The common and superficial femoral are mobilized, and tapes are placed about them. By elevating them slightly, the origin of the profunda comes into view laterally and posteriorly to the common just proximal to the superficial femoral. Dissection of the origin of the profunda femoris should be carried out carefully to avoid injuring collaterals coming off at that level, as well as one or two branches of the satellite veins crossing the anterior portion of its initial segment. It is best to divide the latter and ligate them if mobilization of the profunda is difficult.

Exposure of Proximal Popliteal Artery. The surgeon stands at the opposite side of the table for the approach to the popliteal artery.

The skin incision is made in the lower third of the thigh anterior to the sartorius muscle and is extended close to the medial aspect of the knee. The deep fascia anterior to the sartorius muscle is opened, and the muscle is detached from the vastus medialis and retracted posteriorly and medially. The posterior edge of the vastus medialis muscle is identified and retracted anteriorly. The tendon of the adductor magnus is divided close to its insertion on the femur.

The popliteal artery is identified by palpation as the most superficial structure palpable through this exposure.

The overlying fascia is incised, and the adipose tissue, usually present at this level, is dissected until the vascular bundle is reached.

The sheath of the artery is opened. At this level, a network of venules surrounding the artery is almost always present and requires careful dissection from the arterial wall. This venous network is separated from the arterial adventitia, and the various branches are divided and ligated. The popliteal vein is then separated from the artery. This separation sometimes may be quite difficult because of the intimate connection between the two vessels. In separating them, it is important to avoid injuring any of the genicular branches of the popliteal artery. The latter is freed over a length of approximately 1½ to 2 inches, and tapes are placed around it.

Should the proximal popliteal artery appear markedly sclerotic and unsuitable for anastomosis to the graft, it is then necessary to extend the exposure to the midpopliteal. To do so, the hamstring muscles and their tendons should be mobilized and retracted posteriorly. Then the medial head of the gastrocnemius muscle should be divided close to the medial condyle of the femur.

The sheath of the popliteal is then opened farther distally. The tributaries of the veins surrounding the artery must be further dissected away from the latter vessel. To facilitate the dissection of the mid-portion of the popliteal, flexion of the knee may be helpful in relaxing the artery, thus allowing it to be readily drawn closer to the superficial level of the exposure.

Harvesting of Saphenous Vein. The saphenous vein may be obtained by means of a long single skin incision from the groin down to below the knee. Our preference is to remove it through multiple incisions, as indicated in Figure 36-7B. Using shorter skin incisions offers the advantage of satisfactory healing with less danger of skin necrosis.

The dissection of the saphenous vein is performed from the groin distally. The saphenofemoral junction is carefully mobilized, the vein is divided close to the femoral, and the proximal end is doubly ligated. A small atraumatic bulldog clamp is placed on the distal end. The tributaries are ligated with fine 5-0 or 6-0 silk close to their entrance into the main trunk, care being taken not to impinge on the wall of the latter. By careful dissection distalward and by elevating progressively the main trunk of the saphenous vein, all tributaries are identified and ligated.

Below the knee, bifid trunks are usually present and should be ligated and divided approximately 1 inch beyond their junction. They are removed, with the main trunk to be used for an angioplastic procedure designed to enlarge the vein for the proximal anastomosis (see below).

Before the vein is removed, placement of a marking suture of fine arterial silk through the adventitia may be useful for indicating its longitudinal position when it is placed through the tunnel (Fig. 36-8). Through the distal end of the divided vein, a small cannula is passed into it for irrigation with heparinized saline to expel any possible liquid blood or clots. The vein is then removed from its bed and placed immediately into a basin containing heparinized saline or heparinized whole blood at a temperature of 4° C or cold Hanks' solution. The cannula is left in place

---

*See Chapter 20 for exposure of the femoral artery.

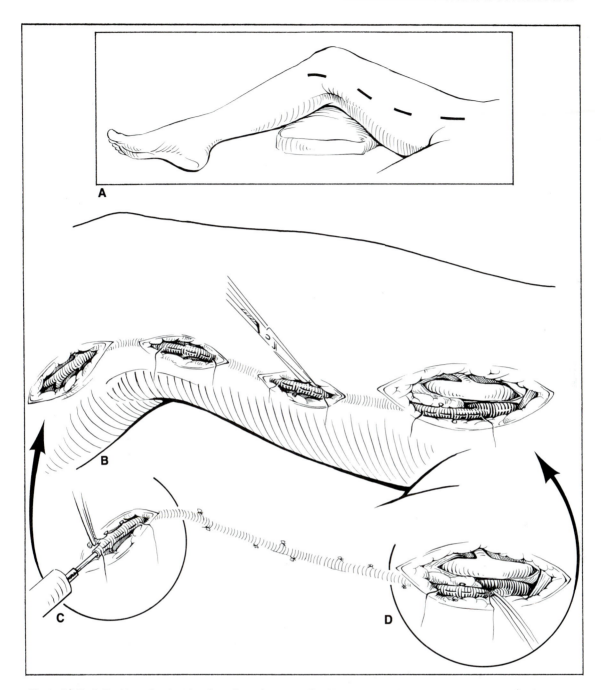

Figure 36-7. A. Position of patient for above-knee femoropopliteal bypass graft. **B,C,D.** Note the interrupted skin incisions for harvesting the saphenous vein from the thigh and upper leg. Alternatively, a single long incision may be used.

to indicate the distal end of the graft, which has to be reversed when implanted into the artery.

Recent studies have emphasized the role of optimum conditions for preparing the vein to prevent structural changes by suggesting the use of a balanced salt solution with a 10% serum at 4° C and with a pH adjusted to 7.0.[27] Based on these data, these studies would indicate that structural alterations resulting from the type of handling of the vein may determine its ultimate biologic fate, although this remains to be proven.

Developing Tunnel for Graft. Before passing the graft from the femoral to the popliteal area, it is necessary to develop a tunnel that parallels the natural course of the arterial tree. It follows over the adductor longus tendon and Hunter's canal beneath the sartorius muscle. A variety of hollow tunnelers* have been described and are available for devel-

---

*Any of these tunnelers is satisfactory, provided one avoids trauma and twisting of the graft.

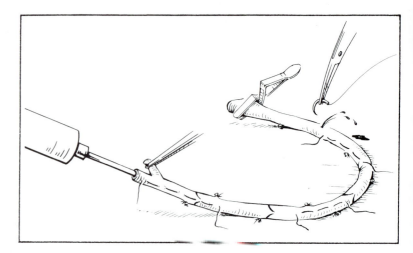

Figure 36-8. Flushing and distension of the saphenous vein. Note the direction of valves and silk marking along the axis of the vein.

oping a passage for the graft.[28,29] Once the instrument has passed in the subsartorial region and the tunnel is developed, it is necessary to complete and enlarge the passage with digital dissection to destroy any strands of tissue that might interfere with the passage of the graft or produce a stricture through the tunnel. A Penrose tubing or umbilical tape is then threaded through it to facilitate the placing of the graft later.

Handling of Vein Graft. The vein graft should be handled with extreme care. Application of arterial clamps on the trunk for any reason should be avoided to prevent injury to the intima or tears of branches at their junction with the wall of the vein. The ends of the graft may be clamped, provided they are later cut away. The vein should not be allowed to dry out either while additional branches or rents are being repaired or while the anastomoses are being performed.

The tributaries should be grasped by the end with a fine hemostat and sufficient traction applied upward. A fine 5–0 or 6–0 ligature is used to ligate the tributary at a point 1 or 2 mm distal to its junction with the main trunk. The ligature should not be placed too close to the wall, but neither should it be placed too far away from the junction with the main trunk.

As mentioned above, the vein is placed in Hanks' solution and gently distended with heparinized saline and again after it is removed so that remaining holes can be identified and closed with fine sutures, using horizontal mattress stitches. Any stricture should be carefully examined and adventitia removed, using a small pair of Metzenbaum scissors for its trimming from the vein. After the length of the graft has been checked for adequacy, it is replaced in the heparinized saline solution.

Implantation of the graft may be started in either the popliteal or femoral artery. My (H.H.) preference, with few exceptions, was to proceed from the proximal to the distal anastomosis, in the direction of the arterial flow, although other surgeons always do the distal anastomosis first, since it is usually the most difficult.

Arteriotomy of Common Femoral Artery. Administration of heparin before applying vascular clamps is routine. A sharp No. 15 knife blade is used for a longitudinal arteri-

otomy into the anterior wall of the artery. Angled Potts scissors are used to enlarge the arteriotomy. If the edges of the latter are calcified and the atheromatous intima exceeds the cut edge, it is best to excise it by using arteriotomy scissors.[30] (See Chapter 21.) If the artery is diseased, we use a No. 15 blade to make the incision. The anastomotic opening of the artery should be long in relation to the diameter of the vessel and a 2:1 arteriotomy-to-vessel diameter ratio is recommended.

The reversed saphenous vein is then brought into the field. Its distal end becomes proximal for the anastomosis (Fig. 36-9). It is enlarged, using a T incision to form a cobra-mouth anastomosis. The right-angled tips of the two sides of the divided posterior wall are cut away. Double-armed sutures are placed through the distal angle, with the needles going from the outside to the inside and then from the inside to the outside of the arteriotomy. Then a similar double-armed suture is passed through the proximal angle of the graft from outside to inside and from inside to outside through the end of the arteriotomy.

A running suture is used for approximating the edge of the vein to that of the arteriotomy, starting from the distal angle toward the proximal. After completion of one half of the anastomosis, the edge of the vein graft and that of the opposite side of the arteriotomy are separated for inspection of the inside of the lumen of the artery and of the appearance of the completed suture. A similar running suture is carried out from the distal end to the proximal for the other half of the anastomosis. The two sutures are tied together, thus completing the implantation of the graft (Fig. 36-9B).

The graft is then distended by injecting heparinized solution into it to test for leaks from it or from the anastomotic site.

A tunneler is then placed under the sartorius muscle and is brought out from the popliteal into the femoral area. The graft is attached at the end of the tunneler and is pulled through to the popliteal space. The black silk marker thread on the vein graft should help to orient the direction of the vein and thus avoid its twisting (Fig. 36-9C,D).

Implantation of Graft into Popliteal Artery. After it has been ascertained that the graft is properly oriented, it is important that it be placed posterior to the saphenous nerve.

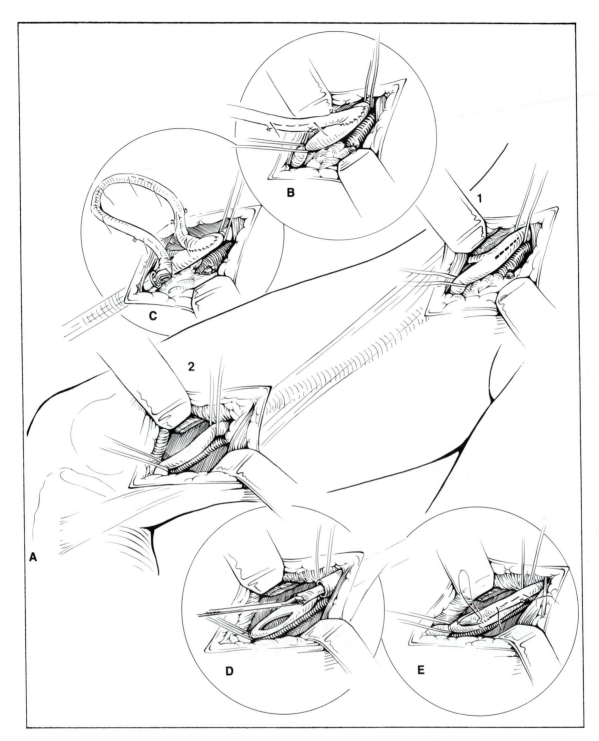

Figure 36-9. A. Diagram indicating completed exposure of the common femoral (*1*) and midpopliteal (*2*) arteries. **B.** Proximal anastomosis of the vein into the common femoral artery. **C.** Vein is pulled through the tunnel. Note the silk marking in the adventitial coat of the vein. **D.** Graft is brought into the popliteal space. **E.** Distal anastomosis of the graft is being completed.

Before starting the distal anastomosis, one should ascertain the proper length of the graft to avoid redundancy. The vein wall opposite to that of the artery is split in a fashion similar to that for the proximal end. After the corners are cut off, the graft is anastomosed to the arteriotomy of the popliteal artery. Its length, like that for the femoral artery, should be at least twice its diameter. The graft is attached by double-armed needles at its proximal angle and then in a similar fashion at its distal angle. The anastomosis is completed first in the center, since the ends are the most difficult and most critical to attach. The alternative is to start with the lateral edges of the graft, working from the proximal to the distal end. The anastomosis of the medial edges is then performed in a similar fashion (Fig. 36-9E).

Before completing this anastomosis of the graft into the popliteal artery, routine distal flushing of the latter and then of the graft is carried out by releasing the respective occluding clamps in the proper sequence.

Figures 36-10 and 36-11 show successful saphenous venous femoropopliteal bypasses, 1 year after surgery.

Below-Knee Procedure (Fig. 36-12)

When the proximal and middle popliteal segments are unsuitable for implantation of the graft because of occlusion or marked stenosis, its infragenual portion, often uninvolved, may be selected for the distal anastomosis.

With the knee moderately flexed and supported by a rolled sheet placed under it, a vertical incision of the skin is made just behind the posteromedial surface of the tibia. Care must be taken to avoid injuring the greater saphenous vein during the skin incision.

The crural fascia is opened along its fibers, its distal attachments are separated from the semitendinosus and gracilis tendons, and the latter are mobilized proximally. The medial head of the gastrocnemius muscle is retracted posteriorly to expose the popliteal artery and vein and poste-

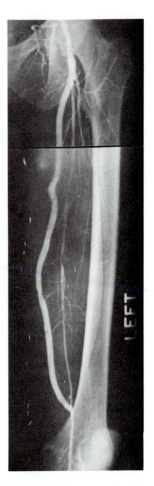

Figure 36-11. Saphenous vein femoropopliteal bypass in a 58-year-old diabetic patient with gangrenous lesions of two toes and severe rest pain. Arteriogram taken 1 year postoperatively. Note minor redundancy of the graft. Healing of lesions occurred shortly after reestablishment of arterial flow.

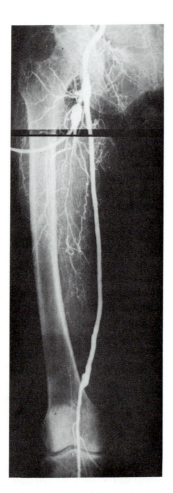

Figure 36-10. Saphenous vein femoropopliteal bypass for occlusion of the superficial femoral and proximal popliteal arteries in a 54-year-old woman with ischemic lesions of the toes. Arteriogram taken 1 year postoperatively.

rior tibial nerve as these structures cross the popliteus muscle posteriorly.

It should be noted that the distal popliteal artery has few branches below the inferior geniculate arteries, that atheromatous plaques are rarely present at this level, and that the arterial wall is more suitable for graft implantation.

The tunneling for the bypass from the femoral triangle to the infragenual popliteal is carried out through Hunter's canal, the upper popliteal space, and then through the infragenual region behind the popliteus muscle. Although the exposure, as described, requires three separate incisions (see Fig. 36-12), it may also be carried out by only two incisions, using the upper femoral and a long medial one starting from the lower third of the thigh and extending all the way into the upper third of the leg 4 to 5 inches below the knee. In this technique, it may be necessary to divide the tendons of the semitendinosus, gracilis, and sartorius muscles. Further exposure may be obtained by dividing the medial head of the gastrocnemius muscle. Except for the medial head of the gastrocnemius muscle, none of the other tendons are reconstructed at the end of the procedure.

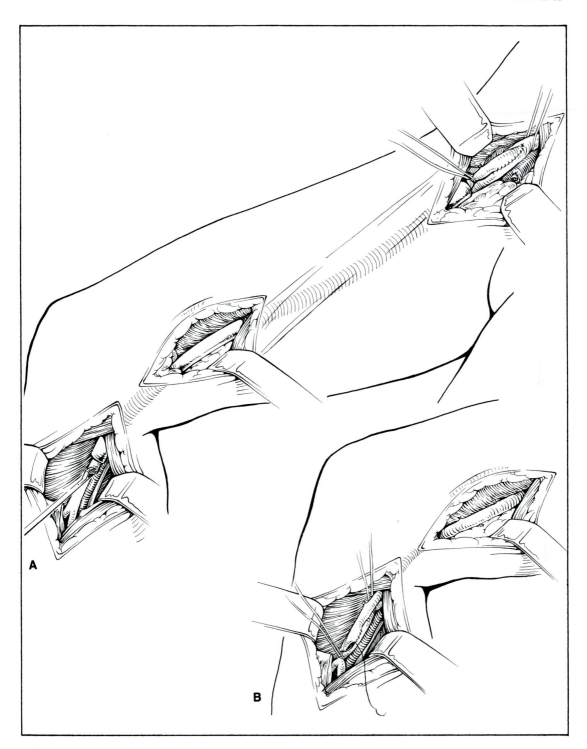

Figure 36-12. A. Three separate skin incisions along the vascular axis used for implantation of a saphenous vein below the knee, **B.**

Because of occasional anatomic variations of the soleus in its proximal portion, it sometimes may be necessary to detach the latter from the tibia to expose the distal popliteal artery at its bifurcation.

The first structure coming into view is the tibial nerve, which is closely associated with one or two popliteal veins accompanying the popliteal artery. After dissection and displacement of the tibial nerve and popliteal veins medially toward the surgeon, the popliteal artery is mobilized, freed, and brought out to a more superficial level. In doing so, it may be necessary to mobilize and sever one or more communicating venous tributaries connecting the two popliteal veins.

Anastomosis of the vein graft into the distal popliteal

proceeds then in a fashion similar to that in the above-knee procedure. Its implantation, however, is somewhat more difficult than in the supragenual region and requires more painstaking attention to all technical details to safeguard against any pitfalls or complications.

Anatomic Variations, Pitfalls, and Safeguards

Anatomic Considerations of Popliteal Bifurcation

Anatomic variations in the division of the popliteal artery (Fig. 36-13), although infrequent, may be encountered in its infragenual portion. Recognition of such variations may

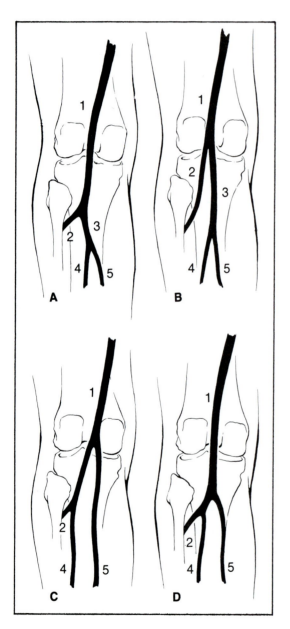

Figure 36-13. Patterns of popliteal division into its branches: (*1*) popliteal, (*2*) anterior tibial, (*3*) posterior tibial or tibioperoneal trunk, (*4*) peroneal artery, and (*5*) posterior tibial. **A.** Pattern 1. **B.** Pattern 2. **C.** Pattern 3. **D.** Pattern 4. (See text for details.)

assume important significance in the techniques used for anastomosing a vein graft into the popliteal artery or its branches. The localization of these branches by a good arteriogram is essential to preoperative planning.

Morris et al.[31] and Bardsley and Staple[32] evaluated the variations in branching of the popliteal artery, based on several hundred arteriograms. From these studies it is possible to describe four main patterns of branching of the popliteal artery (see Fig. 36-13). In approximately 90% of the cases, the *most common pattern* consists of the popliteal artery division more than 1 cm below the joint space into the anterior tibial and the tibioperoneal trunk, with the peroneal artery arising from the latter as a branch. A *second pattern* consists of a high division of the popliteal artery, usually behind the knee-joint space. A *third pattern* consists also of a high division of the popliteal, as in pattern 2, but the peroneal arises from the anterior tibial. A *fourth pattern* consists of a trifurcation at a normal level but with the peroneal arising from the anterior tibial.

Although other minor variations are also described, from a surgical point of view it is well to remember that the normal pattern is present in almost 90% of the extremities. In patterns 2 and 3, instead of the infragenual popliteal, two tibial branches are present.

Limitations Inherent in Veins as Grafts

Limitations in the use of the saphenous vein may be related to the following factors: (1) reduced diameter, below 3.5 mm, (2) inadequate length, (3) mural alterations of the vein due to dilatation or previous thrombosis, (4) irreducible small diameter after attempted dilatation, or (5) absence of the saphenous vein because of previous stripping.

Preoperative Saphenous Phlebography

Clinical assessment of the saphenous vein for use as a bypass is not always possible. To obviate this uncertainty, preoperative phlebography or duplex ultrasonography of the saphenous vein may help in determining its anatomic state, including its diameter, suitable length, valve competency, and venous anomalies, as well as the location of the latter.[33,34]

Pitfalls in Preparing the Vein Graft

Figure 36-14A1 indicates the placement of a ligature around a tributary, about 1 mm away from the main trunk. Figure 36-14A2 depicts the transection of the tributary after its ligation, and Figure 36-14A3 shows the length of its stump.

Figure 36-14B1 indicates the use of a suture ligature, using a fine half-circle needle and 5–0 suture material. Figures 36-14B2 and B3 show the two steps for completing this figure-eight suture ligature. Figures 36-14A and B depict the correct methods for ligating tributaries.

Figure 36-14C depicts improper ligatures of tributaries. Figure 36-14C1 shows a too-long stump of a tributary, resulting in its dilatation. Figure 36-14C2 indicates a thrombus formation in the cul-de-sac, resulting from the improper length of the ligated tributary. Figure 36-14C3 shows a ligature impinging on the wall of the vein, resulting in stenosis of the vessel at that level. Sometimes the stenosis may result from some of the adventitia of the main vessel being caught in the ligature. Eliminating the point of constriction

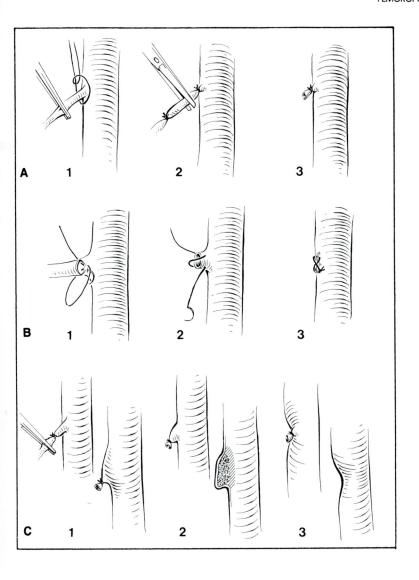

Figure 36-14. Diagrams depicting pitfalls related to improper ligation of tributaries of the main vein.

caused by the poorly placed ligature can sometimes be achieved by cutting away the adventitia at that level very carefully with a fine pair of scissors.

Pitfalls Resulting from Incorrect End-to-Side Anastomosis

Figure 36-15A1 shows the two sutures at each end of the vein and arteriotomy. Figure 36-15A2 indicates completion of one row of anastomosis carried out in the direction of the arrow. The second row is started from the end of the previous one and is continued toward the first suture line. Figure 36-15B1 indicates completed anastomosis of the graft into the artery, showing a slight ballooning of the vein cuff. Figures 36-15A1 and B1 depict the correct appearance of an end-to-side anastomosis.

Figure 36-15B2 shows bites too large in the vein graft, resulting in a stenosis of the graft anastomosis. This is an incorrect implantation into the artery. Figure 36-15B3 is another example of bites too large into the host artery, resulting in a stenosis of the latter at the anastomosis site. Figure 36-15B4 indicates an acute angle of implantation,

with bites too large into the artery, also resulting in a stenosis of the artery.

The latter three types of anastomoses are incorrect. They can be prevented by avoiding bites too large into either the vein graft or host artery. These pitfalls may be prevented by excising some of the adventitia around the anastomosis.

Angioplastic Technique for Improving Graft Diameter

Although the distal anastomosis of a reversed saphenous vein is usually technically satisfactory because of its maximum width at that level, the proximal anastomosis, because of the smaller diameter of the vein, may result in a critical area of narrowing. Royle[35] described an improved technique for preparing the distal end of the reversed saphenous vein used for the proximal anastomosis (Fig. 36-16). The vein with a tributary is cut in a longitudinal direction, as indicated by the dotted line in Figure 36-16A1. Excess vein is excised to fit the arteriotomy. The corners of the opened vein are cut away (Fig. 36-16A2). After the adventitia around the edges of the vein has been trimmed away (Fig. 36-16A3),

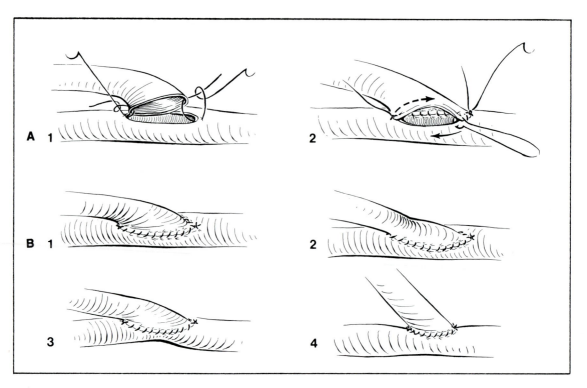

Figure 36-15. Diagrams depicting the correct end-to-side anastomosis and pitfalls resulting from incorrect end-to-side anastomosis. (See text for details.)

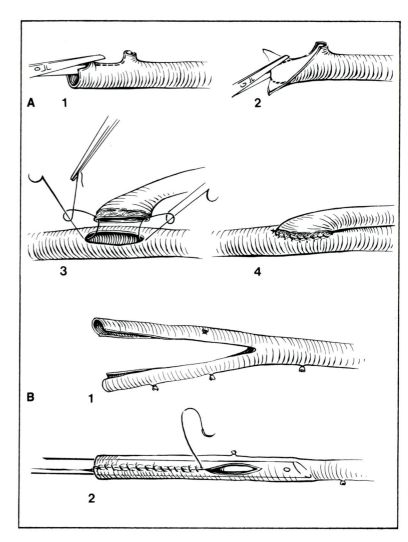

Figure 36-16. A. Diagrams depicting an improved technique described by Royle for preparing the distal end of a reversed saphenous vein for proximal anastomosis. (*From Royle JP: Surgery 60:795, 1966.*) **B.** Angioplastic procedure for a bifid saphenous vein designed to obtain greater length for a proximal anastomosis (Linton's procedure).

the anastomosis is carried out with a continuous suture, as shown in Figure 36-16A4.

Use of a Bifid Saphenous Vein
The two branches of the bifid vein are divided along the inner edges (Fig. 36-16B1). The anterior and posterior walls of the split branches are then sewed together, using fine suture material. This maneuver can be easily achieved by introducing a catheter of an appropriate diameter and suturing the two walls over this stent (Fig. 36-16B2). This angioplastic procedure is designed to obtain a greater length of the vein for a proximal anastomosis.

Figure 36-17A1 indicates the splitting of the vein in the usual fashion and excision of the tips to provide an oval opening for an end-to-side anastomosis.

Techniques for Increasing Vessel Diameter
To achieve a wider diameter, one may excise an area of bifurcation of the vein, as indicated in Figures 36-17B1 and

B2. A variant of this technique for enlarging a diameter is shown in Figures 36-17C1, C2, and C3.

Use of Synthetic Prostheses for Bypass Grafts

The indications for use of a synthetic prosthesis (Fig. 36-18) as a femoropopliteal bypass graft are essentially the absence of available autogenous vein, occasionally in cases of segmental occlusion of the superficial femoral with good popliteal-tibial runoff, and when there is urgent need for salvaging the limb with a questionable saphenous vein. Recently, it has been pointed out that saphenous veins should be spared for future use in these patients with widespread arteriosclerosis in case the need should arise for coronary bypasses.

Experience with some of the newer grafts such as polytetrafluoroethylene (PTFE) and velour Dacron has shown that in the above-knee location, their patency rates and

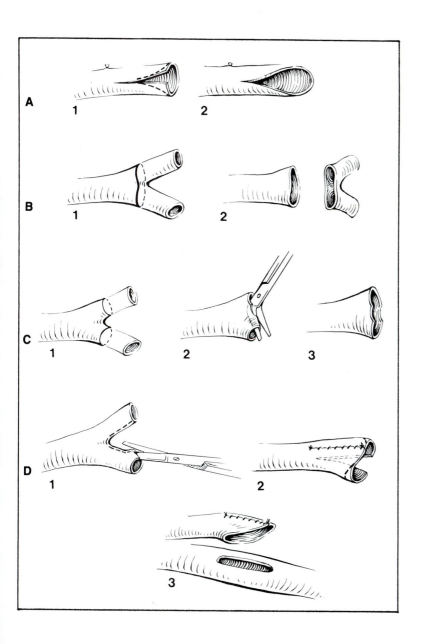

Figure 36-17. Diagrams depicting variants of the procedure for enlarging the diameter of veins, using their bifurcation branches (see text for details).

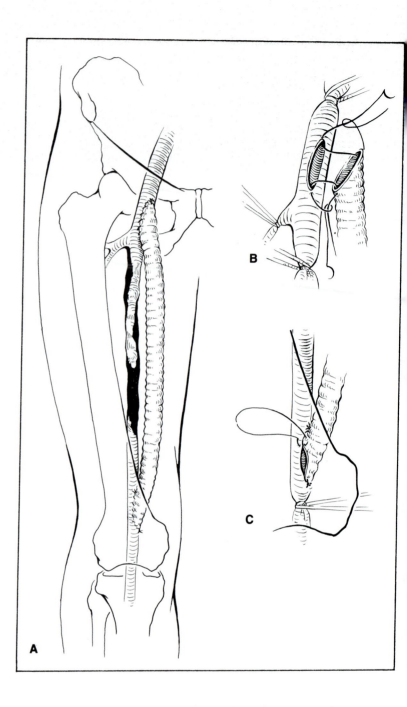

Figure 36-18. Diagram illustrating a synthetic prosthesis in femoropopliteal bypass graft above the knee (see text for details).

durability differ little from those of an autogenous vein. Although a longer-term experience with these newer grafts is not yet available to equate them with the 15- to 20-year statistics of the saphenous vein grafts, recent 3- to 5-year results are nevertheless encouraging. However, their use in the infrapopliteal leg arteries remains less than acceptable, thus leaving the autogenous saphenous vein the graft of choice.

PTFE Bypass Graft
The operative technique for PTFE bypass graft is essentially the same as the standard one described for autologous saphenous vein grafting.

The graft size used generally for a femoropopliteal bypass graft is 6 mm in internal diameter. The shape commonly accepted is a straight tube. Experience with tapered tubes achieves less favorable hemodynamics than with a straight one, and as a result their use is largely abandoned.

The graft is beveled, with the length of the bevel being twice the diameter of the common femoral artery. The implantation of the graft may be started at either the proximal or the distal angle with Prolene 5-0 or 6-0. Care should be taken to avoid a disparity between the length of the bevel and the arteriotomy, which might otherwise result in a stenosis due to suture tension at the level of the anastomosis. It is important to ensure that the graft take off obliquely from the artery to avoid this pitfall. After its anastomosis is completed, the proximal clamp is momentarily opened to flush the graft.

The subsartorial tunnel is prepared in the fashion described. The medial edge of the sartorius at the apex of the femoral incision is freed from its posterior connections. Similarly, the proximal angle of the popliteal exposure is enlarged, with the sartorius being retracted medially. A tunneler is introduced into the subsartorial region, with the graft being attached to it in the femoral area and pulled through into the popliteal space. Great care is taken to avoid any twisting or kinking of the graft during the passage through the tunnel. The exact length of the graft is then assessed and is beveled in the appropriate direction for its implantation into the popliteal.

In performing a femoropopliteal bypass procedure, whether one should do the distal or proximal anastomosis first is a matter of personal preference. If distal anastomosis is performed first, it is best to fill the graft with heparinized saline, which is left in the graft until the procedure is completed and bypass circulation restored. Because of its microstructure, the graft requires no preclotting. Air within

the graft can be easily removed before institution of circulation by first releasing the occlusion at one end or the other until the graft fills with blood, since air is immediately displaced through its pores within the graft wall.

Some sweating of serous droplets through the graft wall may be seen when circulation through the graft wall is begun. Such sweating is of no serious consequence and is in no way indicative of possible subsequent seroma formation postoperatively, since the serum protein in the graft wall will clot as soon as the heparin wears off or is neutralized.

After closure of the anastomoses, sometimes needle-hole oozing or bleeding occurs, which can be controlled easily by application of Surgicel and pressure applied on the area for a few minutes. In general, oozing anastomoses are sealed as a result of gentle pressure rather than as a result of the hemostatic quality of the Surgicel (Fig. 36-19A,B).

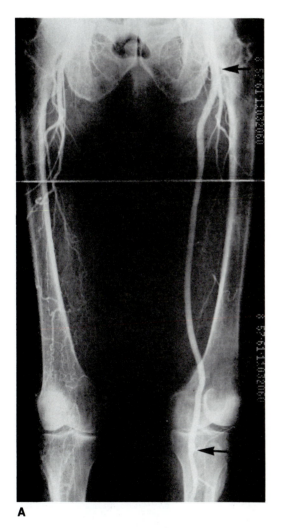

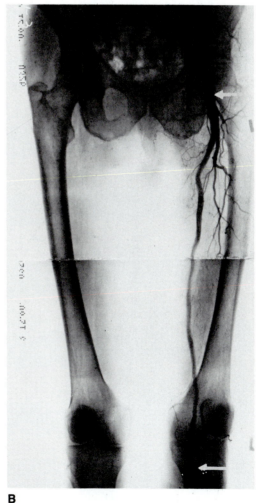

A   **B**

Figure 36-19. A. Left femoropopliteal PTFE 8 mm bypass graft implanted 3 days after an acute femoral and popliteal thrombosis in a borderline diabetic. This arteriogram was done 8 days postoperatively (July 1976). Note the arteriogram on the right side in which there is femoropopliteal occlusive disease for which a right lumbar sympathectomy was carried out 11 years before the left side's acute arterial event. The then acute symptoms improved. Both limbs were salvaged. **B.** The left femoropopliteal bypass graft 5 years (1981) after implantation of PTFE graft. Note some degree of tortuosity and layering of the graft. Clinically, the graft remains patent after 6½ years.

Use of Externally Supported (EXS) Dacron Prostheses
The technique used for implantation in the above-knee femoropopliteal position consists of placing the graft deep, with the length of the anastomosis about 2.5 to 3 times the diameter of the graft (Figs. 36-20 and 36-21). A 6 mm prosthesis is recommended for most patients and a 5 mm for patients with a very small popliteal artery. To reduce the thrombo-

genicity of the fibrin flow surface, it is necessary to inactivate thrombin through the action of heparin-activated antithrombin III in the fourth and final step of the preclotting procedure.[23] Most of the experience with this type of graft has been reported by Kenney, Sauvage, and their group.

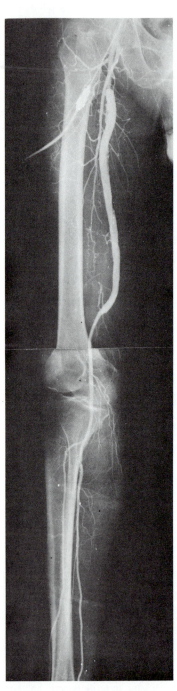

Figure 36-20. Dacron femoropopliteal bypass graft from the superficial femoral to the midpopliteal artery. Note the patency of all three leg arteries. The patient had ischemic and stasis ulcers of the leg, necessitating concomitant ligation and stripping of the saphenous veins. Arteriogram taken 5 years after surgery.

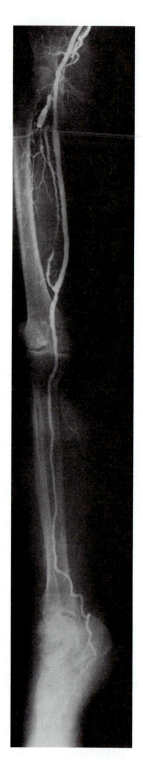

Figure 36-21. Dacron femoropopliteal bypass graft in a 66-year-old nondiabetic woman 6 years after its implantation. Note the patency of the peroneal artery.

The results for above-knee location of this graft are encouraging.

Although the autogenous saphenous vein grafts remain the gold standard of graft materials for lower-extremity bypass procedures, the newer grafts offer a number of advantages as a result of the time saved in preparing the vein graft and their ready availability.

Sequential Grafting

Lack of adequate length of autologous vein and necessity for bypass grafting to distal popliteal or to the infrapopliteal branches (small vessels) has led to the use of either a composite or sequential graft (Fig. 36-22).

A *composite* graft consists of a combined proximal prosthetic (PTFE or Dacron) graft with a distal autologous vein. The prosthetic grafts are attached end-to-side proximally into the common femoral artery and distally into the above-knee popliteal artery. The reversed vein graft is preferably anastomosed first distally into the below-knee popliteal artery or into a leg artery, then the graft is tunnelled in the usual anatomic fashion to above the knee for anastomosis into the popliteal artery below the prosthetic graft.

The *sequential* technique, as defined originally by Edwards et al.,[36] consists of a single graft (vein or PTFE) with multiple anastomoses for the purpose of reducing resistance and increasing flow. In this technique, the proximal and distal anastomoses are performed end-to-side, whereas the middle one or ones are side-to-side.

Both these concepts of composite and single bypass techniques have come to be known as "sequential grafting." Several reports have shown that this concept of sequential bypass provides increased arterial flow, with improved hemodynamic results.

Results of the sequential bypasses have been reported to improve distal perfusion in markedly ischemic limbs, leading to 1 to 8 year patency rates of 76 to 31% respectively.[37] When occlusion of the distal bypass occurs with continued patency of the proximal segment, it is due usually to poor distal runoff. Loss of limb in these cases may occur sometimes with a patent graft.[38] Based on the reported experience, it is reasonable to attempt this technique in well-selected cases for the advantages, as pointed out above, that it offers.

Femoropopliteal Reconstruction in Diabetic Patients

Peripheral arterial disease in diabetics is often associated with, and sometimes dominated by, two other important clinical manifestations: diabetic neuropathy and local infection. Their association, in varying degrees, lends to the lesions a truly characteristic clinical picture, often referred to as the "diabetic foot." The clinical manifestations may thus be conveniently classified under the following four headings: (1) arteriosclerosis obliterans, (2) peripheral neuropathy, (3) infection, and (4) combined lesions.

Accurate diagnosis and prompt treatment of circulatory disturbances seen in the extremities of diabetic patients, therefore, depend on determining the degree of participation of each of these three major causative factors. Thus

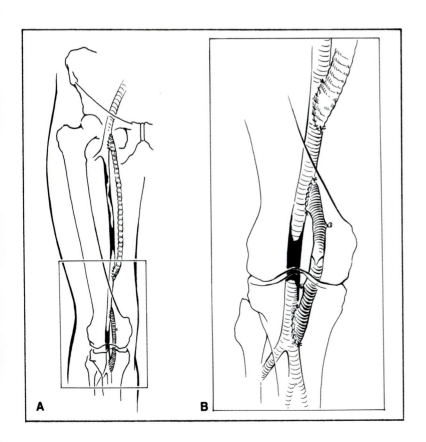

Figure 36-22. Diagram depicting a composite bypass graft, using a synthetic tube for the bypass around the common femoral artery to the midpopliteal artery and a saphenous vein bypass from the mid- to the distal popliteal artery below the knee, **A.** Blowup of the distal anastomoses of the two grafts, **B.**

it is essential to evaluate each patient from this triple point of view before deciding on the course to follow.

Arteriographic patterns of diabetic vs. nondiabetic patients have been reviewed in Chapter 33. Suffice it to state that the majority of the patients with diabetes has more involvement of the distal arterial tree (leg arteries and the popliteal artery) than the nondiabetic patient, in whom the lesions are more proximal but with frequent patent distal vessels. The site and the extent of the arterial lesions in diabetics are the main reasons for their poorer prognosis. Although the inflow tract may be adequate, the outflow tract and the terminal pedal arterial bed in diabetics determine the ultimate prognosis of the viability of tissues.

Careful selection of diabetic patients for reconstructive surgery is essential, although attempts at reconstruction in almost everyone with poor circulation is sometimes rewarding. In contrast, those patients who are initially seen with limited necrotic lesions but with an arteriogram indicating a good or fair runoff should be considered for reconstruction. Those patients who are initially seen with necrosis and infection and whose arteriograms display a distal arterial tree not suitable for reconstructive surgery have borderline indications for surgical reconstruction.

When selection of diabetic patients is based on good runoff of the popliteal and leg arteries, the patency rates of femoropopliteal reconstruction are no different from those obtained in nondiabetics. Wheelock and Filtzer[39] reported their experience with vein grafts in 100 diabetic patients with a 5-year cumulative patency of 72%. Even when cloth bypass grafts were used in diabetics, in the case of unavailability of saphenous vein, Harmon and Hoar[40] presented a 5-year cumulative patency of 59%. The latter results are similar to our own experience of 59.4% patency after 5 years or longer in patients in whom Dacron (Fig. 36-23) bypass grafts were used.[41]

In spite of these cumulative long-term patency percentages in diabetic patients seeming no different from percentages in nondiabetic patients, the former have a poorer prognosis for operative results and long-term survival. Based on his data, Veith[11] has recently reported better results even in diabetics.

Femoropopliteal endarterectomy has yielded generally poor results in this area. However, when endarterectomy is carried out for very short segments with good inflow and outflow tracts, the procedure is beneficial for limb-salvaging purposes. Such cases are best treated today by percutaneous transluminal angiography (PTA).

Associated Intraoperative Measures

The use of antiplatelet agents preoperatively and early postoperatively, before the use of anticoagulation, has been advocated.

Anticoagulation

Before temporary occlusion of the arteries, heparin sodium is administered intravenously, using 5,000 to 7,500 units, the latter being adjusted to the patient's weight. In addition, heparin in solution with normal sodium chloride is used subsequently for periodic irrigation of the graft or the distal arterial tree. Postoperatively, anticoagulants or dextran is

not used unless a specific indication exists. Patency of the graft, as a rule, does not depend on such postoperative measures, although occasionally heparin or dextran may be used for prophylaxis of thromboembolic phenomena. Protamine sulfate may be administered after all occluding clamps are removed if the necessity for reversing the heparin effect is indicated. Otherwise, one should abstain from its routine use. These measures are discussed in Chapter 12.

Intraoperative Arteriography

At completion of the operative procedure, it is essential to evaluate the distal arterial patency. Testing the latter by the quality of backflow, graft pulsation, and Doppler flowmeter, although useful, may sometimes be misleading. If there is any question about outflow, arteriography is indicated. Presence of thrombi, distal anastomosis defect, or an intimal flap, detected intraoperatively by arteriography, can be easily managed or repaired.

However, routine intraoperative arteriography may often be unnecessary and may unduly prolong the operating time. Its use should, therefore, be selective.

Associated Endarterectomy or PTA

If severe plaques in either the femoral or popliteal arteries are present, endarterectomy or PTA may help to avoid narrowing at anastomotic sites.

Complications

Intraoperative and *immediate* postoperative complications include either thrombosis or hemorrhage.

Early Thrombosis

After completion of the anastomoses, pulsation of the graft and distal arteries should be observed while the proximal incision is being closed. The slightest decrease in the pulsation of the graft or of the distal arteries should immediately evoke the possibility of early thrombosis. There are three major areas where thrombosis may originate: (1) the graft, (2) the distal anastomosis, and (3) the runoff.

Thrombosis in the graft may be due to inadequate clearance of fresh blood clots before completing the anastomosis. Accumulation of blood in the graft is a serious pitfall and should be avoided during its implantation. Its palpation between the index finger and the thumb may help to identify the presence of the incipient blood clot. Its immediate recognition and management are essential before closing the operative wounds.

If the distal anastomosis is the site of early thrombotic occlusion, it is usually due to a technical error or to an intimal distal flap. An arteriogram should help to delineate these lesions and provide a precise location for their proper repair.

If leg arterial embolism or thrombosis is suspected, the balloon embolectomy catheter may be useful except for the anterior tibial artery that could not be reached because of its right-angle takeoff from the popliteal artery. It may then require a retrograde thromboembolectomy from the ankle level or direct exposure of this vessel (Chapter 28).

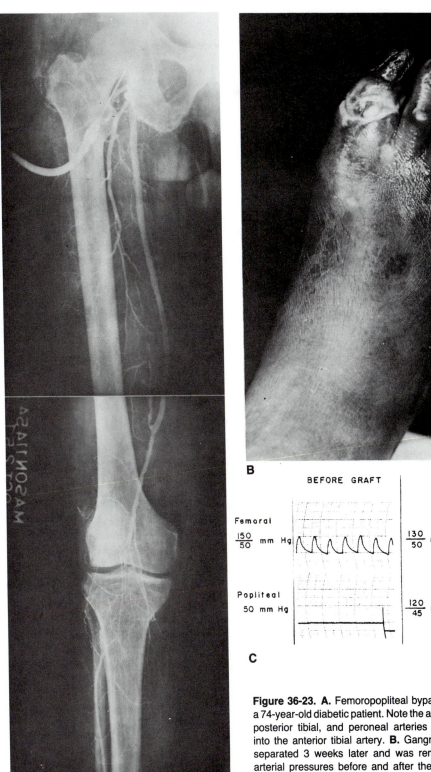

BEFORE GRAFT

AFTER GRAFT

Femoral
$\frac{150}{50}$ mm Hg

$\frac{130}{50}$ mm Hg

Popliteal
50 mm Hg

$\frac{120}{45}$ mm Hg

A

B

C

Figure 36-23. A. Femoropopliteal bypass, using a Dacron graft, in a 74-year-old diabetic patient. Note the absence of the distal popliteal, posterior tibial, and peroneal arteries and reentry of arterial flow into the anterior tibial artery. **B.** Gangrene of the great toe, which separated 3 weeks later and was removed at bedside. **C.** Intra-arterial pressures before and after the femoropopliteal graft. Note restoration of the pulsatile flow in the popliteal artery after graft implantation.

Hemorrhage

Intraoperative bleeding may occur either as a result of an untied small artery or vein branch or of diffuse bleeding from the capillary bed. The former can easily be identified and the vessels ligated. The latter type, commonly associated with heparin overdosage, can be controlled by reversing heparin's effect with protamine sulfate.

Immediate postoperative bleeding, after the wounds have been closed and exclusive of the above factors, may originate from the anastomotic sites or from the graft itself. Early reexploration is mandatory to avoid a tamponade effect from the accumulating blood, which may cause thrombosis of the graft. A few additional sutures of these areas are all that is needed for control of the bleeding.

Hemorrhage occurring in the late postoperative period is usually due to infection or is associated with a false aneurysm. These two points are discussed later in this section.

Postoperative Complications

Lymphorrhea. Inadvertent or unavoidable division of lymphatic vessels in the groin may result in drainage of cloudy watery fluid. If drainage is minimal, the wound may heal spontaneously within 10 days. However, should the drainage be profuse and unyielding to daily dressings, one may have to open the wound and ligate any visible lymphatics or mass-ligate some areas of the subcutaneous tissue. Bed rest with the legs elevated, application of an elastic stocking, and antibiotics should be instituted.

Edema. Edema of the lower extremity is frequently observed, most often after successful reconstructive surgery of the femoropopliteal segment. It usually persists from a few weeks to several months postoperatively. Its mechanism is not entirely elucidated, although several theories have been advanced to account for it, such as deep venous thrombosis, sudden reestablishment of high arterial pressure with a compromised venous return, and postoperative lymphatic abnormalities.

The role of deep venous thrombosis was based more on indirect evidence than on venographic data. The latter usually failed to demonstrate deep venous occlusion. Husni[43] studied this complication in 137 arterial reconstructions of the lower extremity in which phlebograms and pressure studies disclosed normal venous channels and hemodynamics. He believed that the postoperative hyperemia and edema were related to the degree of preexistent ischemia. He concluded that the edema is most probably attributable to an increased hydrostatic pressure and filtration at the capillary end, secondary to an overstretched precapillary arterial tree. On the other hand, Vaughan et al.,[44] using lymphangiograms in 24 patients, found lymphatic abnormalities. Their study established that both superficial and deep lymphatic systems were damaged during the procedures.

Although the mechanism of postarterial reconstructive edema is not entirely elucidated, the available evidence presented by the above and other investigators suggests that a combination of hemodynamic, lymphatic, and other yet unknown factors may account for this complication in the absence of venous thrombosis. Usually, in the mild form, the edema is self-limited after a few weeks. Intermittent daily elevation of the lower extremity above the heart level and use of an elastic support are recommended against the stasis edema.

Infection. Sepsis after a femoropopliteal bypass graft, although more frequently observed in the past, is fortunately seen today in less than 5% of the cases. A detailed account of the management of infection with vascular reconstruction is given in Chapter 43. Prophylactic measures consisting of antiseptic preparation of the skin in the groin for several days preceding surgery and use of antibiotics, especially if foot lesions are present, are of particular importance. If skin infection is present before surgery, the latter should be postponed until the sepsis has been eradicated by local treatment and systemic antibiotics.

Saphenous Neuropathy. A not uncommon complication following a femoropopliteal bypass graft is saphenous neuropathy. The patient complains of pain along the medial aspect in the lower part of the thigh and the medial aspect of the leg. Its distribution coincides with that of the saphenous nerve dermatome. The severity of the pain varies from patient to patient. It may occur spontaneously or may be evoked by pressure on the involved region or may be aggravated by motion and exercise. It may appear as a mild transient discomfort or may assume a burning character or, more rarely, may be persistent and disabling. This pain is related to an operative injury to the nerve or may result from its entrapment in the scar tissue in the lower thigh.

The neuropathy of the saphenous nerve can best be understood from the nerve's anatomic relationship to the femoral and popliteal vessels. It is exclusively a sensory nerve and originates in the distal part of the femoral triangle, lies close to the lateral side of the femoral artery, and thence descends in Hunter's canal with the artery. At this point, it crosses superficially from the lateral to the medial side and then leaves the distal end of Hunter's canal by piercing its aponeurotic roof. From there it passes to the tibial side of the knee and continues distally to the tibial side of the leg, accompanying the saphenous vein. Its terminal branches are distributed to the medial side of the leg and foot down to the level of the medial malleolus.

The anatomic proximity of this nerve to the femoral and popliteal arteries accounts for the possibility of its injury in the course of the bypass procedure or during a thromboendarterectomy.

Management of this neuropathy depends on the severity of the pain. For its mild form, injections of procaine in the area of maximum pain often permanently relieve the discomfort. The injections may have to be repeated several times until therapeutic effect is achieved. In the rare cases of entrapment in the scar, the nerve should be freed from the surrounding fibrous tissue.

Prophylaxis against saphenous neuropathy should be achieved by protecting the nerve from any possible injury during the handling of the adjacent arteries. In closing the popliteal space, particular attention must be paid to the position of the nerve and avoidance of its inclusion in the suture line, either during the approximation of the sartorius to the vastus medialis or during that of the skin.

Late Complications

Graft Thrombosis. Thrombosis of the graft may be related to (1) graft material, (2) proximal or distal progression of the underlying disease, or (3) anastomotic difficulties.

Although considered the best available graft material, autogenous veins are far from being immune to failure because of a number of factors such as graft stenosis, anastomotic stenosis, anastomotic aneurysms, size of the vein, and intimal hyperplasia or valve cusp stenosis. Most of these complicating factors can be identified if patients are followed at frequent regular intervals either by clinical evaluation or especially by Doppler and postoperative arteriograms. Correction of these lesions, preferably before thrombosis occurs, maintains patency in most patients. It has been estimated that the rate of thrombosis in vein grafts is approximately 3% per year.[45] Even after vein and PTFE graft thrombosis has occurred, reoperation is remarkably effective in improving the arterial circulation and salvaging limbs that are threatened by the failure of the arterial reconstruction.[46,47]

Management of late occlusive complications of arterial surgery is considered in Chapter 44.

False Aneurysms. Late occurrence of false aneurysms is observed in both the femoral and popliteal areas, perhaps more frequently in the former location. Their detection and management are discussed in Chapters 52 and 53.

Progression of Arterial Disease. Progression of arterial disease may occur both proximal and distal to the femoropopliteal bypass (Fig. 36-24). Such lesions may be present before the bypass procedure but may remain undetected or hemodynamically not very significant. As the disease progresses, the intimal lesions may increase in size and become significant hemodynamically. In the presence of a decreasing inflow to the graft, it is important to detect such silent lesions first by a noninvasive method and to confirm them by an aortogram. In an angiographic survey of the femoropopliteal segment reported earlier, we found a rather high incidence of 27% of associated aortoiliac lesions.[13] Lesions distal to

the popliteal artery progressing after the implantation of the graft or after an endarterectomy have been demonstrated by a number of investigators.[48,49] The morphology and rate of progression of the distal arterial outflow obstructions can be determined by preoperative and postoperative serial arteriograms (Fig. 36-25). Although progression of the disease either proximally or distally is sufficient to cause late failure of the graft, combined aortoiliac or tibial arteriosclerotic progression provides cumulative reasons for poor late prognosis. Downs and Morrow[50] reported in 1972 on angiographic follow-up assessment of autogenous vein grafts and found proximal disease in 6 out of 56 cases and significant occlusive lesions in the distal outflow in 13 patients. If detected early enough, such lesions are remediable and allow graft salvage.

Degenerative Changes of Graft. Although autogenous venous bypass grafts in the femoropopliteal region have yielded good long-term functional results, a number of these grafts fail because of degenerative changes of the venous tissue itself. DeWeese, et. al.,[51] Szilagyi et al.,[52] and others have shown that these grafts may display histologic changes consisting of progressive thickening of the intima, progressive smooth muscle decrease of the media with an increase of collagen tissue, and increased vascularity extending from the adventitia. These changes are pressure-related, but atheromatous changes have also been observed by a number of investigators in recent years. These atherosclerotic changes are not unlike those observed experimentally in animals as reported by us[53] and other investigators.[54,55] (See Chapter 11 for further details.) Of great significance are the potential causes of graft deterioration when one considers that a third of the lesions observed by Szilagyi et al.[52] were seen over a period of 5 to 10 years. Thus, these defects may threaten the long-term function of the graft.

Half of these defects may be preventable or remediable if detected early enough. Careful technique, avoiding traumatic and suture fibrosis, will prevent some of these complications. However, the intrinsic lesions to which the graft

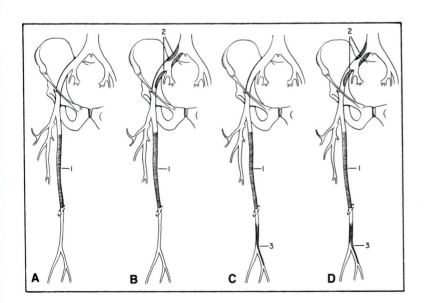

Figure 36-24. Diagram of superficial femoral occlusion (*1*) and involvement of the inflow (*2*) and outflow (*3*) tracts. **A.** Segmental femoral occlusion with normal inflow and outflow tracts. **B.** Inflow stenosis of the iliac arteries. **C.** Outflow stenosis of the popliteal-tibial arteries. **D.** Inflow and outflow tract involvement.

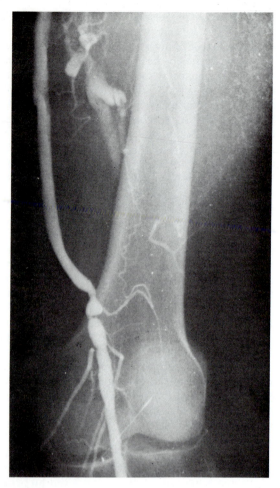

Figure 36-25. Distal anastomosis of a femoropopliteal bypass graft with a marked stenosing plaque of the host popliteal artery distal to the graft.

significant morphologic alterations in the remainder of the neointima of the graft.

The anastomotic neointimal (graft side) and intimal (recipient artery) fibrotic hyperplasia has been observed in autogenous saphenous veins, in such plastic prostheses as Dacron, Teflon, and PTFE, and in endarterectomized arteries. It occurs in many arterial locations—femoropopliteal, infrapopliteal leg arteries, carotid, aortocoronary—but apparently has not been observed in the aortoiliac location.

Failure of arterial grafts may occur early, within 30 days, or late, extending from a few months to a few years.

In the peripheral circulation, it has been estimated that this complication is as high as 7%, whereas in the aortocoronary position, it is as high as 30% at 3-year follow-up. These changes may lead to complete occlusion of the graft whether the intimal hyperplasia occurs proximal to the distal anastomosis or below it.

The pathogenesis of this process, although not entirely understood, implicates a number of potential factors: arterial pressure and flow patterns (hemodynamics), shear stress forces, operative handling of the anastomosis, thrombogenicity of graft, and mechanical mismatch between graft and host artery.[58-61]

Prevention of these lesions is not always achievable because of their multifactorial nature. However, in recent years, use of antiplatelet drugs is claimed to be effective in preventing the anastomotic neointimal fibrous hyperplasia. Evidence that aspirin and dipyridamole inhibit its formation is being presented in increasing experimental and clinical data. The mechanism of action of these drugs is through blocking the production of the prostaglandin endoperoxides PGG_2 and PGH_3 and thromboxane A-2, thus inhibiting platelet aggregation. This effect is achieved only by low concentrations of aspirin. Higher doses of aspirin may actually have the opposite effect by promoting intravascular thrombosis. The administration of both aspirin and dipyridamole has a synergistic effect. This clinical investigation is now in progress. The evidence so far is encouraging. These agents prevent early thrombosis but probably do not prevent intimal hyperplasia.[62]

Endarterectomy of the Femoropopliteal Segment

Since the introduction of interventional radiology for managing stenotic and occlusive lesions of the femoral and popliteal arteries, endarterectomy has generally lost its usefulness in such cases.

However, although PTA results are generally good in a substantial percentage of cases, endarterectomy of a bypass graft may be indicated if the PTA technique fails, since the failure may be due in part to inadequate correction of the small diameter of the vessels.

is susceptible, namely, the intimal thickening and atherosclerosis, are inherent in the new environment into which these grafts are placed.[56,57] Subendothelial hypertrophy and mural layering are a major threat to patency whenever the distal hemodynamics are not satisfactory. Under these conditions, apparently the same process is destined to occur in the autogenous vein graft as has been observed abundantly in synthetic femoropopliteal prostheses.[53-55] Prevention of these degenerative changes may be difficult to achieve. Strict dietary control of lipid levels may delay the onset of this cause of late graft failure. Repeat arteriograms at periodic intervals may help in early detection of these lesions and their repair.

Neointimal (Graft) and Intimal (Recipient Artery) Hyperplasia

In recent years, greater emphasis is being placed on anastomotic intimal hyperplasia as an important factor among the causes of graft failure. Indeed, in addition to progression of arteriosclerosis of the graft itself, much attention is being placed on the suture line reaction, mostly at distal anastomoses. In many instances, these last changes occur without

REFERENCES

1. Humphries AW, deWolfe VG, et al.: Evaluation of the natural history and the results of treatment in occlusive arteriosclerosis involving the lower extremities, in Wesolowski SA, Dennis C (eds): Fundamentals of Vascular Grafting. New York, McGraw-Hill, 1963, p 423.

2. Fontaine R, Kieny R, et al.: Long-term results of restorative-

arterial surgery in obstructive diseases of the arteries. J Cardiovasc Surg 5:463, 1964.

3. Valdoni P, Venturini A: Considerations on late results of vascular prostheses for reconstructive surgery in congenital and acquired arterial disease. J Cardiovasc Surg 5:509, 1964.

4. Gensler SW, Haimovici H, et al.: Study of vascular lesions in diabetic, nondiabetic patients. Arch Surg 91:617, 1965.

5. DeWeese JA, Blaisdell FW, Foster JH: Optimal resources for vascular surgery. Committee on Vascular Surgery. Report of Inter-Society Commission for Heart Disease Resources. Circulation 46:A-305, 1972.

6. Rutkow IM, Ernst CB: Vascular surgical manpower: Too much? Enough? Too little? Unknown? Arch Surg 117:1537, 1982.

7. Dos Santos JC: Sur la desobstruction des thromboses arterielles anciennes. Mem Acad Chir 73:409, 1947.

8. Kunlin J: Le traitement de l'arterite obliterante par la greffe veineuse. Arch Mal Coeur 42:371, 1949.

9. Haimovici H: Hyperemic knee sign. Unpublished data.

10. Veith FJ, Weiser RK, et al.: Diagnosis and management of failing lower extremity arterial reconstructions prior to graft occlusion. J Cardiovasc Surg 25:381, 1984.

11. Veith VJ, Gupta SK, et al.: Progress in limb salvage by reconstructive arterial surgery combined with new or improved adjunctive procedures. Ann Surg 194:386, 1981.

12. Haimovici H: Patterns of arteriosclerotic lesions of the lower extremity. Arch Surg 95:918, 1967.

13. Haimovici H, Steinman C: Aortoiliac angiographic patterns associated with femoropopliteal occlusive disease: Significance in reconstructive arterial surgery. J Cardiovasc Surg 65:232, 1969.

14. Jeger W: Die Chirurgie der Blutgefasse und des Herzens. Berlin, A. Hirschwald, 1913, p 262.

15. Goyanes J: Nuevos trabajos de chirugia vascular, substitucion plastica de las arterias por las venas o arterioplastia venosa, applicada como nuevo metodo, al tratamiento de los aneurismas. El Siglo Med 53:446, 561, 1906.

16. Pringle JH: Two cases of vein grafting for the maintenance of direct arterial circulation. Lancet 1:795, 1913.

17. Bernheim BM: The ideal operation for aneurysm of the extremity. Report of a case. Bull Johns Hopkins Hosp 27:93, 1916.

18. Lexer E: Die ideale Operation des Arteriellen und des Arteriovenosen Aneurysmas. Arch Klin Chir 83:459, 1907.

19. Kakkar VV: The cephalic vein as a peripheral vascular graft. Surg Gynecol Obstet 128:551, 1969.

20. Stipa S: The cephalic and basilic veins in peripheral arterial reconstructive surgery. Ann Surg 175:581, 1972.

21. Tice DA, Santoni E: Use of saphenous vein homografts for arterial reconstruction: A preliminary report. Surgery 67:493, 1970.

22. Ochsner JL, DeCamp PT, Leonard GL: Experience with fresh venous allografts as an arterial substitute. Ann Surg 173:933, 1971.

23. Kenney DA, Sauvage LR, et al.: Comparison of noncrimped, externally supported (EXS) and crimped, nonsupported Dacron prostheses for axillofemoral and above-knee femoropopliteal bypass. Surgery 92:931, 1982.

24. Veith FJ, Gupta SK, et al.: Six year prospective multicenter randomized comparison of autologous saphenous vein and expanded polytetrafluoroethylene grafts in infrainguinal arterial reconstructions. J Vasc Surg 3:104, 1986.

25. Karkow WS, Cranley JJ, et al.: Extended study of aneurysm formation in umbilical grafts. J Vasc Surg 4:486, 1986.

26. Hasson JE, Newton WD, et al.: Mural degeneration in the glutaraldehyde tanned umbilica vein graft. J Vasc Surg 4:243, 1986.

27. Abbott WM, Weiland S, Austen WG: Structural changes during preparation of autogenous venous grafts. Surgery 76:1031, 1974.

28. Lowenberg EL: An instrument to facilitate the long arterial bypass graft. Arch Surg 80:306, 1960.

29. Jackson DR: An improved tunneling device for vascular reconstruction. Surgery 66:807, 1969.

30. Haimovici H: Arteriotomy scissors. Surgery 54:745, 1963.

31. Morris GC, Beall AC, et al.: Anatomical studies of the distal popliteal artery and its branches. Surg Forum 10:498, 1960.

32. Bardsley JL, Staple TW: Variations in branching of the popliteal artery. Radiology 94:581, 1970.

33. Sapala JA, Szilagyi DE: A simple aid in greater saphenous phlebography. Surg Gynecol Obstet 140:265, 1975.

34. Veith FJ, Moss CM, et al.: Preoperative saphenous venography in arterial reconstructions of the lower extremity. Surgery 85:253, 1979.

35. Royle JP: Autogenous vein bypass: An improved technique. Surgery 60:795, 1966.

36. Edwards WS, Gerety E, et al.: Multiple sequential femoral tibial grafting for severe ischemia. Surgery 80:722, 1978.

37. Rosenfeld JC, Savarese RP, et al.: Sequential femoropopliteal and femorotibial bypasses. Arch Surg 116:1538, 1981.

38. Flinn WR, Flanigan P, et al.: Sequential femoral-tibial bypass grafting for limb salvage. Ann Surg 80:722, 1976.

39. Wheelock FC, Filtzer HS: Femoral grafts in diabetics. Arch Surg 99:776, 1969.

40. Harmon JB, Hoar CS Jr: Cloth femoral-popliteal bypass grafts in 29 diabetic patients. Arch Surg 106:282, 1973.

41. Haimovici H: Unpublished data.

42. Stipa S, Wheelock FC: A comparison of femoral artery grafts in diabetic and nondiabetic patients. Am J Surg 121:223, 1971.

43. Husni EA: The edema of arterial reconstruction. Circulation 35,36[suppl 1]:169, 1967.

44. Vaughan BF, Slavotinek AH, Jepson RP: Edema of the lower limb after vascular operations. Surg Gynecol Obstet 131:282, 1970.

45. Darling RC, Linton RR, Razzuk MA: Saphenous vein bypass grafts for femoropopliteal occlusive disease: A reappraisal. Surgery 61:31, 1967.

46. Whittemore A, Clowes AW, et al.: Secondary femoropopliteal reconstruction. Ann Surg 193:35, 1981.

47. Ascer E, Collier P, et al.: Reoperation for polytetrafluoroethylene bypass failure: The importance of distal outflow site and operative technique in determining outcome. J Vasc Surg 5:298, 1987.

48. Morton DL, Ehrenfeld WK, Wylie EJ: Significance of outflow obstruction after femoropopliteal endarterectomy. Arch Surg 94:592, 1967.

49. Couch MP, Wheeler HB, et al.: Factors influencing limb survival after femoropopliteal reconstruction. Arch Surg 95:163, 1967.

50. Downs AR, Morrow IM: Angiographic assessment of antogenous vein grafts. Surgery 72:699, 1972.

51. DeWeese JA, Terry R, et al.: Autogenous venous femoropopliteal bypass grafts. Surgery 59:28, 1966.

52. Szilagyi DE, Elliott JP, et al.: Biologic fate of autogenous vein implants as arterial substitutes: Clinical angiographic and histopathologic observations in femoropopliteal operations for atherosclerosis. Ann Surg 178:232, 1973.

53. Haimovici H, Maier N: Autogenous vein grafts in experimental canine atherosclerosis. Arch Surg 109:95, 1974.

54. Penn I, Schenk E, et al.: Evaluation of the development of athero-arteriosclerosis in autogenous venous grafts inserted into the peripheral arterial system. Circulation 31:192, 1965.

55. Scott HW Jr, Morgan CV, et al.: Experimental atherosclerosis in autogenous venous grafts. Arch Surg 101:677, 1970.

56. Szilagyi DE, Hageman JH, et al.: Autogenous vein grafting in femoropopliteal atherosclerosis: The limits of its effectiveness. Surgery 86:836, 1979.

57. Haimovici H: Ideal arterial graft: An unmet challenge—scope and limitations. Surgery 92:117, 1982.

58. Imparato AM, Bracco A, et al.: Intimal and neointimal fibrous proliferation causing failure of arterial reconstruction. Surgery 72:1007, 1972.

59. Imparato AM, Baumann FG, et al.: Electron microscope studies of experimentally produced fibromuscular arterial lesions. Surg Gynecol Obstet 139:497, 1974.

60. Oblath RW, Buckley FO Jr, et al.: Prevention of platelet aggregation and adherence to prosthetic vascular grafts by aspirin and dipyridamole. Surgery 84:37, 1978.

61. Echave V, Koornick AR, et al.: Intimal hyperplasia as a complication of the use of the polytetrafluoroethylene graft for femoral-popliteal bypass. Surgery 85:395, 1979.

62. Chesebro JH, Clements IP, et al.: A platelet-inhibitor-drug trial in coronary artery bypass operations. N Engl J Med 307:73, 1982.

CHAPTER 37

Small Artery Bypasses to the Tibial and Peroneal Arteries for Limb Salvage

Frank J. Veith, Sushil K. Gupta, and Enrico Ascer

In recent years more aggressive attitudes have evolved concerning the performance of operations designed to salvage patient's limbs when they are threatened by ischemic lesions due to arteriosclerosis below the inguinal ligament.[1] Most of the developments reflecting these attitudes relate to interventions on arteries distal to the popliteal artery. However, some relate also to interventions on arteries between the inguinal ligament and the terminal end of the popliteal artery, and many of the latter deal with improvements in treatment that are possible when a primary arterial procedure has failed.

This chapter deals with limb-salvage bypasses to the tibial and peroneal arteries, that is, so-called distal bypasses to so-called small arteries in the leg and foot. Since these bypasses are required and only justified in patients with threatened lower extremities and critical ischemia,[2] they almost all have multisegment arteriosclerosis, usually with two or three levels of occlusive disease. Accordingly, in any consideration of distal bypasses, one cannot escape the fact that these operations are required in patients with severe generalized atherosclerosis and specifically in patients whose disease involves not only the tibial and peroneal arteries but also often the aorta, the iliac arteries, and the femoropopliteal system as well. Thus many of the points made in the preceding chapter, ''Femoropopliteal Arteriosclerotic Occlusive Disease,'' apply equally well to the present chapter, which is designed to supplement the information provided in Chapter 36.

DEVELOPMENTS LEADING TO SMALL-ARTERY RECONSTRUCTIVE SURGERY

In the last two decades several developments have occurred that have made distal bypasses to even diseased small arteries in the leg and foot possible. One was the evolution

This work was supported in part by grants from the Manning Foundation, the Anna S. Brown Foundation, and the New York Institute for Vascular Studies.

of *arteriographic techniques*, which routinely visualize all patent named arteries in the leg and foot. Only with accurate visualization and definition of all patent arteries and of the extent of occlusive and stenotic disease can bypasses to small distal arteries be planned appropriately.

A second development was the evolution of instruments and methods for performing safe and effective surgery in small vessels. These *specialized vascular techniques* are not truly microvascular since they need not be performed through a microscope, although they may be facilitated with loop magnification and although they draw heavily on the hardware and instruments developed for microvascular surgery. In this regard, fine forceps, Castroviejo needle holders, and fine atraumatic monofilament sutures with small swadged needles are particularly important. Of even greater importance is the realization by the surgeon that these are specialty operations that cannot be performed with standard vascular instruments or techniques but require specialized instruments, training, and methods with meticulous commitment to a myriad of details. A full discussion of all these technical details is beyond the scope of this chapter, which, however, does emphasize those details that are most important. Among the more important technical developments are those that facilitate surgical manipulations (occlusion, arteriotomy, and suturing), even in the presence of severe atheromatous involvement or heavy calcification,[1,3] since many patients requiring these operations will have extensive disease in the patent segment of artery available for anastomosis.

A third development that has contributed heavily to the evolution of limb salvage using small artery distal bypasses and the present aggressive attitudes toward their use is the *in situ vein bypass technique*. This method was first introduced in 1962 by Hall[4] and has recently been popularized and strongly advocated by Leather and his colleagues,[5] who have introduced improved instrumentation for rendering the vein valves incompetent. Although there are theoretic advantages to this form of vein preparation, which will be fully discussed in Chapter 38, its superiority to comparable reversed vein bypasses performed with equal care has yet to be proven in a prospective controlled fashion. Moreover, many patients do not have a vein suitable for an in situ bypass but do have an *ectopic vein* that can be used for a reversed vein bypass (Fig. 37-1). However, the advocates of in situ bypasses deserve credit for promoting the careful semimicrotechniques that make small artery bypasses successful. The increasing acceptance and effectiveness of these very distal procedures are probably due

to this meticulous, careful technique rather than to whether the vein graft is of the in situ or reversed variety. Although in situ vein grafts *may* provide better patency rates than comparably performed reversed vein grafts when a very long graft with a small vein (<3 mm in diameter) is required, this remains to be proven. Moreover, the skilled limb-salvage surgeon should be capable of performing both types of bypass to small arteries since some patients may not be suitable for an in situ bypass and should not be denied an attempt at salvage of a threatened limb.

A fourth development that has contributed to the evaluation and acceptance of small artery bypasses is the *short vein bypass concept*. Traditional practice dictated that all bypasses to the popliteal or more distal arteries should arise from the common femoral artery because of the frequency of disease in the superficial femoral artery. Since 1981 we have advocated use of more distal arteries, when suitable,

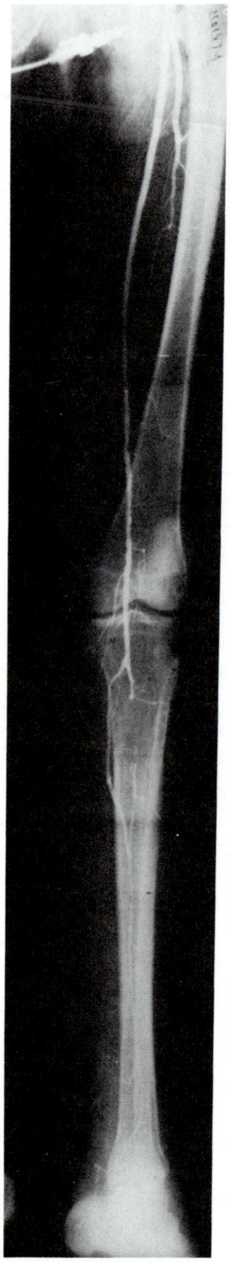

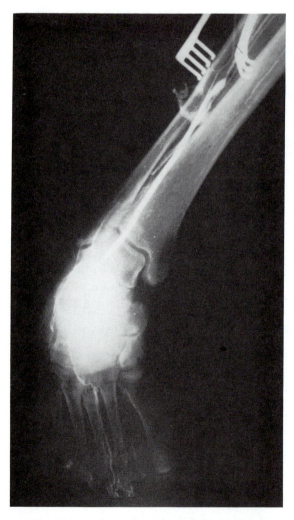

Figure 37-1. Ectopic short-vein graft used to perform a distal popliteal artery to proximal peroneal artery bypass. This patient had no usable vein in the ipsilateral extremity, and his opposite greater saphenous vein had been removed. The graft was from the short saphenous vein in the opposite leg. This arteriogram was performed 4 years after surgery.

Figure 37-2. Intraoperative arteriogram of a short-vein bypass from the anterior tibial artery to the lateral tarsal branch of the dorsalis pedis artery for extensive foot gangrene. The plantar arch is incomplete. The graft was from the opposite leg since all ipsilateral veins had been used for aortocoronary bypass. This graft remains patent more than 3½ years after operation. (*From Veith FJ, Ascer E, et al.: J Vasc Surg 2:552, 1985.*)

as the sites of origin for all lower extremity bypasses.[1,6,7] The superficial femoral, popliteal, and even tibial arteries have been used successfully in this capacity, with long-term patency rates that compare favorably with the standard longer bypasses. The use of shorter vein grafts clearly increases the availability of good quality autologous vein in many patients; it simplifies the operation; it allows the surgeon to avoid obese, scarred, or infected groins; and recently we have presented evidence that short-vein grafts have better patency than comparable long-vein grafts, particularly when the bypass is to a disadvantaged outflow tract (Figs. 37-2 and 37-3).[7,8]

A related development that has contributed to the evolution of small-artery reconstructions has been the realization that *disadvantaged outflow arteries* such as those connecting to incomplete plantar arches, those consisting of isolated or blind segments, and those with considerable disease or heavy calcification can sometimes serve as effective sites for bypass implantation (Figs. 37-2 to 37-6).[1,3,7,8] Thus almost all patients with a threatened limb will have some distal artery that can be used in a limb-salvage effort. This high operability rate is further increased by some of the recent *improvements in anesthesiology and intensive care.* With use of appropriate measures to improve and maintain the function of diseased hearts preoperatively, intraoperatively, and postoperatively, almost all patients, even those with severe heart disease, can, with reasonable safety, undergo even a long operation designed to save a limb.

INTERFACE OF SMALL-ARTERY BYPASSES WITH MORE PROXIMAL REVASCULARIZATION PROCEDURES

Patients requiring distal bypasses frequently have, in addition to proximal occlusions in the infrapopliteal arteries, significant stenotic or occlusive disease involving the distal aorta, the iliac arteries, and the superficial femoral artery or the popliteal artery or both. Sometimes this disease may be segmental in nature so that these patients frequently have an isolated proximal patent segment distal to a hemodynamically significant stenosis or an occlusion. A patent common femoral artery distal to an iliac lesion and outflowing into a normal deep femoral artery or a patent isolated or blind popliteal artery distal to a superficial femoral occlusion and with outflow only through patent collaterals are the two most common isolated segments. Clearly any patient who is a candidate for a small artery bypass should have any correctable more proximal stenosis or occlusion repaired first. Frequently this repair will be enough to obviate the need for the more difficult distal procedure because of the increased distal perfusion obtained from the "trickle-down effect" through collateral arteries. An example of this effect would be a patient with a hemodynamically significant stenosis of the left external iliac artery and occlusions of the superficial femoral, distal, popliteal, and all proximal tibial arteries on the left. If this patient had only severe rest pain in the left foot, it would probably be relieved by an aortofemoral bypass or percutaneous transluminal angioplasty of the iliac artery stenosis. A bypass to the isolated popliteal segment might also be required if the iliac gradient were not large and would probably be required if the patient had significant foot gangrene. In this setting the distal bypass should be performed only if a healed foot could not be obtained by performance of the simpler proximal procedures.

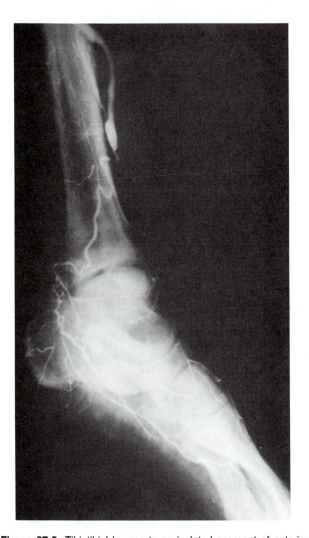

Figure 37-3. Tibiotibial bypass to an isolated segment of anterior tibial artery. This arteriogram was obtained 6 months after operation. (*From Veith FJ, Ascer E, et al.: J Vasc Surg 2:552, 1985.*)

Isolated Popliteal Artery Segment

Many patients who are candidates for a small-artery bypass by virtue of their having a patent tibial or peroneal artery with a continuous lumen extending into the foot will also have an isolated or almost isolated patent popliteal artery segment with flow only into the proximal portion of one tibial artery. The question of what operation to perform is clearly one of *judgment* and depends on many factors, including the quality and anatomy of the superficial veins as demonstrated by venography and duplex ultrasonography, the size and quality of the patent distal small artery, the extent of gangrene or infection in the foot, and, most

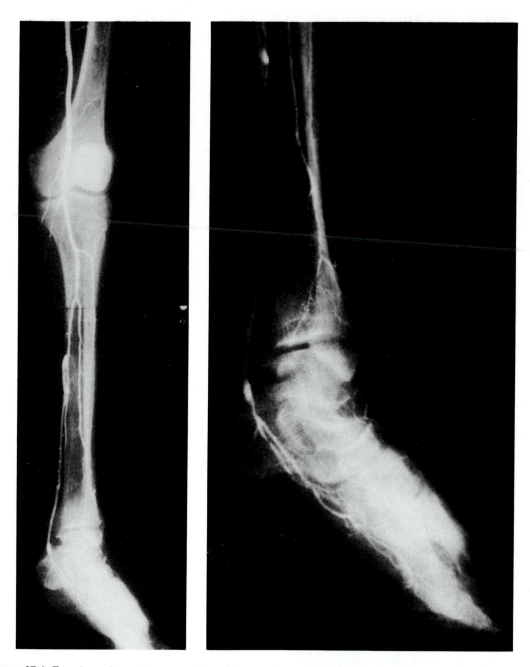

Figure 37-4. Two views of an arteriogram performed 3 years after a posterior tibial-to-posterior tibial bypass. The bypass is inserted into an isolated segment of posterior tibial artery (i.e., the plantar arch is incomplete) and remains patent 6 years after operation. (*From Veith FJ, Ascer, E, et al.: J Vasc Surg 2:552, 1985.*)

importantly, the length and quality of the patent popliteal segment and the collateral arteries that arise from it.[1,9,10] If the popliteal segment is fairly disease free and long (>7 cm) and has good collaterals and if the foot has little if any necrosis, we would advocate performing a femoropopliteal bypass. If on the other hand, the patent popliteal segment was short but still greater than 7 cm in length and had poor collaterals *and* the foot gangrene was extensive, a *sequential* femoro-to-popliteal-to-small-vessel bypass should be performed primarily. If the patent popliteal segment is less than 7 cm in length, a primary small-artery

bypass should be performed, although there may be exceptions. Occasionally after performing a femoropopliteal bypass to an isolated popliteal artery segment, a secondary distal bypass will be required to obtain healing of foot lesions.[1,9]

Judgment in these complex cases depends on these and a number of other variables, as well as on the surgeon's and angiographer's training and experience. It is precisely because of the complexity of this judgment and of the required technical skills to perform the operation that this form of limb-salvage vascular surgery requires special train-

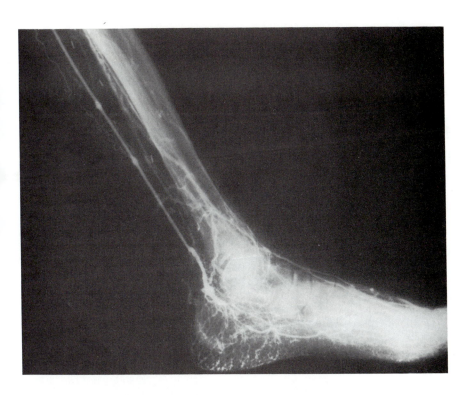

Figure 37-5. Arteriogram after a bypass from the tibioperoneal trunk to the posterior tibial artery at its bifurcation in the foot. Note small size of the vein graft. Despite this size, the graft is patent 3 years after operation. (*From Veith FJ, Ascer E, et al.: J Vasc Surg 2:552, 1985.*)

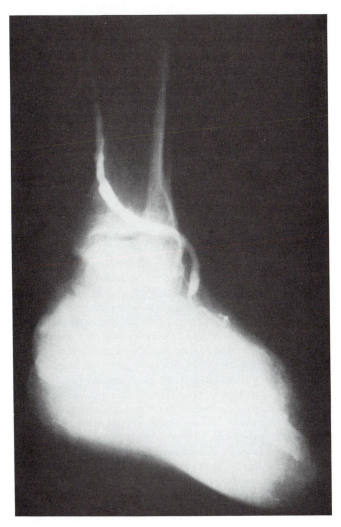

Figure 37-6. Postoperative arteriogram after a short-vein bypass on an isolated segment of dorsalis pedis or lateral tarsal artery that ends in a total occlusion. There is no plantar arch. Despite this lack, the graft is patent 2½ years after operation. (*From Veith FJ, Ascer E, et al.: J Vasc Surg 2:552, 1985.*)

ing, experience, and commitment. It is not a field that is well managed by the occasional or casual vascular surgeon.

INDICATIONS AND CONTRAINDICATIONS

Since bypasses to either of the tibial arteries or the peroneal artery are generally complex, difficult operations with a real incidence of early and late failure and some degree of operative morbidity and mortality, it is my opinion that these operations should rarely, if ever, be performed for *intermittent claudication*. Most patients with this symptom will readily accept the limitations it imposes on their activity if they are told that an operation for claudication does not necessarily lower the risks of subsequent limb loss and that eventual failure of the operation may actually be associated with an increased risk to their limb.

These facts mean that virtually all bypasses to arteries distal to the popliteal should be performed to save a limb that will otherwise be lost because of ischemia. Such critical ischemia is not always easy to determine,[2] since patients with advanced ischemia and limited ischemic rest pain, small patches of gangrene, or ischemic ulceration may occasionally be improved through the use of analgesics and conservative measures, and this improvement may persist for protracted periods despite poor noninvasive indexes.[11] These cases are rare, however; generally, these manifestations, if severe or extensive, will cause limb loss if the circulation is not improved by some form of arterial reconstruction or angioplasty. In cases in which the lesions are limited and the outcome uncertain, a trial period of hospitalization with conservative treatment may be warranted before undertaking a difficult distal bypass.[11] Again, many factors influence this decision, and the experience and judgment of the surgeon are of paramount importance in deciding on the proper course of action. The need for such fine judgment is obviously not required to determine that operation is required for limb salvage when the patient has severe rest pain that interferes with nutrition and sleep or extensive enlarging gangrene or ulceration. It is more important, in the presence of such conditions and any significant distal ischemia as indicated by noninvasive tests, to avoid the performance of local ablative procedures on the toes or foot *without* first performing an appropriate arterial reconstruction, preferably one establishing direct pulsatile arterial flow to the foot. Only in this way will the circulation be adequate to control the necrosis and associated infection and to allow the foot to heal.

Extensive gangrene in the foot, particularly gangrene of the heel, has long been regarded as a contraindication to performing a limb salvage arterial bypass. Increasingly over the years, we have challenged this premise and have been able to show that functional remnants of foot can be obtained even when extensive necrosis and gangrene involve the bones and soft tissues of the forefoot or heel.[1] A healed foot remnant, which can sometimes only be obtained with a split-thickness skin graft, will allow some of these aged, debilitated patients to ambulate far better than a below-knee amputation, even if the forefoot amputation is through the proximal tarsal bones or if the heel amputa-

tion involves the tuberosity of the os calcis and the Achilles tendon.[1]

Similarly, major amputation in preference to limb-salvage arterial reconstruction has been widely advocated for patients who are nonambulatory because of a previous contralateral amputation. However, we have found that these patients need their remaining lower extremity to transfer from bed to wheelchair to toilet and to be cared for by their family at home.[1]

What then are contraindications to limb-salvage distal bypasses? Only such severe organic mental syndrome that the patient is completely out of contact with his environment or gangrene and infection of the midportion of the foot are absolute contraindications to attempts at limb salvage and indications for a primary major amputation. In some other cases, the patient's cardiac status may be so precarious that operative risk for a bypass may be considered excessive. In such instances our practice has been to discuss these risks with the patient and the immediate family and then to let them participate in the amputation vs. limb-salvage decision. Invariably patients will opt for the limb-salvage attempt, even when the risks of failure or death are relatively large, and many of our advances in this field have been prompted by the wishes of courageous patients.

SURGICAL TECHNIQUES

Distal bypasses to small infrapopliteal arteries are usually complex, technically demanding operations. They are time-consuming and require the surgeon to be committed to performing a variety of technical details with patience and expertise. Any flaw in any of these details can jeopardize the success of the procedure. The details that are described below represent one method for performing the operations. Undoubtedly there are other methods for accomplishing the same result. However, the methods presented do work, and the surgeon must remember that, regardless of which methods are used, there is no substitute for care, experience, and commitment to perfection.

Incisions and Approaches

In virtually every instance, there are standard surgical approaches to all infrainguinal arteries, and there are unusual approaches, which can be used when the standard approaches are impossible because of previous operative scarring or infection. Although the deep femoral and popliteal arteries may be used as sites of origin for bypasses to small arteries, in the presence of extensive groin scarring or infection, the second and third portions of the *deep femoral artery* can be approached directly through the medial or anterior thigh to provide an inflow site for a short vein graft to a distal small vessel.[12,13] In similar circumstances when the standard medial approaches to the *popliteal artery* are unusable, we have described lateral approaches to this artery both above and below the knee.[14] In the usual circumstances the surgical approaches to the femoral and popliteal arteries for the performance of distal bypasses are accomplished by the techniques described in Chapters 21 and 36. When the ipsilateral greater saphenous vein in the region of these arteries is to be used for the bypass, the incision is made over the vein (Fig. 37-7A), and the arteries are then reached by raising a subfascial flap.[15]

Tibioperoneal Trunk and Proximal Two Thirds of Posterior Tibial and Peroneal Arteries

These vessels are usually approached through a medial incision below the knee (see Fig. 37-7a). The deep fascia is incised, and the popliteal fossa is entered. The arc of the soleus muscle must be defined and the soleus fibers cut to expose the distal popliteal artery, the tibioperoneal trunk, and the origin of the anterior tibial, the posterior tibial, and the peroneal arteries (Fig. 37-7b to d). Often the arteries are overlaid by the accompanying veins, and division of these veins or their branches is necessary to expose the arterial segment to be used for anastomosis. In Figure 37-7d the anterior tibial vein has been divided to provide arterial exposure.

Direct exposure of the more distal segments of the posterior tibial or peroneal artery is obtained through a medial approach without first exposing the more proximal arteries. The soleus muscle is simply freed by incising its tibial attachments, and the vascular bundles are identified. The peroneal bundle approximates the medial border of the fibula. Once the bundle is found, careful dissection is required to separate the artery from the adjacent veins. No arterial branches, no matter how small, should be ligated or injured.

Anterior Tibial Artery

Except for its proximal centimeter, which can be approached posteromedially, this artery is best approached anterolaterally (Fig. 37-8). The incision is deepened into the muscle layers midway between the two bones. Accompanying veins can be used to trace a path to the artery, and the appropriate segment of artery is isolated by careful dissection, which often requires ligation and division of vein branches (Fig. 37-8c).

Distal Peroneal, Anterior Tibial, Posterior Tibial, and Dorsalis Pedis Arteries

These arteries are best approached through the incisions shown in Figure 37-9. The distal third of the peroneal artery is best accessed by removing a segment of overlying fibula as illustrated in Figure 37-9c. When approaching the distal anterior tibial or dorsalis pedis arteries, a gently curved incision is made, and a short skin and subcutaneous flap with a medial base is raised so that the artery and the anastomosis will be under the base of the flap rather than under the incision in case incisional healing is imperfect (Fig. 37-9f and 37-9g).

Unusual Approaches

In case of medial scarring or infection or both, all three leg arteries can be reached through a lateral approach with fibula resection.[13-16]; the proximal anterior tibial artery can be reached from posteromedially with division of the interosseous membrane[17]; the distal branches of the posterior tibial artery (i.e., the medial and lateral plantar arteries) can be reached in the sole of the foot (Figs. 37-5 and 37-10)[13]; and the terminal branches of the dorsalis pedis artery (lateral tarsal artery and deep plantar arch) can be reached through an appropriate dorsal incision, sometimes with resection of one or more metatarsal bones (see Figs. 37-2 and 37-6).[13] All these vessels have been used successfully as bypass outflow sites (see Figs. 37-2, 37-5, 37-6, and 37-10). Moreover, the distal third of the peroneal artery can be approached and used for anastomosis by making a medial incision and dividing some of the long flexor muscles to aid in exposure. This approach is useful when an in situ vein graft is used.

Graft Tunneling

Bypass grafts are generally brought from inflow sites to outflow sites by subfascial tunnels if possible, minimizing graft exposure if wound breakdown occurs. The tunnels are constructed using a combination of finger and instrument dissection (Figs. 37-7e, 37-8d, and 37-9d). Particular care is required in transversing the interosseous membrane because of the abundance of vessels in the area. This membrane is best divided under direct vision from the front (see Fig. 37-8c). If subfascial planes are not available, subcutaneous tunnels may be used, and they are obligatory for bypasses to the distal anterior tibial and dorsal pedis arteries (Figs. 37-9d and 37-9e).

Vascular Grafts

Clearly, autologous lower-extremity vein represents the best graft with which to perform bypasses to small leg and foot arteries. However, even autologous vein is far from an ideal graft for many reasons. Veins that appear large and healthy when first used may harbor unsuspected defects. Moreover, in some patients even good veins, when used as a bypass, may for unexplained reasons develop focal or diffuse hyperplastic lesions that lead to their ultimate failure.[18] We have observed the inexorable development of such lesions in both reversed and in situ grafts, even when the original operation was smooth and apparently flawless. If the stenosis is focal, detection and correction by percutaneous transluminal dilatation or operative patch angioplasty before graft thrombosis occurs can produce sustained good results.[19,20] If the process is diffuse, detection in the failing state, that is, detection of a lesion before thrombosis occurs, is of little value, and graft occlusion is inevitable. Why some grafts in some patients behave this way remains an unanswered question and an important area for future investigation.

When a patient's ipsilateral greater saphenous vein is absent or too small (i.e., less than 3.5 mm in minimal distended external diameter for femoropopliteal bypasses or less than 3 mm for small-vessel bypasses),[21] the greater saphenous vein from the opposite extremity or the short saphenous vein may be used as the graft. We have found preoperative venography and, more recently, duplex ultrasonography helpful in identifying usable vein segments and predicting their location and size.[22,23] Unless their veins

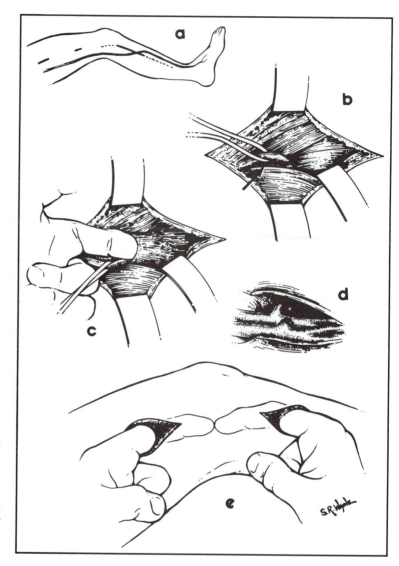

Figure 37-7. Technical steps for the medial approach to lower-extremity vessels, the harvest and preparation of the greater saphenous vein, arterial occlusion and incision, and anastomotic suturing. See text for details. (*From Veith FJ and Gupta SK: Femoral-distal artery bypasses, in Bergan JJ, Yao JST (eds): Operative Techniques in Vascular Surgery. New York, Grune & Stratton, 1980.*)

have been traumatized by previous surgery, most patients will have an adequate vein somewhere in their lower extremities, and this number can be increased by using the distal origin or short-vein graft concept wherever possible.[6-8]

When no usable lower-extremity vein exists, upper-extremity veins (i.e., cephalic and basilic) can sometimes be helpful. However, these veins are generally thin walled, have many fine branches, and, in our experience, often have scarred, recanalized segments from previous venipunctures or intravenous infusions. Two undiseased segments may have to be anastomosed with an oblique union to provide a satisfactory graft.

Prosthetic small artery bypasses have been condemned by some vascular surgeons who have advocated a primary amputation as the treatment of choice when a patient, despite all efforts, truly does not have an autogenous vein graft and requires a bypass to a distal artery.[24] We disagree with this recommendation and will perform a prosthetic bypass with a polytetrafluoroethylene (PTFE) graft in this setting. Even though patency rates of these grafts are far

worse than those for vein grafts, some long-term patency can be obtained, and, more importantly, reasonable late limb-salvage rates can be achieved (see Results p. 512). Although glutaraldehyde-fixed umbilical vein grafts have been advocated as a vein alternative in this setting,[25] the high incidence of aneurysm formation in this graft would seem to preclude its widespread use.[26,27]

Technique for Reversed Vein Graft Preparation

Although the relative merits of in situ and reversed vein grafts are discussed in Chapter 38, it is clear that some patients will have no vein suitable for an in situ graft. These patients usually will have an ectopic segment of usable vein so that all vascular surgeons should be proficient at techniques for harvesting and preparing a standard reversed vein graft. As with all aspects of distal bypass technique, patience and meticulous attention to detail are critical.

As already mentioned, all incisions for approaching the involved arteries should be planned with vein harvest

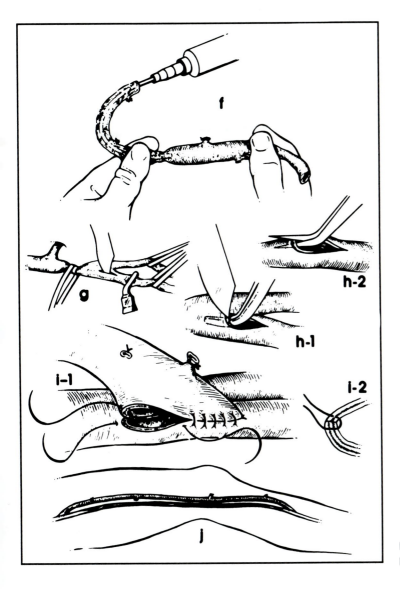

Fig. 37-7 cont'd. For legend see opposite page.

in mind. If the same incision is to be used for both procedures, it should be placed directly over the vein, and a subfascial flap should be raised to access the artery (see Fig. 37-7a). In this way subcutaneous flaps can be avoided, and vein harvest complications minimized. We favor a long incision so that the entire vein can be visualized and trauma to the vein and its branches prevented. In our experience, leaving skin bridges does not eliminate vein-harvest wound complications, although it does make vein harvest more difficult. After the vein is entirely exposed, it is carefully dissected free, and its branches are doubly ligated and divided so as not to cause any constriction by catching excess adventitia from the main vein. When the arterial dissections are completed and the vein graft is removed, all vein-harvest incisions are temporarily closed with skin staples to prevent desiccation of the subcutaneous fat. After completion of arterial anastomoses and reversal of heparin, these incisions are reopened, perfect hemostasis is obtained, and they are meticulously reapproximated in two layers.

As soon as the vein is removed from its bed, it is immersed in 4° C Hanks' solution, a balanced salt solution used in tissue culture. The vein is flushed with the same solution, using a long plastic cannula with a smooth end. This cannula is introduced progressively throughout the length of the vein, which is compartmentalized into 4 to 5 cm segments by gentle finger pressure (Fig. 37-7f). These segments, with the end of the cannula lying within them, are gently distended with Hanks' solution. Any residual unligated branches or vein wall defects can be localized and carefully repaired over the stenting cannula with fine ligatures or 6–0 sutures. In this way, these sutures can obliterate the leaks without narrowing even small veins. The cannula is then advanced until the entire vein has been gently dilated and rendered leak free. Although there may be theoretic reasons to avoid passage of the cannula through the entire lumen of the vein, we believe they are more than compensated for by the frequent nonocclusive intraluminal defects that occur and that can only be detected and eliminated in this way. These defects probably represent segments of recanalized thrombophlebitis. If undetected, they will cause graft failure because the narrowed lumen in such areas is crisscrossed with fibrous strands.

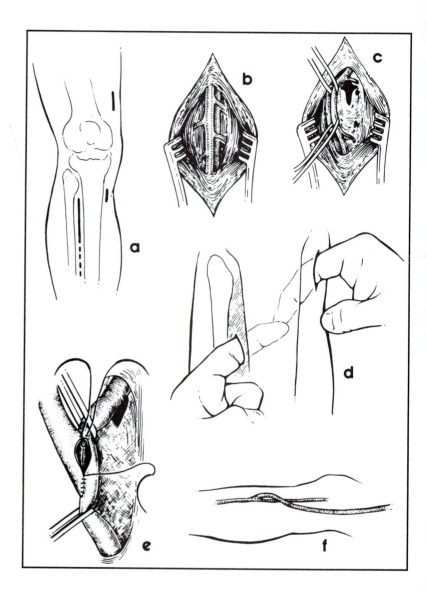

Figure 37-8. Approach to the upper and middle thirds of the anterior tibial artery for performance of a distal bypass. Note details of cruciate incision in interosseous membrane and tunneling of the graft. See text for details. (*From Veith FJ and Gupta SK: Femoral-distal artery bypasses, in Bergan JJ, Yao JST (eds): Operative Techniques in Vascular Surgery. New York, Grune & Stratton, 1980.*)

These segments are detectable because palpation of the vein wall over the cannula reveals thickening or because the cannula's passage is impeded by the fibrous strands. Once the vein is prepared, it is kept immersed in chilled Hanks' solution until and, insofar as possible, during its implantation.

Technique for Occluding, Incising, and Suturing Small Arteries

Although there are many techniques for accomplishing these objectives, the keynote for all is extreme care and delicacy. If techniques and instruments that are used on larger vessels are used on small arteries, injury may occur with untoward results, particularly when disease is present in the segment of vessel being occluded or sutured—a common occurrence in this group of patients.

Arterial Occlusion

Heparin (7,500 IU) is administered intravenously before any arterial occlusion. Heparin (2,500 IU) is then administered after every hour that an artery is occluded. To *occlude*

these small arteries and render the lumen bloodless, simple gentle traction with single- or double-looped silastic vessel loops will often suffice (Fig. 37-7g). Minimal tension that prevents flow into the segment is all that should be used. This technique is particularly useful for soft, normal arteries. A second technique is to use microvascular spring-loaded clips (see Fig. 37-7g), which are also atraumatic. Occasionally these clips may also have to be placed on branches to obtain a dry field. If the vessel is thick-walled, micro-atraumatic clamps similar to those used on larger arteries, but smaller and gentler, are available. Care must be exercised to avoid twisting. If all these techniques fail, an intraluminal balloon catheter (No. 2) may have to be used. However, passage of this or any other catheter into the lumen of these vessels carries considerable risk and should generally be avoided, particularly if the vessel is at all diseased.

Arterial Incision

To gain entrance to the lumen of small arteries I use a new No. 15 scalpel blade (see Fig. 37-7g). Smaller (Beaver) blades are also available. If the artery is normal, a microscissors (Fig. 37-7h-2) may be used. Generally, however, the artery is thick walled or diseased, and use of any scissors

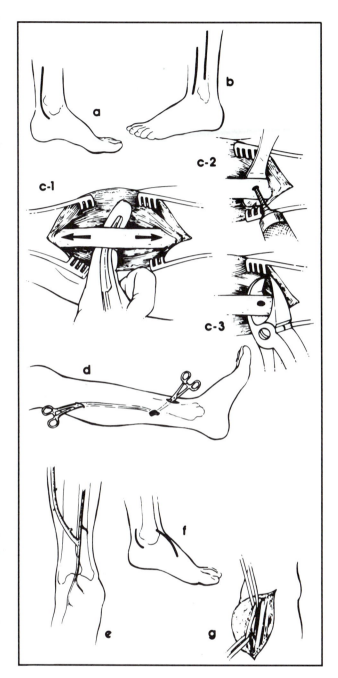

Figure 37-9. Technical details in operations on the distal third of the three leg arteries. See text for details. (*From Veith FJ and Gupta SK: Femoral-distal artery bypasses, in Bergan JJ, Yao JST (eds): Operative Techniques in Vascular Surgery. New York, Grune & Stratton, 1980.*)

the apex (toe) of the anastomosis and the heel. The apex suture is tied and carefully run along both sides of the anastomosis, catching equal small bites of graft and artery (Fig. 37-7i-1 and 37-7i-2). The heel suture is then tied and run similarly to both midpoints of the anastomosis where it is tied. Frequent saline irrigations and optical (loop) magnification may be helpful in *precise* suture placement. One poor stitch at either end of the anastomosis can lead to failure.

After the distal anastomosis is completed, the occlusion is released, and the graft and distal artery are flushed with heparinized saline. The graft is carefully passed through the previously made tunnels to avoid any twists. The proximal graft-to-artery anastomosis is then carried out with the same care, although larger clamps and slightly wider spaced suture bites may be used with the larger vessels.

Calcified Arteries

Even when calcification is extreme, as in some diabetics, arterial occlusion, incision, and suturing can be performed successfully.[1,3] Our technique for dealing with these difficult arteries involves gentle crushing of the calcific deposits with a clamp. The resulting fractured fragments lie within an intact intimal envelope and rarely injure its continuity. If intimal tears occur, they can be repaired with U stitches carefully placed from within the lumen.[3]

After completion of all anastomoses, residual heparin is neutralized with protamine, and careful hemostasis is obtained. Intraoperative angiography to visualize the distal anastomosis and outflow tract may be performed but may be misleading, with both false positive and false negative results. The wounds are closed carefully in layers using meticulous technique.

Foot Debridements and Minor Amputations

If the ischemic foot contains necrotic tissue or undrained infection, the necrotic, infected material should be excised at the conclusion of the small-vessel bypass procedure, and the resulting wound left open. If limited gangrene of the heel or forefoot is present and there is no evidence of infection, the gangrene may be left alone, and it will slowly heal with the improved blood supply. Necrotic toes may have to be excised to achieve a healed foot. If infection is controlled, truly remarkable healing can occur after arterial reconstruction. On the other hand, infection may sometimes preclude healing even with uninterrupted arterial flow to the foot and despite all efforts at local drainage and debridement.[1,9]

The extent of infection and necrosis in the foot can often preclude salvage of all but a small remnant of the midfoot or hindfoot. Despite many opinions to the contrary, we have found such small foot remnants to be remarkably effective in maintaining bipedal ambulation and keeping patients out of nursing homes. Accordingly, we regard these "funny-looking feet,"[28] or foot remnants, worthy of salvage, and almost uniformly the patients agree. Similarly, in many patients, a split-thickness skin graft may be required to obtain a healed foot wound. Even when placed on a weight-bearing surface, these grafts can function extremely well in helping to maintain a patient's effective ambulation.

will produce a jagged arteriotomy with overhanging or undercut intimal layers. We therefore carefully insert a microhemostat into the initial arteriotomy and complete the incision with a knife, cutting between the gently opened blades of the microhemostat (Fig. 37-7h-1). In this way a clean, even incision of all layers is obtained (Fig. 37-7i-1).

Suturing of the graft to the artery is performed under adequate (head-light) illumination, exercising extreme care to see every bite of graft and arterial wall, both from within and without. Double-armed running sutures are placed at

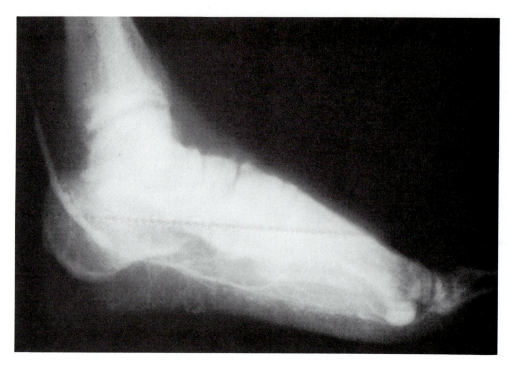

Figure 37-10. Postoperative arteriogram performed 1 year after a bypass to the lateral plantar branch of the posterior tibial artery.

RESULTS

Mortality

With improved anesthetic management and perioperative cardiac monitoring and intensive care, *operative (1 month) mortality* for these small-vessel bypasses has been low, in the 3 to 5% range, despite the facts that advanced coronary atherosclerosis and other diseases are present in most of the patients and that almost no patient was denied operation because of his medical risk status.[1] Most of this mortality is due to perioperative cardiac events, chiefly myocardial infarction, and this event can occur even in patients presumed to be relatively good risks.

In contrast to this low operative mortality, the *late* mortality from intercurrent coronary atherosclerosis in patients undergoing small-vessel bypass for limb salvage is very high. In 5 years, more than 50% of these patients will be dead from causes other than their infrainguinal arteriosclerosis or its treatment.[1] This percentage underscores the facts that patients requiring operations are at the end stage of their life and that the goal of surgical therapy should be palliation.[1]

Morbidity

The morbidity of these operations stems chiefly from the protracted hospital stays that are often required to achieve a healed foot, particularly when gangrene and infection in the foot are extensive. In 7% of our limb-salvage patients, four to seven local operations and 2 to 4 months of hospitalization were required to achieve foot healing.[1] Other factors contribute to this morbidity. Although wound infections involving the bypass are uncommon, occurring in less than 0.5% of our patients undergoing a primary distal bypass, wound problems involving the vein harvest site are common and increase the need for hospital care. These usually respond to conservative measures, although operative debridement and even skin grafting may occasionally be required.

Bypass Patency

Figures for primary patency[*] of bypasses to infrapopliteal arteries vary widely, depending on the graft used, the length of the vein graft,[7,8] the criteria of operability, the operative techniques used, the outflow resistance,[29] the number of patients observed after 2 years, the care during follow-up, and the methods used to determine patency. Although better results have been reported, a primary patency rate of approximately 50% in those patients surviving 5 years would be a reasonable expectation for small-vessel bypasses. Many of the bypasses considered "failures" can be rescued if the threatening lesion can be detected before thrombosis occurs (i.e., in the *failing state*), and be repaired.[19,20,30] Furthermore, 15 to 30% of limb-salvage distal bypasses that thrombose do so without leading to a renewed threat to the limb, probably because the original

---

[*]Primary patency is defined as the duration of bypass patency until the time of graft thrombosis or until the need for a secondary intervention to fix a problem with the arterial reconstruction.

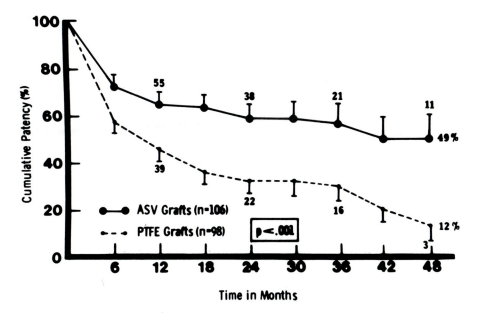

Figure 37-11. Cumulative life-table primary patency rate for all randomized bypasses to infrapopliteal arteries with autologous saphenous vein (ASV) and polytetrafluoroethylene (PTFE) grafts. Number with each point indicates number of grafts observed to be patent for that length of time. Standard error of each point is shown. (*From Veith FJ, Gupto SK, et al.: J Vasc Surg 1:104, 1986.*)

lesion has been healed by virtue of the bypass and remains healed even after it fails.[1]

Patency and Graft Material

Small-artery bypass primary patency has recently been reported from a large randomized prospective comparison of autogenous vein and PTFE grafts.[31] Primary patency at 4 years with vein grafts was 49% ± 10%, whereas with PTFE grafts it was 12% ± 7% (Fig. 37-11). The clear superiority of vein grafts for these operations is thereby established.

Limb Salvage and Palliation

Limb salvage is the parameter that is important to the patient. Limb-salvage rates consistently exceed primary bypass patency rates by 10 to 40% for a variety of reasons, even when the original bypass was performed for critical ischemia. Sustained healing after bypass failure has already been mentioned. The effectiveness of secondary interventions is probably of equal importance. Four-year limb salvage rates for distal bypasses in the cooperative study were 57% ± 10% for vein grafts and 61% ± 10% for PTFE grafts (Fig. 37-12).[31]

Although these figures reflect the fate of the limb in patients who had surgery and survived 4 to 5 years, they do not tell the limb-salvage story in the larger fraction of patients who succumb within that period. The latter parameter is of importance in determining the value or merit of the operations from the patients' perspective. Several years ago we showed that 81 to 95% of patients undergoing these operations and dying within 5 years kept their limb and used it effectively for walking until the time of their death.[1] On the basis of all these data, we concluded that limb-salvage small-vessel bypasses are generally worthwhile and

provide better palliation than the alternative of a major above-knee or below-knee amputation. This is particularly true in light of the fact that more than 25% of our patients are so aged or infirm that they cannot learn to walk with a below-knee prosthesis.[32]

POSTOPERATIVE FOLLOW-UP AND REINTERVENTION

Performance of a successful infrainguinal bypass of any sort does not preclude continuing progression of the atherosclerotic disease process. Moreover, in some patients, although fortunately not in all, the operation initiates the process of *neointimal hyperplasia*. This lesion can involve bypass inflow or outflow tracts if a prosthetic graft is used. If a vein graft is used, it can develop lumen-reducing hyperplastic lesions, which can be focal or diffuse. Any of these processes, as well as *technical imperfections* in the arterial reconstruction, can reduce its flow. This in turn can reduce the hemodynamic therapeutic effectiveness of the procedure and can lead to graft thrombosis. In light of all these processes, plus the advanced stage of the atherosclerosis in patients requiring limb-salvage bypasses to small infrapopliteal arteries, it is not surprising that many of these operations will, with time, fail (thrombose) or develop lesions that reduce their hemodynamic effectiveness.

Failing Graft Concept

We and others have shown that, with frequent careful follow-up examinations by the surgeon and through noninvasive laboratory procedures, it is possible to detect hemodynamically significant lesions that threaten the

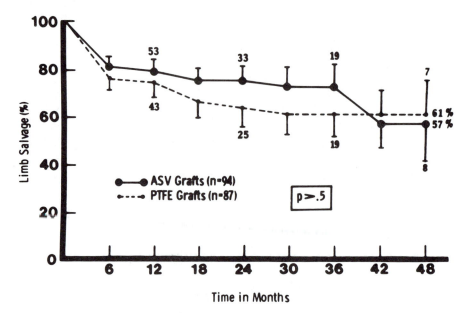

Figure 37-12. Cumulative life-table limb salvage rates for patients with randomized autologous saphenous vein (ASV) and polytetrafluoroethylene (PTFE) grafts to infrapopliteal arteries. All operations represented here were performed to control critical ischemia. Number with each point indicates number of operated limbs observed to be intact for that length of time. Standard error of each point is shown. (*From Veith FJ, Gupto SK, et al.: J Vasc Surg 1:104, 1986.*)

patency of arterial reconstructions before they cause thrombosis.[1,19,30,33-35] These lesions can be in or proximal or distal to the bypass graft. We have shown that these lesions, if left untreated, will invariably result in graft thrombosis.[19] Moreover, we have observed the failing state in arterial reconstructions performed with all types of vein grafts, as well as PTFE grafts, and we and others have been able to show that correction of the responsible lesions before they produce graft thrombosis is both simpler and more effective.[19,20,30] Moreover, healthy segments of vein graft are not damaged by thrombosis and may continue to be useful.

Because of these facts, it is extremely important to observe patients undergoing small-artery bypasses at frequent intervals. The surgeon should perform a careful pulse examination every 6 weeks for the first 6 months after operation. Thereafter the interval between examinations can be increased to 2 to 3 months. Ideally, noninvasive arterial tests should be performed with the same frequency. However, their cost may be prohibitive, and we have usually relied on the surgeon's examination alone for most follow-up. With this modality alone, we have now been able to detect more than 150 failing grafts.

When there is any change in a patient's pulse examination in the involved extremity or if there is any return of symptoms, confirmatory noninvasive studies and arteriography are almost always performed on an urgent basis. If short stenotic lesions are found and they can be treated by percutaneous balloon angioplasty, it is our preferred treatment. If the lesion is an occlusion or is not suitable for angioplasty, a small operation is performed. Usually it takes the form of a vein-patch angioplasty, a short proximal or distal graft extension, or a short-vein bypass of a lesion in the original vein graft.

Failed or Thrombosed Distal Bypasses

Early failure (within 30 days) of a distal bypass is usually associated with some technical imperfection, although rarely it may be due to poor selection of a distal outflow site and extremely high outflow resistance.[36] Invariably if the original operation was for limb salvage, the limb with the failed graft will be threatened again, and urgent reoperation is indicated. The reconstruction is explored by opening the graft by a linear incision in its hood so that the thrombus can be removed with balloon catheters, the interior of the recipient artery can be carefully cleared of clot, and the anastomosis can be clearly visualized.[37,38] Any defect is corrected. The proximal wound is reopened only if necessary. After closure of all arterial and graft openings with fine monofilament sutures, using techniques similar to those already described, intraoperative arteriography of the graft and outflow site is obtained. Any visualized defect is corrected. Distal graft pressure may be measured to rule out inflow gradients. Heparin is reversed. Hemostasis is obtained, and the wounds are closed. Perioperative antiplatelet agents, low-molecular weight dextran, or dicumarol derivatives may be used, although there is no conclusive evidence of their value and all these agents have potential risks and disadvantages.

Late graft failure can occur at any time after 30 days. Failures occurring up to 18 months after operation are generally due to neointimal hyperplasia involving the graft or one anastomosis, usually the distal one. After that time, they are usually due to progression of atherosclerosis. Failures can occur in PTFE grafts to small arteries for no obvious reason, presumably because of this material's greater thrombogenicity. If graft thrombosis occurs several months or years after a small-artery bypass, the patient's foot may have healed and may remain so despite the decreased arterial flow. For that patient, repeat surgery is *not* indicated unless rest pain is truly intolerable even with analgesic medication. If, however, the limb is threatened again, full preoperative arteriography is performed in an attempt to determine the cause of graft failure (e.g., an inflow lesion) but more importantly to determine what patent arterial segments exist for use in the performance of a new bypass. Almost always such segments are present at some level, and we have extensively used the distal deep femoral artery, the popliteal artery, and the same or other infrapopliteal arteries for such *secondary short vein bypasses*. The unusual approaches to these vessels discussed previously are particularly helpful in this regard. Usually, suitable short segments of vein can also be found, but if not, PTFE grafts are a better option than a major amputation.

CONCLUSIONS

Bypasses to small infrapopliteal arteries in the leg or foot can, if performed properly, be useful operations that usually result in limb salvage and help to palliate patients threatened with loss of a lower limb. These operations must be based on accurate preoperative arteriography and should be conducted in centers with individuals who are committed not only to the operative details of the bypass operation but also to the preoperative, intraoperative, and postoperative intensive care required. Moreover, because of the nature of the disease process, ultimate failure of a sizable fraction of these operations is to be expected. Accordingly, diligent follow-up is essential to detect and correct significant lesions in the "failing state," that is, before graft thrombosis occurs. Also important is the commitment to perform difficult repeat operations when failure with graft thrombosis occurs. With these provisos, gratifying results can be obtained in most patients requiring these operations.

REFERENCES

1. Veith FJ, Gupta SK, et al.: Progress in limb salvage by reconstructive arterial surgery combined with new or improved adjunctive procedures. Ann Surg 194:386, 1981.
2. Working Party of the International Vascular Symposium: The definition of critical ischaemia of a limb. Br J Surg 69(suppl):S2, 1982.
3. Ascer E, Veith FJ, White-Flores S: Infrapopliteal bypasses to heavily calcified rock-like arteries. Management and results. Am J Surg 152:220, 1986.
4. Hall KV: The great saphenous vein used in situ as an arterial shunt after extirpation of the vein valves. A preliminary report. Surgery 51:492, 1962.
5. Leather RP, Shah DM, et al.: Infrapopliteal bypass for limb salvage: Increased patency and utilization of the saphenous vein used "in situ." Surgery 90:1000, 1981.
6. Veith FJ, Gupta SK, et al.: Superficial femoral and popliteal arteries as inflow site for distal bypasses. Surgery 90:980, 1981.
7. Veith FJ, Ascer E, et al.: Tibiotibial vein bypass grafts: A new operation for limb salvage. J Vasc Surg 2:552, 1985.
8. Ascer E, Veith FJ, et al.: Short vein grafts: A superior option for arterial reconstructions to poor or compromised outflow tracts. J Vasc Surg 7:370, 1988.
9. Veith FJ, Gupta SK, Daly V: Femoropopliteal bypass to the

10. Davis RC, Davies WT, Mannick JA: Bypass vein grafts in patients with distal popliteal artery occlusion. Am J Surg 129:421, 1975.
11. Rivers SP, Veith FJ, et al.: Successful conservative therapy of severe limb threatening ischemia: The value of nonsympathectomy. Surgery 99:759, 1986.
12. Nunez A, Veith FJ, et al.: Direct approach to the distal two portions of the deep femoral artery for origin or insertion of secondary bypasses. J Vasc Surg. In press.
13. Veith FJ, Ascer E, et al.: Unusual approaches to infrainguinal arteries. J Cardiovasc Surg 28:58, 1987.
14. Veith FJ, Ascer E, et al.: Lateral approach to the popliteal artery. J Vasc Surg 6:119, 1987.
15. Veith FJ, Gupta SK: Femoral-distal artery bypasses, in Bergan JJ, Yao JST (eds): Operative Techniques in Vascular Surgery. New York, Grune & Stratton, Inc., 1980, p 141.
16. Dardik H, Dardik I, Veith FJ: Exposure of the tibial-peroneal arteries by a single lateral approach. Surgery 75:337, 1974.
17. Ascer E, Veith FJ, Gupta SK: Manuscript in preparation, 1989.
18. Szilagyi DE, Smith RF, et al.: The biologic fate of autogenous vein implants as arterial substitutes: Clinical, angiographic and histopathologic observations in femoropopliteal operations for atherosclerosis. Ann Surg 178:232, 1973.
19. Veith FJ, Weiser RK, et al.: Diagnosis and management of failing lower extremity arterial reconstructions. J Cardiovasc Surg 25:381, 1984.
20. Ascer E, Collier P, et al.: Reoperation for PTFE bypass failure: The importance of distal outflow site and operative technique in determining outcome. J Vasc Surg 5:298, 1987.
21. Wengerter K, Gupta SK, Veith FJ: Minimal acceptable distended diameter for infrapopliteal reversed vein grafts. Manuscript in preparation, 1989.
22. Veith F, Moss CM, et al.: Preoperative saphenous venography in arterial reconstructive surgery of the lower extremity. Surgery 85:253, 1979.
23. Franco C, Montefusco C, Veith FJ: Comparison of duplex ultrasonography and contrast venography in preoperative evaluation of superficial veins for use as reversed vein grafts. Manuscript in preparation, 1989.
24. Hobson II RW, Lynch TG, et al.: Results of revascularization and amputation in severe lower extremity ischemia. A 5-year clinical experience. J Vasc Surg 2:174, 1985.
25. Dardik H, Baier RE, et al.: Morphologic biophysical assessment of long term human umbilical cord vein implants used as vascular conduits. Surg Gynecol Obstet 154:17, 1982.
26. Karkow WS, Cranley JJ, et al.: Extended study of aneurysm formation in umbilical grafts. J Vasc Surg 4:486, 1986.
27. Hasson JE, Newton WD, et al.: Mural degeneration in the glutaraldehyde tanned umbilical vein graft: Incidence and implications. J Vasc Surg 4:243, 1986.
28. Ochsner, JL: Personal communication.
29. Ascer E, Veith FJ, et al.: Intraoperative outflow resistance as a predictor of late patency of femoropopliteal and infrapopliteal arterial bypasses. J Vasc Surg 5:820, 1987.
30. Whittemore AD, Clowes AW, et al.: Secondary femoropopliteal reconstruction. Ann Surg 193:35, 1981.
31. Veith FJ, Gupta SK, et al.: Six-year prospective multicenter randomized comparison of autologous saphenous vein and expanded polytetrafluoroethylene grafts in infrainguinal arterial reconstructions. J Vasc Surg 1:104, 1986.
32. Gupta SK, Veith FJ, et al.: Cost analysis of operations for infrainguinal arteriosclerosis. Circulation 66(suppl 2):9, 1982.
33. O'Mara CS, Flinn WR, et al.: Recognition and surgical management of patent but hemodynamically failed arterial grafts. Ann Surg 193:467, 1981.

isolated popliteal segment: Is polytetrafluoroethylene graft acceptable? Surgery 89:296, 1981.

34. Ring EJ, Alpert JR, et al.: Early experience with percutaneous transluminal angioplasty using a vinyl balloon catheter. Ann Surg 191:438, 1980.

35. Smith CR, Green RM, DeWeese JA: Pseudoocclusion of femoropopliteal bypass grafts. Circulation 68(suppl 2):88, 1983.

36. Ascer E, Veith FJ, et al.: Components of outflow resistance and their correlation with graft patency in lower extremity arterial reconstructions. J Vasc Surg 1:817, 1984.

37. Veith FJ, Gupta SK, Daly V: Management of early and late thrombosis of expanded polytetrafluoroethylene (PTFE) femoropopliteal bypass grafts: Favorable prognosis with appropriate reoperation. Surgery 87:581, 1980.

38. Collier PE, Ascer E, et al.: Arterial reconstruction after failed femorotibial or femoroperoneal bypass, in Trout HH, Giordano JM, DePalma RG (eds): Reoperative Vascular Surgery. New York, Marcel Dekker, 1987, p 211.

CHAPTER 38
In Situ Vein Bypass

Robert P. Leather and Frank J. Veith

HISTORICAL DATA

The concept of using the greater saphenous vein as a bypass by rendering its valves incompetent and leaving it within its subcutaneous bed was first introduced by Hall in 1962.[1] It provoked intermittent interest in both the western and the eastern hemispheres and was used and advocated by some vascular surgeons.[2–6] More recently, the in situ vein bypass has gained widespread attention because of the introduction of the concept of producing valvular incompetence by valve incision and the development of effective instruments to accomplish this.[7] This technique, plus the apparently superior results obtained when in situ bypasses are compared to reversed vein bypasses,[8,9] has prompted many vascular surgeons to adopt the in situ vein bypass for all infrainguinal reconstructions wherever possible.[10,11] On the other hand, some surgeons have claimed that in situ vein bypass results appear superior only because they are compared to data from historical controls with reversed vein grafts and that results equally good can be achieved with some of the more modern techniques of reversed vein grafting presented in Chapter 37.[12,13] The only prospective randomized studies of reversed vein grafts and in situ bypasses to date have produced conflicting results,[14,15] probably because of critical differences in the technique used to prepare the in situ conduit.

PRINCIPLES OF THE METHOD

This chapter supplements the material in Chapters 36 and 37. More importantly, it underscores the importance of the in situ vein bypass in the evolution of infrainguinal limb-salvage surgery and describes the techniques for performing it effectively. Clearly the popularity of the in situ vein bypass has prompted many vascular surgeons to attempt limb-salvage arterial reconstructions that previously were being performed in only a few centers. Whether the success of these in situ bypasses, often performed in disadvantaged circumstances, was due to the in situ nature of the bypass

or to the careful semimicrotechniques used by those who have popularized this type of reconstruction remain to be determined. One of the authors of this chapter (RPL) firmly believes that the in situ vein bypass is superior and leads to better vein use; the other author (FJV) believes that it may be better if a long bypass from the upper thigh to the lower leg or foot is required but that this premise has yet to be proven. Moreover, some patients not suitable for an in situ vein bypass will have ectopic vein available (see Chapter 37). Thus for the present, the competent limb-salvage surgeon should be capable of performing both in situ and reversed vein bypasses. Accordingly, this chapter describes the meticulous techniques that make in situ bypasses successful and does not attempt to answer the currently unresolvable question of whether one is better than the other in a patient who could have either type of reconstruction. That question can only be answered by an appropriate prospective randomized study with accurate long-term follow-up.

ADVANTAGES AND DISADVANTAGES

In spite of these conflicting views, it is probable that endothelial preservation is paramount for optimal bypass function. This can be accomplished either by perfusion of the endothelium via the vasa vasorum or by intraluminal flow. In the in situ bypass both these routes are left intact during preparation of the bypass conduit; hence the preservation of this vital determinant is inherent in this technique. Therefore, conceptually, the problem can be viewed as largely logistic; that is, can a vein be harvested without inflicting other critical injuries, and can flow be reestablished before ischemic endothelial damage occurs? At present this goal is most consistently and completely achieved by leaving the vein in situ, provided the valves can be rendered incompetent without causing significant endothelial injury.

In situ vein bypasses, because the veins are left in their normal bed, cannot be twisted as they are placed in a new tunnel, a real threat with reversed vein grafts. However, care must be exercised to avoid twisting of the dissected distal end of the in situ bypass. The in situ bypass is generally a better size match for anastomosis, with the larger end of the saphenous vein available for anastomosis to the femoral artery and the smaller distal end used for the small distal artery. However, we have not found size discrepancy a problem with reversed vein grafts, and occasionally a reversed vein graft will be smaller at its original central end than at its original peripheral end.

Potential *disadvantages* of in situ vein bypasses include the possibility of leaving a partially competent valve, the slightly greater technical complexity, and potential for twisting or kinking at the transition between mobilized and in situ segments. However, the operating time of in situ, as well as reversed bypasses, is more a function of the patient's arterial and venous anatomy and disease than it is of the type of venous conduit preparation chosen for the arterial reconstruction.

PREOPERATIVE ASSESSMENT BY SAPHENOUS PHLEBOGRAPHY

In the early experience, preoperative assessment of the greater saphenous vein was limited to physical examination of its below-knee pathway. Saphenous phlebography was adopted after the encouraging report by Veith et al.[16] of its safety and utility. It has proved invaluable in the preparation of the vein in situ and is mandatory if a valve cutter is to be used safely. Two methods have been used: preoperative phlebography, usually performed the day before surgery, and an intraoperative study, performed in emergency situations or in those patients with impaired renal function.

In more than 300 preoperative phlebograms using a remote vein on the dorsum of the foot of patients who have received heparin pretreatment, venography has proven safe while providing the relevant information for the efficient planning of this procedure.

More recently, transcutaneous mapping of the saphenous vein by B-mode duplex ultrasound has been found to be an equally effective method for determining venous anatomy provided an experienced technician is available.[17] This noninvasive method provides a detailed three-dimensional map of the course of the saphenous vein that may be traced onto the overlying skin. This map aids in the placement of skin incisions and the location of venous access points for instrumentation. Furthermore, it avoids the risks associated with phlebography and can be routinely performed in approximately 30 minutes. Our experience with 345 limbs studied in this way demonstrates that in more than 90% of patients, B-mode imaging, if available, is the optimum technique for venous assessment. In the less than 10% of cases in which complex systems are encountered, we still perform phlebography since it provides additional information for accurate planning of the procedure.

In spite of these considerations, there remain many who are resistant to these preoperative assessments, preferring to determine anatomic variations at operation. However, such attempts to define them by surgical dissection may often be frustrating and ineffective. In addition, they may result in inappropriate excessive dissection, increasing the potential for spasm and other forms of injury to the vein leading to failure and abandonment of the procedure, as well as to an increased incidence of serious wound complications.

EXPOSURE OF SAPHENOUS VEIN

The primary concerns of most surgeons embarking on the use of the saphenous vein in situ for arterial bypass are identification and division of venous valves, as well as location and interruption of the large side branches that become arteriovenous (AV) fistulas when the vein is arterialized. These concerns have led to two technical approaches.

The first method is to expose the vein over its entire length so that all technical maneuvers are in direct view, which is basic to operative surgery. This approach provides familiarity and confidence in performing this new procedure.[11] The alternative method, which we have arrived at through this "open" method, is to use the intraluminal valve cutter on the thigh portion of the vein since it is the largest and least tapered segment.[18] This method allows safe use of this "blind" technique provided the vein is large enough for the cutter to be free-floating, thereby minimizing the potential for endothelial abrasion. As in all surgery there are trade-offs. With the open approach, there is a greater risk of injury to the vein directly and a greater chance of causing spasm and desiccation, in addition to an increase in wound healing problems. With the closed or blind approach it is safe in 90% of cases provided the cutter is used on only the large (>3.5 mm) segment of the vein and that one has precise knowledge of the venous anatomy, gained either by ultrasonic mapping or venography. It is tempting to extend this blind approach to the smaller diameter below the knee portion of the vein. However, this extension exceeds the limit of this approach's safety, since the risk of circumferential abrasion is greatly increased, not only because of decreasing vein size but also because of the propensity of these smaller veins to go into spasm when manipulated. The retrograde valvulotome, because of its minimal potential for endothelial contact, remains the safest instrument for valve incision in small veins.

ANGIOSCOPY

The use of an angioscope has been advocated by some[19] as a means for cutting the valve leaflets under direct vision. Although perhaps comforting, its use is unnecessary since consistently safe and effective valve incision can be produced by the valvulotome or cutter. Furthermore, it is expensive and potentially injurious. The fear of a "missed" valve is more dependent on anatomy and experience than a function of currently available instrumentation.

AV FISTULAS IN IN SITU SAPHENOUS VEINS

The effect of AV fistulas on in situ saphenous vein bypass hemodynamics and patency has been of great concern to some, even to the point of regarding them as a frequent cause of in situ bypass occlusion.[20] From the outset more than 10 years ago, our practice has been to ligate only those fistulas that conduct enough dye during completion angiography to visualize the deep venous system (Fig. 38-1). The vast majority of the residual subcutaneous iatrogenic AV malformations will undergo spontaneous thrombosis. Recently, we have studied more than 200 such bypasses, using duplex ultrasound scanning to assess overall hemodynamic function. The results indicate a steady reduction in fistula flow, with no overall effect on distal perfusion (Fig. 38-2).[21] There is a small group in whom high fistula flow is poorly tolerated, usually in those patients with limited inflow capacity due to proximal stenosis or a small vein (<3 mm outside diameter). In most patients, however, the flow capacity of the in situ conduit far exceeds the sum demanded by the fistula and adequate distal perfusion.

The allegation that fistulas are a potential cause of occlusive bypass failure is not true; rather, the probable cause of failure in this setting is endothelial injury in the distal vein, with that portion of the in situ conduit proximal to the fistula remaining patent because of flow to the fistula. Thus we regard fistulas as at most an annoyance to the patient and the surgeon but not a crucial determinant of thrombosis of the bypass.

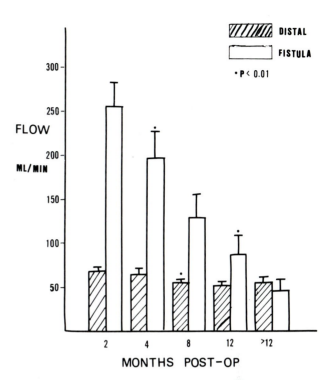

Figure 38-2. Relationship between distal bypass flow and fistula flow.

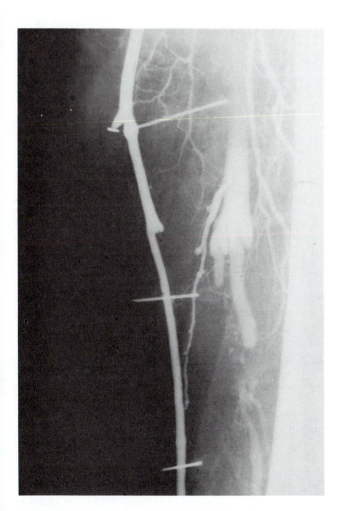

Figure 38-1. Identification of residual AV fistulas by intraoperative angiography using a needle grid.

Technically, the crucial issue in using the greater saphenous vein in situ and the primary reason for its excision and reversal for femoral or distal arterial bypass is to remove the valvular obstruction to arterial flow. In addition, its use in situ entails interruption of the venous side branches, which may become AV fistulas when the vein is arterialized, and the minimal mobilization of its ends for the construction of the proximal and distal anastomoses. The objective is to accomplish this with a minimum of operative manipulation of the vein and especially of the endothelial surface, with particular avoidance of circumferential longitudinal shear. The simplest, most expedient, and least traumatic method of rendering the bicuspid venous valve incompetent is to cut the leaflets in their major axes while they are held in the functionally closed position by fluid or arterial pressure from above. This is the essence of the valve incision technique (Fig. 38-3). Preparation for the operative procedure ideally should include the following:

1. Preoperative arteriography, including the ankle and the foot, with biplane views of the calf, not only to determine the true extent of disease in the vessels but also to accurately differentiate the anterior tibial artery from the peroneal artery
2. Saphenous phlebograms, with biplane views where there are double system variants present or a suitable duplex-generated map
3. Marking the skin with the path of the saphenous vein below the knee
4. Assembling the operating table so that the foot is sufficiently extended to allow performance of all surgical manipulations from the knee down with the surgeon in a

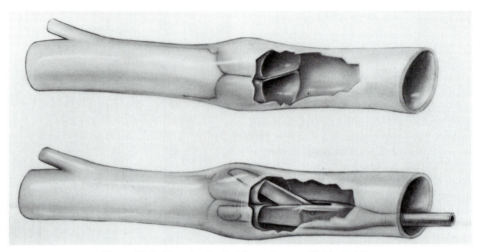

Figure 38-3. Use of valve incision scissors with blunted tips.

comfortable sitting position, with his arms resting on the table for proper use of microsurgical instruments.

In addition, the following equipment is necessary for the optimum performance of tibial artery bypasses:

1. Operating loupes of at least 2.5 power (ideally 3.5 power) with an extended field, that is, a comfortable and easily accommodated field 7 to 8 cm in diameter and comparably deep.
2. Coaxial headlight, which provides ideal illumination required for optimal visual acuity
3. A Doppler ultrasound flow detector with sterile 8 or 10 MHz probe, preferably with a 3 mm tip
4. Microsurgical instruments: forceps, needle holders, and Castroviejo scissors
5. A sterile orthopedic tourniquet cuff for use in place of occlusive vascular clamps or intraluminal balloons for control of calcified tibial vessels
6. Calibrated handleless clips for truly atraumatic control of the saphenous vein and tibial arteries, for example, Yasargil or Weck microclips.
7. Items specific to the in situ procedure in addition to the valvulotomes and the cutter instruments:
   a. A sterile standard IV set
   b. Dextran 40 or 70 in a compliant plastic bag or a similar bag for drawing fresh blood
   c. A pneumatic transfusion cuff
   d. Papaverine hydrochloride 30 mg/ml

After preparation and sterile draping of the entire extremity, warm (37° C) papaverine solution (60 mg/500 ml Plasma-lyte or normal saline) is injected percutaneously into the subcutaneous tissue adjacent to the saphenous vein along its course below the knee.[22]

TECHNIQUES FOR SAPHENOUS IMPLANTATION AND INSTRUMENTATION

The proximal saphenous vein, which lies immediately deep to the superficial fascia, is exposed, and papaverine solution is infiltrated into the surrounding tissue to minimize spasm.

Although the common femoral artery has been considered the proper site for proximal anastomosis of all distal bypasses, there is evidence that use of the superficial femoral artery in some patients within the limb-salvage population is equally satisfactory.[23] Furthermore, technical circumstances such as previous surgical use or exposure of the common femoral artery or its encasement with circumferential calcification make either the profunda femoris artery or the superficial femoral artery valid alternative inflow sources. In spite of its less accessible anatomic location, the profunda femoris artery is usually less invested with thick or calcified plaque than either the common or superficial femoral arteries and, therefore, frequently provides the most satisfactory site for proximal anastomosis. It is best approached from the medial aspect (with the surgeon on the contralateral side of the table) by incision of the subcutaneous tissue immediately lateral to the saphenous vein down to the underlying investing myofascia. Dissection laterally in this fusion plane to the superficial femoral artery is bloodless. The fascia is incised over the superficial femoral artery, and, if it is occluded, a 3 to 5 cm segment can be excised, thus facilitating exposure of the profunda femoris artery. The lateral circumflex femoral vein is divided, and the proximal profunda artery lies immediately deep to it. With the most satisfactory site of proximal anastomosis now determined, the length of the proximal saphenous vein required to reach the site is known. If the common femoral artery is to be used as the inflow source, complete dissection of the saphenous bulb and secure ligation of its branches is carried out. If additional length is required to facilitate anastomosis to the common femoral artery, a portion of the anterior aspect of the common femoral vein is removed in continuity with the saphenous bulb. An alternative to this approach is to preserve an appropriate length of the frequently present anterior branch at the saphenous bulb and to fillet it. The valve leaflets at the saphenofemoral junction are excised, removing only the transparent portion and leaving the usually prominent insertion ridge intact. The second valve invariably present 3 to 5 cm distal to this junction can be incised easily with a retrograde valvulotome through a side branch distal to the valve before the vein is divided, or, alternatively, it can be cut either with scissors or with an antegrade valvulotome through the open end of the vein, as is the valve immediately distal to the medial accessory branch. These valves are identified by gently distending the vein through its open end with dextran or heparinized blood and are cut with scissors, with the thumb and index finger around the shank of the scissor, while the valve is held in the functionally closed position by fluid trapped between the open end of the saphenous vein and the valve.

The plane of closure of the valve cusps is invariably parallel to the skin. This position dictates the orientation of all instruments with relation to the valve cusps.

If a valve cutter cannot be used, the location of the next valve site is determined by advancing a No. 6 French catheter, with the infusion running under 200 mm Hg of pressure until it impacts in the valve sinus. This location is marked on the skin, and the proximal anastomosis is carried out. The saphenous vein is thus arterialized.

If the cutter is to be used, a 3 to 5 cm incision is made 5 mm posterior to the position of the main saphenous vein, which was marked preoperatively on the skin, allowing identification of a predetermined branch seen on the venogram and using it to gain access to the lumen of the saphenous vein. A No. 3 Fogarty catheter is introduced into the saphenous vein through this side branch and is passed proximally, with the leg straightened, to exit through the open end of the vein. The catheter is then divided at an acute angle at the 20 or 30 cm mark, whichever is closest to the open end of the vein. The valve cutter is screwed onto the catheter, and a No. 8 French catheter is then secured to the cutter with a loop of a fine suture. The leading cylinder of the cutter is drawn into the vein, providing a partial obturator obstruction to venous flow while permitting the visualization of the cutting blade and minimal resistance in torque, thus allowing precise orientation of the cutting edges at a 90-degree angle to the plane of closure of the valves, that is, to the plane of the overlying skin surface. The catheter-cutter assembly is then slowly drawn distally while the dextran solution or blood is introduced

through the catheter at 200 to 300 mm Hg pressure, with a pressure seal provided by a 1 mm Silastic rubber vessel loop secured by a small hemostat around the most proximal end of the saphenous vein. This pressurized fluid column snaps each successive valve to the closed position so that the cusps are efficiently engaged by the blades of the cutter (Fig. 38-4). A slight but definite resistance will be felt as the cutter encounters each valve and cuts the leaflets. Greater resistance than this should be managed by turning the cutter 45 degrees and making another attempt at advancement. If this maneuver does not produce the desired result, the cutter should be withdrawn and dismounted, and the area of impaction should be exposed directly. The cutter is advanced through a predetermined safe distance, generally to the knee-joint level, and is then withdrawn to the femoral exposure. The cutter is dismounted, and the catheter is removed from the saphenous vein. Proximal anastomosis of the saphenous vein to the selected inflow artery is performed, and the pulsatile impulse thus provided will make the location of the next competent valve readily apparent.

Continuity incision, exposing the full length of the saphenous vein, is only necessary if the cutter cannot be used and the combination of thick subcutaneous tissue, a small vein, and reduced pulsation due to the presence of an AV fistula makes the valve sites difficult to determine. The remaining valves are incised by means of a retrograde valvulotome introduced through a side branch or the distal end of the vein. This instrument is designed so that it will engage leaflets, center itself, and cut the leaflet in its longitudinal axis. It is then advanced again, carefully rotated through 180 degrees, and withdrawn, thus engaging the remaining leaflet (Fig. 38-5). However, before the cutting force is applied to the valvulotome tip, the valvulotome should be maneuvered toward the center of the vein lumen by depression of the vein itself, allowing division of the remaining leaflet without the risk of entering a side branch, which is invariably present and close to all valve sinuses. In passing the valvulotome intraluminally to and from a valve site, it is important that any pressure on the vein

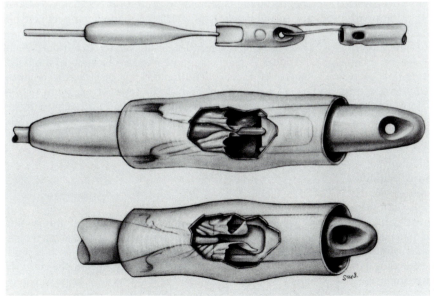

Figure 38-4. Mechanism of action of valve cutter.

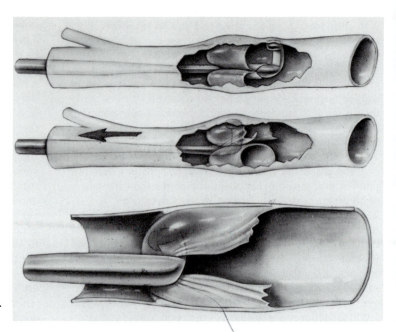

Figure 38-5. Use of modified valvulotome.

wall resulting from the curving path be exerted on the shaft of the instrument rather than on the projecting blade tip. This precaution will lessen the likelihood of the blade becoming lodged in the side branch and lacerating the vein wall. Unobstructed arterial pulsatile flow is thus brought to the desired level. Before transection and mobilization of the distal vein, exposure of the anticipated outflow anastomotic site is carried out. This exposure is desirable not only to minimize the warm ischemia time of the endothelium but also to assess the appropriate bypass length, always allowing an additional 1 to 2 cm so that the manipulated and thus traumatized terminal portion can be excised and discarded.

After completion of the distal anastomosis, flow in the bypass, as well as in the outflow vessel, is confirmed, and a quantitative appraisal is made through use of the sterile Doppler ultrasound probe. A completion angiogram is then performed with radiopaque reference markers (i.e., No. 19 gauge needles in their plastic containers taped to the skin, a radiologic strip marker, or skin clips) to correlate the position of the fistulas as viewed on x-ray film with the surface anatomy.

Most branches of the saphenous vein drain the superficial subcutaneous tissue, and their orifices are generally guarded by a competent valve, thus preventing flow away from the arterialized saphenous vein. Only valveless branches immediately become AV fistulas. However, they are usually small and generally undergo spontaneous thrombosis postoperatively. This thrombotic activity is signaled by the development of superficial phlebitis, the extent of which is determined by the size of this iatrogenic AV malformation. Although occasionally a large area of induration results, it is sterile and self-limiting and invariably resolves within a few days. Even if these superficial veins remain patent, the loss of distal arterial flow is generally small and does not threaten the continued patency of a bypass. As a general rule, only those branches with sufficient flow to allow visualization of the deep venous system with radiopaque dye on the completion angiogram need be ligated.

The normal closing mechanism in a symmetric venous valve is initiated by tension along the leading edge of the valve leaflet caused by expansion of the valve sinus from the raised intraluminal pressures. This tension brings the edge of the leaflet toward the center of the lumen so that flow forces it into the closed competent position. In any segment of vein in which a valve is mechanically opened from below by passage of an instrument (i.e., valvulotome or balloon catheter) in the proximal direction, there is potential for a valve leaflet to be pushed against the wall and to remain temporarily adherent to the valve sinus in the open position. This is most likely to occur in asymmetric valves. In these valves, the normal closing mechanism may not be operative so that the valve may remain open for an indefinite period of time. The subsequent closure, either spontaneous or induced, of the artificially opened valve leaflet by manipulation (e.g., palpation of the pulse in that area) results in partial or even complete obstruction of arterial flow. Therefore, before the operation is completed, deliberate attempts should be made to precipitate closure of any incompletely lysed valves by the following maneuver: with the distal vein open and free flow observed, a sponge is rolled along the in situ conduit from top to bottom. When the cutter is used, the most frequent location of a missed valve is in the segment immediately distal to the point of lowest cutter travel and at the level of exposure of the vein. This segment should be checked routinely with the valvulotome since, in the absence of flow, an undiminished pulse can be transmitted, even through an intact valve in a static hydraulic column.

DISCUSSION

What appears to some as a disadvantage of the in situ technique is that, during preparation of the vein, its endothelial surface remains in constant contact with a static column of blood. However, the flow rate in the normal, nonarterialized saphenous vein is very low, approximately 5 to 10 ml/min. In fact, in some areas the blood is actually stagnant for varying periods. Therefore the presence of a static column of blood in a conduit lined by viable endothelium is a normal physiologic state and does not result in thrombus formation provided that the endothelium has not been damaged. Such an injury is probably due to the shear forces caused by injudicious intraluminal instrumentation. Once endothelial disruption occurs, platelet adhesion and aggregation develop rapidly, particularly in areas of absent or low flow, and this build-up may subsequently jeopardize arterial flow. This build-up may first be detected by the loss or diminution of the pulse distally and by dampening of the Doppler velocity profile. Only temporary improvement follows the passage of the valvulotome to check for a residual valve leaflet. Build-up can also be confirmed by introducing a distal pressure-monitoring catheter and recording the pull-back pressures or by finding a characteristic foamy surface filling defect on the operative angiogram. The simple expedient of assessing flow from the distal divided end of the saphenous vein before construction of the distal anastomosis is very reliable in detecting any proximal hemodynamically significant lesions. If there is steady, undiminished pulsatile flow, it is unlikely that such a lesion is present proximally.

In practice, every effort should be made to prevent intimal injury and its resulting platelet aggregate. Instruments should be passed only when the vein is fully distended, preferably by arterialized blood and pressure, so that contact with the endothelium is prevented as much as possible. Particularly devastating is circumferential shear, especially in the distal mobilized segment, which is smallest in diameter and in which the protective effect of flowing blood through a coincident fistula before completion of the distal anastomosis is absent. Fortunately, with proper care of this critical segment, that is, strict avoidance of instruments exerting circumferential contact, for example, catheters, sounds, dilators, and cylindrical valve cutters or disruptors, this problem is infrequent. When this shear does occur, the span of vein involved is usually short, and it can be easily corrected by removal, under direct vision, of the platelet debris from the area of injured endothelium and with the addition of an autogenous vein patch or by segmental replacement with a fresh segment of vein if the involved area is too long.

In situ vein bypasses require careful preparation. Merely retaining the saphenous vein in situ does not compensate for sustained care, patience, and attention to detail, as well as consistent, meticulous surgical technique aided by optical magnification. Before attempting to adopt this technique, the surgeon should see it performed by an experienced operating team. In addition, familiarity with the use and feel of all instruments should be gained ex vivo on discarded valve-bearing vein segments obtained from aortocoronary bypass procedures, vein-stripping operations, or autopsy specimens.

RESULTS

An in situ bypass was attempted in more than 95% of over 1,000 unselected patients requiring a distal arterial reconstruction for limb preservation. Of these attempts, less than 6% could not be reconstructed by the in situ technique; however, half of them were successfully completed using segments of autogenous vein grafts (a partial in situ bypass). Life-table analysis of secondary patency of bypasses for limb salvage to the popliteal level is shown in Table 38-1 and to the infrapopliteal level in Table 38-2 (Fig. 38-6).

In 1,066 prepared in situ conduits, there were 88 instances of perioperative occlusion or deterioration of graft flow, 64 of which were revised as indicated in Table 38-3. Forty-one of these revisions remained patent longer than 30 days; their subsequent performance has not been significantly different from that of bypasses that did not require revision. The incidence of perioperative occlusion has decreased steadily as greater care and control have been exercised to prevent endothelial injury, particularly in the distal mobilized vein segment. There is ample experimental and clinical evidence that the preservation of endothelial integrity is best achieved by avoidance of the summation of a variety of injuries (i.e., spasm and the subsequent trauma from hydraulic dilatation required for its relief; particularly if a pressure exceeding 300 mm Hg is used; exposure to nonhemic solutions; warm ischemic time exceeding 30 minutes; and the more obvious mechanical trauma of dissection, manipulation, and application of occluding clamps).

Early detection of stenoses and correction of defects of in situ conduits before occlusion occurs can be achieved by a comprehensive follow-up program. Our patients are seen and examined every 3 months for the first 12 months, every 3 to 4 months up to the second year, and every 6 months thereafter. Each examination includes obtaining pulse-volume recordings and segmental pressures and performing audible Doppler assessment along the course of the bypass. More recently, direct visualization of the conduit and estimates of volume flow by duplex ultrasound scanning both at rest and after reactive hyperemia induced by

TABLE 38-1. LIFE-TABLE ANALYSIS OF 285 POPLITEAL IN SITU BYPASSES PERFORMED FOR LIMB SALVAGE

Interval (Months)	Bypasses Entering Interval	Bypasses Failing	Interval Patency (%)	Cumulative Patency (%)
0–1	285	13	95.3	95.3
2–12	257	11	94.9	90.4
13–24	162	6	95.6	86.4
25–36	102	2	97.5	84.3
37–48	56	3	93.9	79.1
49–60	39	0	100	79.1

TABLE 38-2. LIFE-TABLE ANALYSIS OF 632 INFRAPOPLITEAL IN SITU BYPASSES PERFORMED FOR LIMB SALVAGE

Interval (Months)	Bypasses Entering Interval	Bypasses Failing	Interval Patency (%)	Cumulative Patency (%)
0–1	632	29	95.2	95.2
2–12	545	25	94.4	89.8
13–24	318	13	95.0	85.4
25–36	193	7	95.5	81.6
37–48	114	4	95.7	78.1
49–60	70	3	94.3	73.6

3 minutes of tourniquet occlusion have been used and evaluated.

The most sensitive indicator of developing stenosis, exclusive of ultrasound imaging, has been a decreasing slope of the dP/dt segment of the pulse-wave contour, usually accompanied by decreased amplitude of the pulse wave and lowered segmental pressure distally. When possible, examining the patient after he exercises on the treadmill will further increase the sensitivity of these observations and result in earlier detection of these lesions. In addition, duplex ultrasound can identify these lesions before the development of a pressure gradient. These findings are indica-

tions for immediate angiographic examination and operative correction.

Among 1,066 in situ conduits constructed, 69 stenotic lesions have developed in 55 patients. The majority of them occurred within the first 12 months (45 of 69). Twenty-four occurred in the distal mobilized segment, 25 were in the proximal mobilized segment, and 20 were in the midportion of the bypass conduit. They occurred with increased frequency in smaller veins (i.e., 41 [10%] occurred in 412 veins 3.0 mm or less in size, compared with 27 [4%] in 613 veins 3.5 mm or larger). All of these stenoses were treated surgically with vein-patch angioplasty, and all but one remained patent longer than 30 days. Sixty-four residual AV fistulas required ligation, with the patient under local anesthesia, 3 days to 23 months after the initial procedure (6%). There were 62 occlusions within 30 days (immediate patency rate, 94%) and 39 deaths in the same period (surgical mortality, 3.7%).

To prevent these postoperative stenoses we recommend the following:

1. The intraoperative use of papaverine hydrochloride injected percutaneously along the saphenous vein to prevent spasm
2. Rigid control of the pressure used to dilate vein segments
3. Limitation of the warm ischemic time of the mobilized portions of the vein

These measures, together with strict avoidance of mechanical trauma as indicated, are important technical details that affect long-term patency of these bypasses. In addition, the extreme ends of the mobilized segments are maximally exposed to mechanical endothelial trauma. Because this trauma is particularly critical in the divided distal end of small veins, a distal mobilized venous segment, with an

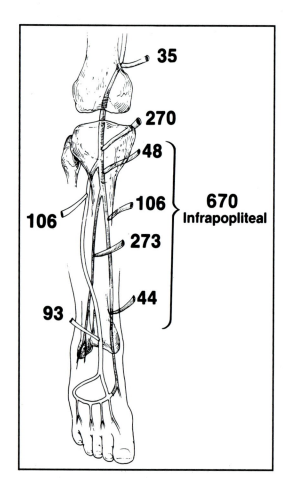

Figure 38-6. Sites of distal anastomosis in 975 in situ arterial bypasses for limb-threatening ischemia.

TABLE 38-3. EARLY (WITHIN 30 DAYS) REVISIONS OF IN SITU CONDUITS

Arteriovenous fistulas	18
Residual valve	11
Distal vein patch	13
Midvein patch	3
Proximal vein patch	2
Distal arterial outflow	11
Proximal arterial inflow	6

excess segment 2 cm long, should be dissected. This excess distal vein segment can then be excised to construct the distal anastomosis with an uninjured vein segment.

CONCLUSIONS

The major advantage of the saphenous vein when prepared in situ for an arterial bypass is the better preservation of a viable, physiologically active endothelium. The ability of such a conduit to maintain satisfactory long-term patency may make it possible to use smaller veins with limited outflow tracts that would otherwise be considered inadequate for use in other methods of reconstruction.

Unquestionably, retaining the vein in situ decreases its accessibility. This procedure requires great care, patience, attention to detail, and meticulous surgical technique. It should not be undertaken without appropriate training. In experienced hands, one can anticipate a patient operability rate of 96%, a vein use rate of 94%, and a cumulative 5-year life-table patency of 74% with femorotibial bypass performed for limb salvage.

REFERENCES

1. Hall KV: The great saphenous vein used in situ as arterial shunt after extirpation of the vein valves. A preliminary report. Surgery 51:492, 1962.
2. Connolly JE, Harris JE, Mills W: Autogenous in situ saphenous vein bypass of femoral popliteal obliterative disease. Surgery 55:144, 1964.
3. May AG, DeWeese JA, Rob CG: Arterialized in situ saphenous vein. Arch Surg 91:743, 1965.
4. Connolly JE, Kwaan JHM: In situ saphenous vein bypass. Arch Surg 117:1551, 1982.
5. Samuels PB, Plested WG, et al.: In situ saphenous vein arterial bypass: A study of the anatomy pertinent to its use as a bypass graft with a description of a new venous valvulotome. Am J Surg 34:122, 1982.
6. Gruss JD, Bartels D, et al.: Arterial reconstruction for distal disease of the lower extremities by the in situ vein graft technique. J Cardiovasc Surg 23:231, 1982.
7. Leather RP, Shah DM, et al.: Instrumental evolution of the valve incision method of in situ saphenous vein bypass. J Vasc Surg 1:113, 1984.
8. Leather RP, Shah DM, Karmody AM: Infrapopliteal bypass for limb salvage: Increased patency and utilization of the saphenous vein used in situ. Surgery 90:1000, 1981.
9. Leather RP, Karmody AM: In situ saphenous vein arterial bypass for the treatment of limb ischemia, in Mannick JA (ed): Advances in Surgery, vol 19. Chicago, Year Book Medical Publishers, Inc, 1986, p 175.
10. Levine AW, Bandyk DF, et al.: Lessons learned in adopting the in situ saphenous vein bypass. J Vasc Surg 2:146, 1985.
11. Fogle MA, Whittemore AD, et al.: A comparison of in situ and reversed saphenous vein grafts for infrainguinal reconstruction. J Vasc Surg 5:46, 1987.
12. Taylor LM, Phinney ES, Porter JM: Present status of reversed vein bypass for lower extremity revascularization. J Vasc Surg 3:288, 1986.
13. Veith FJ, Ascer E, et al.: Tibiotibial vein bypass grafts: A new operation for limb salvage. J Vasc Surg 2:552, 1985.
14. Harris PL, How TV, Jones DR: Prospectively randomized clinical trial to compare in situ and reversed saphenous vein grafts for femoropopliteal bypass. Br J Surg 74:252, 1987.
15. Buchbinder D, Singh JK, et al.: Comparison of patency rate and structural changes of in situ and reversed vein arterial bypass. J Surg Res 30:213, 1981.
16. Veith FJ, Moss CM, et al.: Preoperative saphenous venography in arterial reconstructive surgery of the lower extremity. Surgery 85:253, 1979.
17. Leopold PW, Shandall AA, et al.: Initial experience comparing B-mode imaging and venography of the saphenous vein before in situ bypass. Am J Surg 152:206, 1986.
18. Shah DM, Chang BB, et al.: The anatomy of the greater saphenous venous system. J Vasc Surg 3:273, 1986.
19. Fleischer HL, Thompson BW, et al.: Angioscopically monitored saphenous vein valvulotomy. J Vasc Surg 4:360, 1986.
20. Denton MJ, Hill D, Fairgrieve J: In situ femoropopliteal and distal vein bypass for limb salvage: Experience of 50 cases. Br J Surg 70:358, 1983.
21. Leopold PW, Kupinski AM, et al.: Hemodynamic observations related to in situ bypass arteriovenous fistulae. Vasc Surg 21:265, 1987.
22. LoGerfo FW, Quist WC, Crawshaw HW: An improved technique for endothelial morphology in vein grafts. Surgery 90:1015, 1981.
23. Veith FJ, Gupta SK, et al.: Superficial femoral and popliteal arteries as inflow sites for distal bypasses. Surgery 90:980, 1981.

CHAPTER 39
Extraanatomic Bypasses

Enrico Ascer and Frank J. Veith

Extraanatomic arterial reconstructions were devised to circumvent complex vascular problems when conventional anatomic procedures necessary for relief of severe ischemia were deemed impossible or too hazardous to perform. The concept of extraanatomic bypass was first applied by Freeman and Leeds[1] when they used the superficial femoral artery as a donor to transport blood to the contralateral femoral artery through a subcutaneous, transabdominal pathway. Interestingly, this procedure was described just 3 years after Kunlin[2] reported the first anatomic femoropopliteal bypass operation in 1949. Since then, a multitude of ingenious extraanatomic procedures have been described and widely used with varying degrees of success, to restore an adequate blood supply to both the upper and lower extremities, the brain, and more recently the kidneys. They have been mostly used as primary or secondary operations in patients considered high risk for an abdominal or thoracic operation or in the management of anatomically placed infected grafts. Extraanatomic bypasses such as carotid-subclavian, carotid-carotid, carotid-vertebral, and axilloaxillary have been successfully used for the treatment of brachiocephalic occlusive disease and are described in other chapters.

In this chapter, we focus on *conventional* extraanatomic reconstructions designed to improve lower-limb ischemia, including axillofemoral and femorofemoral bypasses, as well as *extended* extraanatomic bypasses such as axillopopliteal and cross-over femoropopliteal.

CONVENTIONAL EXTRAANATOMIC BYPASSES

Axillofemoral Bypasses

Lewis[3] made an important contribution to vascular surgery in 1959 by demonstrating that the subclavian artery could adapt itself to deliver an adequate blood supply to the lower half of the body without shunting blood away from the ipsilateral arm or cerebral circulation. Blaisdell and Hall[4] in the United States and Louw[5] in South Africa combined this principle with the idea of performing a simpler, quicker, and less risky operation to save ischemic lower limbs in patients too sick to undergo standard aortofemoral procedures. Almost simultaneously, they performed extracavitary bypasses from the axillary artery to the common femoral artery using synthetic graft material. In 1966, Sauvage and Wood[6] modified this procedure by adding a cross-over femoral limb to the axillofemoral graft for the treatment of bilateral lower-limb ischemia, thereby sparing the contralateral axillary artery. One other potential benefit of this cross-over graft is that the flow through the long, vertical portion of the bypass is increased. Whether this configuration minimizes graft thrombosis by the augmentation of blood flow rates remains controversial.

Indications

Axillofemoral bypasses rapidly became an integral part of the overall approach to the management of infected aortic grafts and aortoduodenal fistula complicated by in situ infection. Other local factors known to discourage the use of the aorta as an inflow source in favor of the axillary artery include multiple previous abdominal operations, colostomies and ileostomies, inoperable intraabdominal malignancies, abdominal or pelvic irradiation, and morbid obesity.

Systemic factors, as well, play an important role in the decision to preferentially perform an extraanatomic reconstruction. There is little doubt that a history of recent myocardial infarction, congestive heart failure, inoperable unstable coronary angina, chronic renal failure, advanced malignancy, advanced chronic obstructive pulmonary disease or any other severely debilitating illnesses in patients presenting with threatened, ischemic lower limbs also calls for less invasive procedures. Acute aortic occlusion in high-risk patients is one other common indication for axillofemoral bypasses. Less commonly, axillofemoral bypasses have been used as adjunctive procedures in the nonresective treatment of abdominal aortic aneurysms and in symptomatic iliofemoral occlusion caused by acute aortic dissections.

The safety and ease with which these extraanatomic

operations are performed, coupled with earlier optimistic reports regarding their long-term graft-patency results, encouraged a more lenient attitude toward performing these procedures that included performing them on lower risk patients and ones with claudication. However, the original reports did not differentiate the results obtained with a single operation (primary patency) from those obtained when one or more repeat operations were necessary for continued graft patency (secondary patency).[7,8] They also did not emphasize the frequency, complexity, and number of complications associated with secondary procedures. In fact, a review of our own experience revealed that the cumulative primary patency rate for axillofemoral bypasses was only 47% at 5 years with more than one third of them requiring one or more repeat operations to achieve continued limb salvage.[9] These findings are clearly worse than the ones reported for aortofemoral procedures. When one considers that many patients who carry a prohibitive surgical risk for an abdominal procedure may already have limited ambulation as a result of restricted cardiac or pulmonary capacity, improving their circulation for the purpose of increasing their walking distance would be futile. Therefore we believe that axillofemoral bypasses should be reserved for high-risk patients presenting with severe lower-limb ischemia.

Preoperative Evaluation

Clinical examination of the lower extremities, by noninvasive evaluation of the degree of distal ischemia, and angiographic visualization of the outflow tract are no longer sufficient diagnostic measures to ensure completeness of the preoperative workup. Contrary to widespread belief, the *inflow* tract may harbor hemodynamically significant lesions that escape detection even by a skilled examiner when listening for a supraclavicular bruit or when measuring and comparing upper-extremity blood pressures. Actually, we have shown that occlusive disease of the subclavian or axillary artery can be a cause of axillofemoral bypass failure.[9] More recently, we have prospectively evaluated the incidence of unsuspected inflow disease in candidates for axillofemoral operations. Forty patients underwent angiographic studies of the aortic arch and its branches before axillofemoral bypasses. This study revealed the incidence of significant inflow disease (more than 50% stenosis) was 25%. The consensus that these lesions are more often located on the left side was confirmed by our study; however, a significant number were detected on the right (42% of all lesions). As a result, angiographic assessment of the inflow and outflow tracts should be included as an important component of the preoperative workup.

A Swan-Ganz balloon-tipped catheter inserted to monitor left-ventricular function has been helpful in the perioperative management of these patients.

Technique

Although the basic technical principles involved in the construction of an axillofemoral bypass have remained unchanged since the original report by Blaisdell and Hall,[4] we have added some modifications that we believe are worth describing. This procedure can be entirely performed with the patient under local anesthesia; however, most high-risk patients will tolerate light general endotracheal anesthesia without untoward effects. We now prefer the latter method of anesthesia because it provides a comfortable environment in which the surgeon can perform careful dissections, tunnelings, and meticulous anastomoses, and it gives the anesthesiologist optimal control for monitoring the patient's blood pressure and respiratory function.

Axillounifemoral Bypass

With the patient in the supine position, the donor upper extremity is abducted to 90 degrees, and a cannula is routinely inserted in the contralateral radial artery for continuous blood pressure monitoring. The infraclavicular incision starts approximately 2 cm lateral to the costoclavicular joint and is extended toward the deltopectoral groove for approximately 5 to 6 cm, forming a 35-degree angle with the clavicle (Fig. 39-1, *insert*). The incision is then deepened through the pectoral fascia, displaying the pectoralis major muscle fibers, which are split horizontally along the entire length of the incision. At this point, placing a self-retaining retractor gives adequate exposure for incising the clavipectoral fascia.

After this procedure is accomplished, the pectoralis minor muscle can be readily identified and isolated by blunt dissection. Although the operation may proceed by laterally retracting this muscle, exposure of the second portion of the axillary artery is greatly facilitated by division of the pectoralis minor muscle at the coracoid process. The axillary artery is best localized by palpation of a strong pulse underneath the deep clavipectoral fascia. Awareness of the surrounding structures in this anatomic plane is of the utmost importance to prevent potentially disastrous complications. At this level, the axillary artery is guarded superiorly by the brachial plexus and inferiorly and slightly anteriorly by the axillary vein (see Fig. 39-1). Mobilization of the artery from the loose periadventitial attachments is initiated at the junction of its first and second portions at the medial border of the pectoralis minor muscle. The axillary artery is encircled with a Silastic sling and is gently lifted from its bed to facilitate its circumferential dissection and to isolate its branches. Proximally, the axillary dissection is carried 1 to 2 cm past the origin of the thoracoacromial trunk, and distally it is dissected to the point where the crossing neural branches form the median nerve. After completion of the axillary dissection, attention is turned to the outflow tract.

Selection of the anastomotic outflow site is primarily based on preoperative angiograms. When the runoff from the common femoral artery is unimpeded, this vessel is approached using the standard vertical groin incision, with care taken to leave the deep femoral artery undisturbed for possible future use. However, if the origin of the deep femoral artery is stenosed, the dissection is extended to include its proximal portion. Here it is necessary to ligate and transect a crossing tributary of the deep femoral vein, thus allowing the placement of the distal anastomosis across the stenotic segment of the deep femoral artery. Whenever possible, rather than performing a local endarterectomy, we prefer to fashion the distal end of the graft into a patch to widen the narrowed segment. This technique avoids

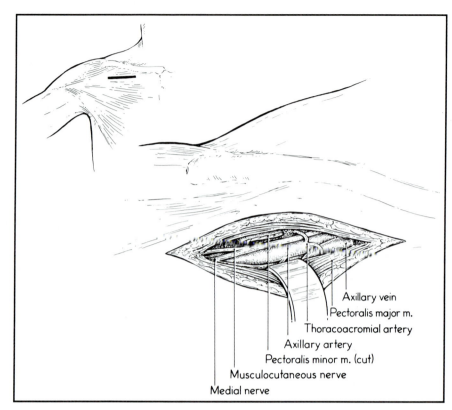

Figure 39-1. Insert illustrates position of the shoulder and the line of incision for exposure of the axillary artery. Note the angle formed by the incision and the lower border of the clavicle. Larger diagram shows the topographic anatomy of the axillary artery and surrounding structures after transection of pectoralis minor muscle.

Axillary vein
Pectoralis major m.
Thoracoacromial artery
Axillary artery
Pectoralis minor m. (cut)
Musculocutaneous nerve
Medial nerve

the problem of dealing with the distal end of an endarterectomized segment, which can be a factor leading to turbulence and graft thrombosis, particularly when the occlusive process is extensive.

When groin infection, multiple previous groin dissections, or significant disease of the proximal arteries is present, one may avoid the troublesome area and select instead, a direct approach to the distal two thirds of the deep femoral artery through an incision in the midthigh along the medial border of the sartorius muscle.

After both arterial dissections are completed, the connecting tunnel is initiated at each end by finger dissection. The upper end of the tunnel is paved under the pectoralis major muscle and between the transected portions of the pectoralis minor muscle and then subcutaneously toward the posterior axillary line. The lower end of the tunnel begins subcutaneously at the superior edge of the incision and moves upward and laterally in the direction of the posterior axillary line, staying medial to the anterosuperior iliac spine. A slightly curved, hollow tunneler is passed from the lower to the upper incision to bridge the remaining distance and is kept in place to transport the graft after the proximal anastomosis is completed. Efforts should be made to avoid making counterincisions when constructing the tunnel because they have been identified as possible culprits for graft infection.

Because the axillary anastomosis and the positioning of the proximal portion of the graft are usually more demanding than the distal anastomosis, we elect to perform this part first to have the freedom to maneuver the graft. Systemic heparinization is accomplished before cross clamping. Proximal and distal control of the axillary artery flow is obtained through the use of atraumatic vascular clamps

rather than by pulling on double-looped Silastic slings. In this manner, undue tension on the donor artery, which can cause severe spasm with diminished flow to the upper extremity, is minimized. A longitudinal incision, 1.8 to 2 cm long, is performed in the anteroinferior border of the second portion of the axillary artery. Six-millimeter polytetrafluoroethylene (PTFE) grafts were selected for most of our bypasses. The proximal end of the graft is cut sharply with scissors and is measured to fit the arteriotomy exactly. A running, four-quadrant suture technique, beginning at the toe of the end-to-side anastomosis, is then performed using monofilament 6-0 sutures. To avoid mechanical obstruction of the artery due to shoulder motion (Fig. 39-2A and A'), this long, oblique anastomosis allows for an intentional slight redundancy of the axillofemoral graft (Fig. 39-2B and B'). After this procedure, the graft is filled with a crystalloid solution to test the integrity of the proximal anastomosis and to assist in passing it through the tunneler to avoid torsion, kinking, or excessive tension.

Attention is then turned to the recipient artery. After gaining proximal and distal control with atraumatic vascular clamps, a 1.7 to 2.0 cm arteriotomy is performed at the appropriate site. The distal end of the graft is tailored to fit this opening, and the anastomosis is likewise performed with a four-quadrant running suture technique beginning at the heel of the anastomosis. At the completion of the bypass, the heparin is reversed with protamine sulfate according to the activated clotting time.

Axillobifemoral Bypass

In addition to the technical details previously mentioned for axillounifemoral bypass, dissection of the contralateral femoral artery and creation of a subcutaneous, suprapubic

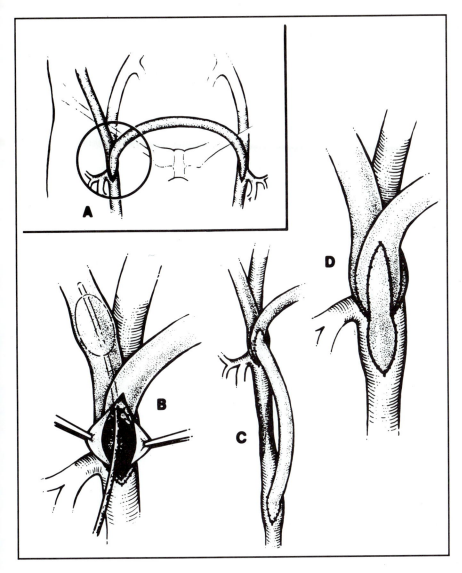

Figure 39-5. A. Diagram depicts several advantages of our axillobifemoral bypass configuration in the management of occluded grafts. A single opening over the graft-to-graft anastomosis allows thrombectomy of both limbs of the bypass, **B;** it can be used as an inflow site for a distal extension, **C,** or it can be carried across the stenotic outflow and repaired with a patch, **D.**

operation to salvage the contralateral limb.[9] Finally, this approach not only shortens the operative time in these high-risk patients, but it also avoids placing the asymptomatic limb in jeopardy because of early or late failure of what would amount to a prophylactic portion of a bilateral procedure.

Results

Our operative mortality (30 days) has been low considering the poor general status of these patients. In a series of 56 patients, it was 5.3%, and all deaths were caused by myocardial infarctions. The severity of the underlying diseases was clearly reflected in the 5-year cumulative survival rate of only 43%.[9]

The most common cause of axillofemoral graft failure is "spontaneous thrombosis," which occurs most frequently in the first year of graft implantation. It remains controversial whether external compression (e.g., tight belts, sleeping on the side of the graft) contributes to graft thrombosis. When no obvious cause of graft failure can be identified, these bypasses respond favorably to repeated attempts at simple thrombectomy. Progression of distal disease followed by progression of inflow disease is another important cause of graft failure, whereas intimal hyperplasia has been a rare finding during repeat surgery.

The reported cumulative patency rates for axillofemoral bypasses have varied from approximately 35 to 76% at 5 years.[10,11] This wide variation could point out the lack of standardization in the reporting of results. The former figure indicates the results obtained with a single operation, whereas the latter reflects the multiple repeat operations needed to maintain graft patency. We were first to call attention to this notable issue by distinguishing primary from secondary patency rates for axillounifemoral and axillobifemoral bypasses. In our experience, the 4-year primary patency rate for the unifemoral procedure was 44%, and it was 50% for the bifemoral (not statistically significant). Interestingly, an aggressive approach during repeat operations improved the results to 71% and 77%, respectively. Comparable limb-salvage rates were 73% and 89%, respectively.[9]

Recently, improved primary patency results (80% at 7 years) have been reported by Sauvage and colleagues,[12] using 8 mm externally supported Dacron grafts.

Failed Vs. Failing Grafts. Contrary to general belief, detection of hemodynamically compromised PTFE grafts due to an inflow or outflow stenosis before actual graft thrombosis is possible and preferable because it allows precise identification of the causative lesion.[13,14] Thus far, we have detected and treated 13 failing axillofemoral bypasses by percutaneous transluminal angioplasty (5 cases), a graft extension (6 cases), or a simple patch (2 cases). These procedures were easier to perform when compared to repeat operations on thrombosed grafts, since there was no propagation of clot into the patient's own arteries. More importantly, our patency results for failing PTFE grafts after a single intervention are strikingly superior to those obtained with repeat operations on grafts that had already thrombosed (81% vs. 33% at 2 years). Therefore, the reappearance of ischemic manifestations, diminished or absent graft pulse, or deterioration of noninvasive parameters is a signal that should alert one to obtain angiographic studies to detect a failing graft. The recent addition of duplex scanning as an integral part of postoperative graft surveillance has increased our ability to diagnose failing grafts and, in many cases, to distinguish a failing from an occluded graft. This differentiation is particularly useful in patients whose limbs are not threatened. Angiography may be avoided if the graft has failed and the limb is unthreatened, in which case repeat operation should not be undertaken. However, angiography is mandatory if the presence of a still-patent but failing graft is confirmed because treatment will be greatly simplified and far more effective if carried out before graft thrombosis occurs.

Complications. Axillofemoral bypasses have not been spared from any complication occurring with other prosthetic bypasses such as hematoma, seroma, and false aneurysm. Fortunately, these problems are rare (1 to 2%). The graft infection rate is approximately 1.5%, increasing to 2.7% after multiple repeat operations.[14] Injury to the brachial plexus, due either to direct trauma during exposure of the axillary artery or to excessive abduction of the arm, is also a rare occurrence.

Femorofemoral Bypasses

Although Freeman and Leeds[1] first described the cross-over femorofemoral bypass for unilateral iliac occlusive disease, it was Vetto, in 1962,[15] who popularized this concept by performing subcutaneous cross-over femorofemoral grafts in 10 patients with acceptable limb-salvage results. This short, suprapubic graft rapidly emerged as the least controversial of all extraanatomic bypasses, and several clinicians have since confirmed its long-term durability.

Indications
The long-term primary patency rates for cross-over femoral grafts are superior to those obtained with axillounifemoral reconstructions. Thus high-risk patients who are

initially seen with unilateral, limb-threatening ischemia due to iliofemoral occlusive disease should preferentially be treated by using the former procedure if the adequacy of the contralateral inflow system is confirmed by angiographic and hemodynamic criteria. For this same reason, one can broaden the indications for this operation by including better-risk patients and patients in whom the ischemic process results in disabling claudication alone.

Femorofemoral bypasses are a satisfactory option for patients who develop severe leg ischemia after transfemoral placement of an intraaortic counterpulsation balloon but who are too unstable to have it removed.[16] Simple crossover extension grafts can also be successfully performed in patients already subjected to unilateral aortofemoral or axillofemoral procedures who now have become symptomatic in the contralateral limb. Failed attempts at thrombectomy of a unilaterally occluded aortobifemoral graft also warrant placement of a cross-over femoral graft to avoid a difficult abdominal repeat operation.

Inflow Arteries
Concern has been raised regarding the possibility of impaired distal perfusion in the donor limb after placement of a femorofemoral bypass. However, experimental data published by Ehrenfeld and his colleagues[17] demonstrated that a *normal* donor artery, when challenged with an arteriovenous (AV) fistula, can deliver up to 10 times its resting flow rates without diverting blood away from the distal arterial segment ("steal" phenomenon). This physiologic adaptive response to an increased flow demand may be impaired in the presence of a narrowed inflow vessel. Therefore complete preoperative angiographic studies of the inflow and outflow tracts with biplane films are important to rule out obstructing lesions. In cases in which the donor artery is diffusely narrowed or if it harbors a stenosis more than 25% in diameter, the hemodynamic significance of these lesions should be assessed during angiography by measuring pressures across the lesion. Pressure gradients higher than 10 to 15 mm Hg indicate that it is a critical stenosis. When no pressure gradient is elicited at rest, yet the stenosis appears suspicious, an intraarterial injection of a peripheral vasodilator is warranted. It will challenge the stenosis by decreasing the outflow resistance and increasing flow rates. However, markedly diseased outflow vessels may mask the hemodynamic significance of an inflow lesion even when vasodilators are used. Therefore it is good practice to measure intraoperative pressures after the graft is in place and to be prepared to use an alternate inflow site when unacceptably high gradients are identified.

In some high-risk patients in whom critical stenoses of the inflow tract were detected (with or without pharmacologic manipulation), we have staged the performance of a percutaneous transluminal angioplasty followed by a crossover femoral graft in preference to an axillounifemoral bypass. Our experience with 35 of these tandem procedures is promising, yielding a 4-year graft patency rate of 68%.

Techniques
Although the cross-over femorofemoral bypass graft can be performed entirely with the patient under local anesthesia, we prefer to use light general anesthesia for the reasons

previously described. The operative technique for this procedure has not changed significantly since its description by Vetto.[15] We too prefer the inverted C configuration for a primary cross-over graft since we often extend the anastomosis into the deep femoral artery. Six-millimeter PTFE grafts have been used in all our cases, although it has been reported that Dacron grafts function equally well.

Both femoral arteries are exposed through standard longitudinal groin incisions and are connected via a suprapubic subcutaneous tunnel. Digital dissection should be used when creating the tunnel to prevent inadvertent penetration into the abdominal cavity or the bladder. It is important that the anastomosis of the graft to the low-pressure recipient femoral artery be carried out before its anastomosis to the donor artery. This preference is based on the observation that suture leakage in the graft may be significant under normal arterial pressure and anticoagulation. In this manner, not only is blood loss diminished, but the period of occlusion of the donor artery is minimized.

Generally, this operation is simple and can be expeditiously performed. At times, however, the femoral arteries may harbor a thick anterior plaque or may be heavily calcified. Because these two factors can significantly add to the complexity of the procedure, judicious technique should be used to ensure turbulence-free circulation into the outflow vessels. In these circumstances, ample exposure of the femoral artery and its bifurcation is necessary to permit adequate reconstruction of a possibly damaged lumen. Excessive tension should not be applied to the side branches because it may induce separation of the thickened plaque from the arterial wall. Also, one should not be tempted to perform a femoral endarterectomy since the disease process may extend well into the deep femoral artery, making appropriate repair difficult to accomplish. Instead, the edges of the plaque should be anchored to the arterial wall with interrupted U stitches, and the distal end of the graft should be tailored as a patch over this repair.

We have previously described our technique for overcoming circumferentially calcified arteries that cannot be occluded or entered with an ordinary scalpel or Potts scissors.[18] By partially fracturing the calcified artery with a hemostat clamp at 3 to 4 mm intervals, the artery is rendered suitable for occlusion, incision, and suture placement (Fig. 39-6). Intimal damage can occur in approximately 30% of the cases subjected to the fracture technique; however, adventitial perforation is uncommon. When careful repair of any existing intimal flap is undertaken, as shown in Figure 39-7, acceptable short-term and long-term results can be expected despite this seemingly traumatic approach.

If any question remains about the technical perfection of the bypass or if the preoperative angiogram has failed to demonstrate the runoff vessels at least to the knee level, a completion angiogram must be obtained. Intraoperative duplex scanning may also be helpful in ruling out technical defects, although at this point the angiogram continues to be the gold standard.

Results

Reports of operative mortality ranging from 2 to 15% reflect differences in patient populations rather than the complexity of the procedure.[10,19] Similarly, long-term patient survival has varied from 42 to 80% at 5 years.[10,19]

Although the graft-patency results published to date have not distinguished primary from secondary results, it is widely accepted that these operations are less likely to require multiple thrombectomies than axillofemoral bypasses. Our published 5-year graft-patency rate for femorofemoral bypasses is 83%.[20] However, others have found somewhat lower patency rates (70%).[19] Several factors could have influenced these differing results, including the indica-

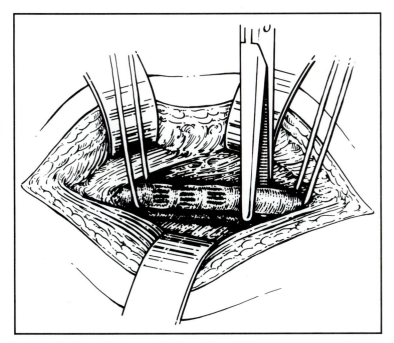

Figure 39-6. Fracture technique used with a calcified artery. The artery is partially fractured at 3 to 4 mm intervals with a hemostat clamp, allowing for occlusion, incision, and suture placement. (*From Ascer E, Veith F, et al.: Am J Surg 152:221, 1986.*)

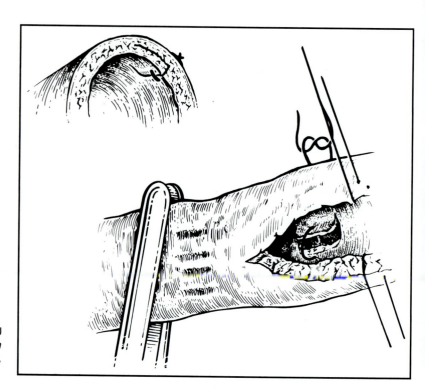

Figure 39-7. Placement of interrupted U stitches to tack down the intimal flap. (*From Ascer E, Veith F, et al.: Am J Surg 152:221, 1986.*)

tions for surgery (claudication vs. limb salvage), the morphology of the runoff vessels, the type and diameter of the graft and the surgeon's philosophy toward an aggressive repeat operation. Nevertheless, femorofemoral bypasses are now established procedures for limb salvage and disabling claudication.

EXTENDED EXTRAANATOMIC BYPASSES

The idea of crossing multiple joints with synthetic conduits crystalized with the reports of Smith and his colleagues (1977)[21] and Veith and his associates, 1978.[22] Until then the concept of extended extraanatomic bypasses was not applied, even though many patients with threatened limbs would not have been able to ambulate with a prosthesis after major primary or secondary amputations. The latter report demonstrated satisfactory early graft patency and limb-salvage results with axillopopliteal, cross-over axillopopliteal, and cross-over femoropopliteal bypasses that supported their continued use. Clearly, the advent of the PTFE graft played an important role in the successful outcome of these types of bypasses since its thrombotic threshold is higher than that of Dacron grafts.

Axillopopliteal Bypasses

The limb-salvage results obtained from using the axillary artery as an inflow site for standard extraanatomic bypasses in poor-risk patients were sufficiently good to motivate us to extend these procedures further—to the level of the knee or beyond.[22]

Over the last 12 years we have performed more than 60 straight axillopopliteal or sequential axillofemoral-popliteal bypasses using 6 mm PTFE grafts. A number of different bypass configurations were used to overcome the various complexities often encountered in these patients such as scarring due to multiple repeat operations, local infection, or marked arterial occlusive disease. We have not hesitated to perform cross-over bypasses or to use unusual approaches to the infrainguinal arteries. Often, it has been necessary to expose either the above-knee or below-knee popliteal arteries through a lateral, virginal approach to allow or facilitate the performance of an axillopopliteal bypass.[23] Furthermore, we have ventured to use, in six instances, one of the infrapopliteal vessels as a sequential bypass when the outflow from the popliteal artery was compromised by extensive disease.

Selection Criteria
Thus far, our criteria for selecting high-risk patients for axillopopliteal bypasses has included the following:

1. Severe atherosclerotic occlusive disease of the common, superficial, and deep femoral arteries
2. Failed aortofemoral bypass with disease progression into the deep femoral artery
3. Insufficient hemodynamic and clinical improvement after an axillofemoral bypass
4. Groin sepsis from a previously infected graft in patients in whom a standard obturator canal bypass was not possible because of multiple cardiac risk factors or morbid obesity

These procedures were limited to patients with limb-threatening ischemia.

Preoperative Evaluation

The same clinical and diagnostic protocol described previously for conventional extraanatomic bypasses is followed to prepare patients for the extended procedures.

Techniques

The basic principles regarding positioning of the patient on the operating table, type of anesthesia, exposure of the axillary artery, performance of the proximal anastomosis, and creation of the tunnel from the infraclavicular region to the lower abdomen remain similar to those described for axillofemoral bypasses.

The choice of the surgical access to the recipient arteries and the corresponding tunnelings depends on the presence or absence of infection or scar tissue. In primary, uncomplicated cases, the above-knee or below-knee popliteal arteries are exposed through standard medial approaches, and the tunnels follow an anatomic, subsartorial route.

When the ischemic limb is opposite to the axillary inflow site, a cross-over bypass operation is necessary. The graft should not be tunneled across the chest or the midabdomen because this route may complicate unanticipated abdominal or chest operations. Rather, the tunnel is formed from the axillary artery to the ipsilateral groin and is brought to the contralateral groin through a subcutaneous, suprapubic approach.

In cases of densely scarred or infected groins, the tunnel is created away from the area in question, even as far as lateral to the anterosuperior iliac spine, and then is carried subcutaneously, straight down to the level of the mid thigh where it is gradually curved toward the medial aspect of the lower thigh. At this level, the popliteal fossa is entered,

and the tunnel follows the anatomic route of the popliteal artery to the elected site of graft insertion.

Lateral Approach to the Popliteal Artery. When infection or previous multiple repeat operations make the standard medial approach to the popliteal artery not feasible, the popliteal artery can be safely reached through a lateral approach.

The lateral approach to the *above-knee popliteal artery* consists of a 7 to 10 cm lateral skin incision along the groove formed by the iliotibial tract muscle and the biceps femoris muscle at the lower third of the thigh (Fig. 39-8). This incision is deepened through the lateral intermuscular septum to allow entry into the popliteal space and isolation of the popliteal artery. Caution should be used not to injure the common peroneal nerve and adjacent veins (Fig. 39-9).

Lateral exposure of the *below-knee popliteal artery* is somewhat more complex than for the above-knee popliteal artery. A 10 to 12 cm skin incision is made over the lower border of the upper fibula (see Fig. 39-8). This incision is deepened through the subcutaneous tissue and superficial muscle attachments to the fibula, allowing identification of the common peroneal nerve as it traverses the neck of this bone (Fig. 39-10). Then the nerve is dissected free so it can be retracted and protected from harm, and the biceps femoris tendon is divided. The ligamentous attachments of the fibula head are incised, and the upper fourth of the fibula is bluntly freed from its muscular and ligamentous attachments, staying as close to the bone as possible. A retractor is placed deep to the fibula to protect underlying structures, and one or two holes are drilled in the bone at the selected site of transection. Through these holes, a rib shears can

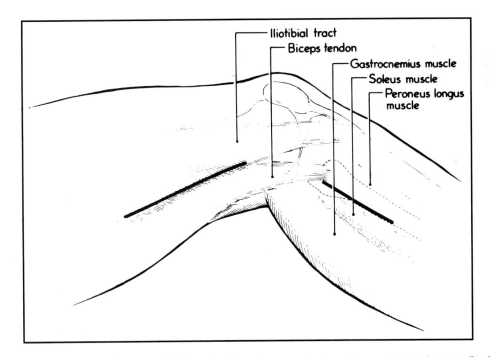

Figure 39-8. Incisions in lateral aspect of thigh and calf to gain access to above-knee and below-knee popliteal artery. *(From Veith F, Ascer E, et al.: J Vasc Surg 6:120, 1987.)*

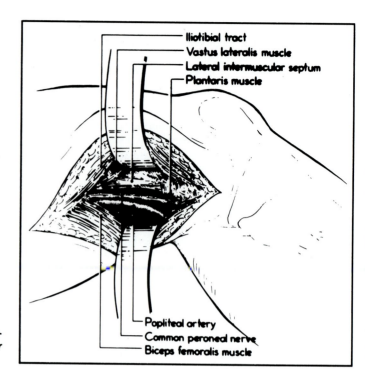

Figure 39-9. Lateral exposure of the above-knee popliteal artery. (*From Veith F, Ascer E, et al.: J Vasc Surg 6:121, 1987.*)

cleanly transect the bone without leaving sharp edges. With the upper fibula removed, the entire below-knee popliteal artery, tibioperoneal trunk, anterior tibial artery, and the orgins of the peroneal and posterior tibial arteries lie just deep to the excised bone and can easily be dissected from their adjacent veins (Fig. 39-11).

Tunnelings for bypasses performed through the lateral approach are preferentially constructed in a subcutaneous plane.

We now prefer to use externally supported prosthetic grafts for all our extended bypasses, particularly when the pathway of the graft is tortuous or is through scarred tissue.

Results

Operative Mortality. Despite a multitude of risk factors, the operative mortality (1 month) was only 6% in our reported series.[24]

Patency and Limb-Salvage Results. The cumulative patency rates for our initial 34 PTFE axillopopliteal bypasses

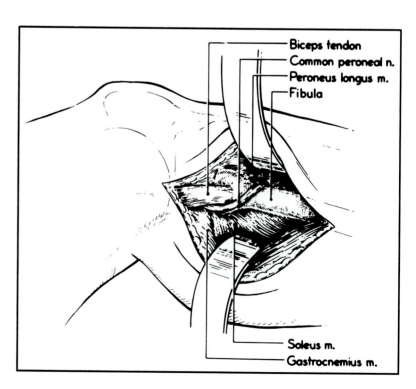

Figure 39-10. Lateral exposure of upper fourth of fibula before its resection. Note position of common peroneal nerve, which must be protected from injury. (*From Veith F, Ascer E, et al.: J Vasc Surg 6:122, 1987.*)

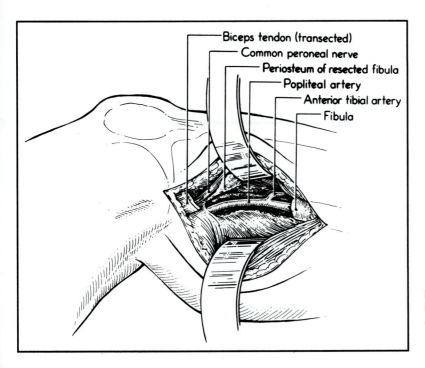

Figure 39-11. Lateral exposure of below-knee popliteal artery and its distal branches after removal of upper portion of fibula. (*From Veith F, Ascer E, et al.: J Vasc Surg 6:122, 1987.*)

Labels in figure:
- Biceps tendon (transected)
- Common peroneal nerve
- Periosteum of resected fibula
- Popliteal artery
- Anterior tibial artery
- Fibula

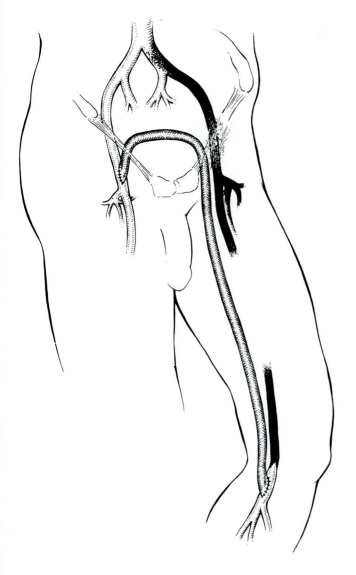

Figure 39-12. Cross-over femoropopliteal bypass in a high-risk patient in whom a standard procedure was not feasible because of extensive ipsilateral iliofemoral occlusive disease.

were 77% at 1 year, 51% at 3 years, and 45% at 5 years. Comparable limb-salvage rates were 86%, 57%, and 57%, respectively. It is of interest to note that the cumulative patient survival rate was approximately 50% at 3 years and that more than 80% of the patients who died during the remote postoperative period had intact limbs at the time of death.

Complications. Ten of the 34 limbs revascularized by axillopopliteal bypass required major amputation after graft thrombosis. In seven instances, this amputation was at the above-knee level and in three instances, at the below-knee level. Six of these patients were not deemed candidates for prosthetic rehabilitation and have been confined to a wheelchair.

No graft infection or any other major complication occurred in this series of cases.

Cross-over Femoropopliteal Bypasses

The contralateral femoral artery may be a suitable alternative for an inflow site whenever the ipsilateral femoral artery cannot be used because of severe occlusive disease or groin infection. Cross-over femoropopliteal or distal bypasses are appropriate options for the high-risk patient with threatened ischemic limbs in whom an aortic procedure is technically difficult or carries too high a morbidity or mortality rate.

Since our preliminary report describing our experience with this newer approach, we have preferentially used it instead of an axillopopliteal bypass. This rationale is based on the superior patency results generated by grafts originating from the femoral artery (femorofemoral bypasses) as compared to those from the axillary artery (axillofemoral bypasses).

Thus far, we have performed 28 cross-over femoropopliteal bypasses (Fig. 39-12), including seven extensions to infrapopliteal vessels. The 5-year cumulative patency rate for the entire series is 52%, with a comparable limb-salvage rate of 68%. The complication rate is small, and continued use of this type of extended approach to limb salvage is justified.

REFERENCES

1. Freeman NE, Leeds FH: Operations on large arteries. Calif Med 77:229, 1952.
2. Kunlin J: Le traitement de l'arterite obliterante par la greffe veineuse. Arch Mal Coeur 42:371, 1949.
3. Lewis CD: A subclavian artery as a means of blood supply to the lower half of the body. Br J Surg 48:574, 1961.
4. Blaisdell FW, Hall AD: Axillary-femoral artery bypass for lower extremity ischemia. Surgery 54:563, 1963.
5. Louw JH: The treatment of combined aorto-iliac and femoro-popliteal occlusive disease by spleno-femoral and axillo-femoral bypass grafts. Surgery 55:387, 1964.
6. Sauvage LR, Wood SJ: Unilateral axillary bilateral femoral bifurcation graft: A procedure for the poor risk patient with aortoiliac disease. Surgery 60:573, 1966.
7. Ray LI, O'Connor JB, et al.: Axillofemoral bypass: A critical reappraisal of its role in the management of aortoiliac occlusive disease. Am J Surg 138:117, 1979.
8. Logerfo FW, Johnson WC, et al.: A comparison of the late patency rates of axillo-bilateral femoral and axillo-unilateral femoral grafts. Surgery 81:33, 1977.
9. Ascer E, Veith FJ, et al.: Comparison of axillounifemoral and axillobifemoral bypass operations. Surgery 97:169, 1985.
10. Eugene J, Goldstone J, Moore WS: Fifteen year experience with subcutaneous bypass grafts for lower extremity ischemia. Ann Surg 186:177, 1977.
11. Johnson WC, Logerfo FW, et al.: Is axillo-bilateral femoral graft an effective substitute for aortic-bilateral iliac/femoral graft? Ann Surg 186:123, 1977.
12. Schultz G, Sauvage L, et al.: Five to 7 year experience with externally supported dacron prosthesis in axillofemoral and femoral-popliteal bypasses. Ann Vasc Surg 1:214, 1986.
13. Veith FJ, Weiser RK, et al.: Diagnosis and management of failing lower extremity arterial reconstructions prior to graft occlusion. J Cardiovasc Surg 25:381, 1984.
14. Ascer E, Collier P, et al.: Reoperation for polytetrafluoroethylene bypass failure: The importance of distal outflow site and operative technique in determining outcome. J Vasc Surg 5:298, 1987.
15. Vetto RM: The treatment of unilateral iliac artery obstruction with a transabdominal, subcutaneous, femoro-femoral graft. Surgery 52:342, 1962.
16. Alpert J, Goldenkranz R, et al.: Limb ischemia during intra-aortic balloon pumping. Indication for femorofemoral crossover graft. J Thorac Cardiovasc Surg 79:729, 1980.
17. Ehrenfeld WK, Harris JD, Wylie EJ: Vascular "steal" phenomenon. An experimental study. Am J Surg 116:192, 1968.
18. Ascer E, Veith FJ, White Flores SA: Infrapopliteal bypasses to heavily calcified rock-like arteries. Management and results. Am J Surg 152:220, 1986.
19. Brief DK, Brener BJ: Extraanatomic bypasses, in Wilson S, Veith FJ, et al. (eds): Vascular Surgery. Principles and Practice. New York, McGraw-Hill Book Co, 1987, p 414.
20. Ascer E, Veith FJ, et al.: Six year experience with expanded polytetrafluoroethylene arterial grafts for limb salvage. J Cardiovasc Surg 26:468, 1985.
21. Smith RB, Perdue GD, et al.: Management of the infected aorto-femoral prosthesis including use of an axillopopliteal bypass. Am Surg 43:65, 1977.
22. Veith FJ, Moss CM, et al.: New approaches to limb salvage by extended extra-anatomic bypasses and prosthetic reconstructions to foot arteries. Surgery 84:764, 1978.
23. Veith FJ, Ascer E, et al.: Lateral approach to the popliteal artery. J Vasc Surg 6:119, 1987.
24. Gupta SK, Veith FJ, et al.: Five year experience with axillopopliteal bypasses for limb salvage. J Cardiovasc Surg 26:321, 1985.

CHAPTER 40
Bypass Grafts Using the Obturator Foramen

Robert A. Schwartz and Arthur E. Baue

The groin is the most common site of infection after arterial reconstructive surgery. Such infection usually requires removal of the involved segment of the graft and a revascularization procedure in a new clean area if both the patient's life and limb are to be salvaged. When faced with such a problem some years ago, we considered the possibility of creating a tunnel through the obturator foramen so that a new graft could be inserted in the retroperitoneal area from a point proximal to the infection and brought into the thigh through a clean incision and field to the distal uninvolved artery. The infected segment of the graft could then be removed from the groin. This approach was successfully used in two of the first three patients so treated.[1]

Since the initial description of the operative procedure, other surgeons have been able to apply the technique to a variety of clinical situations in which the common femoral artery was unsuitable for bypass:

1. Mycotic aneurysms involving the femoral artery[2]
2. An extensive suppurative epidermoid carcinoma involving the groin[3]
3. Infected prosthetic graft material in the groin[2,4-6]
4. A therapeutic radiation-induced femoral aneurysm[7]
5. Bacterial arteritis of the femoral artery[8]
6. Complex vascular reconstruction in which groin dissection would be hazardous[9]

The long-term patency rates for obturator bypass have been encouraging. Van Det and Brands[9] performed the procedure in 13 individuals and had an 80% cumulative patency rate at 6 years. In their review of the 79 reported cases, satisfactory outcomes occurred in 66 patients.

The complications of the procedure are noteworthy as well. The occurrence of obturator vein injury can be difficult to control. Avoidance of the obturator vessels by precise dissection and localization of the vessels is essential. Inadvertent perforation of the bladder has been remedied by partial bladder retraction.[10] Graft damage and subsequent pseudoaneurysm formation have occurred when the graft is injured in the tunneling process. This can usually be avoided by using tunneling devices that put a minimum of torque on the graft material.

Thus the obturator foramen bypass technique has been demonstrated to be a feasible alternative for bypass grafting from the iliac or aortic vessels to the femoral or popliteal vessels when the groin and femoral triangle are unsuitable for this purpose.

INDICATIONS

A bypass graft through the obturator foramen may be helpful or necessary whenever it would be hazardous or impossible to bring the graft beneath the inguinal ligament and into the groin to revascularize the leg. Specific indications are as follows:

1. Localized infection in the groin segment of a previously placed graft that extends from the aorta to the femoral artery. Such an infection requires removal of this segment of the graft to prevent fatal bleeding from the distal anastomosis that will eventually occur. If the graft is patent, the infection may remain localized in the groin and not ascend the graft. The proximal uninfected segment of the graft above the inguinal ligament can then be used to revascularize the leg by a new segment attached to it and brought through the obturator foramen. If, however, the graft is infected in the groin and is thrombosed, the ascending infection that usually occurs will necessitate removal of the entire graft. (See Chapter 43.)
2. Infection in the femoral region of a femoropopliteal bypass graft, particularly if the graft is of prosthetic material. In such a situation the leg may be salvaged by placing a graft in a clean field from the iliac artery through the obturator foramen to the popliteal artery or to the distal uninvolved segment of the graft, followed by removal of the septic graft in the groin.
3. Extensive tissue and vessel injury in the groin, for which

vascular repair must be carried out with insufficient healthy or clean muscle and skin to cover the repair or assure a clean closed wound.

4. Mycotic aneurysms of the femoral artery.
5. Radiation necrosis of the groin when vascular damage has occurred.
6. Neoplasms involving the groin and the femoral vessels that require an extensive en bloc resection.
7. Carcinoma-induced ulceration involving the femoral vessels.
8. Infected, injured, or exposed femoral vessels caused by ischemia of skin flaps in the groin, as might occur after groin dissection.
9. Revascularization of the leg necessitated by septic lesions of the foot and suppurative lymphadenopathy in the groin.
10. Septic false aneurysms occurring after cannulation or catheterization of the femoral artery.

TECHNIQUE

If the problem in the groin for which an obturator bypass is to be carried out requires attention, particularly when there has been threatening hemorrhage from an infected graft, this is attended to first. Hemorrhage should be controlled by adequate packing if this is satisfactory, by temporary suturing of anastomotic leaks, or, as a last resort, by vessel or graft occlusion. Then, with the patient in the supine position, the groin wound is carefully covered and excluded from the field. Occlusive plastic drapes are ideal for this purpose. Then a clean instrument pack and drapes are used to prepare and drape the abdomen and leg.

An abdominal incision is made initially (Fig. 40-1). Adequate exposure is best obtained by a right paramedian incision with retraction of the rectus muscle laterally. A transverse lower abdominal incision can be used, but exposure is not as good. If it is necessary to expose only the iliac vessels or a patent graft coming down from the aorta and the obturator fossa, this exposure can be accomplished easily by reflection of the peritoneum. If the aorta must be approached, a transperitoneal approach is best. The iliac vessels are exposed initially (Fig. 40-2). If there is a graft coming from the aorta as an aortofemoral prosthesis, the prosthesis is next exposed, and it is determined whether the septic process in the groin, if such has been the case, has extended proximally to this level. The absence of infection in this region is confirmed by the presence of adequate incorporation of the prosthesis by the surrounding tissue and overlying peritoneum without induration, edema, or purulence. If this limb of the graft is occluded and there is infection in the groin, it is best to assume that organisms have already ascended the graft and that the entire graft is infected and must be removed. If there has been no previous retroperitoneal graft, the common iliac artery or aorta is selected for the proximal anastomosis. These vessels are mobilized, and umbilical tapes are placed around them (see Fig. 40-2). When there is minimal iliac arteriosclerotic disease, the common iliac artery can serve well for the proximal anastomosis. The ureter is mobilized and retracted

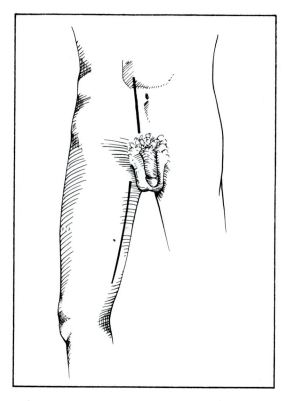

Figure 40-1. Incisions for an obturator foramen bypass graft: a right paramedian incision to expose the aorta and iliac vessels and a posterior-medial incision in the thigh to expose the distal vessels.

to a safe location. The obturator foramen is then located. The obturator fossa is posterior to the superior pubic ramus, and the obturator artery, vein, and nerve pass through it. These vessels and the nerve can and should be visualized (Fig. 40-3).

The origin of the obturator artery is most commonly from the internal iliac artery and can usually be identified coursing downward to the foramen. On occasion, this artery arises from the inferior epigastric artery, and in this situation it may course directly posterior from the inferior epigastric artery over the superior ramus of the pubis down to the obturator foramen. The exact location of the obturator foramen can be determined by following the course of the obturator artery and nerve and by palpation. The nerve, artery, and vein pass through the superior part of the obturator membrane in close apposition to the bony ridge forming the lateral superior margin of the obturator canal. The ventral edge of the obturator fossa is formed by the superior ramus of the pubis, and in this location the vas deferens crosses the pubic ramus.

After exposure of the obturator fossa and determination of its landmarks, an incision is made in the leg to approach the obturator foramen from below. A posterior medial incision is made in the proximal portion of the thigh (see Fig. 40-1). This incision is kept well behind the groin and its septic contents. Exposure and dissection in the thigh are facilitated by placing the leg in a position of slight flexion at the hip and by external rotation. The adductor longus

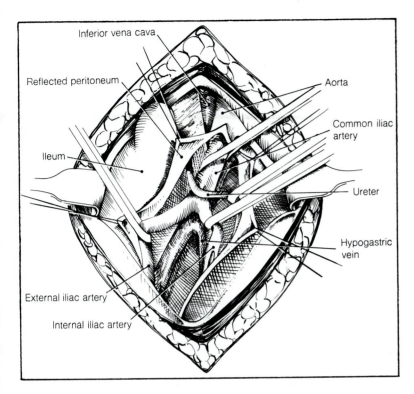

Figure 40-2. Common, external, and internal iliac arteries are exposed in the right lower quadrant for the proximal anastomosis. If there has been a previous graft, it may be used if patent and not infected. This figure illustrates the transperitoneal approach to these vessels.

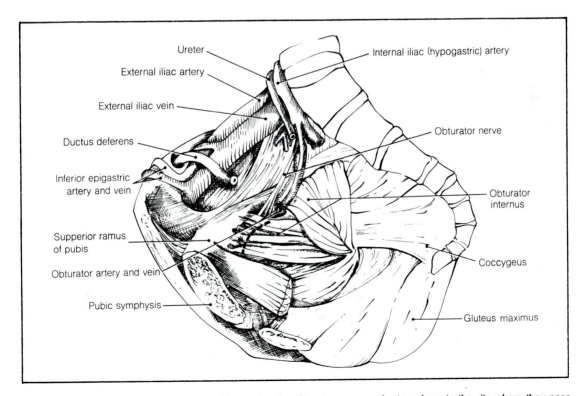

Figure 40-3. The obturator fossa is located by tracing the obturator nerve and artery down to the site where they pass through the foramen just behind the superior ramus of the pubis. The tunnel through the foramen is begun by blunt dissection through the obturator internus muscle medial to the nerve and artery (*dotted line*).

muscle is exposed and retracted laterally, entering the deep space between the adductor longus and the gracilis muscles. The adductor brevis muscle is exposed, and the obturator nerve may be seen lying on this muscle. Blunt finger dissection upward between the adductor longus and brevis muscles will lead to the obturator externus muscle, which covers the inferior aspect of the obturator foramen. Care must be taken not to dissect anterior to the adductor longus muscle, or one will enter the femoral triangle from the medial aspect and contaminate the field.

The obturator foramen is covered below by the obturator externus muscle. Inside the pelvis the foramen is covered by the obturator internus muscle. The tunnel through the foramen should be made some distance from the point through which the obturator vessels and nerve pass to prevent injury to these vessels. This is best done in the extreme anteromedial portion of the foramen or medial and inferior to the vessels (see Fig. 40-3). The inferiorly placed fleshy part of the obturator internus muscle is avoided. After blunt dissection through the obturator internus muscle, an aponeurotic membrane is encountered. The obturator membrane, the tough fascial wall of the foramen, is actually a dense aponeurotic fascia of the muscles and lies between them. It is necessary to incise this membrane by sharp dissection rather than by trying to break through it with a finger (Fig. 40-4). After incision of the membrane, a long sponge forceps, uterine forceps, or preferably a vascular tunneling instrument can be passed through the membrane and, by blunt dissection through the obturator externus, inserted into the thigh incision (Fig. 40-5).

The best site for exposure of the distal vessels—the superficial femoral or the popliteal artery—depends on the patient's disease process. If the superficial femoral artery is patent below the femoral triangle, the thigh incision can be extended inferiorly, and the superficial femoral artery can be exposed from the same incision medial and inferior to the sartorius muscle. Although it is possible to reach the superficial femoral artery by tunneling through the substance of the adductor longus muscle, it is preferable to go farther down the leg to the adductor canal. If the infection in the groin extends along the superficial femoral artery beyond the femoral triangle, this approach must be avoided. If dissected downward, the plane between the adductor longus and brevis will extend to the anterior surface of the adductor magnus and to the more familiar territory of the adductor canal and the superficial femoral artery (Figs. 40-5 and 40-6). The vessel is exposed and mobilized. A graft can then be brought from the pelvic vessels to this location through the obturator foramen tunnel.

If the superficial femoral artery is obstructed or badly diseased, the distal anastomosis should be carried out in the popliteal artery below the adductor canal. Although it is possible to expose the profunda femoris artery through this incision by dissecting medially between the adductor longus and brevis muscles, whether the profunda femoris artery is to be used will depend on the particular patient's situation. If the problem is infection following an aortofemoral bypass graft and the distal anastomosis has been placed just proximal to the division of the common femoral artery into its superficial and deep branches, the profunda femoris artery at its origin will very likely be involved in the septic process, and exposing the vessel a few centimeters down-

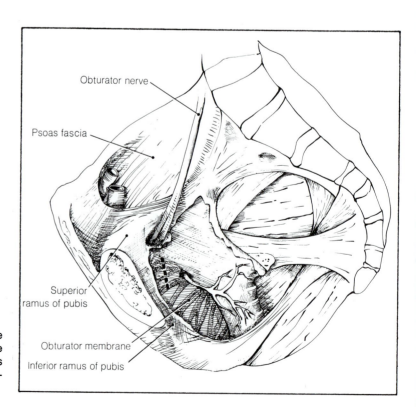

Figure 40-4. The tough obturator membrane is shown with the obturator internus muscle removed. The incision in the membrane is made anteromedially, well away from the obturator nerve, artery, and vein.

Obturator nerve

Psoas fascia

Superior
ramus of pubis

Obturator membrane

Inferior ramus of pubis

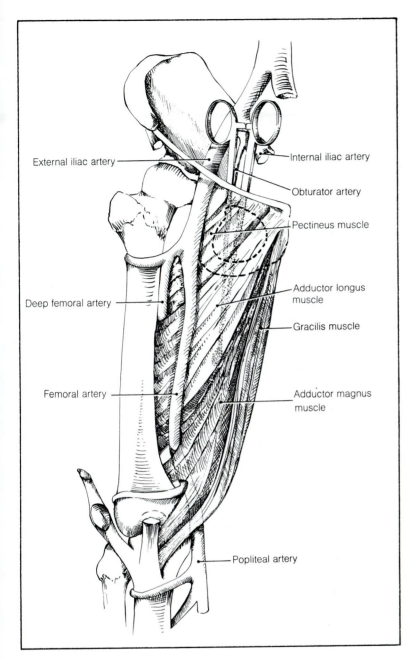

External iliac artery

Internal iliac artery

Obturator artery

Pectineus muscle

Deep femoral artery

Adductor longus muscle

Gracilis muscle

Femoral artery

Adductor magnus muscle

Popliteal artery

Figure 40-5. The tunnel through the obturator foramen into the thigh is completed after blunt dissection through the obturator internus, incision of the obturator membrane, and passage of a sponge forceps or tunneling instrument into the thigh deep to the adductor longus muscle. Continuation of the tunnel below the lower edge of the adductor longus muscle will lead to the adductor magnus muscle and the adductor canal for exposure of the superficial femoral artery. If the tunnel is carried through the adductor magnus muscle, the popliteal space will be entered.

ward would result in contamination of the new graft. If, however, the proximal anastomosis were placed more proximally in the common femoral artery and in the original dissection the profunda femoris and superficial femoral arteries were not exposed, then the profunda femoris artery could possibly be mobilized without entering the septic area and could be used for the distal anastomosis in a patient with an obstructed superficial femoral artery who also has severe popliteal arterial disease. This procedure is technically more difficult, however, and it is best to use the distal superficial femoral or popliteal artery whenever possible. If it is necessary to extend the graft distally to the popliteal artery, it is preferable to use a vein graft from the other

leg since long-term patency will be better than if a cloth or prosthetic graft is used.

Depending on the location of the distal anastomosis, a single incision or two incisions in the thigh may be used. A short upper-thigh incision to begin the tunnel may be combined with a lower-thigh incision to expose the adductor canal. If the popliteal artery is to be used, a second lower incision is preferable. Guida and Moore[8] described making a deeper tunnel through the thigh posterior to the adductor magnus muscle. The tunnel from the obturator foramen is extended by blunt dissection back through the adductor brevis and magnus muscles and then is continued down the thigh between the adductor magnus and the semimem-

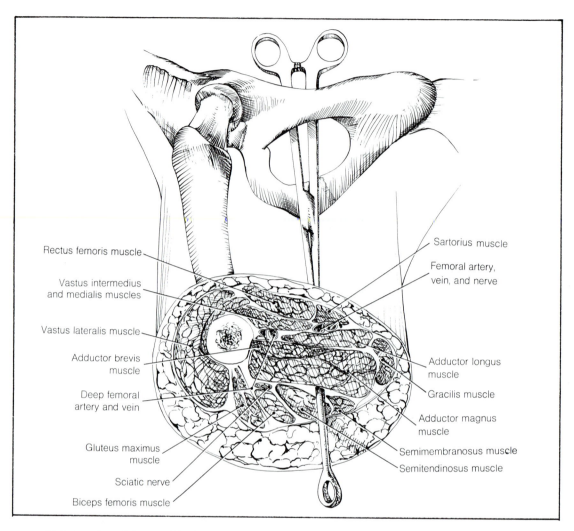

Figure 40-6. Location of the tunnel in the thigh is demonstrated in relationship to the other muscles and the femoral vessels. Usually the tunnel is made deep to the adductor longus and alongside the adductor brevis.

branosus and semitendinosus muscles to enter the popliteal space (Fig. 40-6). This approach avoids the adductor canal and should be considered if infection extends down the superficial femoral artery beyond the apex of the femoral canal.

If the patient has had a previous aortofemoral graft and the infection is indeed localized to the groin, the proximal limb of the graft on that side can be used. Following heparinization of the patient, the proximal graft in the retroperitoneal area is divided. The distal end is ligated; this divided distal end leading to the infected area is excluded from the operative site by suturing soft tissue and peritoneum over it. This procedure excludes it from the clean field and allows its removal later from the groin. Continuity can then be restored by an end-to-end anastomosis of a graft to the proximal limb of the prosthesis. This graft is then brought through the obturator tunnel to the distal femoral or popliteal artery (Fig. 40-7). Usually the distal anastomosis is constructed first. After restoration of flow, careful closure of the peritoneum around the iliac vessels

is carried out. The abdominal and clean thigh wounds are carefully closed and covered. The inguinal area can then be dealt with appropriately. If the problem is a septic graft, the defunctioned limb of the graft can be pulled down and removed, with closure of the femoral artery. This closure should be buttressed with viable tissue such as adjoining fascia, fascia lata, or sartorius muscle. The infected wound is then debrided extensively and packed open or drained. Appropriate antibiotics are continued. Wound care is continued until the groin wound has healed.

CONCLUSIONS

The indications and technique for arterial bypass grafting through the obturator foramen have been described. This approach is useful whenever a graft from the aorta or iliac vessels cannot be brought to the leg through the groin and into the femoral triangle because of infection, tissue necrosis, or injury in the inguinal region.

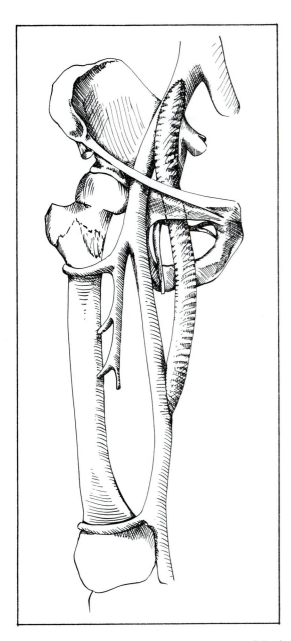

Figure 40-7. Completed obturator foramen bypass graft is shown with the proximal anastomosis to the common iliac artery and the distal anastomosis to the superficial femoral artery in the adductor canal.

REFERENCES

1. Shaw RS, Baue AE: Management of sepsis complicating arterial reconstructive surgery. Surgery 53:75, 1962.
2. Mahoney WD, Whelan TJ: Use of the obturator foramen in iliofemoral artery grafting. Ann Surg 163:215, 1966.
3. Donahoe PK, Froio RA, Nabseth DC: Obturator bypass graft in radical excision of inguinal neoplasm. Ann Surg 166:147, 1967.
4. Mentha C, Launois B, and DeLaere J: Les pontages artieriels iliofemoraux par le trou obturateur. J Chir (Paris) 90:131, 1965.
5. DePalma RG, Hubay CA: Arterial bypass via the obturator foramen. Am J Surg 115:323, 1968.
6. Rudlech M, Gutierrez IZ, Gage AA: Obturator foramen bypass in the management of infected vascular prosthesis. Am J Surg 137:657, 1979.
7. Hegarty JC, Linton PC, McSweeney ED: Revascularization of the lower extremity through the obturator canal. Arch Surg 98:35, 1969.
8. Guida PM, Moore SW: Obturator bypass technique. Surg Gynecol Obstet 128:1307, 1969.
9. Van Det RJ, Brands LC: The obturator foramen bypass: An alternative procedure in iliofemoral artery revascularization. Surgery 89:543, 1981.
10. Sheiner NM, Sigman H, Stilman A: An unusual complication of obturator foramen arterial bypass. J Cardiovasc Surg 10:324, 1969.

CHAPTER 41
Reconstruction of the Profunda Femoris Artery

Henry Haimovici

In the presence of occlusive disease of the superficial femoral artery, the profunda femoris artery (PFA) plays the chief role of collateral channel between the iliac and popliteal arterial systems. Clinical and angiographic data have provided direct and abundant evidence of this significant fact.

Ischemia, both chronic and acute, of the lower extremity, whether due to aortoiliac or femoropopliteal disease, can often be managed only by increasing arterial pressure and flow through this artery. Under these circumstances the profunda femoris is truly the artery of "revascularization" of the leg and foot. Its reconstruction, whether isolated or combined with other procedures, has played an increasing role in the management of occlusive arterial disease of the lower extremity ever since it was emphasized in 1961 by Leeds and Gilfillan[1] and Morris, Edwards, and associates[2] and later by others.[3–7]

SURGICAL ANATOMY

The profunda femoris artery (Fig. 41-1) is a division branch of the common femoral artery and originates usually 3 to 5 cm below the inguinal ligament. Its takeoff from the common femoral artery is, however, variable. In 50% of cases, it is found 3.5 to 5.0 cm below the ligament; in 24%, 5.0 to 8.5 cm below the ligament; and in 25%, under the ligament or above.[7] The PFA, whose caliber at its origin is somewhat less than that of the superficial femoral artery, arises from the lateral and posterior aspect of the common femoral artery. At first it lies lateral to it and then runs behind it and the femoral vein, coursing toward the medial side of the femur. It then passes downward behind the adductor longus muscle, ending at the lower third of the thigh in a branch which pierces the adductor magnus muscle.

Branches of Profunda Femoris Artery

The lateral femoral circumflex artery arises from the lateral side of the PFA, passes horizontally between the divisions of the femoral nerve and behind the sartorius and rectus femoris, and divides into ascending, transverse, and descending branches (see Fig. 41-1). The ascending branch passes upward to the lateral aspect of the hip, the transverse branch passes laterally over the vastus intermedius and thence around the femur, and the descending branch runs downward behind the rectus femoris. One long branch of the latter descends in the muscle as far as the knee and anastomoses with the superior lateral genicular branch of the popliteal artery. This descending branch, often called the artery of the quadriceps, plays a significant role in the anastomotic network of the thigh.

The medial femoral circumflex artery arises most often from the origin of the PFA, although in 25% of the cases it may arise from the posterior aspect of the common femoral artery proximal to the origin of the PFA. It usually winds around the medial side of the femur, passing between the pectineus and psoas major.

The perforating arteries, usually three in number, pass backward, close to the linea aspera of the femur by perforating the tendon of the adductor magnus, thus reaching the back of the thigh. The three perforating arteries give off branches joining with each other both in front of and behind the linea aspera. The termination of the profunda artery, already mentioned, is sometimes called the fourth perforating artery.

The PFA gives off numerous muscular branches for the adductors and the hamstrings. These muscular branches participate actively in the collateral networks of the profunda with the popliteal collaterals.

It should be pointed out that, when the origin of the PFA is under the inguinal ligament, it is the PFA that gives off all the branches that normally arise from the common femoral.

The branches of the PFA present the pivotal anastomotic pathways with those from the iliac above and popliteal below (see Fig. 41-1). The first perforating artery, which gives off branches to the adductors, biceps femoris, and gluteus maximus, provides anastomoses with the inferior gluteal, medial, and lateral circumflex femoral arteries and the second perforating artery. The latter provides anastomosis with the terminal branches of the profunda and the

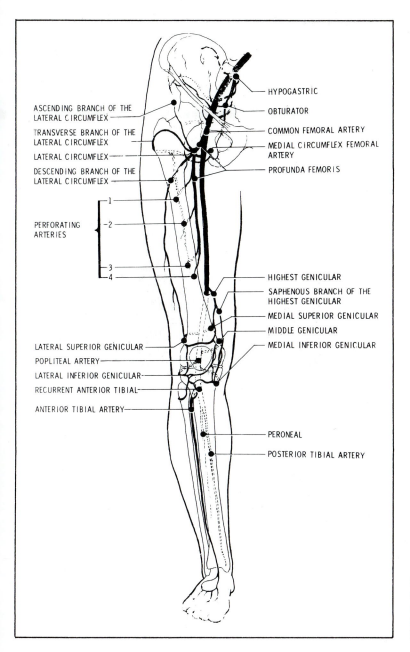

Figure 41-1. Arteries of the lower extremity, with special reference to the profunda femoris artery, its branches, and anastomotic pathways to the iliac and popliteal arteries.

muscular branches of the popliteal. Thus the various anastomoses provide an important chain that extends from the gluteal arteries above to the popliteal and tibial muscular branches below. When the superficial femoral or proximal popliteal artery is occluded, the PFA and its collateral branches enlarge and may transmit pulsatile flow distally. Indeed, this collateral circulation may be so effective that intermittent claudication may sometimes go unnoticed, especially in the presence of short segmental occlusions.

Relations of Profunda Femoris Artery

The PFA lies from above downward on the psoas and pectineus, then on the vastus medialis, adductor brevis, and the adductor magnus. In front, it is separated from the superficial femoral artery by the femoral and profunda veins above and by the adductor longus below. Laterally, the origin of the vastus medialis intervenes between it and the femur.

The PFA's relations with the satellite veins deserve a special mention. The profunda femoral vein in situated posteromedially to it and gives off two or three branches: the external circumflex and the quadriceps vein, which cross the origin of the PFA, often obscuring its origin (see Fig. 41-5). These branches must be divided to expose the PFA as well as some of the more distal branches that join the superficial femoral vein. Of note also are the lymphatic channels, which accompany the PFA and course along its branches to join the lymph nodes in Scarpa's triangle.

Angiographic Data

In contrast to the aortoiliac or femoropopliteal segments, the PFA is rarely involved with arteriosclerosis as an isolated lesion. It is usually associated with either an aortoiliac stenosis or a femoropopliteal segmental occlusion (Fig. 41-2). In a study of 321 femoral arteriograms carried out in 189 patients, I found arteriosclerotic changes of the PFA in approximately one third of the diabetic patients and in only 1 out of 10 nondiabetic patients (Fig. 41-3).[8] In a recent study, King et al.[9] confirmed the statistical significance of diabetes involvement of the PFA. In the former group of

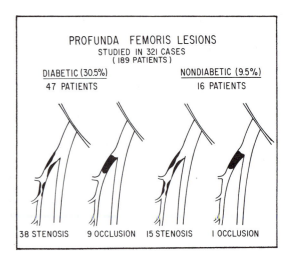

Figure 41-3. Distribution of lesions of the PFA in diabetic and nondiabetic patients.

47 patients, 38 had stenotic lesions involving not only the initial segment but also extending more distally to the first perforating branches and sometimes beyond, and nine cases exhibited complete occlusion least of the initial segment.[8] In contrast, out of 16 nondiabetic patients, 15 had stenotic lesions, and only one a complete occlusion. These data seem to indicate that the PFA is more often involved than the current literature would lead us to believe. Mavor,[10] in his series of 104 cases of arteriosclerotic nondiabetic patients, found the PFA free of disease in all instances. Lindbom[11] noted it in 4 out of 108 cases. In 1970 Frawley and Martin[12] reported PFA lesions in 59% of a series of 110 limbs, investigated by the arteriographic techniques of Beals et al.[13] The latter authors showed that the PFA is best visualized in the lateral projection rather than in the anteroposterior (Fig. 41-4). Using this technique, Martin et al.[14] further reported in 1972 that 77% of 230 patients had reconstructive surgery of the PFA or bypass of lesions proximal to its origin, and all but five had had occlusion of the femoropopliteal segment.

It should be pointed out that there is a significant difference between the diabetic and nondiabetic, the diabetic displaying a greater incidence and more severe lesions than the latter group.[8] This may account, in part, for the poor prognosis of arterial disease in the diabetic as compared with the nondiabetic.

METHODS OF EXPOSURE

Reconstruction of the PFA is indicated either as a sole operative procedure or more often in association with aortoiliac reconstruction or a variant of inflow-type surgery. Irrespective of the procedure or procedures involved in the reconstruction of the PFA, the methods of its exposure remain identical.

Although only the proximal segment of the PFA is involved in the majority of cases (74%), in a number of instances the lesions extend further distally to the second

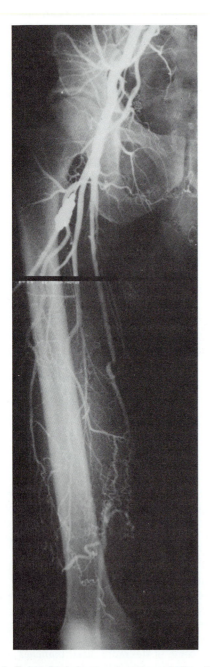

Figure 41-2. Femoral arteriogram showing occlusion of the distal superficial femoral and proximal popliteal arteries and collateralization through the profunda femoris artery (PFA).

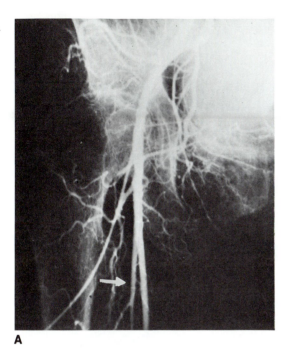
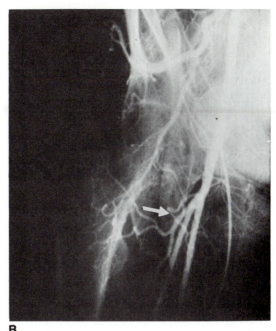

A   **B**

Figure 41-4. Femoral arteriogram. **A.** The PFA (*arrow*) is inadequately visualized in the anteroposterior projection. **B.** Lateral projection shows the profunda and its lateral circumflex branch (not visualized in **A**).

and sometimes the third perforating branches. In the latter case an extended surgical approach may be necessary.

Exposure of Proximal Profunda Femoris Artery

The patient is placed in the supine position with the thigh in slight external rotation and with the knee flexed and supported by a rolled sheet placed under it. The skin incision extends from slightly above the inguinal ligament downward along the course of the femoral vessels for about 15 to 20 cm, the direction of the incision being along the medial border of the sartorius, and slightly convex lateralward. The exposure (Fig. 41-5) is essentially that of a classic approach to the common and superficial femoral arteries. Because the PFA is lateral to the common femoral artery, the lymphoadipose tissue should be avoided to prevent injury to the lymphatics. It is essential to use electrocoagulation if lymphatics are being injured to avoid lymphorrhea postoperatively.

The common and superficial femoral arteries are exposed after opening the arterial sheath, and both of these vessels are retracted medially by means of Vesseloops (Med General, Minneapolis, Minn.). This procedure allows exposure of the origin and the initial course of the PFA.

A fibrous band that usually crosses the origin of the profunda should be carefully dissected and divided. At that point there is also a small vein that lies behind it, and it should be clamped before division of the fibrous band. In lifting up the origin of the PFA, care should be exercised not to injure the posteromedial circumflex artery, which often arises from the common femoral artery or from the PFA near its origin.

The dissection of the PFA is continued downward.

Usually two veins cross the anterior surface of its proximal segment (the lateral circumflex and quadricipital veins). Other veins may cross the artery more distally and should be dealt with similarly.

After division of these venae comitantes, the proximal branches of the PFA can be easily mobilized and placed under the protection of Vesseloops. The origin of the PFA is then freed circumferentially. One should bear in mind that at that point the posterior wall of the vessel is quite weak and injury may occur in its mobilization. The rent usually occurs in the posterior wall and becomes apparent only after releasing the occluding tapes of the common femoral artery.

More distal dissection of the PFA involves retraction of the muscular masses (the sartorius and rectus femoris laterally and the adductor longus medially). This retraction allows this more distal segment of the PFA with its three perforating branches to be exposed in the depths of the space between these muscles.

Exposure of Middle and Distal Profunda Femoris Artery

If exposure of the middle PFA is rendered difficult by the rectus femoris muscle or if the depth of the dissection renders the procedure difficult, use of an extended approach to this vessel is recommended. Hershey and Auer,[15] using the method described by Henry,[16] recommended the use of this approach. In this procedure, the incision begins medial to the anterosuperior iliac spine and extends inferiorly to the medial border of the patella. The deep fascia is divided, and the medial edges of the sartorius and rectus femoris muscles are mobilized and retracted laterally. In

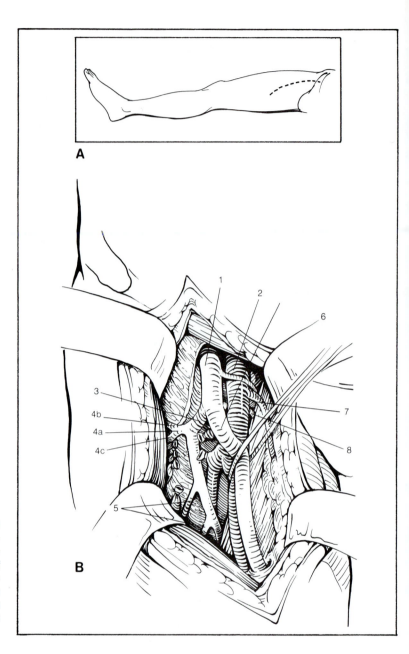

Figure 41-5. A. Exposure of the proximal and middle PFA through an anterolateral approach. **B.** Common femoral artery (*1*); common femoral vein (*2*); proximal segment of PFA (*3*); lateral circumflex trunk (*4a*), ascending branch (*4b*), descending branch (*4c*); first and second perforating branches (*5*); superficial femoral artery (*6*); saphenous vein (*7*); medial circumflex artery (*8*).

the lower portion of the dissection, which is carried out as in the proximal approach, the PFA and its satellite veins are parallel to the superficial femoral artery. In its lower part it passes behind the adductor longus muscle for about 3 to 5 cm. Its exposure at this point is facilitated by the division of these muscle fibers. The most distal portion of the PFA is close to the linea aspera, is covered by the dense insertions of the adductors, and is not accessible by this approach.[15,16]

OPERATIVE PROCEDURES AND INDICATIONS FOR PFA RECONSTRUCTION

The rationale for use of the PFA as a means of revascularizing the lower extremity is based on the well-known fact that in the presence of a segmental occlusion of the superfi-

cial femoral artery the increased blood flow through the PFA often offers enough inflow to the popliteal-tibial vessels that the limb is asymptomatic. However, this situation does not always prevail because the arteriosclerotic process is rarely localized and unifocal. In the presence of multiple arterial lesions, both proximally and distally, involving the PFA as well, reconstruction of the latter is often indicated.

Several operative procedures for PFA revascularization are available, depending on the type of associated lesions:

1. Endarterectomy as a sole procedure
2. Endarterectomy associated with a patch graft
3. PFA endarterectomy associated with inflow reconstructive procedures of the aortoiliac segment
4. In the presence of associated femoropopliteal lesions, reconstruction of the PFA alone or combined with additional revascularization of the distal arterial tree using a bypass graft

The operative procedures designed to achieve patency of the PFA are endarterectomy or thromboendarterectomy, either alone or associated with a patch graft. Figure 41-6 depicts the several possibilities in reconstructing the PFA. Figure 41-6A1 depicts a simple endarterectomy involving the junction between the PFA and the common femoral artery and involving only the initial portion of the PFA up to the level of the first branch. Figure 41-6A2 indicates the technique of the endarterectomy and the type of incision made for the procedure, extending from the common femoral artery to the initial segment of the PFA. Figure 41-6A3 indicates the completion of the procedure in which a patch graft was also used.

Figure 41-6B indicates involvement of the common femoral artery and the initial segment of the PFA. A broken line on Figure 41-6B1 indicates the area of the inflow, which

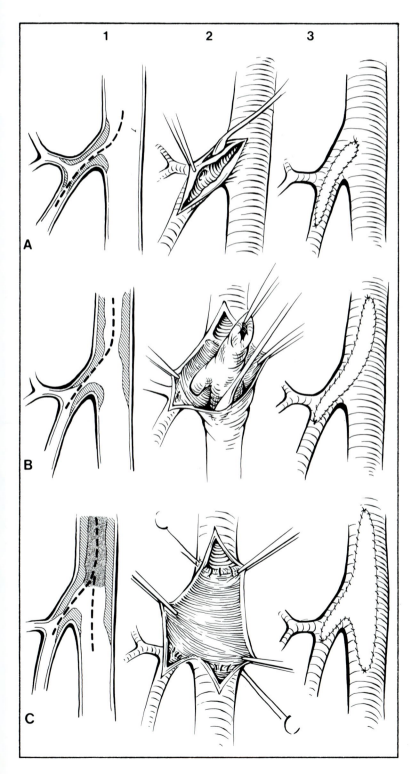

Figure 41-6. Isolated stenosing lesion. See text for details. (*Redrawn in part from Cormier JM: Chirurgie de l'artère fémorale profonde, in Techniques Chirurgicales. Paris, Encyclopédie Médico-Chirurgicale, 1969.*)

is decreased by the atherosclerotic lesions. Figure 41-6B2 shows the completion of the endarterectomy of the common femoral artery proximally and distally: the removal of the atherosclerotic lesion from the initial segment of the PFA and from the initial segment of the superficial femoral. Figure 41-6B3 indicates completion of this procedure in which a patch graft was inserted into the common femoral artery extending into the origin of the profunda.

Figure 41-6C indicates a complete occlusion of the common femoral artery and the initial segment of the PFA.

Figure 41-6C2 shows a completed endarterectomy and indicates the tacking down of the proximal edge of the intima with a few stitches to prevent any flap of this segment. Similarly, tacking with a few stitches was carried out in the distal area of the endarterectomized segment in the superficial femoral artery and in the area of the origin of the first branch and the initial segment of the PFA. Figure 41-6C3 indicates the completion of the procedure with a patch graft, which was used for the hockey-stick arteriotomy necessary in this case because of the presence of lesions,

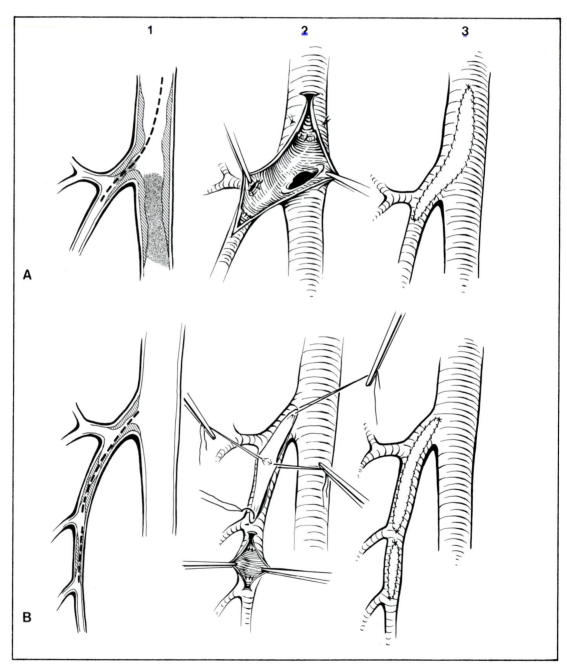

Figure 41-7. More advanced arterial lesion. See text for details. (*Redrawn in part from Cormier JM: Chirurgie de l'artère fémorale profonde, in Techniques Chirurgicales. Paris, Encyclopédie Médico-Chirurgicale, 1969.*)

not only in the initial segment of the PFA but in the initial area of the superficial femoral artery.

The lesions involving the PFA, although localized at the proximal segment in the majority of cases, are often associated with similar lesions of the adjacent common femoral and superficial femoral arteries. Essentially, five typical patterns of arteriosclerotic lesions involving the PFA and the bifurcation of the common femoral artery with its superficial femoral artery may be encountered as depicted in Figure 41-7. Figure 41-7A depicts a more advanced arterial lesion involving not only the common and profunda vessels, but also the proximal superficial femoral artery, which is completely occluded. Although Figure 41-7A indicates that an arteriotomy of the common and profunda vessels may be sufficient to complete the thromboendarterectomy of the superficial femoral artery, it is often necessary to extend the arteriotomy into the superficial femoral artery to ensure complete removal of the plaque and thrombus.

Figure 41-7B depicts a diffuse arteriosclerotic lesion of the PFA beyond the second perforating branch. The endarterectomy may be carried out either by a continuous arteriotomy or by two separate incisions with two separate patch grafts as indicated in Figure 41-7B. However, if the atheromatous lesions involve the entire length of the PFA, it is preferable to have a completely open vessel and continuous patch graft from end to end.

Complete occlusion of the superficial femoral artery with stenosing lesions of the common femoral and profunda femoris vessels are depicted in Figure 41-8A. If a femoropopliteal bypass is also contemplated, the arteriotomy from the common femoral artery to the PFA that was performed for the endarterectomy may be used for implantation of the vein graft into the common and profunda vessels as indicated in Figures 41-8B1 and 41-8B2. The distal anastomosis is carried out in the usual fashion into the popliteal artery.

If, in addition to the occlusion of the inflow tract and the superficial femoral artery, there is occlusion of the PFA, a different approach is indicated. Figure 41-9A depicts occlusion of the iliofemoral artery and aneurysmal dilatation of the common femoral artery, as well as complete occlusion of the superficial femoral artery. The possibility it would be necessary to reconstruct the PFA in the involved area would require a different type of procedure. In a case where the reconstruction of the PFA is obviously necessary, as in the presence of severe ischemia with imminent loss of limb, the modality for revascularizing the PFA would consist of excision of the common femoral aneurysm and, possibly, a femorofemoral bypass graft between the noninvolved femoral artery and the PFA after the ligation of the superficial femoral artery, excluding it from the field.

One of the most common PFA inflow reconstructive procedures is the aortofemoral bypass graft with endarterectomy of the PFA and possible reconstruction of the superficial femoral artery if the outflow is not sufficient to revascularize the leg and foot. Figure 41-10 shows diagrams of an aortofemoral bypass graft and an endarterectomy of the PFA.

Patch Graft Material

PFA reconstruction may require use of autogenous material provided by the saphenous vein or an endarterectomized segment of the superficial femoral artery. In 1966 Waibel[3] reported an autogenous reconstruction of the deep femoral artery in which he used the superficial femoral artery, which

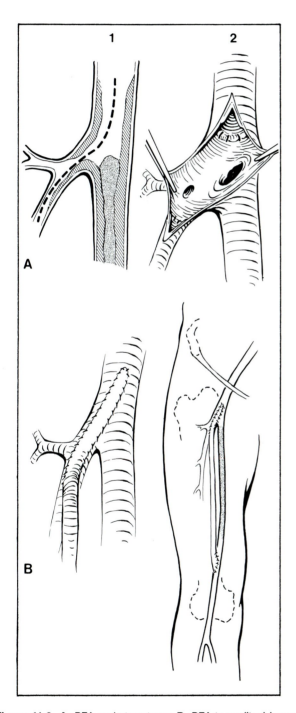

Figure 41-8. A. PFA endarterectomy. **B.** PFA-to-popliteal bypass graft. (*Redrawn in part from Cormier JM: Chirurgie de l'artère fémorale profonde, in Techniques Chirurgicales. Paris, Encyclopédie Médico-Chirurgicale, 1969.*)

had been occluded for patching the endarterectomized PFA. He used two modalities. One consisted of endarterectomy of the superficial femoral artery using the posterior wall resected up to the bifurcation. By this method, he used the autogenous arterial flap of the superficial femoral as a patch for the anterior portion of the open PFA. The other modality consisted of dividing the superficial femoral artery after endarterectomy had been carried out and using an end-to-side anastomosis with the PFA beyond its region. More recently, other surgeons have used the same technique but with some modification of the endarterectomy of the superficial femoral artery and its attachment to the open endarterectomized PFA.[17,18] Alternatives to extended profundaplasty, used by other surgeons include eversion endarterectomy of the superficial femoral and end to side anastomosis to the deep femoral artery. These are variants of the original techniques for providing a patch graft to the PFA to enlarge its diameter.

In summary, the various reconstruction modalities used to provide inflow to the PFA or through the PFA to the more distal portion of the arterial tree have largely been successful, as have reconstructions to correct associated lesions of the superficial femoral and proximal inflow tracts.

Embolism of Common Femoral and Profunda Femoris Arteries

Arterial embolism occurring in patients with preexisting arteriosclerosis is not unusual, especially during the sixth and seventh decades. As one might anticipate, this association may present special diagnostic and surgical problems. The clinical manifestations in these patients depend (1) on the site and extent of the arteriosclerotic occlusion and (2) on the effect that the embolic occlusion will exert on the collateral circulation. If the latter remains largely unaffected, additional manifestations may be mild or moderate. However, should the major collateral pathway be blocked by the embolus, its effect upon the viability of the limb may be disastrous without immediate intervention.

Fig. 41-11 is a diagram of the arterial tree of the right lower extremity, depicting an embolic occlusion of the PFA. The patient, a 74-year-old woman, was seen 8 hours after the acute onset of pain and cyanosis of the entire limb up to the upper third of the thigh. The common femoral pulse was easily palpable, the superficial femoral artery was known to be occluded from previous examination, and it appeared, therefore, that the PFA had been occluded by a recent embolus, the patient having had auricular fibrillation for a number of years. An embolectomy of the PFA through an arteriotomy in the common femoral artery promptly relieved all the ischemic manifestations, since it restored the patency to this vessel and vascularity to the rest of the limb.

In contrast to this case in which the PFA displayed only minimal intimal changes, often the latter vessel is markedly stenosed by large and extensive plaques. In such instances, in addition to the embolectomy, an endarterectomy of the PFA must be carried out to restore its patency since

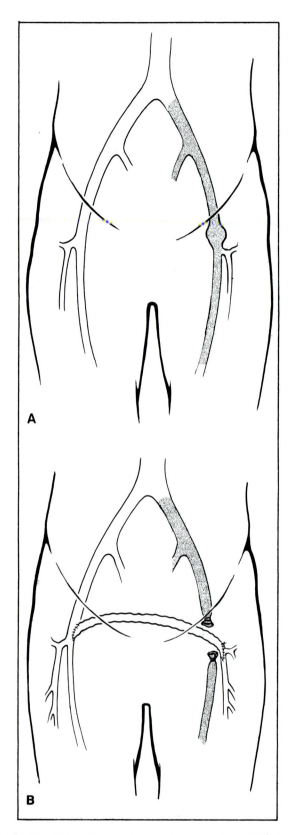

Figure 41-9. Femorofemoral crossover bypass graft for a left iliofemoral occlusion, using the PFA for limb revascularization. (*Redrawn in part from Cormier JM: Techniques Chirurgicales. Paris, Encyclopédie Médico-Chirurgicale, 1969.*)

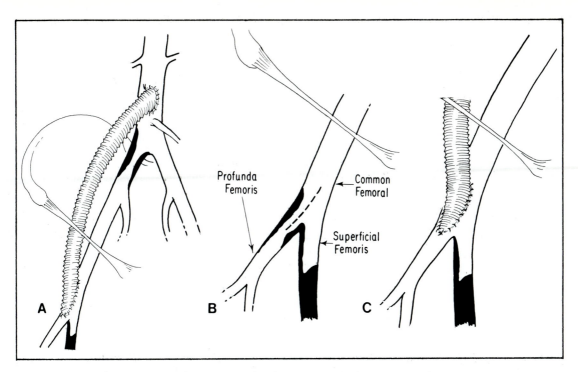

Figure 41-10. A. Aortofemoral bypass graft. **B.** and **C.** Endarterectomy of the PFA.

Profunda Femoris

Common Femoral

Superficial Femoris

A

B

C

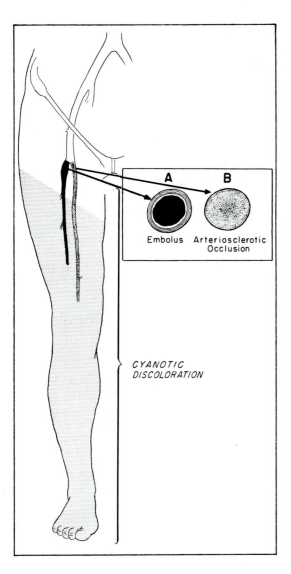

A

B

Embolus

Arteriosclerotic Occlusion

CYANOTIC DISCOLORATION

Figure 41-11. PFA embolectomy. See text for details.

the superficial femoral artery in such cases is completely occluded.

Aneurysms of Common Femoral Artery

Fig. 41-12A depicts an aneurysm of the common femoral artery with thrombosis extending into the origin of the PFA and into the superficial femoral artery, which is com-

pletely occluded. The reestablishment of flow into the PFA is achieved by partial excision of the common femoral artery and the initial segment of the PFA. The superficial femoral artery is transected and ligated. A patch graft is inserted on the common femoral artery and the initial segment of the PFA, thus providing continuity in the lumen between the common femoral artery and the PFA.

Fig. 41-12B indicates a more advanced occlusive process due to the extension of the thrombosis into the superficial

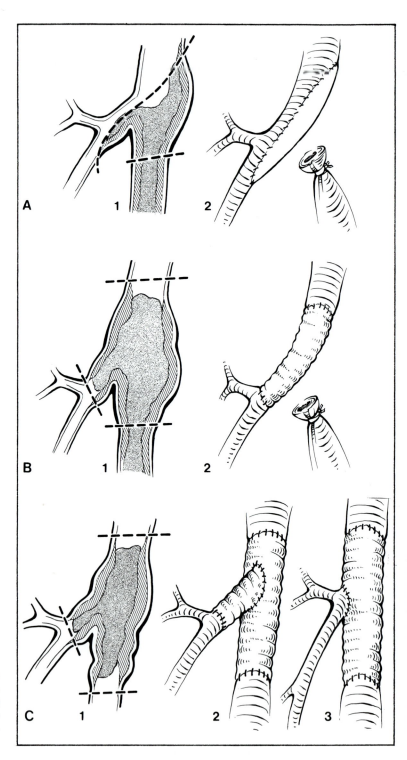

Figure 41-12. Methods of PFA revascularization in the presence of a thrombosed common femoral artery aneurysm. (*Redrawn in part from Cormier JM: Techniques Chirurgicales. Paris, Encyclopédie Médico-Chirurgicale, 1969.*)

and profunda femoral vessels. Flow between the common femoral artery and the PFA is achieved by interposing a tubular graft between the segments of these vessels. The superficial femoral artery is transected and ligated.

Fig. 41-12C, in which the superficial femoral artery is patent, the excision of the aneurysm is repaired by interposing a tubular graft between the common and the superficial femoral vessels. The PFA is reattached to the tubular graft either directly or by interposing a smaller tube between the two.

COMMENT

After completion of the reconstruction of the PFA, it is desirable in all instances to carry out an arteriogram to determine the quality of patency achieved. Since most cases of profundaplasty are combined with proximal reconstruction, the arteriographic evaluation should also include the inflow tract to avoid any possible postoperative complications.

When carried out with careful technique, profundaplasty not only may relieve rest pain and limit the tissue loss but also may often reestablish distal pulsations if the arterial tree distal to the popliteal is still unaffected. In properly selected patients, the overall results of this operation are gratifying, as indicated by several recent publications.

REFERENCES

1. Leeds FH, Gilfillan RS: Revascularization of the ischemic limb. Arch Surg 82:25, 1961.
2. Morris GC Jr, Edwards W, et al.: Surgical importance of the profunda femoris. Arch Surg 82:32, 1961.
3. Waibel PP: Autogenous reconstructions of the deep femoral artery. J Cardiovasc Surg 7:179, 1966.
4. Wesolowski SA, Martinez A, et al.: Indications for aortofemoral arterial reconstruction: A study of borderline risk patients. Surgery 60:288, 1966.
5. Strandness DE: Functional results after revascularization of the profunda femoris artery. Am J Surg 119:240, 1970.
6. Cohn LH, Trueblood W, et al.: Profunda femoris reconstruction in the treatment of femoropopliteal occlusive disease. Arch Surg 103:475, 1971.
7. Cormier JM: Chirurgie de l'artère fémorale profonde, in Techniques Chirurgicales. Paris, Encyclopédie Médico-Chirurgicale, 1969, sec. 43,070.
8. Haimovici H: Patterns of arteriosclerotic lesions of the lower extremity. Arch Surg 95:918, 1967.
9. King TA, DePalma RG, Rhodes RS: Diabetes mellitus and atherosclerotic involvement of the profunda femoris artery. Surg Gynecol Obstet 159:553, 1984.
10. Mavor GE: Pattern of occlusion in atheroma of lower limb arteries. Br J Surg 43:352, 1956.
11. Lindbom A: Arteriosclerosis and arterial thrombosis in lower limb. Acta Radiol 80(suppl):1950.
12. Frawley JE, Martin P: Quoted in reference 14.
13. Beals JSM, Adcock FA, et al.: The radiological assessment of disease of the profunda femoris artery. Br J Radiol 44:854, 1971.
14. Martin P, Frawley JE, et al.: On the surgery of atherosclerosis of the profunda femoris artery. Surgery 71:182, 1972.
15. Hershey FB, Auer AI: Extended surgical approach to the profunda femoris artery. Surg Gynecol Obstet 138:88, 1974.
16. Henry AK: Extensile Exposure, 2nd ed. Baltimore, The Williams & Wilkins Co, 1957, p 227.
17. Rollins DL, Towne JB, et al.: Endarterectomized superficial femoral artery as an arterial patch. Arch Surg 120:367, 1985.
18. Feldhaus RJ, Sterpetti AV, et al.: A technique for profunda femoris artery reconstruction: Hemodynamic assessment and functional results. Ann Surg 203(4):390, 1986.
19. Feldhaus RJ, Sterpetti AV, et al.: Eversion endarterectomy of the superficial femoral artery and end-to-side anastomosis to the deep femoral artery: An alternative to extended profundoplasty. Am J Surg 150:748, 1985.

CHAPTER 42
Popliteal Artery Entrapment Syndrome

George J. Collins

The clinical and anatomic features of popliteal artery entrapment were initially described in 1879 by T. P. Anderson Stuart while he was still a medical student in Edinburgh, Scotland.[1] However, almost a hundred years elapsed before Love and Whelan coined the phrase "popliteal artery entrapment syndrome."[2] Since then numerous descriptions of popliteal artery entrapment syndrome have appeared; entrapment of the popliteal artery is now widely recognized as one of the causes of intermittent claudication and threatened limb loss in young people. Popliteal artery entrapment syndrome is intriguing because it arises from a congenital anomaly that rarely produces symptoms until several years later in life. It rarely affects women and, in contrast to most arterial disorders, is not related to cigarette smoking. Clinically, popliteal artery entrapment syndrome closely resembles adventitial cystic disease of the popliteal artery.[3] Other disorders that must be considered in the differential diagnosis in a patient suspected of having popliteal artery entrapment syndrome are arteriosclerosis obliterans, Buerger's disease, nonvasculogenic claudication, compression of the distal superficial femoral artery as it exits the adductor canal,[4] and adventitial cystic disease of the popliteal artery.[3]

ETIOLOGY

Popliteal artery entrapment syndrome is caused by an abnormal relationship of the popliteal artery to the muscular structures around the knee. Whereas it is important to recognize that compression of the distal superficial femoral artery as it exits the adductor canal causes symptoms similar to those of popliteal artery entrapment,[4] the "adductor canal syndrome" is not formally included as one of the variants of popliteal artery entrapment syndrome. Rare cases have been reported in which both the popliteal artery and vein were entrapped.[5] Isolated cases of tibial nerve entrapment[6] and popliteal vein[7] entrapment have also been reported.

Although detailed classifications do exist and mixed variants occur,[8] one is better served by developing an understanding of the usual anatomic variants associated with popliteal artery entrapment than by attempting to memorize all of the variants that have been reported. One needs to have working knowledge of only four major variants.[9,10] These variants, described under anatomic considerations, are illustrated in Figure 42-1.

ANATOMIC CONSIDERATIONS

Normally the popliteal artery exits the adductor hiatus and courses downward and laterally toward the middle of the popliteal space to lie between the medial and lateral heads of the gastrocnemius muscle. The principal anatomic abnormalities that cause entrapment of the popliteal artery are as follows.

Type 1: The medial head of the gastrocnemius muscle arises normally (immediately above the medial femoral condyle), but the popliteal artery, instead of passing between the two heads of the gastrocnemius muscle, courses medial and deep to the medial head. The artery is grossly deviated in a medial direction and entrapped in its deep position beneath the medial head of the gastrocnemius muscle.

Type 2: The medial head of the gastrocnemius muscle arises more laterally than usual. The popliteal artery takes a relatively straight course downward but still passes medial and deep to the medial head of the gastrocnemius muscle.

Type 3: The popliteal artery also has a relatively straight course downward, but it is compressed as it courses medial and deep to an accessory slip of the medial head of the gastrocnemius muscle. This accessory slip of muscle arises more laterally than the major portion of the medial head of the gastrocnemius muscle.

Type 4: The popliteal artery descends in a relatively straight line but is compressed as it passes deep to the popliteus muscle or a fibrous band in the

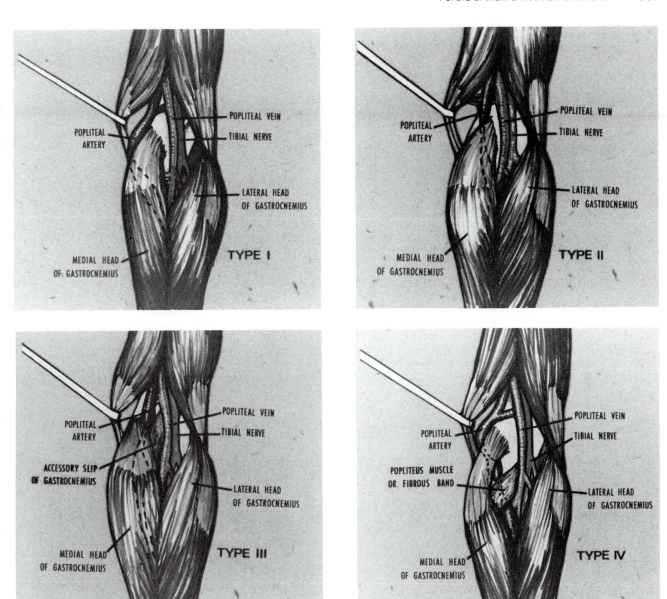

Figure 42-1. The four common variants of popliteal artery entrapment.

same location. In this variant, the artery may also lie medial and deep to the medial head of the gastrocnemius muscle as it does in the type 1 variant.

CLINICAL FEATURES AND DIAGNOSIS

Popliteal artery entrapment syndrome should be suspected in any young person who complains of intermittent claudication or who has developed an acute symptomatic occlusion of the popliteal artery. Popliteal artery entrapment syndrome is rare in patients younger than their teens and is equally rare in patients over 50 years of age. Most of the reported cases cluster in the under 30 age group. Peculiarly, symptomatic patients seem to have the sudden, rather than gradual, onset of intermittent claudication; symptoms are frequently brought on by some unusually strenuous type of physical activity. After symptoms of intermittent claudication begin, they are generally reproducible, as in patients with arteriosclerosis. Unusual features such as claudication while walking but not while running, claudication beginning immediately with the first steps, and claudication primarily involving the foot rather than the calf have been reported, but most patients with popliteal artery entrapment syndrome behave just as arteriosclerotic patients do, with claudication relating to the type and duration of exercise. Since the remainder of the vasculature is normal, the thigh and buttocks are spared in popliteal artery entrapment syndrome, with claudication confined to the calf and foot.

Some patients remain asymptomatic until they develop an acute occlusion of the popliteal artery or thromboembolic complications of a poststenotic popliteal artery aneurysm. When this occurs, it should be remembered that poststenotic dilatation and aneurysm formation are natural consequences of years of compression of the popliteal artery. In patients with acute complications, the usual signs and symptoms of ischemia including pain, pallor, paresthesias, paralysis, and poikilothermia develop. Since these signs and symptoms are nonspecific, only a high index of suspicion will lead to the diagnosis of popliteal artery entrapment syndrome in patients presenting with such findings.

Physical findings are nonspecific in patients with popliteal artery entrapment syndrome. Even in the type 1 variant, which represents the most extreme degree of arterial deviation occurring in this syndrome, the medial deviation of the artery cannot be discerned by physical examination, and patients who have not developed a complication usually have normal resting popliteal and pedal pulses. Loss of pedal pulses with active plantar flexion or passive dorsiflexion of the foot should arouse suspicion of the syndrome in symptomatic patients, but some normal individuals will also lose pulses with these maneuvers. Hyperabduction of the knee may also cause obliteration of pulses in patients with popliteal artery entrapment. The true value of this test is not known. A false negative test will occur if distal pulses have been reconstituted via collaterals in a patient with a total occlusion of the popliteal artery.

The above maneuvers tighten the gastrocnemius muscle, thereby reproducing the effects of exercise in patients who complain of intermittent claudication but have no symptoms or physical findings at rest. The finding of a popliteal artery aneurysm or the absence of pedal pulses in a relatively young person should raise suspicion of popliteal artery entrapment syndrome.

Treadmill examination with ankle/brachial pressure ratios before and after exercise is useful, as it further increases one's suspicion of the syndrome when positive and points to other diagnoses when negative. An extended treadmill test may be positive in young athletic patients even when a standard treadmill test is negative.[11] The standard treadmill test is performed over 3 minutes at 3 mph and no grade. The extended treadmill test is performed at 4.2 mph and a 10-degree grade. The test is continued until claudication occurs or is discontinued at 10 minutes in the absence of symptoms.

Contrast-enhanced computerized axial tomography has recently been reported as a useful adjunct in the diagnosis of popliteal artery entrapment.[12] However, there is limited experience with this technique and arteriography remains the gold standard for diagnosing popliteal artery entrapment syndrome. In almost all cases the arteriogram will provide enough supporting evidence that one can be confident of the diagnosis preoperatively. The most classic arteriographic abnormality is an exaggerated medial deviation of the artery as seen in the type 1 variant (Fig. 42-2).

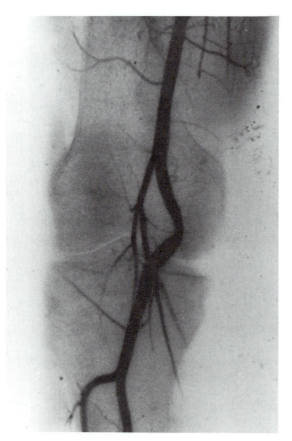

Figure 42-2. In the type 1 variant of popliteal artery entrapment syndrome, there is marked medial deviation of the popliteal artery.

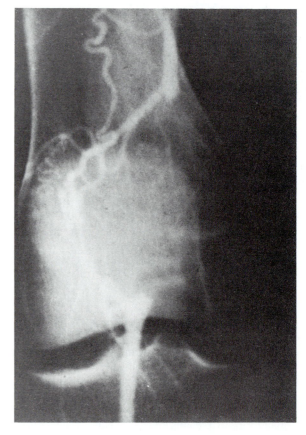

Figure 42-3. An example of occlusion of the midpopliteal artery with preservation of runoff via collaterals.

A lesser degree of medial deviation is seen in the type 2 variant. In some cases the artery will not be deviated at all, and other arteriographic signs must be used to confirm the diagnosis. Among these signs are poststenotic dilatation in an otherwise normal appearing artery, the presence of a popliteal artery aneurysm in a relatively young patient, and occlusion of the popliteal artery in its midportion (Fig. 42-3). Occlusion of the midportion of the popliteal artery is often accompanied by the development of large collaterals. The arteriographic study can be augmented with active plantar flexion and passive dorsiflexion views if the diagnosis is not apparent from routine views. If popliteal artery entrapment is present, these views may magnify subtle degrees of medial deviation. One or the other view (or both) may demonstrate a cutoff of contrast or narrowing of the contrast column at the level of popliteal artery entrapment (Fig. 42-4). Biplanar views are useful when standard anteroposterior views are nondiagnostic. Both lower extremities should be examined in all suspected cases because bilaterality is present in more than 25% of cases.[9] Arteriographically and clinically, popliteal artery entrapment can be mimicked to a degree by adventitial cystic disease of the popliteal artery. However, adventitial cystic disease is more classically associated with a smooth tapered stenosis resulting in an "hourglass" or "scimitar" deformity than with either total occlusion or subtotal occlusion and poststenotic dilatation.

Although the diagnosis of popliteal artery entrapment is never absolutely confirmed before operation, the history and physical findings supported by treadmill testing and appropriate arteriographic studies will lead to the correct diagnosis in almost all cases. The precise anatomic variant can frequently be predicted from the arteriogram and will be confirmed at the time of operation.

TREATMENT

Because popliteal artery entrapment syndrome results from a congenital anomaly, there is no effective medical treatment. Following asymptomatic patients with known popliteal artery entrapment may lead to tragic, irreversible complications. Thus barring unusual risk factors, all patients with the syndrome are candidates for surgery regardless of the presence or absence of symptoms. Particular attention should be paid to the asymptomatic limb in patients with unilateral symptoms because of the high incidence of bilaterality.[9] Elective decompression should be performed before the onset of any permanent structural damage to the artery.

In uncomplicated cases without structural damage to the popliteal artery, simply dividing the obstructing muscle or fibrous band often provides a cure. Care must be taken, however, to dissect completely down to the level of the adventitia so that no potentially obstructing fibers are left behind.

When complications of popliteal artery entrapment have already occurred, appropriate vascular surgical corrective techniques are used. In acute thrombotic occlusion of the popliteal artery, division of the compressing muscle or fibrous band and balloon catheter thrombectomy may be sufficient treatment. An operative arteriogram is recommended, however, to rule out a fixed stenosis or intimal injury. If either is found, it should be treated at the time of thrombectomy. Aneurysms of the popliteal artery must be treated by inflow and outflow ligation and interposition vein grafting or vein bypass. Chronically occluded short segments of popliteal artery can be treated effectively by thromboendarterectomy and vein patch angioplasty in some instances but are most commonly, and perhaps most confidently, treated by short segment vein bypass. Longer segment occlusions are treated by standard bypass techniques. Autogenous saphenous vein from the ipsilateral extremity is the preferred arterial substitute for use in bypassing lesions in the popliteal artery.

Whether or not to replace or bypass an arterial segment when the only arterial abnormality is a very minor degree of poststenotic dilatation is always a difficult decision, since the natural history of such minor lesions is not known. Because these lesions can be followed after decompression both clinically and by noninvasive techniques, it seems prudent not to intervene unless major changes have occurred. Certainly, a significant residual stenotic lesion should not be left behind, nor should one leave behind what is clearly a popliteal aneurysm. Unfortunately, more precise guide-

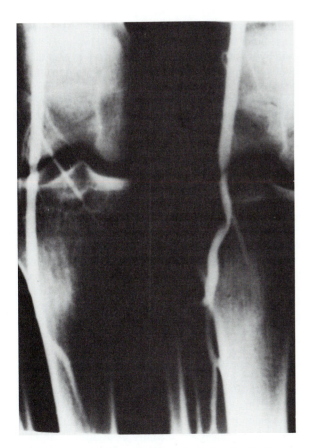

Figure 42-4. Active plantar flexion and passive dorsiflexion views may demonstrate arterial compression (*right*) even when the usual anteroposterior views show no arterial deviation. Note that compression is below the level of the joint line.

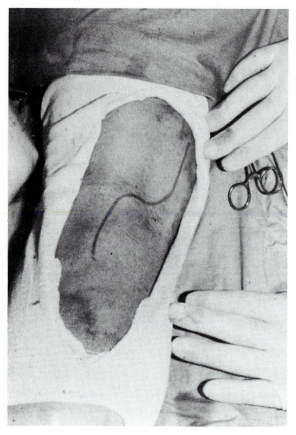

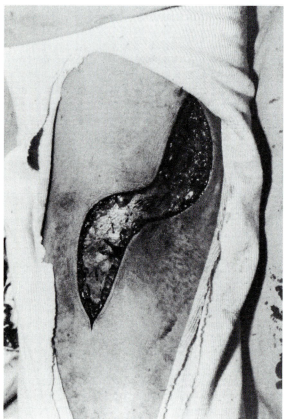

Figure 42-5. The S-shaped incision gives excellent exposure from the posterior approach.

lines are not available, and clinical judgment is required for each case.

The anatomy of the popliteal space is best visualized from the posterior approach. The standard incision for treating popliteal artery entrapment is S-shaped with the upper vertical limb on the medial aspect of the thigh, the horizontal limb in the center of the popliteal crease, and the lower vertical limb at the junction of the outer and middle one third of the calf (Fig. 42-5). Flaps are raised as necessary, but this should be done with caution to prevent healing problems. A deep dissection plane at the level of the muscle fascia should be used when these flaps are raised. When it is known that a vein graft will be needed, it is easier to harvest the graft while the patient is still supine. When total occlusion of the popliteal artery has occurred and it is known with certainty that bypass is required, the medial approach to the popliteal space is an acceptable alternative. In this setting the precise cause of the occlusion need not be defined to achieve a satisfactory result. However, one must be certain not to entrap the conduit while bypassing the obstructed artery.

The musculocutaneous branch of the sural nerve lies just subfascial in the operative field; injury to it should be avoided. The first major structure encountered as one enters the popliteal space proper is the tibial nerve. Great caution should be exercised in dissecting around it because even minor trauma may result in a disabling, prolonged neuropraxia. If the nerve is cut, permanent neurologic impairment manifested by foot drop will result. The lesser saphenous vein should be preserved if possible. However, there is generally no morbidity from dividing the lesser saphenous vein for exposure or from harvesting a portion of it for arterial repair.

The anatomic abnormality causing popliteal artery entrapment will be readily apparent in most instances. In some cases, however, one will be confused by not finding anything abnormal at first glance. This occurs most frequently with the type 3 and 4 variants, as accessory slips of the medial head of the gastrocnemius muscle and obstructing fibrous bands can arise at a surprisingly low level.[13] Another perplexing feature occasionally encountered is that the area of anatomic compression of the artery does not seem to conform precisely to the area of arteriographic abnormality. This is especially true when plantar flexion and dorsiflexion views are needed for diagnosis. When the anatomic abnormality is not readily apparent, one must explore both more proximally, searching for adductor entrapment, and more distally, searching for compression of the popliteal artery at a lower than expected level.

CONCLUSIONS

Excellent results will usually be obtained if patients with popliteal artery entrapment are operated on before complications have occurred. Patients who present with claudication but no popliteal artery injury or occlusion can be expected to resume unlimited activity. Conversely, popliteal artery entrapment is truly limb threatening, and some patients with acute thromboembolic popliteal artery or infrapopliteal artery runoff occlusions or both will lose their leg despite heroic attempts at revascularization. Similarly, chronic midpopliteal artery occlusions, even with preserved runoff, present greater than expected challenges in some cases. Patients whose legs are successfully revascularized remain at risk of developing complications related to the arterial substitute for the remainder of their lives. The key to successful management of popliteal artery entrapment syndrome lies in early recognition and operative correction before the onset of structural arterial damage or thromboembolic complications.

REFERENCES

1. Stuart TPA: A note on a variation in the course of the popliteal artery. J Anat Physiol 13:162, 1879.
2. Love JW, Whelan TJ: Popliteal artery entrapment syndrome. Am J Surg 109:620, 1965.
3. Flanagan DP, Burnham SJ, et al.: Summary of cases of adventitial cystic disease of the popliteal artery. Ann Surg 189:165, 1979.
4. Lee BY, La Pointe DG, Madden JL: The adductor canal syndrome. Am J Surg 123:617, 1972.
5. Rich NM, Hughes CW: Popliteal artery and vein entrapment. J Surg 113:696, 1967.
6. Podore PC: Popliteal entrapment syndrome: A report of tibial nerve entrapment. J Vasc Surg 2:335, 1985.
7. Connell J: Popliteal vein entrapment. Br J Surg 65:351, 1978.
8. Insua JA, Young JR, Humphries JW: Popliteal artery entrapment syndrome. Arch Surg 101:771, 1970.
9. Whelan TJ Jr: Popliteal artery entrapment syndrome, in Haimovici H, (ed) Vascular Surgery. New York, McGraw-Hill, 1976, p 493.
10. Rich NM, Collins GJ, et al.: Popliteal vascular entrapment. Arch Surg 114:1377, 1979.
11. McDonald PT, Easterbrok JA, et al.: Popliteal artery entrapment syndrome, clinical, noninvasive, and angiographic diagnosis. Am J Surg 139:318, 1980.
12. Williams LR, Flinn WR, et al.: Popliteal artery entrapment: Diagnosis by computed tomography. J Vasc Surg 3:360, 1986.
13. Haimovici H, Spraygren S, Johnson F: Popliteal artery entrapment by fibrous band. Surgery 72:789, 1972.

CHAPTER 43
Infected Prosthetic Arterial Grafts

Jerry Goldstone

Prosthetic grafts were first successfully used for arterial reconstruction more than 30 years ago. As with other new advances, many complications were subsequently recognized, but infection involving an aortic prosthesis is surely among the most serious and feared. This complication is fortunately uncommon, since few, if any, other surgical infections have as high a morbidity or mortality. Furthermore, prosthetic graft infections may be insidious in onset, occurring up to several years after the original arterial reconstruction. Thus graft infections are typically difficult diagnostic and therapeutic problems that require prolonged and expensive hospitalization. Nevertheless, sufficient experience has been accumulated so that the principles of management are becoming more clearly defined, and a successful outcome can be anticipated in the majority of patients.

MAGNITUDE OF THE PROBLEM

The incidence of graft infection reported in the literature ranges from less than 1% to more than 6%.[1-10] Mortality rates for infected aortic grafts range between 40% and 75%, and limb loss ranges between 20 to 50% in most series. In contrast, infection involving femoropopliteal grafts has an associated mortality of only about 10%, although the rate of limb loss is substantially higher. The higher mortality of aortic graft infections is due to the consequences of sepsis, complications of multiple operations, and hemorrhage from anastomotic dehiscence and graft-enteric fistulas and erosions.

PATHOGENESIS OF AORTIC GRAFT INFECTION

Plastic arterial prostheses can be considered to be multifibered or porous foreign bodies. After contamination has occurred, organisms are harbored indefinitely because the bacteria continue to reside in the interstices of these knitted and woven fabric grafts. Although the bacteria have no significant adverse effects on the fabric prosthesis, the infec-

tion tends to spread to involve the host tissue incorporating the graft, and ultimately destroys the anastomosis between the graft and the host artery. The destruction of the anastomosis leads to the formation of a false aneurysm, with its potential consequences of disruption and hemorrhage. The infection involves the pseudointimal lining of the prosthesis much less commonly.

There are many potential causes of aortic graft infection, some proved by clinical observation, others suggested by scientific experiments, and others representing hypothetical ways in which a prosthesis may become contaminated. It is generally believed that graft contamination occurs most commonly at the time of graft implantation.[11] Contamination can occur in several ways. Improper sterilization of the graft or surgical instruments, or a break in sterile technique are obvious sources of direct contamination during an operation, but these are unlikely to occur in modern operating rooms.

Grafts may also be contaminated by direct contact with the patient's skin. Despite meticulous surgical preparation of the skin, large numbers of bacteria will remain on the skin surface, the skin edges, and within dermal appendages.[12] Staphylococcal species are normal inhabitants of the skin as well as the organisms most often responsible for graft infection. This is probably why the risk of graft contamination from the skin appears to be greater when the graft is placed in a superficial location such as the femoral or popliteal region where skin contact with the graft during implantation is more likely.

Infected lymph glands or channels are another source of organisms that can lead to direct graft contamination. Infected lymph can contaminate a newly implanted graft by two mechanisms: by bathing the graft when lymphatic channels are transected at the time of arterial reconstruction and by transporting bacteria into the bloodstream through lymphaticovenous communications, thereby permitting hematogenous seeding of a graft.[13] These mechanisms are particularly important in patients with groin incisions when infection or gangrene is present distally in the limb and the draining lymphatic channels carry bacteria. Transection of periaortic lymphatics during surgical exposure may play a similar role.

The development of a wound infection adjacent to a vascular graft can lead to infection of the graft by direct extension of the infection. This may also be a factor in the high incidence of infections involving grafts entering or leaving the femoral triangle because wound healing complications are common in this area. Direct infection of an aortic graft by contamination of the perigraft region can also occur secondary to wound dehiscence or the development of colon ischemia postoperatively. Another causative factor is postoperative blood or serum collections that can cause graft infection by producing dead space and a favorable medium for bacterial growth around the graft.

Another potential source of contamination of aortic grafts is the laminated thrombus or atheromatous debris present in aneurysms or atherosclerotic vessels. Several authors have reported a high incidence of positive bacterial cultures from such vessels.[14–16] For example, Macbeth et al. reported a 43% incidence (38 of 88 cases) of positive cultures taken from arteries during routine, clean, elective arterial reconstructive procedures.[15] *Staphylococcus epidermidis*, an organism increasingly recognized as being involved in prosthetic graft infections, accounted for 71% of the positive cultures in this series. It is interesting that three graft infections developed during the course of Macbeth et al.'s study (0.9%), and all occurred in patients whose arterial cultures were positive at the time of the original operation. In each case the organism subsequently cultured from the infected graft was the same as that cultured at the original operation, and in each case this organism was *S. epidermidis*. Therefore it is possible that organisms residing in the wall of the abdominal aorta may be a source of graft contamination.

The performance of concomitant intraabdominal surgical procedures in association with clean vascular grafting operations has frequently been implicated as a source of contamination and subsequent graft infection.[17] Because the consequences of aortic graft sepsis are so grave, *in general* the potential risk of contaminating a freshly implanted graft far outweighs the potential benefit that might accrue from a prophylactic, incidental appendectomy, cholecystectomy, or any additional procedure that violates the gastrointestinal or genitourinary tracts.

Although contamination of prosthetic grafts probably occurs at the time of implantation in most instances, hematogenous seeding of the prosthesis is the most likely explanation for at least some late infections.[18] Transient bacteremias are common in humans even after trivial manipulation of mucous membranes. It has been demonstrated in laboratory animals that newly implanted Dacron aortic grafts can easily be infected via the bloodstream. The fresh intimal surface of a fabric graft is a suitable site for circulating bacteria to settle and establish an infection, and this susceptibility persists as long as the neointimal covering is incomplete. The healing time and completeness of the neointimal lining vary with the type of graft, but the period of susceptibility to infection by intravenous bacteria is at least 1 year in dogs.[19] Furthermore, neointimal surfaces are dynamic, undergoing constant change, so that new or persistent neointimal defects may permit bacterial seeding of a graft

and the establishment of a late clinical graft infection at any time after implantation. An alternative explanation is that the *perigraft* tissues are seeded by blood-borne bacteria and the adjacent prosthesis becomes secondarily infected.

A common feature in most reported series of aortic graft infections is repeated operations for complications of graft limb thrombosis, false aneurysm, or stenosis. This was thought to be a potential contributing factor in 37 of 92 (40%) vascular graft infections reported by Reilly et al.[20] and in 12 of 27 patients (46%) reported by Goldstone and Moore.[5] Presumably graft contamination occurred during the secondary or tertiary arterial operations in at least some of these patients.

BACTERIOLOGY OF GRAFT INFECTIONS

Historically, *Staphylococcus aureus* has been the most frequent microorganism responsible for arterial graft infections. This was reemphasized by Liekweg and Greenfield, who summarized all published cases of vascular prosthetic infection up to 1977 and noted 50% of them to be due to *Staphylococcus aureus*.[7] However, they found an increasing incidence of gram-negative bacterial infections. This gradual change in the microbiology of graft infections has also been noted by several other authors. In addition to more gram-negative infections, there is an increasing frequency of mixed infections involving both aerobic and anaerobic organisms. In the series of 22 graft infections reported by Conn et al., multiple organisms were involved in 13 infections (59.1%).[3] Of the 92 aortic graft infections treated at the University of California, San Francisco before 1984, two to six different organisms were cultured in 29 patients. It is of interest that although preoperative cultures (wound, sinus tract, etc.) yielded two or more organisms in 24 patients, the results of cultures taken intraoperatively were frequently different. The correlation between preoperative and intraoperative cultures was only 72%. This has important implications for the selection of the optimal perioperative antibiotic regimen.

There has also been an increased recognition of graft infections caused by coagulase-negative *S. epidermidis* (also referred to as *S. albus*). This component of normal skin flora was the predominant organism in late postoperative (> 3.5 months) graft infections in one series reported in 1974, accounting for 50% of infections involving aortofemoral grafts.[5] In a more recent review of similar cases, Bandyk et al. documented *S. epidermidis* as the infecting organism in 60% (18 of 30) of their cases.[21] The emergence of this organism of relatively low virulence as an important pathogen in vascular surgery is not surprising since it is a well-recognized organism associated with infection of prosthetic heart valves, cerebrospinal fluid shunts, hip prostheses, and other implanted foreign bodies. In addition, *S. epidermidis* is the organism most frequently isolated from aortic aneurysm mural thrombus, diseased arterial walls, and groin lymph nodes during clean, elective vascular operations.[14–16,22]

Although most graft infections are now due to *S. aureus*, *S. epidermidis*, and gram-negative enteric organisms, it is possible for any organism to infect a graft and a broad spectrum have been reported, including mycobacteria and fungi.

In our own series of infected aortic grafts (now totaling 106), all cultures were negative in over 40% of the patients. There are several possible explanations for this surprising observation. First all patients were given high-dose parenteral antibiotics at the time of treatment, and most were referred from other institutions where they had also received intensive antibiotic therapy. Improper handling of culture specimens, including delays in getting the material from the operating room to the microbiology laboratory, probably accounted for at least some negative cultures because many of our patients were operated on as emergencies during weekends, nights, and holidays. Failure to use the proper culture media and failure to observe the cultures for a sufficiently long period of time are other factors that could have resulted in negative cultures. The importance of these technical details was emphasized in a recent report in which it was noted that cultures of perigraft tissue or fluid were positive in only 2 of 18 cases (11%), whereas cultures of the graft fabric in broth confirmed *S. epidermidis* infection in 15 cases (83%).[21] It has also been recently discovered that most bacteria are buried in an anionic matrix biofilm on the graft surface. Special techniques are required to dislodge some bacterial species from the graft fabric, and this is postulated as one reason for negative cultures as well as for the late clinical appearance and inherent antibiotic resistance of many of these infections.[23] Despite negative cultures in many of our patients, we are convinced, based on clinical grounds, that each patient did indeed have an infected aortic graft. Therefore, the surgeon managing a patient with a potentially infected aortic graft should not insist on a positive culture to establish the appropriate diagnosis. The corollary of this is obvious: negative cultures do not exclude the diagnosis of prosthetic arterial graft infection.

CLINICAL MANIFESTATIONS OF GRAFT INFECTION

An infection involving an aortic prosthetic graft can be classified as either a perigraft infection (PGI) or a prosthetic or aortoenteric fistula (AEF). The vast majority of patients in the PGI group present with some evidence of infection, most commonly involving the groin incision of an aortofemoral graft. Szilagyi et al. reported that 77% of 40 graft infections occurred in the groin.[10] This was also true in 77% (20 of 27) of the graft infections reported by Goldstone and Moore.[5] In these and other series, the femoral infections most often involved the distal portion(s) of aortofemoral graft limbs, thereby setting the stage for the spread of infection proximally to include the body or shaft of the graft itself. The infection usually appears to be clinically localized. Signs may include incisional swelling or mass, with or without erythema, pain, or drainage. Often these areas will break down and spontaneously drain purulent material, rarely with associated hemorrhage. Subsequently a draining sinus often develops, and there may even be exposure of the underlying graft. Another common manifestation of graft infection is the appearance of a false aneurysm. This

occurred in 13.5% of the patients in the series reported by Reilly et al.[20] and in about 10% of those in the collected review by Liekweg and Greenfield.[7] Systemic sepsis, hemorrhage, graft occlusion, and septic emboli are distinctly less common. Patients who have a perigraft infection without an enteric fistula can also present with upper gastrointestinal hemorrhage, presumably as a result of stress- or infection-induced gastritis, duodenitis, or ulceration. This occurred in 9.4% of our patients with PGI.[24]

In contrast, upper or lower gastrointestinal bleeding is the *most* common manifestation of aortic or graft-enteric fistulas, occurring in at least two thirds of the patients. However, approximately one third of the patients with a fistula present with evidence of graft infection only and no evidence of bleeding. Of those patients who do bleed, approximately two thirds bleed acutely, and about half of these acute bleeding episodes are massive. Chronic gastrointestinal bleeding, extending over weeks to months, occurs in the remaining one third of bleeding patients. The pattern of gastrointestinal bleeding tends to correlate with the type of fistula, either anastomotic or paraprosthetic. In our recent review of this subject, acute hemorrhage among patients with aortointestinal fistula was usually associated with an anastomotic fistula, whereas paraprosthetic fistulas often did not bleed at all or bled chronically.[24] Thus, there is a spectrum of gastrointestinal tract involvement by prosthetic graft infection. The pathologic interaction may be direct (fistula formation and gastrointestinal bleeding), indirect (gastrointestinal bleeding without a fistula), or occult (fistula formation with no gastrointestinal bleeding). Localized sepsis or systemic infection probably plays an important causative role in the development of gastrointestinal bleeding in the absence of a vasculoenteric fistula.

Clinical manifestations of infection involving grafts entirely within the abdomen (i.e., aortoaortic or aortoiliac) are often subtle, consisting only of malaise, low-grade fever, mild leukocytosis, or an elevated erythrocyte sedimentation rate. A false aneurysm at an aortic anastomosis may also indicate graft sepsis and can occasionally be detected by physical examination. A high index of suspicion is essential for the early diagnosis of any infected graft; this is most important in patients whose graft is not superficial (i.e., intraabdominal).

The interval between graft insertion and the first manifestation of graft infection varies considerably from a few days to several years (156 months is the longest interval reported). Although in some series the majority of patients with graft infections manifested obvious signs of infection in the immediate postoperative period, only 13 of the 104 aortic graft infections treated at our institution were diagnosed within the first postoperative month. The mean interval between original grafting operation and onset of clinical manifestations for patients with aortoenteric fistulas was 33 months (range, 2 weeks to 156 months), whereas for patients with perigraft infection alone, the interval was 25 months (range, 3 days to 144 months). For patients with grafts confined to the abdomen (aortoaortic and aortoiliac), the mean interval between original graft insertion and onset of graft sepsis was 49.6 months (range, 2 weeks to 99 months), whereas for aortofemoral grafts the interval averaged 32.9 months (range, 2 weeks to 99 months). These data indicate that a substantial proportion (36%) of aortic graft infections are recognized within 1 year of graft implantation, but the risk of infection persists for many years, probably indefinitely.

DIAGNOSIS OF GRAFT INFECTION

Infection of a prosthetic vascular graft is a diagnosis that is frequently difficult to establish. This often leads to considerable delay before the problem is recognized and treatment is instituted. Delay adversely affects outcome and significantly increases morbidity. Therefore, a high index of suspicion must be maintained when evaluating a patient suspected of harboring a possible graft infection. The most important guideline to be followed when interpreting the results of diagnostic tests is that although a positive result is significant, *a negative result does not exclude a graft infection.* If the clinical setting is appropriate and all the tests are negative or nonspecific, exploration of the graft is mandatory to provide the definitive information concerning a possible graft infection.

Perigraft Infection (PGI)

The diagnosis of an infected graft is most commonly made by the appearance of the involved wound or subcutaneous portion of the graft.[2,5,7,20] The typical appearance has been described above. This accounts for the vast majority of patients with perigraft infections, but in some cases (probably no more than 10 to 15%), the infection will be entirely occult and will be discovered only at the time of exploration for false aneurysm repair or graft limb occlusion.

In contrast to the frequent occurrence of signs of localized infection, signs of systemic infection or sepsis (fever, leukocytosis, bacteremia, hypotension) are much less common and were present in only 34 of 71 patients (48%) with perigraft infections in our series.[20,24] Fully 56 (78.9%) of these 71 patients had none or only one of these signs of sepsis. Thus the patient with a perigraft infection is usually readily diagnosed by physical examination alone (if the groin is involved) and rarely demonstrates toxic manifestations of the infection. A far more difficult diagnostic challenge among these patients is the assessment of the extent of involvement of the graft by the infection.

Aortoenteric (AEF) or Graft-enteric Fistulas

The diagnosis of a vasculoenteric fistula is considerably more difficult to establish preoperatively than that of a perigraft infection. We found that although the clinical presentation was suggestive of a fistula in two thirds of patients with AEF, in less than one third was the correct diagnosis made preoperatively.[20] There are several reasons for this. First, the process involves the retroperitoneal graft segment and is inaccessible to physical examination and to most other investigative modalities. Localized wound changes are less common and when present are not helpful in detecting the *fistula.* Second, a certain number of these patients

are unstable and are therefore unable to undergo a thorough evaluation preoperatively. Finally, a significant number of fistula patients in our series presented with evidence of a graft infection without bleeding and as a result were never investigated for the presence of a fistula because it was not suspected.

Evidence of sepsis or systemic infection is much more common among patients with AEF (72%) than among patients with PGI, and the severity of the infection is often worse. This fact can be very useful in the evaluation of patients with suspected or established aortic graft infection.

Diagnostic Modalities

When aortic graft infection or aortoenteric fistula is suspected but unconfirmed, a variety of investigative methods may be used to firmly establish the diagnosis. If a fistula is suspected, the most successful diagnostic technique is upper gastrointestinal endoscopy.[25–29] A positive study result directly visualizes the fistula or demonstrates bleeding from the distal duodenum with an entirely normal esophagus, stomach, and proximal duodenum. However, it is essential that the study be thorough and include the third and fourth portions of the duodenum because the likelihood of a falsely negative examination result increases if the study is incomplete.[27–29]

If a perigraft infection is suspected, the most informative test will be either computed tomographic (CT) scanning or magnetic resonance imaging (MRI). CT scanning is particularly helpful because it can directly assess the retroperitoneum and perigraft space. CT abnormalities that have been correlated with graft infection include perigraft fluid collections, loss of tissue planes around retroperitoneal structures, and the presence of perigraft air.[30–33] When contrast-enhanced CT scanning is performed, false aneurysms and graft limb occlusion can also be detected. Additionally, the ability of CT scanning to simultaneously assess the entire peritoneal cavity and thus provide information on other possible diagnoses makes this the initial technique of choice when aortic graft infection is suspected. MRI may be superior to CT scanning because of its extreme sensitivity to changes in perivascular tissues and its ability to detect perigraft fluid collections. Any fluid seen around a graft more than 3 months after graft implantation is abnormal and should alert the clinician to the possibility of an infected graft. (Fig. 43-1).

Ultrasonography has not been as useful as CT scanning, particularly in assessing the retroperitoneum, because the resolution of nonvascular structures is not nearly as good. There is often a significant problem with overlying bowel gas and increased body size. Interpretation of a study obtained in the early postoperative period is very difficult. However, the ready availability, noninvasive nature, and low cost of this test make ultrasonography the technique of choice for the initial assessment of any collection or mass involving a superficial or subcutaneous portion of a graft.[34]

An additional application of these imaging techniques is their use to guide needle aspiration of perigraft collections.[34,35] This can provide crucial information in the determination of the significance of any abnormality seen

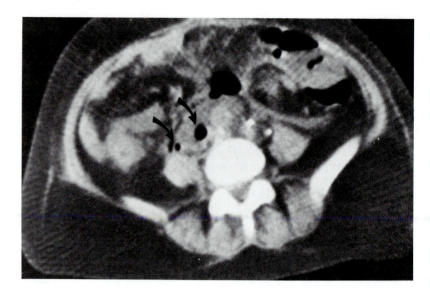

Figure 43-1. CT scan showing gas bubbles (*dark arrows*) within poorly defined fluid collection surrounding aortic graft, and poorly defined tissue planes.

on the scan. Because some graft infections do appear in the early postimplantation period, it may be difficult to decide, based on the appearance of the scan alone, whether a collection is infected or just residual from the operation. Only recently has data on the normal CT appearance of

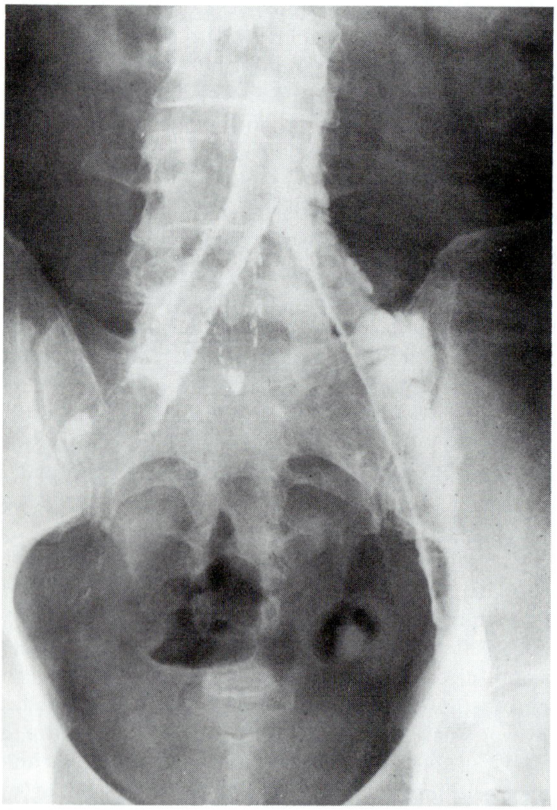

Figure 43-2. Sinogram, performed through draining sinus in left groin, clearly outlines both limbs and the body of aortobifemoral bypass graft, documenting the extent of graft involvement by infection. (*From Reilly LM, Goldstone J: The infected aortic graft, in Bergan JJ, Yao JST (eds): Reoperative Arterial Surgery. Orlando, Fla., Grune & Stratton, 1986, pp 231–253.*)

graft incorporation following uncomplicated aortic reconstruction become available.[36] Therefore, perigraft fluid aspiration offers considerable promise in the diagnosis of early or occult graft infections.

Contrast sinography should be performed whenever there is an open, draining wound. It can be helpful in determining whether a wound infection is superficial or extends deeply enough to involve or surround the graft in question. It can also provide important information about the extent of the graft involved by the infectious process, whether it is confined to the groin, to one graft limb, or involves the body of the graft (Fig. 43-2). Sinography also occasionally demonstrates an occult fistula.

Radionuclide scans using indium 111–labeled leukocytes or platelets or gallium 67 citrate are sometimes helpful in diagnosing graft infections.[37–39] Indium scans appear to be the most sensitive but are normally positive for up to 3 months after graft implantation and are therefore not useful diagnostically in the early postoperative period.

All patients with either a confirmed or a suspected graft infection must undergo angiography. Although rarely establishing the diagnosis of a graft infection, it occasionally will demonstrate a false aneurysm suggestive of an underlying graft complication. Additionally, angiography is mandatory in planning the subsequent arterial reconstruction because it allows identification of the type and location of the proximal anastomosis, and the availability of the superficial femoral and profunda femoris arteries for new graft implantation or as autogenous conduits. In addition, the angiographic localization of the distal graft anastomoses is especially important to avoid contamination of the new graft during subsequent limb revascularization. Therefore, the angiographic study must visualize the entire graft, the native vessels, and the runoff in the legs (Fig. 43–3).

Extent of Graft Involvement

Not every graft infection involves the entire implanted prosthesis, and therefore in some cases partial graft excision should be adequate treatment. An increasing number of reports in the literature of successful treatment of limited

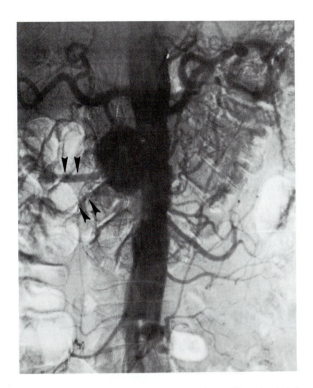

Figure 43-3. Preoperative aortogram in patient with perigraft infection shows large anastomotic false aneurysm extending above renal arteries. Note two right renal arteries arising from pseudoaneurysm (*dark arrows*). The left renal artery is occluded. This study demonstrates the value of preoperative angiography in planning surgical treatment of an infected aortic graft. (*From Reilly LM, Goldstone J: The infected aortic graft, in Bergan JJ, Yao JST (eds): Reoperative Arterial Surgery. Orlando, Fla., Grune & Stratton, 1986, pp 231–253.*)

graft infection using graft limb excision or continuous antibiotic irrigation of the infected segment support this concept.[40,41] However, there is great difficulty in accurately determining the exact extent of the graft infection by noninvasive or minimally invasive methods. Ultrasonography, CT, and MRI scanning, labeled leukocyte scans, and contrast sinography have all been used to determine whether a given graft infection is limited or extensive. Unfortunately, the only absolutely reliable method of determining the extent of graft infection is operative exploration and inspection of the prosthesis. A portion of graft that is well incorporated by fibrous connective tissue and is not surrounded by dark or turbid fluid is not likely to be infected. In our series only one third of patients treated for a localized graft infection by limited graft removal were treated successfully. The remaining two thirds of these patients either died of persistent sepsis or later required complete graft excision. Therefore, at the present time none of the noninvasive diagnostic modalities should be the *only* basis for a decision to treat a patient for a limited graft infection.

TREATMENT

The successful treatment of a prosthetic aortic graft infection requires adequate preparation of the patient for the procedure, accurate planning of the reconstruction, total excision of the infected graft, and meticulous attention to the details of the operative technique. Control of anastomotic or gastrointestinal bleeding, when present, is the first priority, and often determines whether or not a staged approach can be used and the order of the stages. Control of the infection is also a priority when significant systemic or local sepsis is present. This may require incision and drainage of an abscess. Antibiotics should be administered intravenously in high doses. Broad-spectrum antibiotic coverage should be used because the infections are now commonly gram-negative or mixed, because there may be an occult enteric fistula, and because wound drainage cultures do not correlate with intraoperative cultures, as noted previously. Antibiotics should of course cover any organisms recovered from the blood or from aspirated perigraft collections. The antibiotic regimen should be implemented well in advance of the operative procedure, as soon as the patient is admitted to the hospital. In most cases at least a 2-week postoperative course of antibiotics is required for adequate treatment.

Most patients are clinically stable enough to undergo thorough evaluation and optimization of their cardiopulmonary, hematologic, and metabolic functions. However, some patients are severely compromised nutritionally and immunologically by the chronic infection, usually more than their clinical appearance would suggest. For these patients, hyperalimentation is an important adjunct to operative therapy. In patients who are stable, hyperalimentation should be implemented preoperatively and continued well into the postoperative period, but definitive treatment should not be delayed excessively because delays are often associated with sudden deterioration of the patient and the need for emergent operation.

Arterial Reconstruction Materials

Autogenous tissue is the only material that can be safely used if the new arterial reconstruction must traverse the infected field.[42,43] Autogenous tissue may be used as the following:

1. Patch material for angioplasty at the site of a previous end-to-side anastomosis. Saphenous vein or endarterectomized superficial femoral artery (SFA) are the most common donor sites for patch material.
2. Conduits, which may be constructed by endarterectomy of the previously bypassed native vessels and used in situ. For example, aortoiliac or aortofemoral endarterectomy may be used to restore lower limb perfusion after removal of an infected end-to-side aortic bypass graft. The presence of degenerative or aneurysmal changes in the native arterial segments is a contraindication to endarterectomy.
3. Arterial or venous autograft replacement of the infected graft may also be performed.[43] The arterial autograft can be obtained from the iliofemoral system or superficial femoral artery. Patency can be restored by endarterectomy if the vessels are occluded. The venous autograft is usually harvested from the greater saphenous system, and larger vessels can be constructed by sewing two segments of saphenous vein together in a side-by-side manner.

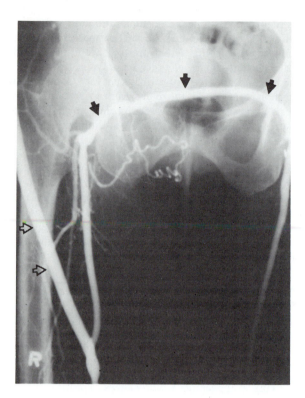

Figure 43-4. Postoperative arteriogram shows extracavitary reconstruction using prosthetic axillo-distal-superficial femoral graft (*open arrows*) that provides retrograde flow into autogenous femoral-femoral bypass (*dark arrows*). In this case, both femoral anastomoses are end-to-end. (*From Reilly LM, Goldstone J: The infected aortic graft, in Bergan JJ, Yao JST (eds): Reoperative Arterial Surgery. Orlando, Fla., Grune & Stratton, 1986, pp 231–253.*)

Prosthetic grafts should be used only outside the infected field. Unless a limited graft infection has been established, it is safer to assume that the entire graft is infected, even if the manifestation of the infection involves only one area of the graft. Therefore, "the infected field" is considered to be any anatomic location containing the graft. The most common method for restoring extremity flow in patients with infected aortic prostheses is an axillobifemoral bypass graft. The superficial or profunda femoral arteries are preferred as the recipient artery for the axillofemoral graft, but occasionally the popliteal artery must be used. Composite reconstructions using both prosthetic and autogenous material may be used if a portion of the revascularization (crossfemoral graft) will be in the infected field, but the remainder will not (axillofemoral graft) (Fig. 43–4). This is the usual situation when aortobifemoral grafts are involved.

Operative Management: General Principles

The operative treatment of an infected aortic graft consists of two phases: revascularization and infected graft removal. A variety of approaches to reconstruction are available. Graft excision alone, without any revascularization, is feasible in some patients, such as those with a chronically oc-

cluded graft and viable limbs or previous amputation, or those with end-to-side bypass grafts whose native vessels have remained patent. For the most part, however, arterial reconstruction will be required to maintain adequate lower extremity perfusion. Delay in the performance of arterial reconstruction should be avoided because it is associated with a greater incidence of limb loss.[10,42,45,46]

Graft excision and endarterectomy of previously bypassed native vessels may be performed for any infected aortic graft, as long as the original disease was occlusive, not aneurysmal, and the original anastomoses were not end to end. Graft excision and remote prosthetic reconstruction outside the infected field is the most common method of reconstruction for an infected aortoiliac graft. Graft excision and composite (prosthetic and autogenous) reconstruction is the safest method of reconstruction for infected aortofemoral grafts.

Although there is considerable debate about the necessity for and the proper timing of the arterial reconstruction,[20,29,44–46] when the patient with an infected graft is stable and has no bleeding manifestations of a fistula (or at most intermittently guaiac-positive stools), optimum operative treatment is staged,[47] with lower extremity revascularization performed first, followed in 3 to 6 days by excision of the infected graft. Antibiotic coverage is maintained during this interval and adjusted according to operative culture data. There is justifiable concern about the risk of infecting the new reconstruction, particularly if it is prosthetic, during the interval before the old infected graft is removed. To date the reported incidence of this situation is low, around 15 to 20%,[20,44,45] except for one series in which the incidence was 43%.[46] These recurrent infections seem to be relatively easily managed but some extremity amputations have been required. Because a staged operative repair seems to have a lower mortality (26% vs. 43% in our series) than the traditional method (infected graft removal followed immediately by limb revascularization), we currently favor this technique for the majority of patients who require revascularization. The operative stress is reduced for both patient and surgeon because both stages of the procedure can be conducted deliberately, without concern for prolonged limb ischemia and the hazards of excessive anticoagulation.

If the patient is not stable or has had a significant bleeding episode, both graft excision and revascularization are performed as a single stage under the same anesthetic. Again, unless there is active and uncontrollable bleeding the arterial revascularization is performed first. If bleeding is too rapid to permit this, transabdominal graft removal and fistula closure (if present) is performed first. The patient is then reprepped and redraped and the revascularization is performed with an entirely new set of instruments, unless the revascularization is to be achieved with only autogenous vessels, in which case both phases can be performed synchronously.

The most important feature of infected aortic graft excision is the management of the aortic stump. The leading cause of perioperative and late deaths among patients with AEF in our series has been aortic stump disruption. There were nine such disruptions; five occurred with recurrent fistulas, and only 1 patient survived.[24] When aortic continuity can be preserved using autogenous patching, the risk of subsequent aortic disruption seems to be almost eradicated. This may be due to the preservation of perfusion, and therefore nutrition, of the aortic wall. However, when proximal infection and a previous end-to-end anastomosis necessitate aortic division, stump disruption is a significant threat. The importance of adequate resection and wide debridement of the proximal anastomotic site and adjacent infrarenal aorta cannot be overemphasized.[15] An adequate length of aorta must be available to allow this debridement and subsequent aortic closure without tension in noninfected tissue. The aorta should be closed with monofilament synthetic suture, using a double row technique. This may require temporary suprarenal or supraceliac aortic cross-clamping and may occasionally require renal artery relocation. Jejunal serosal patching of the aortic stump and anterior spinal ligament or omental reinforcement of stump closure have not yet proved beneficial in reducing stump disruption.[48–50] In Macbeth et al.'s series, all of the aortic stumps that disrupted had positive bacterial cultures[15] suggesting a difference between graft infection with and without aortic wall infection. Gram stain and culture of the aortic wall margin should be performed, and if results are positive, further resection should be carried out. If this is not possible, then a prolonged course of antibiotics is warranted.[15] If the aortic stump disrupts and the patient survives, it may be reasonable to plan a prolonged period of retroperitoneal irrigation with antibiotics or povidone-iodine solution.

The management of the infected femoral wounds is also important. All necrotic and infected tissue should be debrided and the wounds packed open with antibiotic-soaked dressings. If there is an autogenous conduit in the infected field, the subcutaneous tissue layers should be loosely approximated to cover the conduit, and the rest of the wound is left open and dressed with antibiotic-soaked bandages. Occasionally, coverage of exposed vessels with free or rotated muscle flaps is necessary to ensure wound healing and eradication of infection.

Operative Management—Technical Details

Infected Aortoiliac Graft

The available options for a single stage reconstruction of an infected aortoiliac graft are patch angioplasty and graft removal, native vessel endarterectomy (thromboendarterectomy, TEA) and graft removal, or extraanatomic bypass with graft removal. Patch angioplasty or TEA and graft removal can only be performed if the original anastomoses were performed end to side, the native vessels were not divided, and the original disease was occlusive, not aneurysmal. For either of these approaches, the patient is prepared and draped as for a standard transabdominal aortic reconstruction. Because infection may have seriously weakened the proximal aortic anastomotic line, it is advisable with any graft infection to gain supraceliac control of the aorta before mobilization of the graft itself. Through a transcrural approach, the supraceliac aorta is mobilized enough to allow clamping if it should later become necessary. Attention is then turned to the previously placed graft. The graft is dissected from the surrounding capsule and

proximal and distal control of the native aorta and distal iliac vessels is obtained. The end-to-side graft is then detached, taking care to leave no sutures or prosthetic graft fibers. If endarterectomy is employed, we prefer a semiclosed technique, beginning at the aortotomy, and finishing at the site of each previous iliac anastomosis. The use of hand-held arterial strippers or the air-driven oscillating loop stripper facilitates the performance of endarterectomy without requiring additional arteriotomies. The arteriotomies are closed with an autogenous patch, most commonly, in these cases, of saphenous vein or endarterectomized superficial femoral artery. Only monofilament polypropylene sutures are used in the presence of infection. Occasionally, the occlusive disease is mild enough to allow patch angioplasty without associated endarterectomy. The abdomen and retroperitoneum are irrigated with antibiotic solution, but no drains are used unless there is frank abscess formation. The midline incision is closed, with the liberal use of retention sutures. The skin edges are loosely approximated with a few sutures and the rest of the wound is packed with antibiotic-soaked dressings.

If a single stage extraanatomic bypass and infected graft removal is planned, the patient is prepared and draped for both axillobifemoral bypass and transabdominal aortic exposure. The axillofemoral and crossfemoral grafts are prosthetic, either of externally supported Dacron or polytetrafluoroethylene (PTFE); this procedure is performed in the standard manner. At its completion, the wounds are securely closed and sealed with occlusive dressings. If there is concern about competitive flow threatening the patency of the new bypass, occluding vascular clamps are left in place on the common femoral arteries *proximal* to the new anastomotic sites. This prevents flow to the extremities from the in-line infected graft. The wounds are securely closed around these clamps and sealed and draped in such a manner that a nonscrubbed assistant can remove them from beneath the drapes after the abdominal portion of the procedure has been completed. Attention is then turned to the transabdominal removal of the infected graft, which proceeds as described above. After the infected graft is removed and the native vessels are oversewn, the occluding clamps preventing competitive flow are removed from the common femoral arteries. It is advisable to maintain retrograde flow in at least one hypogastric artery if these vessels were patent before infected graft removal to ensure adequate colonic blood flow.

Staged repair of an infected aortoiliac graft consists of prosthetic axillobifemoral bypass, followed within 3 to 6 days by transabdominal removal of the infected graft. The techniques do not differ from those described above. However, in this approach competitive flow can only be prevented by ligating the common femoral or external iliac arteries proximal to the anastomotic sites of the axillobifemoral bypass. Before this is done, consideration must be given to the ultimate perfusion status of the sigmoid colon, after the in-line graft has been removed.

Infected Aortofemoral Graft

The operative approach to the treatment of the infected aortofemoral graft is especially challenging because the presence of infection in the femoral regions precludes safe placement of new prosthetic material in these areas. The one-stage and two-stage options for the treatment of an infected aortofemoral graft are the same as those for an aortoiliac graft. If patch angioplasty and infected graft removal or endarterectomy and infected graft removal are planned, the operative technique is the same as that described above. If either one-stage or two-stage extraanatomic bypass and graft removal are planned, the prosthetic axillofemoral graft must not traverse the previous groin incisions, and the crossfemoral graft must be autogenous or routed circuitously to the distal superficial, profunda femoral, or popliteal artery.

The two-stage axillobifemoral bypass and graft removal is performed in the following manner. The patient is prepared and draped for a standard axillobifemoral bypass, but the legs are prepped at least to the knees, and to the ankles if long segments of the saphenous vein will be needed. If neither groin is obviously involved by the infection, the superficial femoral arteries are patent bilaterally, and the blood pressure is equal in both arms, the right side is chosen for the axillofemoral bypass. There are two reasons for this choice: First, the left subclavian artery is more commonly affected by atherosclerosis than is the right. Second, if the patient becomes a candidate for delayed aortic prosthetic reconstruction,[51] this is often performed through a left thoracoretroperitoneal approach and a left-sided axillofemoral bypass would have to be divided. If only one leg has a patent SFA, the axillofemoral bypass is brought down on this side. If one groin is obviously involved by the infection, the contralateral side is chosen for the axillofemoral bypass (provided there is no arm blood pressure differential), regardless of the status of SFA. In this case the profunda femoral artery (PFA) will be the site of the distal anastomosis.

The axillary artery and the selected site for distal implantation of the prosthetic axillofemoral bypass (the SFA or PFA) are exposed simultaneously. The approach to the femoral vessel is through an incision along the lateral border of the sartorius muscle, placed at the junction of the upper third and the middle third of the thigh. The artery is then approached lateral to and distal to the previous area of dissection and infection. Externally-supported Dacron or PTFE is preferred for the conduit. The proximal and distal anastomoses are constructed using monofilament polypropylene suture. An occluding vascular clamp is left in place on the proximal SFA or PFA to prevent competitive flow; these two incisions are closed in layers and sealed with occlusive dressings. The wounds are redraped to allow later removal of the occluding clamp as described above. The autogenous conduit to be used for the crossfemoral graft, either saphenous vein or endarterectomized occluded SFA, is now dissected. As much conduct is mobilized as possible before the femoral incisions are reopened, particularly if the conduit-harvesting incisions are near the new prosthetic graft. These incisions are then closed and sealed with occlusive dressings. The previous femoral incisions are then opened, and the graft limbs and the native vessels are dissected free. With proximal and distal control of the common, superficial, profunda femoral arteries, and the graft limb, the anastomoses are detached. Each graft limb is mobilized as far proximally as can be safely reached through the groin

incisions, suture-ligated, and tucked up high into the retroperitoneum. This will facilitate later transabdominal graft removal. The autogenous conduit is then anastomosed to the native artery. When this anastomosis has been completed, the clamp preventing retrograde flow from the axillofemoral graft is removed by an unscrubbed assistant. This establishes flow into the femoral vessels. The autograft is brought across to the contralateral groin through a previously placed subcutaneous, suprapubic tunnel and is anastomosed in a similar manner to the native artery. One or both of these anastomoses between the autograft and the distal common femoral artery frequently have to be performed in an end-to-end manner. The groin wounds are then debrided thoroughly and irrigated with antibiotic solution. A few sutures are placed to loosely approximate the subcutaneous tissue over the conduit; the remainder of the wounds are packed with antibiotic-soaked dressings.

The second stage of this procedure is performed 3 to 6 days later, using the technique described for the transabdominal removal of an infected aortoiliac graft. If the treatment sequence is performed in a single stage (sequential treatment), the technique is also the same.

There has been an improved outcome among patients treated for aortic prosthetic graft infection when the management principles outlined above are used. In our experience with 104 patients treated for aortic graft infection, overall mortality including both perioperative and late-related deaths was 26.9%.[47,52] Patients with aortoiliac graft infections have a significantly greater mortality (50%) than patients with infected aortofemoral grafts (21%). This may be a result of the high incidence of associated enteric fistulas among the former group (65.4%), when compared with aortofemoral graft patients (32.4%). Sixty-one percent of the fatalities occurred among patients with AEFs. The mortality among infected aortic graft patients with AEFs was 36%, compared with only 17% among patients with PGI and no fistulas. In contrast, the risk of a major amputation (below-the-knee or higher) was only 7.7% if the patient had an infected aortoiliac graft, but 28.2% if an infected aortofemoral graft was being treated. Staged treatment sequence resulted in fewer amputations.

Recurrent or persistent infection was a significant problem in patients with infected aortic grafts in either location (27%). Persistent infection was associated with a poor prognosis, especially if it involved aortic stump sepsis (80 to 90% mortality), or incomplete graft excision (34% mortality). Thirteen patients developed infection involving the newly placed extraanatomic bypass (an overall incidence of 13%), but this represents 20% of the patients at risk for such an infection (those whose new bypass was at least partially prosthetic). Most of these new infections involved the axillofemoral graft in its proximal or midportion. These new graft infections were relatively easy to treat and did not cause any additional deaths but did lead to two amputations.

Infected Infrainguinal Bypass Grafts

Infections involving infrainguinal bypass grafts are probably more common that those involving aortic grafts. Durham et al. recently reviewed this subject and found an average infection rate of 2.3% (range 0.65 to 12.0%).[53] The same pathophysiologic factors cited above for aortic grafts are believed to be involved in the development of infrainguinal graft infections. The higher incidence in this latter group probably reflects a higher incidence of infected lesions on the distal extremity.

A majority (55%) of infrainguinal graft infections involve the proximal (femoral) anastomosis, with the distal anastomosis involved in nearly one third of reported cases. Staphylococcal species are most commonly the organisms implicated with an increasing incidence of gram-negative and mixed infections now being reported, similar to the changing bacteriology of aortic graft infections.

The consequences of infrainguinal graft infection are not as serious as those of aortic graft infection. Reported mortality rates range from 0 to 33% but average only 9.1%. The amputation rate, however, is much higher, averaging 69.7% in Durham et al.'s review.[52]

The adequate treatment of infrainguinal prosthetic graft infection depends on several factors, including anastomotic involvement, the presence of systemic sepsis, patency of the graft, viability of the limb, the status of the distal arterial bed, and the availability of an adequate autogenous conduit. Local treatment, consisting of drainage, debridement, systemic and topical antibiotics, with or without skeletal muscle coverage, is occasionally successful. It should only be attempted if the graft is patent, the infection is limited, and signs of systemic sepsis are absent.

Partial graft excision may be appropriate for patients with a thrombosed graft, a viable limb, and a localized infection confined to the midportion of the graft without anastomotic involvement.

Most patients are best managed with total graft excision combined with either concomitant lower extremity revascularization or primary amputation. Some patients will have a viable limb after infected graft removal and therefore do not require immediate revascularization. If the distal vessels are not adequate for arterial reconstruction or if life-threatening infection is present, primary lower extremity amputation should be performed. It is probably best in these circumstances to remove the entire infrainguinal prosthetic bypass because problems with amputation stump healing are much more common when portions of the arterial prosthesis are allowed to remain.

Prosthetic Graft Infection in other Locations

Any prosthetic arterial graft can become infected. Extremity grafts used for dialysis access are especially susceptible because of the regular needle punctures required for dialysis. Heterografts (bovine carotid artery) are essentially collagen tubes with an overlying Dacron mesh. Infection tends to cause dissolution of these grafts, and hemorrhage is a frequent presenting manifestation. Infection of short grafts in the neck used to bypass occluded or stenotic carotid or subclavian arteries have also been reported. No report of an infection involving only a renal or visceral arterial prosthetic graft has been identified. Perhaps these grafts are able to resist infection because of their very short length and the ability of true endothelium to grow 2 to 2.5 cm into each end, resulting in total or near total endothelialization.

The management guidelines for infection of prosthetic grafts elsewhere are applicable to the treatment of infections in these other locations (arm, neck, etc.). Although some grafts will be salvaged with nonoperative methods, most grafts will require total removal to permanently cure the infectious process.

CONCLUSIONS

Infections involving prosthetic arterial grafts continue to be challenging both for the patient and the surgeon. Preventive measures including perioperative prophylactic antibiotics and meticulous surgical technique are warranted to reduce the incidence of this dreaded complication to a minimum. An aggressive diagnostic and therapeutic approach is necessary to minimize morbidity and mortality. Factors associated with a favorable prognosis for survival and cure of infection include prompt surgical treatment, complete graft removal, staged graft removal and revascularization, and autogenous reconstructions when feasible. Long-term survival with freedom from infection (i.e., cure), is now an attainable goal in most patients.

BIBLIOGRAPHY

1. Bouhoutsos J, Chavatzas D, et al.: Infected synthetic arterial grafts. Br J Surg 61:108, 1974.
2. Bunt TJ: Synthetic vascular graft infections. I. Graft infections. Surgery 93:733, 1983.
3. Conn JH, Hardy JD, et al.: Infected arterial grafts: Experience in 22 cases with emphasis on unusual bacteria and techniques. Ann Surg 171:704, 1970.
4. Fry WJ, Lindenauer SM: Infection complicating the use of plastic arterial implants. Arch Surg 94:600, 1967.
5. Goldstone J, Moore WS: Infection in vascular prostheses: Clinical manifestation and surgical management. Am J Surg 128:225, 1974.
6. Hoffert PW, Gensler S, Haimovici H: Infection complicating arterial grafts. Arch Surg 90:427, 1965.
7. Liekweg WJ Jr, Greenfield LJ: Vascular prosthetic infections: Collected experience and results of treatment. Surgery 81:335, 1977.
8. Wilson SE, VanWagenen P, Passaro E Jr.: Arterial infection, in Ravitch MM, Steichen FM (eds): Current Problems in Surgery. Chicago, Year Book Medical Publishers, 1978, pp 6–89.
9. Jamieson GG, DeWeese JA, Rob CG: Infected arterial grafts. Ann Surg 181:850, 1975.
10. Szilagyi DE, Smith RF, et al.: Infection in arterial reconstruction with synthetic grafts. Ann Surg 176:321, 1972.
11. Goldstone J, Effeney DJ. Prevention of arterial graft infections, in Bernhard VM, Towne JB (eds): Complications in Vascular Surgery, 2nd ed. New York, Grune & Stratton, 1985, pp 487–98.
12. Cruse PJE, Foord R: The epidemiology of wound infection. A 10-year prospective study of 62,939 wounds. Surg Clin North Am 60:27, 1980.
13. Rubin JR, Malone JM, Goldstone J: The role of the lymphatic system in acute arterial prosthetic graft infections. J Vasc Surg 2:92, 1985.
14. Ernst CB, Campbell C, et al.: Incidence and significance of intraoperative bacterial cultures during abdominal aortic aneurysmectomy. Ann Surg 185:626, 1977.
15. Macbeth GA, Rubin JR, et al.: The relevance of arterial wall

microbiology to the treatment of prosthetic graft infections: Graft infection vs. arterial infection. J Vasc Surg 1:750, 1984.

16. Williams RD, Fisher FW: Aneurysm contents as a source of graft infection. Arch Surg 112:415, 1977.

17. Krupski WC, Mitchell RA, et al.: Appendicitis and aortofemoral graft infection. Arch Surg 114:969, 1979.

18. Malone JM, Moore WS, et al.: Bacteremic infectability of vascular grafts: the influence of pseudointimal integrity and duration of graft function. Surgery 78:211, 1975.

19. Moore WS, Malone JM, Keown K: Prosthetic arterial graft material. Influence on neointimal healing and bacteremic infectability. Arch Surg 115:1379, 1980.

20. Reilly LM, Altman H, et al.: Late results following surgical management of vascular graft infection. J Vasc Surg 1:36, 1984.

21. Bandyk DF, Berni GA, et al.: Aortofemoral graft infection due to Staphylococcus epidermidis. Arch 119:102, 1984.

22. Scobie K, McPhail N, et al.: Bacteriologic monitoring in abdominal aortic surgery. Can J Surg 22:368, 1979.

23. Bandyk DF: Vascular graft infection. Epidemiology, bacteriology and pathogenesis, in Bernhard VM, Towne JB (eds): Complications in Vascular Surgery, 2nd ed. New York. Grune & Stratton, 1985, pp 471–85.

24. Reilly LM, Goldstone J, et al.: Gastrointestinal tract involvement by prosthetic graft infection: The significance of gastrointestinal hemorrhage. Ann Surg 202:342, 1985.

25. O'Donnell TF Jr, Scott G, et al.: Improvements in the diagnosis and management of aortoenteric fistula. Am J Surg 149:481, 1985.

26. Champion MC, Sullivan SN, et al.: Aortoenteric fistula. Incidence, presentation, recognition, management. Ann Surg 195:314, 1982.

27. Bunt TJ. Synthetic vascular graft infections. II. Graft-enteric erosion and graft-enteric fistulas. Surgery 94:1, 1983.

28. O'Mara CS, Williams GM, Ernst CB: Secondary aortoenteric fistula. A 20-year experience. Am J Surg 142:203, 1981.

29. Kleinman LH, Towne JB, Bernhard VM: A diagnostic and therapeutic approach to aortoenteric fistulas: Clinical experience with twenty patients. Surgery 86:868, 1979.

30. Brown OW, Stanson AW, et al.: Computerized tomography following abdominal aortic surgery. Surgery 91:716, 1982.

31. Haaga JR, Baldwin GN, et al.: CT detection of infected synthetic grafts: Preliminary report of a new sign. AJR 131:317, 1978.

32. Mark A, Moss AA, et al.: CT evaluation of complications of abdominal aortic surgery. Radiology 145:409, 1982.

33. Kukora JS, Rushton FW, Cranston PE: New computed tomographic signs of aortoenteric fistula. Arch Surg 119:1073, 1984.

34. Gooding GAW, Effeney DJ, Goldstone J: The aortofemoral graft: Detection and identification of healing complications by ultrasonography. Surgery 89:94, 1981.

35. Cunat JS, Haaga JR, et al.: Periaortic fluid aspiration for recognition of infected graft. AJR 139:251, 1982.

36. Qvarfordt PG, Reilly LM, et al.: Computed tomographic assessment of graft incorporation following aortic reconstruction. Am J Surg 150:227, 1985.

37. Lawrence PF, Dries DJ, et al.: Indium 111-labeled leukocyte scanning for detection of prosthetic vascular graft infection. J Vasc Surg 2:165, 1985.

38. Serota AI, Williams RA, et al.: Uptake of radiolabeled leukocytes in prosthetic graft infection. Surgery 90:35, 1981.

39. Causey DA, Fajman WA, et al.: Gallium 67 scintigraphy in postoperative synthetic graft infections. AJR 134:1041, 1980.

40. Kwaan JHM, Connolly JE: Successful management of prosthetic graft infection with continuous povidone-iodine irrigation. Arch Surg 116:716, 1981.

41. Knight CD, Farnell MB, Hollier LH: Treatment of aortic graft infection with povidone-iodine irrigation. Mayo Clin Proc 58:472, 1983.

42. Ehrenfeld WK, Wilbur BG, et al.: Autogenous tissue reconstruction in the management of infected prosthetic grafts. Surgery 85:82, 1979.

43. Seeger JM, Wheeler JR, et al.: Autogenous graft replacement of infected prosthetic grafts in the femoral position. Surgery 93:39, 1983.

44. Trout HH III, Kozloff L, Giordano JM: Priority of revascularization in patients with graft enteric fistulas, infected arteries, or infected arterial prostheses. Ann Surg 199:669, 1984.

45. Yashar JJ, Weyman AK, et al.: Survival and limb salvage in patients with infected arterial prostheses. Am J Surg 135:499, 1978.

46. Turnipseed WD, Berkoff HA, et al.: Arterial graft infections. Delayed vs. immediate vascular reconstruction. Arch Surg 118:410, 1983.

47. Reilly LM, Stoney RJ, et al.: Improved management of aortic graft infection: The influence of operation sequence and staging. J Vasc Surg 5:412, 1987.

48. Shah DM, Buchbinder D, et al.: Clinical use of the seromuscular jejunal patch for protection of the infected aortic stump. Am J Surg 146:198, 1983.

49. Goldsmith HS, de los Santos R, et al: Experimental protection of vascular prosthesis by omentum. Arch Surg 97:872, 1968.

50. Iliopoulos JI, Pierce GE, et al.: Transmesocolic omentoplasty. Surg Gynecol Obstet 157:282, 1983.

51. Reilly LM, Ehrenfeld WK, Stoney RJ: Delayed aortic prosthetic reconstruction after removal of an infected graft. Am J Surg 148:234, 1984.

52. Reilly LM, Goldstone J: The infected aortic graft, in: Bergan JJ, Yao JST (eds): Reoperative Arterial Surgery. Orlando, Fla., Grune & Stratton, 1986, pp 231–253.

53. Durham JR, Rubin JR, Malone JM: Management of infected infrainguinal bypass grafts, in: Bergan JJ, Yao JST (eds): Reoperative Arterial Surgery. Orlando, Fla., Grune & Stratton, 1986, pp 359–373.

CHAPTER 44
Reoperations for Early and Late Occlusive Complications of Arterial Surgery

John J. Bergan, Wesley S. Moore, and Henry Haimovici

Management of occlusive complications of vascular reconstruction presents difficult problems that tax the ingenuity and capabilities of the surgeon. Although there are many factors common to the management of occlusive complications of all vascular operations, this chapter is divided into sections dealing separately with each type of reconstruction.

FAILURE OF CAROTID BIFURCATION ENDARTERECTOMY

Acute Occlusion

Etiology
Acute carotid artery thrombosis after bifurcation endarterectomy may be due to technical error or accumulation of platelet thrombus. If the distal portion of the endarterectomy is improperly managed, an intimal flap may be left to act as a valve obstructing the flow of blood. This will produce stasis followed by acute thrombosis (Fig. 44-1).

Management
If acute thrombosis of the carotid artery is recognized at the operating table, immediate thrombectomy with correction of the technical error is indicated. Acute postoperative occlusion may be silent or will cause a neurologic deficit. Management of this complication is controversial, but most authorities agree that the patient should be returned immediately to the operating room for thrombectomy and correction of the defect.

Prevention

Optimally, the surgeon should prevent postoperative thrombosis during the primary procedure. This is best accomplished by insisting upon direct visualization of the distal end point of the endarterectomy. Gentle mechanical irrigation of the intimal end point with heparinized saline enables the surgeon to ascertain that the distal end point is firmly adherent to the media. Finally, operative angiography, intraoperative ultrasonography, or angioscopy may provide assurance that a satisfactory technical result has been achieved. The incidence of an unsatisfactory end point has been reported to be as high as 20% and in our series is between 5 and 10%. However, the incidence of postoperative thrombus was 0 in 100 consecutive patients studied with routine postoperative angiography.

Recurrent Carotid Artery Stenosis or Late Occlusion

Etiology
The most frequent cause for recurrent stenosis or occlusion of a carotid artery reconstruction is intimal and subintimal fibrosis at the distal end point of the endarterectomy. Other causes of recurrent stenosis are fibrous tissue organization of an intimal flap left from the initial operation and recurrent atherosclerosis.

Diagnosis
The diagnosis of recurrent stenosis or occlusion may not be made in the absence of recurrent symptoms unless patients are routinely followed with noninvasive studies or carotid angiography. A patient with recurrent stenosis may again have transient ischemic attacks or even a completed stroke. On the other hand, recurrent stenosis or occlusion may be entirely asymptomatic and go undiagnosed. Therefore a duplex scan should be performed postoperatively, at 6 months, and yearly at the anniversary of the operation.

Management
Recurrent stenosis, whether discovered incidentally or by a recurrence of the patient's symptoms, is best treated by operative repair. Failure to do this places the patient at the same risk that existed before the initial operation. The absolute indication for reintervention in the asymptomatic patient is the recurrence of stenosis that reaches 75% or greater.

The major technical difficulty encountered during oper-

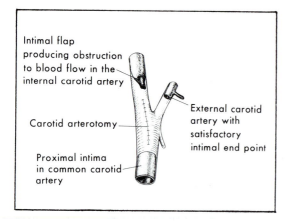

Figure 44-1. Carotid bifurcation endarterectomy in which the distal intima was improperly managed. The intimal flap can act as a valve obstructing blood flow, which may lead to thrombosis. Note particularly the limited extent of the arteriotomy.

ative repair occurs when dissecting out the common carotid bifurcation from surrounding scar tissue. In addition to the difficulty in mobilizing the artery from scar tissue and the jugular vein, the vagus and hypoglossal nerves may be incorporated into the scar tissue, resulting in potential injury to these structures during reoperation.

The dissection is best begun at the most proximal portion of the cervical common carotid artery since this is an area that may not have been previously dissected at the time of the original operation and might, as a result, be a more easily identified and mobilized vessel. After the proximal common carotid artery is mobilized, providing proximal control, dissection is continued to the carotid bifurcation. Mobilization of a previously dissected artery is best accomplished by sharp dissection. The appropriate zone of dissection is identified by applying lateral traction to the artery and countertraction to the surrounding fibrous tissues. Using a scalpel with a No. 15 blade, a groove between the artery and fibrous tissue is incised first on one side of the artery and then on the opposite side. By alternating sides, circumferential skeletonization of the artery encased in scar tissue can be accomplished (Fig. 44-2). As the carotid bifurcation is approached, mobilization is continued up on both the external and internal carotid arteries. Particular care is taken with the external carotid artery because of the accompanying branches, particularly the superior thyroid artery. Once the carotid bifurcation has been mobilized, the dissection is carried up the internal carotid artery well beyond the area of narrowing, so that angioplastic repair can be accomplished.

The decision whether an internal shunt is to be used can often be based on what was required at the time of the original operation. If the patient required an internal

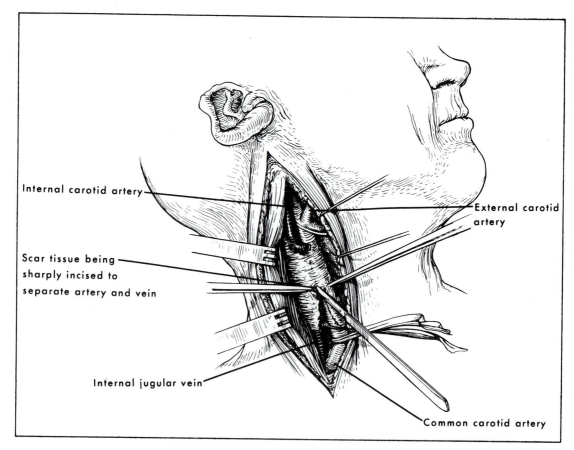

Figure 44-2. Previously operated carotid artery bifurcation encased in scar tissue. The use of sharp dissection to define the plane between the artery and the surrounding scar tissue is demonstrated.

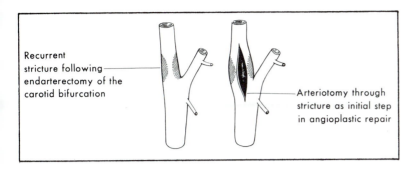

Recurrent stricture following endarterectomy of the carotid bifurcation

Arteriotomy through stricture as initial step in angioplastic repair

Figure 44-3. Recurrent stricture of the first portion of the internal carotid artery. An arteriotomy is made in the common carotid artery extending through the stricture up to a relatively normal portion of the internal carotid artery. This is the initial step in angioplastic repair of the lesion.

shunt then, it would probably be wise to employ a shunt again. On the other hand, if the surgeon does not know what was used or wishes to perform the operation in the absence of a shunt, we recommend measurement of the internal carotid artery back pressure as an index of tolerance to temporary occlusion. The patient is put under general anesthesia with maintenance of normal blood pressure and PCO_2. If the back pressure is 25 mm Hg or greater, cross-clamping can be performed and a shunt is unnecessary.

The arteriotomy is made in the common carotid artery and extended up onto the internal carotid artery through the area of stricture. The stenosis can be patched open, using either autogenous vein or a prosthetic patch, depending on the preference of the surgeon (Figs. 44-3 and 44-4). A polytetrafluoroethylene (PTFE) patch is readily available and easy to use.

A vein patch has the advantage of being autogenous tissue, tending to remain relatively pliable, with the same characteristics as the arterial wall. However, it is somewhat more difficult to use as a patch because of the thinness of the wall and the tendency to roll when sutures are being applied. For this reason, external jugular vein should not be used as patch material. Because ankle vein has a tendency to rupture, it should not be used either.

Angioplasty as well as the original operation should be carried out under adequate anticoagulation with heparin.

We administer 10,000 units of aqueous heparin intravenously before the occluding clamps are applied. After the angioplasty is completed, an operative arteriogram, ultrasonography, or angioscopy is performed.

FAILURE OF AORTOILIAC OR AORTOFEMORAL BYPASS GRAFTS

Acute Thrombosis

Etiology
Acute postoperative occlusion of a graft originating from the abdominal aorta is due to technical error. The most common error is an unsatisfactory distal anastomosis producing a compromise of the runoff flow. Other mechanisms of acute occlusion are unrecognized thrombus in the graft, which may embolize distally, or thrombus that has formed in the distal circulation, a consequence of inadequate heparinization.

Diagnosis
The diagnosis of acute graft thrombosis in the postoperative period can be made by a loss of peripheral pulses, or a failure to achieve optimum distal Doppler pressures. Sudden deterioration of perfusion in the distal extremity is a sign of graft, limb, or distal thrombosis.

Management
As soon as acute thrombosis is recognized, 10,000 units of aqueous heparin is given to prevent propagation of thrombus. The patient is returned to the operating room for graft thrombectomy and correction of the technical error that led to acute thrombosis. If the distal anastomosis was made to the external iliac artery, the abdomen must be reopened to explore the anastomosis, perform balloon catheter thrombectomy, and to inspect the runoff vessels. If the graft extends to the common femoral artery, graft thrombectomy can be performed by exposing the distal graft limb in the femoral incision of the involved extremity. It is unusual for both limbs of a bifurcation graft to undergo acute thrombosis, and reexploration of the appropriate groin may be all that is necessary. We have found it expedient to perform a transverse graftotomy just proximal to the femoral anastomosis so that the graft can be disobliterated by retrograde passage of an embolectomy catheter through an incision that will also provide the opportunity to inspect directly the orifices of the superficial and profunda femoris arteries (Fig. 44-5).

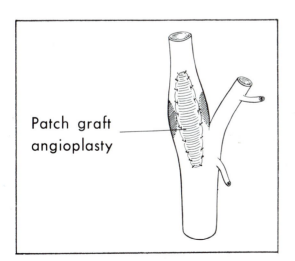

Patch graft angioplasty

Figure 44-4. Arteriotomy through the strictured segment is closed, using patch graft angioplasty. In this manner, the lumen of the internal carotid artery is restored to normal caliber.

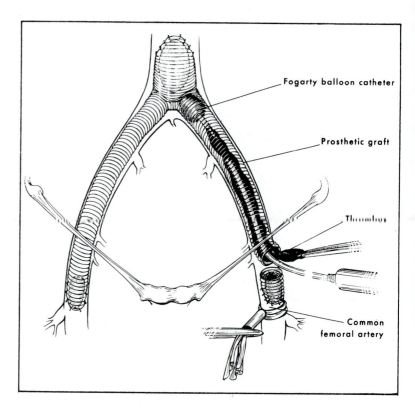

Fogarty balloon catheter

Prosthetic graft

Thrombus

Common femoral artery

Figure 44-5. Transverse graftotomy is made at the distal extent of the occluded limb of a bifurcation graft. This permits retrograde passage of a Fogarty embolectomy catheter for disobliteration of the graft limb. Following thrombectomy, a direct inspection of the distal anastomosis can be accomplished through the graftotomy. Angioscopy is a useful adjunct to ensure total clearing of thrombus from the graft limb.

Direct internal inspection will determine where the technical error occurred that led to graft thrombosis. If the technical error consists of a compromised lumen, the anastomosis may have to be redone. If the reason for thrombosis is simply propagation of thrombus within runoff vessels or unrecognized thrombus in the graft, removal of these thrombotic or embolic debris by balloon catheter may be all that is required. The transverse graftotomy is closed and flow is reestablished.

Prevention
Because compromising the runoff vessels during distal anastomosis is the most common cause for graft thrombosis, one method to prevent lumen compromise is to place intraluminal polyethylene tubes in the superficial or profunda femoris vessels, or both, at the initial stages of the anastomosis and to remove the tubes just before the anastomosis is completed (Fig. 44-6). In this manner there is no chance that a poorly placed suture can compromise the lumen, since the lumen is being held widely open by an internal stent. With these tubes in place, intermittent irrigation with heparinized saline solution prevents intravascular thrombosis, which eliminates another potential cause of acute graft thrombosis. While this technique is quite effective, it is somewhat cumbersome and should not be used routinely. Careful aspiration of each limb of the graft for thrombus or accumulated blood before passing the graft in the retroperitoneal tunnel helps to prevent unrecognized clot in the graft limb. It is our practice, before flushing the distal vessels at the time of completion of the anastomosis, to put a clamp on the most distal extent of the graft to prevent retrograde flow of blood into the graft. Blood flow may be initially started within the common femoral artery or

external iliac artery before blood flow is begun within the graft. As soon as the anastomosis is secure, the distal clamp can be removed, allowing the retrograde flow of blood to push air out of the graft through the interstices. Then, by releasing the proximal clamp on the abdominal portion of the graft, blood flow through the graft is established.

Late Graft Thrombosis

Etiology
The most frequent cause of late graft failure is either progression of occlusive disease at the profunda femoris origin in a patient with an occluded superficial femoral artery, a false aneurysm at the anastomosis, or graft elongation and kinking.

Diagnosis
The diagnosis of recurrent stenosis or graft occlusion can be made by the return of claudication and loss of previously palpable pulses. The status of the reconstruction, whether recurrent stenosis or total occlusion, can be ascertained with aortofemoral angiography after measurement of distal limb pressures. A CT scan will further clarify the cause of graft limb occlusion.

Management
Aortoiliac Bypass Thrombosis

FAILURE OF ONE GRAFT LIMB. This is the most usual mode of presentation, since it is unlikely that both limbs will fail simultaneously. Several approaches are available for the management of this problem. The most direct means of

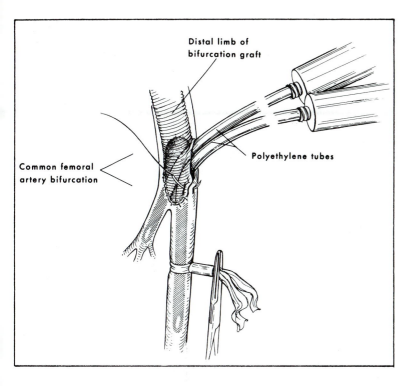

Figure 44-6. Distal anastomosis of a bifurcation graft to the common femoral artery is performed over polyethylene tubes that are inserted into the superficial and profunda femoris branches. In this manner the orifices of the runoff vessels are kept open by the presence of this inlying stent. The polyethylene tubes also provide a vehicle for injection of heparinized saline to prevent distal thrombosis during the performance of the anastomosis.

correcting the occlusion is to extend a new graft limb down to the common femoral artery. One can utilize a suprainguinal, oblique, retroperitoneal exposure of the thrombosed limb of the graft (Fig. 44-7).

Once the involved limb of the graft is identified and mobilized, the graft limb is divided and thrombectomy accomplished by passing a balloon catheter in a retrograde fashion and removing the thrombus (Fig. 44-8). If it is a relatively acute occlusion, the thrombus will come out with ease. If the thrombosis is ancient, it may be easier to carry the dissection back to the bifurcation of the graft, obliquely clamp the body of the graft, and divide the occluded limb just distal to the bifurcation. This provides access to carry out thrombectomy at the origin of the occluded limb. A

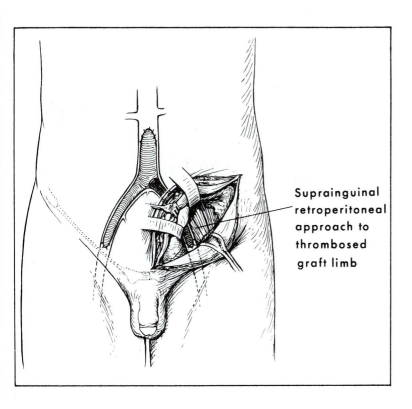

Figure 44-7. Suprainguinal, oblique, retroperitoneal approach to expose an occluded limb of a bifurcation graft.

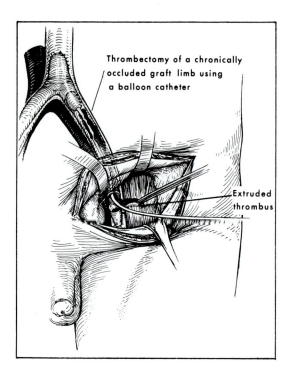

Figure 44-8. Distal extent of the occluded limb is divided and a balloon catheter is inserted in a retrograde manner so as to carry out thrombectomy of the chronically occluded graft limb.

new graft limb of appropriate size can be sutured to the stump end of the bifurcation graft. The new limb is passed through the retroperitoneum and into an area prepared by exposure of the common femoral bifurcation (Fig. 44-9). This approach has the advantage of being direct, and

it avoids a laparotomy. However, if technical difficulties are encountered during graft thrombectomy, or if the common portion of the bifurcated graft is quite high on the aorta, it may be difficult to achieve accessibility through this limited retroperitoneal exposure.

Because of difficulties with graft limb replacement as described above, an alternative treatment is to perform a femoral-to-femoral crossover bypass graft. If the opposite graft limb is widely patent and functioning well, this approach is a satisfactory method of dealing with unilateral graft occlusion (Fig. 44-10). Laparotomy can be avoided, and the operation can be performed in new anatomic areas, obviating the need to redissect fibrosed tissues. The disadvantage of this technique is that the opposite femoral artery must be exposed on a side that is now functioning well. The risk of introducing complications in a normally functioning limb must be considered.

A third alternative for managing unilateral graft occlusion is by total transabdominal replacement of the graft with extension to the groin. This is the most direct approach to the problem; however, it requires laparotomy with transabdominal dissection and should be used selectively when total graft replacement is mandatory.

FAILURE OF BOTH GRAFT LIMBS. The failure of both limbs of a bifurcation graft is a relatively rare complication. However, when it occurs, bilateral femoral false aneurysms should be suspected. If a proximal false aneurysm is also present, the graft must be replaced in its entirety.

Aortofemoral Bypass Graft Occlusion

FAILURE OF ONE LIMB OF GRAFT. In this instance a femoral approach for performing retrograde thrombectomy of the

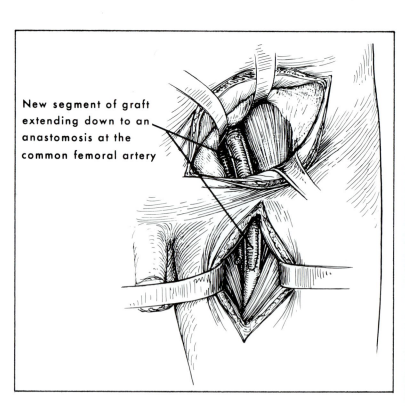

Figure 44-9. Following thrombectomy of the proximal extent of the occluded limb, a graft extension is sutured into place and passed through the retroperitoneal exposure into a femoral incision where it can be anastomosed to the common femoral artery.

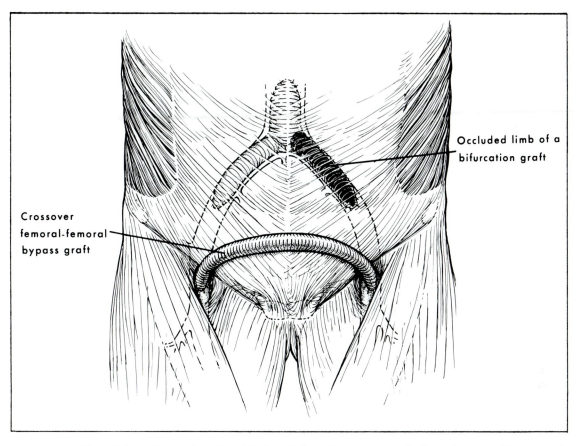

Occluded limb of a bifurcation graft

Crossover femoral-femoral bypass graft

Figure 44-10. Method of treating a unilateral graft limb occlusion with a crossover of a femoral-to-femoral bypass graft extending from the patent side to the occluded side. The crossover may be C-shaped as illustrated or S-shaped and originating from a patent graft limb.

graft with correction of the outflow tract can be an entirely satisfactory means of reestablishing blood flow. The inguinal incision is reopened and dissection is carried down to the graft. Upon incising the fibrous tissue capsule surrounding the graft, a plane between the graft and the fibrous tissue capsule is easily developed (Fig. 44-11). Once the graft is mobilized, dissection is carried distally onto the femoral artery. Sharp dissection in the plane between the fibrous tissue and the femoral artery and its branches is the preferred method of mobilizing this previously dissected vessel.

For ease of identification, it is often best to begin distally on the superficial femoral artery in a previously undissected area to identify this vessel, and then carry the sharp dissection of the surrounding fibrous tissue back to the common femoral artery (Fig. 44-12). Particular care must be taken during the sharp dissection of the profunda femoris artery to avoid dividing significant branches such as the lateral and medial circumflex femoral arteries. After the superficial femoral and profunda femoris arteries are identified and mobilized, dissection is continued back onto the common femoral artery to gain proximal control of this vessel should it still be patent proximal to the graft. The thrombosed graft can now be divided immediately proximal to the femoral anastomosis. The distal portion of the graft is then longi-

tudinally incised to expose the orifices of the outflow vessels and to determine the reason for obstruction.

If it appears that there is fibrosis or progressive disease in one or both runoff vessels, the arteriotomy should be continued onto either the superficial femoral or profunda femoris artery, or both, to split open the stenotic areas and permit angioplastic repair (Fig. 44-13). A short segment of 10 mm graft is suitably beveled for anastomosis to the newly opened femoral artery bifurcation. By appropriate beveling of the graft, the stenotic orifices of the runoff branches can be patched open. This angioplastic technique will ensure an open runoff for the disobliterated graft. We prefer to do the anastomosis over intraluminal tubes placed in either or both runoff branches (Fig. 44-14). This technique assures a technically perfect anastomosis and prevents compromise of the runoff vessels. The intraluminal tubes are also a means of back-bleeding control and obviate the need for vascular clamps that might compromise the runoff vessels by fracturing an atheromatous plaque. Finally, with the tubes in place, intermittent irrigation with heparinized saline can be used to prevent intravascular thrombosis.

An alternative method of angioplastic repair is to use an autogenous patch for the profundaplasty, divide the proximal common femoral artery, and perform an end-to-end anastomosis between the distal graft and the common

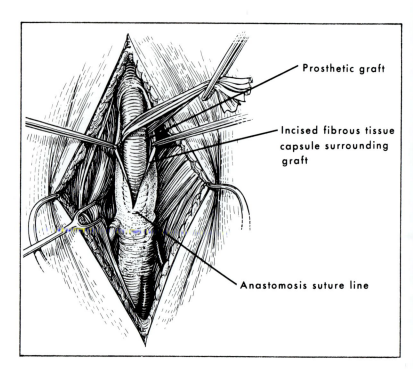

Figure 44-11. Common femoral bifurcation with an occluded graft limb anastomosed to the vessel. An incision is made over the fibrous tissue capsule at the distal extent of the graft to develop the potential space around the graft to mobilize the prosthesis and gain distal control.

femoral artery. Autogenous patch material can come from the adjacent saphenous vein or from suitable preparation of a chronically occluded segment of superficial femoral artery. If the superficial femoral artery is chronically occluded, this is the material of choice. A segment of occluded superficial femoral artery of sufficient length is removed and opened longitudinally. An endarterectomy of the diseased intima is performed and the autogenous strip of arterial adventitia is used for patch material. The long-term patency using autogenous arterial patch is better than the patency obtained with Dacron angioplasty.

After the anastomosis or patch angioplasty has been completed, attention is turned to disobliteration of the proximal portion of the graft. If the occlusion is recent, the clot

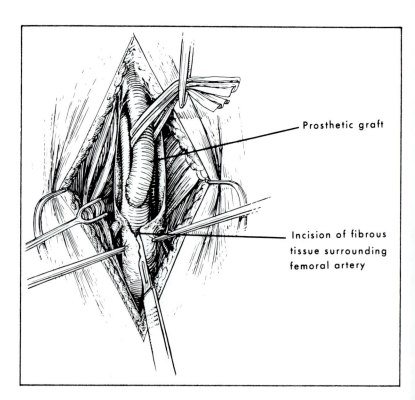

Figure 44-12. Femoral bifurcation is dissected free of surrounding scar tissue, using sharp dissection to establish the plane between the artery and surrounding fibrous tissue.

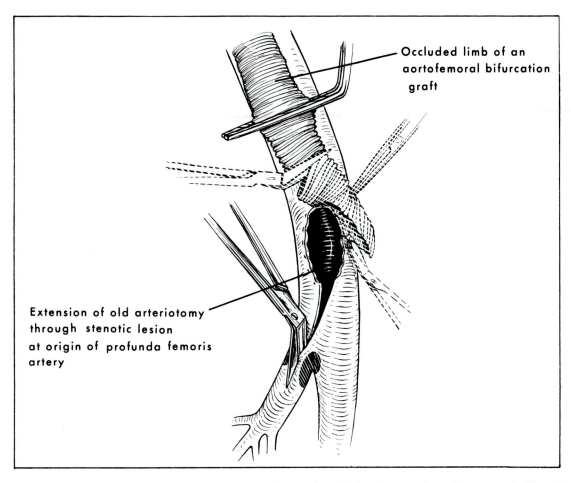

Occluded limb of an
aortofemoral bifurcation
graft

Extension of old arteriotomy
through stenotic lesion
at origin of profunda femoris
artery

Figure 44-13. Detachment of the distal anastomosis of the occluded limb of an aortofemoral bypass graft. The old arteriotomy is extended distally through a stenotic lesion at the origin of the profunda femoris artery so that a new anastomosis can serve as a patch angioplasty of the lesion which led to late occlusion.

can be easily removed with an embolectomy balloon catheter (Fig. 44-15).

After successful removal of the clot and reestablishment of good inflow, an arteriogram of the graft should be obtained. This can best be performed by passing a small catheter into the graft and securing it in place with the appropriate transverse and tangential placement of clamps to prevent blood from leaking around the tube (Fig. 44-16). Retrograde injection of contrast medium provides excellent visualization. An arteriogram will show whether all thrombus has been removed. If the thrombus has not been suitably removed, additional passes of the Fogarty catheter may be required. If the thrombus is old, additional maneuvers may be required to carry out effective thrombectomy. We use an endarterectomy stripper that will fit within the graft. By passing the Fogarty catheter through the loop of the endarterectomy stripper, the catheter can then be advanced well onto the common portion of the graft; the balloon is inflated and then pulled back to impact the orifice of the limb and provide inflow occlusion. The endarterectomy stripper can then be passed into the limb and used to loosen any debris, hypertrophied pseudointima, or areas of disrupted intima that are only partially adherent to the graft

wall (Fig. 44-17). When the graft wall has been suitably scraped clean of adherent debris and pseudointima, the balloon catheter can be pulled down to remove the debris loosened by the stripper.

Once adequate inflow has been obtained, the patient should be given a small dose of heparin to prevent intraluminal thrombosis of the newly constituted graft limb. We have found that 3500 units of aqueous heparin administered intravenously provides enough time to perform the graft-to-graft anastomosis between the constituted aortofemoral graft and the new segment of graft anastomosed to the femoral artery. Once these anastomoses are completed, another operative arteriogram is obtained to document the adequacy of the outflow angioplasty. This technique avoids the need for laparotomy and gives the opportunity to correct the outflow lesion that led to the thrombosis.

An alternative method of therapy, in the case of unilateral graft thrombosis, is to perform a crossover femoral-to-femoral bypass in the manner previously described. The final alternative is transabdominal replacement of the occluded graft limb. This has been the standard method of treatment, but it requires laparotomy and dissection through a previously operated area.

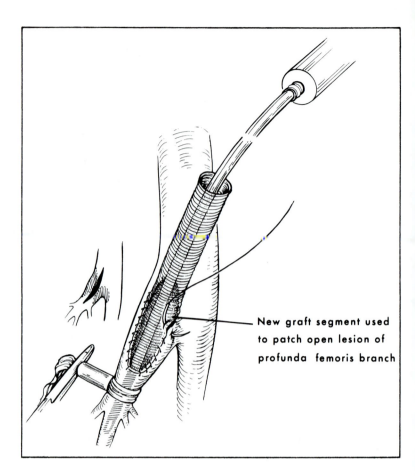

Figure 44-14. Free segment of graft is suitably beveled and anastomosed to the new common femoral arteriotomy over a polyethylene tube used as a stent to maintain the profunda femoris branch in an open position. The beveled end of the graft will serve as an angioplasty for the stenotic lesion at the origin of the profunda femoris artery.

New graft segment used to patch open lesion of profunda femoris branch

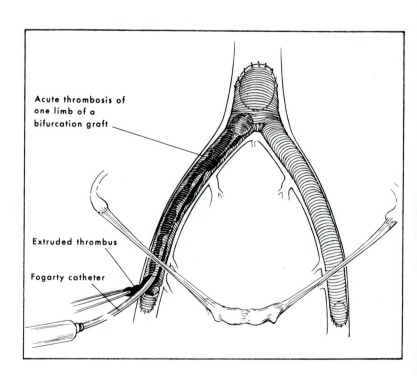

Acute thrombosis of one limb of a bifurcation graft

Extruded thrombus

Fogarty catheter

Figure 44-15. Method of passing a balloon catheter up the occluded limb of an aortofemoral bypass graft. The occluded limb is disobliterated by using the balloon catheter to extrude thrombus material.

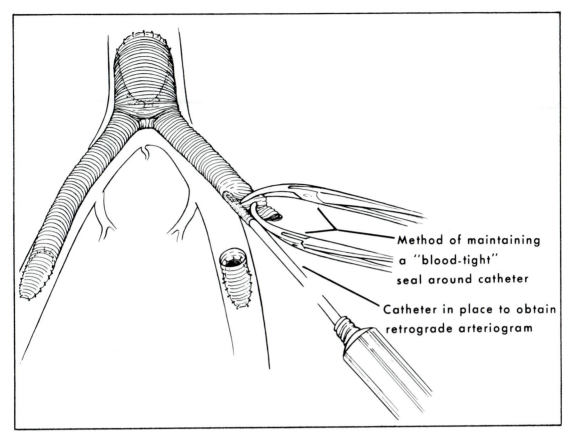

Figure 44-16. Method of holding a catheter in the limb of the graft following removal of thrombus to obtain a detailed arteriogram of the proximal system.

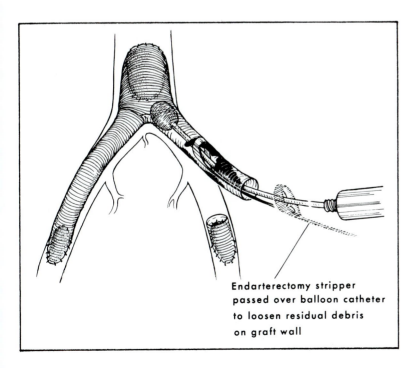

Figure 44-17. Should residual debris be adherent to the graft wall, as documented on arteriography, an endarterectomy stripper can be passed over the balloon catheter and used to scrape the wall of the graft of any residual thrombus material. Hemostasis is maintained by inflating the balloon catheter to prevent the rush of blood down the partially cleared graft limb.

BOTH LIMBS OF GRAFT THROMBOSED. In this case, the best method of management is transabdominal replacement of the entire graft, with bilateral femoral angioplasty to correct the compromised outflow.

Failure of Axillofemoral Bypass Graft

Acute Occlusion

Etiology. Acute occlusion of an axillofemoral bypass graft may be caused by the following:

1. Unrecognized thrombus within the graft at the time flow was initiated
2. Technical errors related to the construction of either the proximal or distal anastomosis
3. Unrecognized rotation or twist of the prosthesis in the subcutaneous tunnel
4. Competitive flow through the patient's own iliofemoral system so as to reduce the flow rate and induce thrombosis of the prosthesis
5. Inadequate runoff due to extensive disease in the branches of the femoral artery or unrecognized thrombosis or distal embolization

Diagnosis. The diagnosis of acute graft thrombosis is made by loss of pulsation in the subcutaneous graft.

Management. Once the diagnosis of acute occlusion is made, systemic anticoagulation is obtained with 10,000 units of aqueous heparin administered intravenously. The patient is then returned to the operating room for graft thrombectomy and correction of the technical error that caused thrombosis. It is usually necessary to reopen both the axillary and the femoral incisions. Because of the extensive length of the prosthesis, thrombectomy is best carried out from both ends. Thrombectomy can be performed through transverse graftotomy incisions, using a large Fogarty balloon catheter. After thrombectomy is completed, the inside of the distal anastomosis is inspected through the graftotomy site for any obvious technical errors. If none are found, the graftotomies are closed and flow is reinstituted. Following reinstitution of flow, an arteriogram, taken through a needle in the graft, should reveal any technical error in association with the distal anastomosis. If the distal anastomosis and runoff vessels appear satisfactory, a proximal graft angiogram should be obtained, with the film placed to visualize the entire length of the prosthesis to determine whether there is a kink or twist in the prosthetic graft.

Prevention. Prevention of unrecognized thrombus within the graft can be achieved by carefully aspirating the entire length of the prosthesis after preclotting of the interstitial spaces of the graft is accomplished. With a clamp placed at the proximal anastomosis, the graft can be aspirated and all free blood removed. Kinks and twists of the prosthesis in the subcutaneous tunnel can be prevented by using a tunneling device connecting the axillary and femoral incisions. With the tunneler in place, the graft can be pulled through to maintain proper orientation. Intraoperative angiography as soon as the distal anastomosis is completed

will prevent graft thrombosis from unrecognized technical errors associated with the distal anastomosis or the presence of thromboembolic material in the runoff vessels.

Late Occlusion

Etiology. The late thrombosis rate of the axillofemoral bypass is considerably higher than an aortofemoral bypass. The primary reason is that the prosthesis is quite long and the flow rate through this long plastic graft is relatively slow. In addition to the natural propensity of this type of reconstruction for late occlusion, several other factors may account for late failure. These include:

1. Extension of occlusive disease in the area of the distal anastomosis. This can be in the form either of progressive atheromatous degeneration or proliferation of fibrous scar tissue in association with the anastomosis.
2. Disruption of pseudointima, poorly adherent to the prosthesis, resulting in a pseudointimal slough with occlusion of the distal anastomosis.

Diagnosis. The diagnosis of late occlusion is readily made from recurrence of symptoms and a loss of pulse along the course of the subcutaneous graft.

Management. Management of chronic occlusion of an axillofemoral bypass graft is directed toward reestablishing the flow through the prosthesis as well as correcting any lesions associated with the distal anastomosis which may have resulted in graft thrombosis. If the time interval between graft thrombosis and operation is relatively short, it is feasible to perform graft thrombectomy and reuse the original prosthesis. If the time interval is more than a few days, it is often easier to replace the prosthetic graft.

Initially the femoral incision is reopened, and dissection is carried down to the prosthetic graft. A transverse graftotomy is made close to the distal anastomosis. The distal thrombus is mechanically removed, and a Fogarty thrombectomy catheter is used to clear the runoff vessels. Once thrombectomy is accomplished and good back-bleeding is established, the caliber of the runoff vessels is measured by introducing either arterial dilators or arterial catheters of progressively larger size. If the caliber of the runoff vessels is adequate, no further modification of the distal anastomosis is necessary. Back-bleeding is easily controlled by insertion of an appropriately sized arterial catheter, which not only prevents back-bleeding but also permits introduction of heparinized saline solution during the next phase of the operation.

After satisfactory outflow is reestablished, a large balloon thrombectomy catheter is inserted into the proximal portion of the graft and several passes are used to disobliterate the previously placed prosthesis. If satisfactory inflow is obtained in this manner, a catheter is inserted into the graft and a retrograde arteriogram is obtained to determine that the graft has been completely evacuated of clot. If irregularities are noted on the arteriogram or if satisfactory inflow is not obtained, the axillary incision is reopened to expose the proximal portion of the prosthesis. This is easily mobilized to the axillary artery and can be divided, leaving a small proximal cuff comprising the anastomosis to the axillary artery. This segment is disobliterated to clear the orifice of the axillary artery, and bleeding is controlled with a clamp. A new prosthesis can then be pulled into place by suturing it to the old prosthesis. By pulling the old prosthesis out, the new prosthesis is drawn into the tunnel. Graft-to-graft anastomoses constructed both proximally and distally complete the procedure. Flow is reinitiated, and operative angiography is obtained to ensure that there is both good inflow and outflow.

Prevention. It has previously been reported that the best patency rates with axillofemoral grafts have occurred with knitted rather than woven grafts, and in combination with a crossover femorofemoral graft limb. The addition of the femorofemoral graft limb effectively doubles the flow rate through the long segment of the graft. Of more importance is the adequacy of the associated profundaplasty that is done to ensure adequate outflow. Similarly, the crossover limb, if done, must be taken off as low as possible to ensure that the greatest volume of blood passes through the axillary to femoral graft segment.

FAILURE OF A CROSSOVER FEMOROFEMORAL BYPASS GRAFT

Acute Occlusion

Etiology
Acute postoperative occlusion of a femorofemoral bypass graft is rare. It may be caused by technical error in one or both anastomoses or by failure to recognize occlusive disease in the iliac system on the donor side.

Diagnosis
The diagnosis of acute occlusion is made by loss of the easily palpable subcutaneous pulse in the suprapubic area, combined with evidence of vascular insufficiency of the recipient extremity.

Management
As soon as the diagnosis is made, 10,000 units of aqueous heparin should be administered intravenously. The patient should then be returned to the operating room where both groins are reexplored and the anastomoses checked for technical error. If technical error is present, this should be corrected and the quality of correction verified by operative angiography. If acute occlusion is caused by inadequate inflow on the donor side due to proximal iliac disease, the treatment of choice is the addition of an axillofemoral graft to the cross-leg bypass graft. This is one means of achieving adequate inflow, assuming that the patient is not a reasonable candidate for intraabdominal vascular reconstruction.

Prevention
Technical error of the anastomosis can be prevented by careful attention to detail during the performance of the procedure, combined with intraoperative angiography to verify the technical result before completing the operation. To prevent acute occlusion due to inadequate inflow, the proximal arterial tree is carefully assessed, primarily by careful scrutiny of a translumbar aortogram.

Late Occlusion

Etiology
Late failure of a femorofemoral crossover bypass can result from progression of disease in the donor iliac system or from atheromatous or fibrotic changes in one or both anastomoses. Donor limb failure is uncommon, but occlusion of the recipient profunda femoris artery is to be expected.

Diagnosis
The diagnosis of late failure can be made by a return of lower-extremity symptoms, loss of the subcutaneous graft pulse, or both.

Management
Careful evaluation of the patient's functional status is in order since there may have been enough internal development of collateral circulation to minimize symptoms. However, if the patient's symptoms justify vascular reconstruction, angiographic evaluation should be performed to document the basis for late failure. A CT scan should be done to determine a proximal atheromatous embolic source. If late failure is due to progression of iliac artery disease on the donor side, inflow can be reestablished by an axillary-to-femoral bypass graft. The femorofemoral bypass is divided, leaving a small distal segment of graft attached to both femoral arteries. Thrombectomy of these distal segments is performed to assess the adequacy of outflow. If the outflow is adequate, an axillofemoral graft with femorofemoral crossover is performed. Both distal anastomoses are attached to the preserved distal segments of old graft. This obviates the need to dissect out the femoral arteries.

If the late failure is due to outflow occlusion, the femoral bifurcation on both sides must be dissected out, the graft detached, the cause of the occlusion determined, and further angioplastic procedures performed. This usually requires an extension of the angioplasty onto the profunda femoris branch so that a new anastomosis will effect an angioplasty on one or both extremities of the bypass.

FAILURE OF FEMORODISTAL RECONSTRUCTION

Acute Occlusion

Etiology
Acute occlusion in a femorodistal reconstruction is caused by technical error. The type of error is related to the type of reconstruction. When a saphenous vein is used to bypass an occluded superficial femoral artery, an inadequate saphenous vein or failure to reverse the saphenous vein so as to put the valves in proper direction of flow is the error that is specific for this type of procedure. More commonly, an iatrogenic entrapment may have been produced. Errors that are general to all types of bypass grafting include technically inadequate anastomoses or improper placement of

the graft, resulting in acute angulation or twisting. Unrecognized thrombus in the graft or runoff vessels is another major cause of acute occlusion when using a bypass technique. Finally, slow flow in a vasoconstricted distal arterial bed is another major factor leading to occlusion.

Diagnosis

The diagnosis of acute occlusion following femorodistal reconstruction is made by loss of peripheral pulses that were previously palpable, the failure of expected peripheral pulses to return following operation, or acute deterioration in the perfusion of the foot during the postoperative period as demonstrated by distal Doppler pressures.

Management

As soon as the diagnosis is made, 10,000 units of aqueous heparin is administered intravenously and the patient is returned to the operating room for reexploration. Thrombectomy of the reconstruction is accomplished with a Fogarty balloon catheter placed initially through an arteriotomy in the proximal portion of the reconstruction. In this manner, only the inguinal incision need be reopened. If the thrombectomy is satisfactory, an arteriogram should be performed through a catheter placed into the reconstructed segment via the open arteriotomy. The arteriogram will document the course of the bypass or the appearance of an endarterectomized segment. In addition, the quality of the distal anastomosis can be ascertained and the presence of any debris or thrombotic material within the runoff vessels can be visualized. Once these conditions are corrected, the arteriotomy is closed and flow is reestablished. An alternative school of thought holds that the distal anastomosis must be explored to remove embolic debris, new thrombus, or correct anastomotic stricture. This is always necessary if the distal anastomosis is to a tibial vessel.

Prevention

Operative angiography should be routinely performed during femorodistal reconstruction. The arteriogram will document any unsuspected technical errors that can be corrected before the patient leaves the operating room. If saphenous veins are used, careful preparation of the vein is indicated, with debridement of the periadventitial tissue to permit maximum expansion of the saphenous vein. Some surgeons use electromagnetic flowmeters to document satisfactory flow through the reconstruction. When flow is inadequate or when there is no dramatic increase in flow after papaverine administration, further investigation is warranted. Duplex scanning is an alternative intraoperative inspection technique.

We have found it helpful to perform the distal anastomosis as the initial part of the bypass procedure. This can be done with bright illumination, magnification, and use of 7–0 suture material.

Late Failure of Femorodistal Reconstruction

Etiology

Failure of the femorodistal reconstruction is relatively common when compared with aortofemoral reconstruction. The 5-year patency rate is reported to vary from 40 to 70%, depending on the technique of reconstruction. The longest patency rates occur with saphenous vein bypass, and the poorest with prosthetic grafting. Causes for late occlusion include progression of distal disease in a runoff segment, including development of anastomotic hyperplasia, fibrosis of retained valve cusps, atheromatous degeneration of vein segments, and opening of arteriovenous fistulas in in situ bypasses.

Diagnosis

Late failure of femorodistal reconstruction is usually associated with the return of symptoms and is confirmed by the loss of previously palpable distal pulses and a marked decrease in Doppler ankle pressures.

Management

The patient should be carefully scrutinized with regard to the functional disability associated with late failure. If there is a threat of limb loss or severely limited walking ability, further reconstruction should be considered. Angiography, beginning with the aortoiliac system and including detailed runoff films of the popliteal and tibial vessels, is of utmost importance. If proximal disease has developed in the interval, proximal reconstruction should be performed initially and may be the only procedure necessary to restore good functional result. If no proximal disease is present, then distal reconstruction is the only option. If a saphenous vein was previously used, then the opposite saphenous vein should be available and would be the graft material of choice. Inspection of the prior intraoperative angiogram may reveal a new outflow in another tibial vessel or more distally in the vessel used.

Extremely poor pedal outflow seen on the prior intraoperative angiogram may signal inability to perform a repeat vascularization.

Either autogenous vein or PTFE may be used for reoperation in the management of late femoropopliteal graft thrombosis. Once a proximal site for anastomosis is prepared, the distal site is dissected. Usually the distal popliteal segment, the tibioperoneal trunk, or posterior tibial artery is necessary for the distal anastomoses. In any event, an incision is made below the knee; this will obviate the need to redissect the area of previous popliteal mobilization. After a satisfactory distal segment is obtained, femorotibial reconstruction can be performed.

REMOVAL OF A THROMBOSED GRAFT

Early thrombosis of a prosthetic or tissue graft material is often amenable to repair by thrombectomy. In contrast, late thrombosis is rarely successfully managed by simple thrombectomy alone, and may require replacement with a new graft. This can be carried out either while leaving the thrombosed graft in place or after removing it from its tunnel. Unfortunately, mobilizing and removal of an old thrombosed graft is usually extremely difficult because of its firm attachment to its tunnel.

The reason for this difficulty lies essentially in the biologic response of the graft and host tissues interaction. Indeed, in the healing process of any graft, especially a prosthetic one, an outer layer of tissue—a perigraft capsule—is formed in addition to the development of an inner-layer capsule (pseudointima). Prosthetic grafts, homografts, and heterografts act as foreign bodies. One of the host's reactions to a foreign body is encapsulation with fibrous tissue. This is also true, perhaps to a lesser extent, for autogenous veins.

Because of this encapsulating scar the graft becomes firmly attached to the surrounding host tissues of the tunnel. All prosthetic and tissue grafts display this biologic reactivity to a lesser or greater extent. Thus, heterografts and homografts may present a more pronounced reaction than velour, Dacron, PTFE, and umbilical veins, to name only a few of the currently used grafts. The perigraft response appears to become increasingly more pronounced with passage of time after implantation. Attempts at removing such grafts at a late postimplantation period, whether in the femoropopliteal (above or below knee) or in the axillofemoral position, are met with the evolutionary changes of the graft and its resultant firm attachment to the tunnel.

TECHNIQUE

The present report describes a simple procedure for the removal of such a graft. The principle of the technique is

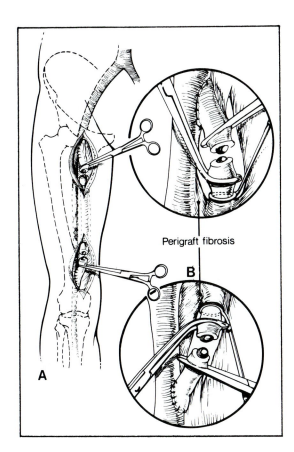

Figure 44-18. A. Diagram of a thrombosed femoropopliteal bypass graft. Note exposure of the two anastomotic areas and transection of graft. **B.** Distal and proximal ends of divided graft, magnified. See text for details.

directed to disrupting mechanically the perigraft fibrous capsule by means of an external ring passed around the graft. To this end the use of an endarterectomy ring or an external varicose vein stripper is quite effective.

The procedure (Fig. 44-18) consists of the following steps:

1. Exposure of the two anastomotic areas of the graft, femoral and popliteal, axillary and femoral, as the case may be.
2. Transection of the proximal and distal ends of the graft 2 to 3 cm from the anastomosis.
3. Clamping of the residual stubs after carefully removing the thrombi.
4. Placing the ring of an appropriate diameter (2 to 3 mm narrower than the divided graft) around one end of the graft.
5. Grasping the graft firmly with a Kelly or Kocher clamp after the ring is placed about 2 cm above its cut end.
6. Advancing the handle of the stripper or of the endarterectomy ring along the graft until it reaches the other end. If the handle of the ring is not long enough to encompass the entire length of the graft, then introduction of the ring through the other divided end will be sufficient to dislodge the remainder of any graft in the positions mentioned above.
7. After completion of the procedure, the graft is easily mobilized and removed from the original tunnel.

Consistent retrieval with ease of such grafts may be thus achieved. After removal of the old graft, a new one is placed through the same tunnel and is implanted end-to-end into the two residual stubs of the previous graft.

BIBLIOGRAPHY

Ascer E, Collier P, et al.: Reoperation for polytetrafluoroethylene bypass failure: The importance of distal outflow site and operative technique in determining outcome. J Vasc Surg 5:298, 1987.

Bandyk DF, Kaebnick HW, et al.: Durability of the in situ saphenous vein arterial bypass: A comparison of primary and secondary patency. J Vasc Surg 5:256, 1987.

Bartlett ST, Olinde AJ, et al.: The reoperative potential of infrainguinal bypass: Long-term limb and patient survival. J Vasc Surg 5:170, 1987.

Becquemin JP, Melliere D, et al.: Late occlusion of aortobifemoral grafts. J Cardiovasc Surg 28:12, 1987.

Bernhard VM, Ray LI, et al.: The reoperation of choice for aortofemoral graft occlusion. Surgery 82:867, 1978.

Brewster DC, Meier III GH, et al.: Reoperation for aortofemoral graft limb occlusion: Optimal methods and long-term results. J Vasc Surg 5:363, 1987.

Cohn LH, Moore WS, et al.: Extraabdominal management of late aortofemoral graft thrombosis. Surgery 67:775, 1970.

Cohen JR, Mannick JA, et al.: Recognition and management of impending vein-graft failure. Arch Surg 121:758, 1986.

Dbornikova V, Elfstrom J, et al.: Restenosis and occlusion after carotid surgery assessed by duplex scanning and digital subtraction angiography. Stroke 17:1137, 1986.

Donaldson MC, Louras JC, et al.: Axillofemoral bypass: A tool with a limited role. J Vasc Surg 3:757, 1986.

Flinn WR, Harris JP, et al.: Reoperation for failed femoral-popliteal or tibial grafts with expanded polytetrafluoroethylene prosthesis, in Greenhalgh RM (ed): Femoro-distal Bypass. London, Pitman Books, 1981, p. 173.

Flinn WR, Harris JP, et al.: Results of repetitive distal revascularization. Surgery 91:566, 1982.

Fulenwider JT, Smith III RB, et al.: Reoperative abdominal arterial surgery—A ten-year experience. Surgery 93:20, 1983.

Green RM, Ouriel K, et al.: Revision of failed infrainguinal bypass graft: Principles of management. Surgery 100:646, 1986.

Haimovici H: Removal of a thrombosed graft. Surg Gynecol Obstet 156:800, 1983.

Imparato AM, Bracco A, et al.: Intimal and neointimal fibrous proliferation causing failure of arterial reconstructions. Surgery 72:1007, 1972.

Katz MM, Jones GT, et al.: The use of patch angioplasty to alter the incidence of carotid restenosis following thromboendarterectomy. J Cardiovasc Surg 28:2, 1987.

Malone JM, Goldstone J, et al.: Autogenous profundaplasty: The key to long-term patency in secondary repair of aortofemoral graft occlusion. Ann Surg 188:817, 1978.

Malone JM, Moore WS: Aortoiliac and aortofemoral grafts: Management of early and late occlusive complication, in Haimovici H (ed): Vascular Emergencies. Norwalk, CT: Appleton-Century-Crofts, 1982, p 441.

Moore WS, Hall AD, et al.: Late results of axillary-femoral bypass grafting. Am J Surg 122:148, 1971.

Mozersky DJ, Summer DS, et al.: Disease progression after femoro-popliteal surgical procedure. Surg Gynecol Obstet 135:700, 1972.

Oblath RW, Green RM, et al.: Extraanatomic bypass of the abdominal aorta: Management of postoperative thrombosis. Ann Surg 187:647, 1978.

Plecha FR, Pories WJ: Intraoperative angiography in the immediate assessment of arterial reconstruction. Arch Surg 105:902, 1972.

Quinones-Baldrich WJ, Ziomek S, et al.: Primary anastomotic bonding in polytetrafluoroethylene grafts? J Vasc Surg 5:311, 1987.

Schwarcz TH, Yates GN, et al.: Pathologic characteristics of recurrent carotid artery stenosis. J Vasc Surg 5:280, 1987.

Szilagyi DE, Elliott JP Jr, et al.: A thirty-year survey of the reconstructive surgical treatment of aortoiliac occlusive disease. J Vasc Surg 3:421, 1986.

Towne JB, Bernhard BM: Technique of intraoperative endoscopic evaluation of occluded femoral grafts following thrombectomy. Surg Gynecol Obstet 148:87, 1979.

Veith FJ, Gupta SK, et al.: Management of early and late thrombosis of expanded polytetrafluoroethylene (PTFE) femoral-popliteal bypass grafts: Favorable diagnosis with appropriate reoperation. Surgery 87:581, 1980.

Veith FJ, Weiser RK, et al.: Diagnosis and management of failing lower extremity arterial reconstruction prior to graft occlusion. J Cardiovasc Surg 25:381, 1984.

Wesolowski SA: Long-term behavior of tissue and prosthetic implants for arterial reconstruction, in Haimovici H (ed): Vascular Surgery: Principles and Techniques. New York, McGraw-Hill Book Co., 1976, p 67.

Yao JST: Postoperative evaluation of graft failure, in Yao JST (ed): Complications in Vascular Surgery. Orlando, Fla., Grune & Stratton, 1985, p 1.

CHAPTER 45
Thoracic Aortic Aneurysms

Joseph S. Coselli and E. Stanley Crawford

Aneurysms of the thoracic aorta are the result of medial degenerative disease, dissection, autoimmune disorders, mycotic processes, trauma, atherosclerosis, and syphilis. Aneurysms resulting from trauma are discussed elsewhere in this text, and in Western civilization, syphilis has become a distinctly rare cause of aortic aneurysm. In the thoracic aorta, atherosclerosis is more commonly superimposed on aneurysms of other etiologies rather than the underlying cause. The most common cause for thoracic aortic aneurysm remains medial degenerative disease, a process that tends to involve multiple segments of the aorta, is associated with dilatation, mural lacerations, dissection, rupture, and death.

METHODS OF STUDY

Most aneurysms of the thoracic aorta are evident by plain roentgenography examination of the chest. They present as mediastinal widening or masses, with those involving the ascending and transverse aortic arch located in the middle and right-upper mediastinum and those involving the distal arch and descending thoracic aorta located to the left of the midline. This method of examination does not precisely localize the lesions nor does it differentiate between aneurysm, aortic tortuosity, and other diseases. Moreover, acute dissection and the aortic root dilatation, as commonly found in Marfan's syndrome, may not be evident by this method of study because of insufficient increase in aortic diameter in the former and the incorporation of the aortic shadow within the cardiac silhouette in the latter. For this reason, many patients with Marfan's syndrome have screening chest x-rays interpreted as normal, only to have aneurysm of the aortic sinus segment confirmed by other study methods. Aortography is the most precise method for diagnosing and evaluating the extent of disease. Aortography also provides information regarding branch vessel involvement by aneurysm or associated occlusive disease.

Computed tomography (CT) has proved valuable in both diagnosis and follow-up in patients with small aneurysms followed nonoperatively. These studies are standardized in measurement, allowing serial examinations to be compared. While aortography delineates the arterial lumen, CT scanning demonstrates the full transverse extent, which is particularly valuable in partially "clot-filled" aneurysms. Additionally, the true and false lumens in patients with aortic dissection are readily identified. The principal limitation of this method is that it does not provide information regarding associated branch lesions, collateral circulation, and runoff in major branches. Consequently, we reserve this method to evaluate the extent of those lesions that are partially clot-filled, the result of dissection, and for postoperative follow-up.

Magnetic resonance imaging (MRI) is a valuable diagnostic tool with capabilities similar to those of CT. As experience with MRI grows, its role is certain to expand. Ultrasonography is a satisfactory method of study for aneurysms of the abdominal segment of the aorta, but it is not currently sufficiently developed for clinical use in the study of lesions in the thoracic aorta.

ANEURYSMS OF THE SINUS OF VALSALVA

Aneurysms of the sinus of Valsalva are rare and usually of congenital origin. These result from lack of fusion of the aortic tissues above with the aortic valve annular tissue below because there is a structural defect in the tissues that bridge the two, that is, a congenital absence of fibroelastic tissue. This permits gradual dilatation and aneurysm formation that has the capability of slowly burrowing within the wall of the heart.[1,2] These lesions have a high incidence in males. The aneurysms formed are initially of little physiologic significance and produce no symptoms early in their course, with the diagnosis often made in this early stage by aortography performed in the study of other conditions. Late in their course, as in all forms of aortic aneurysm, rupture eventually occurs.[3] Typically this complication is likely to develop in a patient's early thirties. Depending

591

on the location of the aneurysm, rupture occurs into one of the heart chambers, usually on the right side into the atrium or ventricle, producing a left-to-right shunt. When this occurs, heart failure rapidly ensues; unless successfully treated by operation, the condition leads to death within 1 year. The right coronary sinus is involved in about 70% of cases, with rupture into the right ventricle most common. The noncoronary sinus is involved in 20% of cases, and rupture usually is into the right atrium. Involvement of the left coronary sinus with rupture into the left atrium is quite rare.[4]

Clinical Manifestations

The symptoms produced by this condition are typically those of acute congestive heart failure, suddenly occurring in a young adult who was previously healthy. Physical findings include an enlarged heart, parasternal murmurs, heart failure, a left-to-right shunt by cardiac catheterization, and the characteristic aortographic findings of sinus aneurysm with fistulous connection to either the right ventricle or the right atrium (Fig. 45-1).[3,4]

Treatment

The treatment, which is curative in nature, is early operation. Various procedures have been employed; however, the method currently used is that first reported by Shumacker is 1965.[5] This procedure consists of exposing the aortic defect through an incision made in the proximal ascending aorta via a median sternotomy and using cardiopulmonary bypass. Once exposed, the defect can be closed without injury to the aortic valve. Closure may be accomplished either by direct suture or by the insertion of a Dacron patch, depending on size and the need to avoid deformity of the aortic valve. Associated ventricular septal defects are common, and these are repaired during the same operation. The results of treatment are good, with survival and permanent correction of abnormalities achieved in most cases.[3,4]

ANEURYSM AND COARCTATION OF THE AORTA

Although various theories exist regarding causation, the etiology of typical coarctation of the aorta is considered congenital. The most common site for coarctation is at the level of attachment of the obliterated ductus; however, in rare instances it may be either above or below the patent ductus arteriosus. In the "preductal" configuration and occasionally in the other forms, intractable cardiac failure develops early in infancy and results in death unless emergency repair is undertaken. Improvement in neonatal intensive care management and the use of prostaglandin E_1 infusion have allowed stabilization of these infants for emergency operative repair.[6] Balloon dilatation angioplasty may also have a role in early stabilization, buying time for the very sick infant, but should be followed by surgical

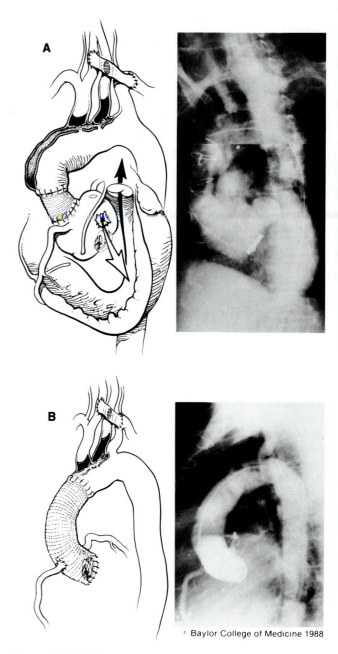

Figure 45-1. **A.** Illustration and aortogram of rupture of aortic sinus aneurysm into the right ventricle 5 years after graft replacement of ascending aorta and separate aortic valve replacement. **B.** Treatment consisted of composite valve graft replacement.

intervention before restenosis or aneurysmal dilatation.[7] The optimum surgical procedure for correction of coarctation of the aorta in the neonatal period has remained controversial.[8] Wide application of the subclavian flap angioplasty procedure introduced by Waldhausen and Nahrwold in 1966 has gained wide acceptance among surgeons for repair of aortic coarctation in infancy.[9] Aortoplasty using prosthetic materials, particularly Dacron, has also been extensively utilized.[10,11] A recognized complication of repair of aortic coarctations using synthetic patches has been the late development of aneurysm at the site of patch repair. A report by Bergdahl and Ljungqvist pointed out late aneurysm formation in the aortic wall opposite the patch graft secondary to medial degeneration, with disintegration and fragmentation of the elastic lamella and degeneration of the muscle fibers in the central portion of the media.[12] Late aneurysm formation has also been reported, with similar histology, on the ipsilateral side of a prosthetic patch graft repair.[13]

Rarely, fusiform aneurysms of the descending thoracic aorta are associated with coarctation.[14] The majority of fusiform aneurysms are located distal to the coarctation and are considered poststenotic in origin (Fig. 45-2). In rare instances, the aneurysm occurs proximal to the coarctation, and in such cases has a propensity to involve the distal transverse aortic arch (Fig. 45-3). Both of these lesions are considered to be due to medial degenerative changes within the aortic wall. In either event, treatment is graft replacement, replacing the aneurysm and relieving the coarctation.

Another complication of aortic coarctation is aortic dissection; this is usually a late complication in the older patient.[14] In most instances, the dissection arises proximal to the congenital defect and progresses in an antegrade fashion. In a minority of cases, the dissection originates distal to the congenital defect and extends distally. The presence of medial degeneration and long-term hypertension probably contribute to the occurrence of this complication. The dissection in general does not pass through the fibrotic changes at the site of coarctation. Treatment required for dissection is based on the segment of aorta involved with the essential features described elsewhere in this chapter, but complicated by the necessity for concomitant treatment of the coarctation. Dissection is less common today

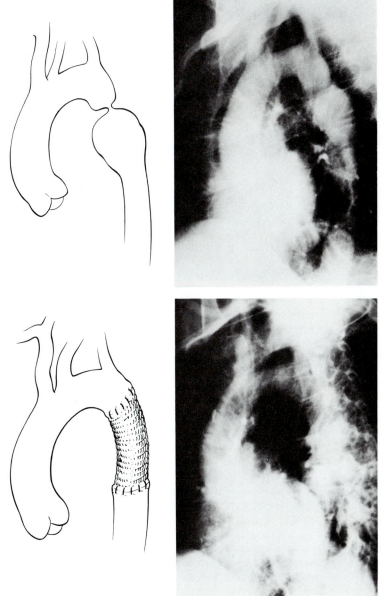

© Baylor College of Medicine 1982

Figure 45-2. Example of treatment of patient with poststenotic (coarctation) aneurysm of the proximal descending thoracic aorta. Top drawing and aortogram show location of coarctation and distal aortic dilatation. The bottom drawing and aortogram were made following replacement by Dacron tube graft.

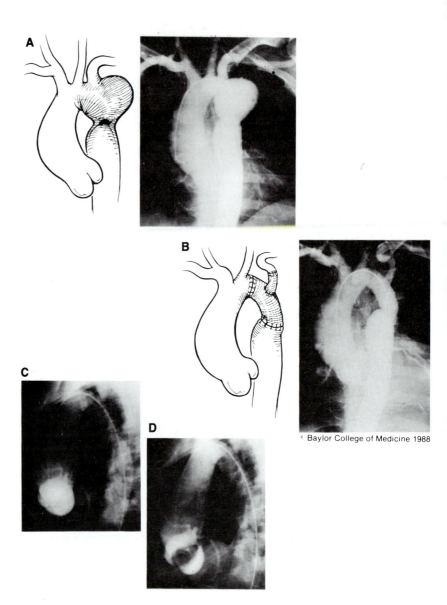

ᶜ Baylor College of Medicine 1988

Figure 45-3. Illustration and aortogram of patient with an aneurysm proximal to coarctation of descending thoracic aorta (**A**). Illustration and aortograms showing postoperative repair with Dacron tube graft replacement of aorta and separate graft replacement of proximal left subclavian artery (**B** to **D**).

because of the popularity of early surgical correction of coarctation.

AORTITIS

Two unusual causes for aneurysms of the aorta are giant cell arteritis (temporal arteritis) and Takayasu's arteritis. In either case, any or all segments of the aorta may be involved with both true thoracic aortic aneurysms and dissecting aneurysms occurring.

Giant cell arteritis is a systemic disease occurring more frequently in women and usually in patients 55 years or older.[15] Histologically, there is transmural chronic inflammation of the aorta and its branches with a large number of giant cells associated with medial degeneration and destruction. This condition leads to the development of both aneurysm and stenosis of the thoracic aorta, lesions which can be successfully treated surgically.[16]

Takayasu's disease also occurs more frequently in women but in a younger age group, usually teenagers and young adults.[17] It is characterized histologically by trans-

mural involvement with adventitial fibrosis, degeneration, disintegration of the media, and intimal cellular proliferation with fibrosis. Generally there is a cellular infiltration concentrated in the media consisting primarily of lymphocytes with occasional histiocytes and plasma cells.[18] This inflammatory process also produces both stenotic and aneurysmal lesions. In addition to being associated with brachiocephalic, aortic, and visceral arterial obstruction, Takayasu's disease is noted for the frequent presence of aneurysms of the coronary, internal mammary, vertebral, carotid, and axillary arteries as well as of the thoracic and abdominal aorta.[19] The pulmonary artery is involved in 50% of cases.

Causes of death for patients with aortitis include stroke, renal failure, hypertensive heart disease, and importantly, rupture or dissection of aortic aneurysms.[20] Although the role for operation of the cerebral vascular component of this disease is not well defined, the aneurysmal manifestations carry the same risks as those of medial degeneration and atherosclerotic lesions and should be treated surgically based on their own merit to prevent rupture and dissection. Surgical treatment is by graft replacement with techniques appropriate for the involved segment (Fig. 45-4).[21]

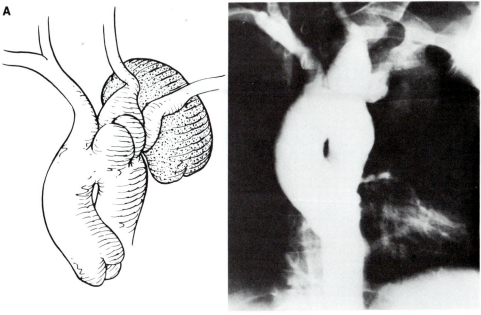

©Baylor College of Medicine 1982

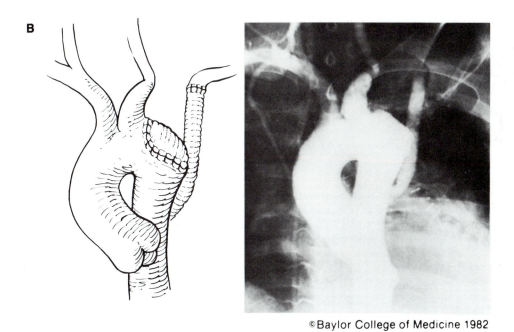

©Baylor College of Medicine 1982

Figure 45-4. A. Multiple sacciform aneurysms arising in the distal arch in a patient with Takayasu's aortitis. **B.** Treatment involved patch graft replacement of the aneurysm and placement of an aortosubclavian bypass graft.

INFECTION

The term *mycotic aneurysm* is commonly used to describe aneurysm formation resulting from infectious destruction of an arterial wall and includes both bacterial and fungal infections. Syphilitic aneurysms are rare because of the ef-

fectiveness of antibiotic therapy administered in the early stages of the disease; however, when present, they generally arise in the ascending aorta and tend to be saccular in nature with a peculiar propensity to erode bone. Aneurysms that are caused by pyogenic infection result from infection of the aortic wall and destruction of aortic tissue.

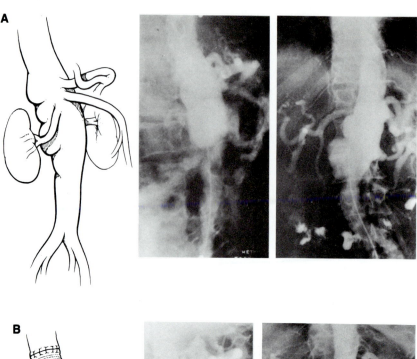

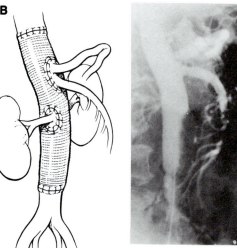

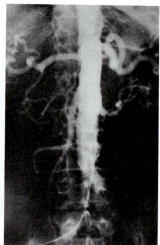

Figure 45-5. A. Illustration and aortogram of patient with mycotic aneurysm of the aorta opposite the origin of the visceral arteries caused by *Staphylococcus epidermidis* and producing complete right renal artery obstruction. **B.** Treatment involved graft replacement after 1 week of intravenous antibiotics, which were continued for 1 month postoperatively, and then indefinitely with oral therapy.

ᶜ Baylor College of Medicine 1988

They are the result of direct extension or embolic seeding from bacterial endocarditis or septicemia to previously normal aorta, to areas of atherosclerosis, or to established atherosclerotic aneurysm. Sources of such septicemia include infection at other sites (i.e., skin, lung, teeth, genitourinary tract) or contaminated intravenous sites. Patients who are susceptible to bacterial endocarditis generally have chronic cardiac valvular disorders; however, the remainder have normal valves and develop acute bacterial endocarditis as a result of the arterial or aortic infection. Other risk factors have included the presence of malignant neoplasms, chronic steroid therapy, diabetes, and a wide variety of debilitating disorders without cardiac valvular defects.

The clinical manifestations of mycotic aortic aneurysms include pain, fever, hoarseness, and a history of previous febrile illness. Organisms that are frequently identified include *Staphylococcus* species, *Streptococcus* species, *Salmonella, Escherichia coli,* and others.[22] The most common sites for mycotic aortic aneurysms, which tend to be saccular in nature, are the aortic arch and the thoracoabdominal aorta at the level of the diaphragm or the region posterior

to the visceral vessels (Fig. 45-5). Successful treatment involves early diagnosis, the institution of broad-spectrum antibiotics, and aggressive surgical intervention.[23] Excision, wide debridement, and extraanatomic bypass are the important principles of treatment in the presence of extensive contamination. However, when mycotic aneurysms involve the aortic arch and thoracoabdominal aorta, extraanatomic bypass is generally not feasible; in situ Dacron graft replacement after wide excision has been undertaken with satisfactory results.[24] Such patients should be treated preoperatively and postoperatively with high doses of specific antibiotics based on both blood and aortic wall cultures. A lifelong course of oral suppressive antibiotics is recommended to reduce chances of recurrence.

ANEURYSMS OF THE ASCENDING AORTA

Aneurysmal involvement of the ascending aorta is due to medial degeneration or dissection in over 95% of cases. These frequently coincide with dissection occurring in an aortic wall compromised with medial degenerative changes. Although atherosclerotic intimal disease may be superimposed on these entities, it is only very rarely the primary cause of aneurysms in this region.[25]

Medial Degeneration

The term *medial degeneration* as it is used here includes the pathologic terms *mucoid degeneration, myxomatous degeneration,* and *cystic medial necrosis.* All refer to the same processes affecting the aortic wall and vary only in degree and extent of involvement.[26] Aneurysms of this etiology may be limited, or they can be diffuse with the entire aorta involved and dilated, that is, "mega aorta."

Aneurysms of the ascending aorta resulting from medial degeneration may involve only the tubular ascending aorta, the segment between the coronary sinuses and the transverse aortic arch. However, the entire aortic root is frequently affected with similar pathologic changes found not only in the wall of the tubular portion but also in the aortic valve leaflets, aortic valve annulus, and the coronary sinus portion. Progressive weakening and dilatation results in aneurysm formation with rupture, dissection, or aortic valve insufficiency with heart failure.[27]

The forces generated by pulsatile aortic pressure and flow produce a variety of lesions when the inner layers of the aortic wall are weakened by degenerative changes. When the intima and internal media break and separate, they may do so in either a linear or stellate fashion. If the process is identified early or is arrested in this state, a "mural laceration" is produced. With continued tearing, dissection and a false channel develop within the media. In either case, the strength of the outer layers is attenuated and is subject to further dilatation, with the former producing a saccular aneurysm. The natural history of each is continued expansion and eventual rupture.[28]

An aortic root aneurysm can rupture into the pericardial sac, which surrounds the heart and ascending aorta, producing immediate cardiac tamponade and death, or a communication may develop with the right ventricle, right atrium, or pulmonary artery, resulting in a large left-to-right shunt with congestive heart failure and death.

With generalized aortic root dilatation, as occurs in Marfan syndrome, medial degeneration, and aging, there is a widening of the annulus, elongation of the commissures, and an inadequate amount of valve leaflet tissue for coaptation during diastole. The result is aortic valvular insufficiency that may be tolerated for extended periods but ultimately leads to congestive heart failure and death.[29]

The patterns of the pathologic changes described occur in two separate clinical situations. First the disease may appear in a younger age group, usually under the age of 30 years, or secondly in an elderly population. In the former, the changes represent the cardiovascular manifestations of Marfan syndrome, which is a hereditary disorder of connective tissue. In addition to the aortic involvement, a variety of anomalies involving the skeleton and eyes are part of the syndrome. In this group, death usually results from cardiovascular complications and occurs in 50% of the patients by the age of 32.[30] In the older group, although the progression is slower, the complications are similar and the pathology equally as lethal.

Treatment of Medial Degeneration

Operation is the treatment of choice for medial degeneration. Historically, a variety of techniques have been employed including valvuloplasty, aortoplasty, wrapping of the aorta, and prosthetic graft replacement with and without valve replacement. Aortoplasty and valvuloplasty fell into early disfavor because of the high frequency of early and late recurrence. Separate replacement of the ascending aorta and aortic valve, without treatment of coronary artery sinus involvement, consistently leads to progression and complications from the untreated segment.[31,32] Improved treatment for aneurysm of the ascending aorta with involvement of the sinus portion was introduced in 1968 by Bentall and DeBono[33] with a technique that consisted of direct reattachment of the coronary artery origins to a composite valve graft. This technique offered complete treatment and has been adopted widely with good early and late results.[34-36] Disadvantages of this type of procedure have included bleeding at operation, often necessitating aneurysm wall wrapping of the graft for hemostasis, and the late development of false aneurysms at the suture lines, particularly the coronary artery reattachment anastomosis. Recent modifications have remedied some of the problems associated with composite valve graft replacement.

Operation for ascending aortic aneurysm is performed through a midsternal incision using cardiopulmonary bypass. We prefer to use bicaval cannulation with pump return via cannulation of a common femoral artery. The left ventricle is decompressed through a sump placed through the right superior pulmonary vein. Moderate hypothermia, cold blood cardioplegia, and topical cooling are employed for myocardial preservation.

The technique used varies with the extent of aneurysm involvement and presence or absence of aortic valve disease. Patients without Marfan syndrome who have an isolated aneurysm of the tubular ascending aorta, a competent aortic valve, and a normal sinus segment are treated with simple graft replacement of the tubular ascending aorta (Fig. 45-6). A woven Dacron graft that has been thoroughly coated with 25% human serum albumin and autoclaved at 270°F for 3 minutes is used to render the interstices of the graft impermeable to heparinized blood. Alternatively, a pre-treated albumin-impregnated knitted Dacron tube graft can be used. Patients with ascending aneurysm and aortic valve disease, insufficiency, or stenosis who do not have Marfan's syndrome or sinus enlargement are treated by graft replacement of the ascending aorta and concomitant separate aortic valve replacement (Fig. 45-6E).

In all patients with Marfan syndrome and others with coronary sinus segment enlargement, a composite valve graft prosthesis is inserted for complete aortic root replacement. For reasons previously noted, we no longer use the technique described by Bentall and DeBono.[33] Currently we use techniques designed to avoid tension at the coronary artery reattachment suture lines to avoid early (intraoperative hemorrhage) and late complications (false aneurysm development). These approaches allow intraoperative test-

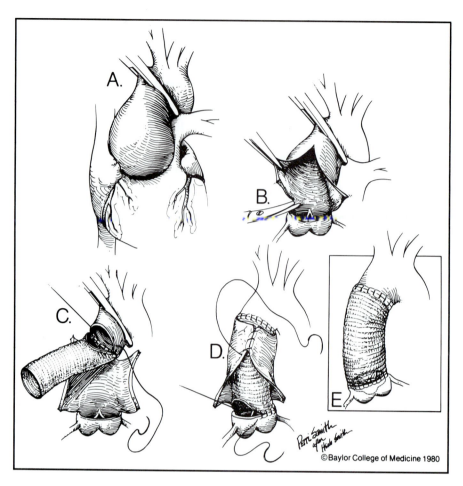

Figure 45-6. Illustration of technique for tubular graft replacement for ascending aortic aneurysm (**A** to **D**) using Dacron tube graft. In the presence of aortic valve disease, prosthetic replacement (**E**) is performed concomitantly.

ing to assure hemostatically secure suture lines and satisfactory exposure to immediately treat leaks with additional direct suture placement without having to resort to wrapping of the graft with the aneurysm wall to achieve hemostasis. Reduction of suture line tension improves hemostasis and prevents later false aneurysm development.

One technique is complete resection of the ascending aortic aneurysm down to within 1 to 2 mm of the aortic valve annulus, leaving a Carrel-type "button" of aortic wall around each of the coronary artery origins. Following insertion of the valve portion of a composite valve graft, the coronary arteries are mobilized for a short distance to allow tension-free attachment to openings made in the side of the composite graft. These anastomoses can be reinforced with Teflon felt for strength and hemostasis. The repair is completed with distal anastomoses using a running suture. Bleeding from the graft portion of the composite valve graft is eliminated by treating the graft with albumin as described. Each suture line is tested for hemostasis immediately after its completion, with placement of additional sutures as needed.

The second method, our currently preferred technique, was first introduced by Cabrol et al.[37,38] who described reattaching the coronary artery origins to a composite valve graft using a separate small Dacron tube graft (the ends of which are first sutured to the aorta around the coronary

ostia) and then attaching the two grafts using openings made in the side of each (Fig. 45-7). This technique also allows tension-free reattachment of the coronary artery origins and accessibility of suture lines to secure hemostasis. Another advantage of this technique is that it can be employed regardless of how far the coronary artery origins are separated from the valve annulus. In the Bentall procedure, if a coronary ostia is too close to the annulus, there is insufficient tissue for "inclusion" reattachment; if the sinuses are too large, tension may be present at the suture line. A technique with a separate Dacron graft to the coronary artery origins allows complete aortic root replacement in all patients with Marfan syndrome, many of whom might otherwise have delayed or inadequate treatment.

We recently used the Cabrol procedure and the Carrel "button" technique in 60 patients each; both techniques provided survival rates of 95%. However, we prefer the Cabrol procedure because it is simple, expeditious, and has general applicability.

Dissection

Aortic dissection begins as an intimal tear and extends as a longitudinal splitting through the media, creating a false channel. In general, the greater portion of a dissection progresses distally, but varying amounts of proximal extension occur in most patients. The intimal tear originates in the ascending aorta (usually 2 to 4 cm beyond the origin of the coronary arteries) in 62% of patients, the arch in 9%, the upper descending thoracic aorta in 26%, and in the abdominal aorta in 3% of patients.[25] It is generally agreed that most patients with involvement of the ascending aorta succumb from complications in the acute phase, within 2 weeks, if left untreated.[39] Acute complications of proximal aortic involvement include rupture into the pericardium, aortic valve insufficiency, coronary artery occlusion, or rupture into the right atrium or right ventricle with a left-to-right shunt. Distal complications include branch vessel occlusion resulting in stroke, visceral or extremity ischemia, and distal aortic rupture, usually into the left chest, although abdominal aortic rupture can occur. Late complications include aneurysm formation from false lumen dilatation, aortic valvular insufficiency, and rupture of the false lumen. A combination of CT scanning and aortography is used to determine the location and full extent of aortic dissection.

Treatment

Emergency operative intervention is undertaken at the time of diagnosis when the ascending aorta is found to be involved. Patients are initially stabilized in an intensive care unit with arterial pressure monitoring and central venous and pulmonary arterial pressure using a Swan-Ganz catheter. Whereas the previously mentioned studies are undertaken to evaluate the aorta, blood pressure is maintained at a tolerated lowered level using sedation, beta blockers, and intravenous sodium nitroprusside infusion.[40,41] Therapeutic goals include replacement of the weakest portion of the aorta, which is usually the site of original intimal

tear in the proximal ascending aorta, prevention of further proximal extension, and treatment of aortic valve or coronary artery insufficiency.

Treatment varies with the extent of dissection and the presence or absence of previous aortic root enlargement. In the simplest case when dissection has occurred in a previously normal aorta and is limited to the tubular ascending portion, simple graft replacement that includes the site of the original intimal tear is accomplished. In acute dissection with friable aortic tissue and danger of laceration from simple crossclamping, the distal anastomosis is accomplished without using a distal aortic clamp by utilizing profound hypothermia and circulatory arrest (see the discussion of transverse aortic arch aneurysm). The ascending aorta is opened, the intimal tear identified, and the tubular ascending aorta resected (Fig. 45-8A to C). The distal aorta is prepared for anastomosis by sandwiching the inner and outer layers between two strips of Teflon felt (Fig. 45-8D). A woven Dacron tube graft treated with albumin is used for replacement. Following completion of the distal anastomosis, the graft is clamped and rewarming is begun while the proximal aorta is similarly prepared just beyond the coronary arteries (Fig. 45-8E).

In the presence of aortic valve insufficiency or sinus segment dilation, we prefer to use a composite valve graft. If the coronary arteries are not involved in the dissection, a smaller Dacron graft is used to reattach their origins as described earlier. However, if the dissection is in close proximity or extends out into the coronary arteries, they are ligated proximally and reconstituted by distal autogenous saphenous vein grafts.

Proximal reconstruction of chronic ascending aortic dissection is based on the principles and techniques outlined for medial degenerative disease. In acute dissection, the distal anastomosis directs flow into the true lumen to control

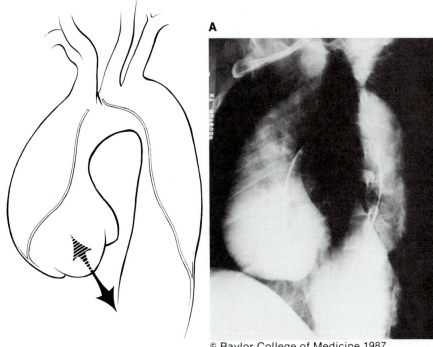

A

© Baylor College of Medicine 1987

Figure 45-7. A. Illustration and aortogram of patient with Marfan syndrome, aortic root aneurysm, and aortic valve insufficiency.

Continued.

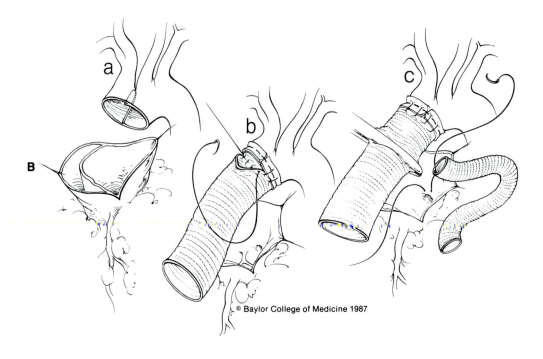

© Baylor College of Medicine 1987

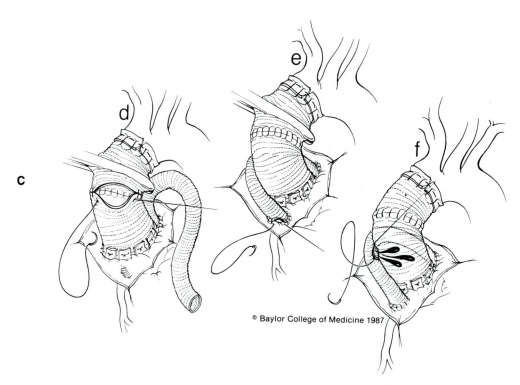

© Baylor College of Medicine 1987

Figure 45-7, cont'd. B and **C.** Illustration of modified Cabrol procedure in treatment of chronic dissecting and nondissecting aneurysm of the proximal ascending aorta. Technique (*a* to *c*) is illustrated using hypothermic circulatory arrest. Distal anastomosis is performed first without aortic clamping to replace all of the ascending aorta. With cardiopulmonary bypass resumed (*d* to *f*) and rewarming begun, the first graft is clamped, the composite valve graft is inserted proximally, and the coronary arteries are reattached using a smaller tube graft.

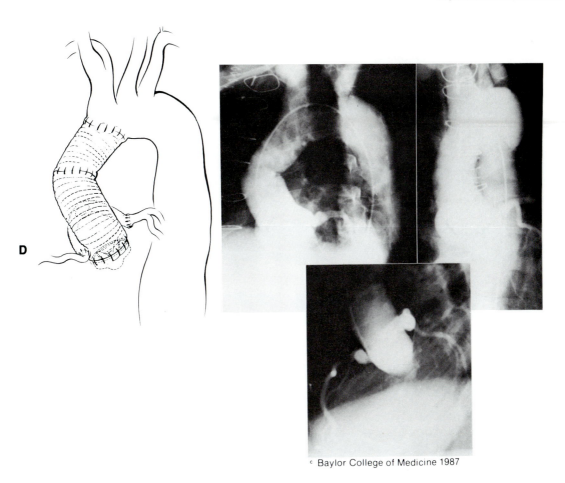

D

Figure 45-7, cont'd. D. Illustration and aortogram made postoperatively demonstrating repair.

progression of dissection distally by reducing the flow and pressure in the false lumen. In the chronic phase, the distal anastomosis is often constructed with flow directed into both the true and the well-established false lumen by resecting a portion of the partition between the two lumens distal to the anastomosis. All patients with dissection are subject to lifelong follow-up of the remaining aorta to detect dilatation of the false channel in an early asymptomatic stage.

TRANSVERSE AORTIC ARCH ANEURYSM

The transverse aortic arch is that segment from which the brachiocephalic arteries arise; aneurysmal involvement of this segment is very variable. Fusiform aneurysms of the ascending aorta can have limited involvement of the aortic arch in the region of the innominate artery, and those of the descending thoracic aorta can have aneurysmal involvement of the distal transverse arch including the left subclavian artery. In some cases, a saccular aneurysm develops opposite the origin of the brachiocephalic arteries; in other cases there is a fusiform aneurysm of the entire aortic arch, sparing the ascending and descending aorta in some, while the entire aorta is diffusely aneurysmal ("mega aorta") in others. Although few dissections originate in the arch, the transverse aortic arch is commonly involved in dissections

beginning in the ascending aorta and occasionally as proximal extension from distal dissections.[42] Aneurysms in this region are usually of medial degeneration in origin when fusiform and atherosclerotic when saccular.[26,43,44]

Complications from aneurysms at this level are generally serious and result from compression of surrounding structures, rupture, or associated disease. The trachea and bronchi, pulmonary artery, and great veins are commonly compressed. Hoarseness from compression of the left recurrent laryngeal nerve is a common first symptom. Rupture occurs into the pericardium with tamponade, into the mediastinum or pleural cavity with fatal hemorrhage, or into the tracheobronchial tree causing drowning. As in other aortic segments, CT scanning and arteriography are the mainstays of diagnosis and evaluation of extent of aneurysm involvement.

Treatment is graft replacement, undertaken electively following diagnosis to avoid the development of complications. Surgical approach depends on the extent of involvement and the need for cardiac and cerebral protection. Patients with distal involvement (the level of the left common carotid or left subclavian arteries and beyond) are approached through the left chest. Proximal aortic control is by simple crossclamp while cardiovascular hemodynamics are controlled with sodium nitroprusside or nitroglycerin infusion. A double-lumen endotracheal tube is used for

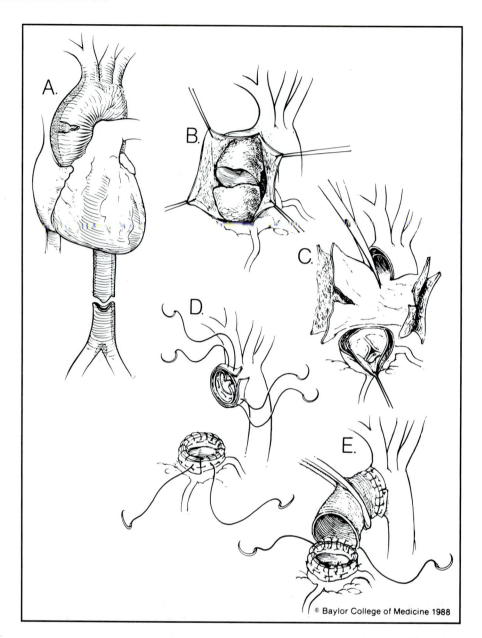

© Baylor College of Medicine 1988

Figure 45-8. Illustration of technique for graft replacement of ascending aorta for acute dissection without involvement of the coronary arteries or aortic valve. All of the involved tubular segment of the ascending aorta **(A** to **C)** is removed, using deep hypothermia and circulatory arrest. Each end of the aorta is reinforced with Teflon felt strips with flow redirected distally into the true lumen **(D).** The proximal portion of repair **(E)** is completed with Dacron, graft clamped, cardiopulmonary bypass is resumed, and rewarming is begun.

selective collapse of the left lung. Saccular aneurysms arising from the lesser curvature of the distal transverse arch that encompass less than 50% of the aortic circumference are treated by Dacron patch graft aortoplasty. Fusiform aneurysms are replaced with tube grafts to which separate side grafts are attached for reconstruction of the left subclavian or left common carotid arteries as needed.

When the vital aortic segment from which the innominate and left common carotid arteries arise is involved, techniques must be employed to protect critical organs, particularly the brain and heart, during the reconstruction period. For such cases we prefer to use circulatory arrest,

which provides a dry, quiet surgical field unencumbered by clamps, bypass grafts, tubes, and reduces blood loss.[45,46] Protection is provided by hypothermia achieved by cardiopulmonary bypass. Temperature is monitored in the nasopharynx, rectum, and esophagus; the cerebral electrical activity is continuously monitored with a 10-lead surface electroencephalogram (EEG). We do not initiate circulatory arrest until the EEG is isoelectric (when the brain temperature is 20 to 21°C).[47-49] This method has protected cerebral function in our most recent 100 cases in which it was used with periods of arrest ranging from 14 to 109 minutes (median, 36 minutes).

Aortic arch aneurysms are preferentially approached through a median sternotomy. However, when multiple previous median sternotomies have been performed in the same patient or large descending aneurysm precludes staged repair, arch replacement can be accomplished through the left chest.[50,51] Hypothermia is obtained with cardiopulmonary bypass by cannulating a femoral artery in the groin and both venae cavae in the chest. In selected cases of reoperation in which safe sternal reentry is not possible, cardiopulmonary bypass is established with the chest closed, using femoral vein-femoral artery cannulation. Median sternotomy is then undertaken only after an appropriate, safe level of hypothermia has been achieved and circulatory arrest initiated.[52,53]

Following exposure, hypothermia, and circulatory arrest, the patient is placed in a steep Trendelenburg position before the aneurysm is opened. This position prevents cerebral air embolism and eliminates the need for unnecessary dissection and clamping of the brachiocephalic vessels. Sacciform aneurysms arising from the transverse arch that involve less than 50% of the aortic circumference are treated by patch aortoplasty using a Dacron patch treated with albumin. Fusiform aneurysms are treated with tube graft replacement with the distal anastomosis performed first

end to end to the proximal descending thoracic aorta. The brachiocephalic vessels are reattached to one or more openings made in the graft (Fig. 45-9) or are replaced with separate smaller grafts if they too are aneurysmal. The graft is flushed of air and debris and clamped just proximal to the innominate artery as cardiopulmonary bypass and rewarming are resumed. The repair is completed with anastomosis to the proximal uninvolved ascending aorta or proximal repair is undertaken based on principles previously outlined for the aortic root disease (Fig. 45-10). Recent evaluation of 626 patients with aneurysm of the ascending aorta or transverse aortic arch revealed a 90% 30-day survival rate in 400 patients without dissection. There were 68 patients with acute dissection and 158 with chronic dissection with a 30-day survival rate of 76% and 89%, respectively.

ANEURYSMS OF THE DESCENDING THORACIC AORTA

Aneurysms of this aortic segment are most commonly secondary to medial degeneration changes, atherosclerosis, and aortic dissection. Other causes include trauma, aortitis, infection, and prosthetic dilatation with coarctation. Trau-

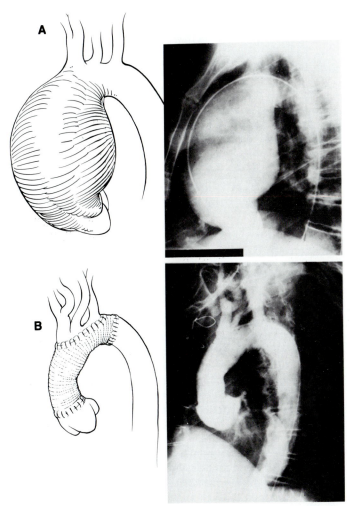

© Baylor College of Medicine 1988

Figure 45-9. A. Illustration and aortogram of patient with fusiform aneurysm involving the ascending aorta and transverse aortic arch. **B.** Postoperative drawing and aortogram showing repair that included reattachment of brachiocephalic arteries to an opening in graft.

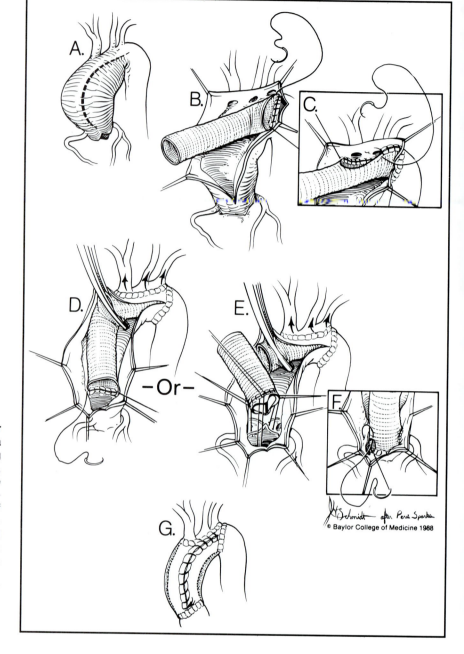

Figure 45-10. Illustration of technique for treatment of aneurysm of ascending aorta and transverse aortic arch **(A to B)**. Using profound hypothermia and circulatory arrest, the distal end-to-end anastomosis to the proximal descending thoracic aorta is performed first. Following this, reattachment of the brachiocephalic arteries **(C)** to an opening in the graft; simple end-to-end proximal anastomosis to the proximal ascending aorta completes the repair **(D)** while the graft is clamped, cardiopulmonary bypass is resumed, and rewarming begun. With coronary artery sinus involvement or aortic valve insufficiency, a composite valve graft **(E to G)** is inserted to complete proximal reconstruction.

matic aneurysms are studied in another chapter; aortitis, infection, and coarctation are discussed separately.

Medial Degeneration

Aneurysms caused by medial degeneration tend to be fusiform, of varying lengths, and frequently have atherosclerosis superimposed. The abdominal aortic segment is involved separately in at least 25% of cases.[44] Less commonly saccular aneurysms occur that tend to be more purely atherosclerotic in origin, with a propensity for development in the lower descending thoracic aorta. The left pleural cavity has the capacity to allow asymptomatic aneurysm expansion for variable periods of time but eventually these lesions produce

pain, dysphagia, hoarseness, hematemesis, or hemoptysis. Death occurs from rupture into the mediastinum, pleural cavity, esophagus, trachea, or bronchus in over 80% of cases within five years of diagnosis.[54,55]

All patients are evaluated preoperatively for concurrent cardiac, renal, and pulmonary disease. Optimal medical management is achieved before surgical intervention. Patients are well hydrated prior to aortography, and operation is delayed for 24 to 48 hours following dye studies in the asymptomatic patient.

Operative treatment is recommended for all symptomatic patients and for all asymptomatic lesions that are twice the size of the normal adjacent aorta (Fig. 45-11). The aorta is approached through a left posterior lateral thoracotomy, usually with resection of the fifth or sixth rib. Double-lumen

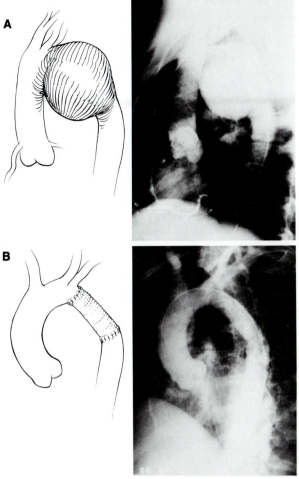

© Baylor College of Medicine 1988

Figure 45-11. Preoperative **(A)** and postoperative **(B)** illustration and aortograms of treatment of patient with fusiform aneurysm of the proximal descending thoracic aorta.

tracheal intubation allows selective collapse of the left lung for improved exposure, and reduces both pulmonary trauma from retraction and cardiac compression. The aneurysm is isolated between clamps and, as at other sites, saccular aneurysms are treated with patch grafts; fusiform lesions are treated with tube graft replacement employing inclusion techniques (Fig. 45-12). Sodium nitroprusside and nitroglycerin infusions are used to maintain normal cardiac hemodynamics. Shed blood from the field is retrieved with an autotransfusion device that provides rapid cell washing and reinfusion.

Dissection

The descending thoracic aorta is involved in most cases of aortic dissection.[42] The origin of dissection is in the proximal descending thoracic aorta in about 26% of cases. When the origin of dissection is in the ascending aorta (62% of patients with dissection), distal extension usually involves this segment. Ascending aortic involvement requires emer-

gent surgical intervention, but most cases arising in the proximal descending thoracic aorta can be initially treated medically with careful monitoring and blood pressure control as described by Wheat.[40,41] Patients who do not respond to this type of therapy, that is, have continued pain, evidence of expansion of the false lumen, symptoms of arterial occlusion, or evidence of leak or rupture, are treated by immediate operation (Fig. 45-13). Surgical treatment is by graft replacement of the weakest aortic segment, that is, the site of intimal tear, usually the very proximal descending thoracic aorta, with restoration of flow back into the true lumen (Fig. 45-14). This is accomplished by sandwiching the two walls at the anatomic site with strips of Teflon felt. The latter decompresses the false lumen, which can relieve arterial branch obstruction and prevent progression of dissection. In the acute setting, extensive aortic replacement is often not required, which has the added benefit of maintaining normal flow through a maximum number of intercostal arteries.

Patients who do respond to initial nonoperative management must continue meticulous control of blood pressure with medications that should include beta blockers. In addition, they should be followed on a regular basis with CT surveillance for dilatation of the false lumen. Over a period of 5 years, at least one third will require surgical intervention. Surgical treatment in these cases is directed toward replacement of fusiform dilatation of the outer lumen of the false channel.

When required, operative treatment entails graft replacement of the dilated segment, which may include all or part of the descending aorta or abdominal aorta. In the chronic state, less attention needs to be directed toward reestablishing a single distal channel. The outer wall of the false lumen in the chronic phase may be strong enough to secure sutures, the walls are frequently too stiff to reapproximate, and the two lumens are often well established. In such instances a wedge of the partition between the two channels is removed distally before distal anastomosis so that flow may be directed down both lumens.

Our recent evaluation of 540 patients with aneurysm of the descending thoracic aorta included 39 patients with acute dissection, 125 patients with chronic dissection, and 376 patients without dissection. They had 30-day survival rates of 67%, 91%, and 22%, respectively.

THORACOABDOMINAL AORTIC ANEURYSMS

Aneurysms that involve the descending thoracic aorta and all or part of the abdominal aorta in continuity, and those that involve the abdominal aortic segment from which the visceral arteries arise are considered together because they require a thoracoabdominal incision for exposure, both require reattachment of visceral arteries, and each has similar operative risks. The frequency of rupture and death in patients who have thoracoabdominal aortic aneurysms is similar to that observed in patients with aneurysms located in other aortic segments. In 94 consecutive patients observed with asymptomatic thoracoabdominal aortic aneurysms in whom operation was not performed, death occurred in 76% within 2 years; half of the deaths were due to rupture

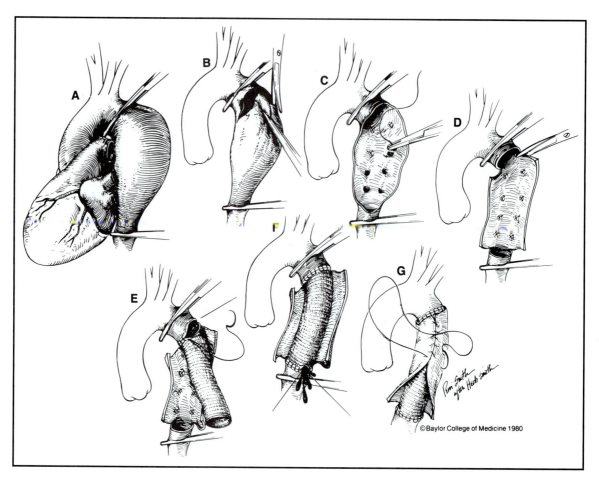

Figure 45-12. Drawings (**A** to **G**) show inclusion technique for graft replacement of descending thoracic aortic aneurysm using simple crossclamping and Dacron tube graft.

regardless of aneurysmal etiology.[56] In contrast, in 604 patients treated surgically, the 30-day, 2-year, and 5-year estimated survival rates are 91%, 70%, and 59%, despite a median age of 66 years at the time of operation.[57]

In recent years diagnosis, extent of disease, and presence or absence of dissection have been facilitated by CT scanning and magnetic resonance imaging. Aortography remains the superior method of determining the presence of associated occlusive disease in the aortic branches.

Operation for these lesions is a formidable undertaking and is generally not recommended for asymptomatic patients with small aneurysms that are less than twice the diameter of the proximal or distal normal aorta. Operation is contraindicated in patients at extreme operative risk from cardiac or pulmonary disease and in whom conditions exist that would produce a limited life expectancy. However, operation is indicated in patients with rupture, with symptoms resulting from aneurysm, and in large aneurysms regardless of symptoms.

Patients are placed in a 60-degree right lateral decubitus position with a beanbag used to maintain this angle. The aorta is approached through a thoracoabdominal incision made over the sixth rib and continued down the abdominal midline in most patients. In patients with aneurysm local-

ized to the lower descending thoracic aorta and below, adequate exposure can be obtained by placing the thoracic component of the incision over a lower rib (sixth to eighth) or interspace. In either case, the diaphragm is split radially to the aortic hiatus and the viscera, including the left kidney, are mobilized by retroperitoneal dissection and retracted to the right. With minimal dissection, the aneurysmal segment is isolated between clamps and opened on the left posterior lateral surface. Back-bleeding from visceral, lumbar, and intercostal arteries that are to be reattached is controlled with balloon catheters. A woven Dacron tube graft is employed for replacement using an inclusion technique (Fig. 45-15). After completion of the proximal anastomosis to the uninvolved proximal aorta using a continuous suture, appropriate openings are made in the graft for reattachment of intercostal and lumbar arteries from T8 to L2, which is also accomplished with a running suture. The visceral arteries are then reattached to openings made in the graft in a similar fashion. When these vessels are widely separated, they are reattached to separate openings; when positioned close together, the island of aorta from which they arise is retained and the arteries reattached as a group. When atherosclerotic occlusive disease is present at the origin of a visceral vessel, an endarterectomy is performed

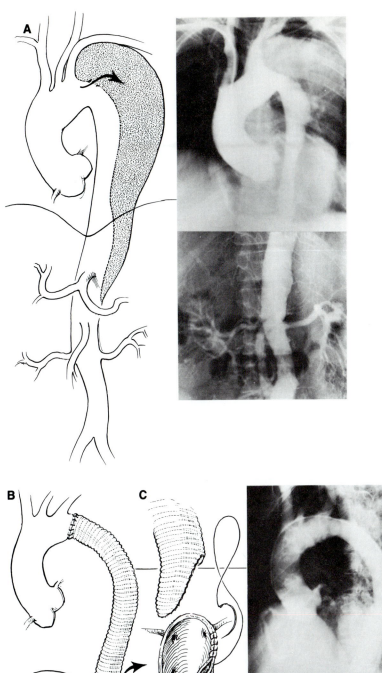

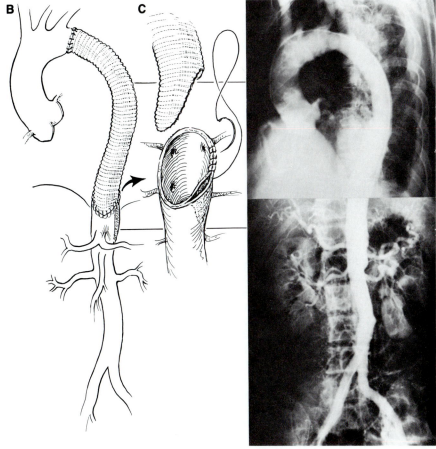

Figure 45-13. A. Preoperative drawing and aortogram of patient with type III aortic dissection and dilatation of the false lumen. **B** to **C.** Postoperative drawing and aortogram show repair that includes preservation of distal intercostal arteries by bevelling the graft and redirection of flow into the true lumen distally.

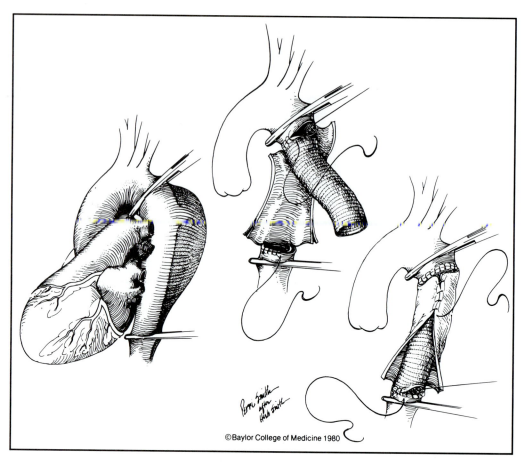

©Baylor College of Medicine 1980

Figure 45-14. Illustration of technique for repair of aortic dissection involving the descending thoracic aorta using Dacron tube graft, proximal and distal clamping, and inclusion technique.

before reattachment. The left renal artery is often widely separated and commonly requires a segmental Dacron tube graft for restoration. As reattachment of these various structures is completed, the proximal clamp is sequentially removed down the graft, restoring flow as distal reconstruction is proceeding. Normal cardiac hemodynamics are volume maintained with sodium nitroprusside infusion upon clamping and venous replacement as the clamp is moved down on the graft or released. Shed blood is washed and reinfused using a rapid cell-saving device. Reconstruction is completed with an end-to-end anastomosis to the distal uninvolved aorta or with the use of a bifurcation graft to the common iliac or common femoral arteries if aneurysmal involvement or associated distal occlusive disease is present. Operation is completed by suturing the aneurysmal wall around the graft and wound closure.

Paraplegia remains a serious complication of extensive aortic replacement. We have recently evaluated the impact of distal aortic perfusion using cardiofemoral bypass without heparin. Using left atrial to common femoral artery bypass, we attempted to maintain a mean distal pressure of 60 mm Hg in 198 patients undergoing descending or

thoracoabdominal aortic replacement while constantly monitoring spinal cord function using somatosensory evoked potentials (SEPs). Satisfactory distal pressures were consistently achieved in only 99 patients, primarily for anatomic reasons such as aortoiliac occlusive disease. The combined use of these modalities resulted in a lower extremity neurologic complication rate no different than simple crossclamping, and SEP monitoring was found to be unreliable in predicting the development of neurologic complications.[57]

There has been a 91% early survival rate in 962 patients treated for thoracoabdominal aortic aneurysms. Death occurs in the perioperative period, most commonly from cardiac, renal, and pulmonary causes.[58] Survival varies little with extent or type of aneurysm. The overall incidence of neuromuscular dysfunction is 12%, one half of this being graded as paraplegia. Of those patients with paraplegia, 85% are able to function independently at 1 year. Of patients with paraparesis, 90% are able to walk with assistance at 30 days with rehabilitation complete in virtually all cases at 6 months.[58] Renal dysfunction requiring hemodialysis occurs in 5% of patients with preoperative renal impairment, the most reliable prediction of postoperative renal problems.

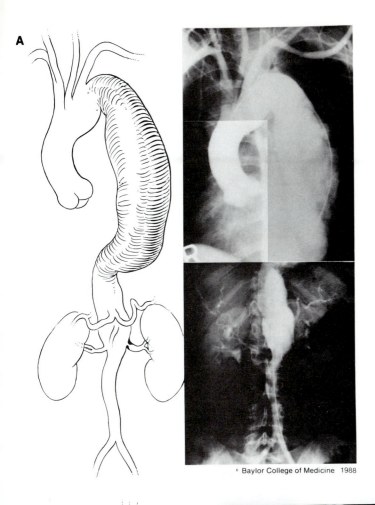

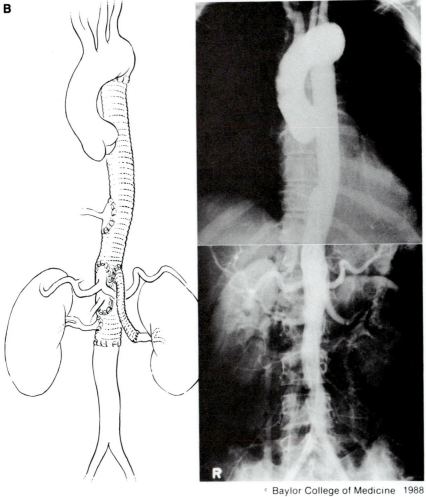

Figure 45-15. A. Illustration and aortogram of patient with diffuse fusiform aneurysm of all the descending and most of the abdominal aorta. **B.** Drawing of repair and postoperative aortogram, showing preservation of reattached intercostal arteries, and reattachment of visceral arteries including separate tube graft reconstruction of left renal artery.

REFERENCES

1. Edwards JE, Burchell HB: The pathological anatomy of deficiencies between the aortic root and the heart, including aortic sinus aneurysms. Thorax 12:125, 1957.

2. Sawyers JL, Adams JE, Scott HW Jr: Surgical treatment for aneurysms of the aortic sinuses with aorticoatrial fistula. Surgery 41:26, 1957.

3. Nowicki ER, Aberdeen E, et al.: Congenital left aortic sinuses, left ventricle fistula and review of aorto-cardiac fistulas. Ann Thorac Surg 23:378, 1977.

4. Meyer J, Wukasch DC, et al.: Aneurysm and fistula of the sinus of Valsalva. Clinical considerations and surgical treatment in 45 patients. Ann Thorac Surg 19:170, 1975.

5. Shumacker HB, King H, Waldhausen JA: Transthoracic approach for the repair of ruptured aneurysms of the sinus of Valsalva. Ann Surg 161:946, 1965.

6. Heyman MA, Berman W Jr, et al.: Dilatation of ductus arteriosus by prostaglandin E_1 in aortic arch abnormalities. Circulation 59:169, 1979.

7. Brandt B, Marvin WJ Jr, et al.: Surgical treatment of coarctation of the aorta after balloon angioplasty. J Thorac Cardiovasc Surg 94:715, 1987.

8. Kopf GS, Hellenbrand W, et al.: Repair of aortic coarctation in the first three months of life: Immediate and long-term results. Ann Thorac Surg 41:225, 1986.

9. Waldhausen JA, Nahrwold DL: Repair of coarctation of the aorta with a subclavian flap. J Thorac Cardiovasc Surg 51:532, 1966.

10. Moore GF, Ionescu MI, Ross DN: Surgical repair of coarctation of the aorta by patch grafting. Ann Thorac Surg 14:626, 1972.

11. Reul GJ, Kabbani SS, et al.: Repair of coarctation of the thoracic aorta by patch graft aortoplasty. J Thorac Cardiovasc Surg 68:696, 1974.

12. Bergdahl L, Ljungqvist A: Long-term results after repair of coarctation of the aorta by patch grafting. J Thorac Cardiovasc Surg 80:177, 1980.

13. McGoldrick JP, Brown IW, Ross DN: Coarctation of the aorta: Late aneurysm formation with Dacron onlay patch grafting. Ann Thorac Surg 45:89, 1988.

14. Abbot ME: Coarctation of the aorta of the adult type. A statistical study and historical retrospect of 200 recorded cases with autopsy of stenosis or obliteration of the descending aortic arch in subjects above the age of two years. Am Heart J 3:392, 1928.

15. Huston KA, Hunder GG, et al.: Temporal arteritis: A 25-year epidemiologic, clinical, and pathologic study. Ann Intern Med 88:162, 1978.

16. Austen WG, Blennerhassett JB: Giant-cell aortitis causing an aneurysm of the ascending aorta and aortic regurgitation. N Engl J Med 272:80, 1965.

17. Lupi-Herrera E, Sanchez-Torres G, et al.: Takayasu's arteritis. Clinical study of 107 cases. Am Heart J 93:94, 1977.

18. Lande A, Berkmen YM: Aortitis: Pathologic, clinical and arteriographic review. Radiol Clin North Am 14:219, 1976.

19. Ishikawa K: Natural history and classification of occlusive thromboaortopathy, Takayasu's disease. Circulation 57:27, 1978.

20. Nasu T: Pathology of pulseless disease, a systematic study and critical review of twenty-one autopsy cases reported in Japan. Angiology 14:225, 1962.

21. Robbs JV, Human RR, Rajaruthnam P: Operative treatment of nonspecific aortitis (Takayasu's arteritis). J Vasc Surg 3:605, 1986.

22. Brow SL, Busuttel RW, et al.: Bacteriologic and surgical determinants of survival in patients with mycotic aneurysms. J Vasc Surg 1:541, 1984.

23. Johansen K, Devin J: Mycotic aortic aneurysms. Arch Surg 118:583, 1983.

24. James EC, Gillespie JT: Aortic mycotic abdominal aneurysm involving all visceral branches: Excision and Dacron graft replacement. J Cardiovasc Surg 18:353, 1977.

25. Roberts WC: Aortic dissection: Anatomy, consequence and causes. Am Heart J 101:195, 1981.

26. Crawford ES, Stowe CL, et al.: Aortic arch aneurysm, a sentinel of tensive aortic disease requiring subtotal and total aortic replacement. Ann Surg 199:742, 1984.

27. Moreno-Cabral CE, Miller DC, et al.: Degenerative and atherosclerotic aneurysms of the thoracic aorta. Determinants of early and late surgical outcome. J Thorac Cardiovasc Surg 88:1020, 1984.

28. Dressler V, McNamara JJ: Thoracic aortic aneurysm. J Thorac Cardiovasc Surg 79:489, 1980.

29. Symbas PN, Baldwin FBJ, et al.: Marfan's syndrome with aneurysm of ascending aorta and aortic regurgitation. Am J Cardiol 25:483, 1970.

30. Murdoch JL, Walker BA, et al.: Life expectancy and causes of death in the Marfan's syndrome. N Engl J Med 286:804, 1972.

31. McCready RA, Pluth JR: Surgical treatment of ascending aortic aneurysms associated with aortic valve insufficiency. Ann Thorac Surg 28:307, 1979.

32. Symbas TN, Raizner AE, et al.: Aneurysms of all sinuses of Valsalva in patients with Marfan's syndrome. Ann Surg 174:902, 1971.

33. Bentall H, DeBono A: A technique for complete replacement of the ascending aorta. Thorax 23:338, 1968.

34. Mayer JE Jr., Lindsay WG, et al.: Composite replacement of the aortic valve and ascending aorta. J Thorac Cardiovasc Surg 76:816, 1978.

35. Kouchoukos NT, Marshall WG Jr, Wedige-Stecher TA: Eleven-year experience with composite valve graft replacement of the ascending aorta and aortic valve. J Thorac Cardiovasc Surg 92:691, 1986.

36. Helseth HK, Haglin JJ, et al.: Results of composite graft replacement for aortic root aneurysm. J Thorac Cardiovasc Surg 80:754, 1980.

37. Cabrol C, Pavie A, et al.: Complete replacement of the ascending aorta with reimplantation of coronary arteries. New surgical approach. J Thorac Cardiovasc Surg 81:309, 1981.

38. Cabrol C, Panie A, et al.: Long-term results with total replacement of the ascending aorta and reimplantation of the coronary arteries. J Thorac Cardiovasc Surg 91:17, 1986.

39. Hirst AE Jr, Johns VL Jr, Kime SW Jr: Dissecting aneurysm at the aorta: A review of 505 cases. Medicine 37:217, 1958.

40. Wheat MW Jr: Acute dissecting aneurysms of the aorta: Diagnosis and treatment. Am Heart J 99:373, 1980.

41. Wheat MW Jr: Acute dissecting aneurysm of the aorta: Medical therapy current status. World J Surg 4:563, 1980.

42. Tharion J, Johnson DC, et al.: Profound hypothermia with circulatory arrest. Nine years' clinical experience. J Thorac Cardiovasc Surg 84:66, 1982.

43. Crawford ES, Saleh SA, Schuessler JS: Treatment of aneurysm of transverse aortic arch. J Thorac Cardiovasc Surg 78:383, 1979.

44. Crawford ES, Cohen ES: Aortic aneurysm: A multifocal disease. Arch Surg 117:1393, 1982.

45. Griepp RB, Stinson EB, et al.: Prosthetic replacement of the aortic arch. J Thorac Cardiovasc Surg 70:1051, 1975.

46. Crawford ES, Snyder DM: Treatment of aneurysms of the aortic arch. A progress report. J Thorac Cardiovasc Surg 85:237, 1983.

47. Woodhall B, Sealy W, et al.: Craniotomy under conditions of quinidine-protected cardioplegia and profound hypothermia. Ann Surg 152:37, 1960.

48. Woodhall B, Reynolds DH, et al.: The physiological and patho-

logic effects of localized cerebral hypothermia. Ann Surg 147:673, 1958.

49. Woodhall B: Experimental and clinical studies in localized cerebral perfusion. Ann Surg 150:640, 1959.

50. Massimo CG, Poma AG, et al.: Simultaneous total aortic replacement from arch to bifurcation: Experience with six cases. Texas Heart Instit J 13:147, 1986.

51. Crawford ES, Coselli JS, Safi HJ: Partial cardiopulmonary bypass, hypothermic circulatory arrest, and posterolateral exposure for thoracic aortic aneurysm operation. J Thorac Cardiovasc Surg 94:824, 1987.

52. Lillehei CW, Todd DB Jr, et al.: Partial cardiopulmonary bypass, hypothermia, and total circulatory arrest. J Thorac Cardiovasc Surg 58:530, 1969.

53. Crawford ES, Crawford JL, et al.: Redo operations for recurrent aneurysmal disease of the ascending aorta and transverse aortic arch. Ann Thorac Surg 40:439, 1985.

54. Bickerstaff LK, Pailrolero PC, et al.: Thoracic aortic aneurysms: A population-based study. Surgery 92:1103, 1982.

55. McNamara JJ, Pressle VM: Natural history of atherosclerotic thoracic aortic aneurysms. Ann Thorac Surg 26:468, 1978.

56. Crawford ES, DeNatale RW: Thoracoabdominal aortic aneurysm: Observations regarding the natural cause of the disease. J Vasc Surg 3:578, 1986.

57. Crawford ES, Mizrahi EM, et al.: The impact of distal aortic perfusion and somatosensory evoked potential monitoring on prevention of paraplegia after aortic aneurysm operation. J Thorac Cardiovasc Surg 95:357, 1988.

58. Crawford ES, Crawford JL, et al.: Thoracoabdominal aortic aneurysms: Preoperative and intraoperative factors determining immediate and long-term results of operations in 605 patients. J Vasc Surg 3:389, 1086.

CHAPTER 46
Thoracoabdominal Aortic Aneurysm

Calvin B. Ernst and Daniel J. Reddy

Thoracoabdominal aortic aneurysms, although relatively uncommon, carry the same risks of expansion, rupture, and distal ischemia from thrombosis or embolus as aneurysms occurring elsewhere. Similarly, these complications are best avoided by timely diagnosis and operation. However, the extent and critical location of thoracoabdominal aneurysms pose unique threats to patients who harbor these lesions and challenges to the vascular surgeon who undertakes their operative management.

The required operative approach to a thoracoabdominal aneurysm carries added risk because the exposure to complete the operation necessitates combined entry into both thoracic and abdominal cavities and division of the left hemidiaphragm. Adding to the operative risk is the need to temporarily occlude the aorta, and the visceral, renal, intercostal, and upper lumbar arteries to permit prosthetic replacement of the thoracoabdominal aorta and restoration of blood flow to each of these important branches. These factors account for the continuing challenges to surgeons treating these patients during the 32 years after Etheredge et al.'s first report of successful replacement of a thoracoabdominal aneurysm.[1]

This chapter addresses the natural history, clinical presentation, diagnosis, and management of atherosclerotic thoracoabdominal aneurysms. Aneurysms of the ascending aorta, aortic arch, those limited to the thoracic or abdominal aorta, dissecting aneurysms, and those occurring as a result of myxomatous degeneration, infection, and trauma are beyond the scope of this chapter.

NATURAL HISTORY

No prospective randomized clinical trial to determine the natural history of treated and untreated thoracoabdominal aortic aneurysms has been reported. One must rely on retrospective reviews to determine the natural history of this pathologic entity. Retrospective reviews of the natural history of atherosclerotic aneurysms occurring in the abdominal, thoracic, or combined thoracoabdominal aorta

have been reported. Szilagyi et al. reported a 19% 5-year actuarial survival rate for untreated patients with infrarenal abdominal aortic aneurysms.[2] The comparable survival rate for patients with aneurysm resection was threefold better than for those not treated. The poor outcome in untreated patients was attributable to aneurysm rupture. Bickerstaff et al. reported on 72 untreated patients with thoracic aortic aneurysms over a 30-year period.[3] The aneurysm ruptured in 18 of 27 patients (67%) with aneurysms in the descending aorta. The overall rupture rate for nondissecting aneurysm was 51%. Crawford and DeNatale studied 94 patients with thoracoabdominal aortic aneurysms and compared the results without treatment to the 579 similar patients who underwent thoracoabdominal aortic aneurysm resection.[4] Sixty-eight percent of untreated patients died; 57% of these deaths were from aneurysm rupture. Only 19% of untreated patients survived 5 years in contrast to 59% of the surgically treated patients.

It is apparent from these and other studies that the natural history of thoracoabdominal aortic aneurysms closely parallels that of aneurysms limited to either the abdominal or descending thoracic aorta. Inexorable aneurysm expansion leading to rupture is likely to occur in a relatively short time after diagnosis unless death occurs from an unrelated cause. If morbidity and mortality rates after operation offer significant benefits over the natural history of the disease, then a policy of elective aneurysmectomy is justified to prevent death from rupture. Encouraged by the excellent results of Crawford and DeNatale, many clinics have undertaken thoracoabdominal aortic aneurysm repair.[4]

ANEURYSM CLASSIFICATION

Experience has shown that the extent of a thoracoabdominal aneurysm is important because it has a bearing on both the operative approach and the outcome after operation. Crawford has developed a classification that stratifies patients into four different types according to aneurysm

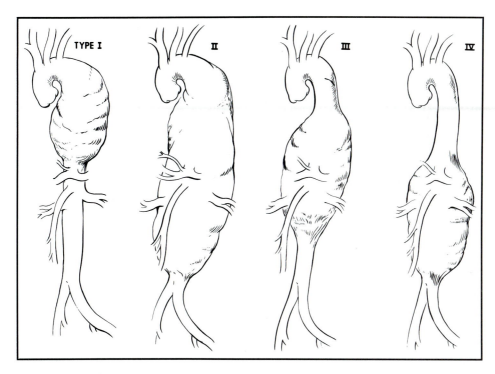

Figure 46-1. Artist's conception of the four types of thoracoabdominal aortic aneurysm. From *left* to *right*: types I, II, III, and IV.

extent.[5] Type I involves most or all of the descending thoracic aorta and upper abdominal aorta, not including the celiac axis. Type II involves most or all of the descending thoracic aorta and most or all of the abdominal aorta. Type III involves the distal half or less of the descending thoracic aorta and most of the abdominal aorta. Type IV involves most or all of the abdominal aorta. Although this classification has yet to be widely adopted, its value is apparent because it provides rational patient selection for risk assessment and operative planning (Fig. 46-1).

CLINICAL PRESENTATION

Thoracoabdominal aortic aneurysms may be asymptomatic for varying periods of time. However, with continuing degeneration of the aortic wall, accelerated by risk factors such as uncontrolled hypertension, aneurysms eventually expand, rupture, embolize, or thrombose. This accounts for the wide array of clinical signs and symptoms associated with their clinical presentation.

Asymptomatic Thoracoabdominal Aortic Aneurysm

Identification of a thoracoabdominal aortic aneurysm is not as straightforward as detection of an asymptomatic abdominal aortic aneurysm that usually is noted by palpation of a pulsatile abdominal mass. Although a large abdominal component of the thoracoabdominal aneurysm may be palpable, this mass is often obscured in the upper abdomen.

This is particularly true if the patient is obese or has a narrow costal margin. Furthermore, the thoracic component is undetectable by physical exam. Some authors have noted that the large size of asymptomatic thoracoabdominal aneurysms, when first recognized, relates to the obscurity of these lesions during development. Many aneurysms are first noted as incidental findings during roentgenography, sonography, or computed tomography (CT) scans of the chest or abdomen or during contrast examinations of the urinary or gastrointestinal tracts.

Symptomatic Thoracoabdominal Aortic Aneurysm

In our experience, 77% of patients (16 of 22) had either ruptured or symptomatic aneurysms at the time of operation. Three patients had frank rupture (13.6%), and another three had a contained rupture (13.6%), for an overall rupture rate of 28%. Crawford et al. reported a rupture rate of 4% and a symptomatic rate of 70% among 605 patients treated by operation.[5] Although sealed ruptures of these aneurysms have been observed, this is an unexpected finding and one cannot assume any safe period after aneurysm rupture that would permit diagnostic testing or temporizing measures.

Symptomatic thoracoabdominal aortic aneurysms may present in a variety of ways but usually are heralded by pain in the back, chest, abdomen, or flank. The differential diagnosis includes the acute surgical abdomen, angina pectoris, acute myocardial infarction, osteoarthritis of the vertebral column, esophagitis with cardiospasm, esophageal perforation, pulmonary embolus, pneumonia, aortic dissection, and urinary colic or sepsis. The pain can be either sharp or dull and is unremitting.

Other less common clinical presentations follow specific complications caused by either compression of adjacent structures by aneurysm expansion, or from branch artery occlusion resulting from thrombosis or emboli originating in the diseased aorta. Renal insufficiency or even renal failure with uremia may be evident secondary to renal artery occlusion. Although spinal cord ischemia with paraplegia or paraparesis is twice as common with dissecting thoraco-abdominal aneurysms, it may occur with atherosclerotic aneurysms as well, secondary to occlusion of critical segmental arterial supply to the spinal cord. In addition to vital organ or spinal cord ischemia, distal arterial embolization of aneurysm contents may result in lower extremity ischemia.

Other unusual clinical presentations include congestive hepatomegaly,[6] compression of the airway of the esophagus, left recurrent nerve palsy with hoarseness, and hemorrhage from either the tracheobronchial tree or the digestive tract. Fischer et al. described three patients with disseminated intravascular coagulation (DIC) occurring as a consequence of extensive thoracoabdominal aortic aneurysms.[7] These patients had a bleeding diathesis and laboratory evidence of thrombocytopenia and elevated fibrin split products. Under these circumstances DIC was thought to be triggered by the large amount of clot forming within the aneurysm.

Associated Aneurysms

Many patients requiring operation for thoracoabdominal aortic aneurysms will have undergone previous vascular operations.[5] Thus the surgeon must search for coexistent or subsequent aneurysm disease during follow-up. Areas of particular concern are the ascending aorta, aortic arch, and visceral, iliac, femoral, and popliteal arteries.

DIAGNOSIS

Whenever a thoracoabdominal aneurysm is suspected, diagnosis must then be confirmed and the aneurysm classified by delineating its extent. This is best accomplished by obtaining one or more of the imaging studies currently available.

Plain roentgenograms of the chest and abdomen taken in multiple planes may be helpful, but provide insufficient information for planning operation. Sonography is of slightly greater value in estimating the size and extent of the abdominal component of a thoracoabdominal aneurysm. Sonograms fail to provide anatomic information regarding aneurysm extension into the pelvis or chest, however.

CT scans enhanced by intravenous administration of contrast media provide excellent assessment of the proximal and distal extents of the aneurysm (Fig. 46-2). Although CT scanning helps to classify aneurysms it fails to yield detailed information regarding the location, number, and patency of visceral and renal arteries. For this reason aortography, either conventional or by intraarterial digital subtraction techniques, is routinely used to define the extent of disease affecting the visceral, renal, and iliac arteries as well as to determine aneurysm size. Combined with CT scans, angiography provides excellent preoperative information (Figs. 46-3 to 46-6). Some authors have suggested that aortography should include selective spinal cord angiograms to identify the critical segmental arterial supply to the cord.[5,8] Such selective angiography might aid revascularization of intercostal and lumbar arteries at the time of the aneurysm resection. For practical reasons, not the least of which is the risk of contrast-induced transverse myelitis, this approach has not gained general acceptance.

Magnetic resonance imaging (MRI) holds promise for diagnosis and classification of thoracoabdominal aortic aneurysms.[9] From transaxial MRI images one may measure aneurysm diameter, identify luminal clot, and atheroscle-

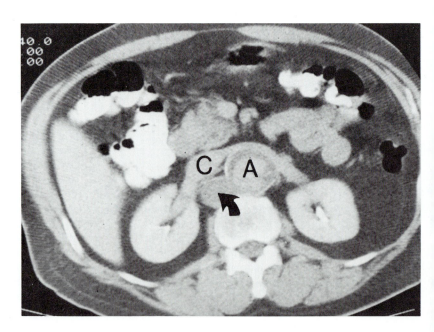

Figure 46-2. Contrast-enhanced transverse CT scan of sealed ruptured Type III thoracoabdominal aortic aneurysm. The *C* overlies the inferior vena cava at the level of the renal veins. The *A* overlies the calcified atherosclerotic aneurysm with luminal clot. The arrow points to the retroaortic hematoma from the right posterior lateral aortic rupture.

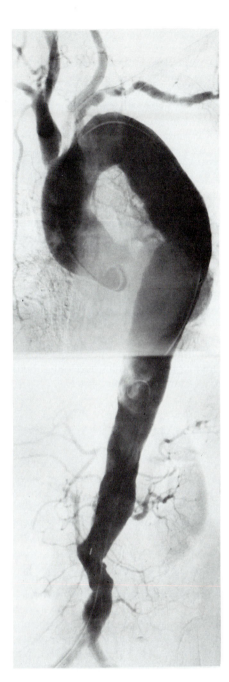

Figure 46-3. Thoracoabdominal aortogram of type I aneurysm involving all of the thoracic aorta and the upper abdominal aorta. A right aortorenal saphenous vein graft is apparent.

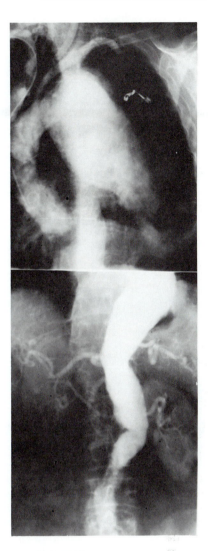

Figure 46-4. Thoracoabdominal aortogram of a type II aneurysm involving all of the descending thoracic aorta and most of the abdominal aorta.

rotic plaque. Parasaggital sections can document the proximal and distal aneurysm extent (Fig. 46-7). MRI has the added advantages of being noninvasive and requiring no contrast media. Avoiding the use of intravascular contrast media precludes contrast-induced renal toxicity in patients with marginal renal function. Currently, it is unclear whether MRI provides the necessary image resolution to determine the size, number, location, and patency of arteries arising from the aneurysm. Without these capabilities, MRI cannot supplant CT scans and aortography. Prospective comparisons with established diagnostic methods are

needed to define the sensitivity, specificity, and utility of MRI in the diagnosis of atherosclerotic thoracoabdominal aortic aneurysm.

MANAGEMENT

Patient Selection

Patient selection for operation is based on risk assessment. All patients who have an estimated life expectancy of 2 or more years are considered candidates for operation. This estimate is based on the severity of coexisting diseases and the likelihood of aneurysm rupture. Elective operation is recommended when the aneurysm diameter exceeds twice the diameter of the undiseased aorta. When the entire aorta is involved, operation is advised when the aneurysm exceeds twice the expected size of the aorta. In our experience, hypertension is the most common associated condition followed by pulmonary, hepatic, cardiac, and cerebrovascular

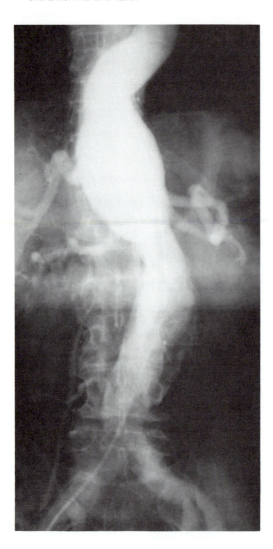

Figure 46-5. Aortogram of a type III thoracoabdominal aneurysm involving the lower portion of the descending thoracic aorta and all of the abdominal aortic and iliac arteries.

diseases. Therefore, particular attention must be paid to the assessment of these organ systems for risk assessment.

Preoperative and operative variables predictive of early mortality (30 day) have been determined by multivariate analysis.[5] The pertinent risk factors identified were patient age, aortic clamp time, and chronic obstructive pulmonary disease. The leading cause of death among 54 of 605 patients who died during the first 30 days after operation was cardiac, accounting for 24 (44%) deaths. Using multivariate discriminant analysis, Goldman et al. identified factors affecting the development of cardiac complications after major noncardiac operations.[10] To specifically evaluate severity of coronary artery disease preoperatively, cardiac imaging with dipyridamole-thallium has proved superior to clinical assessment alone and is safer and more cost effective than coronary angiography.[11] Depending on results of such cardiac evaluation, coronary angiography or coronary revascularization may be required before aneurysm repair, particularly for patients with thallium redistribution, unstable angina, or recent myocardial infarction. Such studies may

also mandate postponement of aneurysm repair in patients with congestive heart failure or serious disturbances of cardiac rhythm until these problems are corrected or improved.

Although use of preoperative spirometry and pulmonary function studies are widely advocated and practiced, no reports are available that document their efficiency in risk assessment for thoracoabdominal aortic aneurysm repair. Crawford advises against elective operation for patients with CO_2 retention or a 1-second forced expiratory volume (FEV_1) of less than 1 L.[5] The FEV_1 should be expressed as a percentage of predicted value adjusted for age, sex, height, and weight.[12] Patients with a FEV_1 less than 75% of the predicted value have an increased risk of postoperative pulmonary complications. Patients with obstructive lung disease may benefit from preoperative pulmonary therapy consisting of cessation of smoking, chest physiotherapy, bronchodilator therapy, and optimal hydration. Patients with restrictive lung disease, characterized by diminished vital capacity, may not benefit from intense preoperative pulmonary therapy.

Renal dysfunction and cerebral vascular arterial occlusive disease must also be considered in preoperative risk assessment. Other conditions of the aged population such as malignant disease of the colon and lung should be sought according to generally accepted practice.

Treatment Options

A variety of surgical options for management of atherosclerotic thoracoabdominal aortic aneurysms have been described. These include (1) aneurysm resection,[13,14] (2) aneurysm bypass with partial aneurysm resection,[15,16] (3) aneurysm exclusion with bypass,[17,18] and (4) aneurysm graft inclusion.[19,20] In the first three operations, visceral and renal artery flow is reestablished by individual grafts originating from the aortic graft. In the fourth operation, developed by Crawford, arterial flow to the visceral and renal arteries is reestablished by direct attachment of arterial orifices to elliptic excisions in the aortic graft. This is accomplished by suturing such anastomoses from inside the opened aneurysm. This technique, because of its simplicity compared to the other procedures, will be described and is the one that we have adopted in our clinical practice.

Operative Technique

Successful operation requires coordinated efforts of anesthetic, surgical, blood bank, and nursing teams. Few other operations require the attention to detail and coordination of such a large and diverse group of professionals. Arterial cannulas are placed in each of the patient's radial arteries for continuous systemic arterial pressure monitoring and to provide fail-safe blood sampling access for arterial blood gas, hemogram, coagulation, and serum electrolyte studies during and after the operation. A pulmonary artery flow-directed balloon catheter is placed percutaneously to monitor pulmonary capillary wedge pressure and to measure cardiac output. Sufficient venous access for fluid and blood

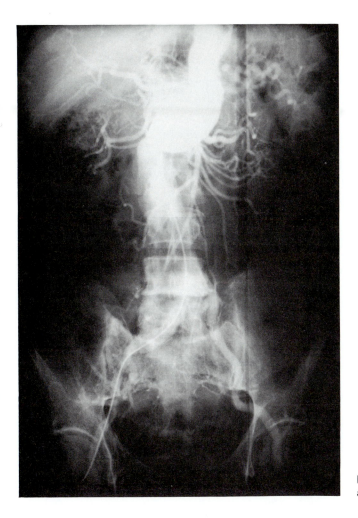

Figure 46-6. Aortogram of a type IV aneurysm involving the entire abdominal aorta.

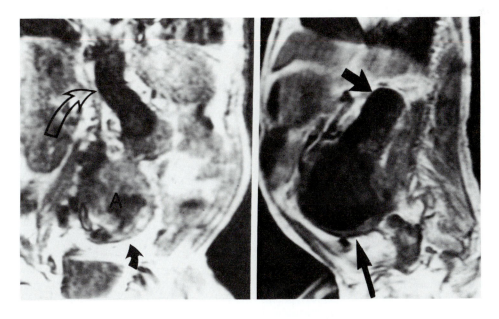

Figure 46-7. Anteroposterior (AP) (*left*) and parasaggital (*right*) magnetic resonance images of a type IV thoracoabdominal aortic aneurysm. In the AP image (*left*) the open arrow shows the proximal extent of the aneurysm. The *A* overlies the large saccular infrarenal component. The closed arrow shows the inferior extent of the aneurysm. In the parasaggital image (*right*), the short arrow shows the proximal extent of the aneurysms and the long arrow shows the distal extent.

administration is secured. It is important to warm intravenous fluids to promote hemostasis and to avoid cardiac arryhmias from hypothermia.

A device for shed blood salvage that permits rapid autotransfusion of large volumes of blood or washed packed red blood cells during the operation is mandatory. Autotransfusion systems that provide washed packed red cells have the theoretical and practical advantages over whole blood salvage systems by avoiding reinfusion of activated protein procoagulants that can lead to DIC.[21] In addition, a blood bank well supplied with cross-matched blood and blood products including fresh frozen plasma and platelets is necessary to supplement any autotransfusion system.

The patient is placed in the right lateral semidecubitus position with the left side turned up 75 degrees. This position is maintained by a beanbag device filled wth plastic spheres that, when evacuated by suction, become rigid and firmly holds the patient in position. General anesthesia is induced before the patient is positioned and a double-lumen endobronchial tube is placed. This tube permits controlled collapse of the left lung during the portions of the operation that require access to the descending thoracic aorta. Reinflation of the left lung without hyperinflation of the right lung can then be done when exposure is no longer necessary.

A posterolateral thoracoabdominal incision is made. For low lesions, the ninth interspace is entered; for higher lesions, the incision is made through the bed of the resected sixth rib. Location of the incision depends on the preoperative assessment of the proximal extent of the aneurysm. The posterolateral approach to the aorta with the left kidney, spleen, pancreas, and left colon reflected to the right provides excellent access to the thoracoabdominal aorta (Fig. 46-8).[20] The left hemidiaphragm is divided radially or circumferentially, the latter providing the theoretical advantage of preserving branches of the phrenic nerve. Although retroperitoneal dissection will lessen the incidence of hypothermia and postoperative third-space fluid accumulations,[22] it limits ability to inspect the intraabdominal viscera. Therefore, we employ a retroperitoneal-transperitoneal approach so the viscera can be inspected at the completion of the operation. This also facilitates assessment of the celiac, mesenteric, and right renal artery pulses following attachment of these vessels to the aortic prosthesis. The retroperitoneal-transperitoneal approach is suitable for all types of thorocoabdominal aneurysms whereas the retroperitoneal approach is reserved for types III and IV aneurysms. No heparin, shunts, bypasses, circulatory arrest, hypothermia, renal cooling, or perfusion are employed. This simplifies the operative technique, reduces blood loss and transfusion requirements, and minimizes postoperative bleeding.[5]

To minimize hypertension and left ventricular strain during aortic crossclamping, an intravenous infusion of 5% sodium nitroprusside is started just before application of the proximal aortic clamp. Closely coordinated efforts between surgeon and anesthesiologist are required to titrate such afterload reduction drugs to avoid iatrogenic hypotension. The aorta is then opened posterolaterally throughout the length of the aneurysm (Fig. 46-8). After opening the aneurysm, balloon catheters are placed in branch ostea to control backbleeding from the celiac axis, superior mesen-

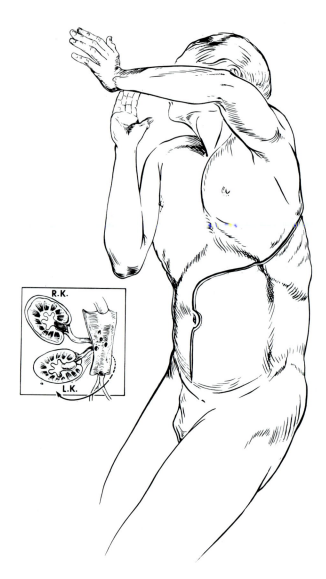

Figure 46-8. Illustration of the operative approach. The patient is in the semidecubitus position and the aorta is approached posteriolaterally. The thoracoabdominal incision is placed from the sixth to eleventh interspace and the diaphragm is divided directly to the aortic hiatus. Dissection is behind the left kidney (*L.K.*), reflecting it anteromedially. Visceral vessel orifices are identified (*insert*) when the aneurysm is opened.

teric, renal, iliac, and intercostal arteries. With type I, II, and III aneurysms, the proximal anastomosis is completed in an end-to-end fashion and identifiable intercostal ostea are replanted to elliptical holes in the graft. The graft is then clamped distal to the reimplanted intercostal vessels and the aortic clamp is slowly removed, restoring intercostal flow.

With the proximal clamp below the attached intercostal arteries, to restore flow and limit spinal ischemia, the mesenteric and renal arteries are reimplanted either individually or together. Usually the celiac, superior mesenteric artery, and right renal arteries can be reimplanted as a button containing all three ostea (Fig. 46-9). Particular attention must be given to selecting a suitable site on the aortic graft

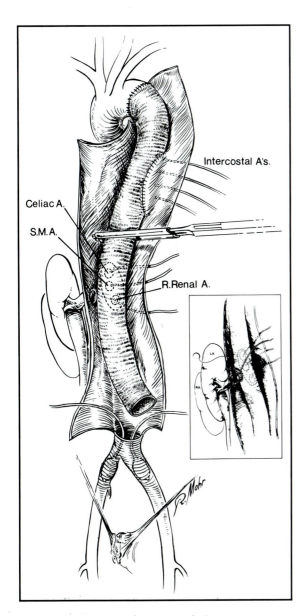

Figure 46-9. Illustration of the operative techniques employed in thoracoabdominal aortic operations. Identified intercostal arteries are reattached and reperfused before completion of the renal and visceral artery anastomoses. The right renal artery, celiac axis, and superior mesenteric artery orifices may be reattached as a unit. Left renal artery reimplantation follows separately (*insert*). Reperfusion of the kidneys and gut precede the distal aortic anastomosis.

for reattachment of the left renal artery to avoid kinking this vessel when the viscera are restored to their normal anatomic positions (Fig. 46-9). Because of this possibility it may be necessary to interpose a 6 mm side limb between the aortic graft and the left renal artery. This is easily accomplished because with this retroperitoneal approach, the left renal artery, unlike the right renal artery, is readily accessible throughout its length. After the left renal reconstruction, the graft clamp is moved distally, slowly restoring flow to the gut and kidneys. After restoring renal blood flow the anesthesiologist administers 5 ml of indicarmine. This dye

is excreted in the urine, coloring it blue. The appearance of blue urine assures the surgeon that at least one kidney is well perfused and producing urine. The distal anastomosis or anastomoses are completed at the aortic bifurcation, iliac or femoral levels, as dictated by the pathologic anatomy.

With type IV aneurysms the procedure may be simplified in some cases by incorporating the visceral, renal, intercostal, and lumbar vessels in the proximal anastomosis. This is accomplished by fashioning the prosthesis as an oval with its toe sutured to the posterior aortic wall above the aneurysm and its heel sutured below the renal arteries on the anterior aortic wall (Fig. 46-10). This modification provides certain advantages of safety and simplicity but should be avoided if the aortic disease makes secure anastomosis unlikely.

Results

Standards to measure results of operation for thoracoabdominal aortic aneurysms have been established by Crawford.[5] No other reports of comparable breadth or length of follow-up are available for comparison; it remains to be seen if others can duplicate Crawford's results of 8.9% operative mortality (30-day) and 60% 5-year survival rates.[5] At the Henry Ford Hospital, over the past 4 years 22 patients have undergone operative repair by the method described. Excluding three patients in extremis with ruptured aneurysm and profound hemorrhagic shock before operation, the operative mortality rate was 26% (5 of 19 patients). All five deaths occurred in patients with symptomatic type II aneurysms. Three of these five deaths occurred in patients with sealed type II aneurysm ruptures. Stratified according to aneurysm type, the mortality rates achieved were: type I (0%), type II (55%, 5 of 9 patients), type III (0%, 0 of 7), and type IV (0%, 0 of 2). All six patients with elective aneurysm repair (three type II and three type III) survived operation.

The major complications following these operations include bleeding, respiratory and renal failure, and spinal cord ischemia. Bleeding occurs from either the surgical incision, the aneurysm sac, any of the anastomoses, or from disorders of coagulation. Bleeding from an injured spleen is generally recognized during operation and is seldom the cause of postoperative bleeding. Coagulopathy usually occurs from dilution of clotting factors associated with massive transfusion or from platelet dysfunction. Liberal and prompt administration of clotting factors and platelets is necessary both during and after operation to avoid this potentially serious complication. Avoiding the use of sodium heparin during aortic reconstruction limits bleeding from the wound, aneurysm sac, and anastomoses. The mechanism for development of postreconstruction coagulopathy is complex, but exacerbating it by use of sodium heparin compounds such problems; consequently, we advise against the use of heparin.

Respiratory complications occur from left lung collapse or atelectasis and from right lung atelectasis associated with the right decubitus position during operation. Care must be taken to avoid injury to pulmonary parenchymal tissue during the dissection of large or adherent aneurysms to

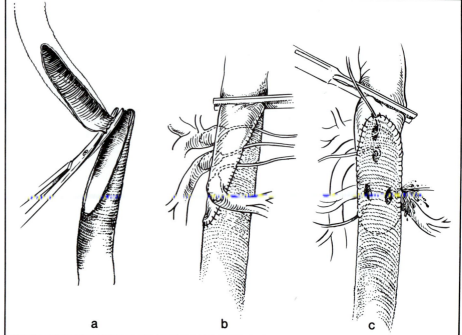

Figure 46-10. Simplified operative technique for a type IV aneurysm. The proximal aortic anastomosis, renal arteries, and visceral arteries are incorporated as a single oval anastomosis. **a.** Aorta is trimmed and prosthesis is cut to match. **b.** Long ovoid anastomosis (viewed from anterior aspect) with occlusion balloon catheters inflated. **c.** Anastomosis viewed from behind with extraction of occlusion catheters and backflushing from visceral vessels.

prevent a persistent bronchopleural fistula or airborne contamination of the wound and prosthesis. Since a high percentage of these patients have chronic obstructive pulmonary disease, pulmonary function should be optimized preoperatively to avoid pulmonary complications and thereby avoid prolonged need for postoperative ventilatory support.

Renal failure, mesenteric ischemia, and lower extremity ischemia seldom occur. In our experience, temporary postoperative dialysis for acute tubular necrosis was required in two of 22 (9.9%) patients. No patient developed permanent renal failure, visceral ischemia, or limb loss.

The major unsolved problem in thoracoabdominal aortic reconstruction is prevention of spinal cord ischemia with resulting paraplegia or paraparesis. This complication has been recognized in experimental aortic reconstruction for more than 75 years.[23] Clinically, paraplegia is unpredictable and has led experienced investigators to conclude that the risk of paraplegia is determined by uncontrollable factors such as the nature and extent of the aneurysm and is not determined by details of operative technique.[24] That the incidence of paraplegia following operations for aortic dissection is twice that observed following operations for atherosclerotic aneurysms supports this view.[5] In addition, the incidence of paraplegia is directly related to size of the aneurysm. Paraplegia incidences for type I, II, III, and IV aneurysms are 8%, 21%, 2%, and 1%, respectively. A type II aneurysm, the most extensive, carries the highest risk of postoperative paraplegia.[5]

Measurement of somatosensory evoked potentials (SEPs) have been suggested as an intraoperative method of detecting cord ischemia to alert the surgeon to the critical intercostal artery blood supply.[25] Although this technique has merit when employed during operations on the descending thoracic aorta, certain limitations such as periph-

eral nerve ischemia during aortic clamping make it impractical and unsuccessful in thoracoabdominal aortic operations.[8] There has been renewed interest in intraoperative spinal fluid manometry and drainage to prolong the safe spinal cord ischemic interval. Although recent data suggest that monitoring and drainage of spinal fluid may increase anterior spinal artery perfusion during aortic clamping,[26,27] efficacy of this modality awaits confirmation by other investigators. Concern also has been expressed that administering sodium nitroprusside for afterload reduction decreases distal aortic pressure, raises spinal fluid pressure, and increases the likelihood of postoperative paraplegia.[28] Other experimental techniques such as electrospinography[29] and regional cord hypothermia[30] are being investigated and await clinical trial. At present, postoperative paraplegia must be considered an unpredictable and unpreventable complication following thoracoabdominal aortic reconstruction.

REFERENCES

1. Etheredge SN, Yee J, et al.: Successful resection of a large aneurysm of the upper abdominal aorta and replacement with homograft. Surgery 38:1071, 1955.
2. Szilagyi DE, Elliott JP, Smith RF: Clinical fate of the patient with asymptomatic abdominal aortic aneurysm and unfit for surgical treatment. Arch Surg 104:600, 1972.
3. Bickerstaff LK, Pairolero PC, et al.: Thoracic aortic aneurysms: a population based study. Surgery 92:1103, 1982.
4. Crawford ES, DeNatale RW: Thoracoabdominal aortic aneurysm: Observations regarding the natural course of the disease. J Vasc Surg 3:578, 1986.
5. Crawford ES, Crawford JL, et al.: Thoracoabdominal aortic aneurysms: Preoperative and intraoperative factors determin-

ing immediate and long-term results of operation in 605 patients. J Vasc Surg 3:389, 1986.

6. Sigal E, Pogany A, Goldman IS: Marked hepatic congestion caused by a thoracoabdominal aneurysm. Gastroenterology 87:1367, 1984.

7. Fischer DF, Yawn DH, Crawford ES: Preoperative disseminated intravascular coagulation associated with aortic aneurysms. Arch Surg 118:1252, 1983.

8. Elliott JP, Szilagyi DE, et al.: Spinal cord ischemia: Secondary to surgery of the abdominal aorta, in Towne J, Bernhard V, (eds): Complications in Vascular Surgery. Orlando, Fla. Grune & Stratton, 1985, pp 291–310.

9. Amparo EG, Higgins CB, et al.: Magnetic resonance imaging of aortic disease: Preliminary results. AJR 142:1203, 1984.

10. Goldman L, Caldera DL, et al.: Multifactorial index of cardiac risk in noncardiac surgical procedures. N Engl J Med 297:845, 1977.

11. Boucher CA, Brewster DC, et al.: Determination of cardiac risk by dipyridamole-thallium imaging before peripheral vascular surgery. N Engl J Med 312:389, 1985.

12. Knudson RJ, Slatin RC, Libowitz MD: The maximal expiratory flow volume curve: Normal standards, variability and effects of age. Am Rev Respir Dis 113:587, 1976.

13. DeBakey ME, Crawford ES, et al.: Surgical considerations in the treatment of aneurysms of the thoracoabdominal aorta. Ann Surg 162:650, 1965.

14. Stoney RJ, Wylie EJ: Surgical management of arterial lesions of the thoracoabdominal aorta. Am J Surg 126:157, 1973.

15. Edmunds LM, Folkman MJ: Aneurysmoplasty and prosthetic bypass for aneurysms of the descending thoracic and thoracoabdominal aorta. J Thorac Cardiovasc Surg 52:395, 1966.

16. Shumacker MB: Innovation in the operative management of the thoracoabdominal aortic aneurysm. Surg Gynecol Obstet 136:793, 1973.

17. Hardy JD, Timmis HH, et al.: Thoracoabdominal aortic aneurysm: Simplified surgical management with case report. Ann Surg 166:1008, 1967.

18. Selle JG, Robicsek F, et al.: Thoracoabdominal aortic aneurysm: A review and current status. Ann Surg 189:158, 1979.

19. Crawford ES: Thoracoabdominal and abdominal aortic aneurysms involving renal, superior mesenteric, and celiac arteries. Ann Surg 179:763, 1974.

20. Crawford ES, Crawford JL: Diseases of the Aorta Including an Atlas of Angiographic Pathology and Surgical Technique. Baltimore/London. The Williams & Wilkins Co., 1984.

21. Orr MD, Blenko JW: Autotransfusion of concentrated selected washed red cells from the surgical field: A biochemical and physiological comparison with homologous cell transfusion. Proceedings of the Blood Conservation Institute, 1978.

22. Williams GM, Ricotta J, et al.: The extended retroperitoneal approach for treatment of extensive atherosclerosis of the aorta and renal vessels. Surgery 88:846, 1980.

23. Carrel A: On experimental surgery of the aorta and heart. Ann Surg 52:83, 1910.

24. Livesay JJ, Cooley DA, et al.: Surgical experience in descending thoracic aneurysmectomy with and without adjuncts to avoid ischemia. Ann Thorac Surg 39:37, 1985.

25. Cunningham JN, Laschinger JC, et al.: Measurement of spinal cord ischemia during operation upon the thoracic aorta. Ann Surg 196:285, 1982.

26. Hollier LH: Protecting the brain and spinal cord. J Vasc Surg 5:524, 1987.

27. Oka Y, Miyamoto T: Prevention of spinal cord injury after cross-clamping of the thoracic aorta. J Cardiovasc Surg 28:398, 1987.

28. Nugent M, Kage MD, McGoon DC: Effects of nitroprusside on aortic and intraspinal pressures during thoracic aortic cross-clamping. (abstract) Anesthesiology 61:68, 1984.

29. Kaschner AG, Sandmann W, Larkamp H: Percutaneous flexible bipolar epidural neuroelectrode for spinal cord stimulation. J Neurosurg 60:1317, 1984.

30. Colon R, Frazier OH, et al.: Hypothermic regional perfusion for protection of the spinal cord during periods of ischemia. Ann Thorac Surg 43:639, 1987.

CHAPTER 47
Abdominal Aortic and Iliac Aneurysms

Norman R. Hertzer

For several reasons, the successful treatment of abdominal aortic aneurysms has served as a benchmark of progress in the field of vascular surgery for more than 3 decades. First, infrarenal aneurysms are common enough to be encountered in every community. Secondly, their risk for sudden rupture and death has been sufficiently documented that the indication for elective resection in appropriate candidates virtually is beyond debate. Moreover, many aspects of their reconstruction directly reflect the stunning advances in anesthetic techniques, prosthetic materials, blood uses, and perioperative monitoring that have taken place since 1950. Finally, the fact that aortic aneurysms tend to occur in older patients who have systemic atherosclerosis makes the management of their associated cardiac and other diseases one of the sternest tests of modern surgical care.

ETIOLOGY

Provided they are not associated with cystic medial necrosis (Marfan's syndrome) or hypertensive dissection, most aneurysms generally are presumed to be atherosclerotic in origin. In addition to the repeated clinical observation that aortic aneurysms and occlusive disease rarely occur simultaneously, however, a number of reports recently have implied that aneurysms might instead be caused by nonatherogenic mechanisms that either prevent collagen cross-linking (copper or amino acid deficiency) or disrupt it (collagenase, protease) within the arterial wall in ways that are as yet poorly understood.[1-4] A few genetic studies also have contributed to speculation about inherent metabolic defects by suggesting that at least some aneurysms represent a recessive chromosomal mutation among selected families in whom conventional risk factors such as hyperlipidemia or tobacco use apparently are absent.[5,6] Conversely, Zarins et al.[7] produced poststenotic dilatation by banding the descending thoracic aorta in primate models and found that collagenase activity in the ectatic segment increased significantly in comparison to that in control animals, a

feature indicating that elevated mural enzyme values may be only one of the secondary consequences of aortic aneurysms.

In a related issue, Swanson et al.[8] concluded that collagen lysis attributed to wound healing and nutritional depletion might be responsible for early rupture of unresected aortic aneurysms in a small series of 10 patients who previously had undergone laparotomy for other indications. Nevertheless, Cohen et al.[9] subsequently demonstrated in rats that surgical trauma without specific injury to the aorta failed to influence its collagenase level. Much is still to be learned about arterial metabolism, but if enzymatic weakening of the aorta were a consistent response to malnutrition or other surgical procedures, rupture would be expected to involve small as well as large aneurysms and would by now be recognized as a common complication in debilitated or postoperative patients. As a practical matter, this does not appear to be the case.

INCIDENCE

According to a survey of the relatively stable population of Rochester, Minn., conducted from 1951 to 1980, the prevalence of abdominal aortic aneurysms apparently is increasing because of either enhanced longevity or improved methods for diagnosis.[10] In this study, Bickerstaff et al.[10] estimated that new aneurysms were approximately four times more common from 1971 to 1980 than they were 20 years earlier, with a consistent ratio between men and women of approximately 4:1. Nearly 65% of these aneurysms were detected during routine physical examinations or on incidental radiographs of the abdomen, and only 13% were ruptured. Taylor and Porter[11] found in their comprehensive review that the specific incidence of aortic aneurysms correlated to a considerable extent with related risk factors and the diligence with which they were investigated. Although abdominal aneurysms have been discovered in only 1.5% of collected autopsy series, they have been found by ultrasound screening to occur in more than 3% of unselected adults, in 5% of patients with coronary disease, in nearly 10% of those patients with peripheral vascular lesions, and in as many as 53% of those patients initially seen with femoral or popliteal aneurysms.

Citing these and similar data, some reports have encouraged the use of routine screening for aortic aneurysms among patients who are especially likely to have them on the grounds that such an approach would prove to be cost effective as well as therapeutically sound. Pasch et al.[12] determined that the length and expense of hospital treatment for ruptured aneurysms were more than twice as high as elective resection and that 2,000 lives and $50 million might have been saved in the United States in 1979 if all ruptured aneurysms had instead been corrected by earlier, planned procedures. Depending on regional charges, Thurmond and Semler[13] calculated that 25 to 50 aortic ultrasound examinations could be performed for the excess cost incurred by a single emergency operation. Accordingly, they concluded that screening measures were justified for any cohort for whom the incidence of unsuspected aneurysms is expected to range from as little as 2 to 4%.

DIAGNOSTIC METHODS

Physical Examination

Although physical examination has been supplanted by more accurate means for measuring abdominal aneurysms, it is still the cornerstone for their initial diagnosis in many patients. The examination should be performed from the right side with the knees of the patient flexed to relax the abdominal muscles. Bimanual palpation is begun to the left of the midline between the xiphoid process and the umbilicus, with the superficial landmarks corresponding to the levels of the renal arteries and the aortic bifurcation, respectively. With one hand compressing the other, both are drawn toward the examiner, first to engage the aorta and then to sweep across its anterior wall. Unless the patient is very obese, the diameter of the normal aorta can usually be felt with this maneuver even if it is tortuous and relatively mobile against the spine. If an aneurysm is suspected, the examining hands must be separated to obtain an estimate of its transverse diameter. Provided the dome of the aneurysm does not extend to the xiphoid process or to the lower rib margin, it probably originates below the renal arteries since 95% of abdominal aneurysms do.[11] Assessment of its distal extent often is less reliable because the bifurcation vessels descend into the pelvis beyond the umbilicus, but large common iliac aneurysms may be palpable. Despite its value as a universal screening study, physical examination no longer provides optimal information about the size or proximal extent of abdominal aneurysms, and it is not sufficiently sensitive to distinguish them from other retroperitoneal masses such as lymphomas, horseshoe kidneys, or even the thickened small bowel mesentery in an overweight man. Therefore most aneurysms should be documented objectively before making any commitment for surgical treatment.

Plain X-ray Films

Since the size of an aortic aneurysm is one of the important criteria determining its management, diagnostic methods must provide a dependable measurement of its maximum diameter. Plain x-ray films represented the only available standard for measurement before the introduction of contemporary noninvasive imaging, and many calcified aneurysms still are discovered during contrast studies of the kidneys or the gastrointestinal tract. A lateral view of the lumbosacral area is necessary, however, to isolate the aorta from the vertebral column directly behind it (Fig. 47-1A). Unfortunately, plain x-ray films are associated with an element of magnification, and only 60 to 70% of aneurysms contain sufficient mural calcification to permit even an estimate of their size.[14,15] For these reasons, lateral roentgenograms have largely been superseded by ultrasonography or computerized scanning for the assessment of aortic aneurysms.

Ultrasonography

For more than 10 years, B-mode ultrasonography has been successfully used for the diagnosis and measurement of infrarenal aneurysms because of its safety, simplicity, moderate cost, and the accuracy of its results. It is particularly useful as a screening examination, even in obese patients, and unlike plain x-ray films or angiography, its reliability is not influenced by either mural calcification or thrombus. Ultrasound studies provide a permanent record of aortic dimensions in both the sagittal (Fig. 47-1B) and the transverse planes. Because of this feature, they are ideal for serial measurements in patients whose aneurysms are too small to warrant immediate resection or in others who are equivocal surgical candidates unless progressive enlargement occurs during observation.[16,17] The only liability of ultrasonography is the fact that it cannot be used originally to assess the suprarenal aorta or the iliac arteries because its images often are obscured by the overlying pancreas and the pelvic viscera.

In their classic articles published in 1966 and 1972, Szilagyi et al.[18,19] confirmed that spontaneous rupture was a frequent complication of aneurysms 6 cm or more in diameter but was a relatively uncommon event for those measuring less than 5 cm. Nevertheless, these traditional guidelines were established on the basis of physical examination and lateral plain x-ray films, both of which tend to overestimate actual aortic size. It is now known that ultrasound results are nearly identical to aneurysm measurements obtained during laparotomy and that these figures are approximately 1 cm smaller than the historic criteria described by Szilagyi and his associates. Accordingly, elective resection should be a serious consideration for aneurysms that are 4 cm in diameter as determined by ultrasonography, and it is firmly indicated for those exceeding 5 cm.[15] This principle also is supported by the work of Darling et al.[20] who discovered that rupture rarely occurred among aneurysms less than 4 cm in diameter in a large series of autopsies.

Computerized Scans

Computed tomographic (CT) scans are more expensive than ultrasonography and offer no real advantages in the investigation of the infrarenal aorta, but they clearly are superior for the diagnosis and measurement of suprarenal and thoracoabdominal aneurysms (Fig. 47-1C), as well as those involving the iliac arteries.[21] Both versatile and convenient, conventional CT scanning is widely available and permits transverse views of long segments of the thoracic and abdominal aorta despite a reasonably low dose of ionizing irradiation. Magnetic resonance imaging (MRI) represents the most recent advance in nonionizing, computer-assisted

interrogation, but unlike standard tomography, it may also be used to study the aorta in the sagittal plane (Fig. 47-1D).[22] Since the protons in flowing blood behave differently when magnetized than do those in static structures (e.g., the aortic wall or mural thrombus), MRI does not require the infusion of contrast medium that is necessary for standard CT imaging.

According to a few reports, CT scanning may add valuable information about symptomatic aneurysms associated with contained rupture (Fig. 47-2A) or proximal dissection.[23,24] In addition, it occasionally demonstrates unexpected features in asymptomatic patients such as periaortic inflammation, horseshoe kidney, or venous

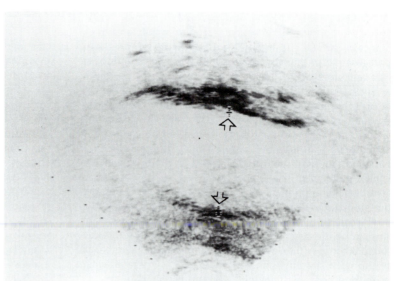

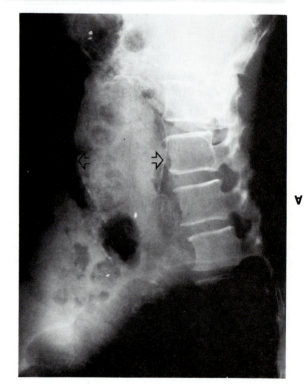

Figure 47-1. Radiographic methods for the diagnosis and measurement of abdominal aortic aneurysms (*arrows*). **A.** Plain roentgenography (with sufficient calcification). **B.** Infrarenal B-mode ultrasonography.

at the time of elective resection.

anomalies (Fig. 47-2B).[25] Surgical candidates with unexplained midscapular pain, preaortic masses on preliminary studies, or atypical features obviously require an intensive preoperative evaluation, but the role of routine imaging must remain in perspective. In the final analysis, most patients with symptomatic infrarenal aneurysms warrant an immediate operation, and *most* truly incidental CT findings would otherwise be recognized and managed appropriately

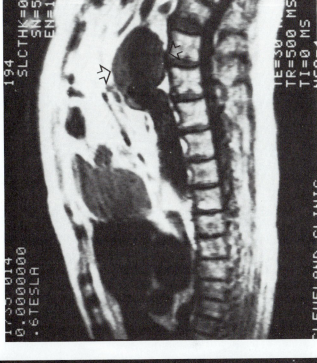

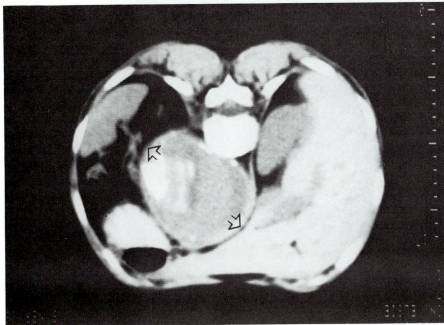

Figure 47-1, cont'd. C. Suprarenal computed tomography. **D.** Nuclear magnetic resonance.

Angiography

Angiography once was considered a prerequisite to the investigation of all abdominal aneurysms, but this approach has received only scattered support since the introduction of modern noninvasive imaging.[26] Although digital subtraction techniques may now be used to eliminate the finite risk for embolization and other complications of Seldinger catheterization, neither method is adequate for the measurement or sometimes even for the diagnosis of aortic aneurysms because of laminated thrombus (Fig. 47-3).[27-29] It is generally agreed that angiography should be reserved for selected patients who have specific indications for it such as suprarenal or multiple aneurysms, associated renal or mesenteric arterial disease, horseshoe kidney, or distal occlusive lesions that might require extension of a replacement graft to the groin or beyond. As is the case with CT scanning, angiography occasionally reveals unanticipated features (e.g., renal polar vessels, a patent inferior mesenteric artery, or small common iliac aneurysms), which might not have been suspected using ultrasonography alone. However, none of these findings is so difficult to identify or manage intraoperatively that it merits routine documentation with contrast studies.[30,31]

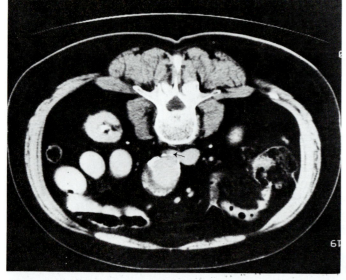
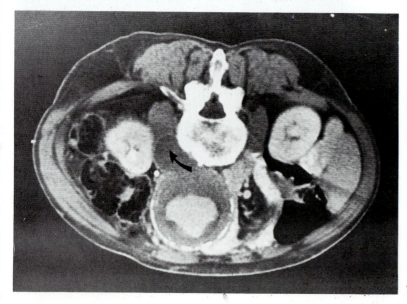

Figure 47-2. Unexpected findings on computed tomographic scans. **A.** Contained aneurysm rupture (arrow). **B.** Retroaortic left renal vein (arrow).

SURGICAL RISK

Ruptured Aneurysms

Abdominal aneurysms occasionally are a source for distal emboli,[32] but their quintessential danger is sudden, exsanguinating rupture. In perhaps the last series of aortic aneurysms for which surgery was not performed because they were collected before surgical treatment became feasible, Estes[33] determined in 1950 that only 19% of 102 patients survived 5 years and that rupture was responsible for 63% of all deaths for which specific causes were known. Two years later, DuBost et al[34] first corrected an infrarenal aneurysm with an arterial homograft, and although fabric materials have proved to be much more durable and convenient, no superior alternative to graft replacement has appeared in the 35 years following this signal report.[35,36] Furthermore, the lethal outcome of ruptured aneurysms has changed very little during that time. Using collected data, Taylor and Porter[11] recently calculated that 50% of patients who experience this catastrophe die before arriving at hospitals. Of those remaining, 24% die before operations can be performed, and another 42% have fatal postoperative complications. Thus the overall mortality for ruptured aneurysms remains nearly 80%.

Operative Mortality

Lawrie et al.[37] have described 61 consecutive patients with ruptured abdominal aortic aneurysms who underwent emergency operations with an early mortality rate of only 15%, a figure comparable to that following the repair of intact symptomatic aneurysms elsewhere.[11] Notwithstand-

ing this remarkable experience, comparable results at virtually every other level of surgical practice have been disappointing. As an example, Table 47-1 contains representative data concerning the operative mortality for ruptured aneurysm resection reported during the past decade from several academic and community centers in the United States and Europe.[38-51] Fatal complications occurred in 26 to 69% of these 905 patients, with a composite mortality rate of 47%. Since the discouraging outcome was relatively similar throughout these series, it may be preordained by factors common to such patients at every hospital.

In fact, several studies have already demonstrated that early mortality after ruptured aneurysm resection correlates directly with a number of independent variables such as patient age, hypovolemic shock or profound anemia on arrival at the hospital, preoperative azotemia, and either a history of previous myocardial infarctions or ischemic

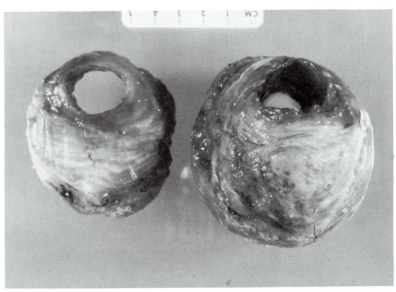

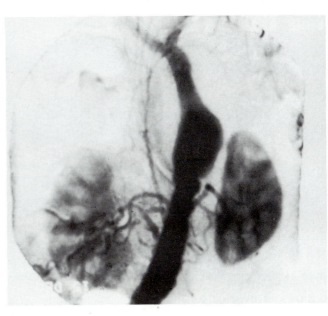

Figure 47-3. A. Intravenous digital subtraction angiogram of an infrarenal aortic aneurysm. **B.** Mural thrombus precluding accurate angiographic measurement.

Asymptomatic Aneurysms

The size of an infrarenal aneurysm at the time of its discovery is the most obvious and immediate criterion with respect to surgical treatment. During a follow-up interval extending as long as 13 years, Szilagyi et al.[18] reported eventual rupture in 20% of unoperated aneurysms ≤6 cm in diameter, compared to 43% of those exceeding 6 cm. Pooled data gathered by Taylor and Porter[11] have since suggested that the annual incidence of rupture is approximately 4% for 5 cm aneurysms, 7% for those approaching 6 cm, and 19% for those 7 cm in diameter. In addition to aneurysm size, Cronenwett et al.[53] also found that both diastolic hypertension and obstructive pulmonary disease were significant covariants predicting subsequent rupture and implied that elective resection of even small aneurysms should be considered in their presence.

Operative Mortality

Representative results for elective resection of infrarenal aortic aneurysms are summarized in Table 47-2. The cited information from the Cleveland Clinic was gathered from 1973 to 1978, but the rest of these data generally have been abstracted to include just those operations performed within the past 10 years if the series from which they were selected encompassed longer study periods. Using routine Swan-Ganz catheterization of the pulmonary artery to monitor volume replacement and pharmacologic manipulation of cardiac performance, Whitemore et al.[54] encountered only a single related death (0.9%) after 110 consecutive procedures. Although a few other respected centers also have had exemplary success, it appears that the acceptable risk for graft replacement of asymptomatic aneurysms currently is in the range of 6% or less. At least in reported patients, the early mortality rates in some community hospitals seem comparable to those in academic units in both the United States and Europe.[58,60] Unfortunately, the results in many areas are unpublished or never have been documented at all.

electrocardiographic changes during resuscitation.[40,42,43] Other important factors related to mortality (i.e., free peritoneal rupture, iatrogenic venous injury), the length of the surgical procedure, and the volume of intraoperative transfusions), however, may in part be influenced by the ability of the surgeon to control the aneurysm safely and to repair it expeditiously.[40,42,52] Furthermore, decisive action by the referring physician is yet another critical element in the management of symptomatic or ruptured aneurysms. In a large series of 152 patients treated in northeastern Ohio, the operative mortality rate more than doubled (from 35 to 75%) when intervention was delayed by an average of more than 2 days because the initial diagnosis was incorrect. It is abundantly clear that the risks of a ruptured aneurysm are multifactorial and that the only way to completely control them is to recognize and resect the aneurysm before this catastrophe can occur.

TABLE 47-1. REPRESENTATIVE OPERATIVE MORTALITY RATES FOR URGENT RESECTION OF RUPTURED INFRARENAL AORTIC ANEURYSMS DURING THE PAST DECADE

Series	Year	No.	Age (Mean)	Mortality (%)
Academic Medical Centers				
Gaylis and Kessler[38]	1980	105	70	58
McCabe et al.[39]	1981	73	73	52
Wakefield et al.[40]	1982	116	69	52
Cleveland Clinic[41]	1983	34	NA*	26
Donaldson et al.[42]	1985	81	70	43
Community Hospitals				
Cleveland Vascular Registry[43]	1982	152	69	38
Botsford et al.[44]	1983	13	66	69
Lawler[45]	1984	43	70	39
Wilcox[46]	1985	16	NA	56
Abernathy[47]	1986	57	NA	47
International Results				
Hepp et al.[48] (West Germany)	1981	44	NA	52
Postier et al.[49] (Ireland)	1982	82	NA	56
Ruberti et al.[50] (Italy)	1985	77	NA	48
Serrano Hernando et al.[51] (Spain)	1985	71	23	43
Total		916		47

* NA, data not available.

TABLE 47-2. REPRESENTATIVE OPERATIVE MORTALITY RATES FOR ELECTIVE RESECTION OF ASYMPTOMATIC INFRARENAL AORTIC ANEURYSMS DURING THE PAST DECADE

Series	Year	No.	Age (Mean)	Mortality (%)
Academic Medical Centers				
Whittemore et al.[54]	1980	110	68	0.9
Brown et al.[55]	1981	422	71	2.4
Crawford et al.[56]	1981	273	NA*	2.6
McCabe et al.[39]	1981	364	66	2.5
Cleveland Clinic[41]	1983	350	NA	5.1
Yeager et al.[57]	1986	97	NA	4.1
Community Hospitals				
Bottsford et al.[44]	1983	53	68	5.6
Cleveland Vascular Registry[58]	1984	840	NA	6.5
Wilcox[46]	1985	86	NA	5.8
International Results				
Hepp et al.[48] (West Germany)	1981	41	NA	0
Postier et al.[49] (Ireland)	1982	142	NA	5.1
Reddy et al.[59] (South Africa)	1985	160	67	4.4
Ruberti et al.[50] (Italy)	1985	216	NA	4.6
Serrano Hernando et al.[51] (Spain)	1985	89	61	6.7
Total		3,243		4.4

* NA, data not available.

Aged Patients

Despite the conventional wisdom that most aneurysms more than 4 cm in diameter on ultrasound examination should be resected, there always has been an understandable reluctance to recommend elective treatment to asymptomatic patients 75 to 80 years of age or older. A number of studies addressing this issue have concluded that chronologic age is an arbitrary consideration that does not necessarily reflect the patient's physiologic status, that the operative risk in many older individuals is equivalent to that of other elective patients during the same era, and that the aged are least able to withstand emergency procedures if rupture should occur during expectant care.[61–64] Furthermore, late survival after successful resection in older patients also has been shown to be comparable to that of a general population of the same age.[61,63] Although such observations are valid, none of these series was prospectively randomized. Accordingly, it is reasonable to assume that their patients represented the most acceptable surgical candidates. Only Esselstyn et al.[61] described the course of similar patients who were denied elective resection within the same study period, and although 67% of them died during a maximum follow-up interval of nearly 10 years, 63% of these deaths were unrelated to aneurysm rupture.

Surgical indications that are unnecessarily restrictive probably are applied to elderly patients with aortic aneurysms by many referring physicians and surgeons who have little personal experience with aortic reconstruction in this or any other age group. Previous myocardial infarction, angina pectoris, hypertension, renal or pulmonary dysfunction, and a host of other problems anticipated with advancing age should be interpreted as a reason to investigate their specific severity in detail, rather than as an absolute contraindication to a planned operation irrespective of aneurysm size. In many cases, objective studies will determine that graft replacement can be safely performed with reasonable precautions. Nevertheless, Plecha et al.[65] calculated that the early mortality rate of elective aneurysm resection among those from 75 to 90 years of age (11%) was twice that (5.6%) of younger patients in northeastern Ohio, and others have demonstrated that certain critical risk factors are prohibitive.[66,67] Bernstein et al.[16,17] found under some circumstances that reassessment with serial ultrasound scans to detect progressive aneurysm enlargement is a rational alternative to immediate intervention, but they also emphasize that resection may become unavoidable if expansion does occur.

LATE SURVIVAL

Despite standardizing both cohorts for age, cardiac status, blood pressure, and renal function, Szilagyi et al.[16] established that the 5-year survival rate was substantially better among patients with asymptomatic aneurysms who underwent resection (53%) than in those who did not (19%).

TABLE 47-3. REPRESENTATIVE 5-YEAR CUMULATIVE SURVIVAL RATES AFTER RESECTION OF INFRARENAL AORTIC ANEURYSMS

Series	Year	No.	Age (Mean)	Cumulative 5-Year Survival (%)
DeBakey et al.[69]	1964	1,432	NA*	58†
Szilagyi et al.[18]	1966	434	NA	49†
Cleveland Clinic[70]	1980	286	66	68
Courbier et al.[71]	1980	100	67	64†
Whittemore et al.[54]	1980	110	68	84†
Crawford et al.[56]	1981	816	65	63
Fielding et al.[72]	1981	296	67	65
Kövecker et al.[73]	1981	91	67	55†
Soreide et al.[74]	1982	200	62	71†
Hollier et al.[75]	1984	1,087	68	67
Ruberti et al.[50]	1985	413	65	49
Total		5,265		61

* NA, Data not available.
† Includes operative mortality.

Even discounting operative mortality, however, 5-year survival for all surgical patients still was approximately 20% (actuarial) below that expected for the normal population. Considering longevity from yet another perspective, Burnham et al.[68] compared the median life expectancy after aneurysm resection in North Carolina to the comparable figure anticipated for other persons of similar ages in the same state. They found that surgical patients lived from 5 to 11 fewer years than the control groups and that survival was equivalent only between those more than the age of 75. As shown in Table 47-3, most long-term studies using life-table data have confirmed the fact that aortic aneurysms are not the only features adversely influencing survival in the patients who have them.

Associated Coronary Disease

According to a recent review of the literature summarized in Table 47-4, associated coronary disease is suggested by traditional criteria in nearly 50% of patients with abdominal aortic aneurysms and is responsible for about half of all perioperative and late deaths.[76] Brown et al.[55] reported an early mortality of only 3% among patients suspected to have coronary involvement, whereas others have found that operative risk is 10% or more in this group even at referral centers.[41,57,73,77] Goldman et al.[67] defined a number of factors, including age above 70 years, congestive heart failure, atrial or ventricular arrhythmias, and recent myocardial infarction, which collectively appear to predict cardiac complications after aortic and other major operations. Applying this index to a series of 167 aneurysm resections, Reddy et al.[59] encountered five fatal myocardial infarctions (45%) in a small subset of 11 patients in whom they were most likely to occur. Several large surveys have proved that the safety of vascular and other noncardiac surgical procedures in candidates who have had previous coronary bypass is comparable to that among patients with no evidence of ischemic heart disease at all.[41,78–80] Other investigations have demonstrated that aortic replacement can be

TABLE 47-4. COLLECTED DATA CONCERNING ASSOCIATED CORONARY DISEASE IN PATIENTS WITH ABDOMINAL AORTIC ANEURYSMS[76]

Coronary Data	Eligible Patients	Range (%)	Mean (%)
Associated coronary disease			
Clinically suspected	4,263	31-70	47
Angiographically serious	375	—	59
Operative mortality	4,013	0.9-10	4.6
No coronary disease	368	0-1.6	1.1
Suspected disease	376	3.5-8.9	5.1
Prior coronary bypass	224	0-1.8	0.4
5-Year mortality	3,755	16-40	32
No coronary disease	629	16-28	22
Suspected disease	637	34-55	44
Prior coronary bypass	119	25-34	28

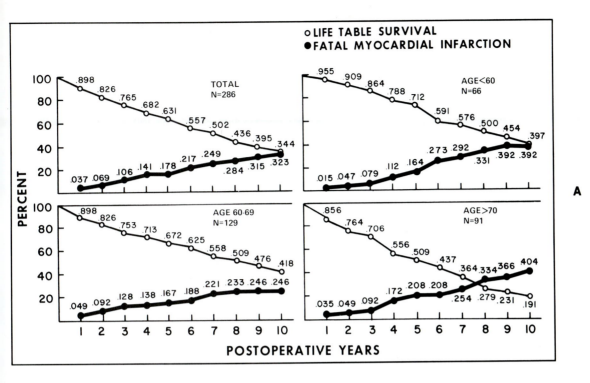

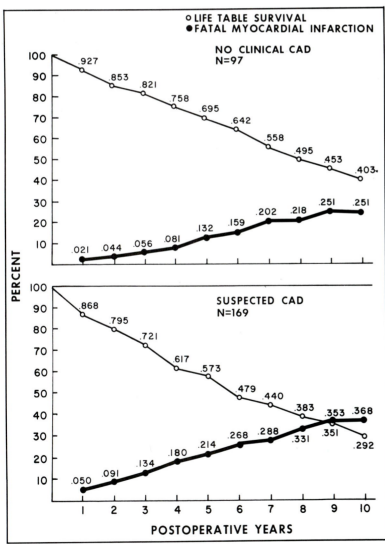

Figure 47-4. Cumulative 10-year survival rate and the incidence of fatal myocardial infarction after successful aortic aneurysm resection in 286 patients at the Cleveland Clinic. **A.** Age at operation. **B.** Associated coronary artery disease (CAD).

performed with acceptable results provided myocardial performance is closely monitored and appropriately maintained.[54,55,57,81–83] Although Kalman et al.[84] reported that pulmonary wedge pressure measurements were not always adequate for this purpose, a conservative approach would have obvious advantages in comparison to coronary bypass if operative risk were the only consideration.

As indicated in Table 47-4, however, late survival also is limited in patients with associated coronary disease, and it cannot realistically be improved by temporary precautions taken only at the time of aortic reconstruction. Like DeBakey et al.[69] almost 20 years earlier, Crawford et al.[55] and Hollier et al.[75] have reaffirmed that the presence of atherosclerotic heart disease substantially reduces actuarial 5 year survival after successful aneurysm resection. Late results after operations at the Cleveland Clinic are illustrated in Figure 47-4 and have been revised to a minimum follow-up interval of 10 years subsequent to their original publication in 1980.[70] Longevity generally could be correlated with age in all 286 operative survivors (Fig. 47-4A), but the cumulative incidence of fatal myocardial infarction was relatively constant in all groups. Incidental coronary disease thus appears to be relatively more ominous when it is a precocious finding in younger patients with aneurysms, a feature that also was noted by Reigel et al.[85] and is consistent with the demographic observations of Burnham et al.[68] in North Carolina. Excluding 20 patients who eventually received myocardial revascularization, both late survival and the cardiac mortality rate were significantly worse ($P \leq 0.05$) in the cohort recognized to have coronary involvement (Fig. 47-4B).

The Cleveland Clinic Experience

Tomatis et al.[86] and Blombery et al.[77] have also used cardiac catheterization during the evaluation of patients with aortic aneurysms, but probably the largest prospective investigation of this kind was conducted at the Cleveland Clinic from 1978 to 1982.[87–89] Coronary angiography was performed in a series of 1,000 patients under consideration for elective peripheral vascular procedures, and in an attempt to enhance operative risk as well as late survival, those patients with severe, surgically correctable coronary artery disease (CAD) were advised to undergo myocardial revascularization. The study group included a total of 263 entrants who were initially seen with abdominal aneurysms, 246 of which were confined to the infrarenal aorta. Table 47-5 contains a summary of the angiographic classification

of associated coronary disease in all 263 patients according to the clinical terms defined in the original report of this work. Severe CAD, usually representing ≥70% stenosis in multiple vessels, was identified in 50% of the patients who had traditional indications of coronary involvement, compared to 20% of those who did not. Moreover, coronary bypass was feasible in 42% and 19% of these two subsets, respectively.

Seventy (28%) of the 246 patients who had infrarenal aneurysms received myocardial revascularization, with four early deaths (5.7%), a figure that is similar to the mortality rate of 5.2% among 1,086 patients 65 years of age or older in the multicentered Coronary Artery Surgery Study (CASS).[90] Of the 66 remaining patients in this subset, 56 eventually underwent aneurysm resection, with a single fatal stroke (1.8%). In comparison, there were nine deaths (4.4%) in a total of 204 patients for whom aortic reconstruction was performed, including two (2.6%) of the 78 with normal coronary arteries or only mild to moderate CAD. Five-year survival and the cumulative cardiac mortality are illustrated for each angiographic classification in Figure 47-5.[91] Ten deaths directly related to aneurysm resection or ligation were omitted from these data, but the risk associated with coronary bypass itself was not. Late survival in the bypass subset (75%) was similar to patients who had only trivial CAD (79%), was superior ($P = 0.0001$) to those with severe, uncorrected CAD (29%), and was consistent with the 5-year survival (71%) reported for older patients with peripheral vascular disease in the CASS survey.[92]

Noninvasive Cardiac Assessment

Several current methods for noninvasive cardiac assessment provide objective information that can be used to select patients for coronary angiography and other precautions at the time of aortic replacement. Although standard stress testing often is not feasible in aged patients or in those with intermittent claudication, even modest treadmill exercise may provoke ischemic electrocardiographic changes in the presence of serious coronary involvement.[93,94] Pasternack et al.[95] employed gated pool angiocardiography in 50 patients scheduled for elective aneurysm resection and found that perioperative myocardial infarctions occurred in 20% of the group with ejection fractions of 36 to 55%, as well as in 80% of those patients who had even worse ventricular function. Two studies by Boucher et al[96,97] and another by Cutler and Leppo[98] have demonstrated that the

TABLE 47-5. INCIDENCE OF ASSOCIATED CORONARY DISEASE DOCUMENTED BY ANGIOGRAPHY IN 263 PATIENTS WITH ABDOMINAL AORTIC ANEURYSMS AT THE CLEVELAND CLINIC[87]

Angiographic Classification	Clinical Coronary Disease					
	None		Suspected		Total	
	No.	%	No.	%	No.	%
Normal coronary arteries	11	9	5	4	16	6
Mild to moderate CAD*	60	47	17	12	77	29
Advanced but compensated CAD	31	24	46	34	77	29
Severe CAD						
Correctable	24	19	57	42	81	31
Inoperable	1	1	11	8	12	5

* CAD, Coronary artery disease

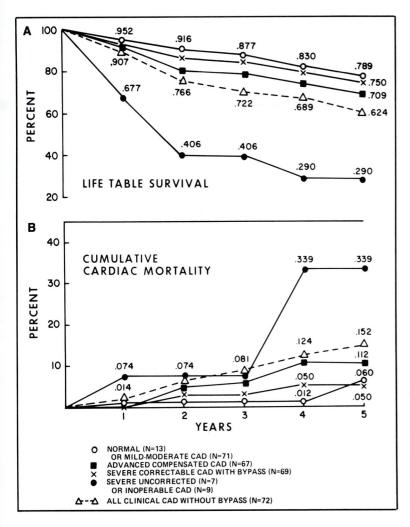

Figure 47-5. Cumulative 5-year survival, **A**, and cardiac mortality, **B**, according to the angiographic classification of associated coronary artery disease (CAD) in 246 patients evaluated because of infrarenal aortic aneurysms at the Cleveland Clinic.

results of dipyridamole-thallium myocardial imaging correlated directly with the risk for cardiac complications after vascular surgical procedures. In a collected series of more than 400 patients with peripheral vascular disease who had some type of preoperative screening, the incidence of postoperative cardiac events was only 6% when noninvasive assessment was normal in comparison to 33% when it was not.[76] Although long-term data are not available, this trend also has obvious implications concerning late survival and cardiac mortality.

A number of algorithms have been suggested for the management of associated coronary disease in patients with aortic aneurysms or other peripheral vascular lesions.[99,100] Noninvasive cardiac assessment is essential to each of them, and the only equivocal issues seem to be whether it should be used to survey all surgical candidates (including those who are asymptomatic) and whether coronary angiography should empirically be considered for patients with convincing clinical indications of myocardial ischemia. At the very least, objective screening should be performed for patients who are suspected of having coronary disease by conventional criteria, and angiographic documentation could then be obtained in those who have positive noninvasive tests.

TECHNICAL CONSIDERATIONS

Elective Resection

Preliminary Dissection

Although an infrarenal aneurysm may be exposed through a transverse "chevron" approach above the umbilicus with division of both rectus muscles, a vertical incision from the xiphoid process to the pubis is usually preferred because it facilitates access to the distal iliac segments and, if necessary, to the suprarenal aorta near the diaphragmatic crus. The retroperitoneum is incised in the avascular fibroareolar plane slightly to the right of the midline to reflect the duodenum, the mesentery of the small intestine, and the ureter from the aorta and the common iliac artery on that side. This dissection should not be performed anterior to the aorta to avoid the thick sigmoid mesocolon, branch vessels of the inferior mesenteric system, and the pelvic nerves responsible for sexual function in men, which should remain undisturbed in their course across the left common iliac artery.

If the common iliac arteries are unremarkable, they may subsequently be occluded by atraumatic vascular clamps with a minimum of manipulation. When they contain additional aneurysms or posterior wall calcification that could be disrupted by vertical compression, circumferential control at the origins of the external iliac and hypogastric arteries may be advisable. In many patients, these two vessels are more suitable for clamping than the common iliac artery itself, particularly when the common iliac vein is densely adherent to it. If an iliac vein is injured during the dissection, minor tears usually respond to a single fine suture or to tamponade by the overlying artery once tension has been released. Larger lacerations, however, are only made worse by further retraction, and some venous injuries are corrected most expeditiously by clamping the common iliac artery, with the patient receiving regional heparin, and transecting and elevating it to permit direct repair of the bleeding site.

Irrespective of the size of the aneurysm, virtually all of the infrarenal aorta should be replaced to preclude further dilatation that might require a difficult repeat surgery in the future. The left renal vein crosses anteriorly at the level that proximal control traditionally is obtained, but if it cannot be identified in this area, it must be assumed to occupy an anomalous position behind the aorta (Fig. 47-2B) where it could be torn posterior to the neck of the aneurysm.[101] Even in its usual location, the left renal vein often interferes with the exposure of a juxtarenal aneurysm. In this situation, the vein either may be mobilized by dividing its adrenal and gonadal branches, or, provided these tributaries are preserved for collateral venous outflow, it may be divided near its junction with the inferior vena cava.[102,103] Although ligation apparently is safe in most patients, it should be used judiciously because venous stasis and functional loss in the left kidney have been reported as a complication.[104,105]

Graft Replacement

Once a fabric bifurcation graft of appropriate diameter has been preclotted and systemic heparin has been administered, the iliac vessels are clamped before the proximal aorta to prevent distal embolization during direct manipulation near the neck of the aneurysm. The aneurysm then is opened along its right anterolateral margin to avoid the pelvic nerves to the left of the midline, and all mural thrombus is evacuated to identify the lumbar arteries along its posterior wall. Several studies have demonstrated that bacterial organisms (70% of which are Gram positive) may be cultured from the aneurysm contents in 10 to 15% of patients, but possibly because prophylactic antibiotics are always used, this finding rarely has serious consequences.[106–108] Calcified plaque is stripped from the lumbar ostia before they are secured with nonabsorbable sutures. If there is vigorous collateral bleeding from the inferior mesenteric artery, it also may be ligated within the aneurysm sac. If retrograde bleeding is unimpressive, however, this vessel should be preserved until another assessment of its functional importance can be made after the hypogastric circulation has been restored.

As illustrated by the schematic examples in Figure 47-6, the proximal anastomosis generally is oriented with the suture line parallel to the plane of the occluding clamp. Provided there is a sufficient length of infrarenal aorta above the aneurysm, it may be transected beyond a horizontal

clamp to facilitate circumferential exposure (Fig. 47-6A). In the presence of a large aneurysm or a short neck, access below even a vertical clamp is so confined that the posterior wall should be left intact and the anastomosis performed using the interpolation method (Fig. 47-6B) introduced by Creech[109] in 1966. According to the experience clearly described by Crawford et al.,[110] juxtarenal aneurysms extending to the level of the renal arteries may not be suspected preoperatively unless a lateral aortogram is available. They obviously require suprarenal clamping, either at the crus of the diaphragm or near the origin of the superior mesenteric artery above the left renal vein, to construct an anastomosis incorporating normal aorta whenever they occur (Fig. 47-6C). A continuous 3-0 polypropylene suture probably is used at most centers, and if necessary it can be reinforced with a strip of Teflon felt to save the time required for the placement of interrupted mattress sutures tied over individual pledgets.[111]

As shown in Figure 47-7, several alternatives are available for the distal reconstruction. If both iliofemoral segments are normal or nearly so, a tube graft terminating at the aortic bifurcation (Fig. 47-7A) is both safe and durable in selected candidates.[112] Nevertheless, many patients already have associated common iliac aneurysms or such generalized arteriomegaly that they could reasonably be expected to develop these aneurysms in the future.[113–115] For this reason, it often is appropriate to perform the anastomosis of each graft limb near the origins of the external iliac and hypogastric arteries (Fig. 47-7B), especially in patients who are relatively young when their aortic aneurysms are discovered. Distal control of large iliac aneurysms that fill the presacral pelvis may be difficult to obtain without excessive retraction and the risk for iatrogenic embolization. Under these circumstances, either the sigmoid colon or the cecum can be reflected medially to isolate the external iliac and hypogastric arteries beyond the aneurysm for clamping and subsequent revascularization (Fig. 47-7C). Prograde flow should always be restored first to the hypogastric artery as yet another precaution to prevent lower-extremity emboli. It is comparatively unusual for advanced external iliac occlusive disease to occur in conjunction with aortic aneurysms, but when it does, the graft may be extended to the level of the common femoral artery below the inguinal ligament (Fig. 47-7D).

Before heparin anticoagulation is reversed with protamine sulfate, each femoral pulse is palpated to confirm that the distal graft anastomosis is widely patent. If the pulse is absent or fails to meet expectations, a transverse incision should be made in the graft limb to assess the lumen near the suture line and to introduce an embolectomy catheter beyond it. Once an obstructing intimal flap or thrombus has been corrected, the graft is repaired, and flow usually may be restored to the leg without exploring the ipsilateral groin. If inspection or Doppler auscultation indicates that the foot is ischemic despite the presence of a normal femoral pulse, however, the groin must be opened to pass smaller balloon catheters into the superficial femoral and profunda femoris arteries. Operative angiography is indicated if this approach does not improve the situation, and complementary lumbar sympathectomy also must be considered if "trash foot" caused by emboli in the plantar

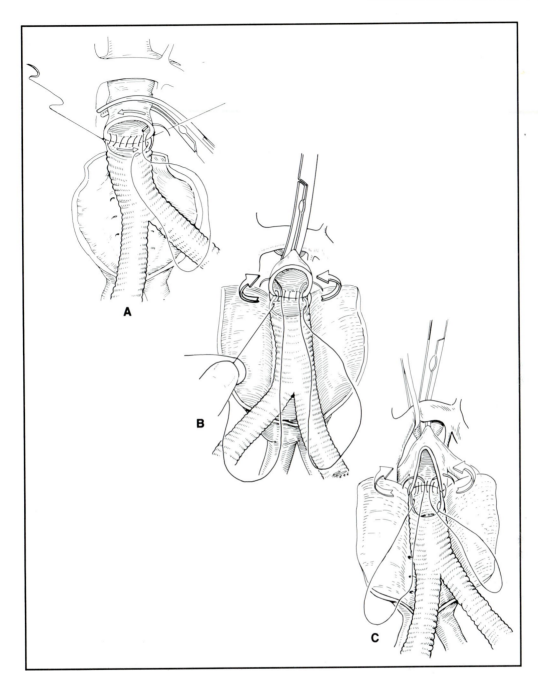

Figure 47-6. Proximal graft anastomosis during aortic aneurysm resection. **A.** Aorta transected (*horizontal clamp*). **B.** Posterior wall intact (*vertical clamp*). **C.** Juxtarenal aneurysm.

arch is suspected. Using several precautions to prevent stasis thrombosis and iatrogenic embolization of mural clot or atheromatous debris, Imparato[116] encountered severe lower-extremity ischemia in only 0.6% of a series of 700 aortic aneurysm resections.

Although Ernst et al.[117,118] discovered postoperative signs of mucosal ischemia through colonoscopy in nearly 7% of patients after the resection of intact aneurysms, Schroeder et al.[119] reported that transmural intestinal injury was limited to 0.5% of 3,092 patients who required aortic

replacement in Denmark from 1975 to 1981. Serious ischemia involving the descending colon and rectum is unlikely to occur if flow is restored to at least one of the hypogastric arteries, but innovative measures sometimes are necessary to accomplish this objective in the presence of saccular common iliac aneurysms (Fig. 47-8A). Revascularization of a patent inferior mesenteric artery should be performed if the sigmoid colon remains ischemic after hypogastric reconstruction or if there is objective evidence of inadequate collateral circulation in the mesocolon.[118] In either case,

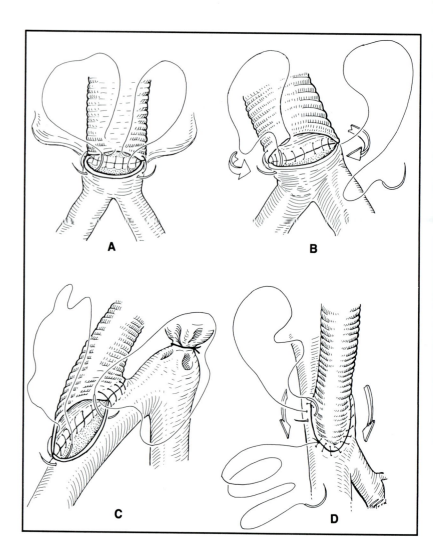

Figure 47-7. Distal graft anastomosis during aortic aneurysm resection. **A.** Tube replacement. **B.** Common iliac reconstruction. **C.** External iliac extension. **D.** Aortofemoral bypass.

this vessel should be reimplanted into the aortic graft from within the aneurysm sac or with the use of a Carrel patch (Fig. 47-8B).

Retroperitoneal Closure

Humphries et al.[120] concluded 25 years ago that an infrarenal prosthetic graft must be separated from the duodenum and other viscera by secure closure of the retroperitoneum to reduce the late risk for an aortoenteric fistula. The unresected aneurysm sac should be coapted snugly over the new graft, imbricating one leaf over the other if the sac is relatively large in comparison to the graft itself. Small aneurysms and those located near the aortic bifurcation often are inadequate for coverage of the proximal anastomosis, the most common site for subsequent fistulas because the duodenum is a retroperitoneal organ at the same level. Under these circumstances, a flap of the sac may be rotated to protect the anastomosis before routinely approximating the remainder of the aneurysm (Fig. 47-9).[121] Lymphoareolar tissue may be used as additional protection for the proximal aorta, and the posterior parietal peritoneum is closed over the distal graft. Finally, a pedicle of viable omentum can instead be mobilized and delivered through an avascular rent in the transverse mesocolon to seal the retroperitoneal

defect.[122] This approach is especially useful when additional renal or mesenteric grafts have been performed in conjunction with aortic replacement and might be compromised by closure of the aneurysm sac.

Ruptured Aneurysms

The cardinal principles of ruptured aneurysm resection include urgent transfer to the operating room without unnecessary studies once the diagnosis seems unequivocal, maintenance of muscular tamponade until the last possible moment before laparotomy is begun, and expeditious control of the proximal aorta to permit further resuscitation. The patient is prepared and draped while still awake, and the abdomen is entered through a long midline incision after rapid intubation and the induction of anesthesia. The supraceliac aorta may be clamped by employing the method described by Veith et al.,[123] but simple manual compression against the spine at the level of the diaphragmatic crus ordinarily is sufficient to reverse hypotension and preclude additional blood loss while the duodenum is reflected from the neck of the aneurysm and a straight clamp is applied to the infrarenal aorta. Several techniques for proximal con-

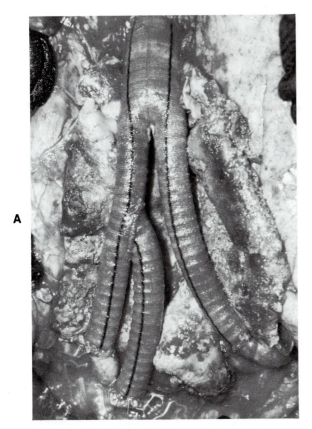

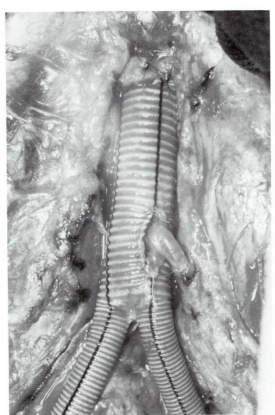

Figure 47-8. Preservation of sigmoid colon perfusion during abdominal aortic reconstruction. **A.** Revascularization of at least one hypogastric artery. **B.** Carrel implantation of the inferior mesenteric artery.

trol using large balloon catheters inserted either percutaneously or intraoperatively also have been described.[124–126] Each may be advantageous under specific circumstances, but they all share a common liability. They take *time*, and wasted time often leads to fatal complications.

Unless they contain aneurysms themselves, the iliac arteries should be clamped with a minimum of dissection to prevent retrograde bleeding, as well as venous or ureteral injuries that can occur when the pelvis is obscured by a large retroperitoneal hematoma. A small amount of heparin (3,000 IU) may be administered regionally or intravenously before aortic clamping to protect the legs from stasis thrombosis, but some surgeons may prefer to omit anticoagulation entirely in patients with ruptured aneurysms. The aneurysm should be replaced with a tightly woven Dacron graft terminating at the aortic bifurcation whenever possible. Once distal flow has been restored, heparin is reversed completely with protamine sulfate, but transfusions of fresh frozen plasma and platelets also may be required to obtain adequate hemostasis.

Aortic Fistulas

Spontaneous aortovenous fistulas represent an unusual example of contained aneurysm rupture. They usually involve the inferior vena cava, but there have been scattered reports of fistulas into retroaortic left renal veins and the common iliac veins as well.[127–133] Although typical features were present in only three of the six patients described by Baker

et al.,[128] classic findings include an abdominal thrill and a continuous bruit, tachycardia, anasarca or lower-extremity edema, and depressed renal function with oliguria and hematuria. The early mortality rate associated with urgent surgical treatment appears to be 20% or more, probably because extensive blood and fluid replacement often is poorly tolerated in the presence of hyperdynamic congestive heart failure. Intraoperative pulmonary embolization may be caused by loose mural thrombus unless compression with sponge sticks or some other method is used to interrupt flow in the vena cava while the aneurysm is opened and evacuated. Once under control, the fistulae should be closed from within the aneurysm before a conventional graft is constructed.

Primary aortoenteric fistulas are so rare as to be anecdotal.[134] They usually are initially seen with herald gastrointestinal bleeding before exsanguinating hemorrhage, and although angiography performed during one of these episodes may be diagnostic (Fig. 47–10), endoscopic studies clearly are preferable during periods of quiescence. Unlike secondary fistulas related to previous aortic grafts, there is reasonable evidence that infection is not the principal etiologic factor causing primary duodenal fistulas and that proximal aortic ligation and extra-anatomic bypass are not mandatory in their treatment.[135] In this respect, Pfeiffer[134] collected a total of 21 patients who were managed successfully with direct aortic grafting and lateral repair of the duodenum.

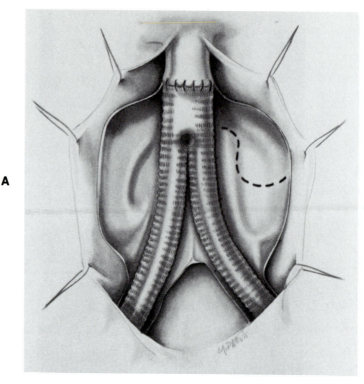

A

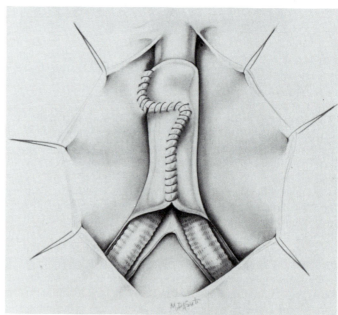

B

Figure 47-9. Tailoring the aneurysm sac to cover the proximal graft anastomosis. **A.** Design of the rotated cuff. **B.** Completed closure.

Related Complications

Either renal failure or the rare catastrophe of spinal cord ischemia can occur in conjunction with elective aortic operations, but both are much more commonly encountered after a prolonged period of hypotension following aneurysm rupture.[136–145] McCombs and Roberts[137] found that the incidence of acute renal failure was 10 times higher in patients who had ruptured aneurysms (21%) than in those who did not (2.5%), with a related mortality rate of approximately 50% in each group. Although maintenance hemodialysis has greatly enhanced the management of postoperative fluid overload, the composite mortality of oliguric renal failure still is discouraging because it often represents only one of many simultaneous complications in older patients with multiple risk factors. Bartlett et al.[140] recently reported early survival in only 31% of such patients despite continuous arteriovenous ultrafiltration and exemplary nutritional support. Although the circumstances leading to renal failure frequently are beyond control in patients who sustain sudden aneurysm rupture, thorough preoperative hydration and intraoperative volume replacement are essential to prevent parenchymal injury in elective surgical candidates.

Spinal cord ischemia occurred after only 0.25% of 3,164 infrarenal aortic procedures performed by Szilagyi et al.[144]

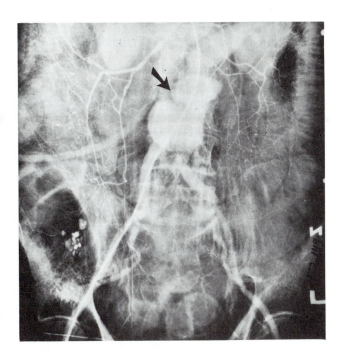

Figure 47-10. Angiographic confirmation of a primary aortoenteric fistula, with extravasated contrast medium in the duodenum (*arrow*) during a late aortogram phase.

and, like renal failure, was 10 times more common in patients with ruptured aneurysms. According to several case reports, the severity of the neurologic injuries comprising this syndrome range from regional motor or sensory deficits in the lower extremities (with occasional spontaneous recovery) to permanent paraplegia and the loss of bowel and bladder control.[141–143] All are presumed to be complications of hypotension among a few patients in whom the artery of Adamkiewicz (arteria magna radicularis), providing segmental circulation to the anterior spinal artery, takes its origin from the abdominal aorta at an unusually low level. Connolly[145] has suggested that selective angiograms should be obtained in an effort to identify the arterial supply to the spinal cord so that revascularization could at least be attempted during elective operations. Others seem to agree, however, that the exceedingly low incidence of spinal complications does not justify the intrinsic risk of this uncertain approach and that cord ischemia remains an unpredictable and essentially unpreventable event in isolated patients.[142,144]

SPECIAL PROBLEMS

Inflammatory Aneurysms

Approximately 5% of infrarenal aortic aneurysms are associated with dense, invasive fibrosis throughout the retroperitoneal space, which commonly incorporates the duodenum, the ureters, the inferior vena cava, and other major veins (Fig. 47-11). Goldstone et al.[146] were among the first to describe the idiopathic inflammation in the thickened aneurysm wall, the glistening sheets of desmoplastic tissue surrounding it, and the risk for duodenal and venous injuries unless these structures are avoided during resection and graft replacement. Several studies have since confirmed that inflammatory aneurysms usually are quite large and often are symptomatic by the time they are discovered.[147–149] These lesions may be suspected on the basis of preoperative weight loss, an elevated erythrocyte sedi-

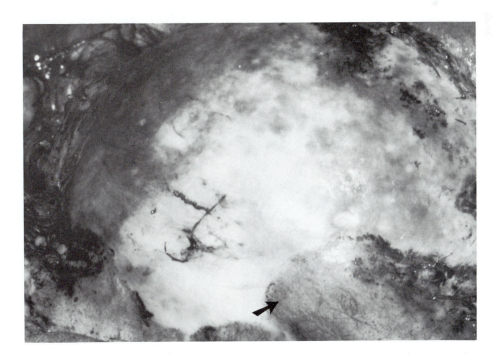

Figure 47-11. An inflammatory (or "white") aneurysm of the infrarenal aorta with fibrous incorporation of the adjacent duodenum (*arrow*).

mentation rate, the typical periaortic capsule demonstrated by computed tomography, or medial deviation of entrapped ureters rather than the lateral displacement that otherwise would be expected with a conventional aneurysm.

The fibrous response frequently does not extend above the left renal vein or beyond the origins of the external iliac and hypogastric arteries, but Crawford et al.[147] still found it necessary to obtain supraceliac control to construct the proximal aortic anastomosis without disturbing the duodenum in about half of the patients they reported. Ureterolysis, however, was rarely required in their extensive experience because the obstructive signs of retroperitoneal inflammation tended to subside after these aneurysms were repaired. Although Savarese et al.[149] concluded that the impressive size of many inflammatory aneurysms suggests that they are less likely to rupture than standard atherosclerotic aneurysms, rupture through the relatively thin posterior wall is known to occur.[146–148] Therefore elective resection is indicated to prevent this complication, as well as to correct the gastrointestinal and urinary symptoms that may precede it.

Complementary Procedures

Since chronic intestinal ischemia is comparatively unusual, renal artery revascularization is the most common additional vascular procedure performed in conjunction with aortic aneurysm resection.[150] Provided the kidney is large enough to warrant salvage rather than nephrectomy, complementary bypass is clearly necessary in hypertensive patients who have renal artery stenosis associated with elevated ipsilateral renin activity on selective assay. Revascularization also seems appropriate to preserve renal mass among those patients having advanced, bilateral arterial lesions as well as deteriorating kidney function, conceding that azotemia in the presence of only unilateral renal artery stenosis probably is related to superimposed parenchymal disease as well.[151] Finally, some patients who are asymptomatic or have hypertension that is adequately controlled by medical means are considered candidates for simultaneous renal grafting at the time of aneurysm resection simply because incidental renal artery stenosis has been documented by preoperative angiography. It is in this group that the merit of complementary bypass is open to speculation. Although Stewart et al.[152] and Brewster et al.[153] reported fatal complications in just 3 to 5% of their series, other data suggest that the early mortality rate of synchronous renal revascularization often is twice that of aortic replacement alone.[150,151] Considering its added risk, therefore, strictly prophylactic renal artery bypass should only be performed at most centers in patients with indisputable high-grade stenosis.

The left renal artery arises from the posterolateral wall

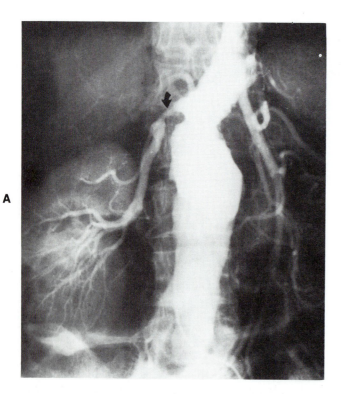
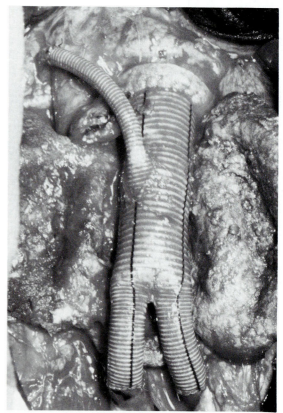

Figure 47-12. Simultaneous renal revascularization during aortic aneurysm resection. **A.** Preoperative angiogram demonstrating severe stenosis of the right renal artery (*arrow*) supplying a solitary kidney. **B.** Surgical reconstruction.

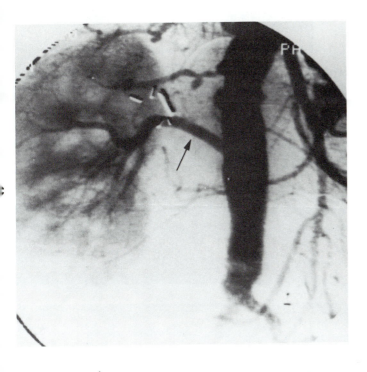

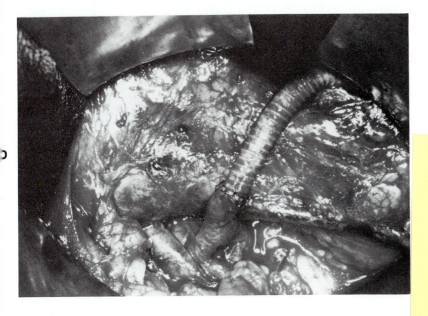

of the aorta and may be exposed by dividing the gonadal and adrenal veins to mobilize the left renal vein. The right renal artery can be isolated anteriorly before it passes behind the inferior vena cava in some slender patients (Fig. 47-12), but this approach may not provide sufficient length for the application of a distal clamp and a spatulated end-to-end anastomosis between the renal artery and a branch graft that was attached to the aortic prosthesis before aneurysm resection. Accordingly, it often is convenient to reflect the duodenum and ascending colon medially to expose a long segment of renal artery near the hilum of the kidney as a preliminary step in the operation. The graft may then be drawn into this area to complete the renal artery bypass

after the a[...]
to the ver[...]
47-12D). P[...]
arteries, t[...]
their revas[...]

Cholecystectomy

Asymptomatic cholelithiasis is by far the most common nonvascular abdominal finding in patients who require aortic reconstruction, occurring at a rate reported to range from 5 to 20%.[150,154,155] Although open intestinal operations at the time of aneurysm resection generally have been condemned because of their perceived risk for graft infections,

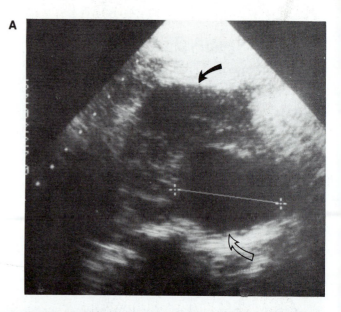

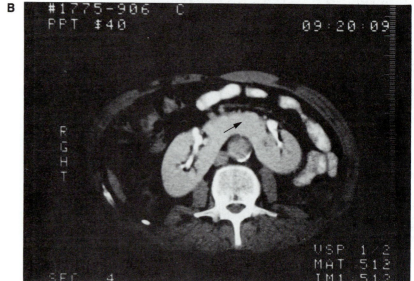

Figure 47-13. Radiographic features of an incidental horseshoe kidney. **A.** Retroperitoneal mass (*dark arrow*) anterior to the aortic aneurysm (*open arrow*) on ultrasonography. **B.** Computerized tomogram at the level of the isthmus (*arrow*).

Ouriel et al.[154] and String[155] have recommended complementary cholecystectomy in appropriate candidates to prevent subsequent complications. In these two studies, 3 of the 28 (11%) patients with gallstones who only underwent aortic replacement developed postoperative cholecystitis, with one related death (4%). Simultaneous cholecystectomy was performed in 34 others, but one early graft infection (3%) was documented in this group. Citing the incidence of contaminated bile (33%) and the fact that iatrogenic graft infections may not be recognized for months or even years, Fry and Fry[156] reserve simultaneous aortic replacement and cholecystectomy for the few patients for whom urgent aneurysm resection is necessary in the presence of symptomatic biliary disease.

Horseshoe Kidney

Since the incidence of horseshoe kidney is only 1:1000 within the general population, it is an exceedingly unusual consideration in random patients with aortic aneurysms.[157] Resection and graft replacement are complicated by several features of this rare anomaly, including fusion of the lower poles of the kidneys anterior to the distal aorta, medial effacement of the collecting systems and ureters, and most importantly, atypical renal arteries that may arise from either the aorta or its bifurcation vessels. A number of reviews[157–160] have established that there are four principal types of vascular anatomy associated with horseshoe kidneys: normal renal arteries to each lobe; normal renal arteries with an accessory iliac branch to the isthmus; duplicate main renal arteries on one or both sides with two additional branches to the isthmus; and, multiple vessels originating throughout the terminal aorta. Connelly et al.[160] estimated that 60% of reported patients had anomalous arterial circulation for which at least segmental renal revascularization may be necessary during aneurysm resection. Therefore preoperative angiograms should be obtained whenever a horseshoe kidney is suspected on the basis of other diagnostic studies performed to evaluate the aneurysm (Fig. 47-13).

When a transabdominal incision is used, the neck of

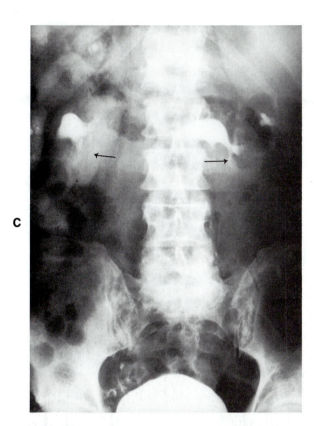

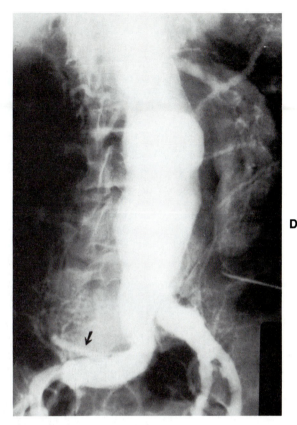

Figure 47-13, cont'd. C. Effacement (arrows) of the renal pelvices demonstrated by intravenous pyelography. **D.** Angiogram demonstrating an accessory renal artery (arrow) near the aortic bifurcation.

the aneurysm can be isolated safely above the isthmus of the kidney, provided the effaced renal pelvis on each side is protected from injury. The aortic bifurcation and the proximal common iliac arteries usually can be identified by retracting the isthmus or, if it is merely a fibrous band, by dividing it to facilitate exposure.[158,160] Whenever the isthmus is thickened and appears to contain functioning parenchyma, it should be preserved by directing the aortic graft through the aneurysm sac behind it. A patch of native aorta containing any anomalous main renal arteries always should be reimplanted into the prosthesis, and every reasonable attempt should be made to salvage branch vessels near the bifurcation as well. Nevertheless, Cohn et al.[157] demonstrated almost 20 years ago that minor ischemia of the isthmus could be tolerated and presumably replaced by scar tissue. Most recently, Morin and Johnston[161] used a retroperitoneal thoracoabdominal approach through the left flank to enter the aneurysm posteriorly, an innovation that may simplify the management of multiple renal arteries in some patients with horseshoe kidneys in the future.

Surgical Alternatives

Extraperitoneal exposure of aortic aneurysm through a left-flank incision extended into either the bed of the eleventh rib or the tenth intercostal space also has been advocated as an alternative to conventional resection in patients with severe cardiac or pulmonary disease because it appears to

be associated with less blood loss, fluid replacement, and interference with respiration.[162-164] For obvious reasons, a posterolateral approach may also be useful in selected candidates with specific technical indications such as morbid obesity, multiple previous laparotomies, intestinal or urinary stomas, and recognized juxtarenal or inflammatory aneurysms. The left kidney may be reflected anteriorly to obtain suprarenal control of the aorta, but this procedure usually is unnecessary when infrarenal grafting is performed (Fig. 47-14A). Distal exposure of the right common iliac artery and its bifurcation is comparatively restricted, but provided the hips of the patient have not been excessively rotated, these vessels may be isolated through a separate extraperitoneal incision in the lower abdomen on the contralateral side.[163] Using this approach in a total of 77 complicated patients, Shepard et al.[163] and Sicard et al.[164] reported only one operative death (1.3%).

Extraanatomic bypass in conjunction with induced thrombosis of the infrarenal aorta initially was proposed as a compromise procedure that appeared feasible for patients who otherwise were considered prohibitive risks for the surgical treatment of large aneurysms.[165-167] After construction of an axillobifemoral graft, the aneurysm was occluded by one of several methods: ligation of the aorta below the renal arteries through a short, upper-abdominal incision; ligation of the common iliac arteries using a bilateral extraperitoneal approach; or ligation of the iliofemoral segments in the groins with subsequent transcatheter embolization of biologic glue or other thrombogenic materials to

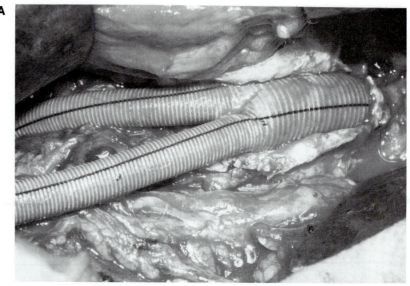

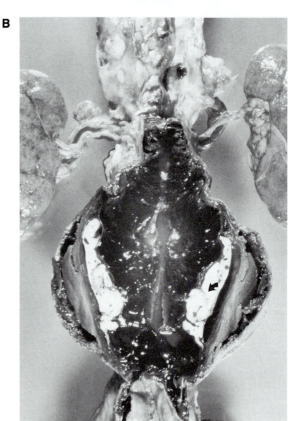

Figure 47-14. Proposed alternatives to conventional transabdominal resection of infrarenal aortic aneurysms in high-risk patients. **A.** Left retroperitoneal approach for direct reconstruction. **B.** Therapeutic embolization with biologic glue (*arrow*) in conjunction with axillobifemoral bypass.

obliterate all outflow vessels from the aneurysm (Fig. 47-14B). Despite its conceptual advantages, however, nonresective treatment has largely been abandoned for several reasons. First, its operative mortality rate was far from negligible (10 to 30%) among the patients in whom it seemed to be appropriate.[167–169] Inahara et al.[168] and Hollier et al.[170] eventually demonstrated that the early risk of direct aortic reconstruction could be limited to a figure approaching 5% even among "poor-risk" groups when extensive precautions were followed. Finally, Lynch et al.[171] collected 206

patients who received nonresective treatment and found that rupture still occurred in 20% of those patients in whom the aneurysm neck had not been formally ligated through an abdominal incision.

Isolated Iliac Aneurysms

The vast majority of atherosclerotic common iliac aneurysms occur in continuity with larger, more obvious aneurysms of the abdominal aorta. According to McCready et al.,[172] the relative incidence of isolated iliac aneurysms in comparison to aortic aneurysms is only 0.9% at the Mayo Clinic and does not exceed 2% in other published series. Because they are confined to the pelvis and may be difficult to feel during physical examination, iliac aneurysms often are either quite large or symptomatic before they are discovered. Only 36% of the 44 iliac aneurysms collected from the literature by Lowry and Kraft[173] were palpable, but 60% of them subsequently ruptured with a relative mortality rate of 52%. Since isolated hypogastric aneurysms are even less likely to be suspected during routine examination, 57% of those described by Brin and Busuttil[174] already had ruptured (26%) or had caused symptoms referable to local compression of the urinary tract, the lumbosacral nerves, or the pelvic veins. For whatever reason, the external iliac arteries almost never contain aneurysms, a feature that has surgical importance because it implies that there virtually always is an uninvolved outflow target for replacement grafting above the inguinal ligament even in patients who have multiseg-mental aneurysms in the abdomen, as well as in the lower extremities.

Unilateral resection and graft replacement of common iliac aneurysms through either a transabdominal or flank incision has been reported.[172,173] Considering their frequent association with infrarenal aortic aneurysms and the fact that many iliac aneurysms are bilateral, however, it seems reasonable to reconstruct most of them with a standard bifurcation prosthesis (Fig. 47-15) to prevent the development of additional aneurysms in the aortoiliac segment in the future. Hypogastric aneurysms may represent an exception to this approach because they are especially uncommon and their treatment rarely involves any type of revascularization. Irrespective of whether they occur in conjunction with other abdominal aneurysms or as isolated lesions, large hypogastric aneurysms generally are corrected by proximal ligation and endoaneurysmorrhaphy with ligation of all outflow vessels to eliminate further compression of adjacent structures in the pelvis.[174–176]

A

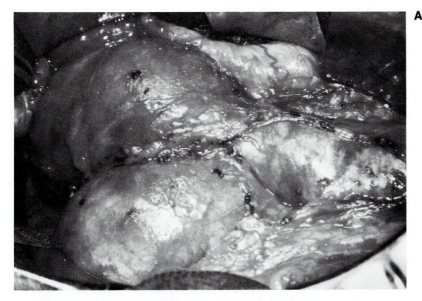

B

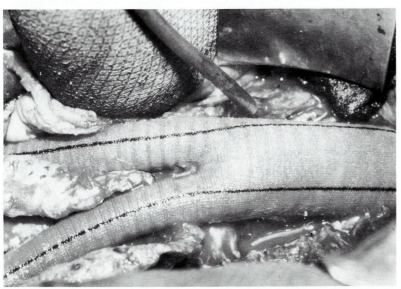

Figure 47-15. Bilateral common iliac aneurysms, **A,** excluded with an aortobifemoral Dacron graft, **B.**

ACKNOWLEDGEMENT

Mr. Robert Reed provided the surgical illustrations.

REFERENCES

1. Bergan JJ: A personal view of abdominal aortic aneurysms. Br J Surg 71:297, 1984.
2. Busuttil RW, Abou-Zamzam AM, Machleder HI: Collagenase activity of the human aorta. Arch Surg 115:1373, 1987.
3. Cohen JR, Mandell C, et al.: Altered aortic protease and anti-protease activity in patients with ruptured abdominal aortic aneurysms. Surg Gynecol Obstet 164:355, 1987.
4. Tilson MD. Further studies of a putative cross-linking amino acid (3-deoxypyridinoline) in skin from patients with abdominal aortic aneurysms. Surgery 98:888, 1985.
5. Tilson MD, Seashore MR: Human genetics of the abdominal aortic aneurysm. Surg Gynecol Obstet 158:129, 1984.
6. Norrgard Ö, Rais O, Ångquist KA: Familial occurrence of abdominal aortic aneurysms. Surgery 95:650, 1983.
7. Zarins CK, Runyon-Hass A, et al.: Increased collagenase activity in early aneurysmal dilatation. J Vasc Surg 3:238, 1986.
8. Swanson RJ, Littooy FN, et al.: Laparotomy as a precipitating factor in the rupture of intra-abdominal aneurysms. Arch Surg 115:299, 1980.
9. Cohen JR, Perry MO, et al.: Aortic collagenase activity as affected by laparotomy, cecal resection, aortic mobilization, and aortotomy in rats. J Vasc Surg 1:562, 1984.
10. Bickerstaff LK, Hollier LH, et al.: Abdominal aortic aneurysms: The changing natural history. J Vasc Surg 1:6, 1984.
11. Taylor LM, Porter JM: Basic data related to clinical decision-making in abdominal aortic aneurysms. Ann Vasc Surg 1:500, 1986.
12. Pasch AR, Ricotta JJ, et al.: Abdominal aortic aneurysm: The case for elective resection. Circulation 70:1, 1984.
13. Thurmond AS, Semler HJ: Abdominal aortic aneurysm: Incidence in a population at risk. J Cardiovasc Surg 27:457, 1986.
14. Brewster DC, Darling RC, et al.: Assessment of abdominal aortic aneurysm size. Circulation 56:164, 1977.
15. Hertzer NR, Beven EG: Ultrasound aortic measurement and elective aneurysmectomy. JAMA 240:1966, 1978.
16. Bernstein EF, Dilley RB, et al.: Growth rates of small abdominal aortic aneurysms. Surgery 80:765, 1976.
17. Bernstein EF, Chan EL: Abdominal aortic aneurysm in high-risk patients. Outcome of selective management based on size and expansion rate. Ann Surg 200:255, 1984.
18. Szilagyi DE, Smith RF, et al.: Contribution of abdominal aortic aneurysmectomy to prolongation of life. Ann Surg 164:678, 1966.
19. Szilagyi DE, Elliott JP, Smith RF: Clinical fate of the patient with asymptomatic abdominal aortic aneurysm and unfit for surgical treatment. Arch Surg 104:600, 1972.
20. Darling RC, Messina CR, et al.: Autopsy study of unoperated abdominal aortic aneurysms. The case for early resection. Circulation 56:161, 1977.
21. Gomes MN, Hufnagel CA: CT scanning: A new method for the diagnosis of abdominal aortic aneurysms. Cardiovasc Surg 20:511, 1979.
22. Dinsmore RE, Liberthson RR, et al.: Magnetic resonance imaging of thoracic aortic aneurysms: Comparison with other imaging methods. AJR 146:309, 1986.
23. Johnson WC, Gale ME, et al.: The role of computed tomography in symptomatic aortic aneurysms. Surg Gynecol Obstet 162:49, 1986.
24. Jones CS, Reilly MK, et al.: Chronic contained rupture of abdominal aortic aneurysms. Arch Surg 121:542, 1986.
25. Williams LR, Flinn WR, et al.: Extended use of computed tomography in the management of complex aortic problems: A learning experience. J Vasc Surg 4:264, 1986.
26. Baur GM, Porter JM, et al.: The role of arteriography in abdominal aortic aneurysm. AM J Surg 136:184, 1978.
27. Wheeler WE, Beachleyb MC, Ranniger K: Angiography and ultrasonography. A comparative study of abdominal aortic aneurysms. AJR 126:95, 1976.
28. Williamson C, Ameli FM, et al.: The role of intravenous digital subtraction angiography as an adjunct to a computed tomography in the preoperative assessment of patients with abdominal aortic aneurysm. J Vasc Surg 6:26, 1987.
29. Turnipseed WD, Acher CW, et al.: Digital subtraction angiography and B-mode ultrasonography for abdominal and peripheral aneurysms. Surgery 92:619, 1982.
30. Bell DD, Gaspar MR: Routine aortography before abdominal aortic aneurysmectomy. A prospective study. AM J Surg 144:191, 1982.
31. Couch NP, O'Mahoney J, et al.: The place of abdominal aortography in abdominal aortic aneurysm resection. Arch Surg 118:1029, 1983.
32. Lord JW Jr, Rossi G, et al.: Unsuspected abdominal aortic aneurysms as the cause of peripheral arterial occlusive disease. Ann Surg 177:767, 1973.
33. Estes EJ Jr: Abdominal aortic aneurysm: A study of 102 cases. Circulation 2:258, 1950.
34. DuBost EC, Allary M, Oeconomos N: Resection of an aneurysm of the abdominal aorta. Re-establishment of the continuity by a preserved human arterial graft with result after 5 months. Arch Surg 64:405, 1952.
35. Dhillon JS, Randhawa GK, et al.: Late rupture after Dacron wrapping of aortic aneurysm. Circulation 74:11, 1986.
36. Kwaan JHM, Dahl RK: Fatal rupture after successful surgical thrombosis of an abdominal aortic aneurysm. Surgery 95:235, 1984.
37. Lawrie GM, Morris GC Jr, et al.: Improved results of operation for ruptured abdominal aortic aneurysms. Surgery 85:483, 1979.
38. Gaylis H, Kessler E: Ruptured aortic aneurysms. Surgery 87:300, 1980.
39. McCabe CJ, Coleman WS, Brewster DC: The advantage of early operation for abdominal aortic aneurysm. Arch Surg 116:1025, 1981.
40. Wakefield TW, Whitehouse WM Jr, et al.: Abdominal aortic aneurysm rupture: Statistical analysis of factors affecting outcome of surgical treatment. Surgery 91:586, 1982.
41. Diehl JT, Cali RF, et al.: Complications of abdominal aortic reconstruction. An analysis of perioperative risk factors in 557 patients. Ann Surg 197:49, 1983.
42. Donaldson MC, Rosenberg JM, Bucknam CA: Factors affecting survival after ruptured abdominal aortic aneurysm. J Vasc Surg 2:564, 1985.
43. Hoffman M, Avellone JC, et al.: Operation for ruptured abdominal aortic aneurysms: A community-wide experience. Surgery 91:597, 1982.
44. Bottsford JE Jr, Bearden RC Jr, Bottsford JG: A 10 year community hospital experience with abdominal aortic aneurysms. J SC Med Assoc 79:57, 1983.
45. Lawler M Jr: Aggressive treatment of ruptured abdominal aortic aneurysm in a community hospital. Surgery 95:37, 1984.
46. Wilcox DD: Abdominal aortic aneurysm resection: A 10-year community hospital experience. Conn Med 49:428, 1985.
47. Abernathy CM Jr, Baumgartner R, et al.: The management of ruptured abdominal aortic aneurysms in rural Colorado. JAMA 256:597, 1986.
48. Hepp W, Vollmar JF, Krier S: Aneurysms of the infrarenal abdominal aorta: Principles and results of surgical treatment. Int Surg 66:203, 1981.

49. Postier R, Hyland J, et al.: The treatment of aortic aneurysms: The results in 436 consecutive patients. Ir Med J 75:279, 1982.

50. Ruberti U, Scorza R, et al.: Nineteen year experience on the treatment of aneurysms of the abdominal aorta: A survey of 832 consecutive cases. J Cardiovasc Surg 26:547, 1985.

51. Serrano Hernando FJ, Martin Paredero V, et al.: Abdominal aortic aneurysms. Results of surgical treatment. J Cardiovasc Surg 26:539, 1985.

52. Hiatt JCG, Barker WF, et al.: Determinants of failure in the treatment of ruptured abdominal aortic aneurysm. Arch Surg 119:1264, 1984.

53. Cronenwett JL, Murphy TF, et al.: Actuarial analysis of variables associated with rupture of small abdominal aortic aneurysms. Surgery 98:471, 1985.

54. Whittemore AD, Clowes AW, et al.: Aortic aneurysm repair. Reduced operative mortality associated with maintenance of optimal cardiac performance. Ann Surg 192:414, 1980.

55. Brown OW, Hollier LH, et al.: Abdominal aortic aneurysm and coronary artery disease. A reassessment. Arch Surg 116:1484, 1981.

56. Crawford ES, Saleh SA, et al.: Infrarenal abdominal aortic aneurysm. Factors influencing survival after operation performed over a 25-year period. Ann Surg 193:699, 1981.

57. Yeager RA, Weigel RM, et al.: Application of clinically valid cardiac risk factors to aortic aneurysm surgery. Arch Surg 121:278, 1986.

58. Hertzer NR, Avellone JC, et al.: The risk of vascular surgery in a metropolitan community. J Vasc Surg 1:13, 1984.

59. Reddy E, Robbs JV, Rubin J: Abdominal aortic aneurysm resection—operative risk and long-term results. S Afr Med J 67:921, 1985.

60. Lundell L, Norbäck: Abdominal aortic aneurysm—results of treatment in nonspecialized units. Acta Chir Scand 149:695, 1983.

61. Esselsytn Jr CB, Humphries AW, et al.: Aneurysmectomy in the aged? Surgery 67:34, 1970.

62. Baker WH, Munns JR: Aneurysmectomy in the aged. Arch Surg 110:513, 1975.

63. O'Donnell TF, Darling RC, Linton RR: Is 80 years too old for aneurysmectomy? Arch Surg 111:1250, 1976.

64. Harris KA, Ameli FM, et al.: Abdominal aortic aneurysm resection in patients more than 80 years old. Surg Gynecol Obstet 162:536, 1986.

65. Plecha FR, Bertin VJ, et al.: The early results of vascular surgery in patients 75 years of age and older: An analysis of 3,259 cases. J Vasc Surg 2:769, 1985.

66. Nel CJC, Snyman JH, Linde SP: Selective management of abdominal aortic aneurysms. S Afr J Surg 24:68, 1986.

67. Goldman L, Caldera DL, et al.: Multifactorial index of cardiac risk in noncardiac surgical procedures. N Eng J Med 297:845, 1977.

68. Burnham SJ, Johnson G Jr, Gurri JA: Mortality risks for survivors of vascular reconstructive procedures. Surgery 92:1071, 1982.

69. DeBakey ME, Crawford ES, et al.: Aneurysm of abdominal aorta. Analysis of results of graft replacement therapy 1 to 11 years after operation. Ann Surg 160:622, 1964.

70. Hertzer NR: Fatal myocardial infarction following abdominal aortic aneurysm resection. Three-hundred forty-three patients followed 6–11 years postoperatively. Ann Surg 192:667, 1980.

71. Courbier R, Jausseran JM, et al.: Long term survival after abdominal aortic aneurysmectomy. J Cardiovasc Surg 21:135, 1980.

72. Fielding JWL, Black J, et al.: Diagnosis and management of 528 abdominal aortic aneurysms. Br Med J 283:1, 1981.

73. Köveker G, deVivie ER, et al.: Early and long-term results after surgical treatment of abdominal aortic aneurysm. Thorac Cardiovasc Surg 29:394, 1981.

74. Soreide O, Lillestol J, et al.: Abdominal aortic aneurysms: Survival analysis of 434 patients. Surgery 91:188, 1982.

75. Hollier LH, Plate G, et al.: Late survival after abdominal aortic aneurysm repair: Influence of coronary artery disease. J Vasc Surg 1:290, 1984.

76. Hertzer NR: Basic data concerning associated coronary disease in peripheral vascular patients. Ann Vasc Surg 1:617, 1987.

77. Blombery PA, Ferguson IA, et al.: The role of coronary artery disease in complications of abdominal aortic aneurysm surgery. Surgery 101:150, 1987.

78. Crawford ES, Morris GC Jr, et al.: Operative risk in patients with previous coronary artery bypass. Ann Thorac Surg 26:215, 1978.

79. Reul GJ Jr, Cooley DA, et al.: The effect of coronary bypass on the outcome of peripheral vascular operations in 1,093 patients. J Vasc Surg 3:788, 1986.

80. Foster ED, Davis KB, et al.: Risk of noncardiac operation in patients with defined coronary disease: The coronary artery surgery study (CASS) registry experience. Ann Thorac Surg 41:42, 1986.

81. Roizen MF, Beupre PN, et al.: Monitoring with two-dimensional transesophageal echocardiography. Comparison of myocardial function in patients undergoing supraceliac, suprarenal-infraceliac, or infrarenal aortic occlusion. J Vasc Surg 1:300, 1984.

82. Gewertz BL, Kremser PC, et al.: Transesophageal echocardiographic monitoring of myocardial ischemia during vascular surgery. J Vasc Surg 5:607, 1987.

83. Ruby ST, Whittemore AD, et al.: Coronary artery disease in patients requiring abdominal aortic aneurysm repair. Ann Surg 201:758, 1985.

84. Kalman PG, Wellwood MR, et al.: Cardiac dysfunction during abdominal aortic operation: The limitations of pulmonary wedge pressures. J Vasc Surg 3:773, 1986.

85. Reigel MM, Hollier LH, et al.: Late survival in abdominal aortic aneurysm patients: The role of selective myocardial revascularization on the basis of clinical symptoms. J Vasc Surg 5:222, 1987.

86. Tomatis LA, Fierens EE, Verbrugge GP: Evaluation of surgical risk in peripheral vascular disease by coronary arteriography. A series of 100 cases. Surgery 71:429, 1972.

87. Hertzer NR, Beven EG, et al.: Coronary artery disease in peripheral vascular patients. A classification of 1,000 coronary angiograms and results of surgical management. Ann Surg 199:223, 1984.

88. Hertzer NR, Young JR, et al.: Late results of coronary bypass in patients with peripheral vascular disease, I. Five-year survival according to age and clinical cardiac status. Cleve Clin Q 53:133, 1986.

89. Hertzer NR, Young JR, et al.: Late results of coronary bypass in patients with peripheral vasscular disease, II. Five-year survival according to sex, hypertension, and diabetes. Cleve Clin J Med 54:15, 1987.

90. Gersh BJ, Kronmal RA, et al.: Coronary arteriography and coronary artery bypass surgery: Morbidity and mortality in patients age 65 years or older. A report from the coronary artery surgery study. Circulation 67:483, 1983.

91. Hertzer NR, Young JR, et al.: Late results of coronary bypass in patients with infrarenal aortic aneurysms. The Cleveland Clinic Study. Ann Surg 205:360, 1987.

92. Gersh BJ, Kronmal RA, et al.: Long-term (5 year) results of coronary bypass surgery in patients 65 years old or older: A report from the Coronary Artery Surgery Study. Circulation 68:190, 1983.

93. Arousa EJ, Baum PL, Cutler BS: The ischemic exercise test in patients with peripheral vascular disease. Implications for management. Arch Surg 119:780, 1984.

94. von Knorring J, Lepäntalo M: Prediction of perioperative car-

diac complications by electrocardiographic monitoring during treadmill exercise testing before peripheral vascular surgery. Surgery 99:610, 1986.

95. Pasternack PF, Imparato AM, et al.: The value of radionuclide angiography as a predictor of perioperative myocardial infarction in patients undergoing abdominal aortic aneurysm resection. J Vasc Surg 1:320, 1984.

96. Boucher CA, Brewster DC, et al.: Determination of cardiac risk by dipyridamole-thallium imaging before peripheral vascular surgery. N Engl J Med 312:389, 1985.

97. Eagle KA, Singer DE, et al.: Dipyridamole-thallium scanning in patients undergoing vascular surgery. JAMA 257:2185, 1987.

98. Cutler BS, Leppo JA: Dipyridamole thallium 201 scintigraphy to detect coronary artery disease before abdominal aortic surgery. J Vasc Surg 5.91, 1987.

99. Nicolaides AN, Salmasi AM, Sonecha TN: How should we investigate the arteriopath for coexisting lesions? J Cardiovasc Surg 27:515, 1986.

100. Hertzer NR: Clinical experience with preoperative coronary angiography. J Vasc Surg 2:510, 1985.

101. Giordano JM, Trout HH III: Anomalies of the inferior vena cava. J Vasc Surg 3:924, 1986.

102. James ED, Fedde CW, et al.: Division of the left renal vein: A safe surgical adjunct. Surgery 83:151, 1978.

103. Adar R, Rabbi I, et al.: Left renal vein division in abdominal aortic aneurysm operations. Arch Surg 120:1033, 1985.

104. Andersen JC, Sjolin SU, Holstein P: Ligation of the renal vein during resection of abdominal aortic aneurysm. J Cardiovasc Surg 27:454, 1986.

105. Lord RSA: Trial clamping before division of the left renal vein. Surgery 91:409, 1982.

106. Ernst CB, Campbell HC, et al.: Incidence and significance of intra-operative bacterial cultures during abdominal aortic aneurysmectomy. Ann Surg 185:626, 1977.

107. McAuley CE, Steed DL, Webster MW: Bacterial presence in aortic thrombus at elective aneurysm resection: Is it clinically significant? Am J Surg 147:320, 1984.

108. Schwartz JA, Powell TW, et al.: Culture of abdominal aortic aneurysm contents. An additional series. Arch Surg 122:777, 1987.

109. Creech O Jr: Endo-aneurysmorrhaphy and treatment of aortic aneurysm. Ann Surg 164:935, 1966.

110. Crawford ES, Beckett WC, Greer MS: Juxtarenal infrarenal abdominal aortic aneurysm. Special diagnostic and therapeutic considerations. Ann Surg 203:661, 1986.

111. Hertzer NR: Teflon reinforcement of an uninterrupted aortic anastomosis. Surg Gynecol Obstet 157:480, 1983.

112. Glickman MH, Julian CC, et al.: Aortic aneurysm: To tube or not to tube. Surgery 91:603, 1982.

113. Tilson MD, Dang C: Generalized arteriomegaly. A possible predisposition to the formation of abdominal aortic aneurysms. Arch Surg 116:1030, 1981.

114. Hollier LH, Stanson AW, et al.: Arteriomegaly: Classification and morbid implications of diffuse aneurysmal disease. Surgery 93:700, 1983.

115. Plate G, Hollier LA, et al.: Recurrent aneurysms and late vascular complications following repair of abdominal aortic aneurysms. Arch Surg 120:590, 1985.

116. Imparato AM: Abdominal aortic surgery: Prevention of lower limb ischemia. Surgery 93:111, 1983.

117. Hagihara PF, Ernst CB, Griffen WO: Incidence of ischemic colitis following abdominal aortic reconstruction. Surg Gynecol Obstet 149:571, 1979.

118. Ernst CB: Prevention of intestinal ischemia following abdominal aortic reconstruction. Surgery 93:101, 1983.

119. Schroeder T, Christoffersen JK, et al.: Ichemic colitis complicat-

ing reconstruction of the abdominal aorta. Surg Gynecol Obstet 160:299, 1985.

120. Humphries AW, Young JR, et al.: Complications of abdominal aortic surgery. Arch Surg 86:43, 1963.

121. Hertzer NR: A rotated aneurysm cuff for separation of aortic graft and duodenum. Surg Gynecol Obstet 147:84, 1978.

122. Bunt TJ, Doerhoff CR, Haynes JL: Retrocolic omental pedicle flap for routine plication of abdominal aortic grafts. Surg Gynecol Obstet 158:591, 1984.

123. Veith FJ, Gupta S, Daly V: Technique for occluding the supraceliac aorta through the abdomen. Surg Gynecol Obstet 151:427, 1980.

124. Sensenig DM: Rapid control in ruptured abdominal aneurysms. Arch Surg 116:1034, 1981.

125. Hyde GL, Sullivan DM: Fogarty catheter tamponade of ruptured abdominal aortic aneurysms. Surg Gynecol Obstet 154:197, 1982.

126. Berkowitz HD, Roberts B: New technique for control of ruptured abdominal aortic aneurysm. Surg Gynecol Obstet 133:107, 1971.

127. Hardy JD, Timmis HH: Abdominal aortic aneurysms: Special problems. Ann Surg 173:945, 1971.

128. Baker WH, Sharzer LA, Ehrenhaft JL: Aortocaval fistula as a complication of abdominal aortic aneurysms. Surgery 72:933, 1972.

129. Mohr LL, Smith LL: Arteriovenous fistula from rupture of abdominal aortic aneurysm. Arch Surg 110:806, 1975.

130. Dardik H, Dardik I, et al.: Intravenous rupture of arteriosclerotic aneurysms of the abdominal aorta. Surgery 80:647, 1976.

131. Suzuki M, Collins GM, et al.: Aorto–left renal vein fistula: An unusual complication of abdominal aortic aneurysm. Ann Surg 184:31, 1976.

132. Merrill WH, Ernst CB: Aorta–left renal vein fistula: Hemodynamic monitoring and timing of operation. Surgery 89:676, 1981.

133. Celoria GM, Friedmann P, et al.: Fistulas between the aorta and the left renal vein. J Vasc Surg 6:191, 1987.

134. Pfeiffer RB Jr: Successful repair of three primary aortoduodenal fistulae. Arch Surg 117:1098, 1982.

135. Daugherty M, Shearer GR, Ernst CB: Primary aortoduodenal fistula: Extra-anatomic vascular reconstruction not required for successful management. Surgery 86:399, 1979.

136. Chawla SK, Najafi H, et al.: Acute renal failure complicating ruptured abdominal aortic aneurysm. Arch Surg 110:521, 1975.

137. McCombs PR, Roberts B: Acute renal failure following resection of abdominal aortic aneurysm. Surg Gynecol Obstet 148:175, 1979.

138. Bush HL Jr: Renal failure following abdominal aortic reconstruction. Surgery 93:107, 1983.

139. Ostri P, Mouritsen L, et al.: Renal function following aneurysmectomy of the abdominal aorta. J Cardiovasc Surg 27:714, 1986.

140. Bartlett RH, Malt JR, et al.: Continuous arteriovenous hemofiltration: Improved survival in surgical acute renal failure? Surgery 100:400, 1986.

141. Golden GT, Sears HF, et al.: Paraplegia complicating resection of aneurysms of the infrarenal abdominal aorta. Surgery 73:91, 1973.

142. Ferguson LRJ, Bergan JJ, et al.: Spinal ischemia following abdominal aortic surgery. Ann Surg 181:267, 1975.

143. Grace RR, Mattox KL: Anterior spinal artery syndrome following abdominal aortic aneurysmectomy. Arch Surg 112:813, 1977.

144. Szilagyi DE, Hageman JH, et al.: Spinal cord damage in surgery of the abdominal aorta. Surgery 83:38, 1978.

145. Connolly JE: Prevention of paraplegia secondary to operations on the aorta. J Cardiovasc Surg 27:410, 1986.

146. Goldstone J, Malone JM, Moore WS: Inflammatory aneurysms of the abdominal aorta. Surgery 83:425, 1978.

147. Crawford JL, Stowe CL, et al.: Inflammatory aneurysms of the aorta. J Vasc Surg 2:113, 1985.

148. Pennell RC, Hollier LH, et al.: Inflammatory abdominal aortic aneurysms: A 30-year review. J Vasc Surg 2:859, 1985.

149. Savarese RP, Rosenfeld JC, DeLaurentis DA: Inflammatory abdominal aortic aneurysm. Surg Gynecol Obstet 162:405, 1986.

150. Bickerstaff LK, Hollier LH, et al.: Abdominal aortic aneurysm repair combined with a second surgical procedure—morbidity and mortality. Surgery 95:487, 1984.

151. Tarazi RY, Hertzer NR, et al.: Simultaneous aortic reconstruction and renal revascularization: Risk factors and late results in 89 patients. J Vasc Surg 5:707, 1987.

152. Stewart MT, Smith RB III, et al.: Concomitant renal revascularization in patients undergoing aortic surgery. J Vasc Surg 2:400, 1985.

153. Brewster DC, Buth J, et al.: Combined aortic and renal reconstruction. Am J Surg 131:457, 1976.

154. Ouriel K, Ricotta JJ, et al.: Management of cholelithiasis in patients with abdominal aortic aneurysm. Ann Surg 198:717, 1983.

155. String ST: Cholelithiasis and aortic reconstruction. J Vasc Surg 1:664, 1984.

156. Fry RE, Fry WJ: Cholelithiasis and aortic reconstruction: The problem of simultaneous surgical therapy. J Vasc Surg 4:345, 1986.

157. Cohn LH, Stoney RJ, Wylie EJ: Abdominal aortic aneurysm and horseshoe kidney. Ann Surg 170:870, 1969.

158. Bietz DS, Merendino KA: Abdominal aneurysm and horseshoe kidney: A review. Ann Surg 181:333, 1975.

159. Lobe TE, Martin EW Jr, et al.: Abdominal aortic surgery in the presence of a horseshoe kidney. Ann Surg 188:71, 1978.

160. Connelly TL, McKinnon W, et al.: Abdominal aortic surgery and horseshoe kidney. Report of six cases and a review. Arch Surg 115:1459, 1980.

161. Morin JF, Johnston KW: Thoracoabdominal retroperitoneal approach for repair of abdominal aortic aneurysm associated with horseshoe kidney. Ann Vasc Surg 2:82, 1988.

162. Williams GM, Ricotta J, et al.: The extended retroperitoneal approach for treatment of extensive atherosclerosis of the aorta and renal vessels. Surgery 88:846, 1980.

163. Shepard AD, Scott GR, et al.: Retroperitoneal approach to high-risk abdominal aortic aneurysms. Arch Surg 121:444, 1986.

164. Sicard GA, Freeman MB, et al.: Comparison between the transabdominal and retroperitoneal approach for reconstruction of the infrarenal abdominal aorta. J Vasc Surg 5:19, 1987.

165. Berguer R, Schneider J, Wilner HI: Induced thrombosis of inoperable abdominal aortic aneurysm. Surgery 83:425, 1978.

166. Leather RP, Shah D, et al.: Nonresective treatment of abdominal aortic aneurysms. Use of acute thrombosis and axillofemoral bypass. Arch Surg 114:1402, 1979.

167. Karmody AM, Leather RP, et al.: The current position of nonresective treatment for abdominal aortic aneurysm. Surgery 94:591, 1983.

168. Inahara T, Geary GL, et al.: The contrary position to the nonresective treatment for abdominal aortic aneurysm. J Vasc Surg 2:42, 1985.

169. Schwartz RA, Nichols WK, Silver D: Is thrombosis of the infrarenal abdominal aortic aneurysm an acceptable alternative? J Vasc Surg 3:448, 1986.

170. Hollier LH, Reigel MM, et al.: Conventional repair of abdominal aortic aneurysm in the high-risk patients: A plea for abandonment of nonresective treatment. J Vasc Surg 3:712, 1986.

171. Lynch K, Kohler T, Johansen K: Nonresective therapy for aortic aneurysm: Results of a survey. J Vasc Surg 4:469, 1986.

172. McCready RA, Pairolero PC, et al.: Isolated iliac artery aneurysms. Surgery 93:688, 1983.

173. Lowry SF, Kraft RO: Isolated aneurysms of the iliac artery. Arch Surg 113:1289, 1978.

174. Brin BJ, Busuttil RW: Isolated hypogastric artery aneurysms. Arch Surg 117:1329, 1982.

175. Kasaulke RJ, Clifford A, et al.: Isolated atherosclerotic aneurysms of the internal iliac arteries. Report of two cases and review of the literature. Arch Surg 117:73, 1982.

176. Perdue GD, Mittenthal MJ, et al.: Aneurysms of the internal iliac artery. Surgery 93:243, 1983.

CHAPTER 48

Management of Impotence Associated with Aortoiliac Surgery

Ralph G. DePalma

Impotence associated with aortoiliac occlusive disease was first recognized by Leriche,[1] who listed it as the initial symptom of the syndrome that bears his name. Impotence after aortoiliac surgery can be caused by failure to achieve adequate perfusion of the corpus cavernosum[2,3] or by disruption of genital autonomic nerves.[4-6] Modern techniques of aortoiliac reconstruction have evolved that minimize these problems.[7-10] These methods of aortoiliac revascularization are refinements offering preservation of sexual function in certain patients and the prospect of restoration of sexual function in others. The anatomy and physiology of male erectile function is a complex subject and has been recently reviewed.[11] This chapter discusses management of impotence associated with aortoiliac surgery.

APPROACH TO PATIENTS WITH AORTOILIAC DISEASE AND SEXUAL DYSFUNCTION

Vasculogenic impotence can be due to a variety of causes, which are listed in Table 48-1. Each factor, either singly or in combination, can contribute to erectile failure. Clearly, in middle-aged or elderly men afflicted with aortoiliac disease, complex interactions between vascular, neurogenic, hormonal, and psychogenic factors also contribute to erectile failure. Emsellem and I[12] have described a sequence to delineate the causes of erectile failure. This sequence initially uses noninvasive vascular tests of estimates of penile perfusion, including penile brachial indexes and pulse volume recording. Concomitantly, neurologic testing using pudendal evoked potentials and measurements of bulbocavernosus reflexes are also obtained. Subsequently, it is possible to observe pharmacologically produced erections using intracorporal papaverine injection.[13] These procedures give an objective estimate of the functional capacity of penile arterial supply and venous competency. In the absence of erection after intracorporal papaverine injection and after vascular laboratory findings indicating inadequate penile perfusion, angiography can be recommended. In spite of these comprehensive investigations, it is not always possible to assign a single cause to impotence in each individual, although in many instances objective evidence of dysfunction is obtained.

It is also not possible to predict with absolute certainty whether aortoiliac surgery will cause impotence or other sexual dysfunctions, nor to ascertain whether potency will be restored by operative or angioplastic interventions. For these reasons, objective measurements should be obtained when the patient voices sexual concerns preoperatively. Even when such concerns are not voiced, the surgeon should inquire about the patient's sexual activity and interest. If these appear important to the patient, the surgeon may wish to obtain preoperative vascular laboratory studies or neural testing. When sexual activity appears to be an overriding concern, sexual function may require additional preoperative documentation. A sleep laboratory study with nocturnal penile-tumescence and rigidity monitoring can also be recommended.[14] When nocturnal rigidity is marginal or poor, the patient can be further counseled preoperatively.

For reasons as yet unknown, the frequency of impotence increases with aging. The incidence of impotence in American males, according to Kinsey's 1948 data,[15] rises in an exponential fashion from 1% at age 45 to about 65% at age 80. It has been suggested that the development of arteriosclerotic occlusive disease associated with aging might play a role and that this phenomenon is vasculogenic in nature.[16] However, our laboratory studies have shown that many men beyond the seventh decade exhibit normal noninvasive studies, as well as normal testosterone levels, while complaining of impotence. More data are needed to understand this problem fully; it is probable that other undefined factors exist.

FUNCTIONAL NEUROVASCULAR EVALUATION

It is useful to detail the sequence of testing used for a neurovascular assessment of impotence because it provides an objective estimate of preoperative or postoperative dys-

TABLE 48-1. PROVISIONAL CLASSIFICATION OF VASCULOGENIC IMPOTENCE

Arterial
Large vessels: aorta and branches to division of internal iliac artery
Small vessels: proper pudendal artery and branches
Combined: embolization from aneurysm, ulcerated plaque, or postoperative

Cavernosal
Fibrosis: idiopathic or postpriapic
Peyronie's disease: deformity or venous leakage
Refractory states: diabetes, antihypertensive therapy, hormonal abnormalities

Venous
Congenital: cavernosus-spongiosus leak
Acquired: cavernosal leak syndrome (venous insufficiency)

functions in men with aortoiliac disease. When impotence is a chief complaint, noninvasive estimates of penile perfusion are obtained by measurements of the penile brachial blood pressure index (PBPI) and recording of pulse wave forms using penile plethysmography.[17] At the time of the initial examination, patients are questioned about risk factors for atherosclerosis that might contribute to arterial disease. Simultaneous noninvasive vascular examination of the lower extremities is also conveniently performed at this time. Penile perfusion pressures are obtained by means of a 10 kHz Doppler probe placed over the corpus cavernosum and angled 30 degrees proximally, maximizing signal detection. A penile cuff is inflated to above systolic pressure, and the returning signal is detected in the arteries proximal to the glans as the cuff is deflated. The pressure is noted, and penile-brachial blood pressure indexes are calculated for each side. During the same examination all peripheral pulses are palpated, and the ankle-to-brachial pressure indexes are recorded. Normal penile brachial pressures are usually 1.0, although function has been reported with ratios as low as 0.6.

The penile systolic pressure is obtained in our laboratory with a pneumographic plethysmographic cuff containing a transducer. This same cuff is then inflated to mean brachial arterial pressure (diastolic blood pressure plus one third of pulse pressure). Wave forms are recorded on a polygraph at a chart speed of 25 mm/sec. Wave-form amplitude greater than 6 to 30 mm and a systolic upstroke rate of 4 to 6 mm are considered normal. Marked flattening of the wave form, with delayed upstroke greater than 6 mm, and rounded wave forms or wave forms that vary from beat to beat are considered abnormal.

The pneumoplethysmographic recording of penile pulse volume offers the following advantages: The cuff measures the pulsation in all the arteries as it compresses spongy penile tissue, which tends to absorb ultrasonic signals. In contrast to pneumoplethysmographic recordings of the lower extremities, as the cuff is inflated, wave forms tend to be well maintained because the arteries are not compressed against bone. Possibly reactive hyperemia accompanies cuff occlusion, adding to functional estimates of blood vessel tone.

This method of plethysmographic recording, along with PBPI has been used to document preoperative and postoperative changes after aortoiliac reconstruction.[18] Favorable changes correlate with return of erectile function. Pneumoplethysmographic recordings are useful in defining borderline cases in which the PBPI ranges from 0.6 to 0.7.[17] An abnormal penile pneumoplethysmographic recording correlates well with the complaint of impotence and suggests proximal arterial compromise.

To assess neural elements in erectile failure and to detect coexisting neurologic disorders (apart from overt diabetic peripheral neuropathy[19]), pudendal as well as the extremes of both responses can be measured conveniently using a modification of methods described by Haldeman et al.[20] These examinations detect subtle changes requiring measurements beyond the capabilities of ordinary physical examination. Somatosensory evoked potentials from the dorsal penile area and posterior tibial nerve stimulation are obtained, as is measurement of the bulbocavernosus reflex (BCR). Previous methods for recording the BCR intervals used electrical stimulation of the dorsal penile nerve with electromyographic recordings obtained by needle electrodes inserted in the bulbocavernosus muscle in the perineum. The technique as now modified uses surface electrodes that make measurements more comfortable and more widely applicable. Table 48-2 summarizes the time intervals obtained from normal controls in our laboratory.[12] Values above the mean plus three standard deviations are considered abnormal.

After these investigations, the vascular components causing erection can be evaluated further through the use of intracorporal papaverine injection to stimulate artificial erection.[13] Currently I use an initial intracorporal dose of papaverine ranging from 15 to 30 mg. Before the injection is administered, informed consent about the risk of priapism is obtained from the patient; all patients are required to remain under clinical observation for several hours. It is important to select reliable candidates for artificial erection, and, in general, men are discouraged from using this occasion for intercourse. The observation of artificial erection provides an opportunity to time the onset and duration of erection and to observe its quality. When the artificial erection lasts more than 5 hours or becomes painful, immediate treatment is needed. The prolonged erection is treated with aspiration of cavernosal blood and intracorporal injection of 1 to 3 mg of dilute metaraminol. A normal erection stimulated by papaverine rules out proximal arterial insufficiency. With venous insufficiency an adequate though transient erection occurs. This phenomenon, called cavernosal

TABLE 48-2. PUDENDAL EVOKED POTENTIAL CONTROL DATA*

	Mean ± SD[†]	±3 SD
Lumbar potential	13.2 ± 0.96	16.1
Cortical potential	40.1 ± 1.9	45.9
Central conduction time	27.0 ± 1.7	32.1
Bulbocavernosus reflex time	30.6 ± 1.9	36.2

* The control group, ages 22 to 54 years (mean 33 years), consisted of 21 subjects reporting normal potency. Data are expressed in milliseconds.
† SD, standard deviation.

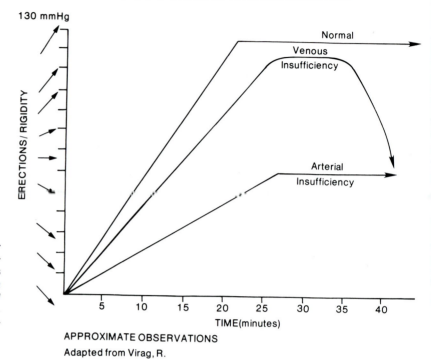

Figure 48-1. Penile responses after intracorporal papaverine injection in healthy patients and in patients in states of venous and arterial insufficiency. (*From DePalma RG: Anatomy and physiology of male sexual function, in Giordano JM, Trout HH III, DePalma RG (eds): Basic Science in Vascular Surgery. New York. Future Publishers, 1988.*)

leak syndrome, is associated with concomitant bounding pulse wave plethysmographic patterns and normal arterial brachial indexes. When this combination exists, venous leakage is probably the main pathophysiology. Figure 48-1 illustrates types of artificial erection responses obtained in patients in various states of venous and arterial insufficiency.

In men with severe occlusive aortoiliac disease, two or more injections of papaverine in increasing dosages up to 60 mg fail to produce erections. Under these circumstances, as well as for conventional indications, angiographic investigation is recommended. When stigmata of large-vessel disease such as claudication, decreased pulses, or an aneurysm exist, conventional aortoiliac angiography using the Seldinger technique is recommended as the first procedure. When the major vessels are normal, to detect the subset of patients with pudendal or distal disease, highly selective pudendal angiography is required. This procedure was originally performed by our group with the patient under epidural anesthesia as described by Ginestie and Romieu[21] and Juhan et al.[22] to avoid spasm of the small penile vessels. However, with the use of nonionic contrast media and sedation, adequate studies can now be obtained without the need for anesthesia. The presence of atherosclerotic debris in the aorta or iliac arteries or severe proximal involvement contraindicates highly selective pudendal angiography because extensive catheter manipulation might cause embolization.

Our data indicate that men with aortoiliac disease are rarely initially seen with the chief complaint of impotence. Among 495 men examined in our vascular laboratories at George Washington University Hospital, only 25 exhibited mainstem aortoiliac disease. Three occult aortic aneurysms,

however, were detected solely as a result of the patient's complaint of impotence and its subsequent investigation. Thus we estimate that approximately 5% of men are initially seen with impotence as a chief complaint associated with or manifested by vascular lesions of the aortoiliac segment.

Most patients with aortoiliac obstructive disease or aneurysmal disease are referred to the vascular surgeon for relief of ischemia or repair of potentially lethal aneurysms. Here, in addition to limb salvage and extension of life, the concern will be mainly preservation of sexual function. As mentioned in the section on approach to patients, a need exists to elicit a history of sexual function, as well as an expression of sexual interest on the part of the patient and, if applicable, his partner. It must not be assumed that advanced age represents lack of sexual interest; preoperative inquiries are usually well accepted by most men. In addition, the refinements in technique that preserve internal iliac flow are important in avoiding later claudication or postoperative cord or lumbar plexus ischemia. It is desirable to ensure, whenever possible, perfusion of at least one of the internal iliac arteries.

RECONSTRUCTIVE TECHNIQUES IN AORTOILIAC DISEASE

Table 48-3 summarizes large-vessel reconstructions that have been used for treating impotence in patients with aortoiliac disease. These operations are the same as those used for lower-extremity revascularization or aneurysm repair. The selection of a particular option or combination of options depends on individual patterns of atherosclerotic involvement. Transluminal angioplasty is emerging as an

TABLE 48-3. LARGE VESSEL RECONSTRUCTIONS FOR TREATING IMPOTENCE

Aortoiliac or aortofemoral bypass
Aortoiliac endarterectomy
Internal iliac endarterectomy or bypass
Femorofemoral reconstruction
Transluminal angioplasty
Profundaplasty in conjunction with other inflow procedures

effective method for treating iliac occlusive disease.[23] When impotence exists, this technique is applicable not only to the common iliac but also to the external iliac arteries. For example, one physiologic mechanism causing erectile failure is a steal that occurs through the superior and inferior gluteal arteries to supply the legs, which causes reduced penile perfusion. Pelvic steal can be suspected clinically when the erection is lost during the first motions of intercourse. Such men may report that they can function in the supine but not in the superior position. A mechanism of pelvic steal with external iliac stenosis is illustrated in Figure 48-2.

Aortoiliac reconstruction that restores or maintains sexual function involves refinement of established principles of aortoiliac surgery. These principles use dissections that preserve, insofar as possible, both arterial and neural elements of the erectile process.[7-10] Operations are planned to restore or maintain internal iliac flow, to avoid atheroembolism into the internal iliac arteries, especially during flushing, and to remove from the aorta atheromatous material that might later escape into the pelvic circulation. The plan of reconstruction to achieve these goals is based on the pattern of aortoiliac atherosclerotic occlusive or aneurysmal disease. With occlusive disease, the external iliac arteries are usually involved. Aortofemoral bypass can thus cause failure of retrograde pelvic perfusion through the diseased external iliac arteries. This situation can be avoided by adding an extra graft limb to perfuse the internal iliac artery.

When possible, in younger men I favor aortoiliac thromboendarterectomy. The operative findings of discrete seg-

mental involvement proximal to the common iliac bifurcation with soft atheromatous lesions and minimal calcification constitute an ideal situation for this procedure. The intrarenal aortic segment is approached through the right side, sparing the inferior mesenteric artery and the associated neural plexi. Mobilization of the vessels should be minimized. Successful proximal thromboendarterectomy maintains axial flow to both internal and external iliac arteries and is an excellent option in situations in which this operation can be performed.

Femorofemoral bypass avoids an aortoiliac dissection completely. This procedure can be combined with a transluminal angioplasty of a donor iliac vessel that contains plaque. At the time of angiography, pressure gradients across common or external iliac arteries should be obtained to assess plaque hemodynamic significance. It is essential that the donor artery be free of lesions that cause a pressure gradient. Although femorofemoral bypass might offer slightly less long-term patency than aortofemoral bypass, it is a useful operation with minimal interference of existing sexual function and a frequent return to normal function.[18]

In the case of late failure of femorofemoral bypass, aortoiliac reconstruction can be performed as a second stage procedure. I rarely recommend axillofemorofemoral bypass because of its poor long-term patency and the need for frequent repeat operations. Flannigan and associates,[24] however, showed that axillofemorofemoral bypass combined with profundaplasty restored sexual function through collaterals arising from the profunda femoris artery even when both internal iliac arteries were believed occluded. It is therefore important to obtain good profunda inflow by extending graft limbs onto these vessels when they are involved with atherosclerosis, not only from the standpoint of limb preservation but also for improvement of pelvic and genital blood flow.

It has been known since 1969 that changes in sexual function after abdominal aortic operation are minimized when aortoiliac anastomoses can be performed proximal to the bifurcation of the common iliac artery.[2] Unfortunately, the usual patterns of atherosclerotic obstructive disease do not permit common iliac anastomoses. A variety of techniques exist to deal with these situations, including

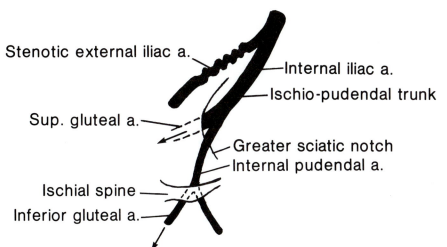

Figure 48-2. Internal pudendal artery steal in oblique view. Superior and inferior gluteal arteries provide lower-limb collateral vessels.

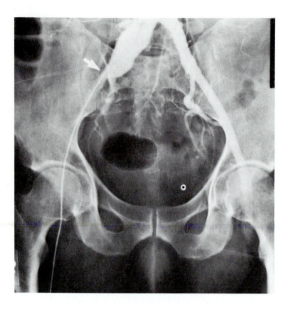

Figure 48-3. Aortogram showing right iliac component of an aorto-iliac aneurysm in a potent 54-year-old man.

tailoring the graft to provide internal iliac perfusion by using an extra limb or combining the operation with an internal iliac endarterectomy and a side-to-side anastomosis with the graft limb.

In patients with abdominal aneurysms, those who are preoperatively impotent almost always remain postoperatively impotent. Those patients who are potent preoperatively commonly remain potent after nerve-sparing operations and judicious efforts to achieve normal internal iliac perfusion. Bilateral isolated internal iliac occlusion is rare, but when it does occur, these men are initially seen with a primary complaint of impotence. I have found this pattern of isolated internal iliac atherosclerosis three times in the last decade, although more cases have been reported by Michal et al.[10] in an Eastern European population. In these instances internal iliac endarterectomy can be performed through a retroperitoneal approach. I use a paramedian incision with medial reflection of the perineal contents. This approach yields excellent exposure of the internal iliac bifurcation, including the superior gluteal artery and the ischiopudendal trunk. Visualization of the distal pelvic vessels through a conventional midline incision for abdominal aortic reconstruction is difficult. In this approach, these vessels can be conveniently exposed by dividing the peritoneum lateral to the cecum on the right side and the descend-

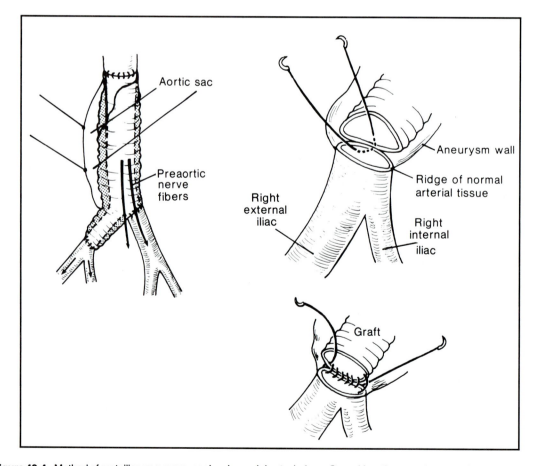

Figure 48-4. Method of aortoiliac aneurysm repair using an inlay technique. Sexual function remains normal postoperatively.

TABLE 48-4. PREOPERATIVE AND POSTOPERATIVE ERECTILE FUNCTION (AFTER AORTOILIAC REVASCULARIZATION)

Status		Average Age (Range)	No.	Comments
Preoperative	Postoperative*			
Potent	Impotent	51, 55, 65, 72	4	3 emergencies 1 elective operation with internal iliac aneurysm
Impotent	Impotent	64.6 (49–79)	52	3 aneurysms discovered during impotence screening 1 previous radical prostatectomy
Potent	Potent	57.0 (39–71)	28	27 elective operations 1 emergency axillofemorofemoral bypass 1 failure to achieve orgasm after colonic surgery
Impotent	Potent	58.0 (38–69)	37	All elective reconstructions; includes 2 internal iliac endarterectomies

* Status 6 months to 1 year postoperatively.

ing colon on the left side. Lateral retraction of the inferior portion of the midline incision provides convenient access to the internal iliac artery and its branches.

Figure 48-3 illustrates a common angiographic pattern in aortoiliac aneurysmal disease in a 54-year-old man with normal sexual function. Preoperative aortography helps plan the pelvic part of the reconstruction and also detects anomalous renal arteries, horseshoe kidney, or abnormal ureters. I recommend obtaining an aortogram before aneurysm reconstruction. Figure 48-4 illustrates the technique that preserves the nerves at the aortic bifurcation and achieves blood flow in both internal iliac arteries. Occasionally, aneurysmal involvement of the internal iliac artery itself requires correction, which can be quite difficult. Intraluminal suture of the aneurysm will minimize disturbance of collaterals. However, when internal iliac aneurysms exist, postoperative impotence can occur in spite of conscientious attempts to achieve penile perfusion. Recognition preoperatively of internal iliac artery aneurysms is therefore important.

POSTOPERATIVE MANAGEMENT

Table 48-4 summarizes my results in cases of aortoiliac reconstruction when attempts were made to preserve or restore sexual function. When patients complain of postoperative impotence, the same sequence of testing used preoperatively can be applied postoperatively. In some of these men, abnormal penile evoked potentials and pudendal evoked potentials are seen even in the presence of noninvasive laboratory studies demonstrating normal penile perfusion. This combination of findings demonstrates neural compromise as a cause of impotence. Some of these men respond to intracorporal papaverine injections with improved erectile function and return periodically for these injections, which help to maintain potency.

In patients with postoperative neurogenic impotence or in patients in whom small vessel penile disease coexists with aortoiliac disease, it is important to recommend penile

prostheses. Other postoperative dysfunctions after aortoiliac reconstruction include complete failure of ejaculation, retrograde ejaculation, or the capacity to stimulate an erection but not to sustain it for orgasm. The latter complaint is rare but vexing. To minimize these neurologic sequelae it is important to use nerve-sparing dissections, avoiding sympathectomy and resection of aortic tissue. Neural disruptions can be quite distressing because they render even treatment with penile prosthetic implantation less than optimal. Once a neural dysfunction has existed for more than 6 months, little improvement can be expected.

When postoperative sexual function is a concern in any patient requiring aortoiliac surgery, irrespective of arteriographic appearance, penile prostheses should be discussed with the patient preoperatively. At the present, one cannot unerringly predict or guarantee maintenance of erectile function or return of erectile function after aortoiliac operations. Therefore use of a penile prosthesis after aortoiliac surgery that fails to preserve or restore sexual function is an important and humane management option.

REFERENCES

1. Leriche R: Des obliterations arterielles hautes (obliteration de la terminasion de l'aorte) comme causes des insuffisances circulatoires des membres inferieurs. Bull Mem Soc Chir 49:1404, 1923.
2. May AG, DeWeese JA, Rolo CG: Changes in sexual function following operation on the abdominal aorta. Surgery 65:41, 1969.
3. Queral LA, Whitehouse WM, et al.: Pelvic hemodynamics after aorto-iliac reconstruction. Surgery 86:799, 1979.
4. Sabri S, Cotton LT: Sexual function following aortoiliac reconstruction. Lancet 2:1218, 1971.
5. Weinstein MH, Machleder HI: Sexual function after aortoiliac surgery. Ann Surg 181:787, 1974.
6. Whitelaw GP, Smithwick RJ: Some secondary effects of sympathectomy with particular reference to disturbance of sexual function. N Engl J Med 254:120, 1951.
7. DePalma RG, Levine SB, Feldman S: Preservation of erectile

function after aortoiliac reconstruction. Arch Surg 113:958, 1978.

8. DePalma RG, Kedia K, Persky L: Vascular operations for preservation of sexual function, in Bergan JJ, Yao JST (eds): The Surgery of the Aorta and its Body Branches. New York, Grune & Stratton, 1979, p 277.

9. DePalma RG: Aorto-iliac dissection principles, in Zorgniotti A, Rossi G (eds): Vasculogenic Impotence. Springfield, Ill., Charles C Thomas, Publisher, 1980, p 299.

10. Michal V, Kramar R, et al.: Aorto-iliac occlusive disease, in Zorgniotti AW, Rossi G (eds): Vasculogenic Impotence. Springfield, Ill., Charles C Thomas, Publisher, 1980, p 203.

11. DePalma RG: Anatomy and physiology of male sexual function, in Giordano JM, Trout HH III, DePalma RG (eds): Basic Science in Vascular Surgery. New York, 1988, Futura Publishers, p 669.

12. DePalma RG, Emsellem HA, et al.: A screening sequence for vasculogenic impotence. J Vasc Surg 5:228, 1987.

13. Virag R, Virag H: L'epreuve a la papaverine intracaverneuse dans l'etude de l'impuissance. J Mal Vasc 8:293, 1983.

14. Karacan I, Aslan C, Hirskowitz M: Erectile mechanisms in man. Science 220:1080, 1983.

15. Kinsey AC, Pomeroy WB, Martin CE: Sexual Behavior in the Human Male. Philadelphia, WB Saunders Co, 1984.

16. Virag R, Bouilly P, Frydman D: Is impotence an arterial disorder? A study of arterial risk factors in 440 impotent men. Lancet 1:181, 1985.

17. Stauffer D, DePalma RG: A comparison of penile-brachial index (PBI) and penile pulse volume recordings (PVR). Bruit 17:29, 1983.

18. Merchant RF Jr, DePalma RG: The effect of femorofemoral grafts on postoperative sexual function: Correlation with penile pulse volume recordings. Surgery 90:962, 1981.

19. Ellenberg M: Impotence in diabetes: The neurologic factor. Ann Intern Med 75:213, 1981.

20. Haldeman S, Bradley WE, et al.: Potential evoked responses. Arch Neurol 39:280, 1982.

21. Ginestie JF, Romieu A: Radiologic exploration of impotence. The Hague, Martinus Nijhoff, 1978.

22. Juhan CM, Hughet JF, et al.: Classification of internal pudendal artery lesions in 100 cases, in Zorgniotti AW, Rossi G (eds): Vasculogenic Impotence. Springfield, Ill., Charles C Thomas, Publisher, 1980, p 169.

23. Goldwasser B, Carson CC III, et al.: Impotence due to the pelvic steal syndrome: Treatment by iliac transluminal angioplasty. J Urol 133:860, 1985.

24. Flannigan DP, Schuler JJ, et al.: Elimination of iatrogenic impotence and improvement of sexual function following aorto-iliac revascularization. Arch Surg 117:544, 1982.

CHAPTER 49
Visceral Artery Aneurysms

Ronald W. Busuttil and Julie A. Freischlag

Aneurysms of the visceral arteries are a heterogeneous group of lesions that can affect most of the splanchnic arteries. In general, their causes, modes of presentation, natural history, and preferred methods of management are varied and must be individualized for the specific situation. Although once considered rare, they are now more commonly encountered, and approximately 2,400 have been reported in the literature. In many cases, these lesions are initially seen with catastrophic, life-threatening bleeding, which requires immediate decisive intervention,[1] whereas in others, an arteriogram for an unrelated process may disclose the presence of an asymptomatic visceral artery aneurysm, which then taxes the most experienced surgeon in planning a treatment strategy. The purpose of this chapter is to review the major pathologic and clinical characteristics of visceral artery aneurysms and to discuss the various treatment options.

ANEURYSMS OF THE SPLENIC ARTERY

Splenic artery aneurysms are the most frequent visceral artery aneurysms and account for more than 50% of these lesions.[2] The true incidence of splenic artery aneurysms is unknown in the general population, but it is estimated, based on autopsy reports, to vary from less than 1 to 10%. These figures reflect the age and sex of the group being studied, as well as the care exercised by the pathologist in looking for the aneurysms. Splenic artery aneurysms rank third after aortic and iliac lesions as the most common intraabdominal aneurysm.

The majority of splenic artery aneurysms occur in women, and several large series report the female predominance over males is a ratio of 4:1.[3–5] With the exception of cerebral artery aneurysms, in which female occurrence out-numbers male by 1.2:1, males have a greater incidence in other aneurysmal disease, including that seen in all other splanchnic vessels. The peak incidence of splenic artery aneurysms is in the sixth decade of life.

Approximately one third of splenic artery aneurysms will be multiple, and most occur at arterial bifurcations in the distal third of the artery. If the cause is portal hypertension, the aneurysms will uniformly be of a saccular configuration and often occur in terminal branches of the splenic artery.

Although there is no unanimity of opinion as to the pathogenesis of splenic artery aneurysms, arteriosclerosis is generally cited. Stanley and Fry,[5] in a report of 60 patients with splenic artery aneurysms, argued that the common histologic finding of atherosclerosis represents a secondary event rather than the initiating cause of most visceral artery aneurysms. In support of this hypothesis, they presented pathologic studies showing localization of calcific arteriosclerotic changes in aneurysms without involving adjacent vessels, as well as data revealing arteriosclerotic changes in some, but not all, aneurysms in which multiple lesions existed. The general incidence of calcification present in splenic artery aneurysms is 80%.

A classification of etiologic factors in the genesis of splenic artery aneurysms proposed by Stanley and Fry[5] is shown in Table 49-1. Although arterial dysplasia has been implicated as a cause of splenic artery aneurysm formation, this has not been proven. However, there is circumstantial evidence to support this hypothesis insofar as there is an association and high incidence of renal artery fibrodysplasia and extracranial carotid dysplastic changes in those patients with splenic artery aneurysms when compared to the normal population.[6,7]

There is a proven association between splenic artery aneurysms and portal hypertension,[2,8,9] and aneurysms were found in 7 to 20% of patients with portal hypertension for which angiography was performed.[10] Dilatation and aneurysmal changes were believed to be sequelae of the hyperkinetic splenic circulation, which is associated with excessive blood volume and increased velocity flow rates. These hyperdynamic changes, coupled with a high resistance to splenic artery outflow, are likely to result in aneurysmal changes. Splenic artery aneurysms after splenic vein thrombosis, however, are rare. Although hormonal perturbations are frequently seen in patients with advanced cirrho-

TABLE 49-1. ETIOLOGY OF SPLENIC ARTERY ANEURYSMS

	No.	%
I. Arterial dysplasia	8	13.3
II. Portal hypertension with splenomegaly	6	10
III. Focal arterial inflammatory processes	3	5
IV. Female patients: ill-defined pathogenesis	35	58.3
V. Male patients: ill-defined pathogenesis	8	13.3

From Stanley JC, Fry WJ: Surgery 76:898, 1974.

sis, the lack of aneurysmal change affecting other visceral arteries lessens the likelihood that hormonally induced vasculopathy is a major cause of these lesions.

Occasionally, splenic artery aneurysms are attributed to primary arterial injury or involvement with an inflammatory process originating in the pancreas or in a penetrating gastric ulcer.[11] In cases related to pancreatitis, the disease has been long-standing and usually involves a chronic relapsing pattern or pseudocyst formation. The natural history of these aneurysms portends a poor prognosis since gastrointestinal hemorrhage occurs in up to 50% of cases and mortality is double that seen for ruptured bland aneurysms (50% vs. 25%). Trauma, usually penetrating, can cause splenic artery aneurysms and was the cause of death by delayed rupture of President James A. Garfield, who died 2 months after being shot by an assassin.[3] Other inflammatory lesions such as periarteritis nodosa have been associated with splenic artery aneurysms and should be investigated when aneurysms are small and multiple.

Arterial degeneration has been implicated as the cause of splenic artery aneurysms in pregnant women. In this group of patients, there is an increased incidence of splenic artery aneurysm, which is further aggravated in grand multipara. In a series published by Busuttil and Brin,[3] 50% of the patients with symptomatic splenic artery aneurysms had had more than six term pregnancies. Other reports have stated a similar association with multigravida women.[5,6,8] This frequency is approximately six times what one would expect in the normal population. The exact role of pregnancy in the formation of splenic artery aneurysms is believed to be related to alterations in the elastin component of the media of the arterial wall, which may be altered hormonally in pregnancy. Repeated pregnancy may cause medial degeneration, allowing aneurysmal formation. Also, the increased vascularity causing relative portal congestion in pregnancy may also lead to aneurysmal changes in the splenic artery.[3] Aneurysmal rupture in pregnant women has a high incidence of mortality for both the mother and the fetus.[8,12]

Atherosclerosis as the sole etiologic factor in splenic artery aneurysm formation may occasionally be seen in males. These patients often have other sites of diffuse atherosclerotic involvement; however, there is no known association between splenic artery aneurysms and aneurysms affecting the aorta or peripheral vessels.

Clinical manifestations of splenic artery aneurysms are rare. When symptoms do occur, they are usually nonspecific, but the most frequent complaint is recurrent left upper-quadrant pain, occasionally radiating to the left scapula

or flank. At times, pain be exacerbated by exercise.[4] In a series of 100 patients with splenic artery aneurysms reported by Trastek and associates,[6] only 17% were asymptomatic. Since these aneurysms are small (usually less than 2 cm), a pulsatile mass or bruit is uncommon. The diagnosis of splenic artery aneurysms may be suggested by the presence of a curvilinear signet ring-like calcification seen in the left upper quadrant of an abdominal roentgenogram. The differential diagnosis for left upper-quadrant oval calcifications includes a tortuous splenic artery, renal artery aneurysm, tuberculous mesenteric lymphadenopathy, and cysts of the liver, spleen, kidney, or adrenal gland. The presence of multiple calcifications is suggestive of splenic artery aneurysms.

Angiography is still the preferred method of diagnosis when a splenic artery aneurysm is suspected. Experience with computerized tomographic scanning or nuclear magnetic resonance is too sparse at present to identify the role of these modalities. Figure 49-1 shows a typical asymptomatic splenic artery aneurysm in a cirrhotic patient with portal hypertension. Not only is angiography the definitive means of diagnosis, exclusive of laparotomy, but its use has brought about a reassessment of the mortality associated with splenic artery aneurysms. Although early reviews suggested an extremely high risk of rupture, it is now realized that many asymptomatic aneurysms were over-looked, and a disproportionately large number of ruptured aneurysms were reported. In the UCLA series,[3] aneurysm rupture occurred in only 1 out of 10 patients, which is similar to that reported for the Mayo Clinic (9.2%)[13] and the University of Michigan (6.6%).[4]

Rupture is the most devastating complication seen with splenic artery aneurysms and usually causes free intraperitoneal hemorrhage (80%). Aneurysms greater than 2 cm in diameter are more prone to burst. Although 80% of these lesions are calcified, calcification does not provide protection against this complication. In 20 to 30% of cases, delayed rupture may occur.[4-6] In this situation, the hemorrhage

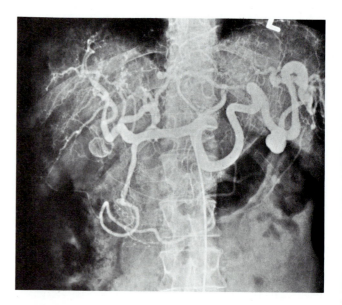

Figure 49-1. Splenic artery aneurysm in a cirrhotic patient.

will be contained within the lesser sac as an expanding hematoma and will be accompanied by severe left upper-quadrant and epigastric pain, which may mimic other intra-abdominal catastrophes. When the hematoma bursts into the free peritoneal cavity, shock occurs. This constellation of symptoms has been called the "double-rupture phenomenon." Occasionally the hematoma may leak through the foramen of Winslow, resulting in lower abdominal pain. Only rarely will splenic artery aneurysms rupture into adjacent viscera or the splenic vein. This rupture may be more common in the inflammatory aneurysms previously discussed. Mortality after rupture of splenic artery aneurysms has improved for nonpregnant patients and is about 5% in recent series.[6] However, death is common after rupture in both the pregnant patient and her fetus and occurs in 75% and 95% respectively.[3] Free intraperitoneal rupture is the rule in pregnancy.

The treatment of patients with known splenic artery aneurysms is dictated by several factors, including age, sex, presence of symptoms, size, and cause of the aneurysm. In general, surgery is seldom required; however, elective repair in good-risk patients is advocated for all patients who are symptomatic (less than 20% of cases) and for women who are pregnant or of child-bearing age. Asymptomatic aneurysms greater than 2 cm in diameter should be repaired because of their increased risk of rupture.[3,6] Patients with aneurysms associated with pancreatitis or pseudocyst formation should have aggressive surgical therapy, which often warrants pancreatic resection. In the poor-risk patient, splenic artery aneurysm control may be obtained with coil or balloon occlusion.[9]

The choice of operation is determined by the location of the aneurysm. If the lesion is in close proximity to the spleen, aneurymal excision with splenectomy may be required; however, attempts at splenic preservation are justified in the young patient. In the series reported by Trastek and associates,[6] 82% of patients had excision with splenectomy, 17% had excision without splenectomy, and only 1% had ligation and exclusion. If located near the celiac axis, aneurysmectomy or proximal and distal ligation with obliteration of all feeding vessels alone may be performed. In this situation, splenectomy is not necessary. The patient with portal hypertension presents an unusually difficult problem because of the extensive collaterals; thus transcatheter embolization may be preferred in this setting.

HEPATIC ARTERY ANEURYSMS

Since Wilson[14] described the first hepatic artery aneurysm in 1819, this lesion has become the second most commonly described splanchnic aneurysm and accounts for 20% of all visceral artery aneurysms. Its exact incidence is unknown; however, as is true for splenic artery aneurysms, the more liberal use of angiography has disclosed a greater incidence of hepatic artery aneurysms than was previously believed.[15]

There are several causes of hepatic artery aneurysms, and these are listed in Table 49-2 in order of frequency.[16] In most series, arteriosclerosis accounts for up to one third of these lesions.[2,4,17] Whether arteriosclerosis is primary

TABLE 49-2. ETIOLOGY OF HEPATIC ARTERY ANEURYSMS

Arteriosclerosis
Medial degeneration
Trauma
Mycotic
Congenital defects

or secondary is difficult to determine. Medial degeneration has been recognized more recently as an etiologic factor, accounting for 25% of hepatic artery aneurysms. It appears that medial degeneration occurs more commonly in dissecting aneurysms. Trauma accounts for approximately 20% of these aneurysms and is increasing.[17–19] Both blunt and penetrating injuries have been implicated, with the former associated with intrahepatic predominance (Fig. 49-2). Despite the decline of mycotic hepatic aneurysms since 1960, 10 to 15% still have an infectious cause.[3,4,19] Whereas 20 years ago endocarditis was the inciting factor, today illicit drug abuse is the most common cause of mycotic hepatic artery aneurysms. Congenital defects contribute to the remainder of hepatic artery aneurysms and include diseases such as Ehlers-Danlos syndrome and periarteritis nodosa. These latter aneurysms are more apt to be multiple, smaller, and solely intrahepatic (Fig. 49-3).[3,19]

Eighty percent of hepatic artery aneurysms are extrahepatic.[4] Of these, approximately 60% involve the common hepatic artery, 30% the right hepatic artery, 5% the left hepatic artery, and 5% both hepatic arteries. The reason for the predilection for the right hepatic artery is unknown, although traumatic injury is more apt to involve the right system. Most hepatic artery aneurysms are symptomatic. Patients may complain of right upper-quadrant abdominal pain radiating to the back that is unrelated to food ingestion.[16] Bruits and palpable masses are rare. Compres-

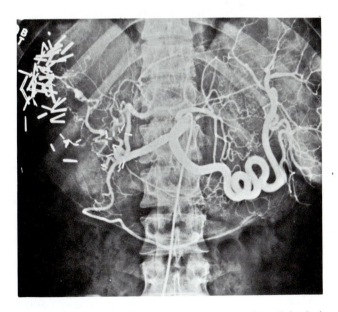

Figure 49-2. Right hepatic artery aneurysm after blunt abdominal trauma.

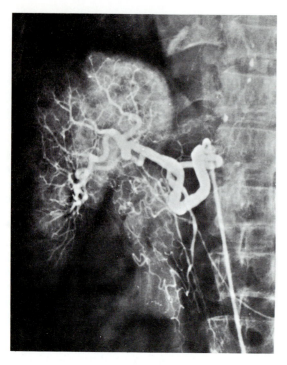

Figure 49-3. Multiple hepatic artery aneurysms in a patient with polyarteritis nodosa.

sion and obstruction of the biliary ducts can produce biliary colic and jaundice. Erosion into the biliary tree causes hemophilia, with the classic triad of gastrointestinal bleeding, biliary colic, and jaundice.[15] Occasionally, large common hepatic artery aneurysms may rupture freely into the peritoneal cavity or erode into the duodenum or portal vein, causing portal hypertension.

Early reports[4] suggested that rupture occurred in 44% of all hepatic artery aneurysms. More recent series[3] have reported a lower rate of about 20 to 30%. Among patients in the UCLA series[3] who had hepatic artery aneurysms, 30% suffered rupture, and there was a 100% mortality. When rupture occurs, there are usually no prodromal symptoms.

Because of the propensity to rupture, hepatic artery aneurysms should be treated once they are discovered. A major problem arises in that diagnosis is difficult until symptoms occur. Noninvasive tests, including ultrasound, radionuclide scans, and gastrointestinal barium studies, have not been very useful. In one report,[20] computed tomography (CT) was found to be useful. Angiography remains the only definitive test, both for diagnosis and for planning of the operative approach.

Exclusive of small, multiple asymptomatic intrahepatic aneurysms that may be treated conservatively, excision or obliteration of all hepatic artery aneurysms appears to be the management of choice unless some compelling circumstances preclude operative intervention.[17] If the aneurysm is located in the common hepatic artery, proximal and distal ligation is possible in most instances without causing hepatic

ischemia.[3,19] In this situation, sufficient collateral blood flow to the liver through the gastroduodenal artery will be provided. For aneurysms involving the proper hepatic artery, simple ligation will usually interfere with hepatic perfusion; thus reconstruction should be performed using saphenous vein or prosthetic material.[18] In certain cases of large saccular aneurysms, aneurysmorrhaphy may be used. Similar methods are used for the treatment of right- or left-branch hepatic arteries. Hepatic resection may be required in rare circumstances to control intrahepatic aneurysms. This situation usually arises with hemorrhage uncontrollable by other means.[2,17] Angiography with selective embolization has emerged as an important adjunct for the treatment of patients with intrahepatic aneurysms.[19,20] This procedure has proven particularly suited to the patient who is initially seen with hemobilia after either blunt or penetrating trauma. Embolization with Gelfoam, Ivalon or Gianturco coils has been described with good results in selected patients.[19,21,22] Using the guidelines mentioned previously, survival of patients with hepatic artery aneurysms has improved and should exceed 75%.[18,22]

CELIAC ARTERY ANEURYSMS

Aneurysms of the celiac trunk are uncommon and comprise only 4% of all visceral artery aneurysms.[18] Shumaker and Sidreys[23] performed the first resection of a celiac aneurysm in 1958. The cause of these aneurysms depends on the era of reporting. Of those lesions described before 1950, most were of infectious origin, with *Treponema pallidum* being the causative organism. In more recent years, medial degeneration and arteriosclerosis are more common causes. The role of arteriosclerosis as a primary or secondary event in celiac aneurysm pathogenesis is undetermined. However, there seems to be a greater association with celiac aneurysms and other peripheral aneurysms, a correlation not seen in other visceral lesions.[18] Congenital and traumatic causes have occasionally been cited in the literature.[2]

Most of these lesions are asymptomatic, and more than 90% are discovered incidentally during aortography for other causes. In symptomatic patients, complaints of upper abdominal discomfort, early satiety, or, rarely, intestinal angina may be reported.[4,24] Masses or bruits are rarely found. Rupture occurs in about 15% of cases and is usually intraperitoneal with a resultant high mortality.[2]

Once an aneurysm is discovered, it should be repaired. Aneurysmectomy with reconstruction is the preferred surgical approach (Fig. 49-4).[24] Because of inadequate exposure, particularly in the large patient, a thoracoabdominal approach may be preferred, with reflection of the spleen, pancreas, and left colon to the right. Simple ligation has been reported[17]; however, this procedure may be fraught with subsequent hepatic ischemia. In circumstances in which a central reconstruction is not possible because of technical reasons, ligation with distal bypass to either the common hepatic or splenic arteries is preferred. Overall, survival after operative intervention for celiac aneurysms has approached 90%.

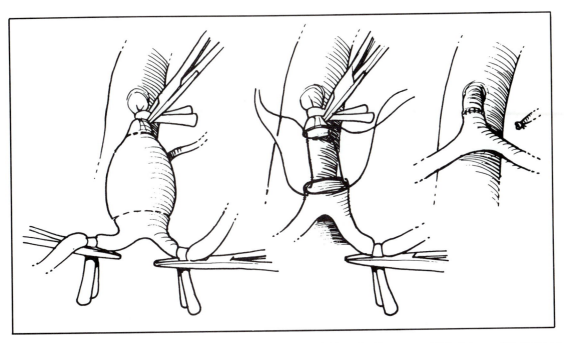

Figure 49-4. Repair of celiac artery aneurysm. (*From Haimovici, H: Vascular Surgery and Principles and Techniques. New York, McGraw-Hill Book Co., 1976.*)

GASTRIC, GASTROEPIPLOIC, GASTRODUODENAL, AND PANCREATICODUODENAL ANEURYSMS

Aneurysms of the gastric, gastroepiploic, gastroduodenal, and pancreaticoduodenal arteries, as well as aneurysms of the jejunal and ileal branch arteries, occur much less frequently than other visceral aneurysms. Less than 100 of these lesions in the aggregate have been reported.

Gastric and gastroepiploic aneurysms in many cases are acquired lesions secondary to an adjacent inflammatory process. Medial degeneration and arteriosclerosis have also been identified.[4] Patients with these aneurysms most often are initially seen with rupture into the gastrointestinal tract (70%) or freely into the peritoneal cavity (30%). Occasionally, a "double-rupture phenomenon" may occur. In most cases, patients are seen with acute bleeding, and the diagnosis is not made preoperatively. Most aneurysms are small (1 cm or less) and are difficult to identify. Operative treatment should include ligation or wedge gastric resection if the aneurysm is adherent to the stomach.[4]

Aneurysms of the gastroduodenal and pancreaticoduodenal arteries have the greatest lethal potential of visceral artery aneurysms. Since many of these are pancreatitis related, there is a male predominance.[25] A history of long-standing pancreatitis with or without pseudocyst formation has been reported in 60% of patients with gastroduodenal artery aneurysms and in 30% of patients with pancreaticoduodenal artery aneurysms.[26-31] Rupture is the most common presenting symptom and occurs in more than 50% of gastroduodenal and 90% of pancreaticoduodenal artery aneurysms.[4,18] When these lesions rupture, they may do so into the gastrointestinal or biliary tract (65%) or into the peritoneal cavity (35%).[28,31,32] Mortality is in excess of 50% after rupture. Preoperative arteriography is important in management, and some authors have recommended intraoperative angiography.[27,28]

Treatment of both gastroduodenal and pancreaticoduodenal aneurysms is surgical. Asymptomatic lesions should be ligated or embolized. A difficult surgical problem arises when the aneurysm is in close proximity to a pancreatic pseudocyst. In this situation, it is difficult to determine if one is dealing with an aneurysm or with erosion of a vessel secondary to the inflammation. Angiography is often useful in directing therapy. Although some surgeons have advocated drainage of the pseudocyst after ligation of the aneurysm,[28,29] we would recommend definitive resection of the involved pancreas, along with the aneurysm. In the rare case, this patient will also require pancreaticoduodenal resection. It is our concern that the incidence of recurrent bleeding and erosion is too high without extirpative therapy.

Jejunal and ileal artery branch aneurysms are uncommon but are the most frequent source of bleeding cited as the cause of "abdominal apoplexy."[33] The cause is believed to be congenital and secondary to medial degeneration.[34] Diagnosis is usually made in the asymptomatic patient during routine angiography. Rupture is unheralded.[18,34] Management consists of elective ligation if the aneurysm is found, since the risk of rupture is 10 to 30%.[34] Rarely will a concomitant bowel resection be needed.

SUPERIOR MESENTERIC ARTERY ANEURYSMS

Superior mesenteric artery aneurysm is the third most common lesion and comprises approximately 8% of all visceral artery aneurysms. The first successful surgical repair was performed by DeBakey and Cooley in 1949.[1] Since then, more than 100 cases have been reported.

Fifty to sixty percent of these aneurysms are mycotic in origin, and there is a high association in patients with bacterial endocarditis or intravenous drug abuse.[2,3,35] Organisms that are frequently found include staphylococcus (both coagulase positive and negative), nonhemolytic streptococcus, and occasionally Gram-negative enteric bacteria. In the majority of cases, the proximal part of the artery is involved, although extension can occur into branches, including the middle colic and jejunal arteries. Other less frequent causes include arteriosclerosis, trauma, and medial degeneration.[36]

Although most superior mesenteric artery aneurysms are discovered incidentally during angiography (Fig. 49-5), many will produce symptom complexes of abdominal pain and intestinal ischemia. The latter is obviously apparent in lesions that propagate thrombus. Rupture, either freely or into the gastrointestinal tract, is uncommon. In approximately one third to one half of patients with a superior mesenteric artery aneurysm, a pulsatile mass may be palpated.[4] This aneurysm can be distinguished from an abdominal aortic aneurysm by the former's greater degree of mobility.

Definitive diagnosis can be accomplished by angiography and in some cases by CT. Operative intervention is indicated for all patients who are acceptable risks and must be individualized. Frequently, simple ligation may not be satisfactory because of inadequate collateral flow; thus bypass is indicated. Because of the high likelihood of a mycotic origin, autogenous tissue reconstruction with saphenous veins should be used, and long-term specific antibiotics should be administered. Aneurysmorrhaphy can be used to preserve arterial collateral flow in suitable lesions.[37] In patients who are initially seen with acute thrombosis of a superior mesenteric artery aneurysm and intestinal ischemia, revascularization should precede bowel resection.

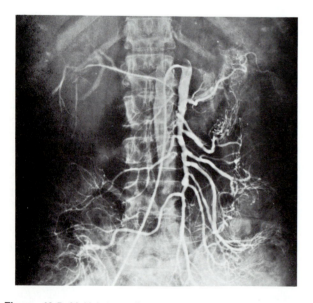

Figure 49-5. Multiple superior mesenteric artery aneurysms in asymptomatic patient.

INFERIOR MESENTERIC ARTERY ANEURYSM

Only 16 aneurysms of the inferior mesenteric artery have been reported in the literature.[38,39] The cause is primarily arteriosclerosis, with periarteritis nodosa, Takayasu's arteritis, dissection, and infection being implicated in a few cases. These aneurysms are usually found incidentally, although a few patients may initially be seen with epigastric pain or with a pulsatile abdominal mass. Rupture may occur, and gut ischemia may result if there is concomitant disease of the superior mesenteric artery or celiac axis or both.[38] Treatment is ligation; however, revascularization is indicated if backbleeding from the inferior mesenteric artery is poor when resection of the aneurysm is undertaken.[39]

RENAL ARTERY ANEURYSMS

Aneurysms affecting the renal arteries are frequently included in a discussion of visceral aneurysms since there is a degree of commonality in their pathogenesis and clinical manifestations with other aneurysms involving the gut, spleen, and liver. However, there are also several distinct differences that merit special consideration.

Renal artery aneurysms, like all visceral artery aneurysms, are receiving increasing attention because of the more frequent use of aortography and renal arteriography in patients with hypertension. In general, one can expect to discover these lesions in less than 1% of the population who undergo renal arteriography.[40] This incidence may be higher in symptomatic patients; however, most renal aneurysms are asymptomatic when discovered.[41,42]

A classification of renal artery aneurysms has been proposed by Poustasse[43] and is based on both pathogenetic and morphologic characteristics of these lesions. The four types of renal artery aneurysms, in order of frequency, include (1) saccular, (2) fusiform (Fig. 49-6), (3) dissecting, and (4) intrarenal microaneurysms (Fig. 49-7).

Saccular aneurysms are the classic renal artery macroaneurysms that occur at branch points. They are most likely due to medial degeneration, with arteriosclerosis occurring as a secondary event. The lack of arteriosclerosis in other vascular beds supports this hypothesis. In most cases, secondary calcification occurs, initially seen as a signet ring, which must be distinguished from splenic artery aneurysms. However, the peak incidence of renal artery aneurysm occurrence (between the fifth and seventh decades) is similar to when arteriosclerosis becomes manifest. This is dissimilar to splenic artery aneurysms, which tend to occur in a younger group. Similar to splenic lesions, calcification in saccular aneurysms has not been proven to offer protection from rupture. Most of these lesions are 1.5 cm or less in diameter. The incidence of rupture is greater once the lesion has reached a diameter greater than 2 cm, and surgical intervention has been recommended at this stage.[43]

Fusiform aneurysms are found in younger patients and are associated with fibromuscular dysplasia. In most cases, the aneurysms develop as a poststenotic dilatation. They occur more commonly in females and involve the right renal artery more frequently. They are the most frequently

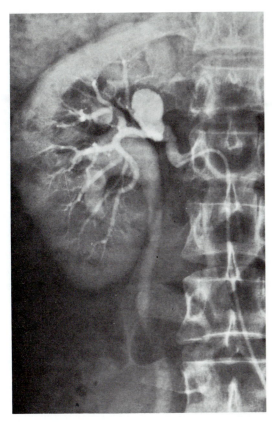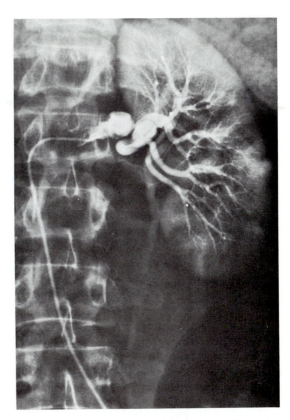

Figure 49-6. Bilateral renal artery aneurysms in a hypertensive female with fibromuscular dysplasia.

encountered aneurysms in the pediatric patient[44] and are associated with hypertension in 80% of patients. Most of these aneurysms are small (less than 5 mm in diameter) and frequently multiple. Branch point occurrence is rare.

Dissecting renal artery aneurysms can arise secondary to aortic dissection or as a primary phenomenon due to either a spontaneous tear of the intima at the site of a mural fibrodysplasia or to trauma. The right renal artery is more commonly involved as is the proximal part of the artery. Stanley and Whilhouse[45] have proposed that abnormalities in the vasa vasorum of these vessels predisposes to rupture and arterial wall hemorrhage, which initiate the dissection. Unlike other renal artery aneurysms, dissecting aneurysms often are initially seen with the acute onset of flank pain, which can resemble renal colic. In other cases, hypertension may be the only clue, with the diagnosis made later by angiography. Of all renal artery aneurysms, the dissecting type is a true surgical emergency since a delay in treatment may result in a loss of kidney function.

The fourth type of renal artery aneurysm is the intrarenal. This type arises from a variety of causes, which include trauma, congenital arterial wall defects, or collagen vascular disease, particularly polyarteritis nodosum.[46,47] In polyarteritis nodosum, the lesions are often bilateral and affect the hepatic artery as well.[48]

Most renal artery aneurysms, exclusive of the dissecting type, are asymptomatic. The diagnosis should be suspected if a signet ring calcification is seen on a plain abdominal roentgenogram; however, only 25% of the lesions will have calcium in the wall.[49] Confirmation is obtained by selective arteriography. Some patients will complain of flank or abdominal pain. If the aneurysms are large, they may partially or wholly obstruct the collecting system, resulting in renal colic or hematuria.[38] Renal artery thrombosis more frequently occurs with dissecting aneurysms and occasionally with stenosis associated with fusiform aneurysms.

An association exists between hypertension and renal artery aneurysms. In a series reported by Soussou and associates,[47] all patients with renal artery aneurysms had hypertension. Several other studies[40,49,50] have shown an association of 50 to 75%. The mechanism of the hypertension is unclear but appears to relate to renal ischemia and elevated renal vein renin levels. Inferentially, the role of hyperreninemia has been validated by the observation that only those patients with elevated renin are cured of hypertension after surgical repair of the aneurysm.

Rupture of renal artery aneurysms is distinctly unusual, and reports indicate an incidence of less than 1%.[51] There is no recent evidence to suggest that asymptomatic renal artery aneurysms in childbearing women have the same propensity for rupture as do splenic artery aneurysms. Thus reconstruction of the former lesions in these circumstances should be considered only after very careful evaluation.

The indications for repair of renal artery aneurysms include the following:

1. Symptomatic aneurysm
2. Renal artery aneurysm associated with hypertension

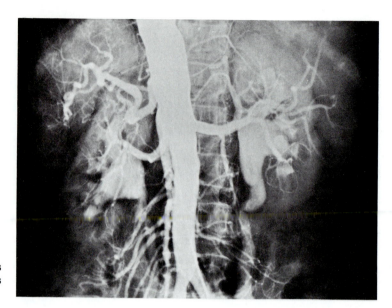

Figure 49-7. Multiple intrarenal aneurysms in the right kidney of a patient with periarteritis nodosa.

3. Aneurysms greater than 1.5 cm in diameter that have been documented as increasing in size[40,43]
4. Asymptomatic small renal artery aneurysms that may be implicated in thromboembolism and deterioration of kidney function.[40,51]

Repair of renal artery aneurysms should be individualized to each patient depending on the location of the aneurysm, the presence or absence of hypertension, and the status of renal function. Repair can be performed by tangential aneurysmectomy and primary arteriography in select cases when the aneurysm is extrarenal.[52] Saphenous vein angioplasty may also be used in selected cases of extrarenal artery aneurysm repair.[42] However, bypass grafting using saphenous vein (preferred) or prosthetic material is the procedure of choice if the aneurysm has caused dissection of the renal artery[46] or if the aneurysm is located close to the renal parenchyma.[47] Nephrectomy is rarely indicated. However, those patients with end-stage renal disease and hypertension may be candidates for nephrectomy.[48] Ex vivo repair has also been described for some renal artery aneurysms that are difficult to expose in order to facilitate a more accurate reconstruction.[53]

REFERENCES

1. DeBakey ME, Cooley DA: Successful resection of mycotic aneurysm of superior mesenteric artery: Case report and a review of the literature. Am Surg 19:202, 1953.
2. Graham JM, McCollum CH, DeBakey ME: Aneurysms of the splanchnic arteries. Am J Surg 140:797, 1980.
3. Busuttil RW, Brin BJ: The diagnosis and management of visceral artery aneurysms. Surgery 88:619, 1980.
4. Stanley JC, Thompson NW, Fry WJ: Splanchnic artery aneurysms. Arch Surg 101:689, 1970.
5. Stanley JC, Fry WJ: Pathogenesis and clinical significance of splenic artery aneurysms. Surgery 76:898, 1974.
6. Trastek VF, Pairolero PC, et al.: Splenic artery aneurysms. Surgery 91:694, 1982.
7. O'Hara PJ, Ratliff NB, et al.: Medial agenesis associated with multiple extracranial peripheral and visceral arterial aneurysms. J Vasc Surg 2:298, 1985.
8. Barrett J, Caldwell BH: Association of portal hypertension and ruptured splenic artery aneurysm in pregnancy. Obstet Gynecol 57:255, 1981.
9. Prosbt P, Castaneda-Zuniga WR, et al.: Nonsurgical treatment of splenic artery aneurysms. Diagn Radiol 128:619, 1978.
10. Feist JG, Gajaraz A: Extra- and intrasplenic artery aneurysms in portal hypertension. Diagn Radiol 125:331, 1977.
11. Gadacz TR, Trunkey D, Kieffer R: Visceral vessel erosion association with pancreatitis. Arch Surg 113:1438, 1978.
12. O'Grady JP, Day EJ, et al.: Splenic artery aneurysm rupture in pregnancy: A review and case report. Obstet Gynecol 50:627, 1977.
13. Spittel JA, Fairbairn JF, et al.: Aneurysms of the splenic artery. JAMA 175:452, 1961.
14. Wilson J: Lectures on the blood, and on the anatomy, physiology and surgical pathology of the vascular system of the human body. Papers read before the Royal College of Surgeons. London, 1819.
15. Harlaftis NN, Akin JT: Hemobilia from ruptured hepatic artery aneurysm—report of a case and review of the literature. Am J Surg 133:229, 1977.
16. Guida PM, Moore SW: Aneurysm of the hepatic artery: Report of the five cases with a brief review of the previously reported cases. Surgery 60:299, 1966.
17. Hetzler PT, Thiele BL: Hepatic artery aneurysms. Surg Rounds 32:69, 1986.
18. Rutherford RB: Vascular Surgery. Philadelphia, WB Saunders Co, 1984, p 798.
19. Mathisen DJ, Athanasoulis CA, Malt BA: Preservation of arterial blood flow to the liver: Goal in treatment of extrahepatic and post-traumatic intrahepatic aneurysms of the hepatic artery. Ann Surg 196:400, 1982.
20. Kibbler CC, Cohen DL, et al.: Use of CAT scanning in the diagnosis and management of hepatic artery aneurysm. Gut 26:752, 1985.
21. Goldblatt MB, Goldin MBB, Shaft MI: Percutaneous embolization for the management of hepatic artery aneurysms. Gastroenterology 73:1142, 1977.
22. Keehan MF, Kistner RL, Banis J: Angiography as an aid in

extraenteric gastrointestinal bleeding due to visceral artery aneurysm. Ann Surg 187:357, 1978.

23. Shumacker HB Jr, Siderys H: Excisional treatment of aneurysm of celiac artery. Am J Surg 148:885, 1958.

24. Haimovici H, Sprayregen S, et al.: Celiac artery aneurysmectomy: Case report with review of the literature. Surgery 79:592, 1976.

25. Spanos PK, Kloppedal EA, Murray CA III: Aneurysms of the gastroduodenal and pancreaticoduodenal arteries. Am J Surg 127:345, 1974.

26. Eckhauser FE, Stanley JC, et al.: Gastroduodenal and pancreaticoduodenal artery aneurysms: A complication of pancreatitis causing massive gastrointestinal hemorrhage. Surgery 88:335, 1980.

27. Verta MJ Jr, Dean RH, et al.: Pancreaticoduodenal arterial aneurysms. Ann Surg 186:111, 1976.

28. Stanley JC, Frey CF, et al.: Major arterial hemorrhage—a complication of pancreatic pseudocysts and chronic pancreatitis. Arch Surg 111:435, 1976.

29. Gangahar DM, Carveth SW, et al.: True aneurysm of the pancreaticoduodenal artery: A case report and review of the literature. J Vasc Surg 2:741, 1985.

30. Harris RD, Anderson JE, Coel MN: Aneurysms of the small pancreatic arteries: A cause of upper abdominal and intestinal bleeding. Radiology 114:17, 1975.

31. Janne P, Bremen J, Bremer A: Aneurysm of the gastroduodenal artery as a cause of hemobilia. Am J Surg 133:633, 1977.

32. Mandel SR, Jaques PF, et al.: Nonoperative management of peripancreatic arterial aneurysms—a 10-year experience. Ann Surg 205:126, 1987.

33. Buchler PK, Dailey TH, Lazarevic B: Spontaneous rupture of colic-artery aneurysms: Report of two cases. Dis Colon Rectum 19:671, 1976.

34. McNamara MF, Griska LB: Superior mesenteric artery branch aneurysms. Surgery 88:625, 1980.

35. Christophe C, Burnist W, et al.: Ruptured mycotic aneurysm of the superior mesenteric artery secondary to bacterial endocarditis in a 6-year-old girl. Radiology 15:202, 1985.

36. Gebauer VA: Aneurysm of the superior mesenteric artery: Its diagnosis and clinical significance. ROFO 141:529, 1984.

37. Olcott C, Ehrenfeld WK: Endoaneurysmorrhaphy for visceral artery aneurysms. Am J Surg 133:636, 1977.

38. LeBas P, Batt M, et al.: Aneurysm of the inferior mesenteric artery associated with occlusion of the celiac axis and superior mesenteric artery. Ann Vasc Surg 1:253, 1986.

39. Graham LM, Hay MR, et al.: Inferior mesenteric artery aneurysms. Surgery 97:158, 1985.

40. Hageman JH, Smith RF, et al.: Aneurysms of the renal artery: Problems of prognosis and surgical management. Surgery 84:563, 1978.

41. Cummings KB, Lecky JW, Kaufman JJ: Renal artery aneurysms and hypertension. J Urol 109:144, 1973.

42. McCarron JT Jr, Marshall VF, Whitsell JC: Indications for surgery on renal artery aneurysms. J Urol 114:177, 1975.

43. Poutasse EF: Renal artery aneurysms. J Urol 113:443, 1975.

44. Stanley JC, Fry WJ: Pediatric renal artery occlusive disease and renovascular hypertension. Arch Surg 116:669, 1981.

45. Stanley JC, Whilhouse WM Jr: Renal artery macroaneurysms, in Bergan JJ, Yao JST (eds): Aneurysms: Diagnosis and Treatment. New York, Grune & Stratton, Inc, 1982, p 417.

46. Kaufman JJ, Coulson WF, et al.: Primary dissecting aneurysm of renal artery: Report of a case causing reversible renal hypertension. Ann Surg 177:259, 1973.

47. Soussou ID, Starr DS, et al.: Renal artery aneurysm—long-term relief of renovascular hypertension by in-situ operative correction. Arch Surg 114:1410, 1979.

48. Charron J, Belanger P, et al.: Renal artery aneurysm—polyaneurysmal lesion of kidney. Urology 5:1, 1975.

49. Gil Montero G, Bagley M: Renal vascular hypertension secondary to renal arterial aneurysm. Urology 6:647, 1975.

50. Cummings KB, Lecky JW, Kaufman JJ: Renal artery aneurysms and hypertension. J Urol 109:144, 1973.

51. Stanley JC, Rhodes LE, et al.: Renal artery aneurysms significance of macroaneurysms exclusive of dissections and fibrodysplastic mural dilations. Arch Surg 110:1327, 1975.

52. Cifarelli F, Choon SS, et al.: Aneurysm of a polar renal artery. Surgery 78:660, 1975.

53. Gaylis H, Lissoos I: Aneurysms of the renal artery with a case of extra-corporeal repair. S Afr Med J 49:1963, 1975.

CHAPTER 50
Isolated Iliac Artery Aneurysms

Henry Haimovici

The majority of iliac aneurysms are associated with those of the abdominal aorta and, therefore, are not included in this chapter. (See Chapter 47.) Only isolated iliac aneurysms are considered here.[1-5]

INCIDENCE

An isolated iliac aneurysm is a rare vascular entity. In one of the earliest comprehensive reports, published in 1961, Markowitz and Norman[3] dealt with 30 patients collected from the Columbia Presbyterian Medical Center. They included the common, external, and internal iliac arteries as a group. The true incidence of isolated iliac aneurysm is quite small and has been considered 1.5% of that of an abdominal aortic aneurysm. More recently, Lowry and Kraft[2] published eight cases encountered in a 10-year period and reviewed 36 cases from the literature.

The *natural course* of an isolated iliac aneurysm is toward progressive enlargement and rupture, often without much in the way of warning symptoms, with incidence of rupture ranging from 18% reported by Markowitz and Norman to 50% reported by Lowry and Kraft. Diagnosis of an isolated artery aneurysm is rendered extremely difficult because of its insidious onset and its often deep pelvic location. As these aneurysms enlarge, especially those of the hypogastric artery, they produce symptoms of compression on the intrapelvic structures, notably the lumbosacral plexus, urinary bladder, or bowel. If the significance of these symptoms is realized, the diagnosis can often be made by careful pelvic examination through the rectum or vagina. Iliac aneurysms may rupture into the retroperitoneal space of the pelvis or, more rarely, into the rectum or sigmoid colon (Fig. 50-1). Symptoms preceding or appearing after rupture consist of abdominal and back pain in the majority of patients. Pain follows the sciatic distribution and is accompanied by straight leg–raising weakness, reflex changes, and sensory impairment. When the symptoms appear abruptly, the clinical features closely resemble the sciatica of a ruptured intervertebral disc.[6] Rectal examination discloses pel-

vic pulsation, and x-ray films often confirm a calcific rim in the wall of the aneurysm.

Most, if not all, patients are men who have associated cardiovascular and hypertensive disease. The average diameter of iliac aneurysms ranges from 7.5 to 8.5 cm. Approximately 50% of those isolated iliac aneurysms previously reported were located in the common iliac artery, with the remainder involving the internal iliac artery.[2,3]

SURGICAL MANAGEMENT

Surgical management of iliac aneurysms is based on general principles of adequate exposure, isolation of the artery, excision, and interposition of a graft. Any one of several surgical techniques may be applied, depending on the size of the aneurysm and its relationship to the adjacent vein and the abdominal aorta: (1) total excision of the aneurysm, (2) partial excision of the sac, and (3) bypass graft combined with exclusion of the aneurysm. For a small isolated lesion of either the common or external iliac artery, an extraperitoneal approach is desirable and may often be adequate. However, should there be any evidence of aortic or large pelvic mass, a transperitoneal approach is indicated. Mortality after elective surgery for iliac artery aneurysm is less than 10%, in contrast to the operative mortality of 52% for ruptured cases.[2] Awareness of iliac aneurysms and their usual propensity to enlarge and rupture is the best approach to early diagnosis and prevention of the high mortality. B-mode ultrasonography and pelvic examination should be helpful in confirming their diagnosis. Elective repair should be carried out without delay.

Aneurysm of Common Iliac Artery

Through a transperitoneal exposure using a medial xiphopubic laparotomy, the distal portion of the abdominal aorta below the inferior mesenteric artery is mobilized. The posterior wall of the aorta is freed, care being taken to avoid

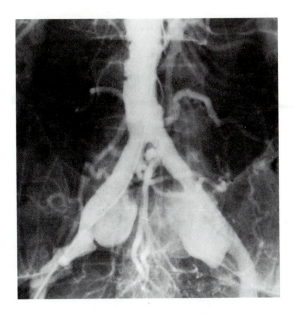

Figure 50-1. Aortogram depicting bilateral iliac aneurysms.

injuring the vena cava. Next is the exposure of the iliac arteries. On the right, this is accomplished by retracting the cecum and terminal ileum and, on the left, the sigmoid colon, after which the posterior parietal peritoneum is incised along the iliac axis. Then the origins of both the external and internal iliac arteries are mobilized.

Depending on the degree of its adhesion to its satellite vein, the aneurysm may be mobilized and separated completely from it or may be handled by opening the aneurysm, evacuating the thrombi, and controlling the bleeding from inside the sac by suture ligatures of the ostia of the collaterals (Fig. 50-2).

In the first instance, a 10 mm woven or knitted Dacron graft is inserted end-to-end between the two transected ends of the common iliac and its bifurcation (Fig. 50-2A).

In the second instance, the implantation of the graft is carried out by the intrasaccular method (Fig. 50-2C). If the proximal and distal ends of the aneurysm are not transected completely, the posterior row of the anastomosis is sutured through the undivided posterior wall in a fashion similar to that indicated for an abdominal aortic aneurysm. (See Chapter 47.)

Figure 50-2. Iliac aneurysms and the methods for their replacement with grafts. **A**1. Isolated common iliac aneurysm. **A**2. Its replacement with an end-to-end prosthetic graft. **B**1. Aneurysm of common and external iliac arteries. **B**2. Replacement with a prosthetic end-to-end graft. Note ligation of the divided internal iliac artery. **C**1. After partial excision of the aneurysmal sac of a common and external iliac aneurysm, prosthetic graft implantation was carried out by the intrasaccular method, using an end-to-end procedure. **C**2. The residual aneurysmal sac surrounding the prosthetic graft was sutured around the latter. Note ligation of the divided internal iliac artery.

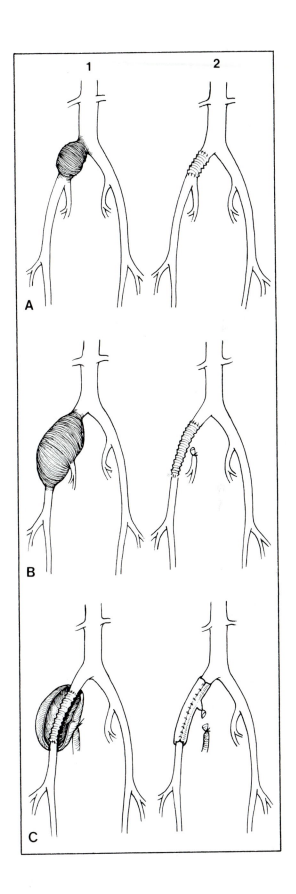

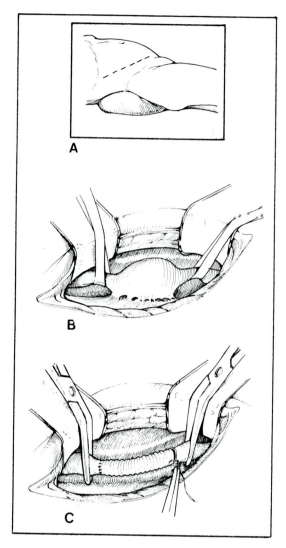

Figure 50-3. A. Position of the patient and the line of abdominal skin incision for an extraperitoneal approach to the iliac arteries. **B.** Isolation of the proximal and distal arterial tree to the iliac aneurysm. **C.** Implantation of graft after complete excision of the aneurysm.

The most serious complication to avoid in mobilizing the iliac aneurysm is injury to the adjacent iliac vein or origin of the inferior vena cava and to the ureter.

Aneurysm of External Iliac Artery

Exposure of an external iliac aneurysm by an extraperitoneal approach is adequate, easy, and safe. (For details of exposure, see Chapter 17.) The aneurysm is mobilized after gaining control of the common, internal, and distal external iliac arteries just above Poupart's ligament. Then, depending on the degree of adhesion between the aneurysm and adjacent structures, the lesion is excised either completely or partially, and a graft is interposed by the end-to-end procedure (Fig. 50-3).

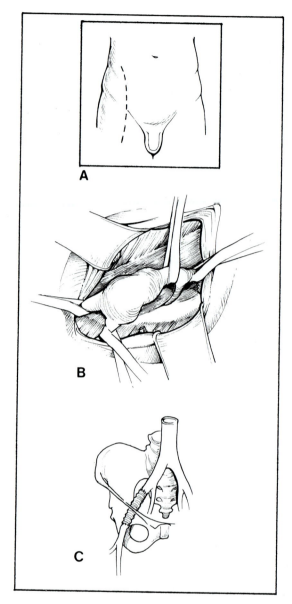

Figure 50-4. Iliofemoral aneurysm. **A.** Line indicating combined abdominal and groin skin incision for exposure of the aneurysm. **B.** Note mobilization of the iliofemoral aneurysm and the ends of transected Poupart's ligament. **C.** Iliofemoral graft in place above and below Poupart's ligament.

Iliofemoral Aneurysm

If the external iliac aneurysm extends beyond Poupart's ligament, a combined iliac and femoral approach through a single incision is indicated (Fig. 50-4). The ligament is divided for the exposure, mobilization, and implantation of the graft, but it is reconstructed at the end of the procedure.

Combined Common and External Iliac Aneurysms

An extraperitoneal approach to a combined common and external iliac aneurysm is often feasible if the proximal segment of the common iliac artery is uninvolved. Otherwise, a transperitoneal approach is used. Control of the proximal segment of the common iliac artery, of the distal external iliac artery, and of the internal iliac artery is achieved by observing the precautions mentioned previously for the isolated segments. In the event that the aneurysm is densely adherent to the adjacent vein, an intrasaccular procedure is carried out. In the presence of a bilateral iliac involvement, a transperitoneal approach is obviously indicated, with reconstruction of at least one of the internal iliac arteries to avoid large bowel ischemia.

Aneurysm of the Internal Iliac Artery

The location of an internal iliac aneurysm within the pelvis often precludes an early diagnosis. As it enlarges, it produces pressure symptoms, distorting one or both ureters, the bladder, urethra, or rectum. The aneurysm may be first noted during a rectal or vaginal examination as part of an evaluation for gastrointestinal or genitourinary symptoms.

Management of the unilateral nonruptured internal iliac (hypogastric) aneurysm, and especially that of bilateral lesions, should be performed through a transperitoneal approach. Clamping the origin of the common iliac artery and the external iliac artery close to the origin of the hypogastric artery is first carried out. Dissection of the aneurysm may be extremely laborious, and an attempt at excising the whole aneurysm or dissecting all the branches in the pelvic depth may be troublesome. After gaining control of the segment of the hypogastric beyond the aneurysm, the anterior wall is excised, and control of backbleeding is achieved by suture ligation of the ostia of the branch vessels, using the obliterative aneurysmorrhaphy technique. The distal end of the aneurysm is then oversewn.

In the presence of ruptured hypogastric artery aneurysm, the reported mortality rates are high, ranging from 29 to 80%.

Ligation of the hypogastric artery may suffice for small aneurysms but is inadequate for aneurysms compressing adjacent viscera. Complete resection of large hypogastric aneurysms may be difficult and dangerous because of the close proximity of the ureters, bowel, and other major vessels. The best way to deal with such an aneurysm is by ligating it, removing the laminated thrombi, excising most of the aneurysmal wall, and performing an obliterative aneurysmorrhaphy.

REFERENCES

1. Baron HC: Isolated aneurysm of internal iliac artery. NY State J Med 1884, 1979.
2. Lowry SF, Kraft RO: Isolated aneurysms of the iliac artery. Arch Surg 113:1289, 1978.
3. Markowitz AM, Norman JC: Aneurysms of the iliac artery. Ann Surg 154:777, 1961.
4. Silver D, Anderson EE, Porter JM: Isolated hypogastric artery aneurysm. Arch Surg 95:308, 1967.
5. Wirthlin LS, Warshaw AL: Ruptured aneurysms of the hypogastric artery. Surgery 73:629, 1973.
6. Chapman EM, Shaw RS, Kubik CS: Sciatic pain from arteriosclerotic aneurysm of pelvic arteries. N Engl J Med 271:1410, 1964.

CHAPTER 51
Peripheral Arterial Aneurysms

Henry Haimovici

HISTORICAL BACKGROUND

Because of the greater accessibility of peripheral aneurysms, the history of their surgical treatment antedated that of intraabdominal and intrathoracic aneurysms. The earliest procedure, ligation of the artery performed either proximal or distal or both to the aneurysmal sac, was applied by a number of surgeons during the eighteenth and nineteenth centuries. Anel[1] used a ligature as near the sac as possible to prevent rupture of a traumatic brachial aneurysm. John Hunter[2] applied the high ligation method in the management of a popliteal aneurysm in the canal that bears his name. Astley Cooper, in 1817, ligated the bifurcation of the aorta for a rapidly expanding left iliac aneurysm. He had already carried out a similar procedure for the common carotid artery a few years before.[3]

In 1888, Matas[4] introduced his classic procedure of endoaneurysmorrhaphy in a case of traumatic aneurysm of the left brachial artery. In this instance he placed the ligatures immediately above and below the sac, which was then opened. The thrombi were then evacuated and the orifices of supply vessels closed in the sac itself. Matas stated, "It is accomplishing this last result that we had an opportunity for observing the advantages gained by the improved technique of the present day."[4] This technique, which he subsequently modified and improved by maintaining the arterial continuity, is still used today, either alone or in combination with other reconstructive procedures.

Excision of an aneurysm with reestablishment of arterial continuity by means of a graft, today's mainstay of vascular repair, was first carried out in 1906 by Goyanes,[5] who resected a popliteal aneurysm and replaced it with the adjacent popliteal vein. Lexer, in 1907, excised a fusiform aneurysm of the iliac artery and restored the arterial continuity by means of a long venous autograft.[6] This method of restoring arterial continuity was used during World War I by Lexer,[7] Subbotitch,[8] and others.

The present era, however, dates back to 1951, when Dubost, of Paris, first excised an abdominal aortic aneurysm,

with graft replacement,[9] and thus paved the way for its application to all aneurysms.

Peripheral aneurysms are recognized with increasing frequency as a result of the extended life span for older-age-group patients, who are more prone to arteriosclerosis, the most common cause of aneurysms. It behooves physicians to detect the aneurysms before their potential serious and disabling complications occur, so that reconstructive arterial surgery can be applied electively and successfully.

ANEURYSMS OF THE LOWER EXTREMITY

Aneurysms of the lower extremity originate infrequently in the femoral, most often in the popliteal, and very rarely in the tibial arteries.

Irrespective of the involved arterial segment, the common denominator of all aneurysms is the underlying weakness of the arterial wall, induced by arteriosclerotic, mycotic, syphilitic, traumatic, or dissecting lesions. By far the most common or almost exclusive cause is arteriosclerosis. Mycotic aneurysms usually follow septic emboli and are rare. The role of syphilis, significant in the past, is uncommon today. Acute trauma usually produces a false aneurysm or arteriovenous fistula rather than a typical aneurysm. Primary dissecting aneurysms of the peripheral arteries, often following trauma, are extremely rare.[10]

If untreated, these peripheral aneurysms may result in a high incidence of arterial thrombosis and of gangrene leading to amputation or even death. Although they may also rupture, this is a rare complication in contrast to that occurring in abdominal or thoracic aneurysms (Table 51-1).

Femoral Aneurysms

The *incidence* of femoral aneurysms is about one third of all peripheral aneurysms and is only 14.3% of popliteal aneurysms (Table 51-2). Primary femoral aneurysms usually

670

TABLE 51-1. COMPLICATIONS OF ANEURYSMS: RELATIVE INCIDENCE

	Rupture	Thrombo-embolism	Compression
Abdominal			
Aorta	Frequent	Occasional	Rare
Iliac	Frequent	Occasional	Rare
Peripheral			
Femoral	Rare	Frequent	Occasional
Popliteal	Rare	Frequent	Occasional
Tibial	Rare	Frequent	Occasional

are of arteriosclerotic origin and are fusiform in shape. Their diagnosis can be made by palpation along the course of the femoral artery axis. Physical examination often permits accurate assessment of location and extent, along with the patency of the vessel. Plain roentgenograms may assist in delineating the extent of the lesion. More accurate evaluation is provided by B-scan ultrasound and arteriography. Ultrasound scan,[17,18] a noninvasive and painless method, is being used widely in delineating both femoral and popliteal aneurysms, as well as other peripheral arterial aneurysms. However, arteriography should be used for accurate visualization of the peripheral vessels when palpation indicates that arterial flow is diminished distal to the aneurysm. It thus provides precise knowledge of the associated vascular lesions, especially if occlusive arterial disease is suspected (Figs. 51-1 and 51-2). Pappas et al.[19] showed that the percentages of the various locations of the aneurysms along the femoral artery were as follows: common femoral, 27; superficial, 26; iliofemoral, 14; femoral-popliteal, 13; and profunda femoris, 1. In 19% the exact location was not ascertained. Femoral aneurysms were bilateral in 36[19] to 47%.[20] Multiple aneurysms in various sites are encountered in about two thirds of the cases.[19,20] The most commonly associated aneurysms are located in the aorta, popliteal artery, and iliac artery, in that order.

The clinical picture is variable. About one third of these aneurysms are asymptomatic, one third expand or rupture, 16% present as acute thrombosis, and 16% as chronic thrombosis.[20] Associated peripheral occlusive arterial disease or coexisting occlusion of a popliteal aneurysm may further complicate the clinical picture. Obviously, in such instances, arteriography is essential to delineate not only the state of the femoral aneurysm but also that of the distal arterial tree. In addition to expansion or rupture or acute or subacute thrombosis, other complications are often due to local pressure symptoms from nerve and vein compression and thrombosis with pulmonary embolism. Except for 29% of asymptomatic limbs, Cutler and Darling[20] found that about 70% of their cases presented rather urgent or emergent indications for repair. The exact incidence of these complications varies with reported series but is generally high. The consensus in recommending an aggressive approach in the management of femoral aneurysms is based on the high complication rate. From all evidence, it appears that when asymptomatic aneurysms are excised and replaced with grafts, the results are excellent, requiring no amputation. This is in contrast to those that are symptomatic because of various peripheral complications leading to poor patency of the graft or poor outflow, which results in failure in the majority of cases, leading to amputation. Management of femoral aneurysms consists essentially of resection and graft replacement. Because of the easy accessibility of these lesions, surgical correction is simple and ideal and should take place before complications occur, especially thrombosis, the incidence of which ranges between 26 and 32%.[19,20]

Surgical Technique

The lower region of the abdomen, the groin, and the thigh down to the knee are prepared and draped in the usual manner. A slightly curved incision, with the concavity medialward, is made over the aneurysm, extending both proximal and distal to it. The exposure should be sufficiently long to allow cross-clamping of the uninvolved arteries and should first be carried out distal to the aneurysm to avoid dislodging emboli.

The approach to a femoral aneurysm should include exposure of the distal segment of the external iliac if the aneurysmal sac extends under Poupart's ligament. Otherwise, only a division of the latter may be necessary to obtain

TABLE 51-2. SITES OF EXTRAPOPLITEAL ANEURYSMS ASSOCIATED WITH 553 POPLITEAL ANEURYSMS

	Gifford et al.[11]	Baird et al.[12]	Crichlow and Roberts[13]	Wychulis et al.[14]	Buda et al.[15]	Chitwood et al.[16]	Totals	Percent
Thoracic aorta	2	—	—	14	4	—	20	8.0
Abdominal aorta	8	6	6	53	9	8	90	34.8
Common iliac	4	7	—	28	—	1	40	16.0
Internal iliac	—	—	—	7	2	—	9	3.5
External iliac	—	—	—	2	10	—	12	4.8
Common femoral	9	—	4	40	7	1	61	22.8
Superficial femoral	—	4	—	4	10	—	18	6.9
Abdominal visceral arteries	—	—	—	1	3	—	4	1.6
Dorsalis pedis	1	2	—	—	—	—	3	1.2
Cerebral	—	—	—	—	1	—	1	0.4
Totals	24	19	10	139	46	10	258	100.0

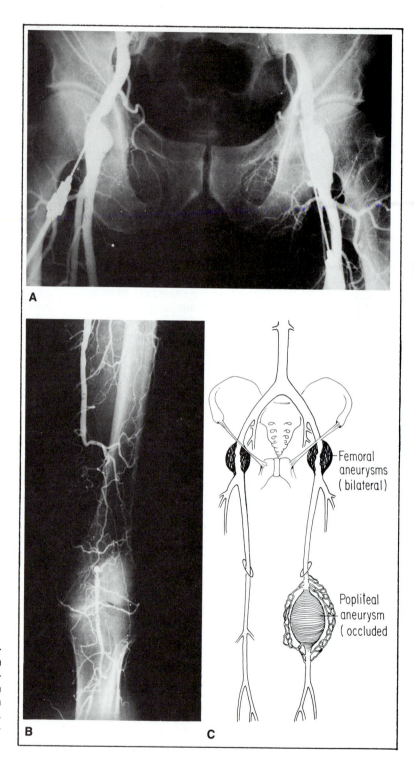

Figure 51-1. A. Bilateral femoral arteriogram showing aneurysms of the common femorals in a 66-year-old man. **B.** Arteriogram in the same patient, showing occlusion of the left popliteal artery, found at operation to be a thrombosed popliteal aneurysm. **C.** Diagram depicting the composite arteriographic findings in **A** and **B.**

exposure of the distal end of the external iliac. The next step consists of mobilizing the superficial femoral, distal to the aneurysmal sac. This is followed by exposing the posterolateral aspect of the aneurysmal sac and the profunda femoris.

Pitfalls to avoid in freeing the aneurysmal sac are injuries to the femoral nerve laterally and the femoral vein medially. If dense adhesions exist between the aneurysm and the adjacent structures, it is best to excise only the anterior wall of the aneurysmal sac and reestablish continuity of the arterial flow by intrasaccular reconstruction.

If the sac is just above the bifurcation of the femoral, the distal anastomosis is carried out into the common stump of the superficial and profunda femoral vessels.

In the case of involvement of the superficial femoral, the profunda femoris is transected and reanastomosed into

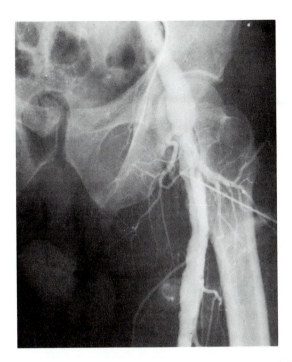

Figure 51-2. Femoral arteriogram depicting diffuse aneurysmal dilation of the common and superficial femoral arteries in a 52-year-old man. One year later a popliteal aneurysm developed on the same side, as depicted in Figure 51-7.

aneurysm need not be excised completely in the presence of dense adhesions to the adjacent structures. If the profunda femoris has to be transected, it is advantageous to leave a portion of the back wall of the aneurysm in continuity with the profunda femoris in order to facilitate its suturing to the prosthetic graft. Restoration of arterial flow via the profunda femoris is essential. The graft most commonly used is 6 to 8 mm in diameter and consists of polytetrafluoroethylene (PTFE) or Dacron or autogenous vein graft.

In the presence of a thrombosed aneurysm involving the origin of both the superficial and profunda, a thrombectomy of the latter should be performed before reanastomosing it to the prosthesis. Since it is not unusual to find atheromatous plaques at the origin of the profunda, it is often necessary to carry out a thromboendarterectomy that may extend to the first or second perforating branches. This is especially imperative in the event of coexisting occlusive arterial disease of the superficial femoral artery. (See Chapter 28.)

The results of excision of the aneurysm with autogenous vein or prosthetic graft replacement are generally excellent.[12,19,20] Thus Cutler and Darling[20] reported 83% graft patency at 5 years but a much poorer prognosis if the superficial femoral is occluded and the patency of the profunda is not maintained for long periods. The key to good long-term results depends, among other factors, on the continued patency of the profunda femoris.

Popliteal Aneurysms

Of the peripheral aneurysms, popliteal aneurysm is by far the most common. As in the case of the femoral artery in Scarpa's triangle, the popliteal has less protection by muscles and is subject to frequent bending. In the presence of arteriosclerotic changes, frequent flexion of the knee is

the graft, which is implanted into the superficial femoral (Fig. 51-3).

Although endarterectomy or thrombectomy may be used occasionally in small aneurysms, the most adequate procedure is excision and restoration of blood flow with insertion of a prosthesis or a vein autogenous graft. The

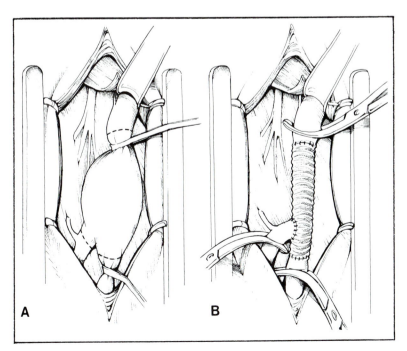

Figure 51-3. A. Diagram illustrating an aneurysm of the common femoral artery involving the origin of the superficial and profunda vessels. Note the lines of transection of the common, superficial, and profunda femorals. **B.** Diagram showing replacement of the aneurysm with a tubular graft and implantation of the profunda into the side of the plastic tube.

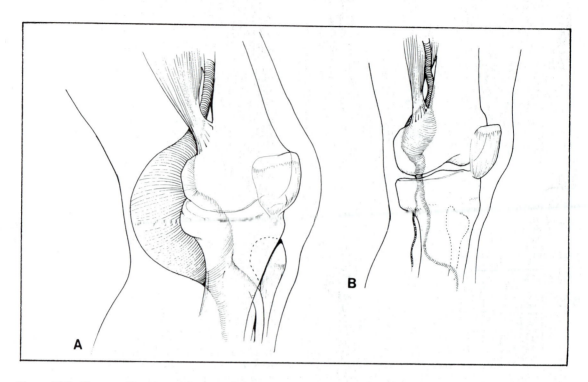

Figure 51-4. Diagrams illustrating the role of poststenotic dilatation in the development of popliteal aneurysms distal to the tendinous hiatus of the adductor magnus. **A.** Large fusiform aneurysm of the entire popliteal artery. **B.** Smaller fusiform popliteal aneurysm with a normal distal artery.

TABLE 51-3. POPLITEAL ANEURYSMS: CLINICAL FEATURES AND COMPLICATIONS

Authors	No. of Patients	No. of Limbs	Male/ Female	Bi-lateral	Extra-popliteal Aneurysm	Diabetes	Thrombosis Acute	Thrombosis Chronic	Embo-lism	Gan-grene	Rupture
Gifford et al.[11] (1953)	69	100	66/3	31	24	1	20	8	14	20	16
Edmunds et al.[22] (1965)	82	98	81/1	26	12	4	23	36	—	12	4
Baird et al.[12] (1966)	36	51	33/3	15	19	3	22	7	17	14	3
Crichlow and Roberts[13] (1966)	42	48	42/0	6	10	—	11	5	19	4	3
Wychulis et al.[14] (1970)	152	233	148/4	89	69	52	65	—	23	28	6
Evans et al.[23] (1971)	36	56	36/0	20	18	2	20	15	15	4	15
Buda et al.[15] (1974)	64	86	62/2	22	46	—	15	39	11	—	5
Hardy et al.[24] (1975)	23	31	21/2	8	10	—	11	10	3	4	2
Towne et al.[25] (1969)	80	115	75/5	36	—	—	33	14	5	—	2
Chitwood et al.[16] (1978)	26	35	25/1	11	11	—	—	7	5	5	—
Inahara and Toledo[26] (1978)	30	40	28/2	14	19	2	11	7	—	2	1
Totals	640	893	617/23	278	249	64	231	148	112	90	46

recognized as a factor predisposing one to dilatation of the vessel. The possibility that poststenotic dilatation plays a role in the development of popliteal aneurysms is supported by observations that these aneurysms arise distal to points of external compression of the artery by the tendinous hiatus of the adductor magnus in the lower medial thigh and possibly at the level of the arcuate popliteal ligament behind the knee.[21] The popliteal aneurysmal sac is almost always elongated and fusiform, tapering distally until it resumes a normal size (Fig. 51-4 and Tables 51-2 and 51-3).

Anatomic Forms

Morphologically, popliteal aneurysms may be divided into three types, according to their location:

1. Proximal: often multilobular, usually large, and occupying the area behind the condyles of the femur (Figs. 51-5, 51-6, and 51-7)

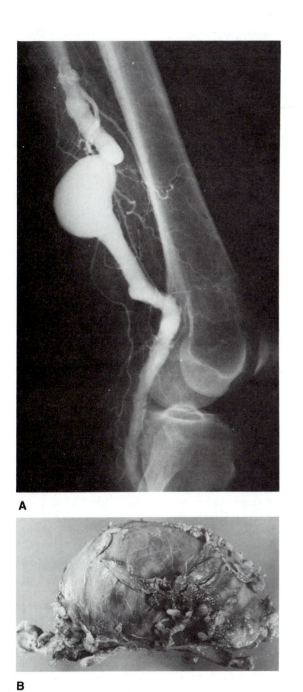

A

B

Figure 51-5. A. Arteriogram of a popliteal aneurysm. **B.** Specimen of the aneurysm removed at surgery, extending from midthigh to just above the knee joint. Note the marked disparity in size between the lesion and that depicted by the arteriogram.

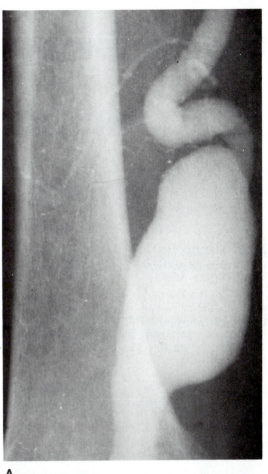

A

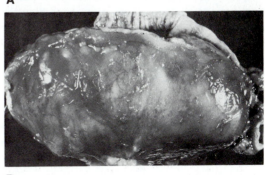

B

Figure 51-6. A. Arteriogram indicating a popliteal aneurysm with marked tortuosity of the proximal popliteal at its junction with the superficial femoral. **B.** Note the large size (14 cm long) of the specimen removed at surgery. See cross section in Figure 51-11.

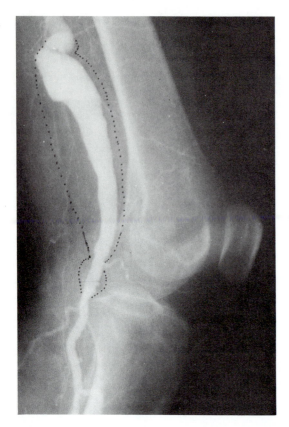

Figure 51-7. Arteriogram depicting a popliteal aneurysm of the same patient having the diffuse femoral aneurysm in Figure 51-2.

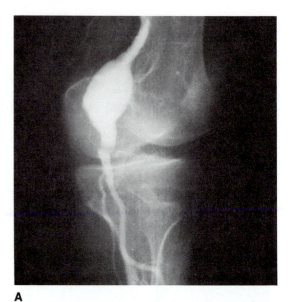

A

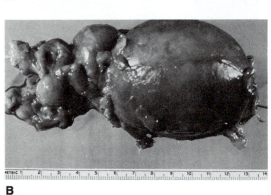

B

Figure 51-8. A. Arteriogram depicting a middle popliteal aneurysm. **B.** Specimen removed at surgery. Note the disparity between the arteriogram and the size of the specimen.

2. Middle: extending both proximally and distally around the knee joint space (Fig. 51-8)
3. Distal: usually smaller than the preceding two forms (Figs. 51-9 and 51-10)

The proximal type may be palpated both from the medial aspect of the lower third of the thigh and from the posterior. The second and third types can be palpated only from the posterior aspect of the popliteal space. The proximal form is usually a large mass containing both laminated and recent thrombi and may develop serious complications (Fig. 51-11). The smaller aneurysms are often silent and may not become clinically conspicuous until they thrombose. Their onset may be an acute occlusion with severe ischemia of the limb. When gangrene develops, its cause may become evident only after examination of the amputated leg.

Associated Cardiovascular Lesions

Popliteal aneurysms, like similar lesions elsewhere, are associated with a high incidence of coexistent cardiovascular diseases, of which arterial hypertension is present in almost one of two patients. Preexisting occlusive arterial disease in approximately 60% of the involved limbs (acute and chronic thrombosis) is an important feature of this aneurysm (Table 51-3). In most of these patients, the nature of the occlusion is considered to be arteriosclerosis obliterans, but in some others it is difficult to determine whether the occlusion is a complication of the aneurysm due to thromboem-

bolism or whether it is a result of coexisting atherosclerotic occlusion. Another important feature of this lesion is the presence of bilateral popliteal aneurysms in a large percentage of cases. Aneurysms at other arterial locations are frequently associated with those of the popliteal, the most common being in the abdominal aorta (34.8%) and femoral, common, and superficial (29.7%) (Tables 51-2 and 51-3).

Diagnosis

Diagnosis of a popliteal aneurysm is usually made by a careful inspection and palpation of the popliteal space. An expansile, pulsatile mass in the popliteal space is the characteristic finding. Aneurysms that are occluded by thrombus are felt as firm, often rather hard, nonpulsatile masses. In these cases the differential diagnosis must consider the presence of benign tumors, such as lipomas and fibromas, and synovial herniations (Baker's cysts). In such cases, to rule out a nonvascular lesion of the popliteal space, one can make the differential diagnosis by B-scan ultrasound (Fig. 51-12). This noninvasive technique has proved helpful in delineating the lesion and differentiating it from other popli-

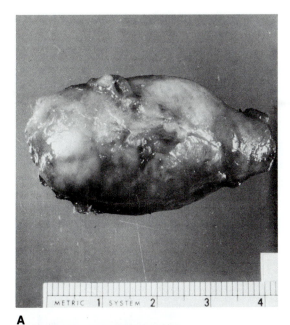

A

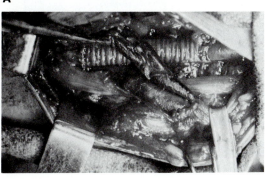

B

Figure 51-9. A. Specimen of a middle popliteal aneurysm. **B.** Its replacement with a Dacron tubular graft.

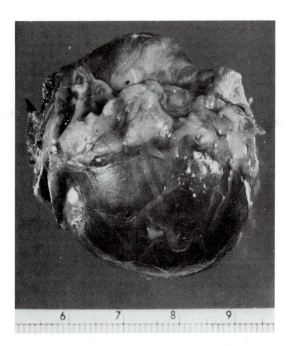

Figure 51-10. Specimen of a small popliteal aneurysm that presented as an acute occlusion of the vessel, producing severe ischemia of the leg and foot. Treatment consisted of lumbar sympathectomy combined with a popliteal graft.

teal masses. However, arteriography may be necessary for assessing the condition of the leg and foot arteries.

Operative Technique and Repair of Aneurysm

Management of popliteal aneurysms consists ideally of resection of the lesion with reestablishment of the continuity of the arterial tree, either with prosthetic material or with a vein.

Five main surgical modalities or variations thereof are available:

1. Complete excision of the aneurysm with graft interposition replacement. This is mostly applicable in small aneurysms.
2. Exclusion of the aneurysm, with ligation both proximal and distal to the sac, combined with a saphenous vein or prosthetic bypass graft.[27]
3. Partial excision of the sac with preservation of collaterals by intrasaccular suture of the ostia and implantation of a graft as an end-to-end intrasaccular procedure.
4. Use of the Matas operation of obliterative endoaneurysmorrhaphy without insertion of a graft. Lord,[28] in

35 Matas procedures carried out without any additional graft, reported loss of only two limbs, which were not salvageable anyway because of marked preoperative ischemia.[28]
5. Lumbar sympathectomy may be used as an adjunctive procedure with any of the above-mentioned modalities, its scope being to provide better collateral flow in the presence of distal occlusive disease of the leg not amenable to direct surgical reconstruction.[29]

Operative Approaches

A popliteal aneurysm may be approached with the patient in three different positions: (1) *medial* aspect of the thigh and leg, (2) *posterior* aspect of the popliteal space, and (3)

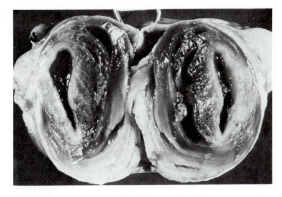

Figure 51-11. Cross section of the popliteal aneurysm shown in Figure 51-6B, indicating thick laminated thrombi resulting in a narrow lumen.

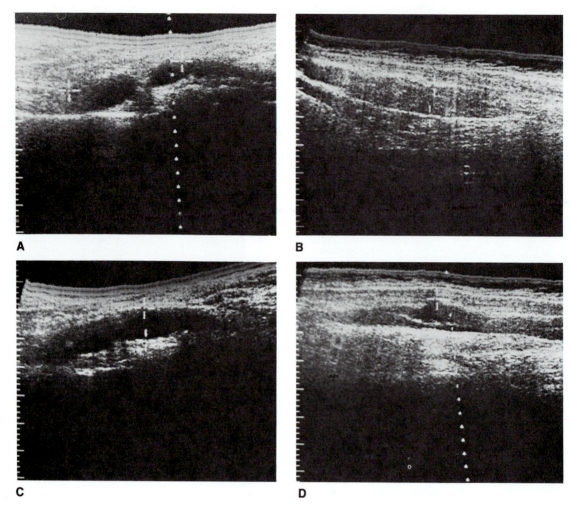

Figure 51-12. Sonograms of popliteal and superficial femoral arteries of both lower extremities. All sonograms are in sagittal views. **A.** Left popliteal aneurysm. Length between the two marks is 8.4 cm. Diameter at its widest point is 2 cm. **B.** Left superficial femoral artery aneurysm. Diameter at its largest point is 2 cm. **C.** Right popliteal aneurysm. Diameter is 2 cm. **D.** Right superficial femoral artery aneurysm. Diameter is 2.2 cm. Note that the left popliteal and superficial femoral aneurysms were thrombosed, and the right popliteal and superficial aneurysms were patent. (*Courtesy of Ruth Rosenblatt, M.D.*)

lateral position with the affected lower extremity down on the table with the opposite leg flexed.

The medial and posterior exposures (Fig. 51-13) have different indications according to the location and size of the aneurysm. The lateral exposure, in our experience, is rather cumbersome and is no longer used by us.

Medial Approach. The patient is placed in the supine position, the lower extremity in slight external rotation with the knee in 30-degree flexion and supported by a rolled sheet. The skin incision is made in the lower third of the thigh, extending toward the midthigh proximally and along the anterior border of the sartorius muscle medial to the knee. After the deep fascia is opened, the sartorius muscle is retracted medially and posteriorly. The popliteal space is entered below the adductor magnus tendon. The sartorius, semimembranosus, gracilis, and semitendinosus muscles may have to be transected near the tibia if better exposure of the aneurysm and the distal popliteal is indicated.

The superficial femoral may have to be exposed if the aneurysm originates distal to the foramen of the adductor magnus. The distal portion of the popliteal below the aneurysm must be mobilized and tape placed about it before handling of the aneurysm per se. If the aneurysm can be mobilized easily from the adjacent structures, it can be excised and a graft inserted in the usual fashion. Otherwise, any of the other modalities as described above should be used to restore continuity to the arterial flow.

Posterior Approach. A long S-shaped skin incision is made, with the superior limb of the incision placed more medially. The advantage of this incision vs. the one described above is that no muscles are transected for exposure of the vessels (Fig. 51-13B).

The popliteal fascia is opened, care being taken to avoid the sciatic or the tibial branch of the latter. The nerve at this level crosses from the medial to the lateral side and superficially to the popliteal artery, giving off several

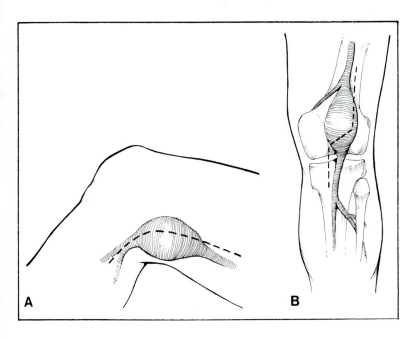

Figure 51-13. Diagrams of approaches to the popliteal artery. **A.** Medial. **B.** Posterior.

branches on its way. A Vesseloop is placed about it, and it is retracted out of the operative field.

Distal control of the aneurysm is first obtained below it by retracting the head of the gastrocnemius muscle. The popliteal vein can be freed at this level and preserved.

Proximal control is obtained after retracting the biceps femoris muscle laterally and the hamstring muscles medially. The popliteal artery above the aneurysm is first identified by palpation, and then mobilized and separated from the adjacent popliteal vein. This vein is often firmly attached to the aneurysm and may not be easy to separate, in which case it may have to be sacrificed between two ligatures. This is especially true in the presence of a large aneurysm. The latter is then excised either completely or partially, as described above.

After the proximal anastomosis is completed first, the graft is pulled down under tension and tailored to the correct length before undertaking the distal anastomosis. For the latter, the posterior row is carried out by intraluminal sutures, using 4-0 synthetic suture material. Before the anterior row of sutures is undertaken, the distal clamp is removed to check the runoff. A Fogarty embolectomy catheter is introduced distally to ascertain its freedom from any possible emboli or thrombi.

Closure of the popliteal fascia should be carefully carried out by having the assistant approximate the two edges of the wound to minimize any tension on the suture line. Drainage is not generally used. Application of a posterior padded splint may be more helpful in this approach than in the medial, so that flexion of the knee is avoided, especially when a synthetic graft is used.

Indications for the Type of Repair of Popliteal Aneurysm

Resection of a popliteal aneurysm with end-to-end anastomosis of the cut ends of the artery is feasible in small lesions, provided there is enough arterial length left after its removal.

In larger aneurysms, resection with graft interposition is indicated if the popliteal vein and the branches of the sciatic nerve can be easily freed without injury to them.

Since avoidance of injuries to the collaterals, nerves, and veins may not always be possible, exclusion of the aneurysm with a bypass graft has been increasingly accepted as a better alternative to the aneurysmectomy procedure. The obvious advantages are the avoidance of the above-mentioned complications. However, leaving in place a large aneurysm that causes symptoms of compression of the sciatic nerve and of its branches may not be relieved by the exclusion of the aneurysm alone. In such instances, an obliterative endoaneurysmorrhaphy (Matas procedure) after ligation of the popliteal artery and evacuation of its contents should be added to the exclusion procedure. This should then relieve all symptoms of compression.

The *results* of the repair of the popliteal artery are excellent in uncomplicated cases. The long-term patency of the graft is partly determined by the extent of occlusive disease in the distal vessels. Thus, in two recent statistical studies, 80% of the patients were asymptomatic, and 5 to 8.5% remained symptomatic (intermittent claudication). In complicated cases, the rate of amputation ranged from 10.5 to 16.6%. All popliteal aneurysms, like those of the femoral, should be treated surgically, and arterial continuity should be restored unless contraindicated by the poor medical condition of the patient.

Tibial Aneurysms

Aneurysms of the tibial arteries are usually the result of trauma.[30] Arteriosclerotic aneurysms of these vessels are very uncommon, having been seen by Pappas et al.[19] in only 1% of 72 cases. When trauma is the sole etiologic factor, the result is usually a false aneurysm. True posttraumatic aneurysms of these vessels have rarely been reported. Diagnosis of such lesions can be made by arteriography or rather B-mode ultrasonography. Excision of the lesions with vein graft replacement is the method of choice. Associated necrotic lesions of the toes should be treated by local amputation after repair of the aneurysm.

ANEURYSMS OF THE UPPER EXTREMITY

Aneurysms are found less commonly in the upper extremity than in the lower. The majority of cases are due to arterial trauma and less frequently to mycotic or necrotizing arteritis and arteriosclerosis. The arteries most often involved are the subclavian, axillary, and brachial, and less commonly those of the wrist or hand.

Subclavian Aneurysms

Aneurysms of the subclavian artery may be due to a post-stenotic compression mechanism or to arteriosclerosis.

The *subclavian artery,* which is situated in the narrow, rigid confines of the thoracic outlet, is subject to extrinsic pressure and aneurysm formation. (See Chapter 60.) This mechanism was first described by Halsted,[31] although aneurysms were observed in the latter part of the nineteenth and early part of the twentieth centuries. Thrombosis of the sac and distal embolization are often seen in advanced cases. (See Chapter 61.) Thromboembolism of the upper extremity as a result of compression and damage of the subclavian is most often associated with damage of a cervical rib.[32]

Treatment of this thoracic outlet thromboembolic syndrome consists of removal of the bony structures responsible for the arterial damage, specifically of the cervical rib, together with resection of the aneurysm and restoration of arterial continuity with a saphenous vein or prosthetic graft. In some cases, only decompression of the artery or a cervico-thoracic sympathectomy may be necessary. (See Chapters 60 and 61 for details.)

Atherosclerotic aneurysms involving the subclavian artery may occur either in an anomalous artery or in an otherwise normal subclavian vessel. They are rare. Crawford et al.[33] reported only 3 such cases in a series of 107 peripheral aneurysms. Hobson et al.[34] reported 4 atherosclerotic aneurysms in 3 adult men and reviewed the literature on this subject. They again pointed out the extreme rarity of isolated atherosclerotic lesions of the subclavian in spite of an increasing awareness of these lesions both because of an aging population and better diagnostic methods.

The surgical repair of aneurysms involving the subclavian artery, exclusive of the aortic arch and innominate artery, is essentially similar for those lesions associated with the thoracic outlet syndrome, excluding the abnormal bony structures. A supraclavicular approach with resection of the medial clavicle is used. The resection of the aneurysm with interposition of an autogenous vein graft or a plastic tube is satisfactory.

Axillary Aneurysms

Axillary aneurysms are usually asymptomatic unless ischemic phenomena occur after thromboembolic complications. Those reported in the literature are usually due to open injury in the axilla as a result of a knife or bullet wound. Owing to the close proximity of the cords and divisions of the brachial plexus, neurologic symptoms are not uncommon with axillary aneurysms and vascular injuries. Szuchmacher and Freed[35] reported on two patients, one with a bilateral arteriosclerotic aneurysm and another with an isolated axillary lesion. Both patients were male and had a history of pain, pallor, cyanosis, and loss of power of the forearm. A pulsatile, palpable symptomatic mass was detected in the second patient. Evaluation of the other arterial segments, namely, the aorta and other peripheral vessels, by means of sonography failed to disclose any abnormalities.

The following case of a patient seen in the vascular service at Montefiore Hospital illustrates some of the clinical and operative highlights of an axillary aneurysm.

The patient, a 68-year-old woman, was admitted for a small mass in the right axilla associated with pain of about 4 months' duration. She apparently had noticed this mass for 8 years, but it remained completely asymptomatic until 4 months before, when the pain began. All pulses in the right upper extremity were palpable. Her blood pressure was 122/80 mm Hg. An upper extremity angiogram via a right transfemoral aortogram disclosed the presence of an aneurysm of the distal axillary artery (Fig. 51-14). Surgical excision of the aneurysm was carried out, with the artery repaired by end-to-end anastomosis of the two transected segments. The histologic report of the aneurysmal sac indicated a cystic medial degeneration with intimal sclerosis but with no thrombus. Culture of a specimen from

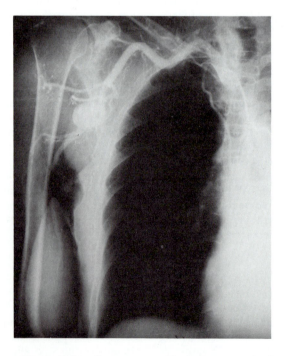

Figure 51-14. Right axillary aneurysm. The lesion was excised, and the two cut ends of the axillary artery were reanastomosed end-to-end. The patient remained free of symptoms postoperatively.

the aneurysmal wall failed to disclose any bacterial growth. The postoperative period was uneventful, and the patient was discharged a week after surgery. Follow-up showed an excellent result.

Comment

This case typifies the long asymptomatic period of axillary aneurysms, especially in the absence of neurologic or thromboembolic manifestations.

Most of the etiologic factors causing axillary aneurysms include infection, periarteritis nodosa, congenital arterial defects, and trauma. The latter remains probably the single most common cause of these aneurysms. However, atherosclerotic degenerative changes have been implicated as an associated factor in many cases. Another significant characteristic is the thromboembolic manifestations that call attention to the lesion in the axillary area. This has been observed by Szuchmacher, as well as by Savelyev, as mentioned in the chapter on arterial embolism of the upper extremity. (See Chapter 28.)

The treatment of these aneurysms is excision and interposition of a graft or ligation with a bypass graft. Associated neurologic manifestations may complicate the management of these lesions and may require repair of the trunks or branches of the brachial plexus.

Brachial Aneurysms

The majority of the brachial aneurysms are the result of trauma. The original case published by Matas and mentioned previously is a classic example of such lesions. Symptoms of the brachial aneurysm include vascular and often neurologic changes characteristic of an upper extremity aneurysm. They may remain silent for some time until thromboembolic or neurologic complications occur. Treatment of choice is excision with a vein graft replacement. Occasionally a combined thoracic sympathectomy may be necessary if distal thrombosis with severe ischemia of the hand is present.

Aneurysms of the Hand

Aneurysms of the hand are less common than the other aneurysms of the upper extremity. Most of the recorded cases occurred after trauma to the ulnar or radial arteries of the level of the wrist.[36-39] Arteriosclerotic aneurysms of the hand are rare.[39] The presenting symptom is a gradually enlarging mass that may be associated with pain and vascular insufficiency. Several reports have been published describing true and false aneurysms, the latter mostly related to blunt trauma. Because of the location in the hand, these aneurysms are seen earlier than those of the axillary or brachial regions.

The diagnosis of an *ulnar aneurysm* is made in the presence of a mass appearing in the hypothenar eminence shortly after the trauma, usually consisting of a blow or stab wound. Pain, coolness, or cyanosis of the medial fingers reflects ischemia of variable degrees. *Radial aneurysm* is diagnosed as a subcutaneous tissue pulsating expansile mass.

Treatment consists of resection of the lesion, with attempted reanastomosis of the ends of the artery, if possible. Otherwise an interposition of an autogenous vein segment is the method of choice. In the event that reconstruction of the arterial tree has been inadequate, a thoracic sympathectomy may be necessary to complete the revascularization of the hand.

EXTRACRANIAL CAROTID ARTERIAL ANEURYSMS

Although carotid arteries are frequently affected by atherosclerosis, aneurysms of these vessels are uncommon as compared with the total number of aneurysms occurring throughout the arterial tree. Houser and Baker[40] found only 8 cervical carotid aneurysms in 5000 angiograms of the cervical and cerebral arteries. In 1962, Beall et al.,[41] in studying a series of 2300 operations for arterial aneurysms, found only 7 extracranial carotid artery aneurysms in a period of 13 years. In 1979, McCollum et al.,[42] from the same institution, were able to collect 37 cases during a 21-year period during which 8500 operations were performed for peripheral artery aneurysms. It would therefore appear that in recent years, greater awareness of these lesions seems to suggest that although rare, they may be less infrequent than indicated in the past.

The *causes* of extracranial carotid aneurysms include arteriosclerosis, previous carotid surgery, trauma, local infection, syphilis, dissecting aneurysms, and congenital conditions. Most common causes today are atherosclerotic, postoperative, and traumatic. They occur most often in the fifth decade of life and involve short segments of the common and internal carotid arteries.

The incidence of false aneurysms after previous carotid operations appears to be on the rise.[43] The anastomotic aneurysms occur at the site of a carotid endarterectomy with a patch graft angioplastic closure or, more rarely, without the latter. Thus, of 44 cases of false carotid aneurysm collected by Busuttil et al.,[44] (see Chapter 49), 30, or 68%, developed this lesion when a patch had been used to close the endarterectomy incision. One of the main factors responsible for these anastomotic aneurysms is suture line infection. These anastomatic aneurysms are prone to cause embolism to the brain. The incidence of syphilitic and mycotic aneurysms has decreased considerably. Today the arteriosclerotic variety is the predominant lesion.

The threat of rupture and embolization from mural thrombi is a compelling indication for surgery even though no symptoms may be present at the time the diagnosis is first made.

Differential diagnosis includes chemodectoma of the carotid body, enlarged lymph nodes, and, more particularly, the buckled or kinked carotid artery. The last condition is more common than are true aneurysms; it occurs almost exclusively in hypertensive women, most often on the right side.[45] A useful maneuver for a differential diagnosis between a buckled artery and a true aneurysm of a common carotid artery is to have the patient inspire and hold his breath. In cases of buckled carotid or innominate artery, the prominent pulsation markedly diminishes or disappears, whereas in cases of aneurysm of the carotid artery, it does not.[45] Angiography may not be necessary because noninvasive evaluation techniques may be helpful in identifying these lesions.

Such aneurysms, in the past, resulted in high mortality rates when left untreated. With increased awareness of their existence, the greatest dangers are rupture and hemorrhage and thromboembolic complications. The last two are the most common and serious threats posed by these extracranial carotid aneurysms.

Definitive surgical treatment is recommended in most cases regardless of symptoms. The first successful surgical treatment of a cervical carotid aneurysm was performed by Sir Astley Cooper in 1808.[46] Proximal ligation remained the most frequent surgical approach to this lesion for more than a century. Dimtza,[47] in 1952, performed the first resection with restoration of continuity by primary end-to-end anastomosis. The first prosthetic graft replacement for this lesion was accomplished by Beall et al.[41] in 1959; an internal shunt was used while a Dacron graft was interposed between the two ends of the common and internal carotid arteries. Partial excision of the aneurysmal sac is recommended, especially if significant inflammation surrounds the aneurysm. Restoration of arterial continuity by interposition graft is the preferred technique. Autogenous saphenous vein, Dacron, and PTFE grafts are the various choices of the conduit for arterial substitution. In anastomotic aneurysms, in up to 50% or more of the cases involving a prosthetic suture line, there was evidence of an infectious process. Because of this important finding, autogenous tissue instead of synthetic material should be chosen for repair. Utilizing an intraluminal shunt in most, if not all, cases of carotid aneurysmectomy is particularly indicated in such procedures, which may be longer than the usual endarterectomy.

Review of the literature indicates that primary anastomosis was possible in 26 of 42, or 62%, of the patients.[48] The morbidity encountered during the postoperative period included cerebrovascular accidents, hypoglossal nerve palsy, recurrent laryngeal nerve palsy, and several other complications related to standard vascular procedures.[48]

In unusual circumstances where repair of the lesion appears too hazardous, carotid arterial ligation may be an alternative. In the face of such a problem, measurement of the stump pressure may serve to assess the safety of carotid ligation. Under these circumstances, full heparinization, beginning intraoperatively, is essential.

MULTIPLE ANEURYSMS

One of the major characteristics of peripheral aneurysms is the presence of multiple similar lesions in various locations of the arterial tree. A number of authors have reported a high incidence of multiple aneurysms associated with femoral, popliteal, or abdominal aortic aneurysms. Crawford et al.,[33] as well as Pappas et al.,[19] reported a 70% incidence of multiple aneurysms (Fig. 51-15). Cutler and Darling[20] reported that of 45 patients with femoral aneurysms, more than half had aneurysms of the distal abdominal aorta. Perhaps a higher incidence would have been

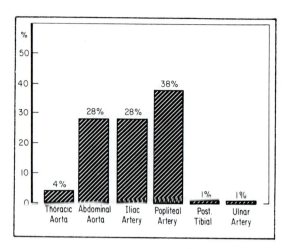

Figure 51-15. Incidence of associated aneurysms in patients with femoral aneurysms. (*Based on data from Pappas G, et al.: JAMA 190:97, 1964.*)

detected had routine arteriography been employed. Among the 37 patients with a common femoral aneurysm reported by Dent et al.,[49] 95% had a second aneurysm, 92% had an aortoiliac aneurysm, and 59% had bilateral femoral aneurysms. Among the 36 patients with a popliteal aneurysm, 78% had a second aneurysm, 64% had an aortoiliac aneurysm, and 47% had bilateral popliteal aneurysm. When a nonpalpable aortoiliac aneurysm in the presence of a peripheral one is suspected, the use of arteriography and sonography cannot be overemphasized.

Surgery for multiple aneurysms should be staged resections, starting with surgery of the most proximal and carrying out procedures on the distal ones in a later stage. Follow-up of these patients with two aneurysms is important, because they may subsequently develop other aneurysmal dilatations of the arterial tree.

MYCOTIC ANEURYSMS

Osler, in 1885, was the first to describe mycotic aneurysms that resulted from septic emboli originating from bacterial endocarditis. The infection reached the vessel either by direct embolic occlusion of the lumen or via the vasa vasorum of the arterial wall. Today the term *mycotic aneurysm* relates to a variety of infected aneurysms. They may be true or false aneurysms, in which the primary infection represents a secondary process of an already existing aneurysmal lesion. Although these aneurysms are relatively uncommon, the high mortality and morbidity rates from hemorrhage and overwhelming sepsis place these lesions in a critical category.[50,51] Infection of surgically induced arteriovenous dialysis fistulas today represents a common form of mycotic aneurysm. These lesions occur in any artery, although there is a predilection for atherosclerotic lesions at the site of branching of these arteries. In the past, before the antibiotic era, the proportion of aortic to peripheral mycotic aneurysms was relatively high. Today, the peripheral arteries are involved in 88% and the aorta in 12% of the cases; these are primarily due to arterial trauma in vascular operations involving peripheral vessels.[52]

With the control of infection and the development of reconstructive vascular procedures, prognosis of mycotic aneurysms has become more favorable. Because of a great tendency to rupture, early recognition and prompt therapy are essential. The nonspecific clinical features make diagnosis rather difficult. An associated history of present or past infection should arouse suspicion of any pulsating or non-pulsating mass, which should be delineated by appropriate sonography and arteriography.

The typical mycotic aneurysm occurs as a rapidly enlarging, warm, tender pulsatile mass in a patient with fever and a history of bacterial endocarditis, rheumatic fever, or some other source of septic embolization or septicemia. Aneurysms can be palpated in 90% of patients if located in the extremities, but rarely if centrally located. A history of recent operative or penetrating trauma to the vessel in question is important, and a systolic bruit may be present. Left untreated, the aneurysm usually ruptures either internally or externally, depending on the status of the surrounding tissues and overlying skin.

If the aneurysm is deeply situated and not palpable, the clinical picture will be that of fever of undetermined cause. Some patients may have malaise, episodes of chills and fever, and increasing weakness over a period of weeks. Fever often persists despite antibiotic therapy.

Mycotic aneurysms may occur in association with petechial skin lesions and septic arthritis due to peripheral emboli originating from an extremity aneurysm. Symptoms of cerebrovascular accident can occur with carotid lesions, and malabsorption symptoms with mycotic aneurysms of the superior mesenteric artery. Sonography and arteriography are essential in delineating and locating the lesions.

Treatment

Two main objectives dominate the management of a mycotic aneurysm: eradication of the infection, which requires excision of the aneurysm, and maintenance of adequate distal circulation. To achieve these two goals, the surgeon must carry out an emergency procedure, which should include certain basic principles: intravenous antibiotics, excision of all infected tissue, wide drainage, vessel ligation as primary treatment if necessary, and bypass grafts before resection of the aneurysm. Synthetic or heterologous grafts are contraindicated. Autologous tissue is the preferred graft. Viable tissue coverage of exposed vessels should be used, and bleeding or thrombosis should indicate persistent infection. The bypass area should be sufficiently extensive so that the anastomosis can be constructed in a more nearly normal segment of the artery. By applying these principles in mycotic aneurysms, the surgeon can achieve a reasonably low morbidity rate. This includes not only the peripheral mycotic aneurysms but the aortic as well, especially since extraanatomic bypass procedures have been employed.

REFERENCES

1. Anel D (1714): As translated by Erichsen JE (ed): Observations on Aneurysm. London, Sydenham Society, 1844, p 217.
2. Hunter J: Cited by Home E (1793), in Erichsen JE (ed): Observations on Aneurysm. London, Sydenham Society, 1844, p 388.
3. Brock RC: The Life and Work of Astley Cooper. Edinburgh and London, Livingstone, 1952, pp 47–55, 50, 57.
4. Matas R: Traumatic aneurism of left brachial artery. Med News 53:462, 1888.
5. Goyanes J: Nuevos trabajos de chirurgia vascular, substitucion plastica de las arterias por las venas o arterioplastia venosa, applicada como nuevo metodo, al tratameiento de los aneurismas. El Siglo Med 53:446, 561, 1906.
6. Lexer E: Die ideale Operation des arteriellen und des arteriovenosen Aneurysma. Arch Klin Chir 83:459, 1907.
7. Lexer E: Zwanzig Jahre Transplantationsforschung in der Chirugie. Arch Klin Chir 138:251, 1925.
8. Subbotitch V: Military experiences of traumatic aneurysms. Lancet 2:720, 1913.
9. Dubost C, Allary M, Oeconomos N: A propos du traitement des anevrysmes de l'aorte. Ablation de l'anevrysme, retablissement de la continuite par greffe d'aorte humaine conservee. Mem Acad Chir 77:38, 1951.
10. Wychulis AR, Kincaid OW, Wallace RB: Primary dissecting aneurysms of peripheral arteries. Mayo Clin Proc 44:804, 1969.
11. Gifford RW Jr, Hines EA Jr, James JM: An analysis and follow-up study of one hundred popliteal aneurysms. Surgery 33:284, 1953.
12. Baird RJ, Sivasankar R, et al: Popliteal aneurysms: A review and analysis of 61 cases. Surgery 59:911, 1966.
13. Crichlow RW, Roberts B: Treatment of popliteal aneurysms by restoration of continuity: Review of 48 cases. Ann Surg 163:417, 1966.
14. Wychulis AR, Spittell JA Jr, Wallace RB: Popliteal aneurysms. Surgery 68:942, 1970.
15. Buda JA, Weber CJ, et al: The results of treatment of popliteal artery aneurysms: A follow-up study of 86 aneurysms. J Cardiovasc Surg 15:615, 1974.
16. Chitwood WR Jr, Stocks LH, Wolfe WG: Popliteal artery aneurysm. Arch Surg 113:1078, 1978.
17. Davis RP, Neiman HL, et al: Ultrasound scan in diagnosis of peripheral aneurysms. Arch Surg 112:55, 1977.
18. Scott WW Jr, Scott PP, Sanders RC: B-scan ultrasound in the diagnosis of popliteal aneurysms. Surgery 81:436, 1977.
19. Pappas G, Janes JM, et al.: Femoral aneurysms. JAMA 190:97, 1964.
20. Cutler BS, Darling RC: Surgical management of arteriosclerotic femoral aneurysms. Surgery 74:764, 1973.
21. Gedge SW, Spittell JA Jr, Ivins JC: Aneurysm of the distal popliteal artery and its relationship to the arcuate popliteal ligament. Circulation 24:270, 1961.
22. Edmunds LH Jr, Darling RC, Linton RR: Surgical management of popliteal aneurysms. Circulation 32:517, 1965.
23. Evans WE, Conley JE, Bernhard V: Popliteal aneurysms. Surgery 70:762, 1971.
24. Hardy JD, Tompkins WC Jr, et al: Aneurysms of the popliteal artery. Surg Gynecol Obstet 140:401, 1975.
25. Towne JB, Thompson JE, et al: Progression of popliteal aneurysmal disease following popliteal aneurysm resection with graft: A twenty year experience. Surgery 99:501, 1969.
26. Inahara T, Toledo AC: Complications and treatment of popliteal aneurysms. Surgery 84:775, 1978.
27. Edwards WS: Exclusion and saphenous vein bypass of popliteal aneurysm. Surg Gynecol Obstet 128:829, 1969.
28. Lord JW Jr: Method of Rudolph Matas for obliterative endoaneurysmorrhaphy for aneurysms of the popliteal artery. Surg Gynecol Obstet 151:663, 1980.
29. Linton RR: The arteriosclerotic popliteal aneurysm: A report of 14 patients treated by preliminary lumbar ganglionectomy and aneurysmectomy. Surgery 26:41, 1949.
30. Carey LC, Stremple JF: An aneurysm of the anterior tibial artery: A case report. Angiology 18:117, 1967.

31. Halsted WS: An experimental study of circumscribed dilation of an artery immediately distal to a partially occluding band and its bearing on the dilation of the subclavian artery observed in certain cases of cervical ribs. Surgery 40:428, 1956.

32. Schein CJ, Haimovici H, Young H: Arterial thrombosis associated with cervical ribs. Surgery 40:428, 1956.

33. Crawford ES, DeBakey ME, Cooley DA: Surgical considerations of peripheral arterial aneurysms. Arch Surg 78:226, 1959.

34. Hobson RW II, Sarkaria J, et al: Atherosclerotic aneurysms of the subclavian artery. Surgery 85:368, 1979.

35. Szuchmacher PH, Freed JS: Axillary aneurysms. NY State J Med 795, 1980.

36. Gaylis H, Kushlick AR: Ulnar artery aneurysms of the hand. Surgery 73:478, 1973.

37. Malt S: An arteriosclerotic aneurysm of the hand. Arch Surg 113:762, 1978.

38. Millender LH, Nalebuff EA, Kasdon E: Aneurysms and thromboses of the ulnar artery in the hand. Arch Surg 105:686, 1972.

39. Thorrens S, Trippel OH, Bergan JJ: Arteriosclerotic aneurysms of the hand. Arch Surg 92:937, 1966.

40. Houser OW, Baker HL Jr: Fibromuscular dysplasia and other uncommon diseases of the cervical carotid artery: Angiographic aspects. Am J Roentgenol Radium Ther Nucl Med 104:201, 1968.

41. Beall AC Jr, Crawford ES, et al: Extracranial aneurysms of the carotid artery: Report of seven cases. Postgrad Med 32:93, 1962.

42. McCollum CH, Wheeler WG, et al: Aneurysms of the extracranial carotid artery. Am J Surg 137:196, 1979.

43. Ehrenfeld WK, Hays RJ: False aneurysm after carotid endarterectomy. Arch Surg 104:288, 1972.

44. Busuttil RW, Davidson RK, et al.: Selective management of extracranial carotid arterial aneurysms. Am J Surg 140:85, 1980.

45. Deterling RA Jr: Tortuous right common carotid artery simulating aneurysm. Angiology 3:483, 1952.

46. Cooper A: Account of the first successful operation performed on the common carotid artery for aneurysm in the year of 1808 with postmortem examination in the year 1821. Guys Hosp Rep 1:53, 1836.

47. Dimtza A: Aneurysm of the carotid arteries: Report of two cases. Postgrad Angiol 7:218, 1956.

48. Rittenhouse EA, Radke HM, Sumner DS: Carotid artery aneurysm: Review of the literature and report of a case with rupture into the oropharynx. Arch Surg 105:786, 1972.

49. Dent TL, Lindenauer SM, et al.: Multiple arteriosclerotic arterial aneurysms. Arch Surg 105:338, 1972.

50. Nabseth DC, Deterling RA Jr: Surgical management of mycotic aneurysms. Surgery 50:347, 1961.

51. Smith RF, Szilagyi DE, Colville JM: Surgical treatment of mycotic aneurysms. Arch Surg 85:663, 1962.

52. Anderson CB, Butcher HR, Ballinger WF: Mycotic aneurysms. Arch Surg 109:712, 1974.

CHAPTER 52
Common Femoral Anastomotic Aneurysms

D. Emerick Szilagyi

The purpose of this chapter is to summarize my observations on the causes, clinical manifestations, and treatment of anastomotic aneurysms in my own series of cases of arterial surgical procedures.[1]

In the clinical experience on which this survey is based, anastomotic aneurysms were the most common, although by no means the most ominous, wound-healing complication seen after arterial reconstructive procedures using synthetic arterial subsitutes. In a series of angiographically followed cases of this type between 1957 and 1974, and comprising 9,561 anastomotic sites, the total incidence of anastomotic aneurysms was 1.7%.[1]

The terminology used for the designation of the pathologic entity under consideration must be clearly defined. As will be seen in the analysis of the etiologic factors, anastomotic aneurysms are usually false aneurysms, but in a significant number of cases the changes seen in the lesion are those of true aneurysms of the parent artery. Because of their frequent occurrence in the common femoral arterial region, where nonanastomotic aneurysms may be observed fairly frequently, the lesions under consideration must be sharply distinguished from pseudoaneurysms due to trauma.

PATHOLOGIC CHARACTERISTICS

True anastomotic aneurysms share the morphologic features of all true aneurysms. These characteristics represent dilatation of the lumen of the recipient parent artery of varying degrees and configurations because of the loss of tensile strength in the arterial wall. In these lesions, unless rupture takes place, there is no extravasation of blood. In contrast, pseudoaneurysms at the anastomotic line are the final morphologic expression of the changes that take place in the evolution of a hematoma originating in a defect in the arterial wall; in the case of anastomotic aneurysms, the defect is located in the suture line. If a break in the continuity of the arterial wall or suture line, usually of small dimensions, does not seal itself spontaneously and

permanently by a healing process, the hematoma to which the disruption of the wall has given rise remains in communication with the arterial lumen. The hematoma itself gradually undergoes fibroblastic organization, which results in the formation of a connective tissue envelope surrounding the central cavity still connected with the arterial lumen. The inherent tendency of this lesion is to enlarge under the force of arterial pressure. As already indicated, when a pseudoaneurysm occurs adjacent to an anastomosis, the first event in the pathologic process is a break in the suture line. The factors leading to this event will be discussed below.

FREQUENCY

The rate of occurrence of anastomotic aneurysms varies markedly according to the anatomic location of the lesion and according to the type of surgical procedure preceding its appearance. Since the technical details of reconstructive vascular surgical procedures vary from one period to another, the incidence of anastomotic aneurysms may also be influenced by the chronology of occurrence. In the past the most striking change in this respect was the abandonment of the use of silk sutures in the construction of vascular anastomoses and the introduction of Dacron suture material in the early 1960s. For the years for which accurate information is available (1957 to 1974),[1] by far the most common anatomic location of anastomotic aneurysm was the common femoral artery, with a per-anastomosis incidence of 3.0%.[*] In the same series of cases, the lesion had an incidence of 1.2% in the iliac artery, 1.1% in the popliteal,

---

[*]The incidence of postoperative complication involving anastomosis can be expressed either by ratio to the number of patients or by ratio to the number of anastomoses. Because every anastomosis is a potential site of such a complication, and because the probability of the occurrence of the complication depends on the number of anastomoses, with respect to a given patient's probability of being involved in such a complication, the expression of frequency in terms of number of anastomoses is more accurate.

0.8% in the carotid, and 0.2% in the aortic areas. There were no anastomotic aneurysms seen in the renal, mesenteric, brachial, and infrapopliteal anatomic regions.

In the series described, therefore, 80% of all the anastomotic aneurysms occurred at the common femoral level. In our current experience the prevalence of the common femoral arterial location is in excess of 90%. Obviously, because of this overwhelming statistical preponderance, the clinical surgeon's attention is focused primarily on the problems related to anastomotic aneurysms at the common femoral level. In this presentation the same trend will be followed. Unless otherwise specifically noted, the following statements refer to common femoral anastomotic aneurysms.

ETIOLOGIC FACTORS

In the search for the factors that lead to the formation of anastomotic aneurysms, the extremely frequent location of these lesions at the common femoral level readily suggests that factors must be at work in this anatomic area that are absent elsewhere.

In the survey mentioned above, we analyzed the possible etiologic factors not only in the 168 cases of anastomotic aneurysms observed after our own surgical procedures but also in 12 referred cases and 30 cases of recurrent lesions—altogether, 205 lesions. The very first question we attempted to answer was the possible effect of the ease with which superficial aneurysms can be detected in comparison with deep-seated lesions. That is to say, we asked whether the frequency with which we detected common femoral aneurysms might not have been due to the ready accessibility of lesions to inspection and palpation, in comparison with anastomotic aneurysms of the aorta or visceral arteries. Since all the cases were followed by periodic postoperative angiographic studies, the effect of this factor could be eliminated with a high degree of certainty. Although some deep-seated anastomotic aneurysmal lesions may have been missed, their number must have been negligible.

The clinical history and operative findings were carefully scrutinized in all 205 cases, and the relevant findings are summarized in Tables 52-1 and 52-2.

The temporal distribution of defective healing is shown in Table 52-1. We defined "defective healing" as a wound complication representing the accumulation of serum, blood, or lymph; shallow necrosis of the skin margin; or infection that did not penetrate below the level of the dermis. The incidence of aneurysmal formation in these cases was three times higher (i.e., 5.8%) than in those with normal healing (1.8%). Moreover, as disclosed in Table 52-1, the increase in the incidence of anastomotic aneurysms occurred preponderantly among patients in whom the lesion made its appearance in the early postoperative period. With the pathologic events that lead to the formation of a false aneurysm kept in mind, the effect of defective healing is readily explained. When improper healing occurs, even in the absence of manifest infection, the sealing of the suture line by deposition of fibrin (an essential part of appropriate healing of the suture line, or the incompletely coapted margins of the arterial wound) is prone to lead to extravasation of blood, hematoma, and eventually false aneurysm formation, as already described. Thus, in a certain number of cases, the formation of a false aneurysm is almost preordained because of the imperfection of subcutaneous healing. Needless to say, the exact identification of this special type of healing defect of the suture line is often very difficult during the time of exploration and repair of a false aneurysm.

It is also difficult to pinpoint with certainty the factors that led to the formation of a false aneurysm in any given case, whether or not the suture line had originally been firmly healed. Among the pertinent factors that we attempted to identify during exploration and repair, listed in Table 52-2, some objective ones can be recognized with precision, such as excessive mechanical stress and hypertension. Suture and graft defects and structural changes in the parent artery were more difficult to ascertain, because the extensive secondary tissue changes surrounding the lesions often obscured the details, and even the nature, of histologic damage at the site of the lesion. The problem was also complicated by the circumstance that at times more than one factor may have been present, so that assigning the respective roles to these factors was difficult. Nevertheless, the categories of etiologic factors listed in Table 52-2 were identified with acceptable clinical accuracy.

The category of mechanical stress included such factors as excessive tension on the shaft of the graft; direct or indirect trauma to the area of anastmosis because of excessive physical activity, usually soon after the original surgical procedure; and excessive bending of the hip joint, likewise usually soon after the surgical procedure. By the term *suture defect*, faulty suturing or defective suture material was meant. "Graft defect" referred to a recognizable flaw in the fabric of the graft, in particular to the disorganization of the textile pattern of the fabric at the suture line.

TABLE 52-1. INCIDENCE OF ANASTOMOTIC ANEURYSMS (205 PATIENTS) AFTER PRIMARY OPERATION WITH AND WITHOUT WOUND COMPLICATIONS ACCORDING TO TIME OF RECOGNITION

Type of Primary Operation	Year of Recognition					
	−0.5 (%)	0.5 to 1.0 (%)	1 to 2 (%)	2 to 5 (%)	5 to 10 (%)	10 to 14 (%)
No wound complication (176 patients)	25.0	11.4	16.5	24.4	14.2	8.5
Wound complication (29 patients)	44.8	10.3	27.6	3.4	13.8	0

TABLE 52-2. ETIOLOGIC FACTORS IN 205 PATIENTS ACCORDING TO TIME OF ONSET OF ANASTOMOTIC ANEURYSM

Time of Onset	No. of Patients	Deficiency in Arterial Wall	Hypertension	Mechanical	Graft Defect	Healing Complications	Endarterectomy	Suture Defect
1–6 mo	56	15	5	10	8	9	4	5
6–12 mo	24	7	7	4	2	1	2	1
1–2 yr	38	15	8	1	3	7	3	1
2–3 yr	17	5	5	4	2		1	
3–4 yr	19	4	5	3	5		2	
4–5 yr	7	1	4		1		1	
5–6 yr	9	4	5					
6–7 yr	11	3	5		2		1	
7–8 yr	7		6		1			
8–9 yr	1	1						
9–10 yr	4	1	2	1				
10–11 yr	3	3						
11–12 yr	5	3	2					
12–13 yr	0							
13–14 yr	4	1	2	1	—	—	—	—
Total	205 (100%)	63 (30.7%)	56 (27.3%)	24 (11.7%)	24 (11.7%)	17 (8.3%)	14 (6.8%)	7 (3.4%)

As a result of growing experience with the exploration and repair of these lesions, our attention was increasingly engaged by the evidence of deficiency in the arterial wall adjacent to the suture line. It was soon recognized that the changes in the arterial wall incident to endarterectomy frequently had an important role in reducing the tensile strength of the arterial wall. A strong impression was also gained that the pathologic deterioration of the arterial wall often manifested itself either in the suture's tearing out of its original position or in the diffuse dilatation of the recipient artery. In the last-named case, one dealt with a true aneurysm of the recipient artery at the site of the anastomosis. True aneurysms are estimated to have been about 20% of the total number of common femoral anastomotic aneurysms, and their proportionate incidence appeared to increase with the lengthening of the postoperative observation period. Unfortunately, no precise statistical data are available in support of this clinical impression.

A careful examination of Table 52-2 suggests that the chronologic distribution of the effects of the etiologic factors enumerated above displays some trends. The mechanical factor exhibits a biphasic distribution, the effect being felt either in the immediate or in the very late postoperative period. The role of healing complications seems to be sharply confined to the immediate and early postoperative periods. The effect of hypertension is prominent in the late and very late years of postoperative observation. The chronologic distribution of the other factors appears to be random. The chronologic spacing of the manifestations brought about by structural weakness of the arterial wall, healing deficiencies, and hypertension corresponds well with the evolutionary pace of the changes caused by these factors.

Although multiple etiologic factors probably are present in most patients, in individual instances certain single events appear to have played a principal role in the pathogenesis of wound-healing complications. The most common operative factor appears to have been the structural deficiency of the parent artery, which was implicated in 30.7% of the patients. In regard to mechanical stress, there is obvious difficulty in singling it out as a single etiologic factor. All the various forces listed above as putting strain on the suture line, as well as the presence of arterial hypertension, produce their effect by impinging on the arterial wall. It follows that the structural state of the arterial wall will ultimately determine the severity of the clinically observed damage. The only exception to this correlation would be the presence of a defective suture line or some flaw in the fabric of the prosthesis. In spite of these problems of interpretation, by a process of judicious exclusion of other possible factors, the cases in which mechanical stress had a primary role were identified with reasonable accuracy.

Hypertension appeared to be an important independent or contributing factor in the development of the structural changes leading to the appearance of anastomotic aneurysms. Arterial hypertension was present in 68.3% of the patients with anastomotic aneurysm, whereas the incidence of hypertension in the patients without this lesion was only 21.3%.

Briefly, the outstanding causative factors that were clearly identified in our study and that together were nearly 80% of the total were structural weakness of the parent artery (30.2%), hypertension (26.8%), mechanical stress (12.2%), and healing defects in the primary wound (9.3%).

TREATMENT

Our concept of managing anastomotic aneurysms of the common femoral artery has been based on the observation that some anastomotic aneurysms appear to be stable and thus devoid of serious clinical risks, whereas others show progressive changes that threaten rupture. Lesions that occur rather late after the original surgical procedure, for example, 2 to 4 years postoperatively, and are less than twice the size of the parent artery in transverse diameter when first noticed, usually require only careful observation by ultrasound image studies and, if an increase in size is noted, by angiography. As many as a third of such lesions will prove to be stable on repeated examination. Contrariwise, a vascular enlargement that arises rapidly, particularly if accompanied by symptoms, may require urgent surgical treatment even if relatively limited in size. If a lesion of this type, because of vagueness of the clinical picture, is treated conservatively, the serial examinations must be closely spaced. Regardless of the postoperative interval of appearance or the original size of the lesion, progressive increase in size always calls for surgical intervention.

Operative Technique

The technical features of repairing anastomotic aneurysms of the common femoral artery, which constitute more than 90% of our clinical experience with this lesion, can be placed in fairly clear-cut categories. These procedures are sketched in Figure 52-1. By far the most common procedure consists of the identification and excision of the aneurysmal sac, together with detachment, resection, and replacement by a new segment of the involved portion of the prosthesis. This technical procedure was carried out most commonly

with an end-to-side anastomosis between the prosthesis and the common or deep femoral artery (Fig. 52-1a). But in an almost equal number of patients, whenever the external iliac artery was already thrombosed, end-to-end anastomosis was used (Fig. 52-1b). In a small group of patients, it was possible to resect the aneurysm and identify and repair the suture defect in the anastomotic line (Fig. 52-1c). In instances in which the external iliac–common femoral trunk was still patent, it is usually possible to repair the arteriotomy site in the common femoral artery with a patch of Dacron fabric or a vein (Fig. 52-1d).

Ligation of the graft limb had to be carried out in those patients in whom no anatomic structures were available to reconstitute an anastomosis between the prosthesis and the femoral arterial trunk. When the external iliac trunk was occluded before the primary operation, both the common femoral artery and the graft limb were ligated (Fig. 52-1e). When adequate collateral circulation existed, the extremity remained viable in such cases, but under emergency conditions, and in the absence of collateral vessels, ligation of the graft led to limb loss in four patients. In 13 instances the reconstitution at the common femoral level was not possible, either because of the danger of infection or because of a lack of suitable tissue for suturing. In these cases the anastomosis was reestablished at a more distal

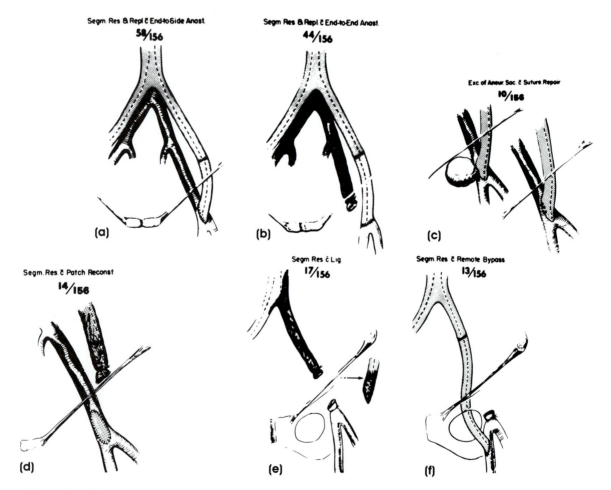

Figure 52-1. Types of surgical repair of anastomotic aneurysms and their incidence.

level by means of an obturator or other type of remote bypass (Fig. 52-1f).

Operative Results

It is obvious that the results of the various types of surgical reconstruction cannot be evaluated comparatively, because they were used according to specific indications in every case. The underlying abnormality calling for surgical intervention being so various, the results are not suitable for comparison.

Another factor affecting surgical procedures, however, is readily identifiable. If one compares the results according to the degree of urgency of the need for treatment, significant differences are noted between the elective surgery group and the emergency surgery group, as clearly shown in Table 52-3. The differences were invariably in favor of the cases in which elective procedures were carried out. This observation provides strong support for a generally aggressive attitude in the therapeutic approach to these lesions, in an attempt to avoid the progression of the lesion to a stage where emergency intervention is necessary.

That the repair of recurrent anastomotic aneurysms was highly successful requires special emphasis. Among 26 patients with one to three recurrences, the artery eventually remained patent, for the duration of observation, in 13; five of the remaining 13 patients retained their limbs, although the repair thrombosed. Thus ultimately 50% had excellent and 70% satisfactory results.

THE PROBLEM OF PREVENTION

It would be highly desirable if one were able to identify some etiologic factors in the causation of anastomotic aneurysms, the avoidance of which would reduce the incidence of this complication.

Surgical technique of the highest order will obviously lessen wound healing complications and avoid the effect of mechanical stress on the suture line that occurs when the prosthetic limb is placed under undue tension. Because hypertension is an important cause of anastomotic aneurysms in patients with reconstructive surgical procedures requiring common femoral anastomosis, medical control of the hypertension assumes particular importance.

Other factors, of course, are beyond the control of the surgeon. Relocating the femoral anastomosis in the pelvis to diminish the risk of unfavorable wound healing and to eliminate mechanical bending stress cannot be favored. (Exploring the femoral bifurcation in all cases of aortoiliac occlusive disease is, however, an essential part of correct surgical management.) Transposing the femoral anastomosis into the pelvis to the level of the external iliac artery to avoid the presumed bending stress in the groin is likewise not justified. If the anastomosis is placed just at or just above the origin of the deep femoral artery, the bending stress on the prosthetic limb is either minimal or nonexistent, even when the thigh is flexed to 90 degrees. The concept of avoiding the increased hemodynamic stress of an end-to-side anastomosis by replacing it with an end-to-end anastomosis between the prosthetic limb and the common femoral artery is not practical, because in many instances such an anastomosis would jeopardize the pelvic circulation.

Avoiding late effects caused by structural deficiency of the parent artery (the common femoral and adjacent external iliac artery) would require a resection of the segment of the common femoral artery that appears to be excessively decayed and its replacement by a sleeve or bifurcation tubular prosthesis. The anastomosis of the iliac limb of the bifurcation prosthesis to this prosthetic sleeve would certainly eliminate the changes subsequent to atherosclerotic degeneration of the common femoral artery. At this time it cannot be said with certainty that the complexity of this approach would be commensurate with the expectable gain in reducing the incidence of anastomotic aneurysm, but its cautious use in certain instances appears to be well justified.

CONCLUSIONS

The most common site of an anastomotic aneurysm in the arterial tree is the common femoral artery, that is, the site of the distal anastomosis of an aortofemoral Dacron bypass. In a large series, this complication developed in 3% of the cases managed by aortofemoral bypass operation with a Dacron graft. The most important causative factors were found to be (1) structural weakness of the parent artery, (2) hypertension, (3) mechanical stress on the suture line, (4) healing complications in the surgical incision, and (5) defects of the prosthesis. None of these factors can be controlled absolutely, but all are subject to possible improvement.

The results of elective surgical treatment were found to be satisfactory. Treatment in the emergency cases gave

TABLE 52-3. OPERATIVE RESULTS IN 129 CASES OF ANASTOMOTIC ANEURYSMS OF THE COMMON FEMORAL ARTERY

	No. of Patients	Patent	Closed Without Amputation[*]	Closed With Amputation[†]	Recurrence	Operative Death
		No. %	No. %	No. %	No. %	No. %
Elective	91	70/76.9	6/6.5	5/5.5	10/11.0	0/9.0
Emergency	38	17/44.7	6/44.7	4/10.5	6/15.8	5/13.1

[*] Operation failed, limb saved.
[†] Operation failed, limb lost.

markedly poorer results. Thus a generally aggressive therapeutic approach is strongly supported by the results. Small lesions, when readily accessible to inspection, may be observed. Large lesions, with dimensions 50% or greater than those of the parent artery, and expanding and symptomatic lesions call for prompt surgical intervention.

REFERENCE

1. Szilagyi DE, Smith RF, et al.: Anastomotic aneurysms after vascular reconstruction: Problems of incidence, etiology, and treatment. Surgery 78:800, 1975.

CHAPTER 53
Extrafemoral Anastomotic Aneurysms: General Considerations and Techniques

Henry Haimovici

Extrafemoral anastomotic aneurysms (AAs), although more uncommon than those of the common femoral artery, have been seen increasingly in recent years, mostly in the last decade, as testified to by a relatively large number of papers on this subject.[1-10] Indeed, these aneurysms are comparatively infrequent when considered in relation to the large number of graft-to-artery anastomoses. They may occur in the extrafemoral area after mostly aortobifemoral and, less often, iliofemoral, axillofemoral, or femoropopliteal bypasses. Their exact cause and pathogenesis in given cases are often a subject of uncertainty. Nevertheless, one fact stands out: the incidence of extrafemoral AAs is less than that of common femoral artery AAs.

This chapter follows one dealing with common femoral AAs, for which a survey was presented by Szilagyi (Chapter 52). He based this survey on his own series of cases, followed between 1957 and 1974 and comprising 9,561 anastomotic sites, in which AAs developed in only 1.7%, a remarkably low incidence.[11] The overwhelming preponderance of AAs in the femoral location (approximately 80%) indicates implicitly that the balance of 20% of the areas in the arterial tree may display similar complications, albeit with serious differences consistent with their mostly inaccessible locations.

Consequently, this chapter, based on the latter group (unlike the preceding chapter), will deal only with certain aspects of this problem, specifically with a few clinical considerations and operative techniques exclusive of those of common femoral AAs.

The arterial site of occurrence of these lesions varies to some extent, as indicated by a review of published papers on this subject. A few large statistical studies (Table 53-1) have reported the frequency of occurrence at the various anatomic sites. These studies reported a cumulative total of 7,366 reconstructive procedures, after which only 308 (4.1%) anastomotic aneurysms developed in 249 (3.4%) patients. Satiani,[6] on the other hand, in a collective review of 444 surgically repaired false aneurysms from 12 reports, found 79% at the femoral level, 10.5% in the aortoiliac area, 6.5% in the popliteal location, and the remaining 4% at miscellaneous areas of the arterial tree. It is only the latter locations, exclusive of the femoral, that will be the subject of description in this chapter.

The causative factors were described in detail in Szilagyi's survey and need not be reviewed here.

NATURAL HISTORY

False aneurysms that appear early, within a month or two of the reconstructive procedure, are generally ascribed to a technical problem involving suture line leakage or infection. Although the initial evolution of AAs remains rather nonprogressive for relatively long periods, it appears that some small AAs, nonprogressive and in an accessible location, could be watched expectantly without undue risk to the patient. According to Thompson et al,[9] the time interval between the original procedure and the diagnosis of false aneurysm has varied from 7 to 84 months. In a collective analysis by Satiani[6] of reports of 486 patients with 585 false aneurysms, the mean interval was 42 months. However, in a substantial number of these patients, the lesion may

TABLE 53-1. INCIDENCE OF ANASTOMOTIC ANEURYSMS (AAs) IN RELATION TO THE TOTAL NUMBER OF PROCEDURES

Author	No. of Procedures	No. of Patients	No. of AAs
Stoney et al.[18]	528	28	32
Sawyers et al.[12]	675	20	20
Sobregrau et al.[16]	619	12	12
Szilagyi et al.[19]	4214	163	205
Starr et al.[17]	1330	26	39
Total	7366	249 (3.4%)	308 (4.1%)

(From Haimovici H: Vascular Emergencies. New York, Appleton-Century-Crofts, 1982.)

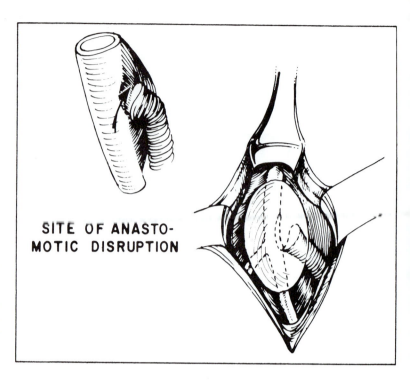

SITE OF ANASTO-
MOTIC DISRUPTION

Figure 53-1. *Left.* Diagram depicting anastomotic disruption between the graft and the host artery, with extravasation of blood localization around it. *Right.* Maturing of the aneurysm is characterized by surrounding fibrous tissues and the presence of communication between the host artery and the hematoma. (*From Haimovici H [ed]: Vascular Emergencies. New York, Appleton-Century-Crofts, 1982.*)

suddenly, at a later phase, evolve at a progressive or rapid pace, often in association with complicating limb-threatening or life-threatening manifestations. Most commonly the aneurysm expands rapidly because of rupture or sepsis, with ischemic symptoms resulting from sudden thrombosis of the host artery and distal embolization from the aneurysmal sac (Fig. 53-1).

Among late complications, diffuse dilatation of the Dacron graft and enteric fistulas have also been reported. According to Thompson et al.,[9] such complications of abdominal aortic reconstructions were encountered in 8.5% of 631 patients, and false aneurysms were the second most common complication after graft occlusion.

Clinical Manifestations

The discussion of clinical pictures in this section will be confined to the AAs located beyond the groin level.

Abdominal Aortic Anastomotic Aneurysms

Clinical manifestations of an aortic AA may remain unrecognized or may be suspected on routine clinical examination or diagnosed after angiography or computed tomography (CT). Awareness of the possibility of such a lesion adjacent to an aortic prosthetic anastomosis is essential in making the diagnosis. Unrecognized, these aortic aneurysms present a progression that may be fatal, as reported by several authors (Olsen et al.[15] and Gardner et al.[16]). If the AA is operated on before rupture or before its erosion into the duodenum, salvage of the patient is still possible. Otherwise, a complicated proximal aortic false aneurysm carries a very poor, if not fatal, prognosis (Olsen et al.[15] and West et al.[17]). By contrast, Carmichael and Barnes[1] reported a case of obstruction of the ureter due to a false aneurysm of an aortic bypass. After revision of the aortic graft anastomosis, the symptoms of pain and ureteral obstruction subsided. Any patient who has had an aortic graft and subsequently has even minor complaints, especially with intermittent gastrointestinal bleeding, should have an immediate angiographic or noninvasive imaging evaluation. If a suspect lesion is detected, emergency surgery may become imperative to avoid a fatal outcome.

Iliac Anastomotic Aneurysms

Iliac AAs occur less frequently than the aortic lesions but carry nearly the same ominous prognosis if not recognized in time. This lesion is usually associated with an aortoiliac or iliofemoral bypass graft. Its clinical behavior is similar to that of abdominal aortic AAs. The arterial enlargement may be accompanied by compression of the adjacent iliac vein and may mimic an iliofemoral vein thrombosis. Any patient who has had an aortoiliac bypass graft and has symptoms of a pulsatile expanding mass should have a CT scan for evaluation of the morphologic features and location of the lesion.

Popliteal Anastomotic Aneurysms

Although much more rarely seen than femoral AAs, those of the popliteal artery are usually associated with a femoropopliteal bypass graft. This lesion is characterized by a pulsatile mass that enlarges progressively. It is felt on the

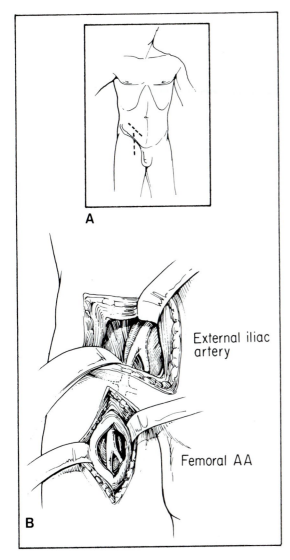

Figure 53-2. A. Lines of abdominal and groin skin incisions. **B.** Retroperitoneal exposure of the external iliac artery and exposure of the right femoral AA below Poupart's ligament.

rysm. The symptoms are usually apparent within 1 to 4 weeks postoperatively.

In septic AA of a bypass, the various conservative attempts at treatment are most often unsuccessful. Exceptions may be found in cases involving autogenous vein grafts, in which such measures occasionally succeed in healing the infected area and salvaging the graft. The procedure that may be tried in such instances, in the absence of host artery disintegration, is direct resuture of the anastomosis with adequate local drainage, copious local irrigations with antibiotic solutions, and use of systemic antibiotics.

In the presence of a prosthetic graft, all conservative measures may fail. Secondary hemorrhage, recurrence of the false aneurysm, and necrosis of the skin prolong the ordeal, and a radical procedure may ultimately become necessary. The aneurysm must then be excised and a new graft implanted into a clean area by means of either an obturator bypass or, preferably, an axillopopliteal bypass.

In *aortic* and *iliac septic aneurysms*, management is different from that of septic aneurysms in the lower extremity and often consists of removal of the aortic graft and ligation of the aorta below the renal vessels. An axillobifemoral bypass graft should precede the ligation of the aorta and removal of the graft. If an associated aortoenteric fistula is present, the prognosis is ominous, in spite of emergency surgical management.

Aortic and iliac AAs may remain unsuspected until the occurrence of a catastrophic rupture either intraperitoneally or into the intestinal tract. The diagnosis, although difficult to ascertain, should be suspected in the presence of intermittent gastrointestinal bleeding or of a pulsating mass in patients who have previously undergone aortic procedures (especially primary aortic aneurysmectomy).

In the *popliteal area*, the lesion, although obvious, has

medial aspect of the lower third of the thigh or in the popliteal space in the upper or distal location below the knee. Routine arteriography or, preferably, CT scan is mandatory in these instances to define and delineate morphologic features.

Anastomotic Aneurysms Associated with Sepsis

Sepsis associated with AA in any location, although uncommon, is a serious complication. A distinction should be made between superficial sepsis, not exceeding the dermis, and deep sepsis affecting the anastomotic aneurysm and its suture line. The former is easily controllable, in contrast to deep sepsis.

Sepsis manifests itself by intermittent bleeding from the area, formation of a hematoma, pus drainage, and lymphorrhea, all of which precede the appearance of the aneu-

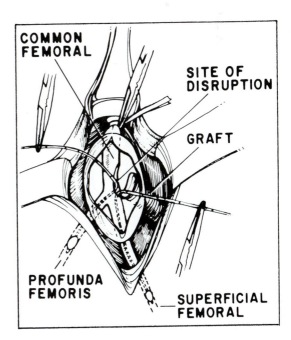

Figure 53-3. Diagram showing the opened aneurysmal sac. Note the intraarterial control with balloon catheters introduced into the outflow arteries of the AA.

been mistaken for an abscess, a true aneurysm, an arteriovenous fistula, and a popliteal pulsating bursa. If in doubt, CT scan and other noninvasive modalities for evaluating the arterial supply should be carried out in all of these instances.

The urgent or emergent nature of these AAs is characterized by the rapid or sudden appearance of pain in the thigh, an expanding mass, or sudden ischemia of the limb. Sudden ischemia is usually due to an acute thrombosis of the aneurysm, affecting the host artery as well. Rupture of the aneurysm may remain unrecognized before operative exposure of the lesion.

OPERATIVE INDICATIONS

Operative indications may depend on the degree of the critical nature of the lesion. Depending on the evolution of the AA, operative indications either assume varying degrees of urgency or are not urgent.

1. In the presence of a small, nonprogressive, asymptomatic lesion in an accessible area, one may adopt an expectant attitude, avoiding an urgent indication on the mere diagnosis of such a lesion. A conservative attitude is justified in the absence of any threatening manifestations.
2. In AAs that slowly enlarge over a period of 1 to 3 years, surgery is best undertaken before complications arise.

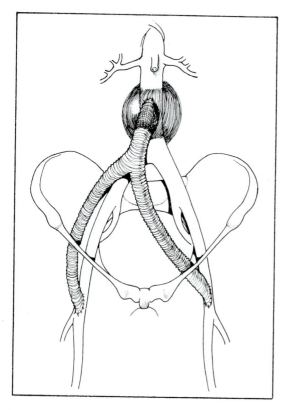

Figure 53-4. Diagram illustrating an aortobifemoral bifurcation graft with a false aneurysm at the aortic anastomosis.

3. In emergency situations, such as recent rapid enlargement, acute pain, sudden thrombosis with distal embolization, rupture with increasing hematoma, or the presence of sepsis, prompt arteriography, noninvasive modalities such as CT scan if necessary, and repair of the lesions appear imperative.
4. Suspicion of an aortic or iliac AA because of a previously implanted aortoiliac graft is a most urgent indication for further diagnostic study. If the diagnosis is confirmed, repair of the lesion is mandatory.

PRINCIPLES OF ARTERIAL REPAIR

The principles and techniques of arterial repair, although applicable to any AA, may vary with the location of the anastomosis. Each major arterial lesion will be illustrated separately.

As stated earlier, the arterial repair of a femoral AA has been described in detail in the Szilagyi chapter (Chapter 52) and need not be repeated here. The principles applied to repair of a femoral AA are similar to those used in repair at other locations, with certain variations. The principles on which the techniques are generally based are (1) *adequate exposure* of the arterial region, (2) *control* of both *inflow* and *outflow*, and (3) *mobilization* of the aneurysm, which may prove to be difficult before the sac can be safely opened (Fig. 53-2). At this point, the contents of the sac may be evacuated and the aneurysmal intrasaccular origins of its collateral vessels can be identified. Fogarty catheters are introduced into these vessels, and the balloons are inflated for control of bleeding (Fig. 53-3). The sac is then mobilized, dissected, and, if possible, excised down to its anastomosis with the vessel to which it is attached (e.g., aorta, iliac artery, popliteal artery). Because the edges of the arteriotomy may show a severe degree of atherosclerotic distintegration, as one would anticipate, their excision may be necessary.

At this point the aneurysm, together with a portion of the old graft, can be removed, followed by interposition of a new segment of the same graft material.

Aortic and Iliac Anastomotic Aneurysms (Fig. 53-4)

The operative field should include exposure of the abdominal aorta and both femoral vessels by means of a long transperitoneal incision, using a xiphopubic approach, and that of both groins.

In the presence of a *nonseptic* aortic aneurysm, the lesion is incised, the thrombi are evacuated, and the site of the disruption is identified. It is best to detach the old graft from the insertion in the aorta. If the edges of the aortotomy have not disintegrated, a new graft may be reattached. Should the edges display marked degenerative changes, it is best to transect the aorta proximally and reattach a graft by an end-to-end procedure (Fig. 53-5). Implantation in the femoral vessels will depend on whether false aneurysms are present distally as well. In that event, the distal aneurysms are also excised and the limbs of the bifurcated

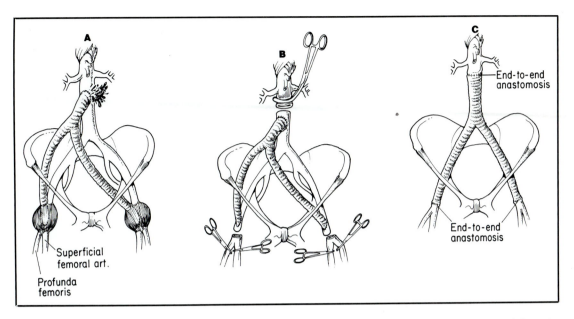

Figure 53-5. **A.** Diagram illustrating an aortobifemoral bifurcation graft with bilateral false femoral aneurysms and disruption of the aortic end-to-side graft anastomosis. **B.** Diagram illustrating the removal of this graft together with excision of the AAs of the femoral arteries. Note also the transection of the abdominal aorta proximal to the original anastomosis. **C.** Insertion of a new aortobifemoral graft in an end-to-end fashion on all anastomotic levels (aorta and residual bifurcation of the femoral arteries).

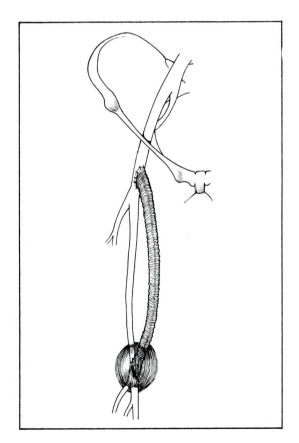

Figure 53-6. Diagram of a false popliteal aneurysm in a femoropopliteal bypass graft.

graft are reattached beyond the original anastomotic areas, preferably into the profunda femoris.

In *septic* aortoiliac grafts with a proximal false aneurysm, the prognosis is poor, especially if recognition is delayed. Management should consist of graft excision and ligation of the aorta below the renal vessels, with axillobifemoral bypass grafts. The latter should be in place before entrance into the abdomen for the procedure.

In the presence of a *septic* iliac aneurysm, besides the above-mentioned procedures, an axillofemoral bypass, instead of an obturator bypass, is preferable.

Popliteal Anastomotic Aneurysms

AAs in the popliteal artery may occur either above or below the knee (Figs. 53-6 and 53-7). Exposure is through a medial approach, either in the lower third of the thigh or in the upper third of the leg. These AAs are by far less frequent than the femoral ones. Management is based on the same principles as those used in management of femoral AAs.

In a *nonseptic* AA of a vein graft, an attempt to resuture the detached end may be carried out if the arteriotomy edges have not disintegrated. In that case, an interposition graft is anastomosed end-to-end to the old detached graft, with an end-to-side anastomosis placed more distally into the popliteal artery or into a major leg artery.

Septic AAs are much less common at this level. If the aneurysm occurs in the presence of a *vein graft*, reattachment of the latter to the old arteriotomy may be attempted.

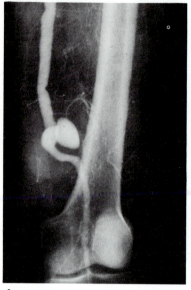
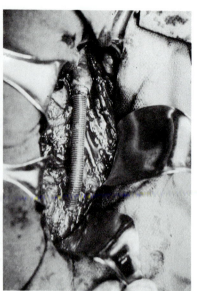

Figure 53-7. A. Femoral arteriogram showing the distal segment of a Dacron femoropopliteal bypass graft performed 8 years before. Note a false anastomotic aneurysm at the site of the graft implantation into the mid-popliteal artery. **B.** After excision of the false aneurysm, a new segment of 10 mm Dacron tube was anastomosed distally into the popliteal artery.

A   **B**

For a *prosthetic graft* aneurysm, the procedure is similar to that for septic femoral AA.

CONCLUSIONS

Although AAs are much less frequent in locations other than the common femoral location, the AAs in the other locations carry an even greater potential for complications, mostly involving aortic prosthetic grafts. As already emphasized, more than one factor participates in the pathogenesis of these AAs. Among the most significant of these factors are degenerative lesions of the host artery, the type of suture material, and the type of construction of the graft-host anastomosis.

Expanding and symptomatic lesions of both the accessible (popliteal) and especially the inaccessible (aortoiliac) vessels call for urgent or emergency surgery to avoid loss of limb and life. This applies particularly to aortic AA grafts, with their potential for rupture retroperitoneally or intraperitoneally or into the duodenum. Elective repair before the latter complications may be successful in 85 to 90% of cases. In contrast, emergency surgery carries a greater challenge and a poorer prognosis, especially in complicated lesions of the aortoiliac segment.

REFERENCES

1. Carmichael DH, Barnes WF: Obstruction of the ureter due to false aneurysm. Surgery 86:769, 1979.
2. Gaylis H: Pathogenesis of anastomotic aneurysms. Surgery 90:509, 1981.
3. Hollier LH, Batson RC, Cohn I Jr: Femoral anastomotic aneurysms. Ann Surg 191:715, 1980.
4. Millili JJ, Lanes JS, Nemir P Jr: A study of anastomotic aneurysms following aortofemoral prosthetic bypass. Ann Surg 192:69, 1980.
5. Nichols WK, Stanton M, et al: Anastomotic aneurysms following lower extremity revascularization. Surgery 88:366, 1980.
6. Satiani B: False aneurysms following arterial reconstruction. Surg Gynecol Obstet 152:357, 1981.
7. Sauvage LR: Graft complications in relation to prosthesis healing, in Haimovici H: Vascular Emergencies. New York, Appleton-Century-Crofts, 1982.
8. Starr DS, Weatherford SC, et al: Suture material as a factor in the occurrence of anastomotic false aneurysms: An analysis of 26 cases. Arch Surg 114:412, 1979.
9. Thompson WM, Johnsrude IS, Jackson DC, et al: Late complications of abdominal aortic reconstructive surgery; roentgen evaluation. Ann Surg 185:326, 1977.
10. Youkey JR, Clagett GP, et al: Femoral anastomotic false aneurysms. Ann Surg 199:703, 1984.
11. Szilagyi DE, Smith RF, et al: Anastomotic aneurysms after vascular reconstruction: Problems of incidence, etiology, and treatment. Surgery 78:800, 1975.
12. Stoney RJ, Albo RJ, Wylie EJ: False aneurysms occurring after arterial grafting operations. Am J Surg 110:153, 1965.
13. Sawyers JL, Jacobs JK, Sutton JP: Peripheral anastomotic aneurysm development following arterial reconstruction with prosthetic grafts. Arch Surg 95:801, 1967.
14. Sobregrau RC, Maldonado CM, et al: Falsos aneurismas en cirugia arterial directa. Barcelona Quir 16:292, 1972.
15. Olsen WR, De Weese MS, Frey WJ: False aneurysm of abdominal aorta: A late complication of aortic aneurysmectomy. Arch Surg 92:123, 1966.
16. Gardner TJ, Brawley RK, Gott VL: Anastomotic false aneurysms. Surgery 72:474, 1972.
17. West UP, Lattes C, Knox WG: Anastomotic false aneurysms. Arch Surg 103:348, 1971.

BIBLIOGRAPHY

Christensen RD, Bernatz PE: Anastomotic aneurysms involving the femoral artery. Mayo Clin Proc 47:313, 1972.

Davis RP, Neiman HL, et al: Ultrasound scan in diagnosis of peripheral aneurysms. Arch Surg 112:55, 1977.

Knox WG: Peripheral vascular anastomotic aneurysm: A 15-year experience. Ann Surg 183:120, 1976.

Moore WS, Hall AD: Late suture failure in the pathogenesis of anastomotic false aneurysms. Ann Surg 172:1064, 1970.

Scott WW, Scott PP, Saunders RC: B-scan ultrasound in the diagnosis of popliteal aneurysms. Surgery 81:436, 1977.

CHAPTER 54
Arteriovenous Fistulas

Peter Gloviczki and Larry H. Hollier

The development of abnormal communications between the arterial and venous system has been the center of interest of surgeons for over two centuries. Depending on the amount of shunted blood that bypasses the capillary circulation, these lesions may be asymptomatic or may have local effects on the surrounding tissues. Arteriovenous fistulas may also have serious consequences for the distal circulation, may cause irreversible pathologic changes in the proximal blood vessels, and in rare cases of large central shunts, they may result in profound circulatory and metabolic alterations.

HISTORICAL NOTE

Guido Guidi (1500–1559), surgeon of the emperor Francis I, is credited with describing the first patient with congenital arteriovenous malformation (AVM) who had pulsating varices (so-called cirsoid aneurysm) of the head.[1]

As early as 1757, William Hunter described a patient with a traumatic arteriovenous fistula,[2] and a detailed analysis of two cases was published in 1764.[3] He not only recognized the characteristic thrill and bruit (which disappeared after compressing the proximal artery or the fistula) but also noted the tortuosity and dilatation of the artery proximal to the "aneurysm by anastomosis," as well as the pulsating, distended superficial vein and a decreased distal arterial pulsation. Early attempts to cure the fistula with ligation of the proximal artery frequently resulted in gangrene of the extremity,[4] but already in 1843, Norris[5] reported on treatment of an arteriovenous fistula by double arterial ligation. The typical "bradycardiac sign," the slowing of the heart rate after compression of the arteriovenous communication, was described first by Nicoladoni[6] in a patient with congenital AVM, and 15 years later, in 1890, by Branham[7] in a patient with acquired arteriovenous fistula. The pathophysiology of arteriovenous fistula was remarkably well documented as early as 1937 by Emile Holman.[8] Experiences from World War II,[9] the Korean conflict,[10] and, most im-

portant, the Vietnam War[11] gave us important information about correct management of traumatic arteriovenous fistulas.

Our knowledge of congenital AVM (Fig. 54-1) is based primarily on the work of Reid,[12] Holman,[8] de Takats,[13] and Coursley et al.[14] Malan and Puglionisi,[15] in landmark articles, summarized the state of the art of congenital angiodysplasias of the extremities, and Szilagyi et al.[16,17] gave us a usable clinical classification and guidelines for management of these lesions. Finally, in the last decade, superselective arterial catheterization was a major advancement; embolization has become an important technique in the treatment of AVMs.[18,19]

ETIOLOGY

Arteriovenous fistulas may be *congenital* or *acquired*. The *congenital* AVMs are not true tumors and represent only an "anomalous development of the primitive vascular system."[13] *Acquired arteriovenous fistulas* are most frequently caused by penetrating injuries; in wartime these are usually due to flying fragments or gunshot wounds,[9–11] whereas among civilian injuries the cause is frequently gunshot or stab wounds and fractures.[20,21] Iatrogenic arteriovenous fistulas have been reported after lumbar laminectomy, orthopedic procedures, diagnostic or therapeutic catheterization, percutaneous biopsies of organs (e.g., kidney or liver), and embolectomy with Fogarty balloon catheters and as a result of mass ligation of artery and vein after splenectomy or nephrectomy.[22–29] Tumors such as hypernephromas or metastases from thyroid carcinomas may also contain arteriovenous fistulas.

Spontaneous major intraabdominal arteriovenous fistulas may develop in patients with atherosclerotic or mycotic aortoiliac aneurysmal disease.[30,31]

Aortocaval fistulas due to abdominal aortic aneurysms and arteriovenous fistulas, the latter created surgically for hemodialysis, as an adjunct to improve patency of distal

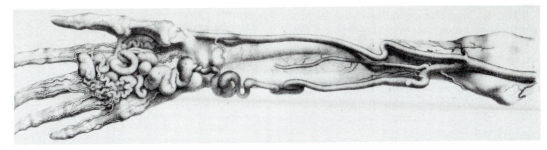

Figure 54-1. Artist's conception of congenital arteriovenous malformation ("cirsoid aneurysm") of the hand. (*From Breschet G: Mem Acad Med (Paris) 3:101, 1833. By permission of the journal.*)

arterial bypasses or venous grafts, or as a treatment option for venous thrombosis, are discussed elsewhere in this book.

PATHOPHYSIOLOGY

According to Holman,[32] all circulatory changes that occur as a result of a congenital or acquired arteriovenous fistula can be explained by a basic hemodynamic principle: "Blood, like flowing water, has an inherent and natural tendency to follow the path of least resistance." The arteriovenous fistula is an abnormal connection between a high-pressure, high-resistance arterial system and a low-pressure, low-resistance, high-capacity venous system. Because of the low resistance, blood preferentially flows through the fistula rather than through the normal capillary bed. Pressure in the artery distal to the fistula decreases; the distal venous pressure increases. These hemodynamic changes lead to the development of increased arterial and venous collateral circulation around the fistula (Fig. 54-2). As a result of increased circulating blood volume, there is a progressive dilatation of the entire circulatory system proximal to the fistula; although cardiac enlargement and venous distension may reverse after fistula closure, irreversible ectasia and

aneurysm formation in the arteries proximal to chronic fistulas may develop. The amount of blood shunted depends on the diameter and type of the fistula and its proximity to the heart.

Whereas many of the congenital AVMs are asymptomatic or cause cosmetic problems or local effects only, the natural history of most acquired arteriovenous fistulas is continuous increase in size and increase in the volume of shunted blood. As a consequence, total blood volume, heart rate, cardiac index, stroke volume, and left atrial and pulmonary artery pressures increase and cardiac failure may develop.

If a significant shunt is closed by external compression, there is an immediate rise in systolic blood pressure, and as a vagal response on the stimulation of baroreceptors in the aorta and cerebral arteries, bradycardia almost instantaneously develops. Cardiac output decreases, and if the closure of the shunt is definitive, total blood volume contracts to normal within a few days.

The metabolic changes that occur as a result of high central shunt have been studied by Davis et al.[33] and by Epstein and Ferguson.[34] It is presumed that the increased venous pressure and the decreased mean arterial pressure, due to the wide pulse pressure, result in decreased renal plasma flow and decreased glomerular filtration rate. As

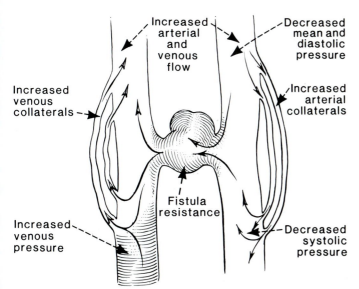

Figure 54-2. Anatomic and hemodynamic changes due to an arteriovenous fistula.

a response, the juxtaglomerular apparatus increases production of aldosterone through the renin-angiotensin system, which subsequently results in increased sodium and water reabsorption and an increase in total plasma volume. The oliguria or anuria that is present in large central shunts can be reversed by closure of the fistula, which produces diuresis, decreases aldosterone secretion, and, within a few days, restores plasma volume to normal levels.

ACQUIRED ARTERIOVENOUS FISTULAS

Incidence and Distribution

Since the diagnosis of an arteriovenous fistula has frequently been made years after the injury, it is difficult to define the true incidence of this lesion. In a review of the literature until 1914, Callander,[35] a student of Halsted, found 447 arteriovenous fistulas and only three of those were congenital. Of 7,500 vascular injuries, 262 patients had arteriovenous fistulas, according to the Vietnam Vascular Registry, which gives an incidence of about 3.5%.[11] An equal number of patients had false arterial aneurysms (3.9%). The incidence of arteriovenous fistula in civilian vascular injuries was similar: 6 of 256 injuries (2.3%) in a review by Patman et al.[20] and 7 of 192 patients (3.6%) in a recent review by Sirinek et al.[36]

Traumatic fistula is most frequent in the lower extremity; in the five largest series of acquired arteriovenous fistulas, over 50% were traumatic fistulas (Fig. 54-3).[9–11,20,37] Of 70 arteriovenous fistulas due to civilian injuries, 13% occurred in the neck between the carotid artery and jugular vein, 12% were carotid-cavernous fistulas, and 17% occurred in the femoral vessels.[21] Within the abdomen, renal arteriovenous fistula is the most frequent, followed by hepatic lesions.

The anatomy of the arteriovenous fistula is determined by the site of arterial and venous injury and by the chronicity of the lesion (Fig. 54-4). False aneurysm develops shortly after the injury as a persisting pulsatile hematoma with arterial and venous connection or as a result of injury to the vessel wall in the proximity of the arteriovenous fistula. Chronic true arterial and venous aneurysms are direct consequences of local and systemic hemodynamic factors, which include increased circulating blood volume, high fistula flow, and increased intravascular pressure, as discussed earlier. The incidence of associated arterial and venous aneurysms ranged from 20 to 60%.[38,39]

Clinical Data

The clinical presentation of a patient with an acquired arteriovenous fistula is usually typical. There is a palpable thrill and a systolic-diastolic machinelike murmur; there may be a pulsatile mass; the superficial veins are distended; the peripheral arterial pulse may be diminished; and there is evidence of penetrating injury or fracture in the proximity of major blood vessels.

In acute arteriovenous fistulas the clinical picture is not always characteristic, and a bruit can be absent in as

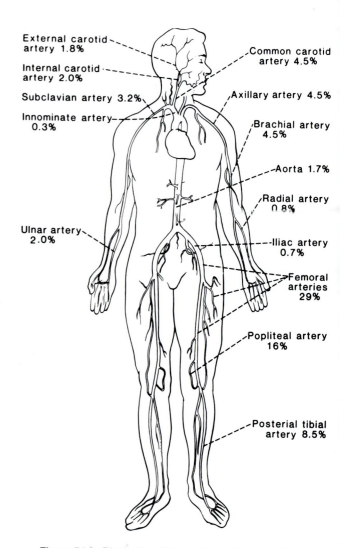

Figure 54-3. Distribution of traumatic arteriovenous fistulas.

many as 45% of the cases. Distal pulses were decreased in only 11% of 70 cases reported by Kollmeyer et al.,[21] and none of the patients with acute fistulas had a positive Branham-Nicoladoni sign.

Although penetrating trauma is the most important cause of arteriovenous fistula, blunt trauma in civilian injuries is a definite etiologic factor. Basilar skull fracture with cranial bruit is pathognomonic of carotid-cavernous fistula. These patients may have pulsatile headache, vision changes, pulsatile exophthalmos, and conjunctival engorgement.[40]

Diagnosis

In patients with chronic arteriovenous fistula, the diagnosis almost always can be made on the basis of history and physical examination alone. Apart from the bruit and thrill, signs of chronic venous stasis, including ulceration, pigmentation, edema, varicosity, and induration, with increased skin temperature at the level of and proximal to the fistula, and signs and symptoms of cardiac failure are

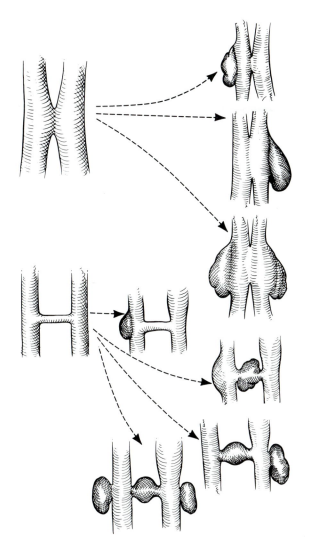

Figure 54-4. Possible anatomic variations of acquired arteriovenous fistulas.

clues to the diagnosis. In long-standing arteriovenous fistulas, if they were present before closure of the epiphyseal plates, the development of bony hypertrophy with elongation of the extremity has been reported.[41] In some patients with chronic fistulas, there is frank aneurysm formation in the arteries proximal to the fistula. As a rare complication of a chronic arteriovenous fistula, subacute bacterial endocarditis may develop.

Patients who have large central shunts, such as an aortocaval fistula, usually have a dramatic presentation, with acute congestive heart failure, abdominal bruit, and wide pulse pressure associated with lower extremity ischemia and edema.[30] In spontaneous iliac arteriovenous fistula, venous stasis or arterial ischemia or both are localized to the affected extremity only.[31]

Noninvasive diagnostic techniques may be necessary to evaluate small arteriovenous fistulas and to determine the amount of shunting and the degree of peripheral ischemia as a result of the "distal" steal. *Segmental limb systolic pressure measurements, pulse-volume recording,* and *Doppler*

examinations are the most valuable diagnostic tools; these tools have recently been evaluated by Sumner[42] and by Rutherford[43] and are discussed in more detail elsewhere in this book.

Segmental limb systolic pressure measurements reveal an elevated systolic pressure proximal to a significant arteriovenous fistula; the pressure may be normal or decreased distal to the lesion compared with the healthy contralateral extremity.

Pulse-volume recordings are elevated proximal to the fistula and show a sharper systolic peak, with a decreased or absent anacrotic notch. Decreased pulse volume may or may not be recorded distally.

Doppler examination seems to be the most valuable noninvasive diagnostic technique. In the proximal artery, it reveals an abnormal velocity waveform with forward diastolic flow instead of a normal triphasic arterial flow. The increase in end-diastolic velocity is proportionate to the decrease in peripheral resistance caused by the arteriovenous fistula. In the proximal veins the Doppler study may reveal a pulsatile flow pattern.

Measurement of *venous oxygen saturation* on the affected extremity proximal to the fistula shows elevated values compared with samples taken from veins of other parts of the body.

Serial angiography is the best and most definitive diagnostic test that delineates anatomy and, as a functional study, gives information on the hemodynamics of the fistula. Although in the cases of low aortic, iliac, or femoral lesions the translumbar approach may be sufficient, in all other patients percutaneous catheterization through the femoral or brachial artery is necessary. Angiography not only localizes the fistula but also reveals arterial and venous aneurysmal changes and may document venous valvular incompetence distal to the fistula. With the Seldinger technique, direct pressure measurements in the artery proximal and distal to the fistula may be possible. Because the diagnosis of an acute traumatic arteriovenous fistula could be missed in 45% of the cases on the basis of physical examination alone,[21] angiography is recommended for every patient with stable hemodynamics who has penetrating injury next to major blood vessels.

Treatment and Results

Disconnection of the arteriovenous fistula and reconstruction of a normal circulation are needed in most cases. Spontaneous cure of small acquired arteriovenous fistulas has been reported[21]; in some types of iatrogenic fistulas, such as those developing after kidney biopsy, spontaneous closure is usual rather than an exception.[26] The majority of acquired arteriovenous fistulas, however, are progressive and require primary surgical treatment.

Hunterian ligation of the artery proximal to the fistula is of historic interest only and should not be used. Quadruple ligation in cases of small distal vessels is still practiced and is acceptable only in distal vessels if the collateral circulation is adequate to prevent distal ischemia.

Figure 54-5 depicts the various possibilities of reconstruction. In spite of an attempt to reconstruct both artery

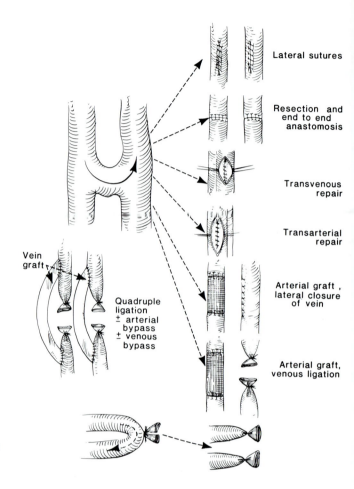

Figure 54-5. Options of surgical treatment for acquired arteriovenous fistulas.

and vein after injury, arterial ligation was still the primary treatment in 52% of 558 patients who had arteriovenous fistula or false aneurysms, according to the Vietnam Vascular Registry. End-to-end anastomosis was done in 25%, vein graft in 10%, and lateral suture in 7% of the arterial repairs. Venous ligation was used in 52% and suture repair in 30% of the cases.[11]

Of 233 patients with traumatic arteriovenous fistula, Linder[39] reported the use of lateral suture repair after division of the fistula in 67% of the cases.

Of 70 arteriovenous fistulas due to civilian injuries, 40% were treated with primary arterial repair by the Parkland group.[20] If lateral repair or end-to-end anastomosis cannot be done, our choice of graft material is the contralateral saphenous vein. Although under exceptional circumstances ligation of major veins can be performed without major consequence or can even be lifesaving for the patient with hemorrhage due to major abdominal trauma, every attempt should be made to reconstruct three important veins: the suprarenal inferior vena cava, the common femoral vein, and the popliteal vein. Prosthetic grafts for popliteal vein replacement have almost uniformly been unsuccessful; therefore contralateral saphenous vein should be used whenever it is necessary. The use of a spiral vein graft is an excellent way to reconstruct short segments of large-caliber veins.[44]

The results of surgical treatment of acquired arteriovenous fistulas are universally good. The overall mortality

rate for 558 arteriovenous fistulas and false aneurysms in the Vietnam Vascular Registry was 1.8%, with a morbidity rate of 6.3% and an amputation rate of 1.7%.[11] Linder[39] reported a cure rate of 96% with only four amputations, which were necessary after quadruple ligation of the vessels.

The complication rate from major intraabdominal arteriovenous fistulas is more significant because of sudden circulatory overload and an increased risk of pulmonary embolization. A recent review of 73 collected cases reported an overall mortality rate of 30% and a morbidity rate of 32%.[30]

Embolization is not as widely used as a treatment option in congenital AVMs. However, in certain types of acquired fistulas, especially in the region of the head and neck, in abdominal viscera, or in fistulas after pelvic fractures, embolization has become an important treatment either alone or as an adjunctive form of surgical treatment.[21] Because the fistula is almost always a single large connection between artery and vein, embolizing particles usually must be larger than those used to obstruct congenital fistulas: detachable balloons, coils, or muscle fragments are used primarily. With detachable balloons alone, Debrun et al.[45] could preserve internal carotid blood flow in 59% of the cases with traumatic carotid-cavernous fistulas. The technique reported by Kollmeyer et al.[21] seems more successful; in high carotid-cavernous fistulas, embolization was preceded by extracranial-intracranial bypass: of six patients treated this way, only one had a transient neurologic deficit.

Arteriovenous Fistula After Lumbar Laminectomy

Arteriovenous fistulas after lumbar laminectomy were reported first by Linton and White[22] in 1945, and the topic was extensively reviewed recently by Quigley and Stoney.[23] The cause of the arteriovenous fistula is usually the bone rongeur, which penetrates the anterior spinal ligament, most frequently at the level of L-4 to L-5, and injures the right common iliac artery and right or left common iliac vein. Arteriovenous fistulas at the L-3 to L-4 and L-5 to S-1 levels have also been reported. Because of retroperitoneal tamponade of the bleeding, this complication usually becomes evident in the postoperative course, sometimes months or even years after the injury. Lower extremity edema, fatigue, signs of congestive heart failure, and systolic-diastolic murmur are clues to the diagnosis, but aortography is recommended to precisely define anatomy and plan surgical correction.

Division of the fistula, venorrhaphy, and direct arterial repair are usually possible. It is sometimes necessary to divide the right common iliac artery to gain better access to the venous repair. Prosthetic graft placement is seldom required, but in rare infected cases the use of in situ autologous material or extraanatomic prosthetic arterial grafting may be needed.

Arteriovenous Fistula After Nephrectomy

The first arteriovenous fistula after nephrectomy was described in 1934 by Hollingsworth,[24] and up to 1984 only 50 cases had been reported.[25] The cause is most frequently the mass ligature of artery and vein, transfixing suture, or local infection. Symptoms, such as pain, palpable mass, elevated blood pressure, and cardiac failure, may develop anywhere from 6 months to 36 years after the operation. An audible bruit at the site of nephrectomy strongly suggests the diagnosis, which is definitively confirmed by angiography. Separate ligature of the artery or vein or transcatheter embolization is the treatment of choice.

Arteriovenous Fistula After Embolectomy with Fogarty Balloon Catheter

Since the first report of an arteriovenous fistula as a complication of the Fogarty embolectomy catheter was described by Lord et al.[27] in 1968, 18 cases had been collected in the literature up to 1985.[28] The number of unreported cases must be much higher, and Schweitzer et al.[29] concluded that 10% of the complications by Fogarty catheters are arteriovenous fistulas. Most of the true arteriovenous fistulas develop distal to the knee, but carotid-cavernous fistulas also have been reported. The causes may be (1) catheters of inadequate size, (2) diseased vessels with atherosclerotic plaques, (3) faulty surgical technique, or (4) multiple attempts to extract emboli, especially in cases of "late" embolectomy.

Although some publications have suggested leaving the arteriovenous fistulas to improve patency, significant arteriovenous fistula should be repaired. The routine use of intraoperative angiogram after embolectomy is recommended.

CONGENITAL ARTERIOVENOUS MALFORMATIONS

Similar to acquired arteriovenous fistulas, congenital AVMs are abnormal communications between the arterial and venous system. These lesions are, however, the result of faulty development of the blood vessels, and the connections between arteries and veins are almost invariably multiple. Progression is mostly the result of hemodynamic factors, and tumorlike behavior with endothelial proliferations is not characteristic.[46]

AVMs are usually present at birth, although signs and symptoms may become manifest only later in life. Hereditary transmisson is exceptionally rare; of 840 cases with vascular malformations, Malan et al.[47] found only seven patients with familial inheritance. The extreme number of clinical presentations explains why so many different names (arteriovenous hemangioma, arteriovenous aneurysm, arteriovenous fistula, cirsoid aneurysm, serpentine aneurysm) and syndromes (Parkes-Weber, Klippel-Trenaunay, Rendu-Osler-Weber) (Table 54-1) have been attached to these lesions.

Classifications

There have been few areas in medicine in which so much confusion and controversy have existed other than in the field of congenital vascular malformations. A plethora of classifications has been suggested, some of those based simply on external appearance of the lesions and on resemblance to fruits, fish, birds, or insects.[48] The most valuable classification systems have been based on morphologic features,[15,49] embryologic development,[16,17] endothelial characteristics and cell biology,[46] hemodynamics, and angiographic appearance.[50,51]

Congenital vascular malformations or angiodysplasias include developmental abnormalities of the arterial, capillary, venous, or lymphatic system. In the case of AVMs, the pathologic vasculature is mixed arteriovenous. Secondary morphologic changes in the feeding arteries and draining veins are the result of hemodynamic factors and depend primarily on the amount of blood shunted through the abnormal vessels.

Malan and Puglionisi[15] divided the AVMs into (1) *truncular arteriovenous fistulas,* local or diffuse, more or less active and (2) *arteriovenous angiomas,* single, polycentric or diffuse, more or less active. On the basis of morphologic variations, further subgroups such as single truncular, plexiform, aneurysmal, or circumscribed were distinguished.

The classification of Szilagyi et al.[16,17] is simpler and is based primarily on the development of the vascular system. Studies by Woollard[52] first shed light on the stages of embryologic development: (1) *the capillary network stage,* which is an undifferentiated interlacing network of primitive blood lakes, (2) *the retiform stage,* when separation of primitive arterial and venous channels develops, and (3) *the stage*

TABLE 54-1. CLINICAL SYNDROMES ASSOCIATED WITH CONGENTIAL VASCULAR MALFORMATIONS (VM)

Syndrome	Inheritance	Type of VM	Location	Characteristic Features	Treatment	Prognosis
Parkes-Weber	No	AVM (intraosseal or close to epiphyseal plate) Port-wine stain	Extremity Pelvis	Soft tissue and bony hypertrophy Varicosity (atypical) Hemangioma	Observation Elastic support Embolization ± excision	Deep diffuse lesions have poor prognosis
Klippel-Trenaunay	No	No or low-shunt AVM Venous or lymphatic VM Port-wine stain	Extremities Pelvis Trunk	Soft tissue and bony hypertrophy Varicosities (lateral lumbar to foot pattern) Hemangioma/lymphangioma	Elastic support Seldor: epiphyseal stapling	Usually good
Rendu-Osler-Weber (hereditary hemorrhagic telangiectasia)	Autosomal dominant	Punctate angioma Telangiectasia AVM	Skin Mucous membrane GI tract Liver Lungs Kidney Brain Spinal cord	Epistaxis Hematemesis, melena Hematuria Hepatomegaly Neurologic symptoms	Transfusions Embolization vs laser treatment ± excision	Good if bleeding can be controlled and no CNS manifestations
Sturge-Weber (encephalo-trigeminal angiomatosis)	No	Port-wine stains	Trigeminal area Leptomeninges Choroid Oral mucosa	Convulsions Hemiplegia Ocular deformities Mental retardation Glaucoma Intracerebral calcification	Anticonvulsants Neurosurgical procedure	Guarded Depends on intracranial lesion
Von Hippel-Lindau (oculo-cerebellar hemangioblastomatosis)	Autosomal dominant	Hemangioma	Retina Cerebellum	Cysts in cerebellum, pancreas, liver, adrenals, kidneys	Excision of cysts	Depends on intracranial lesion
Blue rubber bleb nevus	Autosomal dominant	Cavernous venous hemangioma	Skin GI tract Spleen Liver CNS	Bluish, compressible rubbery lesions GI bleeding, anemia	Transfusions Electrocoagulation Excision	Depends on CNS and GI involvement
Kasabach-Merritt	Autosomal dominant	Large cavernous hemangiomas	Trunk Extremity	Thrombocytopenia Hemorrhage Anemia Ecchymosis Purpura	Compression Transfusion of blood, platelets	Death from hemorrhage or infection
Maffucci (dyschondroplasia with vascular hamartoma)	Probably autosomal dominant	AVM Cavernous hemangioma Lymphangioma	Fingers Toes Extremity Viscera	Enchondromas Spontaneous fractures Deformed, shorter extremity Vitiligo	Orthopedic management	20% chance of malignancy

of gross differentiation with the appearance of mature vascular stems. Although *hemangiomas*, either capillary or cavernous, are developmental abnormalities of the capillary network stage (Fig. 54-6), it is in the retiform stage that arrest in the development results in *congenital arteriovenous fistulas.* Depending on the size of the abnormal communicating vessels and whether or not angiography could demonstrate the exact site of arteriovenous connections, this group has been further subdivided into *microfistulous* and *macrofistulous arteriovenous fistulas.* Abnormal development of stage 3 results in persistence of anomalous vascular channels.

Recent studies of Mulliken et al.[46,53] gave important information on the endothelial characteristics and cell biology of congenital vascular lesions. These authors reserve the term "hemangioma" for those lesions that clinically undergo growth and usually resolution and in the proliferative phase show endothelial hyperplasia; the term "vascular malformation" (like port-wine stains and arteriovenous, venous, or lymphatic malformations) is used for clinically and cellularly adynamic lesions. As opposed to vascular malformations, hemangiomas in the proliferative phase incorporate [³H]thymidine and also have an increased mast cell count.[54]

The classification of Forbes, May, and Jackson,[51] from the Mayo Clinic, is based on hemodynamics and angiographic appearance. Its advantages are that it is simple and it has practical clinical value because, with the clinical picture, it helps to determine treatment and prognosis. Depending on the amount of shunted blood, *high-* and *low-shunt* lesions are distinguished, and the size of the lesion is determined by the volume of blood that enters the feeding vessels. *High-shunt* lesions correspond with macrofistulous AVMs whereas hemangiomas are obviously *low-shunt* lesions. Between these two extremes a whole spectrum of malformations can be found.

Our further discussion is limited to those lesions that have clinical or angiographic evidence of arteriovenous communications and, based on Szilagyi's classification,[16] belong either to the microfistulous or to the macrofistulous arteriovenous fistulas. It should be remembered, however, that over 70% of congenital arteriovenous fistulas are complex vascular malformations that include hemangiomatous elements as well.[17]

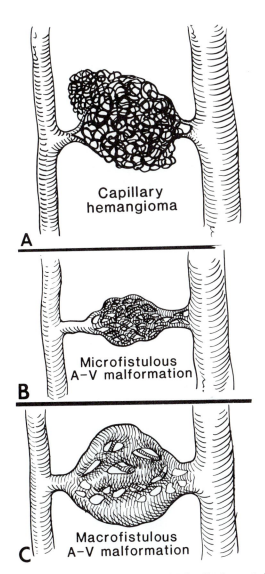

Figure 54-6. A. Capillary hemangiomas. **B.** Microfistulous arteriovenous fistulas. **C.** Macrofistulous arteriovenous fistulas.

Location

Although congenital AVMs can occur almost anywhere in the body, lesions involving the lower extremity are the most frequent (Fig. 54-7). After the extremities, head and neck lesions have the second highest prevalence. Vascular malformations in this area are divided into two groups: *intraaxial* (branches of the internal carotid artery and basilar arteries supplying brain tissue) and *extraaxial* (branches of external carotid artery and those branches of the internal carotid and basilar arteries that supply nonbrain tissue such as dura, bone, or muscle).[19] This distinction is important because the lesions in the two groups are managed differently. AVMs of the spinal cord may have dramatic presentations. Pelvic lesions can be serious management problems, and lesions involving the viscera (lung, gastrointestinal tract, kidneys, and liver) can produce significant symptoms. Lesions in the lung can have either pulmonary arterial or, rarely, systemic blood supply.

Clinical Data

In a recent Mayo Clinic study of 185 patients with congenital AMVs of the extremities and pelvis, there were 100 female and 85 male patients.[55] The median age of the patients when the first lesion was noted was 1.9 years, but the median age at the onset of symptoms was 11 years. No data are available on the natural history because many patients with asymptomatic small lesions never seek medical help. The mean interval between the appearance of the first lesion and the time the first medical examination was done was 12.7 years (median 16.6 years). The most frequent presenting problem was *skin discoloration* (43%), followed by *pain* (37%), a *palpable mass* (35%), and *limb hypertrophy*

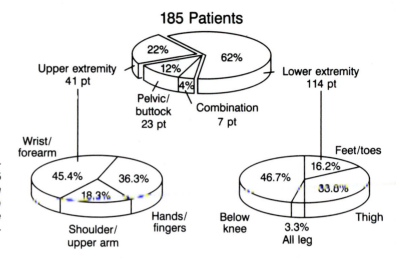

Figure 54-7. Anatomic distribution of congenital arteriovenous malformations in 185 patients. (*From Schwartz RS, Osmundson PJ, Hollier LH: Treatment and prognosis in congenital arteriovenous malformation of the extremity. Phlebology 1:171, 1986. By permission of John Libbey & Co.*)

(34%). Twenty-seven percent of these patients had distended superficial veins, and less than 1% of the patients were completely asymptomatic at the time when medical examination was performed at the Mayo Clinic (Fig. 54-8).

The most frequent abnormality found on physical examination was a *hemangioma* (34%), described usually as "capillary type" (Fig. 54-9). An audible *bruit* was present in 26% of the 185 patients; *ulceration* (Fig. 54-10) and *skin necrosis* were relatively frequent (20%). Increased skin temperature at the level of the lesion, decreased distal pulses, pulsatile veins, and edema of the extremity—with other symptoms of venous hypertension, hyperhydrosis, and hypertrichosis—were additional findings.

The development of soft tissue and bony hypertrophy in association with congenital arteriovenous fistulas, first described by F. Parkes-Weber[56,57] as "hemangiectatic hypertrophy" in 1907 and again in 1918, is still not well understood. Holman's hypothesis that increased arterial flow in the area of the epiphyseal plates is the cause of the overgrowth is hardly acceptable, because nutritive flow in arteriovenous fistulas is always diminished.[20] Venous stasis is another explanation because longer limbs are also seen in

Klippel-Trenaunay syndrome,[58] in which significant arteriovenous shunting is not present. There is some experimental evidence from a small number of animals that venous stasis alone causes bony hypertrophy.[59,60] A tissue growth factor or a complex anomaly in the development of mesenchymal tissue are further possible explanations. The significance of skeletal changes has recently been reconfirmed by Boyd et al.[61]: bony alterations occurred in 34% of 224 vascular malformations, in contrast with only 1% of 356 hemangiomas.

The clinical presentation of AVMs in the head and neck region is determined by the location of the lesion. Occipital dural malformations may be associated with headache, bruit, and seizures; cavernous sinus lesions are associated with retinopathy and vision loss; facial AVMs usually cause cosmetic deformity, mass effect, or bleeding in the tongue or floor of the mouth.[19] Congenital AVMs in the pelvis are more rare than the acquired lesions.[62,63] They may be silent for a long time and be discovered only incidentally during a pelvic examination or computed tomographic (CT) scan or during a laparotomy done for other reasons. Some lesions may cause compression, whereas others may result in vaginal bleeding.

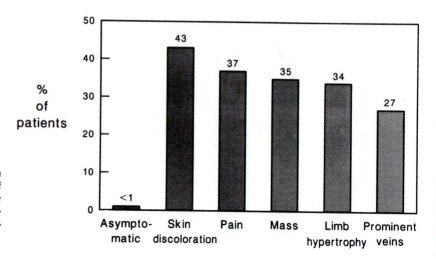

Figure 54-8. Symptoms of 185 patients with congenital arteriovenous malformations of the pelvis and extremities. (*From Schwartz RS, Osmundson PJ, Hollier LH: Phlebology 1:171, 1986. By permission of John Libbey & Co.*)

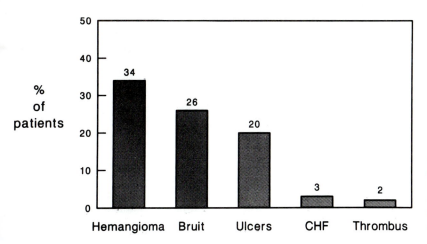

Figure 54-9. Physical findings of 185 patients with congenital arteriovenous malformations of the pelvis and extremities. (*From Schwartz RS, Osmundson PJ, Hollier LH: Phlebology 1:171, 1986. By permission of John Libbey & Co.*)

Diagnosis

The diagnosis of a congenital AVM can usually be made by history and physical examination. Confirmation is generally by angiography. Noninvasive studies, such as *pulse volume recording, sequential limb systolic measurements,* and especially *Doppler examination,* may be useful to diagnose microfistulous, low-shunt lesions not accurately determined by angiography (Fig. 54-11).[64] *Contrast echocardiography* can detect the appearance of indocyanine green on the venous side, after intraarterial injection, and the test is useful to determine residual shunts after surgical excision.[63,65]

Radionuclide scanning of ^{99m}Tc-labeled human albumin can be used to estimate the amount of shunted blood. The labeled 35 μm spheres are injected first into the main feeding artery and then into the vein; radioactivity above the lungs is measured with a gamma camera. Whereas after venous injection, 100% of the isotope is trapped in the lung, the

percentage of radioactivity after arterial injection depends on the arteriovenous shunt flow, which in normal individuals without anesthesia should not exceed 3%.[35] This test is able to estimate local and systemic hemodynamic effects of the arteriovenous shunt and is suitable to monitor the progression of the disease.

These noninvasive examinations, however, do not replace angiography, CT, or nuclear magnetic resonance imaging (MRI).

Angiography
Considerable progress has been made in the field of angiography since Dec. 6, 1933, when Horton and Ghormley[66] first injected 10 ml of thorium oxide (Thorotrast) into the brachial artery of a man to visualize a congenital arteriovenous fistula of the hand. Angiography, complemented by CT with intravenously administered contrast medium or MRI, is today the most important diagnostic test that should

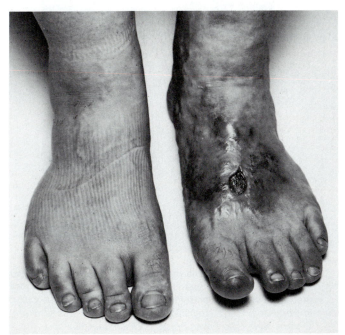

Figure 54-10. Persisting ulcer of dorsum of left foot of 22-year-old woman due to arteriovenous malformation. Repeated embolization and several attempts at skin grafting failed to heal the ulcer.

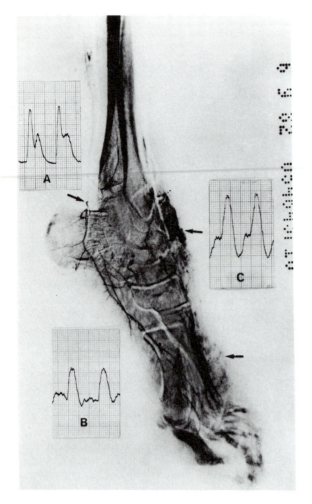

Figure 54-11. Arteriogram of left foot, indicating two areas of angiomas (*arrows*) on lateral side, one at proximal end near ankle and the other at base of fifth toe. **B** and **C.** Doppler ultrasonographic recordings were obtained with probe placed on two angiomatous masses and represented pulsatile waves with contours characteristic of arteriovenous shunts. **A.** Posterotibial arterial pulse wave is distinctly different from those of arteriovenous shunt waves. (*From Haimovici H, Sprayregen S: Arch Surg 121:1065, 1986. By permission of the American Medical Association.*)

be done before any treatment plan is designed. The arteriography is performed with the Seldinger technique, usually through the femoral artery, and selective or superselective catheterization and injections are performed.

With angiography, the size of the feeding arteries can be measured and the size of the arteriovenous shunts (2 mm in large shunts, 100 to 200 μm in small shunts) can be estimated with acceptable accuracy on the basis of appearance time of contrast medium in the vein.[51] The flow volume is determined by the size and rate of opacification of the feeding arteries, whereas the shunt volume can be estimated by the time and appearance of contrast medium in the veins.

On the basis of data from Szilagyi et al.[17] in 1964, in 40% of congenital AVMs the site of shunting cannot be determined with angiography. With the help of superselective angiography of multiple feeding vessels and rapid film-

ing, today this number is probably lower. There are still, however, a considerable number of lesions in which angiography gives only indirect evidence of shunting: early venous filling, increased afferent arterial flow, decreased opacification of the distal arterial tree, pooling of the contrast medium in the area of the fistula, and tortuosity and dilatation of the afferent arteries. In these cases, the diagnosis can be supported further by noninvasive studies.[64]

Computed Tomography

In recent years, CT has made the diagnostic evaluation of patients with congenital AVMs more complete. It delineates the relationship of the lesion to the surrounding tissue. Enhanced with intravenously administered contrast medium, CT provides even better separation of these vascular lesions from adjacent normal tissue. Soft tissue and bone hypertrophy can be accurately documented. Although MRI is gaining increasing popularity, CT scan, because of its easy availability, is still an important diagnostic test in these patients.

Magnetic Resonance Imaging

MRI offers several advantages over other diagnostic modalities and is becoming the complementary technique with angiography to diagnose, follow up, and plan treatment of congenital AVMs.[51,67,68] MRI delineates the relation of AVMs to muscle groups, fascial planes, nerves, and tendons and detects invasion of bone. No contrast medium is needed, no radiation is used, and both sagittal and longitudinal planes can be visualized (Figs. 54-12 and 54-13).

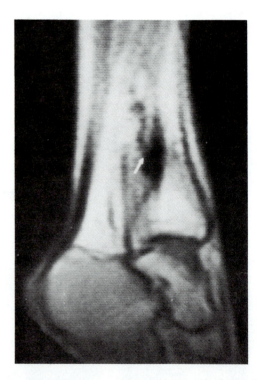

Figure 54-12. Arteriovenous malformation of ankle with serpiginous vessels (*arrow*) clearly seen on partial saturation sagittal magnetic resonance image. (*From Berquist TH: Bone and soft tissue tumors, in Berquist TH (ed): Magnetic Resonance of the Musculoskeletal System. New York, Raven Press, 1987, pp 85–108.*)

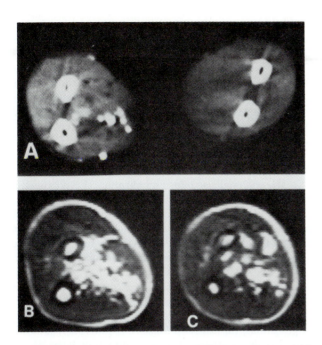

Figure 54-13. Hemangioma of forearm. **A.** Computed tomographic scan with contrast medium shows numerous contrast-filled vessels in forearm. **B** and **C.** Axial magnetic resonance images demonstrate irregular high-intensity lesion with multiple vessels. (*From Berquist TH: Bone and soft tissue tumors, in Berquist TH (ed): Magnetic Resonance of the Musculoskeletal System. New York, Raven Press, 1987, pp 85–108.*)

Treatment and Results

Many congenital AVMs are asymptomatic or have minimal symptoms and require observation only. Because of obvious limitations in the complete cure of these lesions, unless they are small and can be excised *in toto*, it is irresponsible to treat silent and asymptomatic lesions, because any intervention may frequently produce further growth. It is equally important, however, to do everything possible to treat obviously enlarging lesions before significant overgrowth of the extremity or severe disfigurement of the patient develops. In addition, complications of AVMs, such as bleeding, infection, tissue necrosis, and ulcers, need treatment. In rare cases, treatment is indicated because of congestive heart failure, and, in some, secondary aneurysmal changes of the proximal feeding arteries need repair to avoid rupture (Fig. 54-14).

Management of any significant AVM requires teamwork and consultation with the radiologist and the vascular, plastic, or orthopedic surgeon.

Nonsurgical Treatment

Elastic compression, in the form of elastic stocking or garment, is not curative, but it is useful in extremity lesions, not only to compress the hemangioma or the distended superficial veins, but also to give more protection to the extremity to avoid trauma to these vascularized vulnerable lesions.

Laser treatment is becoming increasingly popular for treatment of vascular malformations. The three main types currently in use are the *argon, carbon dioxide,* and *neodymium:yttrium aluminum garnet (Nd:YAG)* lasers. The argon and the Nd:YAG lasers can be used with a flexible endoscope. The Nd:YAG laser, which is used in the treatment of 95% of gastrointestinal lesions, has a deeper penetration, and in contrast to the argon beam, it is not absorbed in the red spectrum and can penetrate blood clot over the vascular malformations. Argon lasers are primarily used for port-wine stains,[69] which are special intradermal capillary malformations, usually in the area of the distribution of the trigeminal nerve or on the lateral aspect of the thigh

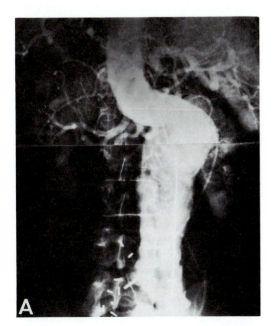
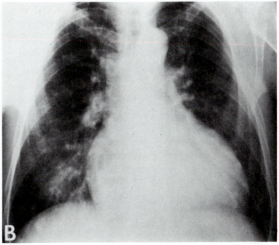

Figure 54-14. A 33-year-old man who required right hip disarticulation for extensive lower extremity arteriovenous malformation. His 12 cm abdominal aortic aneurysm was repaired with a straight aorto–left common iliac dacron graft. **B.** Chest radiograph showing cardiomegaly with pulmonary venous hypertension.

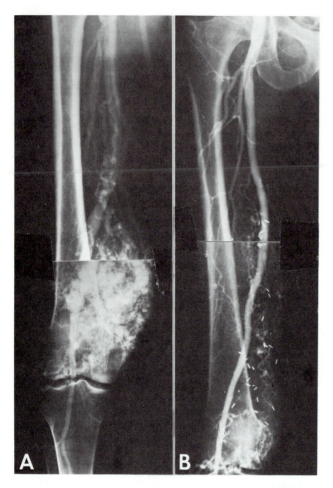

Figure 54-15. A. Large macrofistulous arteriovenous malformation of right thigh of 37-year-old man who had three previous attempts at surgical excision. **B.** Surgical excision and then embolization with 3 mm woolly-tailed coils and Ivalon particles were performed. Angiogram 5 months later shows good result with minimal arteriovenous shunting.

in patients with Klippel-Trenaunay syndrome.[37] Most of the patients, usually adults with purple, well-vascularized lesions, benefit from argon laser treatment, although unacceptable scarring occurs in 5% to 24% of the cases.[48] The use of the laser in larger, high-shunt flow lesions is considered experimental at this time.

Cryotherapy and electrolysis have no proven value in the treatment of AVMs and should be abandoned.

Sclerotherapy can be effectively used in selected low-shunt lesions with the injection of 3% sodium tetradecyl sulfate directly into the lesion.[51] Small amounts of the drug (0.5 to 2.0 ml) are injected during one session after blood has been emptied from the lesion either by aspiration with the syringe or by elevation of the extremity. Compression treatment is necessary after sclerotherapy. The indications for this form of treatment are limited and it should not be used with high-shunt lesions.

Embolization with percutaneous catheterization has become an important treatment option for AVMs, used alone or in combination with surgical treatment (Figs. 54-15 to 54-18).* It requires careful planning, special knowledge of anatomy of the blood vessels, and a radiologist or neuroradiologist who is well trained in selective and superselective catheterization. Congenital AVMs are frequently supplied by several arteries; therefore, catheterization through more than one main artery may be necessary. The aim of the embolization is to stop abnormal shunting at the precapillary or capillary level. Occlusion of the main arterial trunk is a serious error because it makes the AVM inaccessible for further embolization while allowing the AVM to open new distal collateral vessels.

The material used for embolization should therefore be small enough to reach the capillary level but larger than the size of the fistula to avoid pulmonary embolization. Embolizing materials are divided into two groups: temporary and permanent. *Temporary materials* such as *blood clot, gelatin sponge,* or *microfibrillar collagen,* are used for preoperative embolization to decrease operative blood loss, are usually little risk to normal tissues, and dissolve within a few days or weeks. *Permanent materials* used are the *silicon spheres, polyvinyl alcohol particles, stainless steel coils,* or, for large fistulas, the *detachable balloons.* Liquids such as *absolute alcohol* or *bucrylate* are also used, although bucrylate has become less popular recently because of a presumed carcinogenic effect.

Silicon spheres can be accurately sized, but the disadvantage is that a large-diameter catheter is required for delivery. The advantages of *polyvinyl alcohol foam* (Ivalon) are that (1) a smaller catheter can be used and (2) after embolization the size of the particles increases up to 10 times. The particles are injected in the form of a liquid slurry by using a mixture of contrast medium and warm saline solution containing the foam particles, ranging from 100 μm to 1 mm in diameter.[19]

Stainless steel coils with tufted Dacron are adequate to occlude large vessels. Thrombosis, which is enhanced by using the tufted Dacron, can also be augmented by injecting thrombotic materials in addition to the coils.

Embolization is performed in one or, if necessary, in several stages with a continuous fluoroscopically monitored flow-delivery technique using a single-lumen, nontapered catheter, described by Kerber[70] in 1977, to avoid reflux and poor deposition.

Complications can be decreased by careful selection of the embolizing material and embolization technique and by a thorough knowledge of vascular anatomy. Although certain arteries, such as branches of the hypogastric artery, branches of the profunda femoris artery, or certain muscle branches, are ideal for embolization, embolic occlusion of distal arteries of the extremities may, unfortunately, frequently lead to tissue loss or gangrene.

Forbes et al.[19] reported on 31 therapeutic embolizations of 23 patients with extraaxial vascular malformations of the head. Of the nine patients with AVMs, embolization in seven produced excellent results: the degree of obstruction was 80% or more. Two patients with high shunt flow needed combined radiologic-surgical treatment. Beneficial effect from embolization in cases of pelvic congenital AVMs[71] or extremity lesions[18,72] has been reported as well.

---

*References 18, 19, 27, 36, 38, 51, 69–73.

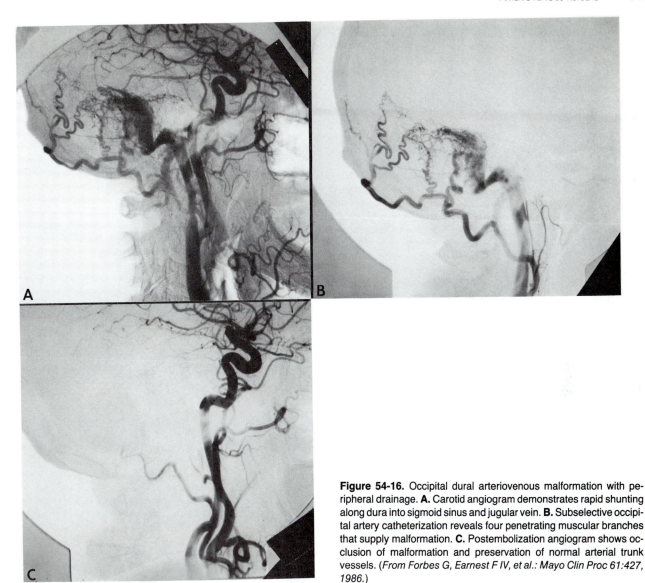

Figure 54-16. Occipital dural arteriovenous malformation with peripheral drainage. **A.** Carotid angiogram demonstrates rapid shunting along dura into sigmoid sinus and jugular vein. **B.** Subselective occipital artery catheterization reveals four penetrating muscular branches that supply malformation. **C.** Postembolization angiogram shows occlusion of malformation and preservation of normal arterial trunk vessels. (*From Forbes G, Earnest F IV, et al.: Mayo Clin Proc 61:427, 1986.*)

Long-term results are, however, still needed to confirm the real value of this procedure.

Surgical Treatment

It is imperative to emphasize that ligation of the proximal feeding vessel alone has no place in the treatment of AVM. It will invariably lead to the development of collateral circulation, and it impedes radiologic embolization as a form of treatment of these lesions. Direct feeding arteries should be ligated only in those rare cases in which immediate complete resection of a localized AVM is possible.

The presence of an AVM alone does not mandate aggressive treatment. This conservative attitude is clearly reflected in the study of Gomes and Bernatz,[74] from the Mayo Clinic: of 80 patients with congenital AVMs of the extremities, surgical excision was attempted only in 10. If surgical treatment is indicated because of rare cosmetic reasons, sudden progression, involvement of adjacent important structures, ulceration of the skin, repeated infection, or bleeding or rarely congestive heart failure, it should be most carefully planned. In our present practice, embolization with or without an attempt at complete surgical resection seems to be the best treatment option. Embolization can be repeated if necessary if the main feeding vessels are left intact.

If excision is contemplated, we avoid staging and make every attempt to perform a resection as complete as possible at one stage. In general, in only about 20% of all AVMs can curative resection be performed.[75] If the lesion is on the extremity, a proximal tourniquet significantly decreases blood loss. Meticulous hemostasis during the procedure is imperative. The use of the cell saver for autotransfusion in these patients has become routine. Cardiopulmonary bypass, temporary circulatory arrest, and hypothermia have been used for excision of large AVMs. Intraoperative Doppler echocardiography has been a useful adjunct to determine the extent of these tumors and to localize the feeding vessels.[76] With the technique of careful serial ligation of all branches of major extremity arteries and veins to interrupt feeding vessels to the AVMs, Vollmar and

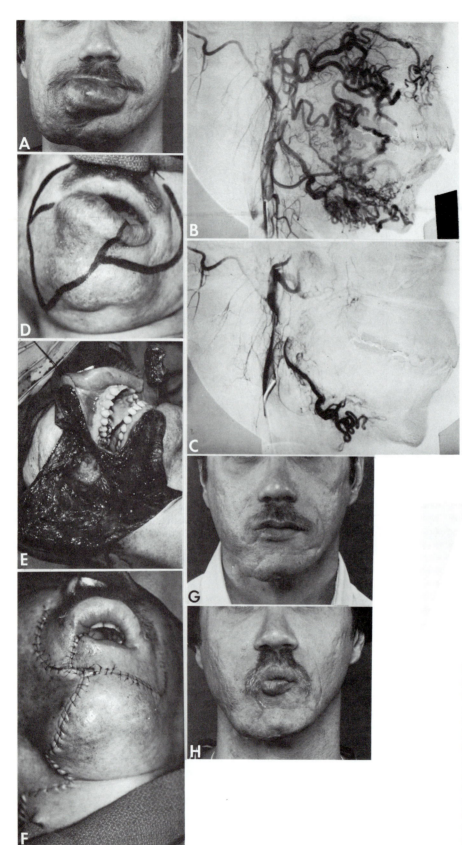

Figure 54-17. A. High-flow arteriovenous malformation. **B.** Clinical impression confirmed by right carotid angiography that shows extensive supply from external system. **C.** Appearance after embolization. **D.** Resection of malformation 48 hours after embolization by using Karapandzic technique of reconstruction. **E.** Lesion excised. **F.** See reconstruction of lip and chin. **G.** Postoperative result. **H.** Function of lips. (*From Forbes G, May GR, Jackson IT: Vascular anomalies in children, in Jackson IT, Mustarde J [eds]: Plastic Surgery in Infancy and Childhood. New York, Churchill Livingstone [in press]*).

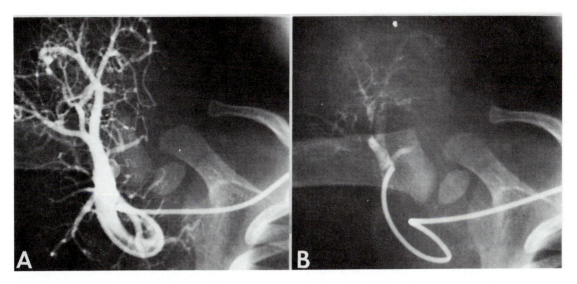

Figure 54-18. A. Angiogram of high-flow arteriovenous malformation of shoulder in child. Lesion is supplied by humeral circumflex arteries. **B.** Postembolization with blood clot; most of arteries are occluded. Lesion was resected 24 hours after embolization. (*From Forbes G, May GR, Jackson IT: Vascular anomalies in children, in Jackson IT, Mustarde J [eds]: Plastic Surgery in Infancy and Childhood. New York, Churchill Livingstone [in press]*).

Stalker[49] reported an improvement in 19 of 21 cases of extremity AVMs, and only two patients needed amputations. We combine this technique with attempts at complete resection, even if large defects are made which need reconstruction with axial or arterialized flaps. The overall experience is, unfortunately, that extensive lesions cannot be excised for cure in the majority of cases. Szilagyi[75] reported poor results in 5 of 8 patients with deep diffuse AVMs who underwent an attempt at surgical resection. Surgery helped in only 1 patient, and the result was clearly worse in 5. Trout et al.[77] attempted surgical treatment of 4 lower extremity AVMs, 2 of which required amputations. In our recent retrospective study,[55] symptomatic patients with surgical excision seemed to do better, most probably because of the larger number of localized lesions than in those treated conservatively. The surgical group of 82 patients included 18 patients who required amputations at various levels of the extremity. Many of these amputations, however, meant cure for the patients and saved them from the long-term morbidity of repeated procedures.

VISCERAL ARTERIOVENOUS MALFORMATIONS

As a result of improvement in diagnostic techniques, especially in selective celiac and superior mesenteric catheterizations, there has been an increased recognition of the importance and frequency of *gastrointestinal AVMs*. The lesions classified as type I by Moore et al.[78] are most probably acquired submucosal AVMs, which develop in elderly patients with valvular heart disease or severe atherosclerosis and are usually located in the terminal ileum, cecum, or ascending colon. The type II lesions are, however, true congenital AVMs and occur mostly in the upper portion of the small bowel in younger patients. The type III lesions

are punctate angiomas, which are the gastrointestinal manifestations of hereditary hemorrhagic telangiectasia (Rendu-Osler-Weber syndrome).

Selective or superselective angiography with magnification is frequently necessary to visualize the lesions, which produce the so-called "tram track" sign, the simultaneous opacification of the feeding artery and the draining vein.

Embolization, endoscopic treatment, and surgical excisions are the options if bleeding does not cease after correction of coagulation abnormalities and transfusion. Embolization, if done, should be performed with extreme caution and with superselective catheterization only; bowel necrosis is a definite possibility.[72] For this reason, endoscopic treatment, with monopolar or bipolar electrocoagulation, heater probe, and especially photocoagulation with the Nd:YAG laser, is gaining increasing popularity. The YAG laser producer thermal destruction of the vascular tissue, even in the submucosa, and produces mucosal ulceration that needs several weeks to heal. It is an effective way, however, to stop bleeding from vascular malformations, although rebleeding rates as high as 25% have been reported. In a series of 59 patients treated with the laser, two cecal perforations required hemicolectomy.[79]

Surgical excision, if the lesion is clearly identified on angiogram, is usually effective.[78] Intraoperative identification of the mucosal AVM may be facilitated by transillumination. Recurrent bleeding, usually from other malformations, can be as frequent as 10%.[80]

Renal AVMs, which are usually located beneath the mucosa of the renal collective system, may result in hematuria or flank pain or may be an incidental finding during renal arteriography done for other purposes. Massive bleeding from renal AVM during pregnancy has been reported.[81]

Transcatheter embolization is the treatment for symptomatic lesions. If it is unsuccessful, partial or sometimes total nephrectomy is necessary.

Hepatic or *splenic AVMs* are extremely rare and may be manifestations of hereditary hemorrhagic telangiectasia (Rendu-Osler-Weber syndrome).[82] Jaundice, significant hepatomegaly, and high shunt volume with cardiac failure have been reported. If the lesions are symptomatic, excision and embolization are the treatment options.

Pulmonary AVMs have an almost 40% chance of being associated with hereditary hemorrhagic telangiectasia. The most frequent symptoms are dyspnea, palpitation, and hemoptysis; 60% of the patients have an audible bruit.[81] Cyanosis and clubbing are additional findings. Patients with hereditary hemorrhagic telangiectasia usually have multiple fistulas. There is an increased rate of fistula growth and increased frequency of complications, especially cerebrovascular accidents.

Angiography confirms multiplicity and identifies blood supply. Surgical excision gives good results and is indicated if the patient is symptomatic and if a single fistula is associated with hereditary telangiectasia and, in the rare cases, with systemic blood supply.[83] Multiple bilateral AVMs with hereditary telangectasia, managed with staged bilateral thoracotomies, have been reported.[84] Patients with multiple bilateral lesions can be effectively treated with embolization with detachable balloons, as reported by Barth et al.[73]

SUMMARY

Because of local effects and systemic hemodynamic consequences, the majority of acquired arteriovenous fistulas, and a smaller number of congenital AVMs, require treatment. Whereas surgical repair of acquired fistulas is rewarding and, except for the large central shunts, has low morbidity and mortality rates, with excellent results, surgical cure of congenital lesions is possible in only about one fifth of the cases. Embolization with or without surgical excision has improved results, especially in the region of the head and neck, pelvis, and certain forms of visceral malformations. The laser is gaining increasing popularity in treating vascular lesions, but, similar to embolization, it still lacks proof of long-term effectiveness. Large high shunt extremity malformations, in spite of the combined radiologic-surgical management, are difficult to control, and in some (fortunately rare) cases amputation is the only alternative.

REFERENCES

1. Virchow R: Pathologie des Tumeurs: Cours professé à l'Université de Berlin, vol. 4. Paris, Germer-Baillière, 1876, p 169.
2. Hunter W: The history of an aneurysm of the aorta, with some remarks on aneurysms in general. Med Observations Inquiries 1:323, 1757.
3. Hunter W: Further observations upon a particular species of aneurysm. Med Observations Inquiries 2:390, 1764.
4. Breschet G: Mémoire sur les anévrysmes. Mem Acad Med (Paris) 3:101, 1833.
5. Norris G: Varicose aneurism at the bend of the arm: Ligature of the artery above and below the sac; secondary hemorrhages with a return of the anurismal thrill on the tenth day; cure. Am J Med Sci 5:28, 1843.
6. Nicoladoni C: Phlebarteriectasie der rechten oberen Extremität. Arch Klin Chir 18:252, 1875.
7. Branham HH: Aneurismal varix of the femoral artery and vein following a gunshot wound. Int J Surg 3:250, 1890.
8. Holman E: Arteriovenous Aneurysm: Abnormal Communications Between the Arterial and Venous Circulations. New York, Macmillan, 1937.
9. Shumacker HB Jr, Carter KL: Arteriovenous fistulas and arterial aneurysms in military personnel. Surgery 20:9, 1946.
10. Hughes CW, Jahnke EJ Jr: The surgery of traumatic arteriovenous fistulas and aneurysms: A five-year follow-up study of 215 lesions. Ann Surg 148:790, 1958.
11. Rich NM, Hobson RW II, Collins GJ Jr: Traumatic arteriovenous fistulas and false aneurysms: A review of 558 lesions. Surgery 78:817, 1975.
12. Reid MR: Studies on abnormal arteriovenous communications, acquired and congenital, I: Report of a series of cases. Arch Surg 10:601, 1925.
13. de Takats G: Vascular anomalies of the extremities: Report of five cases. Surg Gynecol Obstet 55:227, 1932.
14. Coursley G, Ivins JC, Barker NW: Congenital arteriovenous fistulas in the extremities: An analysis of sixty-nine cases. Angiology 7:201, 1956.
15. Malan E, Puglionisi A: Congenital angiodysplasias of the extremities. (Note I: Generalities and classification; venous dysplasias.) (Note II: Arterial, arterial and venous, and haemolymphatic dysplasias.) J Cardiovasc Surg 5:87, 1964; 6:255, 1965.
16. Szilagyi DE, Elliott JP, et al.: Peripheral congenital arteriovenous fistulas. Surgery 57:61, 1965.
17. Szilagyi DE, Smith RF, et al: Congenital arteriovenous anomalies of the limbs. Arch Surg 111:423, 1976.
18. Natali J, Merland JJ: Superselective arteriography and therapeutic embolisation for vascular malformations (angiodysplasias). J Cardiovasc Surg (Torino) 17:465, 1976.
19. Forbes G, Earnest F IV, et al: Therapeutic embolization angiography for extra-axial lesions in the head. Mayo Clin Proc 61:427, 1986.
20. Patman RD, Poulos E, Shires GT: The management of civilian arterial injuries. Surg Gynecol Obstet 118:725, 1964.
21. Kollmeyer KR, Hunt JL, et al.: Acute and chronic traumatic arteriovenous fistulae in civilians: Epidemiology and treatment. Arch Surg 116:697, 1981.
22. Linton RR, White PD: Arteriovenous fistula between the right common iliac artery and the inferior vena cava: Report of a case of its occurrence following an operation for a ruptured intervertebral disk with cure by operation. Arch Surg 50:6, 1945.
23. Quigley TM, Stoney RJ: Arteriovenous fistulas following lumbar laminectomy: The anatomy defined. J Vasc Surg 2:828, 1985.
24. Hollingsworth EW: Arteriovenous fistula of the renal vessels. Am J Med Sci 188:399, 1934.
25. Dzsinich C, Szabó, et al.: Arteriovenous fistula after partial nephrectomy: Successful surgical repair—report of a case. Thorac Cardiovasc Surg 32:325, 1984.
26. Morin RP, Dunn EJ, Wright CB: Renal arteriovenous fistulas: A review of etiology, diagnosis, and management. Surgery 99:114, 1986.
27. Lord RSA, Ehrenfeld WK, Wylie EJ: Arterial injury from the Fogarty catheter. Med J Aust 2:70, 1968.
28. Shifrin EG, Anner H, et al: Arterio-venous fistula in the lower limb in consequence of Fogarty balloon catheter embolectomy: Case report and review of the literature. J Cardiovasc Surg (Torino) 26:310, 1985.
29. Schweitzer DL, Aguam AS, Wilder JR: Complications encountered during arterial embolectomy with the Fogarty balloon catheter: Report of a case and review of the literature. Vasc Surg 10:144, 1976.

30. Astarita D, Filippone DR, Cohn JD: Spontaneous major intra-abdominal arteriovenous fistulas: A report of several cases. Angiology 36:656, 1985.

31. McAuley CE, Peitzman AB, et al.: The syndrome of spontaneous iliac arteriovenous fistula: A distinct clinical and pathophysiologic entity. Surgery 99:373, 1986.

32. Holman E: Abnormal Arteriovenous Communications. Springfield, Ill., Charles C Thomas, Publisher, 1968.

33. Davis JO, Urquhart J, et al.: Hypersecretion of aldosterone in dogs with a chronic aortic-caval fistula and high output heart failure. Circ Res 14:471, 1964.

34. Epstein FH, Ferguson TB: The effect of the formation of an arteriovenous fistula upon blood volume. J Clin Invest 34:434, 1955.

35. Callander CL: Study of arterio-venous fistula with an analysis of 447 cases. Johns Hopkins Hosp Rep 19:259, 1920.

36. Sirinek KR, Gaskill HV III, et al.: Exclusion angiography for patients with possible vascular injuries of the extremities: A better use of trauma center resources. Surgery 94:598, 1983.

37. Vollmar J, Krumhaar D: Surgical experience with 200 traumatic arteriovenous fistulae, in Hiertonn T, Rybeck B (eds): Symposium on Traumatic Arterial Lesions, Uppsala. Stockholm, Försvarets forskningsanstalt, 1968.

38. Shumacker HB Jr, Wayson EE: Spontaneous cure of aneurysms and arteriovenous fistulas, with some notes on intrasaccular thrombosis. Am J Surg 79:532, 1950.

39. Linder F: Acquired arterio-venous fistulas: Report of 223 operated cases. Ann Chir Gynaecol 74:1, 1985.

40. Harris AE, McMenamin PG: Carotid artery-cavernous sinus fistula. Arch Otolaryngol 110:618, 1984.

41. Janes JM, Jennings WK Jr: Effect of induced arteriovenous fistula on leg length: 10-year observations. Proc Staff Meeting Mayo Clin 36:1, 1961.

42. Sumner DS: Diagnostic evaluation of arteriovenous fistulas, in Rutherford RB (eds): Vascular Surgery, 2nd ed. Philadelphia, WB Saunders, 1984.

43. Rutherford RB: Noninvasive testing in the diagnosis and assessment of arteriovenous fistula, in Bernstein EF (ed): Noninvasive Diagnostic Techniques in Vascular Disease, 3rd ed. St. Louis, CV Mosby, 1985, pp 666–679.

44. Gloviczki P, Hollier LH, et al.: Experimental replacement of the inferior vena cava: Factors affecting patency. Surgery 95:657, 1984.

45. Debrun G, Lacour P, et al.: Treatment of 54 traumatic carotid-cavernous fistulas. J Neurosurg 55:678, 1981.

46. Mulliken JB, Glowacki J: Hemangiomas and vascular malformations in infants and children: A classification based on endothelial characteristics. Plast Reconstr Surg 69:412, 1982.

47. Malan E, Sala A, Tardito E: Arteriovenous fistulas, in Haimovici H (ed): Vascular Surgery: Principles and Techniques, 2nd ed. Norwalk, Conn., Appleton-Century-Crofts, 1984, pp 777–794.

48. Rohrich RJ, Spicer TE: Hemangiomas and vascular malformations/lymphedema. Selected Readings Plast Surg 4:1, 1986.

49. Vollmar JF, Stalker CG: The surgical treatment of congenital arterio-venous fistulas in the extremities. J Cardiovasc Surg (Torino) 17:340, 1976.

50. Merland JJ, Riche MC, et al.: Classification actuelle des malformations vasculaires. Ann Chir Plast 25:105, 1980.

51. Forbes G, May GR, Jackson IT: Vascular anomalies in children, in Jackson IT, Mustardé J (eds): Plastic Surgery in Infancy and Childhood. New York, Churchill Livingstone (in press).

52. Woollard HH: The development of the principal arterial stems in the forelimb of the pig, in Carnegie Institution of Washington: Contributions to Embryology, vol 14, No. 70. Publication No. 277. Washington, Carnegie Institution of Washington, 1922, pp 139–154.

53. Mulliken JB, Zetter BR, Folkman J: In vitro characteristics of endothelium from hemangiomas and vascular malformations. Surgery 92:348, 1982.

54. Glowacki J, Mulliken JB: Mast cells in hemangiomas and vascular malformations. Pediatrics 70:48, 1982.

55. Schwartz RS, Osmundson PJ, Hollier LH: Treatment and prognosis in congenital arteriovenous malformation of the extremity. Phlebology 1:171, 1986.

56. Weber FP: Angioma-formation in connection with hypertrophy of limbs and hemi-hypertrophy. Br J Dermatol 19:231, 1907.

57. Weber FP: Haemangiectatic hypertrophy of limbs: Congenital phlebarteriectasis and so-called congenital varicose veins. Br J Child Dis 15:13, 1918.

58. Gloviczki P, Hollier LH, et al.: Surgical implications of Klippel-Trenaunay syndrome. Ann Surg 197:353, 1983.

59. Servelle M: Stase veineuse et croissance osseuse. Bull Acad Natl Med 132:471, 1948.

60. Hutchison WJ, Burdeaux BD Jr: The influence of stasis on bone growth. Surg Gynecol Obstet 99:413, 1954.

61. Boyd JB, Mulliken JB, et al: Skeletal changes associated with vascular malformations. Plast Reconstr Surg 74:789, 1984.

62. Decker DG, Fish CR, Juergens JL: Arteriovenous fistulas of the female pelvis: A diagnostic problem. Obstet Gynecol 31:799, 1968.

63. Pritchard DA, Maloney JD, et al.: Surgical treatment of congenital pelvic arteriovenous malformation. Mayo Clin Proc 53:607, 1978.

64. Haimovici H, Sprayregen S: Congenital microarteriovenous shunts: Angiographic and Doppler ultrasonographic identification. Arch Surg 121:1065, 1986.

65. Pritchard DA, Maloney JD, et al: Peripheral arteriovenous fistula: Detection by contrast echocardiography. Mayo Clin Proc 52:186, 1977.

66. Horton BT, Ghormley RK: Congenital arteriovenous fistulae of the extremities visualized by arteriography. Surg Gynecol Obstet 60:978, 1935.

67. Amparo EG, Higgins CB, Hricak H: Primary diagnosis of abdominal arteriovenous fistula by MR imaging. J Comput Assist Tomogr 8:1140, 1984.

68. Berquist TH: Bone and soft tissue tumors, in Berquist TH (ed): Magnetic Resonance of the Musculoskeletal System. New York, Raven Press, 1987, pp 85–108.

69. Noe JM, Barsky SH, et al.: Port wine stains and the response to argon laser therapy: Successful treatment and the predictive role of color, age, and biopsy. Plast Reconstr Surg 65:130, 1980.

70. Kerber CW: Catheter therapy: Fluoroscopic monitoring of deliberate embolic occlusion. Radiology 125:538, 1977.

71. Kaufman SL, Kumar AAJ, et al.: Transcatheter embolization in the management of congenital arteriovenous malformations. Radiology 137:21, 1980.

72. Gomes AS, Mali WP, Oppenheim WL: Embolization therapy in the management of congenital arteriovenous malformations. Radiology 144:41, 1982.

73. Barth KH, White RI Jr, et al.: Embolotherapy of pulmonary arteriovenous malformations with detachable balloons. Radiology 142:599, 1982.

74. Gomes MMR, Bernatz PE: Arteriovenous fistulas: A review and ten-year experience at the Mayo Clinic. Mayo Clin Proc 45:81, 1970.

75. Szilagyi DE: Vascular malformations (with special emphasis on peripheral arteriovenous lesions), in Moore W (ed): Vascular Surgery: A Comprehensive Review, 2nd ed. New York, Grune & Stratton, 1986, pp 773–790.

76. Cormier JM, Laurian C, et al.: Traitement chirurgical des fistules artério-veineuses congénitales des membres sous contrôle ultrasonographique. Chirurgie 107:424, 1981.

77. Trout HH III, McAllister HA Jr, et al.: Vascular malformations. Surgery 97:36, 1985.

78. Moore JD, Thompson NW, et al.: Arteriovenous malformations of the gastrointestinal tract. Arch Surg 111:381, 1976.

79. Rutgeerts P, Van Gompel F, et al.: Long-term results of treatment of vascular malformations of the gastrointestinal tract by neodymium:YAG laser photocoagulation. Gut 26:586, 1985.

80. Richardson JD, Max MH, et al.: Bleeding vascular malformations of the intestine. Surgery 84:430, 1978.

81. Klimberg I, Wilson J, et al.: Hemorrhage from congenital renal arteriovenous malformation in pregnancy. Urology 23:381, 1984.

82. Burckhardt D, Stalder GA, et al.: Hyperdynamic circulatory state due to Osler-Weber-Rendu disease with intrahepatic arteriovenous fistulas. Am Heart J 85:797, 1973.

83. Dines DE, Arms RA, et al.: Pulmonary arteriovenous fistulas. Mayo Clin Proc 49:460, 1974.

84. Brown SE, Wright PW, et al.: Staged bilateral thoracotomies for multiple pulmonary arteriovenous malformations complicating hereditary hemorrhagic telangiectasia. J Thorac Cardiovasc Surg 83:285, 1982.

PART V
Surgery of Visceral Vessels

CHAPTER 55
Cerebrovascular Insufficiency

Allan D. Callow

INCIDENCE, PREVALENCE, AND COST

For each of the 5 years from 1971 to 1976, stroke incidence in the United States was approximately 407,000.[1] Of these strokes, approximately 300,000 were initial strokes. Age-adjusted stroke incidence of 152 per 100,000 in 1971 declined to 137 per 100,000 by 1976.

Approximately 8% of all deaths reported in the United States are directly due to stroke, and stroke ranks as the fourth cause of death in this country, having recently been displaced from third place by trauma. Two thirds of stroke victims who survive 1 month are permanently disabled to some degree.

In 1950, stroke mortality was approximately 90 per 100,000; in 1982 it had decreased to 35.8 per 100,000, and in a more recent period from 1979 to 1982, age-adjusted stroke mortality had fallen nearly 14% (Fig. 55-1).[2] Declining incidence may be primarily responsible for the declining mortality.[3]

Two million surviving stroke victims in the United States comprise a prevalence rate of 9.7 per 100,000. Of as great concern as the incidence and mortality is the continuing risk for recurrent stroke among survivors. In a recent Framingham Study of 394 stroke victims, 84, or 21%, had second strokes, and 27, or 7%, had third strokes.[4] The leading cause of death among the 30-day survivors of stroke was concomitant cardiovascular disease.

In 1972, the direct costs of stroke in the United States were estimated at $2.03 billion. This amount had increased to $3.26 billion by 1975 and to $6.8 billion by 1985. In 1985 dollars, using 1980 incidence and prevalence figures and including indirect costs, the estimated annual total cost of stroke was $16 billion to $20 billion. Federal and state governments, private insurance companies, patients, their families, and their employers bear this enormous financial burden.[5,6]

ANATOMY AND PHYSIOLOGY

The principal arteries supplying the head and neck are the right common carotid branch of the innominate artery and the left common carotid artery arising directly from the aortic arch (Fig. 55-2). The left common carotid artery may originate from the innominate artery in 8% of individuals.[7,8] The sternocleidomastoid, sternohyoid, sternothyroid, and omohyoid muscles cover the proximal portion of the cervical carotid artery, but as it ascends, it is covered only by the cervical fascia, the platysma, and the skin. A sheath derived from the deep cervical fascia encloses the common carotid artery, the internal jugular vein (lateral to the common carotid artery), and the vagus nerve, which lies between the artery and the vein and deep to both. An important variation is the frequent inclusion of the hypoglossal nerve and the ansa cervicalis within the carotid sheath. The recurrent laryngeal nerve travels obliquely dorsal to the proximal end of the common carotid artery. In approximately 70% of dissections, the carotid bifurcation occurs at the level of the thyroid cartilage. In approximately 15 to 20% the bifurcation occurs between this point and the hyoid bone, and in the remaining 10% of dissections, it occurs at a higher level, still between the hyoid bone and the angle of the mandible. Rarely, the internal and external carotid arteries may originate directly from the innominate artery or from the aortic arch. The dilated first centimeter of the internal carotid artery and the end of the common carotid artery form the carotid bulb. Regulation of the systemic blood pressure through a branch of the hypoglossal nerve occurs here in the carotid sinus.

The *external carotid artery* is a landmark to several nerves. The first is the superior laryngeal nerve, which courses medially and deep to the external carotid artery and is overlain by the lingual, common facial, and superior thyroid veins and by the digastric and stylohyoid muscles.

TABLE 55-1. ANNUAL AVERAGE INITIAL STROKE INCIDENCE RATE PER 100,000

Age at Onset	Male	Female
All ages—crude	148.1	133.8
55-64	341.6	191.1
65-74	658.4	524.2
75-84	1,713.6	1,280.2

From Robins M, Baum HM, in Weinfeld FD (ed): The National Survey of Stroke. Bethesda, Md, Office of Scientific and Health Reports, National Institute of Neurological and Communicative Disorders and Stroke, National Institutes of Health, Public Health Service, 1981.

TABLE 55-2. EFFECT OF STROKE AMONG 30-DAY SURVIVORS

Two thirds are permanently disabled.

One half survive at least 5 years.

One third require prolonged inpatient rehabilitation.

From McDowell FH, Caplan LR (eds): Cerebrovascular Survey Report 1985. Bethesda, Md, National Institute of Neurological and Communicative Disorders and Stroke, National Institutes of Health, Public Health Service, 1985.

It supplies the false vocal cords and other structures of the pharynx.

The second is the hypoglossal nerve, which crosses the main trunk of the external carotid artery and innervates the tongue.

The *internal carotid artery* may begin at various levels from the bifurcation of the common carotid artery. Proximally, it is usually posterior and somewhat lateral to the

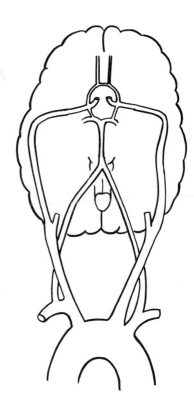

Figure 55-2. The three primary branches of the aortic arch.

external carotid artery, parallel to the internal jugular vein, and partially overridden by the sternocleidomastoid muscle. It is crossed by the hypoglossal nerve and the digastric and stylohyoid muscles. The vagus nerve lies posterolateral to the internal carotid. Near the base of the skull, the vagus,

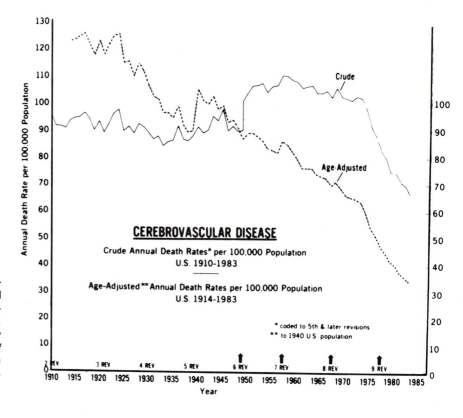

Figure 55-1. Cerebrovascular disease annual crude (1910-1983) and age-adjusted (1914-1983) death rates per 100,000 population, United States. (*From McDowell, FH, Caplan LR (eds): Cerebrovascular Survey Report 1985. For the National Institute of Neurological and Communicative Disorders and Stroke, National Institute of Health, Public Health Service, Bethesda, Md.*)

Rarely, in association with an anomalous subclavian artery, the vertebral artery may arise from the common carotid artery. When one vertebral artery is hypoplastic, the posterior cerebral arteries arise from the terminal portion of the basilar artery. In approximately 20% of individuals, the posterior cerebral artery may be an extension of the internal carotid branch.

The *circle of Willis* is composed of the posterior cerebral arteries arising from the basilar artery (posterior circulation) and of the internal carotid and its two terminal branches, the middle and anterior cerebral arteries (the anterior circulation). The anterior and posterior systems are connected via the two posterior communicating branches of the posterior cerebral arteries. The two hemispheres are connected via the single, transversely situated, anterior communicating artery joining the two anterior cerebral arteries. This vessel completes the circle of Willis (Fig. 55-3).[9,10] This classic configuration, an effective equalizer of flow, occurs in approximately 50% of individuals. Anatomic variations are numerous and are most frequently due to hypoplasia or agenesis of the various communicating arteries. These undetected anatomic variations, compounded by occlusive disease lesions, render the circle of Willis an unreliable provider of collateral circulation (Fig. 55-4).[11]

The *anterior circulation* is composed of the anterior and middle cerebral arteries from which the eyes, the basal ganglia, most of the hypothalamus, the frontal lobe, the parietal lobe, and most of the temporal lobe derive their supply. Approximately 80% of the total supply of blood to the brain comes through the middle cerebral artery, which has been labeled the artery of aphasia and is the one most frequently associated with cerebral infarction. In addition to the circle of Willis, collateral pathways are provided by the leptomeningeal anastomoses, by the network of unnamed vessels in the watershed areas of the anterior, middle, and posterior cerebral arteries, by anastomoses between the anterior and middle meningeal arteries, and by a number

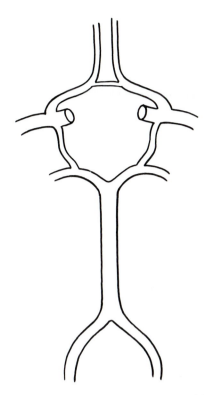

Figure 55-3. Vessels that form the circle of Willis.

glossopharyngeal, accessory, and hypoglossal nerves lie between the internal carotid artery and the internal jugular vein and deep to the artery.

The *vertebral artery* is the first branch of the subclavian artery, but in approximately 6% of cases the left vertebral artery may arise directly from the arch of the aorta. One vertebral artery is frequently larger than the other, and in approximately 65% of these cases, the left one is dominant.

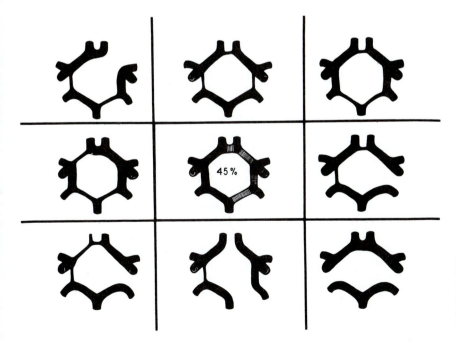

Figure 55-4. Congenital variations consisting of hypoplastic or absent communicating arteries. The incidence of anomalies is approximately 45%. (*Modified from Abrams HL: Angiography, 2nd ed, Boston, Little, Brown & Co, 1961, p 180*).

of named and unnamed cervical branches of the external carotid and vertebral arteries. The functional capacity of these collaterals is not measurable by clinical examination or by conventional diagnostic tools.

Cerebral autoregulation is the ability of the brain to maintain constant flow and is a remarkable feature of the cerebral circulation. Unlike other vascular beds, substantial changes in brain blood flow do not occur with normal physiologic variations in cardiac output, blood pressure, and pulse rate. Except in extreme circumstances such as severe hypovolemia or cardiac failure, perfusion pressure remains constant. This self-regulatory ability of the brain, based on continuous adjustment of the resistance of small cerebral arteries and arterioles, makes induced hypertension during carotid endarterectomy largely ineffective. The arterioles must be supplied with an adequate perfusion pressure if their normal function is to be preserved. Autoregulation is impaired as a consequence of prolonged hypotension, hypertension, hypoxia, and the action of many drugs. Under these abnormal conditions, cerebral blood flow is dependent on perfusion pressure. The localized vasodilatation occurring during hypoxia may not be a compensatory response but rather the result of "cerebral vasoparalysis." Autoregulation is lost, and blood flow changes passively with pressure. Thus, during endarterectomy, systemic arterial blood pressure should not be allowed to fall below the patient's usual level. Prolonged hypoxia is accompanied by a decrease in flow, an increase in viscosity, and sludging. Spasm of the arterioles, unresponsive to usual vasodilating measures, occurs. Uncoupling of the relationship between function and flow occurs; the metabolic demands of the region of hypoxia are low. Normal perfusion pressure restoration results in a local hyperemic state. Luxury perfusion, that is, flow in excess of the need, occurs.[12–15]

CLINICAL PRESENTATIONS AND CAUSES

Intracranial Causes

There are five major causes of stroke: reduced cerebral perfusion, thrombosis of first and second order vessels, embolism from remote or nearby sources, and subarachnoid and intracerebral hemorrhage.

Intracerebral Hemorrhage and Subarachnoid Hemorrhage

During subarachnoid hemorrhage, usually due to rupture of an aneurysm or an arteriovenous (AV) malformation, blood spreads on the brain surface and finds its way around the brain through pathways it shares with the spinal fluid. Usually there is sudden increase in intracranial pressure. By contrast, intracerebral hemorrhage,[16] usually associated with hypertension,[17] occurs directly into the brain parenchyma. Because of leakage of blood, intracerebral hemorrhage may often, but not always, be diagnosed by the presence of blood in the lumbar puncture sample of cerebrospinal fluid. Computed tomographic (CT) scan may reveal the hemorrhage and a shift of midline structures.[18]

Cerebral embolism is the probable cause of stroke in approximately 70% of patients. Thrombotic occlusion and intracerebral hemorrhage account for approximately 20% and 10% respectively. Thus ischemic stroke is the correct diagnosis in four out of five patients and subarachnoid hemorrhage in less than one in 10. A few clinical features may be helpful. Headache at or near onset invariably occurs with subarachnoid hemorrhage but is less frequent with thrombotic stroke and intracerebral hemorrhage. With intracerebral hemorrhage, the signs and symptoms are usually progressive. With extension of the hematoma, headache, vomiting, and changes in consciousness—common in subarachnoid hemorrhage—occur. Loss of consciousness is rare during ischemic stroke unless it is extensive or there is bilateral brain stem involvement. Coexisting diabetes and coronary artery disease strongly suggest artery-to-artery embolus because atherosclerosis of the extracranial vessels is so common in patients with these conditions. On average, 60% of strokes are considered thrombotic, 20% are embolic, 12% are due to intracerebral hemorrhage, and 8% are due to subarachnoid hemorrhage.[19]

A frequent precursor of thrombotic stroke is a transient ischemic attack (TIA). Multiple TIAs are near-certain evidence of the diagnosis. A recent TIA demands urgent evaluation, for it is more ominous than that which occurred weeks to months ago.

Extracranial Causes

Fibromuscular Dysplasia

Fibromuscular dysplasia is a rare fascinating condition of unknown cause with unpredictable consequences. During gross examination, the appearance of the artery may suggest a string of beads because of interposed segments of concentric stenosis and dilatation. Typically, the lesions affect the middle 2 to 3 cm of the cervical internal carotid artery approximately at the level of the second cervical vertebra in an area usually free of atherosclerosis. Elongation and tortuosity of the internal carotid artery may develop.

Four types of fibromuscular dysplasia are recognized: fibroplasia of the intima; hyperplasia and fibromuscular stenosis of the medial layer, plus disruption of the internal elastic membrane and development of focal microaneurysms; subadventitial or perimedial dysplasia in which elastic tissue accumulates between the media and the adventitia; and a type limited to the adventitia, with periarterial fibrosis producing the stenoses. Intimal fibroplasia with its normal media and adventitia accounts for an estimated 5% of cases. There is no gender preference. Fibroplasia of the medial layer is the most common form and occurs more frequently in women.[20] Coexisting fibromuscular disease of the renal and carotid arteries, plus intracranial berry aneurysms, has been reported.[21–23] Most patients with fibromuscular dysplasia remain asymptomatic. Those few who become symptomatic do so for unknown reasons,[24] although embolism, hypoperfusion secondary to critical stenosis, and intracranial fibromuscular dysplasia are possibilities.[20] Fibromuscular dysplasia of the internal carotid artery is not of and by itself an indication for operation. The asymptomatic fibromuscular dysplasia lesion of the internal carotid artery is best left alone despite an incidence in 22% of patients of a completed stroke before presentation.[25] Once fibromuscu-

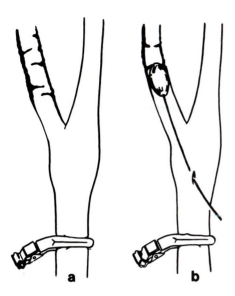

Figure 55-5. Obstruction in fibromuscular dysplasia (a). Disruption of dysplastic lesions with rigid dilator (b).

lar dysplasia becomes symptomatic, it can no longer be considered a benign disease. In one third of patients, the first manifestation is awareness of a carotid bruit, which is an indication for arteriography. In others, it may be a stroke. The discovery of the bruit should lead to angiographic assessment of extracranial intracranial vessels. More information is needed about the natural history of the disorder.

Therapy. Early operations for treatment of fibromuscular dysplasia consisted of resection of a short segment with end-to-end anastomosis, interposition of autogenous saphenous vein, and arteriotomy excision of the areas of thickening, followed by patch angioplasty.[26,27] Except in unusual circumstances, these procedures have been abandoned in favor of graded intraluminal dilatation through a 2 to 3 cm long arteriotomy, beginning in the bulb and extending upward to the first centimeter of the internal carotid artery (Fig. 55-5). To facilitate this procedure, the

internal carotid artery should be dissected free to within a few centimeters of the base of the skull, taking care not to injure the adjacent cranial nerves, IX, X, XI, and XII. The artery is allowed to bleed back from time to time to remove debris and thrombus, and the arteriotomy is closed. Completion angiography is recommended. Systemic heparin is administered during the procedure, followed by aspirin as soon as the patient is able to swallow. Postdilatation neurologic deficits occurred in approximately 5% of 170 operations. One percent of patients died, less than 2% suffered subsequent TIAs, and stroke occurred in an additional 2%.[28]

Recently, balloon catheters inserted over a guidewire through a 1 cm arteriotomy have been used in place of rigid dilators.[29-34]

Coils and Kinks

Coils and loops of the carotid artery are thought to be congenital in origin, probably due to inappropriate elongation of the cervical carotid and innominate arteries during descent of the heart into the mediastinum (Fig. 55-6). They are frequently bilateral and almost never symptomatic, even when a coil has formed a 360-degree loop.[35] Secondary elongation of the carotid artery occurs because of degenerative changes of aging in the arterial wall. This type of tortuosity is rarely responsible for either transient or permanent neurologic deficits unless there is coexisting atherosclerotic disease.[36] Flow reduction may occur with positional changes of the head and neck. Reproduction of neurologic symptoms by positional testing justifies angiographic evaluation of all four extracranial vessels.

Kinking, buckling, or acute angulation is usually a byproduct of atherosclerosis. It occurs at the distal end of the atheromatous plaque. Actual incidence is unknown, for most patients with the condition come to medical attention as a consequence of finding atherosclerotic disease either during physical examination (e.g., through detection of a cervical bruit) or because of neurologic symptoms leading to angiographic evaluation. In all probability, surgical correction of the incidental and asymptomatic carotid kink is not indicated even if on noninvasive testing reduction in flow can be demonstrated by positional changes.[36] The primary indication for correction of the kink is symptomatic

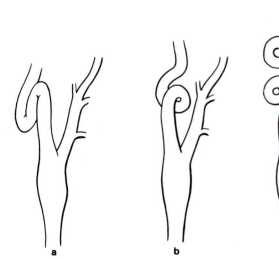
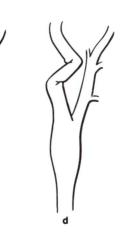

Figure 55-6. Example of sinusoidal elongation (a), single coil (b), double coil (c), and kinking (d) of the internal carotid artery.

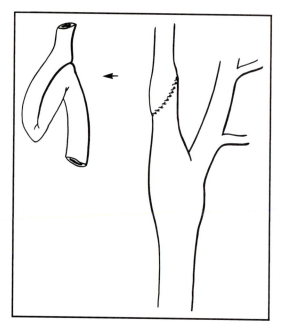

Figure 55-7. Example of surgical correction of a kinked internal carotid artery by excision and oblique end-to-side anastomosis.

internal carotid atherosclerotic occlusive disease and coexisting angulation. Several techniques for shortening the redundant postendarterectomy artery are available (Fig. 55-7). The simplest technique is resection of a portion of the proximal carotid artery and an oblique or elliptical end-to-end anastomosis to the distal end of the carotid bulb.[37–40]

Aneurysms

Although the incidence of carotid aneurysms is extremely low, 37 out of a total of 8,500 aneurysms of all locations,[41] it carries the risk of hemorrhage, thrombosis, embolism, and consequent cerebral complications. The cause may be Marfan's syndrome, various types of arteritis, cystic medial necrosis, or a mycotic or infected aneurysm. The commonest causes are atherosclerosis and trauma. In the older patient with atherosclerosis and hypertension, carotid aneurysms are frequently bilateral. The bifurcation is the usual site. Blunt trauma aneurysms usually occur at the mid and distal portions of the internal carotid artery. False aneurysms also occur after carotid endarterectomy.[42] Epistaxis, bleeding from the ear, rupture, and life-threatening hemorrhage into the oropharynx may occur. Hoarseness is due to compression of the vagus and recurrent laryngeal nerves. Ipsilateral Horner's syndrome is due to cervical sympathetic nerve involvement. False and infected aneurysms are especially likely to rupture.

Diagnosis and appropriate therapy cannot be established without adequate arteriography. Secondary dissection of the aneurysm is usually associated with a fine tapered line of contrast medium, the so-called "string sign."

Surgical removal and restoration of flow either by primary closure or with patch angioplasty in the small saccular aneurysm or resection and interposition of autologous tissue are recommended for aneurysms of the common and proximal third of the internal carotid artery. Complete excision

of a large aneurysm carries with it the threat of associated nerve damage. Aneurysms in the distal portion of the internal carotid artery, particularly if small and asymptomatic, are best left alone, to be followed with serial observation including angiography. If symptomatic, these high aneurysms may be best treated by internal carotid ligation, leaving no cul-de-sac from which emboli may arise, and, if the collateral circulation is inadequate, an extraintracranial bypass graft is indicated.

Restoration operations are reported to be associated with a lower incidence of neurologic deficits of about 10 to 25% as contrasted to 30% with simple carotid ligation.[43] Different series report widely differing results.[44–51]

Spontaneous Dissection

The carotid string sign may also be seen with spontaneous dissection of the cervical internal carotid artery. It is less a marker for a specific disease than it is for narrowing of the lumen as a consequence of hematoma formation. With greater use of angiography, dissection is more frequently seen with trauma such as hyperextension, rotation, and deceleration injuries and blunt and penetrating trauma. Disruption of the intima, with intramural hemorrhage, is probably the common denominator. Complications are cerebral emboli and thrombotic occlusion. Thrombectomy, graded dilatation of the lumen, and segmental resection with interposition grafting have been largely abandoned in favor of heparin followed by warfarin and careful reevaluation. Most dissections managed this way reveal a normal or near normal appearance of angiography at about 1 year. If symptoms develop or if the lumen progressively narrows, operation should be considered.

Given a history of cervical trauma and pain in the vicinity of the carotid artery, with or without swelling and with or without neurologic signs, arteriographic evaluation is indicated. Carotid occlusion and neurologic signs and symptoms may not occur for hours to days after injury. In this situation, anticoagulant therapy carries an unnecessary risk.[52–55]

Atherosclerotic Occlusive Disease

Low Flow. Low flow may be due to reduced blood volume, reduced pump efficiency, and obstruction in the system, as for example, large vessel stenosis. Possibly 20% of TIAs and strokes may have a hemodynamic basis. Poor cardiac function is most often based on congestive heart failure, myocardial infarction, and arrhythmias. Other causes of hemodynamic abnormalities are trauma and overmedication with antihypertensive drugs and diuretics. Reduced cerebral perfusion may also be due to hypovolemia.

Thrombosis. Severe obstruction to blood flow is usually followed by stasis and clot formation. Polycythemia is a rare cause. Atherosclerosis affects the intracranial vessels less often than does chronic hypertension.[56] Reduction of the lumen of the intracranial vessel is a consequence of medial hypertrophy and mural deposition of fibrinoid material. Spontaneous thrombosis is the ultimate event. Thrombosis may also occur with fibromuscular dysplasia, Takayasu's disease, aneurysms, and dissection within the wall, whether spontaneous or secondary to trauma. The most

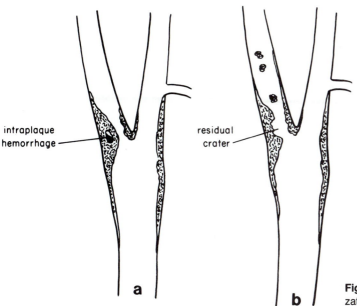

intraplaque
hemorrhage

residual
crater

a

b

Figure 55-8. Representation of an unstable plaque (a), and embolization from it (b).

common cause of thrombosis in extracranial vessels is atherosclerotic plaque, with loss of the antithrombogenic properties of the normal endothelium, followed by ulceration, deposition of fibrin, thrombin, platelets, and clot formation.

Embolism. Thrombosis results in localized obstruction that originates in the affected vessel. Embolism, by contrast, leads to blockage of a vessel remote from the point of origin. Cardiac emboli are responsible for possibly 10 to 15% of cerebral infarcts. Emboli from a mural thrombus of a previous myocardial infarction are usually large, obstruct major cerebral arteries, and are fatal in one third of patients. Embolic fragments from the carotid bifurcation plaque may be the most common cause of cerebral TIAs and strokes. It is estimated that as high as 80% of such ischemic attacks have an embolic cause (Fig. 55-8).[57–66]

MEDICAL TREATMENT FOR TIAS AND STROKE

The pathogenesis, natural history, and management of TIAs and stroke are not substantially different among patients whose symptoms have lasted a few minutes, a few hours, or a few days. Despite the accepted 24-hour time limit allegedly distinguishing TIA from stroke, often it is impossible to identify the precise cause.

Anticoagulant and antiplatelet drugs and, more recently, thrombolytic agents have been used based on the presumption that thrombosis and thromboembolism are the causes of most cerebral ischemic episodes. The objective, of course, is to prevent development or propagation of thrombus and, on a long-term basis, reformation of a nidus of clot in a proximal atherosclerotic vessel. Anticoagulant therapy for TIA has shown neither increased survival rates nor a reduction in incidence of cerebral infarction. Hemorrhagic complications discourage the use of anticoagulants

in progressing and completed stroke. Thrombolytic therapy has several limitations, the most serious being conversion of an ischemic infarct into a hemorrhagic infarct. Generally, irreversible cerebral and vascular changes have occurred in the involved area of the brain by the time the stroke patient is admitted. This is usually more than 1 hour after onset.

Theoretically, antiplatelet agents provide the only way of trying to prevent stroke in the recurrent TIA patient. Thromboxane A_2 enhances platelet aggregation, and prostacyclin inhibits it. How often platelet fibrin aggregates cause cerebral infarction is unknown. One gram of aspirin per day has been shown to reduce both cerebral morbidity and mortality in patients with recurrent TIAs. As little as 325 mg of aspirin reduces the synthesis of platelet-produced thromboxane A_2 without reducing prostacyclin (PGI_2) production by the endothelial cell, but the efficacy of low-dose aspirin is yet to be properly documented. The addition of dipyridamole is no better than aspirin alone. Despite a belief to the contrary, women respond to aspirin as well as men.

In a group of 303 patients randomized between nonsurgical and surgical therapy, 125 underwent carotid endarterectomy and were then given either aspirin or a placebo.[67] In both the nonsurgical and the surgical groups, there were only half as many strokes or deaths among those given aspirin as among those in the placebo cohort. The follow-up period, however, was only 6 months. For patients with TIAs and carotid stenosis of less than 80%, aspirin appears the most effective medical therapy for the prevention of stroke.[68] In patients who continue to experience TIAs despite aspirin and with stenosis of 80% or more, endarterectomy offers greater safety.[69,70] Endarterectomy is the only therapy that removes the atherosclerotic plaque, with its threat of embolization and thrombosis, as well as usually restoring normal flow through the cervical internal carotid artery.[71–73]

CAROTID ENDARTERECTOMY

Despite a recent spate of dissenting opinions, carotid endarterectomy in properly selected patients is a widely accepted, valuable, and time-tested surgical procedure.

Anesthesia Management

The patient with carotid artery occlusive disease sufficiently severe to need carotid endarterectomy usually has multisystem disease and may be receiving a number of medications. Possibly as many as 30% of patients will have a history of coronary disease,[74] and a substantially larger number will have coronary artery disease discovered during investigation despite lack of clinical suspicion.[75] A larger number of patients have coexisting hypertension and some degree of respiratory impairment. Evaluation of cardiac, pulmonary, and renal function, therefore, is mandatory. Postoperative morbidity and mortality are most often due to hypertension, myocardial ischemia, and cardiac arrhythmias. With the exception of diuretics, frequently associated with hypovolemia and hypokalemia, the antihypertensive medicines should be continued, for higher morbidity and mortality rates have been associated with poor blood pressure control.[76] Poor control may lead to hypotension on induction of anesthesia with reduced myocardial and cerebral perfusion. Patients with coexisting disease processes, particularly ischemic heart disease and pulmonary obstructive disease, usually fare better with general than with local anesthesia, because heart rate, blood pressure, oxygenation, and arrhythmias may be better controlled. The best results in terms of mortality and morbidity using local anesthesia do not surpass the best results obtained with general anesthesia.

Of greatest importance is the maintenance of blood pressure at or slightly above normal during carotid cross-clamping because of the possibility of loss of cerebral circulatory autoregulation secondary to regional hypoxia. Because areas of infarction or ischemia are likely serviced by blood vessels already at maximal dilatation, increasing the P_{CO_2}, while possibly increasing total cerebral blood flow, may actually produce an absolute flow diminution to an area of ischemia. The same may be said for artificial elevation of blood pressure, which is unlikely to increase local flow through poorly perfused areas already served by maximally dilated vessels. An increase in perioperative myocardial infarction and mortality has been reported with this maneuver.[77] The use of barbiturates in customary doses in the attempt to decrease cerebral metabolism and thus lessen the influence of reduced perfusion is unsupported by experience. Large doses are required, and the secondary effects may be troublesome. Both vasodilators and vasopressors should be immediately available for administration during the procedure, as well as in the recovery room. For prompt recognition and treatment, continuous indwelling arterial blood pressure monitoring must be performed, not only during the operation but in the recovery room. Routine postoperative ECG monitoring is strongly urged.[78,79]

Cerebral Protection

Patients at high risk for cerebral ischemia during cross-clamping of the carotid artery include those with the following:

1. A history of a previous stroke
2. A positive CT scan for cerebral infarct, whether symptomatic or asymptomatic
3. A residual neurologic deficit at the time of operation
4. Contralateral carotid occlusion or a severe contralateral stenosis
5. Signs and symptoms of coexisting vertebral basilar insufficiency
6. Poorly controlled hypertension

Thus the need for temporary shunting during carotid endarterectomy may vary from zero in the asymptomatic patient with normal collateral circulation to as much as 25% in patients with reduced regional and collateral flow from whatever cause. It is in this latter group of patients that perioperative neurologic deficits may be based on low perfusion pressure. In lower-risk patients the probability is high but impossible to establish that more perioperative neurologic deficits are the consequence of embolization during dissection or after restoration of flow than of cerebral hypoxia. The incidence of perioperative complications also correlates with the neurologic condition of the patient at the time of operation. It is highest in patients with a stroke in evolution, less frequent but still substantial in the patient with a fixed preoperative deficit, and least in the patient with a normal neurologic status.

Routine use of an indwelling shunt is a reliable method for preventing cerebral hypoxia. It permits general anesthesia, maintains adequate carotid flow, avoids a sense of haste during the operation, and eliminates the need for monitoring cerebral blood flow. Its greatest disadvantage is impaired visualization of a long distal extension of the plaque, especially in patients with a short neck or an abnormally high carotid bifurcation, as at the level of C-2. The possibility of embolization of plaque particles and "snowplowing" of the intima during insertion and removal are additional limitations (Fig. 55-9).[80] A second popular method is indirect assessment of the cerebral circulation by measuring internal carotid artery pressure distal to the occluding clamp. The safe level of this so-called back or stump pressure is usually specified as 50 mm Hg.[81]

Occlusion or severe stenosis of the contralateral carotid artery also places the patient at an assumed increased risk. A shunt is used in these patients if the stump pressure is less than 50 mm Hg. If the contralateral internal carotid artery is patent, no shunt is used.[82] Theoretic objections to this technique include the significant number of false negative and false positive measurements when compared to actual blood flow techniques, that although the stump pressure may reflect the collateral circulation, variations in regional blood flow will not be appreciated, and lastly, that the stump pressure is but a single determination subject to significant changes in systemic blood pressure, cardiac output, and oxygenation during operation.

Certainly the efficacy of the collateral circulation is eas-

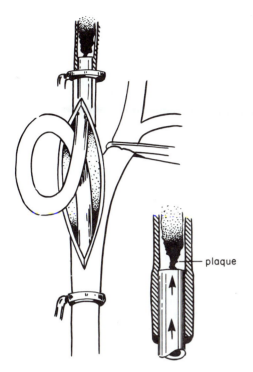

Figure 55-9. "Snowplow" effect of improper shunt insertion. (*Modified from Matsumoto GM, Cossman D, Callow AD: Am J Surg 133:458, 1977.*)

ily and effectively assessed in the awake patient using local or regional cervical block.[83] Constant assessment of the patient's neurologic status is available throughout the operation. Immediate identification of the neurologic deficit at the time of occurrence, with immediate therapeutic intervention, is possible. An additional alleged benefit is the reduction of the cardiac risk factor associated with general anesthesia. One series noted a nonneurologic complication rate for carotid endarterectomy patients under general anesthesia of 12.9%, compared to 2.8% for patients under regional block.[84] The claim, however, that operation in the awake patient is comfortable and safe for both patient and surgeon is not unanimously supported by all who have used it.

Intraoperative ophthalmoplethysmographic techniques to monitor distal internal carotid artery pressure have never gained widespread acceptance. Attempts to reduce the metabolism of the brain with barbiturates based on the assumption that the brain thereby becomes less susceptible to ischemia, attempts to improve collateral flow by induced hypertension, or reduction of intracerebral vascular resistance by induced hypercarbia have been abandoned as ineffective and sometimes dangerous. Hypertension places an additional burden on the myocardium of the patient with coexisting coronary artery disease, and hypercarbia may cause postoperative intracerebral hemorrhage.

Continuous electroencephalographic (EEG) monitoring provides a highly reliable method for assessing cerebral oxygenation. Its use permits general endotracheal anesthesia, which, despite some claims to the contrary, appears the best method for supporting the carotid endarterectomy patient who has actual or suspected coronary artery disease. General endotracheal anesthesia provides good airway control, permits higher Pa_{O_2} levels, better and prompter regulation of the Pa_{CO_2} level, and far better control of cardiac rate and blood pressure than may be possible with regional and local anesthesia. The EEG determines the patient in need of a shunt as well as the patient in whom it may be safely avoided. There is the opportunity for careful, meticulous, and sometimes lengthy performance of the endarterectomy and arteriotomy closure. Without a shunt, unimpaired visualization of the distal end of the plaque is possible, as is meticulous removal of residual remnants, which occasionally persist despite what is considered an adequate dissection. EEG monitoring provides satisfactory protection for all risk categories of patients throughout the operation, irrespective of changes in collateral blood flow secondary to changes in cardiac and respiratory function.

Surveillance is continuous throughout the induction of anesthesia, the operation, and the early postoperative period. Detection of a neurologic deficit need not wait for patient awakening. Provided the depth of anesthesia is not profoundly altered, the EEG is an accurate and highly reliable indicator of cortical perfusion.[85,86] No new perioperative deficit has been seen that was not predicted by the EEG. Although patients with TIAs and old strokes may be initially seen with either normal or abnormal tracings, no prolonged or fixed neurologic perioperative deficit has occurred in my experience without an associated EEG abnormality. The reverse, however, is not true. Focal EEG changes in silent areas, as for example the temporal and frontal lobes, have been seen during operation but with no recorded fixed deficit detectable postoperatively. Thromboembolism from the endarterectomy site or thrombosis is usually indicated by substantial transient or permanent ipsilateral EEG changes occurring suddenly or immediately after surgery.[87] Of 1,262 carotid endarterectomies performed for a variety of indications between 1968 and 1983 with continuous EEG monitoring, the incidence of transient deficits was 2.8%, and the incidence for prolonged deficits was 1.3%. There were six deaths for a mortality rate of 0.48%; each death was due to myocardial infarction, and none was a primary stroke death.[85]

Recently, multiport transcranial ultrasound scanning, measuring velocity and direction of flow, has been introduced to ascertain cerebral perfusion during carotid endarterectomy. Experience is too limited to permit evaluation.[88]

Inasmuch as equally good results in terms of mortality and transient and prolonged neurologic deficits have been obtained with all of the above techniques for cerebral monitoring and cerebral protection, it becomes apparent that the key elements in each are experience, judgment, and meticulous attention to detail. The selection of patients, the application of some form of cerebral protection or monitoring, and the conduct of the operative procedure place the emphasis where it should be, namely on the skill and experience of the team. The given modality may be less important than the care with which it is used.[89–97]

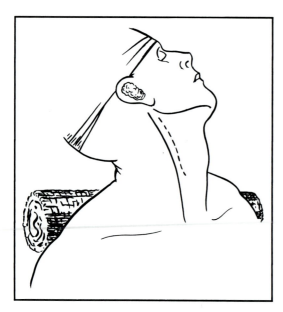

Figure 55-10. For carotid endarterectomy, the shoulders are elevated, and the head is hyperextended and turned away from the operative side. Bone wax is placed in the ear, and the skin incision is made parallel to the anterior border of the sternocleidomastoid muscle. (*Modified from Callow AD, Shepard A, Russell J: Contemp Surg 30:31, 1987.*)

Operative Technique

For carotid endarterectomy, the patient is placed on the operating table with his shoulders elevated by a rolled sheet or towel. The head is slightly hyperextended, turned toward the contralateral shoulder (Fig. 55-10),[98] and secured with a wide band of tape over the forehead to each side of the table. The table is put in a 10- to 15-degree Trendelenburg position to reduce venous pressure in the field and to encourage drainage of blood and irrigating solutions away from the distal end of the endarterectomy.

Although a slightly improved cosmetic result may be obtained with a curvilinear transverse cervical incision following a natural skin crease, wider exposure from the tip of the mastoid along the entire length of the cervical common carotid artery, if necessary, is provided by a vertical approach. The incision is placed along the anterior border of the sternocleidomastoid muscle, which is dissected from the carotid sheath (Fig. 55-11).[98] Lymph nodes and even the tail of the parotid gland, which may be in the field, should be mobilized rather than risk troublesome oozing or a parotid cutaneous fistula or salivary seroma if it is divided.

The carotid sheath is opened, exposing the jugular vein. Its large common facial vein is divided and suture ligated. Several smaller veins may replace the single common facial vein. The facial vein is carefully separated from the hypoglossal nerve, which may traverse the field deep to the vein, especially with an unusually high carotid bifurcation. The point of juncture of the common facial and internal jugular veins serves as a guide immediately deep to which is the carotid bifurcation. The internal jugular vein and the sternocleidomastoid muscle are mobilized lat-

erally. Search for the carotid artery is begun at the common carotid level to lessen the possibility of dislodging friable material within the carotid bulb. Retraction of the internal jugular vein exposes the vagus nerve behind the vein and posterolateral to the common carotid artery and carotid bifurcation.

Dissection is continued upward to the bulb where the external carotid is identified together with its first branch, the superficial thyroid artery. Backbleeding from this area can be controlled with a neurosurgical Heifitz clip or an encircling loop of vessel tape or ligature. The uppermost portion of the internal carotid artery is then mobilized, taking care not to dissect in the vicinity of the carotid bifurcation itself until the internal, external, and distal internal arteries have been identified and encircled with vascular loops. Dissection of the bulb should be delayed until a temporary occluding clamp is placed on the internal carotid artery to prevent upward passage of any dislodged material. The patient is dissected away from carotid artery rather than the carotid artery away from the patient. On call from the anesthesiologist should bradycardia develop, 1 ml of 1% lidocaine is injected in the vicinity of the carotid bifurcation. The glossopharyngeal and the spinal accessory nerves, together with the vagus nerve, are contained within the carotid sheath in a posterior relationship to the artery. In approximately 5% of individuals, the vagus nerve may lie anterior to the internal and common carotid arteries and be mistaken for the ansa cervicalis usually seen in that location (Fig. 55-12).[80] Dividing the structures within the fork of the carotid bifurcation may permit additional mobilization of the artery if downward traction is required and

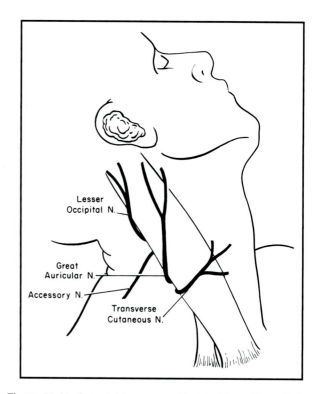

Figure 55-11. Superficial nerves subject to injury. (*From Callow AD, Shepard A, Russell J: Contemp Surg 30:31, 1987.*)

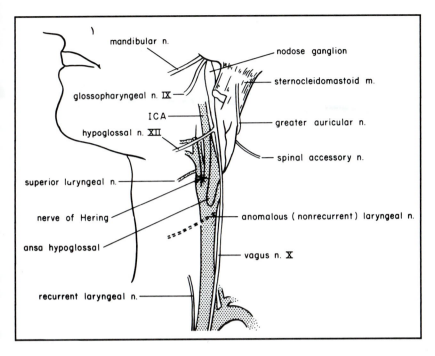

Figure 55-12. Cranial nerves adjacent to the carotid artery. (*Modified from Matsumoto GM, Cossman D, Callow AD: Am J Surg 133:458, 1977.*)

also prevents troublesome bleeding during endarterectomy from the small artery originating at that point. Impairment of carotid body function leading to loss of compensatory respiratory and circulatory responses has been reported with bilateral carotid endarterectomy.

On occasion, the entire extracranial extent of the internal carotid artery must be exposed. This procedure may be necessitated by an abnormally high bifurcation and by an unusually distal extent of the atheromatous process. The skin incision should be extended toward the mastoid process with medial reflection of the hypoglossal nerve. A small artery and vein from the external carotid artery to the sternocleidomastoid muscle pass over the hypoglossal nerve and superficial to the internal carotid artery and form the so-called "carotid sling" (Fig. 55-13). These vessels are quite constant, and their division permits greater displacement of the hypoglossal nerve. If they are torn, there may be troublesome bleeding in an area where hemostatic control is awkward and loss of visibility invites technical error. Cautery should be avoided, and application of hemostatic clamps should be done under good vision. The ansa cervicalis may be divided; the sternocleidomastoid muscle should be mobilized upward, approaching its insertion on the mastoid process with care to avoid injury to the spinal accessory nerve innervating the muscle at that high level. The posterior belly of the digastric muscle becomes visible and, together with the stylohyoid muscle, may be divided without clinical consequence. A long styloid process may be shortened with a bone rongeur. The most distal portion of the cervical internal carotid artery is hidden by the vertical ramus of the mandible. Lesions of the internal carotid artery above a line drawn from the tip of the mastoid process along the lower border of the jaw are no longer considered inaccessible. A number of techniques have been described to deal with this problem, but simple forward subluxation with the patient under general anesthesia provides the

needed exposure and makes any form of osteotomy of the ramus unnecessary (Fig. 55-14). Division of several branches of the external carotid artery permits additional downward traction on the internal carotid artery and gains a few additional millimeters of exposure.

Although the dissection up to this point can be performed without magnifying loops or special lighting, the

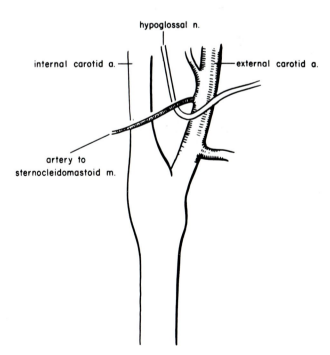

Figure 55-13. The hypoglossal nerve is tethered by vessels from the external carotid artery to the stenocleidomastoid muscle and against the internal carotid artery, forming the "carotid sling."

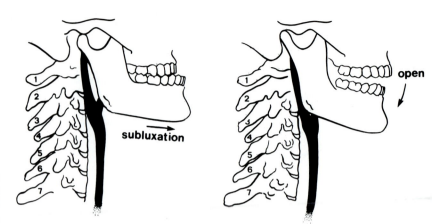

Figure 55-14. Subluxation of the jaw gives an additional several millimeters of exposure of the distal internal carotid artery. The distal carotid artery is hidden with the mouth open.

actual endarterectomy is performed with magnifying loops on the surgeon and the first assistant and a headlight for the surgeon. One unit of low-molecular dextran is administered intravenously for its antiplatelet effect at a rate that will have most if not all of it circulating by the time blood flow is restored to the internal carotid artery. Depending on the patient's weight, 5,000 to 10,000 units of heparin are administered intravenously before cross-clamping of the major vessels. Heparin is not reversed unless troublesome oozing persists. In theory, the laying down of a carpet of platelets after restoration of blood flow may be inhibited by both heparin and dextran. Heparin also possesses an antiproliferative effect against the smooth muscle cell that occurs at low dosage levels, but its effect probably is so evanescent as to have no value. Test occlusion of the internal carotid artery and cerebral perfusion is performed, depending on the surgeon's preference, by measuring carotid back or stump pressure. Neurologic signs and symptoms can be observed in the awake patient, or changes in the electroencephalogram (EEG) can be compared with the preinduction and postinduction baseline tracings. Unilateral loss of fast-wave activity, the disappearance of the fast beta complex, and the appearance of long slow-wave activity and the delta complex, unassociated with changes in cardiorespiratory efficiency and persisting for as long as 1 minute, call for insertion of a shunt. Of the several shunts available, the choice of which one to use is again the surgeon's to make. Whatever the method chosen, the systemic blood pressure must not be allowed to fall below the level present at the time cerebral perfusion was tested. A simple sphygmomanometer cuff is inadequate. An inlying arterial catheter with constant monitoring on a visual display screen is mandatory.

There is no instrument, whether a vessel loop or a

so-called "atraumatic" clamp, that does not impose some injury on the arterial wall. Even a balloon obturator inserted into the lumen may damage the endothelial layer. I favor the small neurosurgical Heifitz clips, which are available in various sizes and configurations (Fig. 55-15).[98] They produce less compression than the thumb-and-finger ratchet-type arterial clamp. Applied with a removable applicator,

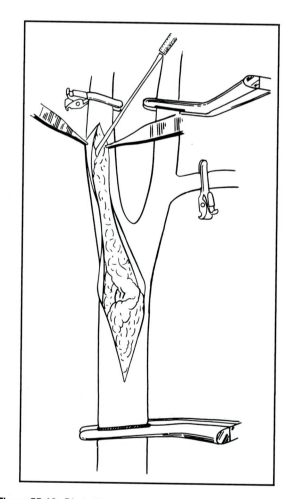

Figure 55-16. Dissection is extended proximally as far as necessary to remove all of the plaque. Edges of arterial wall are gently pushed aside to avoid repeated trauma with forceps. (*From Callow AD, Shepard A, Russell J: Contemp Surg 30:31, 1987.*)

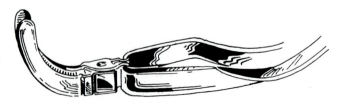

Figure 55-15. Curved Heifitz arterial occluding clip. (*From Callow AD, Shepard A, Russell J: Contemp Surg 30:31, 1987.*)

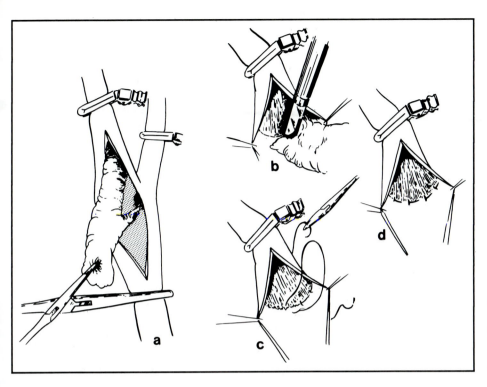

Figure 55-17. The external carotid artery is opened by sharp and blunt dissection (a). Sharp dissection of distal end of plaque (b). Tacking sutures (c). Interrupted suture attachment on completion (d).

Heifitz clips are the least obtrusive of the occluding instruments. The internal carotid artery is first occluded at a point well above the atheroma. The common carotid artery is next occluded with a small angulated ratchet type clamp, applying only sufficient pressure to occlude the vessel and then its external branch. The superior thyroid artery is occluded with a Heifitz clip. The internal carotid artery has much less elastic lamina than the common and external branches and is much more susceptible to clamp damage.

The common carotid artery proximal to the plaque is entered with a scalpel of proper size and configuration. A No. 11 blade is convenient. Angulated Potts scissors extend the incision both in a proximal and distal direction so that the distal end of the atherosclerotic plaque can be visualized (Figs. 55-16[98] and 55-17). In most instances, this plaque can be removed in such a fashion as to obtain "feathering" of the edge. A near-normal artery should be visualized at the cephalad end. The use of "tacking" sutures is in most instances considered to be an indication of an incomplete removal of the offending plaque (Fig. 55-18). Although these sutures may prevent the development of an intimal flap, the disturbance to laminar flow created by the edge encourages local platelet aggregation and possibly dislodgement of small platelet emboli. In addition, the residual atherosclerotic material may enlarge with time and be a cause of recurrent stenosis.

Certain safeguards in the making of the arteriotomy are helpful. The incision should be made precisely in the midline of the internal carotid artery, well away from the crotch, thus making closure easier. A "no touch" technique of dealing with the edges of the internal carotid artery should be followed, for repetitive handling unnecessarily and sometimes dangerously traumatizes the residual wall.

There is some disagreement as to proper depth of the plane of dissection of the plaque, with some advocating

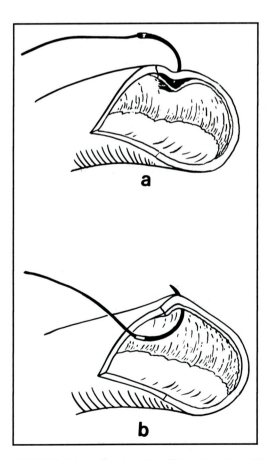

Figure 55-18. Tacking suture technique. Wrong technique (a). Correct technique (b).

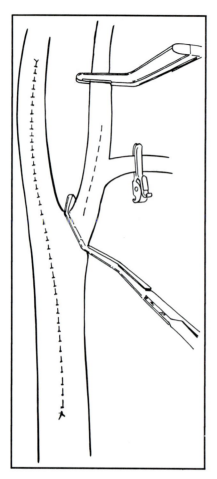

Figure 55-19. A secondary incision may be necessary for a complete external carotid endarterectomy. (*From Callow AD, Shepard A, Russell J: Contemp Surg 30:31, 1987.*)

ment sutures (Fig. 55-21).[98] Sutures are placed extremely closely together to abut rather than evert the edges. Larger bites are required in the common carotid artery with its tougher consistency. Before the last few stitches are applied, all clamps are removed sequentially to allow back bleeding. A final catheter flush with dilute dextran is performed.

After closure, blood flow is restored first to the external and then to the internal carotid artery (Fig. 55-22). A tiny clip is put at each end of the arteriotomy for future reference if necessary. The EEG is closely observed during this period for any changes in the ipsilateral hemisphere. Any perfusion changes call for immediate reopening of the arteriotomy and inspection for red or white thrombus. A patch using proximal saphenous vein is used only for a very small internal carotid artery and for a reentry closure (Fig. 55-23).[98] The once-sutured endarterectomized internal carotid artery is impossible to close a second time with a simple running suture without some eversion and constriction. Cautery for hemostasis is not used in the vicinity of previously identified nerves. The carotid sheath is left open, the subcutaneous tissues are closed with interrupted absorbable sutures, and the skin is closed with carefully applied staples, which are promptly replaced in 2 or 3 days with carefully applied Steristrips.

The EEG electrodes are left in place until the patient is fully awake and a satisfactory neurologic examination can be performed. Should a neurologic deficit appear, the patient is returned to the operating room for exploration of the endarterectomy site. Arteriographic and noninvasive assessment may fail to detect very small imperfections such as platelet aggregates. In addition, the endarterectomy site may appear satisfactory once the offending embolus has departed, but the condition that caused it may still exist. Reentry for correction of this defect is essential.

Some means of completion assessment of the endarter-

that the circular fibers of the media should be left behind. It is my custom to take as much of the media as possible except at the distal 3 to 4 mm of the plaque. Here, the dissection is gradually made more superficial to avoid a ragged end point. At the proximal end, the circumferential plaque is removed for at least 3 to 4 cm into the common carotid artery in an attempt to discourage recurrent disease. The endarterectomy is continued into the orifice and into 1 to 3 cm or more of the external carotid artery as necessary. If disease can still be palpated within it, a second short incision in the external carotid artery is made with the endarterectomy under direct vision (Fig. 55-19).[98]

Under magnification and special lighting, copious quantities of heparinized saline are used to flood the field for removal of "floaters" (Fig. 55-20) or fragments of the media, calcific infiltrates from the plaque into the wall, and shreads of intima and subintimal media, which may be seen to float at the distal end. Despite systemic heparinization and local wash with heparinized saline, oozing from the vasa vasorum, which are now open, may cause red cell and fibrinous material to agglutinate in the field, so the final flushing is performed with dilute dextran solution. The opened artery is filled with dextran, and closure is begun at the distal end using 6–0 to 7–0 synthetic monofila-

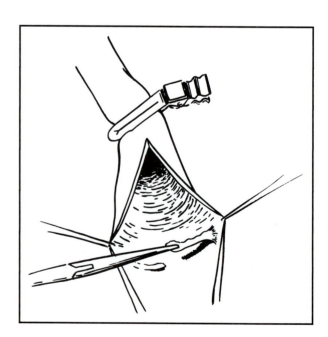

Figure 55-20. Tags or floaters of fragments of plaque and loosened media are removed through meticulous dissection.

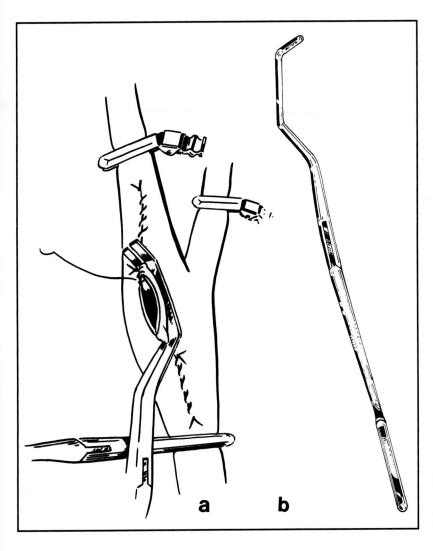

a   **b**

Figure 55-21. Partial restoration of flow (a), with a specially designed clamp (b) during arteriotomy closure. (*From Callow AD, Shepard A, Russell J: Contemp Surg 30:31, 1987.*)

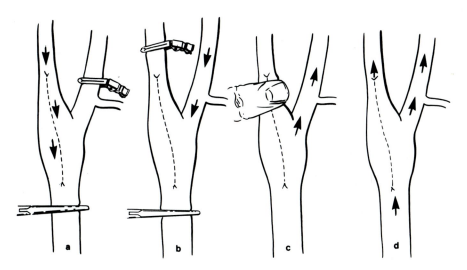

Figure 55-22. Steps in restoring flow on completion of endarterectomy. Temporary inflow to the bulb via the internal carotid artery (a). Flow through the external carotid artery (b). Finger pressure occlusion of the internal carotid with flow via the external carotid artery (c). Flow returned last to internal carotid artery (d).

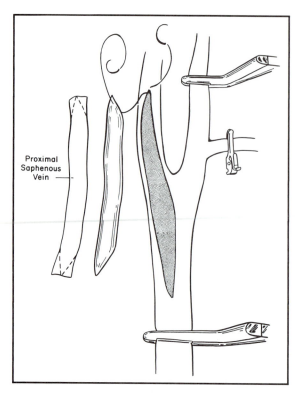

Figure 55-23. The venous patch should be tapered at each end, creating a "tight" fit. Too large a patch will create a bulbous distortion and disturbance in laminar flow. (*From Callow AD, Shepard A, Russell J: Contemp Surg 30:31, 1987.*)

ectomy site is mandatory whether by arteriography or some form of noninvasive scan.

Percutaneous transluminal dilatation in place of endarterectomy has recently been reported.[99,100] During a 5-year period in one series, 16 patients underwent transluminal dilatation for 21 stenoses of the carotid and vertebral arteries. In two patients the procedure was unsuccessful because of the irregularity of the stenosis. Three patients had successful bilateral dilatations. No neurologic complication was observed. All patients received anticoagulant therapy thereafter.[101]

Complications

"Carotid endarterectomy, arguably the least difficult of the arterial reconstructions, is the most unforgiving of operative error or lapse of judgment in patient selection."[102]

The two complications of greatest concern are perioperative stroke and myocardial infarction, and although each may be followed by death, the mortality rate of carotid endarterectomy in many series is under 2%. Overall morbidity is under 4%.[103] The neurologic status at the time of the operation correlates with operative mortality.[104] It is reported as zero in patients with asymptomatic plaques, 1.1% with transient ischemic attacks, and 5.1% in the patient with a fixed neurologic deficit.[105] In a group of approximately 2,300 consecutive carotid endarterectomies distributed in all of the above categories, our mortality rate

at the New England Medical Center, Boston, was 0.8%. Combined transient and prolonged neurologic deficit was 2.8% (Table 55-3).

Probably the most common cause of neurologic deficit is thrombus formation at the operative site, with or without embolization and distal occlusion. Inadequate intraoperative cerebral perfusion ranks as a low second cause. Neurologic deficits are immediately apparent during their occurrence in operations in the awake state or with patients under general anesthesia and continuous EEG monitoring. Immediate inspection of the endarterectomy site is possible.

Neurologic Deficit

For the patient awakening from anesthesia with a neurologic deficit or for one in whom a deficit develops a few minutes to a few hours thereafter, several options may be considered (Fig. 55-24).[106] If the deficit is of a minor degree, the choice often is to provide support without surgical intervention. For the more severe deficit and when thrombosis is suspected, immediate return to the operating room is recommended, for if surgical intervention is to be beneficial, it must be done without delay. Because small shreds of platelet thrombi are not visualized in an apparently normal completion arteriogram, reopening the arteriotomy is indicated. If the deficit is due to distal embolization and there is no residual thrombus at the endarterectomy site, surgical intervention is of no help. Evaluation through noninvasive testing (e.g., bidirectional Doppler) is often helpful in determining the patency of the endarterectomy site.[107,108] If the test remains positive in that there is reduced flow in the carotid artery or the test does not show improvement from preoperative examination, again the patient should be returned to the operating room without the delay of arteriography. If the artery is nonpulsatile, the decision to operate is not difficult; however, one can be misled by an apparent pulse just proximal to an occluded or partially thrombosed artery. It is preferable to open the arteriotomy wound because the postoperative arteriogram may fail to reveal a minimal amount of platelet thrombi.

In the delayed postoperative stroke, i.e., 3 to 10 days later, intracerebral hemorrhage must be considered along with the ever-present possibility of embolization (Fig. 55-25).[106] The former often results in severe deficit and death. Noninvasive testing, CT brain scan, and arteriography are indicated. In one series of 1,800 operations, 44 strokes occurred, 11 due to embolization, 9 to thrombosis, 9 to intracerebral hemorrhage, 8 to hypotensive ischemia, 2 to wound hematoma and shock, and 9 to unknown cause.[109] Of these stroke patients, 14 recovered.

Contralateral hemispheric neurologic deficits in the im-

TABLE 55-3. MORTALITY AND NEUROLOGICAL DEFICITS IN CAROTID ENDARTERECTOMY SERIES: 1958 TO JUNE 30, 1985*

Operations	Deaths		Transient Deficits		Permanent Deficits	
	No.	%	No.	%	No.	%
2274	18	0.8	40	1.7	26	1.1

* New England Medical Center, Boston.

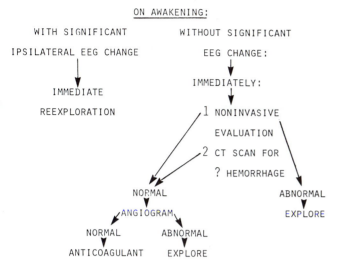

ON AWAKENING:

WITH SIGNIFICANT   WITHOUT SIGNIFICANT

IPSILATERAL EEG CHANGE   EEG CHANGE:

                        IMMEDIATELY:

IMMEDIATE   1 NONINVASIVE

REEXPLORATION   EVALUATION

                          2 CT SCAN FOR

                          ? HEMORRHAGE

              NORMAL   ABNORMAL

                                EXPLORE

              ANGIOGRAM

        NORMAL   ABNORMAL

      ANTICOAGULANT   EXPLORE

Figure 55-24. Algorithm outlining management of neurologic deficits after carotid endarterectomy. (*From Callow AD: Arch Chir Torac Cardiovasc 7:849, 1985.*)

mediate postoperative period that persist after correction of cardiac arrhythmias, pump failure, hypotension, or hypertension or that are not associated with these conditions require urgent arteriography and surgery on the contralateral carotid.

For the patient with a single TIA, observation and administration of antiplatelet agents are usually sufficient, for stroke is uncommon.

Myocardial Ischemia

The coexistence of coronary and carotid artery occlusive disease is now widely recognized. Approximately one third of carotid artery patients have, based on coronary catheter studies, surgically correctable coronary artery disease.[110]

Myocardial infarction is the leading cause of both postoperative and late death after carotid endarterectomy. Among 506 patients with extracranial occlusive disease, 40% had no clinical evidence of coronary atherosclerosis.

Coronary angiography revealed normal coronary arteries in only 7% of the 506 patients, mild-to-moderate disease in 28% and advanced but compensated disease that did not require revascularization in 30%. Severe coronary lesions were documented in 35% of patients initially seen with cerebrovascular disease. The use of combined or simultaneous coronary bypass and carotid endarterectomy is best confined to patients with left main coronary disease and severe multiple lesions with inadequate collaterals and for the patient with unstable angina, assuming, of course, that carotid endarterectomy is necessary. In a prospectively randomized group of 70 patients with unstable coronary disease, 34 underwent combined procedures and 36 a coronary bypass preceding carotid endarterectomy.[111] Surgical strokes or death occurred in 5.9% of patients in the combined operations, compared to 2.8% mortality in patients undergoing coronary bypass without carotid endarterectomy.

Exercise thallium scanning is of great assistance in identifying the patient at coronary risk. In the patient requiring endarterectomy, a normal exercise scan is followed by carotid endarterectomy. If the scan is abnormal, however, coronary angiography is performed, followed by carotid endarterectomy if revascularization is judged not necessary or can be deferred. If myocardial revascularization is needed and if the individual's coronary disease is stable, carotid endarterectomy is performed, followed several days to weeks later by the coronary artery bypass graft. If, however, the coronary artery disease is unstable, this individual is recommended for simultaneous coronary bypass and carotid endarterectomy.[112,113]

Blood Pressure Changes

Among patients receiving surgery for symptomatic carotid occlusive disease and among those patients with chronic hypertension whether well controlled or not, postoperative blood pressure instability is common. The incidence of severe hypertension, often associated with cardiac arrhythmias, is so often followed by serious and indeed lethal complications that adequate blood pressure control should be established before an elective procedure. Although the

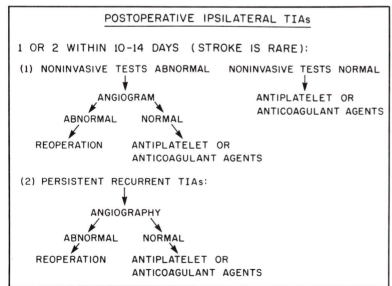

POSTOPERATIVE IPSILATERAL TIAs

1 OR 2 WITHIN 10-14 DAYS (STROKE IS RARE):

(1) NONINVASIVE TESTS ABNORMAL   NONINVASIVE TESTS NORMAL

          ANGIOGRAM   ANTIPLATELET OR
                              ANTICOAGULANT AGENTS
      ABNORMAL   NORMAL

  REOPERATION   ANTIPLATELET OR
              ANTICOAGULANT AGENTS

(2) PERSISTENT RECURRENT TIAs:

          ANGIOGRAPHY

      ABNORMAL   NORMAL

  REOPERATION   ANTIPLATELET OR
              ANTICOAGULANT AGENTS

Figure 55-25. Algorithm outlining management of ipsilateral TIAs after carotid endarterectomy. (*From Callow AD: Arch Chir Torac Cardiovasc 7:849, 1985.*)

exact cause of the blood pressure fluctuations may not be clearly defined, the carotid sinus baroreceptors concentrated at the carotid bifurcation are probably involved. Division or other trauma to the carotid sinus nerve of Hering, which is located between the internal and external carotid arteries, may result in reduced stimulation of the vasomotor center. Systemic hypotension is the interpretation by the brain, resulting in reflex hypertension and tachycardia. A second mechanism may be due to increased intracranial pressure secondary to relief of severe carotid stenosis. Increased capillary permeability in a recent or remote cerebral infarct may result in intracranial edema and hemorrhage. Reflex systemic hypertension occurs and foreshadows impending stroke. If hyperperfusion greatly exceeds need, severe headache unresponsive to usual medications may occur.[13–15,114] Meticulously careful monitoring is required. Intravenous nitroprusside is usually effective.

Hypotension is somewhat less common. It may be due to overmedication, abnormal function of the baroreceptor reflex arc, and other undiscovered causes. In any event, it must be treated to avoid the sequelae usually targeted to the coronary circulation. Infusion of epinephrine and careful monitoring of the blood pressure are usually sufficient.

Peripheral Nerve Damage

The actual incidence of peripheral nerve injury during carotid endarterectomy is unknown, for few are reported. Our early experience at the New England Medical Center is summarized in Table 55-4.

In another series of 450 patients the incidence of damage to the recurrent laryngeal nerve was 30 patients (6.7%) with 26 injuries of the hypoglossal nerve (5.8%), 8 injuries of the marginal mandibular nerve (1.8%), and 8 injuries of the superior laryngeal nerve (1.8%). Not all of them were symptomatic, however. For complete recovery, the mean interval in months varied from 1.4 to 3.4, but recovery was incomplete in approximately 20% of the recurrent laryngeal nerve injuries and in approximately 50% of the superior laryngeal nerve injuries.[115,116] Thus in this group of 450 patients, 60, or 13%, experienced a total of 72 nerve injuries. Approximately two thirds were obvious. One third of the

TABLE 55-4. IMMEDIATE COMPLICATIONS OF CAROTID ENDARTERECTOMY: 1974–1975 SERIES OF 130 CONSECUTIVE CASES*

Complication	No. of Cases	%	Deaths
Peripheral nerve injury (transient)	16	12.3	—
Hypoglossal nerve paresis	11	8.5	—
Vocal cord paresis	3	2.3	—
Cervical branch of the facial nerve paresis	2	1.5	—
Medical complications		6.9	—
Myocardial infarction	3	2.3	2
Pulmonary edema	5	3.8	—
Pulmonary embolus	1		—
Neurologic deaths	0		—

* New England Medical Center, Boston.

recurrent laryngeal nerve injuries would not have been suspected without direct laryngoscopic examination, an important observation when bilateral carotid endarterectomy is indicated. Satisfactory return of function must be objectively demonstrated, for bilateral vocal cord palsy requires tracheostomy.[115,117–119]

Wound Complications

Dehiscence and infection are extremely rare. Hematoma formation, however, is not uncommon. It may follow extubation. Transfixion sutures of the major vessels such as the common facial vein are therefore recommended. Drainage of the surgical site is not required except in a wet field. Hematomas may cause compression of the trachea. They may undergo liquifaction and become a nidus of infection. Hematomas should be promptly evacuated, the area irrigated, a search made for bleeding points, and the incision closed primarily.

Risks and Results

When planning carotid endarterectomy, the surgeon must take into consideration not only the complications of the operative procedure itself but of the arteriogram, the rate of recurrent stenosis, and the quality and duration of life after the operation. At the Mayo Clinic, patients have been placed in one of four groups based on three categories—the neurologic status, the angiographic findings, and coexisting illness such as coronary artery disease.[120] In the first group of neurologically stable patients with no major medical disease and no angiographically defined risk such as intracranial stenosis or thrombus superimposed on the carotid plaque, the combined operative morbidity and mortality rate was 1%. In the neurologically stable patient without major medical disease but with a significant angiographically defined risk (e.g., contralateral occlusion), the morbidity and mortality rate was 2%. In the neurologically stable patient with significant medical risk factors but without angiographically defined risks, the mortality and morbidity combined rate was 7%. In the highest risk patients, those who were neurologically unstable, that is, with waxing and waning TIAs and either with or without coexisting medical diseases or the angiographically defined risk, total morbidity and mortality was 10%.[120]

The higher complication and mortality rates in the neurologically unstable patient were confirmed in Thompson's[121] large experience. Here the mortality varied from zero for the patient with the asymptomatic bruit to 1.1% for the patient with TIAs and to 5.1% for the patient with a frank stroke. In an uncontrolled study of prophylactic endarterectomy that is, for the asymptomatic plaque, followed for 16 years, there was no operative mortality, and 91% of patients remained asymptomatic as contrasted to only 56% in the control group, who were not operated on. The late stroke rate—nonfatal—was 2.3% in the surgical patients and 15% in the control group. In a widely quoted and the only published randomized trial of carotid endarterectomy from the Joint Study of Extracranial Arterial Occlusion,[122] a 12% stroke rate was found in the surgical group and a 27% stroke or death rate. In the nonsurgical group these figures were 13% and 26% respectively. Thus conservative management provided as satisfactory an experience over a follow-up of approximately 4 years as did the surgical group. This study, however, was published between 1962 and 1968 and was based on TIAs among 316 patients. The low operative morbidity and mortality rates currently experienced in most centers largely invalidate that study of 20 years ago.

Patients with the least disease do best in late follow-up. Thompson et al.[123] report that at up to 13 years after surgery, 91% of patients with an asymptomatic bruit were normal neurologically, as were 81% of TIA patients, compared to only 30% of patients with a frank stroke. As might be expected, the incidence of late and permanent strokes correlated with the preoperative neurologic condition. After 5 years the incidence in the frank stroke group was 10.6%, 5.4% in the TIA group, and 4.6% in the asymptomatic bruit patients.[123] Possibly because the asymptomatic bruit patients and the TIA patients lived longer than those with frank stroke, heart disease was the cause of death in 72% of the asymptomatic bruit patients, 61% for the TIA group, and 41% of those with frank stroke.

It is interesting to speculate about what might be the duration and quality of life if the major risk factors could be eliminated. Among carotid endarterectomy patients with coronary artery disease, the 5-year survival rate was 63% for patients without prior coronary bypass and 85% for those with it.[124] These figures are reinforced by a second study in which only 4% of patients undergoing coronary artery bypass either before or after carotid endarterectomy died of myocardial infarction.[125] Thus among some carotid patients, the late cardiac mortality may be sustantially reduced.

Several retrospective studies support the claim that carotid endarterectomy is an effective and durable operation. Among 400 patients followed for 2 years, late stroke occurred in less than 1%, and stroke frequency was less than 2% per year after carotid endarterectomy.[126] Of 146 patients who underwent carotid endarterectomy for symp-

tomatic and contralateral asymptomatic disease during a mean follow-up of 4.3 years and who were on long-term antiplatelet therapy, the cumulative stroke rate by life-table analysis was 17.6% for those who had unilateral carotid endarterectomy and 5.6% for those who had bilateral operations (Fig. 55-26).[127] Comparing follow-up data averaging about 5 years for many series, approximately 10% of patients undergoing carotid endarterectomy for symptomatic disease can be expected to have recurrence of the TIAs and to suffer a stroke rate of approximately 6 to 8%. Of 335 patients during a follow-up period averaging 8.6 years, 38 (11%) developed TIAs of the ipsilateral or operated on artery.[129] Among those same patients, late stroke rate on the side operated on was 7%.[130–135]

Recurrent Stenosis

In the reported incidence of recurrent carotid stenosis varying from less than 3 to 22%, probably less than half are symptomatic (Fig. 55-27).[123,136–146] The need for lifetime follow-up is based on the observation that symptoms in the territory of the ipsilateral hemisphere are usually associated with recurrent disease. Recurrences within the first 24 to 36 months after operation are predominantly of the neointimal fibromuscular hyperplastic type, histologic examination of which reveals stellate or spindle-shaped cells in a homogeneous matrix (Fig. 55-28).[147] It is presumed that these cells originate from residual smooth muscle cells at the endarterectomy site and are stimulated to proliferate by the microthrombus on the injured arterial wall.[148] With the exception of one recent report,[149] reendothelialization of the endarterectomy site has not been demonstrated.[150] Late lesions occurring beyond 2 or 3 years have lipid-laden cells, neovascularization, and hemosiderin, characteristics of atherosclerosis. The discussion continues as to whether the early and late recurrent disease are distinct pathologic entities: a hyperplastic myofibroblastic response to injury or an early phase of atherosclerosis.[151] Recent observations suggest that the primary element in the formation of the recurrent lesion is continuing thrombogenesis, with its con-

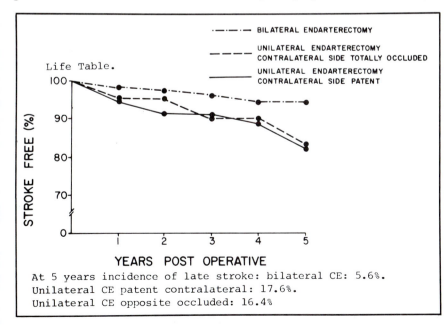

At 5 years incidence of late stroke: bilateral CE: 5.6%.
Unilateral CE patent contralateral: 17.6%.
Unilateral CE opposite occluded: 16.4%

Figure 55-26. Cumulative stroke rate after carotid endarterectomy. (*From Riles TS, Imparato AM, et al.: Surgery 91:258, 1982.*)

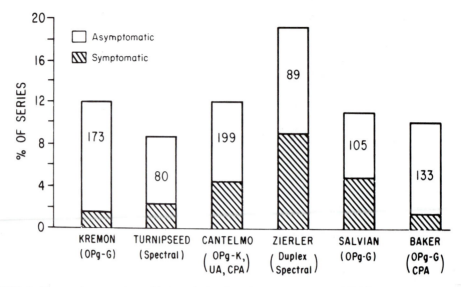

Figure 55-27. Incidence of recurrent carotid stenosis (noninvasive hemodynamics).[140-145] (*Courtesy of TF O'Donnell.*)

tinuing proliferative stimulus to smooth muscle cells and late atherosclerotic degeneration.

Possible risk factors are continued smoking, an ongoing active atherosclerotic process throughout the body, the female sex, hyperlipidemia, and hypertension.

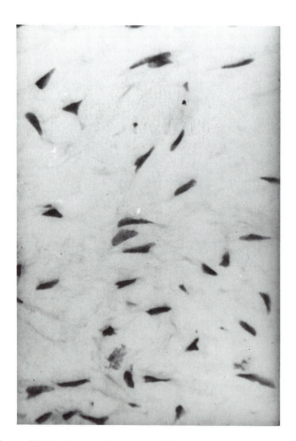

Figure 55-28. Exuberant myointimal hyperplasia removed during second operation 6 months after first endarterectomy. (High magnification; H & E; original magnification ×308.) (*From Callow AD: Arch Surg 117:1082, 1982.*)

Although it is claimed that a venous patch closure of the first endarterectomy prevents recurrences,[152] this has not been established. Eikelboom and associates[153] reported an incidence of 3.5% (2/57) with a vein patch versus 21% (10/48) without it. Restenosis was 24% in the female patients and 7.5% in the male patients. Presumably the venous patch with its antithrombogenic luminal surface retards thrombogenesis at the endarterectomy site and may promote reendothelialization. However, the venous patch surface does not extend around the full circumference of the endarterectomized carotid bulb where thrombogenesis would be as likely to occur as along the arteriotomy suture closure.

Arteriograms of the early recurrent lesion show a smoothly tapered hourglass area of constriction quite unlike the ulcerated irregularity usually seen in the advanced atherosclerotic plaque (Fig. 55-29).[150] Gross examination reveals a smooth glistening whitish surface lacking the characteristic changes of the atherosclerotic plaque, namely ulceration, hemorrhage, thrombosis, and calcification. Because of the dense, firm, and somewhat rubbery inflexible nature of the lesion, the operation is technically more difficult. The usual cleavage plane between the atherosclerotic plaque and the media and adventitia is not present. It is not recommended, therefore, that this early lesion be removed by endarterectomy, but rather than the lumen be opened, and the area of constriction eliminated by insertion of a venous patch. Care must be taken in the surgical approach to the artery to avoid damage to surrounding structures, especially nerves that may be imbedded in scar tissue. Second and third recurrences have been reported. In this instance, excision of the area of carotid involvement and insertion of an interposition saphenous vein graft is recommended. Completion angiography makes it possible to distinguish between a true recurrence or residual disease left at the time of the first operation. Blaisdell and associates[154] found substantial residual deficits in 27%; Flanigan,[155] in 28%, of which 7% required reentry and repair; and Courbier,[156] a 5% reentry and repair rate when defects greater than 30% stenosis were taken as a baseline.[157,158]

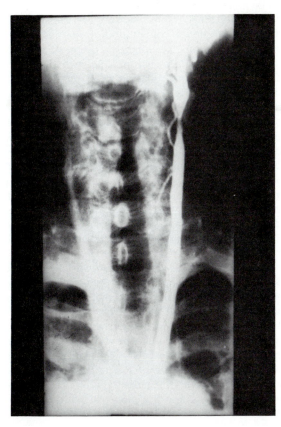

Figure 55-29. Smoothly tapered hourglass constriction characteristic of the early hyperplastic recurrent lesion. (*From Callow AD, O'Donnell TF Jr: Recurrent carotid stenosis: Frequency, clinical implications, and some suggestions concerning etiology, in Bergan JJ, Yao JST (eds): Reoperative arterial surgery. New York, Grune & Stratton, 1986, p 513.*)

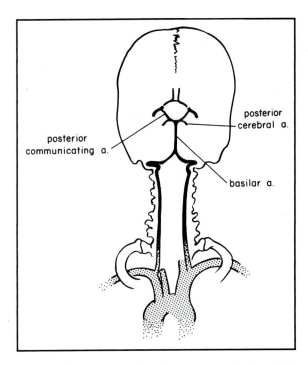

Figure 55-30. Vertebrobasilar and posterior cerebral circulation.

VERTEBROBASILAR ARTERY SYNDROMES

Anatomy

The vertebral arteries are customarily divided into four segments (Fig. 55-30).[159] The first segment consists of its origin from the first portion of the subclavian artery and the first 5 to 7 cm until it enters the foramen in the transverse process of the sixth cervical vertebra. This section has no branches. Branches of the thyrocervical trunk may pass anterior to it at this level. The second section consists of that portion passing through the foramina of the transverse processes up to the axis. The third portion extends from the upper border of the axis through the foramen in the transverse process of the atlas. Here the vessel turns backward and enters the skull through the foramen magnum. At this point it becomes the fourth portion and joins the vertebral artery of the other side to form the midline basilar artery. On the left side the thoracic duct is anterior to the vertebral artery. On the right side the recurrent laryngeal nerve winds around the subclavian artery and rises in the neck parallel with the first few centimeters of the vertebral artery.

Clinical Presentation

The vertebral and basilar arteries supply the pons, thalamus, midbrain, and temporo-occipital portions of the cerebral hemispheres. Vertebrobasilar insufficiency produces symptoms characteristic of involvement of one or both pyramidal tracts of the long sensory tracts and of cranial nerves III to XI. Because the territories served by the posterior circulation include the brain stem, parts of the temporal lobes, and the occipital lobes, each of which contains many anatomic structures serving many functions, TIAs in the vertebrobasilar territory are extremely variable. Signs and symptoms may include the following:

1. Visual field disturbance
2. Amnesia and confusional episodes
3. Diplopia
4. Disturbance of sensation in the face
5. Vertigo
6. Dysphasia and dysarthria
7. Ataxia
8. Hemiplegia and hemianesthesia
9. Drop attacks
10. Headache.

Vertebrobasilar insufficiency has been defined as limited to the clinical presentation of at least two of the following symptoms:

1. Motor or sensory symptoms or both, occurring bilaterally in the same attack
2. Ataxia of gait or clumsiness of both extremities
3. Diplopia
4. Dysarthria
5. Bilateral homonymous hemianopia

Additional signs and symptoms that are compatible but not necessarily diagnostic are as follows:

1. Vertigo
2. Tinnitus
3. Multiple cranial nerve involvement, usually contralateral to the major sensory deficit
4. Motor involvement of the extremities

Dizziness alone is not considered a symptom of vertebrobasilar insufficiency, nor is syncope, certain drop attacks, or transient global amnesia. Following are causes other than vertebrobasilar insufficiency that should be considered[160–162]: cardiac arrhythmias, a reduced ejection fraction, and emboli from various sources; blood dyscrasias, particularly thrombocytosis, sickle cell disease, or hypercoagulability from any cause; intracranial hemorrhage; demyelinating diseases; intracranial tumors, especially at the cerebellopontine angle and of the cerebellum; and labrynthitis and Meniere's disease. The pathophysiology of the vertebrobasilar TIA or stroke must be better defined. The frequent practice of lumping all patients with vertebrobasilar disease into one category must be discouraged.[163]

Several special types of vertebrobasilar insufficiency have been identified that need only be mentioned here:

1. Basilar branch occlusion: high mortality and limited interventional accessibility.
2. Lacunar strokes: small, deep infarcts in the territory of penetrating vessels associated with hypertension and distinguished from atherosclerosis by lipohyalinosis of the arterial wall.
3. Basilar artery stenosis and occlusion: associated with bilateral long-tract signs; poor results were observed in the few cases treated with percutaneous transluminal angioplasty.
4. "Top of the basilar" ischemia: deficits referable to the high brainstem and posterior cerebral artery territories.
5. Cervical vertebral artery disease: the atheroma serves as a nidus for emboli and thrombosis. Despite TIAs, brainstem strokes are uncommon, probably because of the remarkable collateral circulation in these patients. In a survey of more than 100 cases of subclavian steal syndrome, no major brainstem infarctions occurred unless widespread disease of other extracranial or intracranial vessels was present.
6. Intracranial vertebral occlusion: relatively benign with survival of most patients; associated with lateral medullary infarction, posterior inferior cerebellar artery territory ischemia, cerebellar infarction, and hemi-infarction of the medulla.
7. Bilateral vertebral occlusive disease: this carries a prolonged risk of serious and often fatal brainstem or cerebellar infarction; less collateral circulation is available than exists with basilar artery occlusion. An occipital artery bypass to the posterior inferior cerebellar artery may be worthwhile.

Compared to symptomatic carotid occlusive disease, isolated symptomatic vertebral occlusive disease is rare.[164] Of the 4,748 patients in the Joint Study of Extracranial Arterial Occlusion, 10% of patients with cerebrovascular insufficiency showed angiographic evidence of occlusive involvement of the posterior communicating arteries; 17% had subclavian or innominate artery occlusion or stenosis of greater than 30%. Only 168, or 15%, with these lesions fulfilled the criteria of subclavian steal, and of them, 80% had associated lesions of other extracranial vessels. Right vertebral artery stenosis or occlusion occurred in 22%, and left vertebral artery involvement occurred in 28% of all patients.[165] Imparato and Riles,[166] in a series of 1,400 extracranial operations, reported that operations on the vertebral arteries represented only 5.8% of the procedures. Correction of subclavian steal or innominate artery disease was performed in 2.5%, thus indicating the need for specific criteria in patient selection. Subclavian steal may be asymptomatic and appear only as a radiographic phenomenon. In a Houston report of more than 3,000 cerebrovascular operations, only 40 were direct vertebral operations.[167]

In patients with single vertebral occlusions, symptoms of stroke are not as important as they are in the carotid system.[168] Vertebral lesions in combination with carotid lesions, however, result in a greater risk for stroke since posterior cerebral ischemia may occur along with mid and anterior cerebral territory ischemia.[169] When the only angiographic abnormality was subclavian stenosis, completed stroke was extremely rare in 168 patients in a follow-up study of up to 8 years.[170] Coexisting carotid artery disease may produce signs and symptoms of both anterior and posterior circulations.

Diagnosis

Noninvasive studies are of little or no help in assessing the vertebrobasilar circulation. Standard arch arteriography with selective injections of the vertebrals is by far the most reliable modality. A retrograde brachial arterial injection may be needed. Views of the basilar artery are mandatory if vertebral artery surgery is contemplated. CT scan may be required.

Medical Therapy

A decrease in mortality from 43 to 14% was reported with long-term anticoagulant therapy,[171] and stroke incidence decreased from 35 to 15% within 4 years.[162]

Surgical Therapy

Bilateral flow impeding vertebral lesions plus a reasonably satisfactory basilar artery must be visualized by angiography if vertebral surgery is to be done. In the presence of hemodynamically significant carotid lesions, carotid endarterectomy alone may relieve the ischemic signs and symptoms of the posterior territory.

Conditions for which vertebral artery operations are most likely indicated include the following[166]:

1. Severe stenosis or occlusion of both vertebral arteries, with cerebral symptoms and no other accessible extracranial lesions

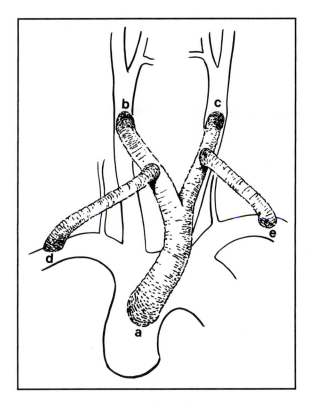

Figure 55-31. A variety of brachiocephalic bypass procedures.

2. Symptomatic bilateral vertebral artery stenoses that have failed to improve after correction of a coexisting carotid lesion
3. Symptomatic bilateral stenoses of the vertebral arteries and bilateral internal carotid artery occlusions
4. Embolization to the brain stem from brachiocephalic vessels

The natural history of patients with vertebrobasilar insufficiency due to atherosclerotic lesions has not been well documented, and unfortunately no randomized prospective studies are available. Available information suggests that the stroke risk for untreated patients with symptomatic vertebrobasilar ischemia is 35% within 4 years of onset of symptoms.[162] Surgical morbidity for patients with angiographically proven significant vertebral or basilar or vertebrobasilar arterial lesions is reported as 5% and surgical mortality as 3%. There is no controlled randomized prospective study of medically treated vs. surgically treated patients.

Crawford, DeBakey, and Fields[172] reported surgical treatment for lesions of the extracranial vertebral artery in 1958, and since that time, many procedures have been used[173–185] (Fig. 55-31).

1. Subclavian vertebral angioplasty
2. Subclavian vertebral endarterectomy
3. Reimplantation of vertebral artery to the carotid artery
4. Carotid vertebral bypass (proximal and distal)
5. Rongeur decompression of the bony canal formed by the transverse processes of the cervical vertebras
6. Extracranial or intracranial bypass

AREAS OF UNCERTAINTY OR CONTROVERSY

Coexisting Coronary and Carotid Occlusive Disease

Consideration of performing simultaneous coronary artery bypass with carotid endarterectomy is not often required, for the number of patients with urgent symptomatic disease in both systems is few. That the morbidity and mortality of such combined simultaneous operations is increased over those that are staged, except for some special situations, is the subject of several reports.[75,186,187] Hence, if surgery on both systems is needed, efforts should be made to stage them so that the system which is symptomatic is operated on first. Although the patient with asymptomatic carotid plaque may be presumed at high risk because of preocclusive stenosis, thrombus superimposed on the stenosis, or severe ulceration, the symptomatic coronary artery disease should be repaired first, and carotid endarterectomy should be performed several days to weeks later. There are instances of exceptionally qualified cardiovascular surgeons located in a few centers who can successfully undertake simultaneous operations.[75,125] However, the average vascular surgeon, lacking high volume and frequent experience, will do much better with staged procedures. The carotid endarterectomy that goes quite successfully during combined operations comes to be at risk of thrombosis by unexpected complications associated with coronary bypass such as inordinate mediastinal bleeding and poor myocardial function.

The Asymptomatic Bruit

Emphasis should be directed more toward the presence of a carotid bifurcation occlusive lesion than to the presence or absence of a carotid bruit. The absence of a bruit indicates little or nothing about the status of the carotid artery, the characteristics of a plaque, or the degree of risk of stroke. The sudden conversion of a stable plaque into one that is unstable is receiving increasing recognition. Intraplaque hemorrhage, presumably from the vasa vasorum, can produce sudden and unpredictable reduction in the size of the lumen and eventual disgorgement of contents.[188] Presently, this event is impossible to prevent or predict. The attendant possibility of cerebral catastrophe lends support to the proponents of prophylactic endarterectomy. On the other hand, the bruit is more a marker for cardiovascular disease and risk of myocardial infarction than for cerebral infarction.[70,189–191]

Approximately 20% of patients with cervical bruits have hemodynamically significant stenosis of the internal carotid artery.[192] Evaluation of the bruit should be undertaken to identify high-grade internal carotid stenoses of 75% or more, the large ulcerated lesion with or without stenosis, and the ominous soft-core plaque. The risk of stroke correlates with the degree of stenosis. Eighty-nine percent of 203 patients followed by duplex scanning who developed either transient ischemic attack (TIA) or stroke experienced stenosis progression to greater than 80%. The risk of neurologic deficit or progression to occlusion was 35% within 6 months and 46% risk at 12 months.[69] Among 294 patients followed noninvasively for a 5-year period, 12% suffered a stroke, only one of which was preceded by a warning transient event. Patients with an initial stenosis in excess of 50% experienced a 17% stroke rate. By life-table analysis, the 5-year stroke rate was 9% for patients with minimal stenosis, 14% for moderate—up to 49% stenosis—and 21% for patients with the greatest amount of stenosis. For individuals over age 70 with hypertension and greater than 50% stenosis, the 5-year stroke rate was 49% or almost 10% per year.[193] Among 500 patients followed noninvasively, the incidence of all cerebral ischemic events in patients with a stenosis of 75 to 100% was 18%. At 1 year, a completed stroke incidence was 5%, and stroke without preceding TIA was 3%.[195] Hertzer et al.[187] in a follow-up study up to 5 years, found freedom from neurologic events was approximately 85% in patients with lesions of 50 to 69% stenosis and without surgery. In contrast, in individuals with stenosis of 70% or greater and without operation, freedom from neurologic events at the fourth- and fifth-year level was 65%. In the patients with lesser stenosis, there was no statistically significant difference in freedom from neurologic events among those who underwent carotid endarterectomy and those who did not. In those patients with greater than 70% stenosis, however, at the fourth year, freedom from neurologic events was 83%. Again among patients with a 70-degree stenosis or greater, cumulative late stroke at the fourth year level was 31% for the nonsurgical carotid patient and only 7% for those patients undergoing endarterectomy. A consistent pattern is emerging that suggests that patients with carotid lesions associated with 75% stenosis or greater may suffer a stroke rate of approximately 5% per year.

Arteriographic demonstration of ulceration is evidence that the simple and presumably stable plaque has undergone degenerative changes, rendering it unstable and highly suspect as a source of emboli. A 7.5% per year stroke risk has been identified with a large or compound ulceration.[195,196]

That prophylactic carotid endarterectomy can be performed with minimal morbidity and mortality in the asymptomatic carotid plaque patient is demonstrated by several reviews reporting morbidity and mortality rates from 0 to 2.3%. The surgical mortality rate of the 426 patients collected from this review was 0.2%, the combined stroke rate was 0.7%, and the overall combined morbidity and mortality rate was 0.9%.[125,197]

The belief that one may reduce the incidence of perioperative stroke by performing prophylactic carotid endarterectomy at the time of some other major procedure has not been reliably confirmed, for as many perioperative strokes occur on the side contralateral to the asymptomatic carotid bruit as on the ipsilateral side.[111,198,199]

There is less and less evidence that the practice of routine prophylactic carotid endarterectomy for asymptomatic carotid disease in the individual who is to undergo major cardiovascular surgery is justifiable. Recent evidence suggests that the risk of perioperative stroke during such major cardiovascular surgery is the same in patients with or without asymptomatic carotid artery disease. In these circumstances, prophylactic carotid endarterectomy before or simultaneously with major cardiovascular surgery in the asymptomatic patient may be of benefit only in preventing late postoperative rather than early perioperative stroke and death.[200,201] Confusion exists about whether to wait for symptoms to develop from an asymptomatic carotid lesion before considering prophylactic operation,[202–204] or to proceed.[197,205] Although randomized prospective studies are underway, definitive data are several years away.

In the meantime, noninvasive assessment of the carotid artery in the patient with an asymptomatic bruit should be performed and repeated at appropriate intervals such as every 6 months. Patients with angiographically confirmed stenosis greater than 75%, with or without ulceration, or a large compound ulceration, with or without substantial stenosis, are, on the basis of current information, at increased risk. This risk is increased by the coexistence of hypertension and age over 70. In the absence of coexisting disease in other systems severe enough to make anesthesia and operative risk excessive and if the documented combined morbidity and mortality of carotid endarterectomy in that institution is less than 3%, prophylactic carotid endarterectomy is recommended.[110,206,207]

Contralateral, or Second-Side, Operation

Even the best of evidence favoring contralateral, or second-side, prophylactic carotid endarterectomy is anecdotal. Contrasting patients with elective contralateral endarterectomy with those who have had observation of the second lesion only, among those who had prophylactic surgery, the cumulative stroke-free percentage was approximately 88% through the seventh year. Among those whose lesion was observed only, the stroke-free percentage fell steadily from 96% at the first year to 64% at the seventh year. Among the surgical patients the cumulative late stroke incidence was 2% through the seventh and eighth years as contrasted to 20% during the same time interval for the nonsurgical patient.[110] Among these same patients (surgical and nonsurgical) the percent of stroke-free patients with contralateral stenosis of less than 50% was 92% at the fifth year and 83% at the seventh year. Those patients with contralateral stenosis greater than 50% had a stroke-free incidence of 80% at the fifth year and approximately 75% at the seventh year. Sobel and Imparato et al.[208] in a retrospective study of contralateral side neurologic symptoms after unilateral carotid endarterectomy, suggest that 11.6% of patients after unilateral carotid endarterectomy will have major neurologic symptoms referable to the asymptomatic nonoperated carotid territory. Of the 11 strokes in the Sobel and Imparato study,[208] none was preceded by a warning TIA, and strokes outnumbered TIAs as the initial symptom. The presence of hypertension showed not only a higher neurologic morbidity but also a higher mortality from unrelated causes in these patients by life-table comparison. In an earlier study[127] of prophylactic endarterectomy for the contralateral side versus observation alone, by life-table analysis the 5-year cumulative stroke rate was 5.6% after bilateral endarterectomy as contrasted to 11.6% in the more recent study. Recognized difficulties that compound the problem are as follows: nonstenotic but ulcerated arteries may produce neurologic events by embolization; occult progression of

TABLE 55-5. 1958 TO 1967 SERIES OF 266 CAROTID ENDARTERECTOMIES

Reason for Surgery	Number of Operations	Improved		Unchanged		Worse		Expired	
		No.	%	No.	%	No.	%	No.	%
TIA	216	188	87	21	10	5	1	1	1
Completed infarct	20	2	10	14	70	3	15	1	5
Acute Stroke	30	8	26	8	26	8	26	6	20

From Callow AD: David M. Hume Memorial Lecture. An overview of the stroke problem in the carotid territory. Am J Surg 140: 181, 1980.

disease in the asymptomatic artery is unknown unless the patient is carefully followed; and widely varying opinions and practices exist concerning postoperative antiplatelet and anticoagulation therapy.[209]

The Acute Stroke and Stroke in Evolution

If there is a place for carotid endarterectomy in the management of acute stroke, it is yet to be defined.[210] An early experience is presented in Table 55-5.[181] Illustrating the improvement in the state of the art in 20 years is a second experience (Table 55-6).[211]

A collective series of all cases of this type published through 1980 documented that 56% of 217 patients were improved, 25% were unchanged, 8% were worse, and only 9% died after operative intervention.[212,213] The surgical mortality of the earlier experience of 20 years ago (see Table 55-5) was 20%, and 26% were made worse by emergency carotid endarterectomy.

There are three problems to consider in the decision-making process concerning surgical intervention. The first is the risk of introducing toxic angiographic contrast agents with their higher incidence of radiographic neurologic complications in this group of patients. The second is the possibility of converting what might become, or is, a dry or ischemic infarct into a hemorrhagic infarct with a greater neurologic deficit, and the third consideration is the greater risk of surgery in any acutely ill individual.[214,215] Uncertainty as to diagnosis, that is, a TIA, a stroke in progress, or a

completed infarct, surrounds the patient with sudden onset of a focal neurologic deficit. In general, the safer management course is to consider the deficit the result of a stroke in progress and to withhold angiographic or surgical intervention because of the high risks and uncertain benefit. Most studies of the acute stroke problem are old and lack the benefit of more recent sophisticated studies such as CT scan and magnetic resonance imaging (MRI). There is little reliable evidence that patients with progressing strokes are substantially benefitted by anticoagulant therapy such as intravenous heparin, warfarin, low-molecular-weight dextran, and the administration of corticosteroids. One must await the results of studies presently underway concerning new treatment modalities.[216]

The patient with a waxing and waning neurologic deficit or a stroke in evolution requires extremely careful evaluation. A very few, unlike the acute stroke patient, may be helped by surgical intervention. The neurologic deficit at onset may be of limited extent but within hours to days may become a major stroke with brief periods of apparent improvement. Recovery, however, remains incomplete. Despite occasional optimistic anecdotal reports, the course of the patient with an acute progressing stroke is unfavorable and usually ends with a permanent fixed deficit of some degree.

The clinician faced with this problem has the choice of administering heparin, surgical intervention, or "general medical supportive therapy." Anecdotal evidence suggests that anticoagulation therapy reduces the incidence of stroke progression and therefore death. Despite its proponents,

TABLE 55-6. EMERGENCY CAROTID ENDARTERECTOMY BASED ON SURGICAL FINDINGS OR PREOPERATIVE NEUROLOGIC STATUS

	Outcome				
	Excellent	Good	Poor	Death	Total
Surgical Findings					
Stenosis	8	11	4	3	26
Occluded (flow restored)	5	11	2	3	21
Occluded (flow not restored)	—	1	5	2	8
Total	13	23	11	8	55
Preoperative Neurologic Status					
TIAS	4	—	—	—	4
Mild deficit	2	2	—	—	4
Moderate deficit	7	14	6	1	28
Sudden severe deficit	1	5	6	7	19
Total	14	21	12	8	55

From Ojemann RG, Crowell RM: Surgical Management of Cerebrovascular Disease. Baltimore, Williams & Wilkins, 1983.

TABLE 55-7. NATURAL HISTORY OF 204 CONSECUTIVE PATIENTS WITH ACUTE ONSET OF PROGRESSING STROKE IN THE CAROTID SYSTEM

Fourteen Days after Onset	
Condition	%
Normal	12
Monoparesis	5
Hemiparesis	69
Dead	14

Modified from Milliken CH: Formal discussion, in McDowell FH, Brennan RW (eds): Cerebral Vascular Diseases. Eighth Princeton Conference on Cerebrovascular Diseases. New York, Grune & Stratton, 1973.

TABLE 55-8. EMERGENCY CAROTID ENDARTERECTOMY

Indications (both must be present)
  1. Unstable lesion
  2. Unstable neurological status
Contraindications (any one, singly or in combination)
  1. Profound neurologic deficit
  2. Altered level of consciousness
  3. Improving neurologic status
  4. Internal carotid artery occlusion

emergency carotid endarterectomy seems indicated only for patients with deficits of a mild-to-moderate degree and no change in level of consciousness—a sign of widespread cerebrovascular involvement. The evolving stroke patient should have the benefit of a CT scan or, if available, MRI as soon as possible after the neurologic evaluation. One may thus possibly exclude intracerebral hemorrhage, lacunar infarcts, and mass lesions such as tumors. Severe hypertension must be controlled and is a contraindication to heparin therapy. If diagnosis cannot be made, arteriography is indicated. The discovery of a critical degree of stenosis or stenosis with ulceration or superimposed thrombus within the lumen of the internal carotid artery requires immediate endarterectomy. In the absence of substantial carotid occlusive disease, hypertension, and CT scan evidence of intracerebral hemorrhage, intravenous heparin administration should be started with the activated partial thromboplastin time elevated to twice normal. The intravenous route is preferable. Should surgical intervention be the choice for a patient with a critical cervical carotid artery lesion, an unstable deficit appropriate to the lesion, and no evidence of intracranial hemorrhage, endotracheal general anesthesia is much preferred over local anesthesia. An intraluminal shunt should always be used, and completion evaluation by angiography or duplex scanning is mandatory (Fig. 55-32).[217] Patients with a fixed neurologic deficit or with changes in the level of consciousness have probably already suffered irreversible cerebral infarction. Reduced to the essential, guidelines for emergency carotid endarterectomy are presented in Table 55-8.

For the present, operations for this condition should be limited to centers of excellence with the facilities and interest for prospective randomized controlled studies. Under the best of circumstances, management of the acute stroke and of the stroke in evolution is a difficult problem, and the introduction of surgical effort further compounds it. Depending on the time of onset of the deficit and the promptness with which the patient can be evaluated and the diagnosis made, surgical intervention may be considered.[102]

REFERENCES

1. Robins M, Baum HM: Incidence, in Weinfeld FD (ed): The National Survey of Stroke. Bethesda, Md., Office of Scientific and Health Reports, National Institute of Neurological and Communicative Disorders and Stroke, National Institutes of Health, Public Health Service, 1981, p I45.
2. McDowell FH, Caplan LR (eds): Cerebrovascular Survey Report 1985. Bethesda, Md, for the National Institute of Neuro-

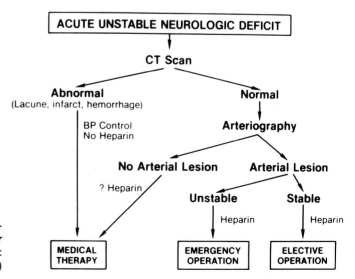

Figure 55-32. Algorithm outlining management of unstable neurologic deficit. (*From McIntyre KE, Goldstone J: Carotid surgery for crescendo TIA and stroke in evolution, in Bergan JJ, Yao JST (eds): Cerebrovascular Insufficiency. New York, Grune & Stratton, 1983.*)

logical and Communicative Disorders and Stroke, National Institutes of Health, Public Health Service, 1985.

3. Callow AD, Mackey WC: The social, economic and personal impact of stroke and its prevention, in Moore WS (ed): Surgery for Cerebrovascular Disease. New York, Churchill Livingstone, 1987.

4. Sacco RL, Wolf PA, et al.: Survival and recurrence following stroke: The Framingham Study. Stroke 13:290, 1982.

5. Hodgson TA, Kopstein AN: Health care expenditures for major disease, in Health: United States—1983. The US Department of Health and Human Services. Public Health Service Pub No 84-1232. Washington, DC, US Government Printing Office, 1983.

6. Whisnant JP, Fitzgibbons JP, et al.: Natural history of stroke in Rochester, Minnesota, 1945 through 1954. Stroke 4:666, 1973.

7. Day AL: Anatomy of the extracranial vessels, in Smith RR (ed): Stroke and the Extracranial Vessels. New York, Raven Press, 1984.

8. Hill EG, McKinney WM: Vascular anatomy and pathology of the head and neck: Method of corrosion casting, in Carney AL, Anderson EM (eds): Advances in Neurology. Diagnosis and Treatment of Brain Ischemia, vol 30. New York, Raven Press, 1981.

9. Greitz T, Lindgren E: Cerebral angiography: Technique of examination, in Abrams HL (ed): Angiography, 1st ed. Boston, Little, Brown & Co, Inc, 1961, p 41.

10. Callow AD, Moran JM, et al.: Patterns of atherosclerosis of extracranial cerebral arteries. Ann NY Acad Sci 149:974, 1968.

11. Abrams HL: Angiography, 2nd ed, vol 1. Boston, Little, Brown and Co, Inc, 1961, p 180.

12. Lassen NA: The luxury-perfusion syndrome and its possible relation to acute metabolic acidosis localized within the brain. Lancet 2:1113, 1966.

13. Leviton A, Caplan L, Salzman E: Severe headache after carotid endarterectomy. Headache 15:207, 1975.

14. Dolan JG, Mushlin AI: Hypertension, vascular headaches, and seizures after carotid endarterectomy. Arch Intern Med 144:1489, 1984.

15. Bernstein M, Fleming JFR, Deck JHN: Cerebral hyperperfusion after carotid endarterectomy: A cause of cerebral hemorrhage. Neurosurgery 15:50, 1984.

16. Caplan LR: Intracerebral hemorrhage. Curr Neurol 2:185, 1979.

17. Fisher CM: The arterial lesions underlying lacunes. Acta Neuropathol 12:1, 1969.

18. Moossy J: Morphology, sites and epidemiology of cerebral atherosclerosis. Res Publ Assoc Res Nerv Ment Dis 41:1, 1966.

19. Mohr J, Caplan LR, et al.: Harvard Cooperative Stroke Registry: A prospective registry. Neurology 28:754, 1978.

20. Effeney DJ, Ehrenfeld WK, et al.: Fibromuscular dysplasia of the internal carotid artery. World J Surg 3:179, 1979.

21. Wylie EJ, Perloff D, Wellington DJ: Fibromuscular hyperplasia of the renal arteries. Ann Surg 156:592, 1962.

22. Stanley JC, Gewertz BL, et al.: Arterial fibrodysplasia: Histopathologic character and current etiologic concepts. Arch Surg 110:561, 1975.

23. Palubinskas AJ, Ripley HR: Fibromuscular hyperplasia in extrarenal arteries. Radiology 82:451, 1964.

24. Effeney DJ, Ehrenfeld WK, et al.: Why operate on carotid fibromuscular dysplasia. Arch Surg 115:1261, 1980.

25. Effeney DJ, Krupski WC, et al.: Fibromuscular dysplasia of the carotid artery, in Wilson SE, Veith FJ, et al.: Vascular Surgery. Principles and Practice. New York, McGraw-Hill Book Co, 1987, p 614.

26. Connett MC, Lansche KM: Fibromuscular hyperplasia of internal carotid artery: Report of a case. Ann Surg 162:59, 1965.

27. Lamis PA, Carson WP, et al.: Recognition and treatment of fibromuscular hyperplasia of the internal carotid artery. Surgery 69:498, 1971.

28. Stanley JC: Extracranial internal carotid artery fibrodysplasia, in Ernst CB, Stanley JC (eds): Current Therapy in Vascular Surgery. Toronto, Brian C Decker, Publisher, 1987, p 17.

29. Smith DC, Smith LL, Hasso AN: Fibromuscular dysplasia of the internal carotid artery treated by operative transluminal balloon angioplasty. Radiology 155:645, 1985.

30. Ehrenfeld WK, Wylie EJ: Fibromuscular dysplasia of the internal carotid artery. Arch Surg 109:676, 1974.

31. Patman RD, Thompson JE, et al.: Natural history of fibromuscular dysplasia of the carotid artery. Stroke 2:135, 1980.

32. Perry MO: Fibromuscular dysplasia. Surg Gynecol Obstet 139:97, 1974.

33. Stanley JC, Fry WJ, et al.: Extracranial internal carotid and vertebral artery fibrodysplasia. Arch Surg 109:215, 1974.

34. Starr DS, Laurie GM, Morris CC: Fibromuscular disease of carotid arteries: Long-term results of graduated intraluminal dilatation. Stroke 12:196, 1981.

35. Weibel J, Fields WS: Tortuosity, coiling, and kinking of the internal carotid artery, I. Etiology and radiographic anatomy. Neurology (Minneapolis) 15:7, 1965.

36. Perdue GD, Barreca JP, et al.: The significance of elongation and angulation of the carotid artery: A negative view. Surgery 77:45, 1975.

37. Cairney J: Tortuosity of the cervical segment of the internal carotid artery. J Anat 59:87, 1924.

38. Quattlebaum JK Jr, Wade JS, Whiddon CM: Stroke associated with elongation and kinking of the carotid artery: Long-term follow-up. Ann Surg 177:572, 1973.

39. Stanton PE Jr, McClusky DA Jr, Lamis PA: Hemodynamic assessment and surgical correction of kinking of the internal carotid artery. Surgery 84:793, 1978.

40. Vannix RS, Joergenson FJ, Carter R: Kinking of the internal carotid artery. Clinical significance and surgical management. Am J Surg 134:82, 1977.

41. McCollum CH, Wheeler WG, et al.: Aneurysms of the extracranial carotid artery. Twenty-one years' experience. Am J Surg 137:196, 1979.

42. Buscaglia LC, Moore WS, Hall AD: False aneurysm after carotid endarterectomy. JAMA 209:1529, 1969.

43. Rittenhouse EA, Radke HM, Sumner DS: Carotid artery aneurysm. Arch Surg 105:786, 1972.

44. Pellegrini RV, Manzetti GW, et al.: The direct surgical management of lesions of the high internal carotid artery. J Cardiovasc Surg 25:29, 1984.

45. Mokri B, Piepgras DG, et al.: Extracranial internal carotid artery aneurysms. Mayo Clin Proc 57:310, 1982.

46. Wylie EJ: Overview: Minisymposium: Unusual problems in carotid surgery. Surgery 93:297, 1983.

47. Busuttil RW, Davidson RK, et al.: Selective management of extracranial carotid artery aneurysms. Am J Surg 140:85, 1980.

48. Chiras J, Marciano S, et al.: Spontaneous dissecting aneurysm of the extracranial vertebral artery. Neuroradiology 27:327, 1985.

49. Kaupp HA, Haid SP, et al.: Aneurysms of the extracranial carotid artery. Surgery 72:946, 1972.

50. Teal JS, Bergeron RT, et al.: Aneurysms of the cervical portion of the internal carotid artery associated with nonpenetrating neck trauma. Radiology 105:353, 1972.

51. Thompson JE, Austin DJ: Surgical management of cervical carotid aneurysms. Arch Surg 74:80, 1957.

52. Ehrenfeld WK, Wylie EJ: Spontaneous dissection of the internal carotid artery. Arch Surg 111:1294, 1976.

53. Fisher CM, Ojemann RG, Roberson GH: Spontaneous dissection of cervicocerebral arteries. Can J Neurol Sci 5:9, 1978.

54. Gee W, Kaupp HA, et al.: Spontaneous dissection of internal carotid arteries. Spontaneous resolution documented by serial ocular pneumoplethysmography and angiography. Arch Surg 115:944, 1980.

55. McNeill DH Jr, Driesbach J, Marsden RJ: Spontaneous dissection of the internal carotid artery. Its conservative management with heparin sodium. Arch Neurol 37:54, 1980.

56. Fisher CM: Lacunes: Small deep cerebral infarcts. Neurology 15:774, 1965.

57. Caplan LR, Hier DB, D'Cruz I: Cerebral embolism in the Michael Reese Stroke Registry. Stroke 14:530, 1983.

58. Fisher CM: Observations of the fundus oculi in transient monocular blindness. Neurology 9:333, 1959.

59. Fisher CM, Pritchard JE, Mathews WH: Arteriosclerosis of the carotid arteries. Circulation 6:457, 1952.

60. Imparato AM, Riles TS, Gorstein F: The carotid bifurcation plaque: Pathologic findings associated with cerebral ischemia. Stroke 10:238, 1979.

61. Denny-Brown D: Recurrent cerebrovascular episodes. Arch Neurol 2:194, 1960.

62. Ehrenfeld WK, Hoyt WF, Wylie EJ: Embolization and transient blindness from carotid atheroma. Surgical considerations. Arch Surg 93:787, 1966.

63. Fields WS, North R, et al.: Joint study of extracranial arterial occlusion as a cause of stroke, I: Organization of study and survey of patient population. JAMA 203:955, 1968.

64. Flory CM: Arterial occlusions produced by emboli from eroded aortic atheromatous plaques. Am J Pathol 21:549, 1945.

65. Hollenhorst RW: Significance of bright plaques in the retinal arterioles. JAMA 178:23, 1961.

66. Russell RWR: Observations on the retinal blood vessels in monocular blindness. Lancet 2:1422, 1961.

67. Fields WS: Medical therapy for transient ischemic attack and stroke, in Ernst CB, Stanley JC (eds): Current Therapy in Vascular Surgery. Toronto, Brian C Decker, Publisher, 1987, p 5.

68. Dyken ML: Anticoagulant and platelet-antiaggregation therapy in stroke and threatened stroke. Neurol Clin North Am 1:223, 1983.

69. Roederer GO, Langlois YE, et al.: The natural history of carotid arterial disease in asymptomatic patients with cervical bruits. Stroke 15:605, 1984.

70. Toole JF, Yuson CP, et al.: Transient ischemic attacks: A prospective study of 225 patients. Neurology (Minneapolis) 28:746, 1978.

71. Carson SN, Demling RH, Esquivel CD: Aspirin failure in symptomatic arteriosclerotic carotid artery disease. Surgery 90:1084, 1981.

72. Fields WS, Lemak NA, et al.: Controlled trial of aspirin in cerebral ischemia. Stroke 8:301, 1977.

73. Fields WS, Lemak NA, et al.: Controlled trial of aspirin in cerebral ischemia, II: Surgical group. Stroke 9:309, 1978.

74. Ennix C, Lawrie G, et al.: Improved results of carotid endarterectomy in patients with symptomatic coronary disease; an analysis of 1,546 consecutive carotid operations. Stroke 10:122, 1979.

75. Cosgrove DM, Hertzer NR, Loop FD: Surgical management of synchronous carotid and coronary artery disease. J Vasc Surg 4:690, 1986.

76. Towne J, Bernhard V: The relationship of postoperative hypertension to complications following carotid endarterectomy. Surgery 88:575, 1980.

77. Keats A: Anesthesia for carotid endarterectomy. Cleve Clin Q 48:68, 1981.

78. Bove EL, Fry WJ, et al.: Hypotension and hypertension as consequences of baroreceptor dysfunction following carotid endarterectomy. Surgery 85:633, 1979.

79. Davies MJ, Cronin KD: Post carotid endarterectomy hypertension. Anaesth Intensive Care 8:190, 1980.

80. Matsumoto GM, Cossman D, Callow AD: Hazards and safeguards during carotid endarterectomy, technical considerations. Am J Surg 133:458, 1977.

81. Hunter GC, Sieffert G, et al.: The accuracy of carotid back pressure as an index for shunt requirement: A reappraisal. Stroke 13:319, 1982.

82. Baker WH: Shunting and nonshunting during carotid artery endarterectomy, in Ernst CB, Stanley JC (eds): Current Therapy in Vascular Surgery. Toronto, Brian C Decker, Publisher, 1987, p 27.

83. Connolly JE: Carotid endarterectomy in the awake patient, in Robicsek F (ed): Extracranial Cerebrovascular Disease. Diagnosis and Management. New York, Macmillan, Inc, 1986, p 289.

84. Peitzman AB, Webster MW, et al.: Carotid endarterectomy under regional (conductive) anesthesia. Ann Surg 196:59, 1982.

85. Callow AD, O'Donnell TF: The detection of cerebral ischemia during carotid endarterectomy by continuous electroencephalographic monitoring, in Greenhalgh RM (ed): Progress in Stroke Research, vol 2. London, Pitman Medical Publishing Co, Ltd, 1982, p 354.

86. Callow AD: The value of electroencephalography for cerebral protection, in Greenhalgh RM (ed): Diagnostic Techniques and Assessment Procedures in Vascular Surgery. London, Grune & Stratton, Inc, 1985, p 129.

87. Sundt TM, Sharbrough FW, Piepgras DG: Correlation of cerebral blood flow and electroencephalographic changes during carotid endarterectomy with results of surgery and hemodynamics of cerebral ischemia. Mayo Clin Proc 56:533, 1981.

88. Bernstein EF, Schneider PA, et al.: Transcranial Doppler in the management of extracranial cerebrovascular disease: Implications in diagnosis and monitoring. J Vasc Surg 7:223, 1988.

89. Callow AD: Cerebral protection during carotid artery surgery, in Wilson SE, Veith FJ, et al. (eds): Vascular Surgery. Principles and Practice. New York, McGraw-Hill Book Co, 1986, p 596.

90. Harris EJ, Brown WH, et al.: Continuous electroencephalographic monitoring during carotid artery endarterectomy. Surgery 62:441, 1967.

91. Padayachee TS, Gosline RG, et al.: Monitoring middle cerebral artery blood velocity during carotid endarterectomy. Br J Surg 73:98, 1986.

92. Trojaborg W, Boysen G: Relation between EEG, regional cerebral blood flow and internal carotid artery pressure during carotid endarterectomy. Electroencephalogr Clin Neurophysiol 34:61, 1973.

93. Waltz AG, Sundt TM Jr, Michenfelder JD: Cerebral blood flow during carotid endarterectomy. Circulation 45:1091, 1972.

94. Baker JD, Gluecklich B, et al.: An evaluation of electroencephalographic monitoring for carotid surgery. Surgery 78:787, 1975.

95. Hertzer NR, Beven EG: A retrospective comparison of the use of shunts during carotid endarterectomy. Surg Gynecol Obstet 151:81, 1980.

96. Thompson JE: Cerebral protection during carotid endarterectomy. JAMA 202:1046, 1967.

97. Fields WS: Selection of stroke patients for arterial reconstructive surgery. Am J Surg 125:527, 1973.

98. Callow AD, Shepard A, Russell J: Technical considerations in performing carotid endarterectomy: Indications for shunt. Contemp Surg 30:31, 1987.

99. Tsai FY, Matovich V, et al.: Percutaneous transluminal angioplasty of the carotid artery. AJNR 7:349, 1986.

100. Freitag G, Freitag J, et al.: Percutaneous angioplasty of carotid artery stenoses. Neuroradiology 28:126, 1986.

101. Kachel R, Ritter H, et al.: Results of percutaneous transluminal dilatation of stenoses of cerebral vessels. Fortschr Geb Rontgenstr Nuklearmed Erganzungsband 144:338, 1986.

102. Wilson SE, Donayre CE, Williams RA: Extracranial carotid artery occlusive disease, in Wilson SE, Veith FJ, et al. (eds): Vascular Surgery. Principles and Practice. New York, McGraw-Hill Book Co, 1987, p 545.

103. DeWeese JD: Long-term result of surgery for carotid artery stenosis, in Bergan JJ, Yao JST (eds): Cerebrovascular Insufficiency. New York, Grune & Stratton, Inc, 1983, p 507.

104. Bernstein EF, Humber PB, et al.: Influence of preoperative factors on late neurologic events after carotid endarterectomy, in International Vascular Symposium Program and Abstracts. New York, Macmillan, Inc, 1981, p 460.

105. Thompson JE: Operative mortality following carotid endarterectomy. Stroke 14:115, 1983.

106. Callow AD: Neurologic deficits after carotid endarterectomy and their management. Arch Chir Torac Cardiovasc 7:849, 1985.

107. Perdue GD: Management of postendarterectomy neurologic deficits. Arch Surg 117:1079, 1982.

108. Rosenthal D, Zeichner WD, et al.: Neurologic deficit after carotid endarterectomy: Pathogenesis and management. Surgery 94:776, 1983.

109. Imparato AM, Riles TS, Ramirez AA: Mechanisms of intraoperative strokes, in Courbier R (ed): Basis for a Classification of Cerebral Arterial Diseases. Amsterdam, Excerpta Medica, 1985, p 87.

110. Moore DJ, Sheehan MP, et al.: Are strokes predictable with noninvasive methods: A 5-year followup of 303 unoperated patients. J Vasc Surg 2:654, 1985.

111. O'Hara PJ, Hertzer NR: Concomitant carotid and coronary arterial occlusive disease, in Ernst CB, Stanley JC (eds): Current Therapy in Vascular Surgery. Toronto, Brian C Decker, Publisher, 1987, p 66.

112. Hertzer NR, Lees CD: Fatal myocardial infarction following carotid endarterectomy. 335 patients followed 6-11 postoperative years. Ann Surg 194:212, 1981.

113. Riles TS, Kopelman I, Imparato AM: Myocardial infarction following carotid endarterectomy: A review of 683 operations. Surgery 85:249, 1979.

114. Reigel MM, Hollier LH, et al.: Cerebral hyperperfusion syndrome: A cause of neurologic dysfunction after carotid endarterectomy. J Vasc Surg 5:628, 1987.

115. Hertzer NR: Postoperative management and complications of extracranial carotid reconstruction, in Rutherford RB (ed): Vascular Surgery, 2nd ed. Philadelphia, WB Saunders Co, 1984, p 1300.

116. Hertzer NR, Feldman BJ, et al.: A prospective study of the incidence of injury to the cranial nerves during carotid endarterectomy. Surg Gynecol Obstet 151:781, 1980.

117. Imparato AM, Bracco A, et al.: The hypoglossal nerve in carotid arterial reconstructions. Stroke 3:576, 1972.

118. Theodotou B, Mahaley MS: Injury of the peripheral cranial nerves during carotid endarterectomy. Stroke 16:894, 1985.

119. Verta MJ Jr, Applebaum EL, et al.: Cranial nerve injury during carotid endarterectomy. Ann Surg 185:192, 1977.

120. Sundt TM Jr, Sandok BA, Whisnant JP: Carotid endarterectomy: Complications and preoperative assessment of risk. Mayo Clin Proc 50:302, 1975.

121. Thompson JE: Carotid endarterectomy, 1982—the state of the art. Br J Surg 70:371, 1983.

122. Fields WS, Maslenikov V, et al.: Joint study of extracranial arterial occlusion. Progress report of prognosis following surgery or non-surgical treatment for transient cerebral ischaemic attacks and cervical carotid lesions. JAMA 211:1993, 1970.

123. Thompson JE, Austin DJ, Patman RD: Carotid endarterectomy for cerebrovascular insufficiency: Long term results in 592 patients followed up to 13 years. Ann Surg 172:663, 1970.

124. Hertzer NR, Loop FD, et al.: Combined myocardial revascularization and carotid endarterectomy: Operative and late results in 331 patients. J Thorac Cardiovasc Surg 85:577, 1983.

125. Bernstein EF, Humber PB, et al.: Life expectancy and late stroke following carotid endarterectomy. Ann Surg 198:80, 1983.

126. Field PL: Effective stroke prevention with carotid endarterectomy: A series of 400 cases with 2 year follow-up. International Vascular Program and Abstracts. New York, Macmillan, Inc, 1981, p 528.

127. Riles TS, Imparato AM, et al.: Comparison of results of bilateral and unilateral carotid endarterectomy 5 years after surgery. Surgery 91:258, 1982.

128. Quinones-Baldrich WJ, Moore WS: Results of medical and surgical therapy for extracranial arterial occlusive disease, in Rutherford RB (ed): Vascular Surgery, 2nd ed. Philadelphia, WB Saunders Co, 1984, p 1322.

129. Lees CD, Hertzer NR: Postoperative stroke and late neurologic complications after carotid endarterectomy. Arch Surg 116:1561, 1981.

130. The Canadian Cooperative Study Group: A randomized trial of aspirin and sulfinpyrazone in threatened strokes. N Engl J Med 299:53, 1978.

131. DeBakey ME, Crawford ES, et al.: Cerebral arterial insufficiency: One to 11-year results following arterial reconstructive operation. Ann Surg 161:921, 1965.

132. DeWeese JA, Rob CG, et al.: Results of carotid endarterectomies for transient ischemic attacks—5 years later. Ann Surg 178:258, 1973.

133. The EC/IC Bypass Study Group: Failure of extracranial-intracranial arterial bypass to reduce the risk of ischemic stroke: Results of an international randomized trial. N Engl J Med 313:1191, 1985.

134. Bouchier-Hayes D, DeCosta A, Macgowan WAL: The morbidity of carotid endarterectomy. Br J Surg 66:433, 1979.

135. Easton JD, Sherman DG: Stroke and mortality rate in carotid endarterectomy: 228 consecutive operations. Stroke 8:565, 1977.

136. McBride K, Callow AD: Recurrent stenosis after carotid endarterectomy—a limited survey, in Bernard VM, Towne JB (eds): Complications in Vascular Surgery. New York, Grune & Stratton, Inc, 1980, p 259.

137. Hertzer NR, Martinez BD, Beven EG: Recurrent stenosis after carotid endarterectomy. Surg Gynecol Obstet 149:360, 1979.

138. Stoney FJ, String ST: Recurrent carotid stenosis. Surgery 80:705, 1976.

139. Cossman D, Callow AD, et al.: Early restenosis after carotid endarterectomy. Arch Surg 113:275, 1978.

140. Kremen JE, Gee W, et al.: Restenosis or occlusion after carotid endarterectomy. A survey with ocular plethysmography. Arch Surg 114:607, 1979.

141. Turnipseed WD, Berkoff HA, Crummy A: Postoperative occlusion after carotid endarterectomy. Arch Surg 115:573, 1980.

142. Cantelmo NL, Cutler BS, et al.: Noninvasive detection of carotid stenosis following endarterectomy. Arch Surg 116:1005, 1981.

143. Zierler RE, Bandyk DR, et al.: Carotid artery stenosis following endarterectomy. Arch Surg 117:1408, 1982.

144. Salvian A, Baker JD, et al.: Cause and noninvasive detection of restenosis after carotid endarterectomy. Am J Surg 146:29, 1983.

145. Baker WH, Hayes AC, et al.: Durability of carotid endarterectomy. Surgery 94:112, 1983.

146. O'Donnell TF Jr, Callow AD, et al.: Ultrasound characteristics of recurrent carotid disease: Hypothesis explaining the low

incidence of symptomatic recurrence. J Vasc Surg 2:26, 1985.

147. Callow AD: Recurrent stenosis after carotid endarterectomy. Arch Surg 117:1082, 1982.

148. Clagett GP, Robinowitz M, et al.: Morphogenesis and clinicopathologic characteristics of recurrent carotid disease. J Vasc Surg 3:10, 1986.

149. Schwarcz TH, Yates GN, et al.: Pathologic characteristics of recurrent carotid artery stenosis. (In press.)

150. Callow AD, O'Donnell TF Jr: Recurrent carotid stenosis: Frequency, clinical implications, and some suggestions concerning etiology, in Bergan JJ, Yao JST (eds): Reoperative Arterial Surgery. New York, Grune & Stratton, Inc, 1986, p 513.

151. Imparato AM: Discussion: Recurrent carotid stenosis (Stoney and String). Surgery 80:709, 1976.

152. Deriu GP, Ballotta EB, et al.: The rationale for patch-graft angioplasty after carotid endarterectomy: Early and long-term follow-up. Stroke 15:972, 1984.

153. Eikelboom BC, Ackerstaff RGA, et al.: J Vasc Surg. (In press.)

154. Blaisdell FW, Lim R Jr, Hall AD: Technical result of carotid endarterectomy. Am J Surg 114:239, 1967.

155. Flanigan DP, Sigel B, Schuler JJ: Intraoperative ultrasonic carotid artery imaging, in Bergan JJ, Yao JST (eds): Cerebrovascular Insufficiency. New York, Grune and Stratton, Inc, 1983, p 343.

156. Courbier R, Jausseran JM, et al.: Routine intraoperative angiography: Its impact on operative morbidity and carotid restenosis. J Vasc Surg 3:343, 1986.

157. Callow AD: Management of recurrent carotid stenosis with some comments on pathology and possible pre-disposing factors, in Greenhalgh RM (ed): Extra-anatomic and Secondary Arterial Reconstruction. London, Pitman Medical Publishing Co, Ltd, 1982, p 252.

158. O'Donnell TF, Erdoes LP, et al.: Correlation of B-mode ultrasound imaging and angiography with pathologic findings at carotid endarterectomy. Arch Surg 120:443, 1985.

159. Berguer R, Bauer R: Vertebrobasilar Arterial Occlusive Disease. New York, Raven Press, 1984.

160. Diaz FG, Ausman JI: Surgical reconstruction of vascular lesions of the vertebral basilar circulation. Curr Conc Cerebrovasc Dis (Stroke) 19(4):19, 1984.

161. Sahs AL, Hartman EC: Fundamentals of stroke care. DHEW Publication (HRA) 76-14016. Washington, DC, US Department of Health, Education and Welfare, 1976.

162. Whisnant JP, Cartlidge NEF, Elvebach LR: Carotid and vertebrobasilar transient ischemic attacks: Effects of anticoagulants, hypertension and cardiac disorders on survival and stroke occurrence—a population study. Ann Neurol 3:107, 1978.

163. Caplan LR: Vertebrobasilar disease. Time for a new strategy. Curr Conc of Cerebrovasc Dis (Stroke) 15(3):11, 1980.

164. Fry, WJ: Vertebral artery reconstruction ACS PGC, in Peripheral Vascular Surgery, Chicago, Year Book Medical Publishers, 1982.

165. Hass WK, Fields WS, et al.: Joint study of extracranial arterial occlusion, II. Arteriography, techniques, sites and complications. JAMA 203:159, 1968.

166. Imparato AM, Riles TS: Surgery of the vertebral and subclavian artery occlusion, in Bergan JJ, Yao JST (eds): Cerebrovascular Insufficiency. New York, Grune & Stratton, Inc, 1983, p 521.

167. Reul GJ, Cooley DA, et al.: Long-term results of direct verteberal artery operations. Surgery 96:854, 1984.

168. Rosenthal D, Cossman D, Callow AD: Results of carotid endarterectomy for vertebrobasilar insufficiency. Arch Surg 113:1361, 1978.

169. Hutchinson EC, Manc MD: Carotico-vertebral stenosis. Lancet 1:2, 1957.

170. Fields WS, Lemak NA: Joint study of extracranial arterial occlu-sion, VII. Subclavian steal—a review of 168 cases. JAMA 22:1139, 1972.

171. Millikan CH, Siekert RG, Shick RM: Studies in cerebrovascular disease, III: The use of anticoagulant drugs in the treatment of insufficiency or thrombosis within the basilar arterial system. Proc Staff Meet Mayo Clin 30:116, 1955.

172. Crawford ES, DeBakey ME, Fields WS: Roentgenographic diagnosis and surgical treatment of basilar artery insufficiency. JAMA 166:509, 1958.

173. Imparato AM: Surgery for extracranial cerebrovascular insufficiency, in Ransohoff J (ed): Modern Techniques in Surgery, Neurosurgery, vol 14. New York, Futura Pub Co, 1979, p 1.

174. Edwards WH, Wright RS: A new surgical technique for relief of subclavian stenosis. Hosp Pract 7:78, 1972.

175. Roon AJ, Ehrenfeld WK, et al.: Vertebral artery reconstruction. Am J Surg 29:138, 1979.

176. Imparato AM: Vertebral arterial reconstruction: A nineteen year experience. J Vasc Surg 2:626, 1985.

177. Edwards WH, Mulherin JL Jr: The surgical reconstruction of the proximal subclavian and vertebral artery. J Vasc Surg 2:634, 1985.

178. Kieffer E, Rancurel G, Richard T: Reconstruction of the distal cervical vertebral artery, in Berguer R, Bauer RB (eds): Vertebrobasilar Arterial Occlusive Disease. New York, Raven Press, 1984, p 265.

179. Berguer R: Distal vertebral by-pass: Technique, the "occipital connection," potential uses. J Vasc Surg 2:621, 1985.

180. Sundt TM Jr, Smith HC, et al.: Transluminal angioplasty for basilar artery stenosis. Mayo Clin Proc 55:673, 1980.

181. Sundt TM Jr, Piepgras DG, et al.: Interposition saphenous vein grafts for advanced occlusive disease and large aneurysms in the posterior circulation. J Neurosurg 56:205, 1982.

182. Callow AD: David M. Hume Memorial Lecture. An overview of the stroke problem in the carotid territory. Am J Surg 140:181, 1980.

183. Humphries AW, Young JR, et al.: Relief of vertebrobasilar symptoms by carotid endarterectomy. Surgery 57:48, 1965.

184. Marshall J: A survey of occlusive disease of the vertebrobasilar arterial system, in Vinken PJ, Bruyn GW (eds): Handbook of Clinical Neurology, vol 11. Amsterdam, North-Holland Publishing Co, 1972.

185. Reivich M, Holling HE, et al.: Reversal of blood flow through the vertebral artery and its effect on cerebral circulation. N Engl J Med 165:878, 1961.

186. Brener BJ, Brief DK, et al.: The risk of stroke in patients with asymptomatic carotid stenosis undergoing cardiac surgery: A follow-up study. J Vasc Surg 5:269, 1987.

187. Hertzer NR, Flanagan RA Jr, et al.: Surgical versus nonoperative treatment of asymptomatic carotid stenosis. Ann Surg 204:163, 1986.

188. Imparato A, Riles T, et al.: The importance of hemorrhage in the relationship between gross morphologic characteristics and cerebral symptoms in 376 carotid artery plaques. Ann Surg 197:195, 1983.

189. Imparato AM: Personal communication: Letter to American Neurological Association, 1986.

190. Callow AD: How should the patient with an asymptomatic carotid bruit be managed? in Najarian JS (ed): Progress in Vascular Surgery. Chicago, Year Book Medical Publishers, Inc, 1987.

191. Wolf PA, Kannel WB, et al.: Asymptomatic carotid bruit and risk of stroke. The Framingham Study. JAMA 245:1442, 1981.

192. Malone JM, Bean B, et al.: Diagnosis of carotid artery stenosis: Comparison of oculoplethysmography and Doppler supraorbital examination. Ann Surg 191:347, 1980.

193. Moore DJ, Miles RD, et al.: Noninvasive assessment of stroke

risk in asymptomatic and nonhemispheric patients with suspected carotid disease: Five-year follow-up of 294 unoperated and 81 operated patients. Ann Surg 202:491, 1985.

194. Chambers BR, Norris JW: Outcome in patients with asymptomatic neck bruits. N Engl J Med 315:860, 1986.

195. Moore WS, Boren CB, et al.: Natural history of nonstenotic, asymptomatic ulcerative lesions of the carotid artery. Arch Surg 113:1352, 1978.

196. Dixon S, Pais SO, et al.: Natural history of nonstenotic asymptomatic ulcerative lesions of the carotid artery. Arch Surg 117:1493, 1982.

197. Thompson JE, Patman RD, Talkington CM: Asymptomatic carotid bruit: Long term outcome of patients having endarterectomy compared with unoperated controls. Ann Surg 188:308, 1978.

198. O'Donnell TF, Callow AD, et al.: The impact of coronary artery disease on carotid endarterectomy. Ann Surg 198:705, 1983.

199. Hertzer NR, Young JR, et al.: Coronary angiography in 506 patients with extracranial cerebrovascular disease. Arch Intern Med 145:849, 1985.

200. Barnes RW, Nix ML, et al.: Late outcome of untreated asymptomatic carotid disease following cardiovascular operations. J Vasc Surg 2:843, 1985.

201. Treiman RL, Foran RF, et al.: Carotid bruit: A follow-up report on its significance in patients undergoing an abdominal aortic operation. Arch Surg 114:1138, 1979.

202. Barnes RW, Liebman PR, et al.: Natural history of asymptomatic carotid disease in patient undergoing cardiovascular surgery. Surgery 90:1075, 1981.

203. Humphries AW, Young JR, et al.: Unoperated asymptomatic significant internal carotid artery stenosis: A review of 182 instances. Surgery 80:695, 1976.

204. Levin SM, Sondenheimer FK, Levin JM: Contralateral diseased but asymptomatic carotid artery: To operate or not? An update. Am J Surg 140:203, 1980.

205. Kartchner MM, McRae LOP: Guidelines for non-invasive evaluation of asymptomatic carotid bruits. Clin Neurosurg 28:418, 1981.

206. Johnson JM, Kennelly MM, et al.: Natural history of asymptomatic carotid plaque. Arch Surg 120:1010, 1985.

207. Levin SM, Sondheimer FK: Stenosis of contralateral asymptomatic carotid artery—to operate or not? Vasc Surg 7:3, 1973.

208. Sobel M, Imparato AM, et al.: Contralateral neurologic symptoms after carotid surgery: A 9-year follow-up. J Vasc Surg 3:623, 1986.

209. Riles TS, Imparato AM, Kopelman I: Carotid artery stenosis with contralateral internal carotid occlusion: Long-term results in fifty-four patients. Surgery 87:363, 1980.

210. Callow AD: Fact or fancy: A 20 year personal perspective on the detection and management of carotid occlusive disease. J Cardiovasc Surg 21:641, 1980.

211. Ojemann RG, Crowell RM: Surgical Management of Cerebrovascular Disease. Baltimore, Williams & Wilkins, 1983, p 26.

212. Goldstone J: Evolving stroke secondary to carotid artery atherosclerosis, in Ernst CB, Stanley JC (eds): Current Therapy in Vascular Surgery. Toronto, Brian C Decker, Publisher, 1987, p 7.

213. Goldstone J, Moore WS: A new look at emergency carotid artery operations for the treatment of cerebrovascular insufficiency. Stroke 9:599, 1978.

214. Wylie EJ, Hein MF, Adams JE: Intracranial hemorrhage following surgical revascularization for treatment of acute stroke. J Neurosurg 21:212, 1964.

215. Maddison FE: Angiographic study of patients with cerebrovascular disease, in Rutherford RB (ed): Vascular Surgery. 2nd ed. Philadelphia, WB Saunders Co, 1984, p 1239.

216. Caplan LR: Treatment of cerebral ischemia—where are we headed? Stroke 15:571, 1984.

217. McIntyre KE, Goldstone J: Carotid surgery for crescendo TIA and stroke in evolution, in Bergan JJ, Yao JST (eds): Cerebrovascular Insufficiency. New York, Grune & Stratton, Inc, 1983, p 213.

CHAPTER 56
Surgery of Celiac and Mesenteric Arteries

Pär A. Olofsson, Daniel P. Connelly, and Ronald J. Stoney

Visceral ischemic syndromes represent a diverse spectrum of disease that presents a challenge in both diagnosis and treatment. *Acute* visceral ischemia represents a medical and surgical emergency in which timely diagnosis and treatment are critical in obtaining bowel salvage and patient survival. *Chronic* visceral ischemia is frequently overlooked in assessing patients with abdominal pain, and a delayed diagnosis subjects the patient to undue suffering, weight loss, and the threat of fatal intestinal gangrene. This chapter reviews the syndromes' historical background and discusses the overall management of patients with both acute and chronic visceral ischemia. The etiology, clinical presentation, diagnostic evaluation, perioperative management, operative techniques, and results of therapy are presented.

HISTORICAL BACKGROUND

Gradual occlusion of one or all of the aortic visceral branches may occur without producing any abdominal symptoms, provided that adequate intestinal blood supply is maintained through the abundant collateral pathways. Chiene,[1] in 1869, noted occlusion of all three major visceral arteries in a patient who had no abdominal symptoms but who died from other causes.

The fact that all three visceral vessels could occlude without universally producing intestinal ischemia or infarction was probably responsible for a great deal of the delay in recognizing chronic visceral ischemia as a distinct disease. In 1894, Councilman[2] proposed that abdominal pain could result from obstruction of the visceral arteries; however, this report was generally overlooked. Indeed, Osler believed that the abdominal complaints of patients with atherosclerotic disease of the visceral arteries was in fact atypical angina pectoris. In 1936, Dunphy[3] reported seven of 12 patients dying of mesenteric infarction who had premorbid complaints consisting of abdominal pain, weight loss, and altered intestinal motility. He correctly established the relationship between chronic visceral ischemia and subsequent

Supported in part by the Pacific Vascular Research Foundation, San Francisco, California.

fatal intestinal gangrene. Mikkelson[4] proposed surgical treatment to relieve intestinal ischemia and coined the term *intestinal angina* in 1957. Within a year, Shaw and Maynard[5] reported two patients with intestinal gangrene successfully treated with thromboendarterectomy and bowel resection. They also described the malabsorption associated with visceral ischemia. In 1959, surgical relief of chronic intestinal ischemia by superior mesenteric endarterectomy was accomplished and thus began the modern management of this disease.[6] Alternative techniques for surgical treatment were introduced in 1962, when Morris and Crawford[7] described retrograde Dacron bypass from the infrarenal aorta, and in 1963, when Fry and Kraft[8] introduced autologous vein bypass in the same position. Antegrade aortovisceral bypass and transaortic visceral endarterectomy were introduced as operative techniques in 1966.[9]

ACUTE VISCERAL ISCHEMIA

Background and Etiology

Early reports of acute mesenteric ischemia noted an extremely high mortality associated with this disease and its treatment. Surgical management by intestinal resection, as reported by Elliott in 1895,[10] remained the definite treatment into the 1950s when the first report on successful revascularization was published.[5] Despite the obvious advantage of this type of treatment, clinical experience was slow to accumulate. The evolution toward revascularization and improved perioperative management and a better understanding of the pathophysiology of acute mesenteric ischemia have been responsible for an overall improved outcome for the patients with this disease.

Acute visceral ischemia results from acute thrombotic occlusion of the major visceral branches of the aorta—the ultimate complication of chronic visceral ischemia due to atherosclerosis—or from embolic occlusion of the superior mesenteric artery. Nonocclusive mesenteric ischemia is usually a manifestation of cardiac dysfunction and is not within the scope of this chapter. Patients with acute ischemia are immediately endangered by the development of irreversible intestinal infarction and gangrene, thus necessitating its early recognition and treatment.

Embolic Occlusion of Superior Mesenteric Artery

Clinical Presentation and Diagnosis

The presentation of patients who sustain embolic occlusion of the superior mesenteric artery is sufficiently distinct to allow its early differentiation from thrombotic occlusion and subsequent early intervention.[11-14] Because of the acute obstruction of mesenteric blood flow, there is insufficient time for the development of protective visceral collaterals. The initial response of the ischemic small bowel is vigorous contraction and spasm. This is perceived by the patient as severe periumbilical abdominal pain frequently associated with gut emptying. At this early stage, peritoneal inflammation is not yet present, and physical examination may demonstrate only active bowel sounds and minimal tenderness. Surgical exploration at this stage has likewise occasionally resulted in a missed diagnosis because the intestines are pale in color and vigorously contracting.[15] Almost all patients have an obvious cardiac source as origin for the embolus, and embolic occlusion of other vascular beds (cerebral, renal, or extremity) is present in approximately one third of the patients with emboli to the superior mesenteric artery.

A plain x-ray film is often obtained to rule out other intraabdominal catastrophes. In acute intestinal ischemia this film might show a gasless abdomen or, later, bowel dilatation. The definite diagnosis is obtained at laparotomy or by preoperative arteriogram. Biplanar arteriograms will demonstrate minimal or no blood flow to the superior mesenteric artery. On the lateral views a patent proximal superior mesenteric artery orifice will be seen, as well as contrast in the first 5 to 7 cm of the vessel, that is, to the level where the embolus usually lodges.

Surgical Treatment

Although nonoperative management with dextran has been described,[16] salvaging both the threatened bowel and the patient requires a timely operation after aggressive resuscitation. Preoperative management with careful monitoring, optimizing cardiac function, controlling cardiac arrhythmias, and instituting appropriate volume replacement, is critical.

The abdominal exploration is usually performed through a midline incision. Characteristically, the duodenum and the first several centimeters of the jejunum are normally perfused and viable, whereas the remainder of the small bowel and right colon show evidence of ischemia. With prolonged ischemia, the bowel begins to manifest evidence of hemorrhagic infarction, with edema, dilatation, and hemorrhage into the mesentery. However, revascularization at this point will allow normal bowel color and motor activity to return.

The point of obstruction can be identified by palpating the superior mesenteric artery. The superior mesenteric artery is exposed by elevating the transverse colon and incising the base of the overlying transverse mesocolon.

A transverse arteriotomy is made in the superior mesenteric artery distal to the middle colic artery. Bidirectional catheter thromboembolectomy is then completed, and the vessel is flushed with a heparin-saline solution. After closure of the arteriotomy with fine interrupted sutures, the bowel is returned to its normal anatomic position for observation. Viability is reassessed after an observation period of 30 to 45 minutes. Areas of obvious gangrene have to be resected. The assessment of bowel viability may be aided by the use of a Doppler probe or by fluorescin injection and inspection under ultraviolet light.[17,18] In the absence of extensive intraabdominal contamination, primary intestinal anastomosis is performed. Before completion of the procedure, a decision has to be made regarding the advisability of a second-look operation. Once a second-look procedure is planned, the subsequent postoperative course should not alter this decision.

Thrombotic Occlusion of Visceral Arteries

Clinical Presentation and Diagnosis

Acute mesenteric ischemia due to thrombotic occlusion of the superior mesenteric or celiac arteries is the consequence of gradual atherosclerotic occlusion of these vessels with superimposed thrombosis. The progressive stenosis of the visceral vessels allows collateral pathways to develop. The collaterals provide a marginal blood supply to the intestines and are responsible for blunting the initial severity of the thrombosis. The symptomatology is similar to that of intestinal ischemia caused by emboli, but its onset is more insidious, and it may initially be intermittent and reminiscent of abdominal angina as first reported by Dunphy.[3]

An aggressive approach and the liberal use of arteriography in those patients who are initially seen with suspected acute bowel ischemia are essential.[19] Aortograms will usually show extensive occlusive disease involving the visceral arteries. Lateral aortography is done to evaluate the origins of the celiac and superior mesenteric arteries. As in embolic occlusion, perioperative monitoring and correction of organ dysfunction, including fluid replacement to normalize metabolic acidosis, are critical.

Surgical Treatment

Since an assessment of intestinal viability is mandatory, the exploration is accomplished through a midline laparotomy. Attention is first directed at determining the extent of the vessel occlusion, as well as the intestinal viability. If acute visceral artery reconstruction is indicated and reasonable, the celiac axis and mesenteric arteries are mobilized for aortovisceral bypass. The superior mesenteric artery frequently has extensive arterial wall plaques, whereas the celiac artery may only have a short segment of orifice occlusion. Exposure of the mesenteric arteries and the technique for reconstruction are described below under Chronic Visceral Ischemia. The risk of contamination from an ischemic or necrotic bowel usually contraindicates the use of prosthetic grafts, and autogenous reconstruction using reversed aortovisceral saphenous vein grafts or visceral thromboendarterectomy is available. If however, intraabdominal contamination is excluded, prosthetic aortovisceral grafts may be used. After revascularization the bowel is observed for viability and is resected as indicated.

CHRONIC VISCERAL ISCHEMIA

Etiology

Atherosclerosis

Chronic visceral ischemia is overwhelmingly (95%) caused by atherosclerosis. One third of the patients have co-existing atherosclerotic disease in the aorta and other aortic branches.[20] In this location, atherosclerosis is usually orificial and most commonly involves the ventral aspect of the suprarenal aorta, frequently forming a homogeneous succulent layer of intimal thickening overlying the orifices of the visceral arteries.[21,22] Multiple involvement of the visceral branches is common. In our series of 73 patients, only one had single-vessel involvement. There is, however, no constant correlation between the number of branches involved and the severity of symptoms. Isolated celiac artery lesions might be symptomatic; on the other hand, lesions of the superior or inferior mesenteric arteries alone rarely cause symptoms. In some cases occlusion of all three branches might be asymptomatic because of a well-developed collateral system.

The physiologic mechanism causing the typical postprandial abdominal pain is probably a discrepancy between the demand for increased intestinal blood flow after food intake and the insufficient inflow caused by the occluding or stenosing lesions and a not fully compensating collateral system. However, this cause is still debated, and a steal phenomenon from the intestine to the gastric circulation has recently been suggested as an alternative.[23]

A rare manifestation of atherosclerosis causing chronic visceral ischemia is dissection of an atherosclerotic aorta involving the orifices of the visceral branches. "Coral reef atherosclerosis," a special form of advanced suprarenal aortic atherosclerosis that obstructs the lumen of the suprarenal aorta and the visceral, renal, and iliac branches singly or together, might exhibit chronic visceral ischemic symptomatology.[24]

Celiac Axis Compression

Atherosclerosis is the most frequently encountered lesion in chronic visceral ischemic syndromes, but other rare causes do exist. The most common of these is the so-called celiac axis compression syndrome, or median arcuate ligament syndrome, originally described by Dunbar et al.[25] The clinical relevance and the pathophysiologic background of this syndrome are still a matter of discussion.[26-29] It is generally presumed to be caused by an anatomic abnormality in the relation between the celiac axis and the median arcuate ligament, resulting in external compression of the celiac axis, which occasionally involves the superior mesenteric artery as well. This presumption is opposed by the fact that celiac artery compression has been demonstrated in asymptomatic patients.[29] In this disease the aorta and its other branches are free from lesions, and the collateral circulation is less evident than in patients with chronic visceral ischemia caused by atherosclerosis.[30]

Other Rare Causes

External compression of the celiac axis has been reported to occur as a rare phenomenon in pathologic processes involving the neural and fibrous tissue surrounding the aorta at this level, that is, neurofibromatosis.[31,32] Spontaneous intimal dissection in the superior mesenteric artery has been reported as another rare cause for symptomatic chronic visceral ischemia.[33] Fibromuscular hyperplasia has been found in the celiac axis and superior mesenteric arteries, but its relation to symptoms of chronic visceral ischemia is not settled.[34] Chronic visceral ischemic syndromes have also been described as a consequence of radiation, systemic lupus erythematosus, rheumatoid arthritis, and allergic vasculitis.[35]

Collateral Pathways

Proximal branches of the major and minor visceral branches are of great importance in preventing bowel ischemia and symptoms in patients with occlusive visceral artery disease. The fact that gradual occlusion of all major visceral branches can occur without causing bowel infarction or ischemic symptoms demonstrates the great capacity of the visceral collaterals. These collateral branches are located beyond the flow-limiting lesions and are capable of enlarging and reversing their flow into the ischemic splanchnic bed.

In celiac axis occlusion the major collateral flow connects the hepatic artery, a major celiac branch, with the superior mesenteric artery through the gastroduodenal artery and the inferior and superior pancreaticoduodenal arteries. Because of its angiographic appearance (a single vessel around the head of the pancreas and the dorsal aspect of the descending duodenum), this collateral pathway is usually termed the pancreaticoduodenal arcade. A less common collateral pathway develops between the middle colic and the dorsal pancreaticosplenic arteries. When the superior mesenteric artery is occluded, the most important collateral pathway is the pancreaticoduodenal arcade connecting the superior mesenteric artery with the celiac axis. The inferior mesenteric artery also provides major collateral blood flow to the superior mesenteric artery through branches of the lower colic and midcolic arteries. In combined celiac axis and superior mesenteric artery occlusion, both can be sufficiently supplied from the inferior mesenteric artery through the marginal anastomotic arteries and the pancreaticoduodenal arcade.

In obstruction of all three aortic visceral branches, one or both internal iliac arteries may provide afferent splanchnic flow through the inferior mesenteric artery and the meandering mesenteric and gastroduodenal collaterals to the entire gut (Fig. 56-1).

Clinical Presentation

Atherosclerosis

Chronic visceral ischemia caused by atherosclerosis usually develops in the fifth through seventh decades (mean age, 59 years), with a sex ratio of three females to one male. A typical postprandial abdominal pain, termed abdominal an-

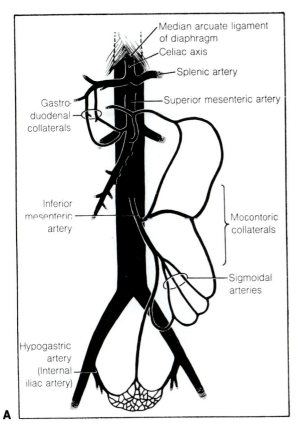
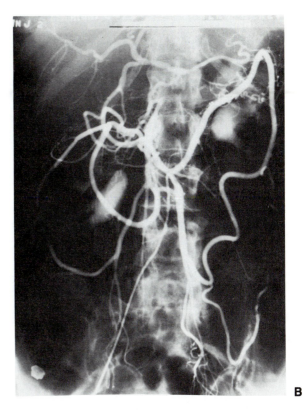

A

B

Figure 56-1. A. The visceral arteries and collateral pathways. **B.** Arteriogram (anteroposterior projection) showing the main collateral pathways—the pancreaticoduodenal arcade, the meandering mesenteric artery (the marginal artery), and branches of the inferior mesenteric artery extending down to the hypogastric artery. (*From Wylie EJ, Stoney RJ, et al.: Manual of Vascular Surgery, vols 1 and 2. New York, Springer Verlag New York, 1980.*)

gina,[4] is the most common symptom in chronic visceral ischemia due to atherosclerosis (90 to 95%). This pain is mostly located in the epigastrium and is of a colicky-cramping or dull-aching character. It typically starts 15 to 30 minutes after food ingestion and lasts for 1 to 3 hours. Significant weight loss is the second most common symptom (79%). It is secondary to the postprandial pain, which causes the patient to ingest smaller meals or fluid only or ultimately to avoid food intake ("food fear").[20] Accordingly, secondary starvation is likely to cause the weight loss rather than malabsorption as originally advocated.[5] Twenty-five percent of the patients are initially seen with ischemia-induced motility disturbances such as nausea and vomiting, diarrhea, or constipation. Physical examination commonly reveals signs of substantial weight loss and advanced systemic atherosclerosis. An epigastric bruit is present in 85% of the patients.[20,36-40]

This symptomatology is not specific, frequently misleading the diagnostic efforts toward gastrointestinal malignancy. Consequently, the patients have very often gone through a complete gastrointestinal work-up, including x-ray examination, endoscopies, computed tomographic (CT) scans, and ultrasounds before he is referred to the vascular surgeon.[20,37,39] However, it must be emphasized that a history based on knowledge and awareness of the disease

would most likely provide sufficient information for a primary, correct diagnosis. Use of aortography, with both anteroposterior and lateral views, is essential to establish the diagnosis and to plan subsequent surgical intervention. The anteroposterior aortogram will disclose the collateral vessels and will additionally allow assessment of the renal arteries and the infrarenal aorta, which frequently have coexisting atherosclerotic disease (see Fig. 56-1B). A lateral aortogram provides visualization of the origins of both the superior mesenteric and celiac arteries (Fig. 56-2).

Celiac Axis Compression

The sex ratio (76% women) is the same in celiac axis compression as in atherosclerosis, but patients with celiac axis compression are generally younger (mean age, 47 years).[30] The symptomatology in celiac axis compression is less characteristic than in visceral ischemia caused by atherosclerosis. Abdominal pain is similarly the most common symptom (100%), but in patients with celiac axis compression, pain is often atypical, and only 37% had postprandial symptoms reminiscent of abdominal angina. The pain is usually epigastric and cramping and in one fourth of the cases is related to different body positions. Weight loss was less frequent (61%) and less pronounced when compared to that of patients with atherosclerosis. Diarrhea and nausea and vomit-

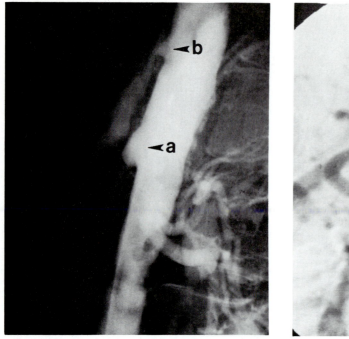
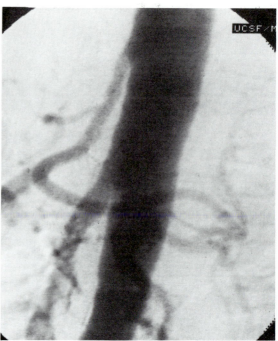

Figure 56-2. A. Aortograms (lateral projection) showing occluded superior mesenteric artery, *a*, and severely stenosed celiac artery, *b*. **B.** Digital subtraction angiography after transaortic visceral thromboendarterectomy. (*From Wylie EJ, Stoney RJ, et al.: Manual of Vascular Surgery, vols 1 and 2. New York, Springer Verlag New York, 1980*).

ing, symptoms of disturbed intestinal motility, were present in 65% of the patients. Twenty-three percent of the patients had a history of a psychiatric disorder or alcohol abuse before the onset of symptoms. Furthermore, a history of previous abdominal operations was common (69%).

As in atherosclerosis, physical findings are rare. Clinical signs of malnutrition are less common and less impressive

in patients with celiac axis compression. Epigastric bruit is common (85%) and typically varies with respiration, being more pronounced during expiration.

Lateral aortographic projections during both inspiration and expiration will unmask the typical lesion in celiac axis compression, allowing its differentiation from atherosclerosis (Fig. 56-3). In 78% of angiographies performed in

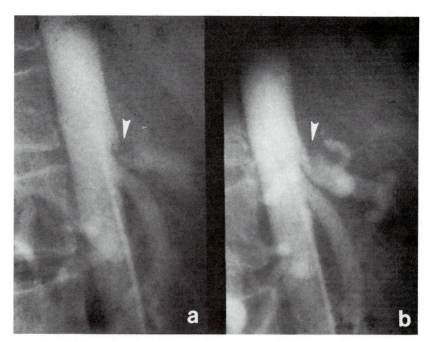

Figure 56-3. Aortograms (lateral view) during *expiration*, **a,** and *inspiration*, **b,** in a patient with celiac axis compression syndrome. (*From Wylie EJ, Stoney RJ, et al.: Manual of Vascular Surgery, vols 1 and 2, New York, Springer Verlag New York, 1980*).

patients with celiac axis compression, a diameter reduction of >50% was found in the celiac axis.[30]

Indications for Surgical Treatment

Atherosclerosis
All patients with a history suggestive of chronic visceral ischemia and a negative gastrointestinal workup should undergo biplanar aortography if the patient is a candidate for visceral artery reconstruction. The aim of the operative treatment is relief of pain, reversal of inanition, and prevention of progress of the disease, which ultimately results in visceral infarction. Because multiple involvement of the visceral arteries is common, many authors suggest revascularization of as many arteries as possible.[36-39] In our experience, the first priority is the celiac axis, and the second, the superior mesenteric artery. This is based on the observation that only postoperative celiac reocclusion was associated with recurrent ischemic symptoms, even when the superior mesenteric artery was patent. Furthermore, persistent occlusion or reocclusion of the superior mesenteric artery has not caused ischemic symptoms, provided that the celiac artery is patent. The only indications for revascularization of the inferior mesenteric artery, which is rarely performed, are distal superior mesenteric artery lesions, failure of previous aortovisceral bypass, or a common celiac and superior mesenteric artery trunk. Concomitant aortic repair including both renal arteries is frequently required because of the extension of advanced atherosclerotic occlusive or aneurysmal disease to the infrarenal aorta.[20]

Exposure and reconstruction of the visceral arteries to improve intestinal circulation are very challenging,[7] and a variety of techniques have been used. The early operative experience in treatment of chronic visceral ischemia included transmesenteric arterial thromboendarterectomy, saphenous vein bypass, arterial autograft, and vessel reimplantation.[5,41-43] In our experience, these procedures had a high rate of early and late failures, which prompted the development of transaortic visceral thromboendarterectomy and antegrade aortovisceral bypass. These are the methods with which we have achieved significantly improved outcome for our patients. The choice of procedure has to be individualized according to the pattern of disease, but generally we perform thromboendarterectomy in patients with relatively low operative risks and when reconstruction of both the celiac axis and the superior mesenteric artery is feasible. This is also the preferred procedure when there is concomitant renal artery or infrarenal aortic disease. Antegrade aortovisceral grafting is reserved for elderly, high-risk patients without significant concomitant renal or infrarenal aortic disease.[9,20-22]

Celiac Axis Compression

Because of the atypical clinical picture, patients who are considered for surgical relief from celiac axis compression should be thoroughly evaluated and carefully selected.

In our experience relief from symptoms was highly likely when the patient was female with a typical postprandial pain pattern and a weight loss greater than 20 pounds.[30]

Perioperative Management

Considering the high incidence of other problems in patients with visceral atherosclerosis (80% smokers, 32% coronary artery disease, 66% hypertension, 36% renal insufficiency), preoperative cardiopulmonary optimization is frequently needed. Because of the commonly present significant weight loss, nutritional repletion should be considered. Antibiotics are regularly started 12 hours before surgery and are continued for 48 hours.

Recent technical advances have provided new possibilities for facilitating these challenging procedures and have improved the patient outcome. Supraceliac cross-clamping is associated with a high incidence of myocardial ischemia, dysfunction, and an increased risk for myocardial infarction. The use of intraoperative cardiac monitoring with two-dimensional transesophageal echocardiography (2D-TEE) have increased our ability to discover and treat cardiac complications at a very early stage.[44] Furthermore, the use of table-fixed self-retaining retractors have significantly improved the exposure and facilitated the reconstruction of the aorta and its branches (Fig. 56-4).[45]

After the reconstruction, intraoperative duplex ultrasound has proven invaluable for assessment of vessel patency and for disclosing technical errors before closure.[46] Before discharge from the hospital, the patients regularly have a digital subtraction arteriogram to determine patency of the reconstruction (see Fig. 56-2B).

Exposure of Mesenteric Arteries

Retroperitoneal Thoracoabdominal Approach
The retroperitoneal thoracoabdominal approach gives an unrestricted exposure of the entire thoracoabdominal aorta, including the major visceral and renal branches.[47,48] The patient is positioned supine on the operating table, and the left chest is elevated 45 degrees. An incision is made in the eighth intercostal space from the posterior axillary fold obliquely across the abdomen to the midline. Following division of the abdominal muscles and retroperitoneal dissection, the peritoneum with its contents is retracted to the right. The left half of the diaphragm is divided circumferentially 2 to 3 cm from its origin to avoid denervation injury of the diaphragm. During the retroperitoneal dissection, the kidney is preferably left in its posterior position. The supraceliac aorta is exposed by dividing the overlying fibers at the midline. Resection of the celiac ganglionic fibers exposes the celiac axis. After elevation of the pancreas, the superior mesenteric artery is exposed. The inferior mesenteric artery is easily reached by further retroperitoneal dissection to the lower part of the abdominal aorta.

A major advantage of this exposure is the simplicity of concomitant reconstruction of renal arteries (one third of patients) or the infrarenal aorta (11%). The thoracoretroperitoneal approach is, however, not possible for all patients because of greater physiologic stress and should be avoided

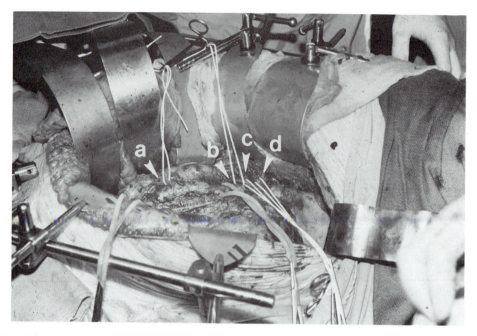

Figure 56-4. Retroperitoneal thoracoabdominal approach and exposure of the entire thoracoabdominal aorta and its major branches (*a*, inferior mesenteric artery; *b*, renal arteries; *c*, superior mesenteric artery; *d*, celiac axis) maintained by a table-fixed self-retaining retractor without any handheld retractors. (*From Wylie EJ, Stoney RJ, et al.: Manual of Vascular Surgery, vols 1 and 2, New York, Springer Verlag New York, 1980*).

in high-risk patients with significant cardiopulmonary disease.[20]

Transabdominal Approach

Transabdominal exposure of the celiac and supramesenteric arteries is performed through an upper two-thirds midline incision.[47,48] The gastrohepatic ligament is divided vertically, starting slightly to the right of the midline from the diaphragm and extending down to the lesser curvature of the stomach. Injuries to the nerve of Latarjet should be avoided. The triangular ligament is divided to allow retraction of the liver to the right. The stomach and esophagus are retracted to the left; then the arcuate ligament and the diaphragmatic crura are divided to provide circumferential exposure to the distal 5 cm of the thoracic aorta. The common hepatic and splenic arteries are freed and elevated from their position at the upper border of the pancreas. After caudad retraction of the pancreas and division and excision of celiac ganglionic fibers, exposure of the entire celiac axis and superior mesenteric artery is obtained.

Techniques for Visceral Artery Reconstruction in Atherosclerosis

Thromboendarterectomy

Since visceral artery thromboendarterectomy aims at removal of both the aortic atheroma and the orifice lesions that cause the visceral artery obstruction, a transaortic endarterectomy is preferred. This procedure requires unrestricted access to the entire thoracoabdominal aorta, and the retroperitoneal thoracoabdominal approach is mandatory, consequently excluding high-risk patients from this type of reconstruction (see Fig. 56-4). The aorta is cross-clamped above and below the major visceral branches, which are temporarily controlled. A U-shaped "trap-door" aortotomy is performed, partially surrounding the orifices of the celiac axis and the superior mesenteric artery. The aortic orifice atheroma is removed, using extraction endarterectomy (Fig. 56-5A and B).[48] If the renal arteries are included in the thromboendarterectomy, the distal portion of the aortotomy is extended to an infrarenal level, allowing en bloc removal of the diseased intima from the aorta and the orifice lesions from all involved branches of the upper abdominal aorta (Fig. 56-6). After checking the back-bleeding from the visceral branches, the aortotomy is closed with a running suture.

When the superior mesenteric artery is totally occluded, a separate longitudinal arteriotomy is created after the aortotomy is closed to allow direct visual control of the distal intimal end point of the occlusion. Furthermore, this allows removal of the "tail-thrombus," which might extend distally to the level of the reentry collateral, that is, 5 to 8 cm from the orifice. The arteriotomy is then closed with an autogenous vein patch to avoid narrowing (Fig. 56-7).

Aortovisceral Bypass Grafting

Aortovisceral bypass grafting can be performed with a variety of arterial substitutes and can be constructed to provide antegrade or retrograde flow. Autogenous vein or artery grafts used in a retrograde orientation with proximal infrarenal anastomosis have been abandoned because of unaccept-

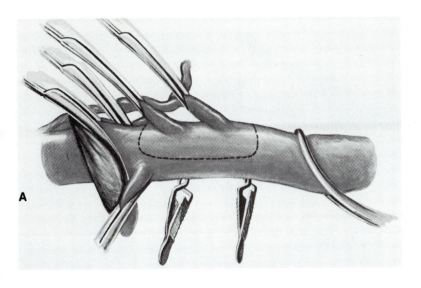

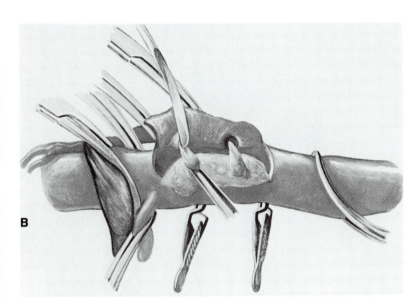

Figure 56-5. "Trap-door" aortotomy, **A,** used for transaortic visceral artery extraction thromboendarterectomy, **B.** (*From Wylie EJ, Stoney RJ, et al.: Manual of Vascular Surgery, vols 1 and 2, New York, Springer Verlag New York, 1980.*)

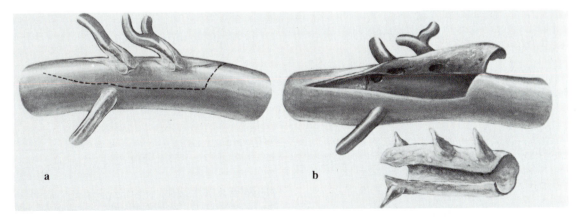

Figure 56-6. "Trap-door" aortotomy extended to include the renal arteries, **A,** for a combined transaortic extraction thromboendarterectomy of the visceral and renal arteries, **B.** (*From Wylie EJ, Stoney RJ, et al.: Manual of Vascular Surgery, vols 1 and 2, New York, Springer Verlag New York, 1980*).

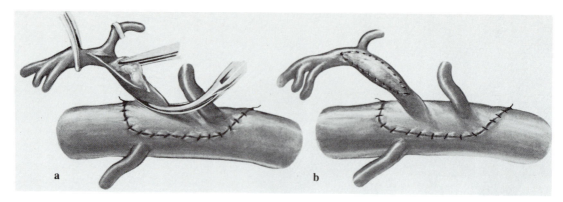

Figure 56-7. A. Separate arteriotomy for thromboendarterectomy of the totally occluded superior mesenteric artery. **B.** Closure of the arteriotomy with a venous patch to avoid narrowing. (*From Wylie EJ, Stoney RJ, et al.: Manual of Vascular Surgery, vols 1 and 2, New York, Springer Verlag New York, 1980*).

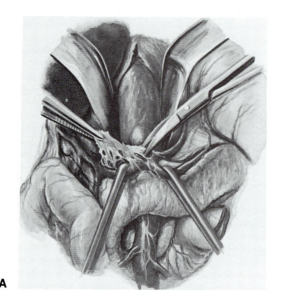

A

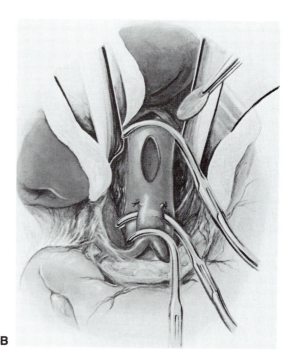

B

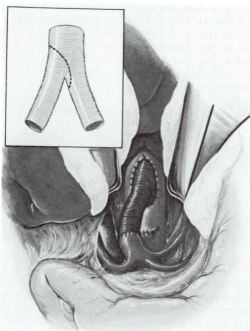

C

Figure 56-8. A. Excision of celiac ganglion fibers for exposure of the celiac axis. **B.** Segmental aortic clamping and aortotomy for proximal anastomosis of aortovisceral graft. **C.** Flanged Dacron graft, cut from a bifurcated graft (*inset*), used for aortoceliac reconstruction with antegrade alignment. (*From Wylie EJ, Stoney RJ, et al.: Manual of Vascular Surgery, vols 1 and 2. New York, Springer Verlag New York, 1980.*)

ably high, early and late failure rates.[34-42] The following basic principles for aortovisceral bypass grafting have been associated with a significantly improved patency and are therefore recommended:

1. An undiseased aortic segment, with little risk for future disease developing at the origin, for the graft to provide durable inflow.
2. An antegrade alignment of the graft to minimize turbulence and kinking.
3. A prosthetic Dacron graft, which is reliable and has no tendency to the degenerative changes observed in vein grafts. A flanged, knitted Dacron prosthesis, cut from a bifurcated graft, is preferred for a single-vessel bypass, and bifurcated grafts (10 × 5 mm or 12 × 6 mm) are used when both vessels are reconstructed.

The transabdominal approach is used. A 3.5 to 5 cm length of supraceliac aorta is controlled between vascular clamps. For celiac axis reconstruction, an elliptical aortotomy is created on the anterior aspect of the aorta for anastomosis of the beveled end of the prosthetic graft. Aortic flow can then be restored and the graft clamped separately. The celiac artery is transected beyond the lesion, and the proximal stump is oversewn; then the distal end is sutured end-to-end to the graft limb (Fig. 56-8A-C).

For combined celiac axis and superior mesenteric artery reconstruction, the aortotomy is placed on the right anterolateral aspect of the aorta, allowing placement of one limb of the graft in a retropancreatic position for end-to-end anastomosis to the divided superior mesenteric artery. The visceral arteries are grafted sequentially to minimize ischemia (Fig. 56-9).

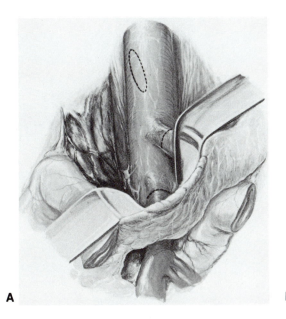
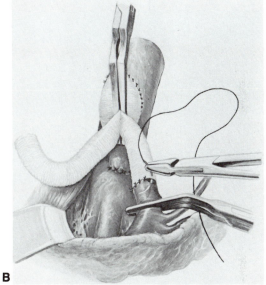
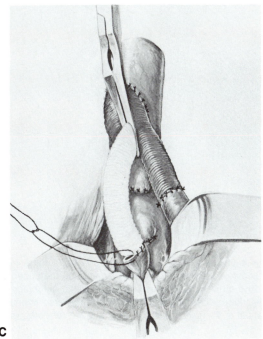

Figure 56-9. A. Exposure of celiac axis and superior mesenteric artery and placement of the aortotomy for combined aortovisceral reconstruction. **B.** Separate clamping of the bifurcated graft restores aortic flow. End-to-end anastomosis between prosthetic graft limb and the transected celiac artery is performed. **C.** Restored flow to the celiac artery and completion of anastomosis between graft and the superior mesenteric artery. (*From Wylie EJ, Stoney RJ, et al.: Manual of Vascular Surgery, vols 1 and 2. New York, Springer Verlag New York, 1980.*)

Results and Complications

Among 74 patients who underwent 76 operations for chronic visceral ischemia between 1959 and 1986, 52 had transaortic endarterectomies, and 24 had antegrade prosthetic bypass grafting.[20] Six perioperative deaths occurred, five in the transaortic group and one in the bypass group. All other patients were discharged cured of symptoms of chronic visceral ischemia and regained their lost weight during follow-up. During late assessment, two patients developed recurrent mesenteric symptoms and were successfully reoperated on. Three other patients expired 2 and 3 years postoperatively from intestinal infarction. All 61 of the 63 patients available at late follow-up (mean 53 months) remained asymptomatic. Thirty-four patients had aortogra-

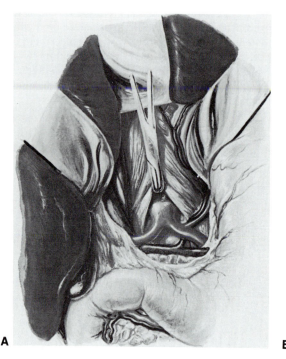

A

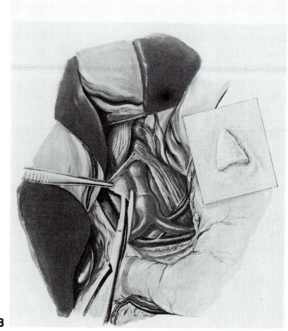

B

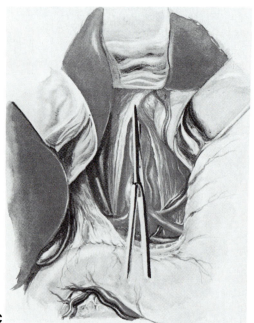

C

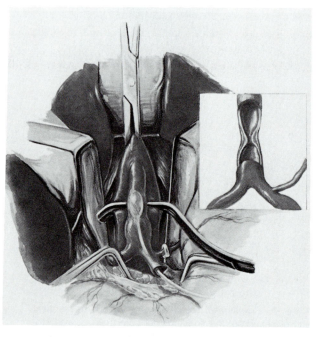

D

Figure 56-10. Technique for exposure in the surgical treatment of celiac axis compression. Right-angle clamp is used to separate the median arcuate ligament and the underlying artery, **A,** before triangular excision of the ligament, **B. C.** Midline division of the muscular fibers of the diaphragmatic crus exposes the celiac origin and the thoracic aorta. **D.** Dilatation of the celiac axis through a transverse arteriotomy in the splenic artery. (*From Wylie EJ, Stoney RJ, et al.: Manual of Vascular Surgery, vols 1 and 2. New York, Springer Verlag New York, 1980.*)

phy at late follow-up, documenting 58 patent reconstructions, two asymptomatic single-vessel stenoses, and one asymptomatic occlusion.

Transaortic endarterectomy and antegrade visceral bypass provide long-term relief from visceral ischemic symptoms and prevent visceral gangrene. The durability of these procedures is attributed to the elimination of turbulent blood flow by the endarterectomy and antegrade graft placement and the elimination of conduit complications inherent in retrograde graft alignment.

Celiac Artery Compression Syndrome

With the exception of patients having multiple prior abdominal operations, a standard transabdominal approach is used. Principally celiac axis compression is treated in three different ways: decompression alone, decompression and dilatation, or decompression and celiac artery reconstruction.

Decompression means resection of the median arcuate ligament and the celiac ganglion fibers. If a flow-limiting fibrotic stenosis has resulted from the compression, it can be dilated by use of retrograde intraluminal graded dilators (Fig. 56-10). This procedure is performed through a transverse arteriotomy in the splenic artery. If dilatation fails to restore good celiac inflow, estimated by Duplex scanning or a residual pressure gradient, aortoceliac bypass is performed. The celiac artery can be reconstructed by a short interposition Dacron graft proximally anastomosed to the celiac axis stump and distally to the divided end of the celiac artery.[49]

Results and Complications

In a series of 51 patients treated between 1964 and 1981, each of the three different principal treatments was used with roughly the same frequency.[30] No mortality occurred. Forty-four patients were available for late follow-up after a mean period of 9 years. Thirty of these patients were cured, and 14 were still symptomatic. The cure rate was higher when decompression was combined with dilatation or reconstruction than when it was used alone (79 and 73% vs. 53% asymptomatic patients). Combined with the fact that decompression alone had a high rate of pressure gradients, these results might suggest that decreased celiac flow really is a significant factor in this syndrome.

REFERENCES

1. Chiene J: Complete obliteration of the celiac and mesenteric arteries. J Anat Physiol 3:65, 1869.
2. Councilman WT: Three cases of occlusion of the superior mesenteric artery. Boston Med Surg J 130:4, 1894.
3. Dunphy JE: Abdominal pain of vascular origin. Am J Med Sci 192:102, 1936.
4. Mikkelsen WP: Intestinal angina: Its surgical significance. Am J Surg 99:262, 1957.
5. Shaw RS, Maynard EP III: Acute and chronic thrombosis of mesenteric arteries associated with malabsorption: Report of two cases successfully treated with thromboendarterectomy. N Engl J Med 258:874, 1958.
6. Mikkelsen WP, Zaro JA: Intestinal angina—report of a case with preoperative diagnosis and surgical relief. N Engl J Med 260:912, 1959.
7. Morris GC, Crawford ES, et al.: Revascularization of the celiac and superior mesenteric arteries. Arch Surg 84:95, 1962.
8. Fry WD, Kraft RO: Visceral angina. Surg Gynecol Obstet 117:417, 1963.
9. Stoney RJ, Wylie EJ: Recognition and surgical management of visceral ischemic syndromes. Ann Surg 164:714, 1966.
10. Elliott JW: Operative relief of gangrene of the intestine due to occlusion of the mesenteric vessels. Ann Surg 21:9, 1895.
11. Bergan JJ: Recognition and treatment of superior mesenteric artery embolization. Geriatrics 24:118, 1969.
12. Bergan JJ: Recognition and treatment of superior mesenteric artery embolization. Surg Clin North Am 47:109, 1967.
13. Bergan JJ, Dean RH, et al.: Revascularization in the treatment of mesenteric infarction. Ann Surg 182:430, 1975.
14. Bergan JJ, Dry L, et al.: Intestinal ischemia syndromes. Ann Surg 169:120, 1969.
15. Wilson GSM, Block J: Mesenteric vascular occlusion. Arch Surg 73:330, 1956.
16. Serjeant JCB: Mesenteric embolus treated with low molecular weight Dextran. Lancet 1:139, 1965.
17. Marfuggi RA, Greenspan M: Reliable intraoperative prediction of intestinal viability using fluorescent indicator. Surg Gynecol Obstet 152:33, 1980.
18. Wright CB, Hobson RW: Prediction of intestinal viability using Doppler ultrasound technique. Am J Surg 129:642, 1975.
19. Wittenberg J, Asthanasoulis CA, et al.: A radiological approach to the patient with acute, extensive bowel ischemia. Radiology 106:13, 1973.
20. Rapp JH, Reilly LM, et al.: Durability of endarterectomy and antegrade grafts in the treatment of chronic visceral ischemia. J Vasc Surg 3:799, 1986.
21. Stoney RJ, Ehrenfeld WK, Wylie EJ: Revascularization methods in chronic visceral ischemia caused by atherosclerosis. Ann Surg 186:468, 1977.
22. Stoney RJ, Olcott C IV: Visceral artery syndrome and reconstructions. Surg Clin North Am 59:637, 1979.
23. Poole JW, Sammartano BS, Boley SJ: Hemodynamic basis of the pain of chronic mesenteric ischemia. Am J Surg 153:171, 1987.
24. Qvarfordt PG, Reilly LM, et al.: "Coral Reef" atherosclerosis of the suprarenal aorta: A unique clinical entity. J Vasc Surg 1:903, 1984.
25. Dunbar JD, Molner RL, et al.: Compression of the celiac trunk and abdominal angina: Preliminary report of 15 cases. AJR 95:731, 1965.
26. Evans WE: Long-term evaluation of the celiac band syndrome. Surgery 76:867, 1974.
27. Brandt IJ, Boley SJ: Celiac axis compression. A critical review. Am J Dig Dis 23:633, 1978.
28. Rogers DM, Thompson JE, et al.: Mesenteric vascular problems—a 26-year experience. Ann Surg 195:554, 1982.
29. Szilagyi DE, Rian RL, et al.: The celiac axis compression syndrome. Does it exist? Surgery 72:849, 1972.
30. Reilly LM, Ammar AD, et al.: Late results following operative repair for celiac artery compression syndrome. J Vasc Surg 2:79, 1985.
31. Snyder MA, Mahoney EB, et al.: Symptomatic celiac artery stenosis due to constriction by the neurofibrous tissue of the celiac ganglion. Surgery 61:372, 1967.
32. Harjola PT, Lahtiharjn A: Celiac axis syndrome: Abdominal angina caused by external compression of the celiac artery. Am J Surg 115:864, 1968.
33. Krupski WC, Effeney DJ, Ehrenfeld WK: Spontaneous dissection of the superior mesenteric artery. J Vasc Surg 2:731, 1985.

34. Pallubinskas AJ, Ripley HR: Fibromuscular hyperplasia in extra-renal arteries. Radiology 82:451, 1964.

35. Williams LF Jr.: Vascular insufficiency of the intestines. Gastroenterology 61:757, 1971.

36. Connolly JE, Kwaan JHM: Management of chronic visceral ischemia. Surg Clin North Am 62:345, 1982.

37. Baur GM, Millay DJ, et al.: Treatment of chronic visceral ischemia. Am J Surg 148:138, 1984.

38. Hollier LH, Bernatz PE, et al.: Surgical management of chronic intestinal ischemia: A reappraisal. Surgery 90:940, 1981.

39. Connelly TJ, Perdue GD, et al.: Elective mesenteric revascularization. Am J Surg 115:497, 1980.

40. Zelenock GB, Graham LM, et al.: Splanchnic arteriosclerotic disease and intestinal angina. Arch Surg 115:497, 1980.

41. Dean RH, Wilson JP, Burko H: Saphenous vein aortorenal bypass grafts: Serial arteriographic study. Ann Surg 180:469, 1974.

42. Stanley JC, Ernst CB, Fry WJ: Fate of 100 aortorenal vein grafts: Characteristics of late graft expansion, aneurysmal dilatation, and stenosis. Surgery 74:931, 1973.

43. Stoney RJ, DeLuccia N, et al.: Aortorenal arterial autografts. Long term assessment. Arch Surg 116:1416, 1981.

44. Sohn YJ, Cronnelly R, et al.: Monitoring with two-dimensional transesophageal echocardiography. Comparison of myocardial function in patients undergoing supraceliac, suprarenal, infraceliac or infrarenal aortic occlusion. J Vasc Surg 1:300, 1984.

45. Stacey-Clear A, Jamieson CW: Omnitract retractor. Br J Surg 74:22, 1987.

46. Okuhn SP, Reilly LM: Intraoperative assessment of renal and visceral artery reconstruction: The role of Duplex scanning and special analysis. J Vasc Surg 5:137, 1987.

47. Stoney RJ, Wylie RJ: Surgical management of arterial lesion of the thoracoabdominal aorta. Am J Surg 126:157, 1973.

48. Wylie EJ, Stoney RJ, Ehrenfeld WK: Manual of Vascular Surgery, vol 1. New York, Springer-Verlag New York, 1980, p 207.

49. Wylie EJ, Stoney RJ, et al.: Manual of Vascular Surgery, vol. 2. New York, Springer-Verlag New York, 1980, p 210.

CHAPTER 57
Renal Artery Reconstruction

Calvin B. Ernst

Reconstruction of a renal artery is an infrequently performed visceral revascularization procedure in most centers in the United States. In some centers, however, renal artery reconstructions compose the majority of visceral revascularization procedures; thus data and experience from these centers of excellence provide the basis of our knowledge of indications for and results of renal artery reconstruction. The most compelling reason for renal artery reconstruction is renovascular hypertension (RVH) resulting from occlusive disease of a renal artery. Other indications for renal artery reconstruction include, in descending order of frequency, renal artery aneurysms, emboli, arteriovenous fistulas, and blunt or penetrating trauma. Renal artery reconstruction for acute occlusion of a previously normal renal artery is usually futile because of irreversible ischemia of the renal parenchyma. Consequently, almost all renal artery reconstructions are performed electively to reverse hypertension or to preserve renal parenchyma.

HISTORY

Richard Bright,[1] in 1827, first reported the relationship between "hardness of the pulse" and "hardening of the kidneys." But almost 50 years elapsed before Mahomed,[2] in 1874, actually measured "high tension in the arterial system" in patients with renal disease. The first suggestion that this renal-related hypertension resulted from a renal pressor substance came in 1898 from Tigerstedt and Bergmann.[3] The seminal report of Goldblatt and colleagues,[4] in 1934, that experimental hypertension could be produced by renal artery constriction provided the connecting link between renal artery disease and hypertension and alerted clinicians to a potentially curable form of hypertension.

In 1938, Leadbetter and Burkland[5] first documented relief of hypertension after nephrectomy for renal artery occlusion due to "a mass of tissue made up chiefly of smooth muscle outlined by elastic lamella." This was the first description of fibromuscular dysplasia of the renal artery.

Enthusiasm among clinicians for surgical treatment of renal hypertension was notably and justifiably dampened by the 1948 report of Smith,[6] who noted that only 19% of 200 hypertensive patients had relief of hypertension after nephrectomy.

Even though Freeman and colleagues[7] first documented, in 1954, the fact that renal artery reconstruction by endarterectomy could preserve renal parenchyma and cure RVH, clinicians remained skeptical and discouraged that a consistently curable form of hypertension had been identified.

With the introduction of aortography by dos Santos and colleagues,[8] in 1929, and further refinement in the early 1950s by Smith et al.,[9] a more selective method of identifying suitable candidates for renal artery reconstruction became available.

Even though aortography provided morphologic confirmation of a renal artery lesion, it became apparent that not all renal artery stenoses caused hypertension.[10] A means of proving the functional significance of a renal artery lesion was necessary, and this was first provided by Howard and associates,[11] in 1954. They documented, by individual ureteral catheterizations, the fact that sodium and water excretion by an ischemic kidney differed both quantitatively and qualitatively from that of the contralateral nonischemic, normal kidney. The "Howard test," although modified and refined, has been abandoned in most centers in favor of comparative measurements of renal vein renin activity, first by comparing renin ratios[12,13] and subsequently by determining renal-systemic renin indexes.[14,15]

Thus experimental hypotheses have become clinical realities. The connection between a renal artery lesion and hypertension has now proved, through refined diagnostic and surgical techniques, to be a consistently curable form of hypertension.

MAGNITUDE OF THE PROBLEM

Renal revascularization is an infrequently performed procedure in comparison with carotid endarterectomy or aortic reconstruction.[16] The reason for the paucity of renal revascularization procedures is that proven renovascular disease may result in RVH among only 35 to 50% of patients.[17] The true prevalence of RVH in an unselected population, therefore, is unknown. Nonetheless, a reasonable estimate of the prevalence of RVH appears to be 1% of unselected hypertensive patients.[17] Since there may be 25 million hypertensive patients in the United States, there are potentially 250,000 with this curable form of hypertension, and a potentially similar number of renal revascularization procedures. Although the precise incidence of RVH among both adults and children remains unknown, it should be noted that RVH outnumbers all other forms of surgically curable hypertension combined, including pheochromocytoma, Cushing's disease, primary aldosteronism (Conn's syndrome) and unilateral renal parenchymal disease. The difference in renal artery reconstructions performed in 1985 (approximately 2000) and the potential need for this operation reflect the nonaggressive approach to identifying patients with surgically curable hypertensive disease.

PATHOPHYSIOLOGY AND CLINICAL CHARACTERISTICS OF RENOVASCULAR HYPERTENSION

Pathology

Stenotic disease of the renal artery and, rarely, isolated renal artery aneurysms induce the most commonly curable form of hypertension. Such lesions result from arteriosclerosis or fibromuscular dysplasia (Figs. 57-1 and 57-2). An arteriosclerotic lesion typically involves the proximal main renal artery or its ostium as an extension of aortic atherosclerosis. Such lesions are similar to atherosclerotic plaques elsewhere in the body and are a consequence of aging. Therefore RVH due to renal artery atherosclerosis occurs in elderly persons, primarily men, and most frequently

involves the left renal artery. Such lesions account for approximately 60 to 70% of cases of RVH.

Renal arterial fibromuscular dysplasia, the second most common cause of RVH, represents a heterogeneous group of diseases of unknown cause and includes intimal fibroplasia, medial fibrodysplasia, and perimedial dysplasia.[18] Fibromuscular dysplasia characteristically involves the mid and distal portions of the renal artery and may extend into the primary branches.

Intimal fibroplasia (5%) occurs equally in both men and women. It is more likely to be found in children and young adults than in older individuals. Medial fibrodysplasia (85%) almost exclusively affects women, usually in their fourth and fifth decades. Although this form may occur as a solitary stenosis, more commonly it appears as multiple tandem stenoses with alternating aneurysmal outpouchings resembling a string of beads (Fig. 57-2). Perimedial dysplasia (10%) often coexists with medial fibrodysplasia and usually affects women in their fourth and fifth decades of life.

Miscellaneous causes of RVH include developmental abnormalities characterized by coarctation of the abdominal aorta, Takayasu's aortitis, renal artery dissections, arteriovenous malformations of the renal parenchyma, and embolic and traumatic lesions.

Physiology

The precise mechanism of hypertension due to a renal artery stenosis remains controversial. Although the exact mechanism of sustained hypertension due to a renal arterial stenosis is unknown, abundant data suggest that renin is important in initiating the hypertension. It appears that both vasoconstrictive and volume-dependent mechanisms are responsible, mediated through the renin-angiotensin-aldosterone axis.

The renin-angiotensin-aldosterone axis is a complex

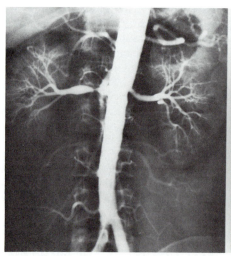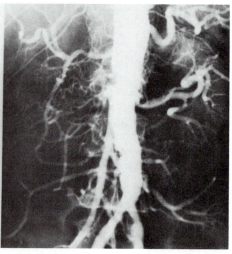

Figure 57-1. Aortograms depicting two types of arteriosclerotic renal artery lesions. *Left. Focal* right renal artery stenosis of proximal main renal artery. *Right. Diffuse* arteriosclerosis involving aorta and its branches. Right renal artery is occluded at ostium. Left renal artery ostial stenosis is an extension of aortic disease.

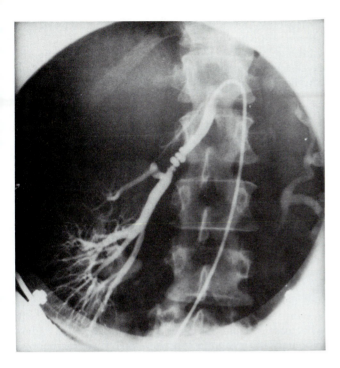

Figure 57-2. Selective right renal arteriogram of typical medial fibrodysplastic lesion. Tandem stenoses involve distal renal artery. Proximal main renal artery appears normal.

homeostatic mechanism that acts to maintain normal blood pressure and blood volume and is closely related to the degree of sodium balance. Specialized cells, probably of smooth muscle origin, located mainly in the walls of the afferent arterioles of the glomerulus, synthesize and store renin. These cells, along with a specialized tubular area marking the transition from the ascending loop of Henle to the distal convoluted tubule, known as the macula densa, constitute the juxtaglomerular apparatus. Contemporary data suggest that renin is released in response to changes in renal artery perfusion pressure and changes in sodium chloride concentration presented to the macula densa.[19] The renal sympathetic nerves, which richly innervate the juxtaglomerular apparatus, may serve to modulate renin release.

Renin, a proteolytic enzyme, acts on a tetradecapeptide (angiotensinogen) made in the liver to produce a decapeptide (angiotensin I). The two terminal amino acids, leucine and valine, are split from angiotensin I by a converting enzyme, found mainly in the lung, to yield an octapeptide, angiotensin II. Angiotensin II, a potent vasoconstrictor, stimulates release of aldosterone from the adrenal cortex and potentiates the effects of circulating catecholamines, resulting in vasoconstriction, sodium retention, and subsequent hypertension. Sustained elevation of arterial blood pressure may reflect a combination of vasoconstrictive (angiotensin II activity) and volume-dependent (aldosterone-induced sodium retention) mechanisms. Intrarenal inhibition of renin release may be through a positive feedback mechanism whereby the increased blood volume and arte-

rial perfusion pressure suppress renin release. Although prostaglandins may also contribute to intrarenal renin regulation, their roles are not as yet defined.

Contemporary data suggest that a hemodynamically significant lesion of the renal artery activates the renin-aldosterone-angiotensin system to produce hypertension. The presence of a renal artery stenosis and hypertension, however, are not necessarily causal, and determination of the functional significance of a stenosis must be based on renin, sodium, and water balance studies.

Clinical Characteristics

Data from the cooperative study of renovascular hypertension provided documentation that there were no clinical characteristics that precisely discriminated between patients with RVH and essential hypertension.[20] However, certain clinical findings suggest a renovascular origin of hypertension. Patients with mild hypertension (diastolic blood pressure less than 105 mm Hg) have only a minimal chance of having RVH, whereas those with diastolic blood pressures greater than 105 mm Hg have a greater chance of having RVH. Therefore, once the hypertensive patient has been identified, severity of hypertension serves as the basis for further investigation. In general, the higher the untreated diastolic blood pressure, the greater the likelihood of a renovascular origin. Patients who would otherwise be operative candidates if a renal artery lesion were found and whose untreated diastolic blood pressure is greater than 105 mm Hg, should undergo intensive study to identify a renovascular origin. A diastolic blood pressure of 115 mm Hg or greater absolutely mandates aggressive investigation.

A typical prototype patient with RVH due to an arteriosclerotic renal artery lesion is a 65-year-old man who has recently been normotensive or whose hypertension has been easily controlled and whose blood pressure now measures 240/140 mm Hg. He may also have retinal hemorrhages, exudates, and papilledema. A typical prototype patient with RVH due to a fibrodysplastic renal artery lesion is a 20-year-old woman who is known to have had normal blood pressure 6 months previously and now has a blood pressure reading of 230/130 mm Hg. She complains of headaches, and her ocular fundi are grade 4 (hemorrhages, exudates, papilledema). Finally, any child with sustained diastolic hypertension deserves thorough study.

The decision to subject the patient to investigative studies, however, depends largely on whether the patient would be an operative candidate if a correctable lesion were found. In general, young hypertensive patients should be thoroughly evaluated and, if a significant renal arterial lesion is documented, must be offered the benefits of surgical treatment. This is particularly true for patients with fibromuscular dysplasia. On the other hand, elderly hypertensive patients with limited life expectancy probably would not be candidates for renal artery reconstruction, because the results of surgical treatment of this problem must be judged against the natural history of generalized symptomatic arteriosclerosis.

DIAGNOSTIC EVALUATION

General

All patients with suspected RVH are thoroughly evaluated for other forms of hypertension and to determine their cardiac and renal function, which may be impaired as a result of the hypertension (Table 57-1). Normal hematologic, serum chemistry, and renal function studies effectively exclude pheochromocytoma, primary aldosteronism, Cushing's disease, and renal arteriolar nephrosclerosis. Any suggestion of significant cardiac compromise by electrocardiogram or symptoms requires further investigation, which may include myocardial performance studies (see Chapter 13).

Currently accepted diagnostic studies for RVH include hypertensive urography, radioisotope renography, determination of renal venous renin activity, split renal function studies, and standard and digital subtraction renal arteriography. Although no single study is diagnostic, renal arteriography is mandatory and is the mainstay of diagnosis.

Intravenous Pyelography

Hypertensive or rapid-sequence urography, because of availability and safety, has been widely employed in the assessment of patients with suspected RVH. Isotope renography adds little or no additional information to urography, and both studies are similarly unreliable for diagnosis of RVH.[21,22] Because of bilateral and segmental arterial involvement among pediatric patients, hypertensive urography has very limited diagnostic reliability. Urography may suggest unilateral renovascular disease documented by (1) delay in the appearance of contrast material within the collecting system of the ischemic kidney in comparison with the normal kidney, (2) differences in renal length, the ischemic kidney being at least 1.5 cm smaller than the normal kidney, and (3) hyperconcentration of contrast material by the ischemic kidney on late x-ray films. Ureteral or renal pelvis indentations due to renal arterial collateral vessels may also be seen, but this is rarely an isolated finding. Size differences have proved to be the most common abnormality. However, in only 25% of children, and in approximately 50 to 70% of adults, has rapid sequence urography shown positive results among those with proven RVH.[21,22] Although an unreliable screening test for RVH, hypertensive urography should be performed to exclude other renal and perirenal causes of hypertension.

Split Function Studies

Bilateral ureteral catheterization with determination of individual kidney excretory function has proved useful in determining the functional significance of a renal artery stenosis in adults. Classically, a patient with a positive study result has a 40% decrease in urine volume, a 50% increase in creatinine concentration, and a 100% increase in para-aminohippurate concentration on the involved side. Dean and colleagues,[23,24] the group with the most experience with split function studies, suggest that these criteria are too rigid, and they have therefore liberalized these criteria and define a positive study result as one in which there is consistent lateralization of each of three samples, with a decrease in urine volume and an increase in para-aminohippurate and creatinine concentrations. However, because of the risks of ureteral catheterization, associated discomfort, and confusing results, the regular use of split function studies is not justified, particularly now that renal vein renin assay is available.

Renin Assays

Excessive renin production by an ischemic kidney may be reflected in increased peripheral and increased renal venous renin activity, although peripheral venous plasma renin activity is neither sensitive nor specific for RVH. Because of the interdependence of renin production and renal sodium balance, the recording of renin secretion in relation to sodium excretion should increase the sensitivity and specificity of peripheral plasma renin analysis in detecting RVH. However, even these refinements in renin measurements have proved not only unreliable but also impractical.[24]

A popular method of detecting hyperreninemic kidneys and determining the functional significance of a renal artery lesion has been to determine individual renal vein renin activities and calculate a ratio that compares the ischemic kidney with the normal kidney.[12] A disparity of 40 to 50% (ratios of 1.4 and 1.5, respectively) in renal vein renin activity between kidneys suggests a functional significance. Although lateralized renin ratios suggest functional significance, no correlation between the degree of elevation of renal vein renin ratios and cure or improvement of patients by renal revascularization has been reported. Elevation of the renal vein renin ratio does appear to discriminate between those benefited by operation and those in whom surgical treatment failed, however.[12,15] Nonetheless, it must be noted that renin ratios have an overall accuracy of only about 80% among patients with proven RVH—those who have benefited from renal revascularization. This lack of sensitivity may be due to many factors, including suppression of renin release by antihypertensive drugs, most nota-

TABLE 57-1. ROUTINE STUDIES OBTAINED IN ALL PATIENTS WITH SUSPECTED RENOVASCULAR HYPERTENSION

Hemogram, including coagulation studies

SMA-12 panel

Serum potassium levels (three)

Urinalysis and culture

Creatinine clearance

Urinary levels of electrolytes, metanephrine, normetanephrine, and 17-OH steroids

Electrocardiogram

Chest x-ray film

Rapid-sequence urography

Renal arteriography

bly beta-adrenergic blocking agents such as propranolol and alpha-methyldopa, poor sampling techniques, and significant collateral blood flow, which may cause renin not to lateralize.[25] Consequently, a patient with a hemodynamically significant renal artery lesion should not be denied the benefits of renal revascularization solely on the basis of a nonlateralizing renal vein renin study.

A renal-systemic renin index (RSRI) that determines individual renin secretory activity has been devised to refine the discriminatory value of renal vein renin studies.[13,15] The RSRI is calculated by subtracting systemic renin activity (inferior vena cava blood renin) from the individual kidney's venous renin activity and dividing the result by the systemic renin activity. Comparisons of renal vein renin activity from an individual kidney should probably not result in an RSRI greater than 0.24. When combined activities of both kidneys are related to systemic activity, the RSRI should not be greater than 0.48. An RSRI greater than 0.48 from an individual kidney or from both kidneys reflects renin production that exceeds hepatic clearance and suggests hyperreninemia. Beneficial responses to unilateral renal revascularization are most likely with an RSRI greater than 0.48 in the ischemic kidney and an RSRI approaching zero in the opposite kidney.[15] These data may not be completely applicable to children, however, because almost all renin data have been compiled from adult RVH patients.

Noninvasive Imaging Studies

Duplex imaging of the visceral vessels, and of the renal arteries in particular, holds promise as a screening test for the absence or presence of a renal artery lesion.[26] Contemporary technology, however, does not provide sufficiently precise resolution of the duplex image to identify renal artery disease consistently. As imaging technology is further refined, reliable noninvasive screening of patients with suspected hypertension of a renovascular origin will become a clinical reality and will provide an inexpensive, widely applicable, much-needed screening test for RVH.

Renal Arteriography

Renal arteriography, either by conventional or digital subtraction techniques, is the only definitive diagnostic RVH study. Arteriography is essential in establishing the morphologic features and anatomic distribution of obstructing lesions, as well as their hemodynamic significance. Any young patient who is otherwise a candidate for renal artery reconstruction, if a renal artery lesion is identified and if diastolic blood pressure is 105 mm Hg or greater, should undergo renal arteriography. The decision to perform arteriography depends on many factors, not the least of which is the experience of the angiographer, but in centers of excellence for managing vascular diseases, morbidity from arteriography is minimal. Among preschool children and infants, general anesthesia may be necessary. In infancy and childhood, flush aortography alone is usually performed. Selective arterial catheterization with oblique filming techniques is reserved for older children and adults.

Intravenous digital subtraction arteriography, because it lacks precise resolution to document subtle renal artery lesions, is not a substitute for conventional arteriography. Further experience with intraarterial digital subtraction arteriography, however, may prove to be superior to conventional arteriography.

Summary

RVH can be determined only in retrospect, after the patient has responded favorably to renal artery reconstruction. Preoperative diagnosis depends on identification of the renal artery lesion and on the determination of its hemodynamic significance by arteriography and of its functional significance by renal venous renin assays. Hemodynamic significance is documented by identifying collateral channels bypassing the stenosis or occlusion. Although functional significance of a lesion cannot be determined by arteriography, identification of a hemodynamically significant fibrodysplastic lesion in a child or a young adult with sustained diastolic hypertension, in whom no other cause for hypertension is apparent, is prima facie evidence for RVH. Renal artery reconstruction is almost universally beneficial in such patients.

Among patients with arteriosclerotic renovascular disease, one must be more circumspect and less aggressively oriented toward renal artery reconstruction. Nevertheless, a hemodynamically significant lesion, which is functionally significant by renal venous renin or split renal function studies, in an individual who is otherwise a candidate for renal arterial reconstruction, demands surgical correction because an excellent outcome can be anticipated among the majority of patients.

OPERATIVE MANAGEMENT

Preoperative Preparation

In addition to the above-mentioned diagnostic studies relating to the hypertension, thorough evaluation of the cardiovascular system is essential to successful management because of the consequences of hypertension as a risk factor for advanced cardiovascular disease (see Chapter 13). This is particularly true for patients with arteriosclerotic RVH. In an analysis of arteriosclerotic patients undergoing operation for RVH, it has been documented that operative deaths occur primarily among those with clinical manifestations of diffuse arteriosclerosis, such as coronary artery disease and myocardial infarction, angina pectoris, or congestive heart failure; extracranial cerebrovascular occlusive disease with stroke or transient ischemic attacks; peripheral occlusive disease with intermittent claudication; or aneurysmal disease of the abdominal aorta.[27] Death after renal artery reconstruction in patients with only focal renal artery stenoses as manifestations of arteriosclerosis or in those with fibromuscular dysplasia is rare.[28]

Antihypertensive medications should be continued throughout the preoperative, operative, and postoperative periods, if necessary, to maintain blood pressure as close to normal as possible. It is a mistake to discontinue antihypertensive drugs for fear of complicating anethestic management during and after operation. For a competent anesthesiologist, antihypertensive drug effects pose few, if any, problems in anesthetic management.

Depending on the cardiac status of the patient, a Swan-Ganz catheter for monitoring cardiac function may or may not be used. Blood volumes among patients with RVH vary depending on preoperative sodium balance and blood pressure control, but they may be either expanded or contracted. Under such circumstances, and particularly among patients with arteriosclerotic RVH, Swan-Ganz catheter monitoring data have proved helpful for optimal perioperative fluid management. All patients, however, must have a radial artery catheter in place to monitor blood pressure.

Surgical Techniques

Before vascular surgery techniques were refined, nephrectomy was the only effective operation for RVH. But over the past two decades, perfection of vascular surgery techniques has relegated the role of nephrectomy, as a form of primary therapy, to historical interest only.

The surgical technique must be tailored to the patient. What may be appropriate for a young female patient with medial fibrodysplasia extending into the primary renal artery branches may not be appropriate for the elderly male patient with renal ostial arteriosclerosis and aortic involvement.

The two preferred renal artery reconstructive procedures are aortorenal bypass, using autogenous saphenous vein, hypogastric artery, or prosthetic materials, and endarterectomy. Whereas aortorenal bypass is applicable to both fibrodysplasic and arteriosclerotic lesions, endarterectomy is possible only for arteriosclerosis. Segmental arterial resection and reanastomosis or renal artery reimplantation into the aorta, local angioplasty, ex vivo reconstruction, primary operative dilation, and hepatorenal and splenorenal bypass are other but less frequently required or used techniques of renal artery reconstruction.

Occasionally, simultaneous renal arterial repair and aortic reconstruction may be necessary. Such simultaneous procedures, however, have consistently significant greater mortality and morbidity rates than renal arterial reconstruction alone and reflect the severity and extent of arteriosclerotic involvement.[27,29] Consequently, unless there are compelling reasons, such as deteriorating renal function or difficult-to-manage RVH, incidental renal artery reconstruction during aortic reconstruction should be avoided. If, however, compelling indications for renal artery reconstruction exist in a high-risk patient who has aortic disease that in itself is not an indication for operation but precludes a satisfactory inflow origin for renal revascularization, hepatorenal bypass and splenorenal bypass are viable alternatives.[30]

Aortorenal Bypass

For an aortorenal bypass procedure, the patient lies supine with a small, folded drape under the flank of the involved side. Inadequate exposure, particularly within the deep retroperitoneum, may compromise the successful completion of what might otherwise be an easy renal revascularization. I prefer transverse abdominal incisions for most renal artery reconstructions (Fig. 57-3). A vertical midline incision is an acceptable alternative and may be preferred when a hypogastric artery segment is used as the aortorenal graft, because such an incision facilitates hypogastric artery harvesting (Fig. 57-4). For right-sided procedures, the transverse incision is made above the umbilicus and extends from the left midclavicular line across both rectus muscles to well within the right flank, where the oblique and transverse abdominal muscles are divided. When one is performing left-sided revascularization procedures, a mirror image of the right-sided incision is used. Bilateral procedures usually entail extending the incision into both flanks.

After the peritoneal cavity is entered, access to the right renal artery is obtained by incising the peritoneum lateral to the ascending colon and mobilizing and reflecting the colon and duodenum to the left as an extended Kocher maneuver. Dissection is continued in an extraperitoneal plane between the colon and the kidney. Gerota's fascia and the capsule of the kidney are not disturbed, lest troublesome bleeding from small extraparenchymal collateral vessels occur. The intestines are retracted medially to the opposite side of the abdominal cavity. In infants and small children, the small bowel may be eviscerated and covered with moist packs.

Initially, the right renal vein is identified at its junction with the inferior vena cava. The proximal vein is dissected about its circumference. Ligation and transection of adrenal branches may facilitate this dissection. The renal vein is then elevated from the underlying tissues by gentle traction on encircling vessel loops or by a vein retractor. The right

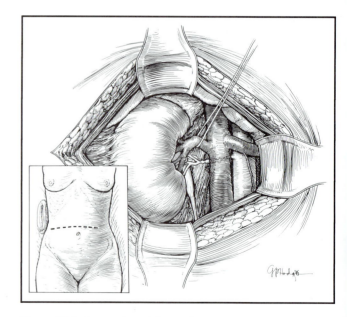

Figure 57-3. Approach to right renal artery through a transverse, supraumbilical incision. Duodenum and ascending colon mobilized by an extended Kocher maneuver provides exposure of right renal artery, vena cava, and aorta. (*From Stanley JC, Ernst CB, Fry WJ (eds): Renovascular Hypertension. Philadelphia, WB Saunders Co., 1984.*)

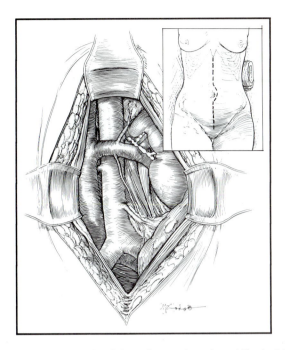

Figure 57-4. Approach to left renal artery through a midline incision. Descending colon and abdominal contents mobilized to the right in an extraperitoneal plane anterior to kidney provides exposure to renal vessels and aorta. Hypogastric arteries are readily accessible. *(From Stanley JC, Ernst CB, Fry WJ (eds): Renovascular Hypertension. Philadelphia, WB Saunders Co., 1984.)*

main renal artery is usually located deep to the renal vein at, or just cephalad to, its superior border. Dissection of the artery is best begun at its midportion just lateral to the vena cava. More distal dissection, if performed first, may lead to troublesome disruption of small arterial and venous branches. Once the vessel is freed from surrounding structures, it is encircled with fine polyethylene tubing (PE-90) or an elastic vessel loop. Gentle traction on the artery facilitates dissection behind the inferior vena cava toward the aorta and distally to its primary branches within the renal hilum. Under some circumstances, the vena cava may be retracted laterally and the right renal artery dissected at its aortic origin. This approach is usually undertaken in the treatment of proximal arteriosclerotic or developmental ostial lesions. Ligation and division of lumbar veins may be necessary to adequately mobilize the vena cava during these dissections.

Exposure of the left renal artery is obtained in a manner similar to that on the right side after the peritoneum is incised laterally and the descending colon is mobilized by dissection within the avascular plane between the bowel and the kidney. Rarely must the spleen be included in the dissection. With reflection of the viscera to the right, the left renal vein, left renal artery, and aorta are readily exposed. With a transverse abdominal incision, minimal retraction is required to maintain this exposure; such retraction is easily obtained by any self-retaining retractor fixed to the operating table. On the left, the adrenal and gonadal veins must frequently be ligated while the left renal vein is mobilized from the underlying aorta toward the kidney.

This facilitates dissection of the left renal artery to within the renal hilum.

After a suitable segment of appropriate renal artery is mobilized distal to the diseased segment, the infrarenal aorta is dissected about its circumference between the renal and the inferior mesenteric arteries. Grafts to the right kidney are usually placed in a retrocaval position, taking origin from a lateral aortotomy. However, placement of right-sided grafts should be individualized. Some lie most comfortably anterior to the vena cava, in which case an anterolateral aortotomy is required. Left-sided grafts may be positioned in front of or behind the left renal vein; this maneuver, too, is individualized on the basis of local anatomy.

When staged bilateral revascularizations are anticipated, aortic mobilization during the first of the two repairs should be limited. The aortic anastomosis should be as proximal on the aorta near the renal arteries as possible, so that during the second procedure, the aortic anastomosis may be constructed distal to the first. By keeping aortic mobilization to a minimum during the first procedure, fibrous scar tissue is minimized and a less tedious dissection is required during the second procedure. Because of the perceived increased morbidity and mortality rates attending simultaneous bilateral bypass procedures, many surgeons prefer staged reconstructions when both renal arteries are diseased; among low-risk patients, however, simultaneous bilateral renal reconstructions may prove to be more efficacious than staged procedures.

Autogenous saphenous vein is the preferred material for aortorenal bypass in adults, in most medical centers. For children, hypogastric artery is preferred because of the propensity of autogenous vein to dilate during late follow-up. However, autogenous hypogastric artery may dilate as well, but with less frequency than vein. In the absence of autogenous saphenous vein, prosthetic material such as knitted Dacron or expanded polytetrafluoroethylene may be used. Suitable segments of autogenous vein are almost always available, with segments of the greater saphenous vein from the groin being used most frequently. Sporadic adverse reports of the use of gonadal, jungular, or iliac venous segments condemn the use of such veins. Saphenous vein segments are carefully procured. The groin incision is made over the course of the greater saphenous vein, which is dissected for 10 to 15 cm. Minimal acceptable internal diameters of veins used for renal revascularization depend on the size of the artery being reconstructed. Veins less than 4 mm in diameter are inadequate for reconstructing main renal arteries, although such small-caliber veins may suffice for replacing or bypassing diseased segmental branches. During graft harvesting, tributaries are ligated and transected in situ, with care being taken not to injure or devascularize the vessel by excessive dissection of the adventitia. Prevention of venospasm by using agents such as papaverine may enhance the endothelial integrity of transplanted vein grafts. Veins should be cautiously irrigated with cold, heparinized blood or balanced salt solution, and distension should be avoided.

After the vein is harvested, systemic anticoagulation is accomplished by intravenous administration of sodium heparin, 100 units per kilogram. The aortic anastomosis is performed first (Fig. 57-5). A side-biting vascular clamp is

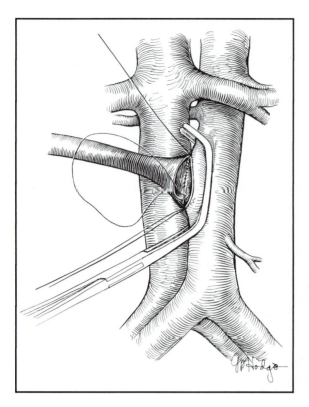

Figure 57-5. Anastomosis of end-to-side vein graft to aorta. Aorta is side clamped. Aortotomy length is two to three times diameter of vein. Graft may be positioned either anterior or posterior to vena cava, depending on local anatomy. (*From Stanley JC, Ernst CB, Fry WJ (eds): Renovascular Hypertension. Philadelphia, WB Saunders Co., 1984.*)

used to partially occlude the aorta midway between the renal vessels and the inferior mesenteric artery. In some instances, total aortic occlusion is necessary. The length of the aortotomy should be approximately two to three times the graft diameter. Excision of a button of aortic tissue is not necessary. The graft is beveled and spatulated, and the aortic anastomosis is performed with a continuous 5-0 or 6-0 polypropylene suture. The aortic clamp is usually left in place during completion of the renal anastomosis. To remove it and place an occluding clamp on the vein graft may injure the conduit and lead to late vein graft stenosis. Attention is then directed to the renal anastomosis. At this time, a 12.5 g dose of mannitol is given intravenously to provide a reasonable diuresis. The proximal renal artery is clamped, transected, and ligated. Microvascular clamps, developing tensions from 30 to 70 mm Hg, are favored for distal renal arterial occlusion. Because of the adequacy of collateral circulation in most cases, an unhurried, precise anastomosis may be performed with little risk of significant renal ischemia. Under such circumstances, normothermic renal ischemic times of approximately 30 to 40 minutes are usually well tolerated. If the renal artery has been totally occluded by the disease process, acceptable normothermic renal ischemic times may be even longer. Nonetheless, in experienced hands, the distal renal anastomosis can usually be constructed within 15 to 20 minutes.

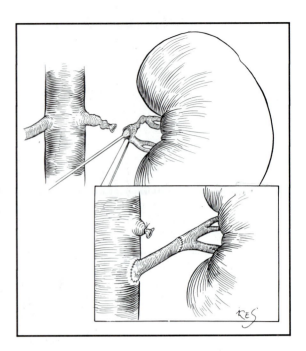

Figure 57-6. Adjunctive arterial dilation of primary renal artery branch using olive-tipped stainless steel dilators. (*From Stanley JC, Ernst CB, Fry WJ (eds): Renovascular Hypertension. Philadelphia, WB Saunders Co., 1984.*)

In revascularizations for proximal main renal arteriosclerotic disease, the distal renal artery is usually of sufficient length so that a microvascular clamp may be applied to the vessel beyond the area of intended anastomosis. In revascularizations for fibromuscular dysplasia with branch arterial involvement, it may be necessary to place microvascular clamps on segmental vessels to provide enough distal main renal artery for an unencumbered anastomosis. In the treatment of fibromuscular dysplasia, it may also be necessary to dilate the main renal artery or its primary branches by using either rigid olive-tipped stainless steel metal dilators or hydrostatic balloon devices (Fig. 57-6). Caution must accompany adjunctive dilation, lest these delicate arteries be perforated or overdistended, with subsequent intimal damage.

An end-to-end vein graft renal artery anastomosis is preferred over an end-to-side anastomosis. In addition to the greater technical ease of this type of reconstruction, its flow characteristics seem to be better when compared with those of end-to-side anastomoses. Renal anastomoses are facilitated by spatulation of the vein graft posteriorly and the renal artery anteriorly (Fig. 57-7). This allows visualization of the artery's interior, so that inclusion of intima with each stitch is ensured. In adults, the anastomosis is usually completed with a continuous 6-0 polypropylene suture. In most pediatric patients, three or four interrupted sutures of 7-0 polypropylene provide for anastomotic growth. In the case of a vessel smaller than 2 mm in diameter, the anastomosis is often accomplished with interrupted sutures about the entire circumference. It is important to realize that spatulated anastomoses ensure ovoid, nonstrictured healing.

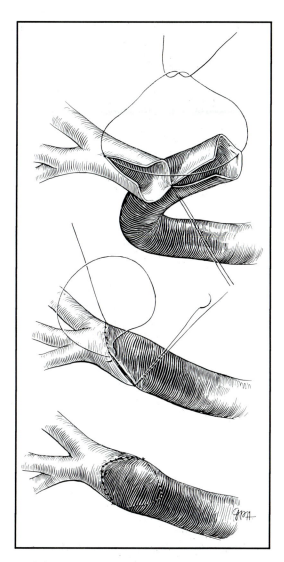

Figure 57-7. Anastomosis of end-to-end vein graft to renal artery. Graft is spatulated anteriorially, and renal artery is spatulated posteriorally. (*From Stanley JC, Ernst CB, Fry WJ (eds): Renovascular Hypertension. Philadelphia, WB Saunders Co., 1984.*)

Management of stenotic disease affecting multiple renal arteries or segmental branches poses a unique problem in renal artery reconstruction. Two alternative revascularization strategies are usually considered. The first involves separate in situ implantations of the renal arteries into the vein graft. This is usually accomplished with one anastomosis as the proximal end-to-side connection and the other as a distal end-to-end anastomosis (Fig. 57-8). The second method entails anastomosis of the involved arteries in a side-to-side manner, with subsequent anastomosis of the vein graft to the common orifice created by the arterial union (Fig. 57-9). The use of these more complicated reconstructions must be individualized and depends as much on the technical ease of completing the procedure as on the disease process being treated. Pliability of autogenous saphenous vein facilitates construction of these complex anastomoses.

After aortic and renal artery clamps are removed and anterograde renal blood flow is reestablished, the heparin effect is reversed with intravenous administration of protamine sulfate. Usually 1.2 mg of protamine sulfate is sufficient to reverse 100 units of sodium heparin, and this is monitored by measuring the activated clotting times. Intraoperative arteriography is seldom necessary, and operative Doppler flow analysis has not been widely employed. However, as such noninvasive techniques are refined, they may become of practical value in confirming the adequacy of anastomoses.

After the abdominal viscera are allowed to assume their normal position, the abdomen is closed in layers with nonabsorable sutures. Interposition of tissue between the bowel and an autogenous tissue graft is not necessary. However, if a prosthetic graft has been employed and it lies immediately adjacent to the duodenum, available retroperitoneal tissue must be interposed between the graft and the bowel.

Aortorenal Endarterectomy

Exposure for endarterectomy differs from that for aortorenal bypass because the juxtarenal aorta must be tediously and carefully dissected and mobilized. The juxtarenal aorta is exposed through either a vertical midline or a supraumbilical transverse incision extending into both flanks. Because success of the operation for either unilateral or bilateral renal endarterectomy depends on visualization of the aortic lumen proximal and distal to the renal artery ostia, midline dissection and mobilization of the aorta must extend from the infraceliac to the infrarenal segment. Dissection of dense neural tissue and division of the left crus of the diaphragm facilitate proximal exposure.

The left renal vein is completely mobilized, which requires ligation and division of the adrenal and gonadal veins. Extensive mobilization of left renal vein facilitates the subsequent aortotomy by retracting the vein caudally, either with a vein retractor or an encircling vessel loop.

Usually, transaortic rather than transrenal endarterectomy is necessary because of the difficulties in removing thickened aortic intima by transrenal exposure. Furthermore, inadequate sharp dissection of the thickened aortic intima through the renal ostium may lead to subintimal aortic dissection. Very localized focal lesions of the renal artery just distal to the renal origin, with minimal aortic involvement, however, may be effectively removed by transrenal endarterectomy and patch graft angioplasty with the use of either saphenous vein or expanded polytetrafluoroethylene (Fig. 57-10). Such focal left renal arterial stenoses may be exposed through the left retroperitoneal approach (see Chapter 18). When one is using the left retroperitoneal approach, the kidney is mobilized and reflected to the right, exposing the aortorenal junction posterolaterally. Through this approach, the deep side-biting aortic clamp includes the renal ostium, as is done for right-sided lesions (Fig. 57-10).

Transaortic renal endarterectomy requires aortic occlusion just proximal to the superior mesenteric artery (SMA) and 3 to 5 cm distal to the renal arteries (Fig. 57-11). The renal arteries are occluded with any small, low-tension clamps. Mannitol and heparin sodium are employed as for aortorenal bypass.

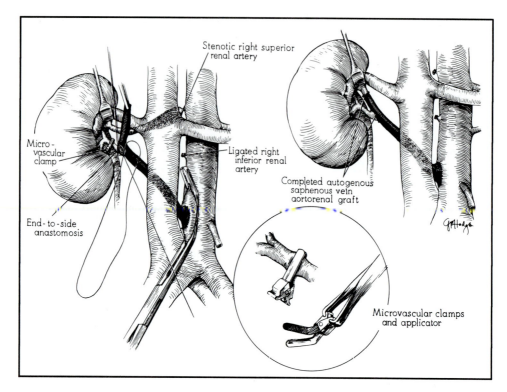

Figure 57-8. Technique of in situ reconstruction of multiple renal arteries. Lower branch is an anastomosed to side-of-vein graft. Upper branch is anastomosed in end-to-end manner to vein graft. Microvascular low tension clamps facilitate repair. (*From Ernst CB, Stanley JC, Fry WJ: Surg Gynecol Obstet 137:1023, 1973.*)

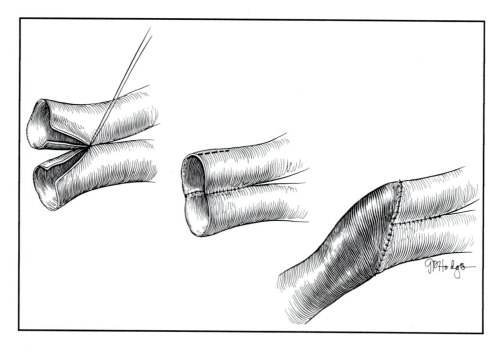

Figure 57-9. Technique of anastomosing renal artery branches in side-to-side manner, followed by end-to-end vein graft to common renal artery orifice anastomosis. (*From Stanley JC, Ernst CB, Fry WJ (eds): Renovascular Hypertension. Philadelphia, WB Saunders Co., 1984.*)

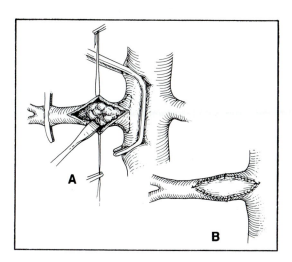

Figure 57-10. Transrenal endarterectomy, which is reserved for focal proximal renal artery arteriosclerosis (see Fig. 57-1, left panel). **A.** Aorta side-clamped and endarterectomy performed. **B.** Patch angioplasty closure.

An 8 to 10 cm anterior aortotomy extends from just to the left of the SMA origin into the infrarenal aorta (Fig. 57-11). A circumferential sleeve of aortic intima is removed along with the renal ostial plaques (Fig. 57-12). The aortic intima is first sharply transected distally and the circumferential plaque is mobilized proximally. In so doing, each

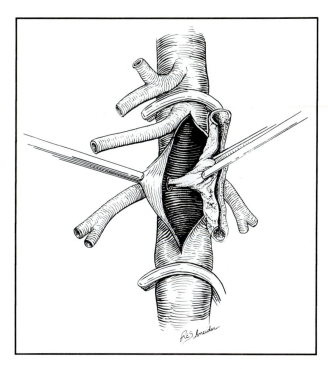

Figure 57-12. Technique of removing aortorenal arteriosclerotic plaque. Traction on transected aortic intima facilitates renal osteum endarterectomy. (*From Stanley JC, Ernst CB, Fry WJ (eds): Renovascular Hypertension. Philadelphia, WB Saunders Co., 1984.*)

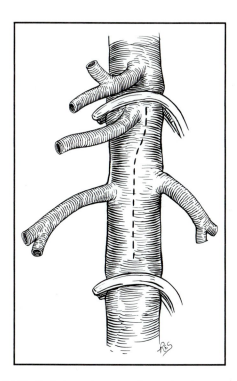

Figure 57-11. Technique of transaortic renal endarterectomy. Aortotomy extends from a point lateral to superior mesenteric artery to below renal arteries. (*From Stanley JC, Ernst CB, Fry WJ (eds): Renovascular Hypertension. Philadelphia, WB Saunders Co., 1984.*)

renal ostium is endarterectomized individually by placing gentle traction on the aortic plaque and pushing the media away from the intima, as with any eversion endarterectomy. The assistant facilitates endarterectomy of the renal ostia by pushing the kidney medially to enhance the renal artery prolapse. As the endarterectomy continues, the atherosclerotic plaque usually separates and breaks cleanly with a well-feathered endpoint. After the plaque is removed from both renal arteries, the circumferential aortic endarterectomy is continued up to, but not including, the SMA ostium. Here, again, the plaque is sharply transected. Residual intimal fragments are carefully removed and the endarterectomized segment is copiously irrigated with heparinized saline solution. The renal artery clamps are transiently released to ensure adequate backbleeding. The vertical aortotomy is then closed with a running 4-0 or 5-0 polypropylene suture without a patch graft. Renal ischemia times rarely exceed 20 to 30 minutes, and as noted above, because of preexisting collateral vessels, such ischemia times are well within safe limits.

Adequacy of the aortorenal endarterectomy is ensured by operative arteriography. The proximal and distal aortic clamps are replaced and 20 ml of contrast material is injected into the isolated aortic segment.[31] Any significant residual renal plaque that is identified on the arteriogram may be removed through a separate transverse renal arteriotomy. If this procedure is necessary, the two aortic clamps are removed and a single aortic side-biting clamp is employed to occlude the proximal renal artery. Closure of the transverse renal arteriotomy is accomplished with 5-0 or 6-0 polypropylene suture without a patch.

As with aortorenal bypass, the heparin effect may be reversed and is monitored by the activated clotting time. The abdominal closure proceeds as with aortorenal bypass reconstruction.

Operative Arterial Dilation

The distal extent and distribution of lesions and the small size of renal and femoral arteries preclude percutaneous transluminal dilation in most children and certainly in infants and preschool children. The role of percutaneous arterial dilation in management of RVH is still evolving, and all experience comparing percutaneous dilation with surgical repair has been restricted to adult RVH. Consequently, the place of this new modality for treatment of pediatric patients is unknown and should be viewed as an experimental procedure. The use of this technique in older children awaits further experience and long-term (more than 5 years) follow-up study in adults.

Open surgical dilation, however, is a procedure that has merit and has been employed successfully both as a primary isolated procedure and as an adjunct to aortorenal bypass.[32,33] Primary dilation is particularly applicable to children with focal renal artery stenoses and when the small size of the renal vessels precludes other forms of reconstruction.[33a]

Exposure of the renal vessels is similar to that used for aortorenal bypass. The renal artery in question must be dissected and mobilized throughout its length, well proximal and distal to the stenotic lesion. After systemic heparin effect is achieved, the proximal renal artery is occluded and a small transverse arteriotomy is made in the normal main renal artery proximal to the stenosis. Backbleeding is usually nonexistent or minimal because of the stenosis. Rigid olive-tipped dilators are gently advanced through the stenosis, the surgeon's left hand guiding the tip by palpating the mobilized renal artery. When the stenosis is encoun-

tered, resistance to the dilator will be felt. With gentle but progressive force, the dilator will be felt to "pop" through the lesion (Fig. 57-13). Once the stenosis is disrupted, backbleeding through the arteriotomy may occur; it can be controlled by occlusion of the distal branch of the renal artery with low-tension microvascular clamps. The dilation is begun with the smallest dilator estimated to pass through the lesion, usually the 0.5 mm dilator. The stenotic area is progressively expanded in 0.5 mm increments by careful passage of increasingly larger dilators through the stenosis. Dilators more than 1.0 mm larger than the diameter of the vessel being dilated should not be used lest overdilation and arterial disruption occur. After adequate dilation, the short arteriotomy is closed with a few 7-0 polypropylene sutures and blood flow is restored.

Operative dilation is also employed in the treatment of tandem lesions in renal artery branches during aortorenal bypass (Fig. 57-6). Under such circumstances, the graded dilators are passed through the open transected distal renal artery into the appropriate renal artery branch before the distal anastomosis of the aortorenal bypass is constructed.

RENAL ARTERY ANEURYSM REPAIR

Indications for Repair

Indications for renal artery reconstruction for renal artery aneurysm cannot be rigidly defined because the natural history and incidence of these lesions are unknown. Since renal artery aneurysms are rarely searched for during routine autopsies, frequency in a relatively unselected population cannot be determined. Increasing use of arteriography has provided an estimate of the incidence of renal artery aneurysms in this highly selected population, however, and has been estimated to approximate 0.09%.[34]

Renal artery aneurysms may result from atherosclerotic or fibromuscular dysplastic disease. The true cause of most

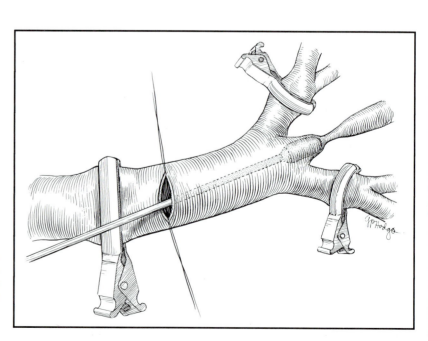

Figure 57-13. Technique of operative dilation of fibrodysplastic branch stenosis. Dilator inserted into main renal artery and through the branch stenosis. Arteriotomy is closed with interrupted sutures. (*From Rutherford RB (ed): Vascular Surgery. Philadelphia, WB Saunders Co., 1984.*)

macroaneurysms is unknown, and arteriosclerosis is usually a secondary process rather than an inciting cause.

The clinical significance of renal artery aneurysms relates to their casual or causal relationship to RVH and to the potential for rupture, with retroperitoneal hemorrhage and loss of a kidney but rarely with loss of life. In one study, rupture occurred among 5.6% of patients.[34] Although death after aneuysm rupture is very rare, pregnant women are particularly vulnerable, having a mortality rate greater than 50%.[35]

Hypertensive individuals who harbor renal artery aneurysms should be thoroughly evaluated for a renovascular origin of the hypertension, as outlined previously. Although the association of hypertension may approach 80%, amelioration of hypertension after aneurysm repair cannot be expected unless a coexisting hemodynamically and functionally significant stenotic lesion is identified and corrected as well.

Complications of renal artery aneurysms to be prevented by aneurysm excision and renal artery reconstruction include rupture, dissection, aneurysm, thrombosis, ureteral obstruction, erosion into an adjacent vein, and renal parenchymal emboli originating from aneurysm thrombus.

Although precise and objective indications for renal artery aneurysm repair are lacking, the following are accepted and justified: symptomatic aneurysms, aneurysms associated with RVH, aneurysms serving as embologenic foci, aneurysms in pregnant or childbearing-age women, dissecting aneurysms, and those documented to be enlarging on serial x-ray studies. Small (<2.0 cm in diameter) aneurysms that do not meet these criteria should be followed up and managed expectantly.[34,36]

Operative Techniques

The objective of renal artery aneurysm repair is excision of the aneurysm with preservation of the kidney. Location, size, and arterial branch involvement preclude recommendations for any single operative approach, and innovation, tailoring the operation to the patient, is important to successful renal artery reconstruction.

Because most renal artery aneurysms involve the bifurcation of the main renal artery, the surgeon must be prepared to repair the involved branches either by in situ or ex vivo reconstructive techniques. Autogenous saphenous vein, because of its plasticity, is preferred for these complex in situ reconstructions[37] (Fig. 57-14).

The three most commonly employed techniques are aneurysm excision plus (1) primary arteriorrhaphy or end-to-end anastomosis (Fig. 57-15), (2) aortorenal grafting (Fig. 57-14), and (3) patch graft angioplasty (Fig. 57-16). Exposure of the renal arteries is obtained as described in the discussion of aortorenal bypass reconstruction. Meticulous surgical technique, systemic heparinization, preocclusion administration of mannitol, low-tension microvascular clamps, fine suture material, and optical magnification are all commonly employed for renal arterial aneurysm repair. Most repairs can be accomplished without removing the kidney from its retroperitoneal position. However, occasionally ex vivo

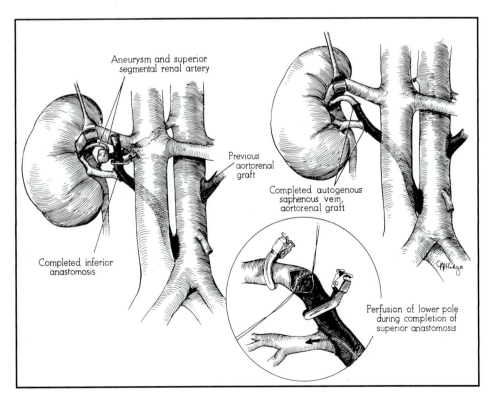

Figure 57-14. Technique of in situ repair of a renal artery aneurysm involving primary branches. (*From Ernst CB, Stanley JC, Fry WJ: Surg Gynecol Obstet 137:1023, 1973.*)

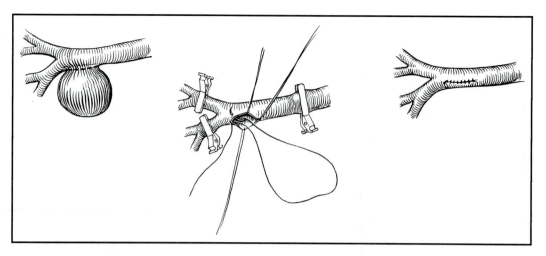

Figure 57-15. Technique of excision of distal main renal artery aneurysm, followed by primary arteriorrhaphy. (*From Bergan JJ, Yao JST (eds): Operative Techniques in Vascular Surgery. New York, Grune & Stratton, 1980.*)

reconstruction may be required, particularly when multiple primary branches are involved in the aneurysmal process.

Results of Renal Artery Reconstruction

Results of renal artery reconstruction depend largely on the overall condition of the patient and on the extent of the disease being treated. Issues that must be addressed are operative mortality rates, postoperative blood pressure responses, preservation and function of the kidney, and durability of the reconstruction.

Mortality Rates

Contemporary overall operative mortality rates for renal artery reconstruction range from 0.9 to 5.4% (Table 57-2). In analyses categorizing patients into specific subgroups—pediatric fibromuscular dysplasia, adult fibrodysplasia, arteriosclerotic focal renal artery disease, and clinically overt generalized arteriosclerosis—the operative mortality rate for all but those patients with generalized arteriosclerosis is zero (Table 57-3). It is apparent that because the results in patients with arteriosclerosis vary and depend on the extent of generalized arteriosclerosis, this category should not be considered as homogeneous.[27]

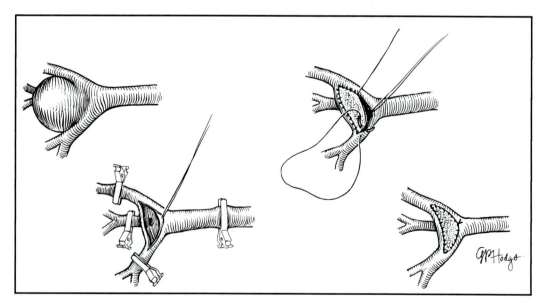

Figure 57-16. Technique of excising aneurysm arising from renal artery bifurcation. Vein patch and angioplasty ensures patulous reconstruction of primary renal arterial branches. (*From Bergan JJ, Yao JST (eds): Operative Techniques in Vascular Surgery. New York, Grune & Stratton, 1980.*)

TABLE 57-2. SURGICAL TREATMENT OF RENOVASCULAR HYPERTENSION

Institution	Time Period	No. of Patients	Ratio of Arteriosclerotic to Nonarteriosclerotic Disease	Operative Outcome (%)*			Surgical Mortality Rate (%)
				Cured	Improved	Failure	
University of California, Los Angeles[‡,49]	1958–1977	503	1.0/2.0	64	23	13	2.1
Baylor College of Medicine[50]	1959–1979	489	3.2/1.0	36	29	35	1.8
University of Michigan[51]	1961–1980	313	1.0/1.5	47	42	11	1.9
Cleveland Clinic[§,52–56]	1962–1978	225	1.5/1.0	50	34	16	3.1
University of Rome, University of L'Aguila[‖,57]	1960–1977	219	4.1/1.0	53	28	19	3.2
University of California, San Francisco[§,58,59]	1958–1977	128	2.0/1.0	39	34	27	1.6
University of Lund, Malmö Sweden[60]	1971–1977	125	1.1/1.0	55	25	20	0.9
Vanderbilt University[22]	1961–1972	122	1.8/1.0	59	31	10	5.4[¶]
Columbia University[†,61]	1962–1976	116	1.3/1.0	66	19	15	1.0
Hospital Alguelongue, Montpellier, France[62]	1965–1976	110	2.3/1.0	55	34	11	1.8
St. Mary's Hospital, London England[63]	Unstated	110	2.4/1.0	37	54	9	Unstated

* Criteria for blood pressure response usually defined in cited publications.
† Series includes 42 nephrectomies.
‡ Series includes 230 primary, secondary, or partial nephrectomies; stated mortality rate is from 1972–1977 experience (142 cases).
§ Data from overlapping publications; not inclusive of entire experience.
‖ Series includes 61 nephrectomies.
¶ Mortality rate from more recent experience was 0.5% among 200 reconstructions, excluding those associated with aortic surgery.
Adapted from Stanley JC, Ernst CB, Fry WJ (eds): Renovascular Hypertension. Philadelphia, WB Saunders Co., 1984, pp 363–371.

TABLE 57-3. SURGICAL TREATMENT OF RENOVASCULAR HYPERTENSION: RESULTS IN SPECIFIC PATIENT SUBGROUPS, 1961–1980*,[51]

Subgroups[†]	No. of Patients	Primary Operative Procedures		Operative Outcome[‡] (%)			Surgical Mortality Rate[§]
		Arterial Reconstruction	Nephrectomy	Cured	Improved	Failed	
Fibrodysplasia, pediatric	34	39	2	85	12	3	0
Fibrodysplasia, adult	144	160	6	55	39	6	0
Arteriosclerosis, focal renal artery disease	64	63	3	33	58	9	0
Arteriosclerosis, overt generalized disease	71	70	6	25	47	28	8.5[‖]

* Represents results of 405 operations (346 primary, 59 secondary).
† See text for subgroup definition.
‡ Effect of operation on blood pressure defined as follows: *cured* if blood pressure readings were 150/90 mm Hg or less for a minimum of 6 months, during which no antihypertensive medications were administered (lower pressure levels were used in evaluating pediatric patients); *improved* if normotensive while receiving drug therapy or if diastolic blood pressure readings ranged between 90 and 100 mm Hg but were at least 15% lower than preoperative levels (none of the improved patients were receiving converting enzyme inhibitors); *failure* if diastolic blood pressures were >90 mm Hg but <15% lower than preoperative levels, or >100 mm Hg.
§ Surgical mortality rate includes all deaths within 30 days of operation.
‖ Four of six deaths in this group were associated with concomitant aortic reconstructive surgery.
Adapted from Stanley JC, Ernst CB, Fry WJ (eds): Renovascular Hypertension. Philadelphia, WB Saunders Co., 1984, pp 363–371.

TABLE 57-4. FIBRODYSPLASTIC RENOVASCULAR HYPERTENSION, ADULTS

Institution	Time Period	No. of Patients	Operative Outcome* (%)			Surgical Mortality Rate (%)
			Cured	Improved	Failed	
University of Michigan[51]	1961–1980	144	55.0	39.0	6.0	0
Baylor College of Medicine[50]	1959–1979	113	43.0	24.0	33.0	0[†]
Cleveland Clinic[‡,53–56]	1962–1977	92	58.0	31.0	11.0	Unstated
University of California, San Francisco[48]	1964–1980	77	66.0	32.0	1.3	0
Mayo Clinic[64]	1968–1975	63	66.0	24.0	10.0	Unstated
Vanderbilt University[§,22]	1962–1972	44	72.0	24.0	4.0	2.3
Columbia University[61]	1962–1976	42	76.0	14.0	10.0	Unstated
University of Lund, Malmö, Sweden[60]	1971–1977	40	66.0	24.0	10.0	0

* Criteria for blood pressure response defined in cited publications.
† No deaths in 100 patients; mortality data on 13 additional patients with associated arteriosclerosis unstated.
‡ Data from overlapping publications, not inclusive of entire experience.
§ Series includes pediatric patients.
Adapted from Stanley JC, Ernst CB, Fry WJ (eds): Renovascular Hypertension. Philadelphia, WB Saunders Co., 1984, pp 363–371.

Blood Pressure Responses

Beneficial blood pressure responses mainly relate to proper patient selection and technical precision in performance of the reconstruction. Overall cure and improvement rates range from 65 to 91% (Table 57-2). Patients undergoing renal artery reconstruction for fibrodysplasia fare better than those with arteriosclerosis (Tables 57-4 and 57-5). Over 90% of patients with fibrodysplasia and focal renal arteriosclerosis can be expected to benefit from renal artery reconstruction.

Preservation of Renal Function

Apart from operative mortality rates and blood pressure responses, preservation or improvement of renal function after renal artery reconstruction has received little attention.

Intuitively, one would expect that improvement in renal blood flow should improve renal function.[38] In many instances, however, improvement in renal function is a consequence of better blood pressure control after renal artery reconstruction.[39] Nonetheless, statistically significant improvement in renal function has been documented among patients with poor function reflected by creatinine clearances of 15 ml/min or less.[40] In addition, among patients with a single functioning ischemic kidney, renal artery reconstruction preserves or significantly improves renal function.[41] Some have cautioned, however, that reconstruction of a unilateral stenosis of the "protected kidney" in an attempt to improve overall function in a severely azotemic patient is rarely beneficial unless both renal arteries are severely stenotic.[24]

TABLE 57-5. ARTERIOSCLEROTIC RENOVASCULAR HYPERTENSION, ADULTS

Institution	Time Period	No. of Patients	Operative Outcome* (%)			Surgical Mortality Rate (%)
			Cured	Improved	Failed	
Baylor College of Medicine[50]	1959–1979	360	34	31	35	2.5
University of Michigan[51]	1961–1980	135	29	52	19	4.4
University of California, San Francisco[59]	1963–1974	84	39	23	38	2.4
Cleveland Clinic[55]	1974–1980	78	40	51	9	2.0
Columbia University[61]	1962–1976	67	58	21	21	Unstated
University of Lund, Malmö, Sweden[60]	1971–1977	66	49	24	27	0.9
Hospital Aiguelongue, Montpellier, France[62]	1965–1976	65	45	40	15	1.1
Vanderbilt University[22]	1962–1972	63	50	45	5	9.0
Indiana University[65]	1973–1978	52	31	61	8	5.8

* Criteria for blood pressure response defined in cited publications.
Adapted from Stanley JC, Ernst CB, Fry WJ (eds): Renovascular Hypertension. Philadelphia, WB Saunders Co., 1984, pp 363–371.

Durability of Renal Artery Reconstruction

Since the initial description of long-term longitudinal arteriographic follow-up of aortorenal vein grafts by Ernst and colleagues,[42-44] several reports have verified the durability of renal artery reconstruction. In contemporary practice, postoperative graft thrombosis is a very rare event. Late stenoses requiring reoperation for recurrent RVH are similarly rare, affecting approximately 5% of grafts on late follow-up.[43,44] Uniform increases in graft size without saccular or concentric configurations have been defined as graft expansion.[42] About 20 to 40% of aortorenal vein grafts undergo expansion. Aneurysmal changes in aortorenal vein grafts, first reported in 1972,[42] affect 5% of such conduits. These alterations occur most frequently among children.[45-47] Because of the yet unknown but worrisome potential problems associated with aortorenal vein grafts in children, autogenous arterial segments, most commonly hypogastric artery, have been employed. Yet, such arterial segments do not appear immune to aneurysmal dilation, either.[46-48]

On balance, renal artery reconstruction has proved to be a durable procedure for the long term extending over 20 years. As such, it has an established place in vascular surgery.

REFERENCES

1. Bright R: Reports of medical cases selected with a view of illustrating symptoms and cure of diseases by a reference to morbid anatomy, vol 1. London, Longman, Rees, Orme, Brown and Green, 1827.
2. Mahomed FA: The etiology of Bright's disease and the prealbuminuric stage. Med Chir Trans 57:197, 1874.
3. Tigerstedt R, Bergmann PG: Niere und Krieslauf. Skandinar Arch Physiol 8:223, 1898.
4. Goldblatt H, Lynch J, et al.: Studies on experimental hypertension. I. The production of persistent elevation of systolic blood-pressure by means of renal ischemia. J Exp Med 59:347, 1934.
5. Leadbetter WF, Burkland CE: Hypertension in unilateral renal disease. J Urol 39:611, 1938.
6. Smith HW: Hypertension and urologic disease. Am J Med 4:724, 1948.
7. Freeman NE, Leeds FH, et al.: Thromboendarterectomy for hypertension due to renal artery occlusion. JAMA 156:1077, 1954.
8. dos Santos R, Lamas C, Caldas P: L'arteriographie des membres d'aorte et de ses branches abdominales. Med Contemp 47:93, 1929.
9. Smith PG, Rush TW, Evans AT: The technique of translumbar arteriography. JAMA 198:255, 1951.
10. Eyler WR, Clark MD, et al.: Angiography of the renal areas including a comparative study of renal arterial stenosis in patients with and without hypertension. Radiology 78:789, 1962.
11. Howard JE, Berthrong M, et al.: Hypertension resulting from unilateral vascular disease and its relief in nephrectomy. Bull Johns Hopkins Hosp 94:51, 1954.
12. Ernst CB, Bookstein JJ, et al.: Renal vein renin ratios and collateral vessels in renovascular hypertension. Arch Surg 104:496, 1972.
13. Judson WE, Helmer OM: Diagnostic and prognostic values of renin activity in renal venous plasma in renovascular hypertension. Hypertension 13:79, 1965.
14. Vaughn ED Jr, Buhler FR, et al.: Renovascular hypertension: Renin measurements to indicate hypersecretion and contralateral suppression, estimate renal plasma flow, and score for curability. Am J Med 55:402, 1973.
15. Stanley JC, Fry WJ: Surgical treatment of renovascular hypertension. Arch Surg 112:1291, 1977.
16. Ernst CB, Rutkow IM, et al.: Vascular surgery in the United States: Report of the Joint Society for Vascular Surgery–International Society for Cardiovascular Surgery Committee on Vascular Surgical Manpower. J Vasc Surg 6:611, 1987.
17. Gifford RW Jr: Epidemiology and clinical manifestations of renovascular hypertension, in Stanley JC, Ernst CB, Fry WJ (eds): Renovascular Hypertension. Philadelphia, WB Saunders Co., 1984, pp 77–99.
18. Stanley JC, Gewertz BC, et al.: Arterial fibrodysplasia: Histopathologic character and current etiologic concepts. Arch Surg 110:561, 1975.
19. Vander AJ: Renin-angiotensin system, in Stanley JC, Ernst CB, Fry WJ (eds): Renovascular Hypertension. Philadelphia, WB Saunders Co., 1984, pp. 20–45.
20. Simon N, Franklin SS, et al.: Clinical characteristics of renovascular hypertension. JAMA 220:1209, 1972.
21. Thornbury JR, Stanley JC, Fryback DG: Hypertensive urogram: A nondiscriminatory test for renovascular hypertension. AJR 138:43, 1982.
22. Foster JH, Dean RH, et al.: Ten years' experience with the surgical management of renovascular hypertension. Ann Surg 177:755, 1973.
23. Davidson J, Lowe B, et al.: Variability of split renal functional studies in essential and renovascular hypertension. Surg Forum 30:574, 1979.
24. Dean RH: Renovascular hypertension, in Moore WS (ed): Vascular Surgery. New York, Grune & Stratton, 1986, pp 561–592.
25. Ernst CB, Daugherty ME, Kotchen TA: Relationship between collateral development and renin in experimental renal arterial stenosis. Surgery 80:252, 1976.
26. Taylor DC, Kettler MD, et al.: Duplex ultrasound in the diagnosis of renal artery stenosis: A prospective evaluation. J Vasc Surg 7:363, 1988.
27. Ernst CB, Stanley JC, et al.: Renal revascularization for arteriosclerotic renovascular hypertension: Prognostic implications for focal renal arterial vs overt generalized arteriosclerosis. Surgery 73:859, 1973.
28. Stanley JC, Ernst CB, Fry WJ: Surgical treatment of renovascular hypertension: Results in specific patient subgroups, in Stanley JC, Ernst CB, Fry WJ (eds): Renovascular Hypertension. Philadelphia, WB Saunders Co., 1984, pp 363–371.
29. Tarazi RY, Hertzer NR, et al.: Simultaneous aortic reconstruction and renal revascularization: Risk factors and late results in eighty-nine patients. J Vasc Surg 5:707, 1987.
30. Moncure AC, Brewster DC, et al.: Use of the splenic and hepatic arteries for renal revascularization. J Vasc Surg 3:196, 1986.
31. Wylie EJ: Surgical treatment of renovascular hypertension: Renal artery endarterectomy, in Stanley JC, Ernst CB, Fry WJ (eds): Renovascular Hypertension. Philadelphia, WB Saunders Co., 1984, pp 309–314.
32. Fry WJ, Ernst CB, et al.: Renovascular hypertension in the pediatric patient. Arch Surg 107:692, 1973.
33. Fry WJ, Brink BE, Thompson NW: New techniques in the treatment of extensive fibromuscular disease involving the renal arteries. Surgery 68:959, 1970.
33a. Ernst CB: Childhood renovascular hypertension, in Kotchen TA, Kotchen TM (eds): Clinical Approaches to High Blood Pressure in the Young. Boston, John Wright. PSE, 1983, pp 151–173.
34. Stanley JC, Rhodes EL, et al.: Renal artery aneurysms. Arch Surg 110:1327, 1975.

35. Cohen JR, Shamash FS: Ruptured renal artery aneurysms during pregnancy. J Vasc Surg 6:51, 1987.

36. Hageman JH, Smith RF, et al.: Aneurysms of the renal artery: Problems of prognosis and surgical management. Surgery 84:563, 1978.

37. Ernst CB, Stanley JC, Fry WJ: Multiple primary and segmental renal artery revascularization utilizing autogenous saphenous vein. Surg Gynecol Obstet 137:1023, 1973.

38. Novick AC, Textor SC, et al.: Revascularization to preserve renal function in patients with arteriosclerotic renovascular disease. Urol Clin North Am 11:477, 1984.

39. Whitehouse WM Jr, Kazmers A, et al.: Chronic total renal artery occlusion: Effects of treatment on secondary hypertension and renal function. Surgery 89:753, 1981.

40. Dean RH, Englund R, et al.: Retrieval of renal function by revascularization: Study of preoperative predictors of outcome. Ann Surg 202:367, 1985.

41. McCready RA, Daugherty ME, et al.: Renal revascularization in patients with a single functioning ischemic kidney. J Vasc Surg 6:185, 1987.

42. Ernst CB, Stanley JC, et al.: Autogenous saphenous vein aortorenal grafts: A ten-year experience. Arch Surg 105:855, 1972.

43. Stanley JC, Ernst CB, Fry WJ: Fate of 100 aortorenal vein grafts: Characteristics of late graft expansion, aneurysmal dilatation, and stenosis. Surgery 74:931, 1973.

44. Dean RH, Krueger TC, et al.: Operative treatment of renovascular hypertension: Results after a follow-up of fifteen to twenty-three years. J Vasc Surg 1:234, 1984.

45. Stanley JC, Fry WJ: Pediatric renal artery occlusive disease and renovascular hypertension: Etiology, diagnosis, and operative treatment. Arch Surg 116:669, 1981.

46. Lawson JD, Boerth R, et al.: Diagnosis and management of renovascular hypertension in children. Arch Surg 112:1307, 1977.

47. Stanley P, Gyepes MT, et al.: Renovascular hypertension in children and adolescents. Radiology 129:123, 1978.

48. Stoney RJ, DeLuccia N, et al.: Aortorenal arterial autografts: Long-term assessment. Arch Surg 116:1416, 1981.

49. Kaufman JJ: Renovascular hypertension: The UCLA experience. J Urol 112:139, 1979.

50. Lawrie GM, Morris GC Jr, et al.: Late results of reconstructive surgery for renovascular disease. Ann Surg 191:528, 1980.

51. Stanley JC, Whitehouse WM Jr, et al.: Operative therapy of renovascular hypertension. Br J Surg (Suppl) 69:S63, 1982.

52. Noble MJ, Pechan BW, et al.: Unpublished data, personal correspondence, 1979.

53. Novick AC, Banowsky IH, et al.: Splenorenal bypass in the treatment of renal artery stenosis. Trans Am Assoc Genitourin Surg 69:139, 1978.

54. Novick AC, Straffon RA, et al.: Surgical treatment of renovascular hypertension in the pediatric patient. J Urol 119:794, 1981.

55. Novick AC, Straffon RA, et al.: Diminished operative morbidity and mortality in renal revascularization. JAMA 246:749, 1981.

56. Straffon R, Siegel DF: Saphenous vein bypass graft in the treatment of renovascular hypertension. Urol Clin North Am 2:337, 1975.

57. Stefanini P, Benedetti-Valentini F Jr, Fiorani P: Selection for surgery and long-term results in renovascular hypertension. Int Surg 63:73, 1978.

58. Lye CR, String ST, et al.: Aortorenal arterial autografts: Late observations. Arch Surg 110:1321, 1977.

59. Stoney RJ: Transaortic renal endarterectomy, in Rutherford RB (ed): Vascular Surgery. Philadelphia, WB Saunders Co., 1977, p 1001.

60. Bergentz SE, Ericsson BF, Husberg B: Technique and complications in the surgical treatment of renovascular hypertension. Acta Chir Scand 145:143, 1979.

61. Buda JA, Baer L, et al.: Predictability of surgical response in renovascular hypertension. Arch Surg 111:243, 1976.

62. Thevenet A, Mary H, Boennec M: Results following surgical correction of renovascular hypertension. J Cardiovasc Surg 21:517, 1980.

63. Snell ME: Renovascular surgery. Br J Hosp Med 24:130, 1980.

64. Hunt JC, Strong CG: Renovascular hypertension: Mechanisms, natural history and treatment. Am J Cardiol 32:562, 1973.

65. Lankford NS, Donohue JP, et al.: Results of surgical treatment of renovascular hypertension. J Urol 122:439, 1979.

CHAPTER 58
Portal Decompression

Allan D. Callow

HISTORICAL BACKGROUND

Despite intense study throughout the world since Whipple, some 40 to 45 years ago, applied the Eck-fistula principle to the treatment of portal hypertension, there has been little if any improvement in the survival of patients with portal hypertension due to hepatic cirrhosis.[1] Cirrhosis (from the Greek *kirrhos*, to describe the yellowish discoloration rather than the hardening of the liver) is the most common cause of portal hypertension in the Western world. Seventy-five percent of patients have a history of alcohol overuse.[2] Cirrhosis as a cause of death has steadily increased in the last two or three decades and is one of six leading causes of death in the United States. For men 35 to 54 years of age, it is the third leading cause.[3]

ANATOMY AND PHYSIOLOGY

The valveless portal vein, approximately 8 cm in length and 1.2 cm in diameter, begins at the confluence of the splenic and superior mesenteric veins deep to the head of the pancreas[3,4] (Fig. 58-1). A network of hilar splenic veins joins short gastric veins near the tail of the pancreas to form the splenic vein with its many small tributaries from the pancreas. The left gastroepiploic vein enters the splenic vein close to the spleen. The inferior mesenteric vein, draining the left colon and rectum, enters the middle third of the splenic vein. The left gastric or coronary vein joins the portal vein near its origin, although it may enter the splenic. A much smaller right coronary vein also enters the portal vein. The portal vein provides approximately two thirds of total hepatic blood flow and approximately 50% of hepatic oxygen need.

The hepatic artery is the second important afferent supply. The common hepatic artery originates from the celiac axis, gives off the right gastric artery, and ascends in the hepatoduodenal ligament to the left of the common bile duct and superior to the portal vein. It forms right and left branches to the left of the main lobar fissure. The portal vein at the same location divides into branches to each lobe.

An increase in portal pressure (from the accepted norm of 5 to 10 mm Hg or 60 to 140 mm of saline solution) with a normal inferior vena cava pressure of 0.5 to 4 mm Hg (or 7 to 55 mm saline solution) results in increased flow through the collateral circulation[5-10] (Fig. 58-2). Portal blood is diverted from the splanchnic to the systemic veins at areas where they are in juxtaposition to one another. These are the submucosa of the esophagus and proximal portion of the stomach, the rectum and its hemorrhoidal plexus, the umbilicus, and retroperitoneal locations involving the duodenal, lumbar, renal, and gonadal venous pathways. Of them all, the gastroesophageal network has been the subject of the greatest attention because of its propensity for bleeding.

Blood from the hepatic artery and the portal venous system mix within the hepatic sinusoid. This mixed blood enters the central vein of the hepatic lobule[6] (Fig. 58-3), passes through several generations of increasingly larger and shorter veins, and ultimately enters the major hepatic veins emptying into the vena cava.

ETIOLOGY AND PATHOPHYSIOLOGY

The commonest cause of portal obstruction in the Western world is cirrhosis of the liver. The three requirements for diagnosis are necrosis of the hepatocyte, fibrous tissue proliferation, and nodular islands of regenerating liver cells. Both micronodular and macronodular types are recognized, but the net result is diversion of blood flow within the liver.

Classification

Several *classifications of portal hypertension* have evolved. Each has limitations. The increasingly popular classification of presinusoidal, sinusoidal, and postsinusoidal is based on

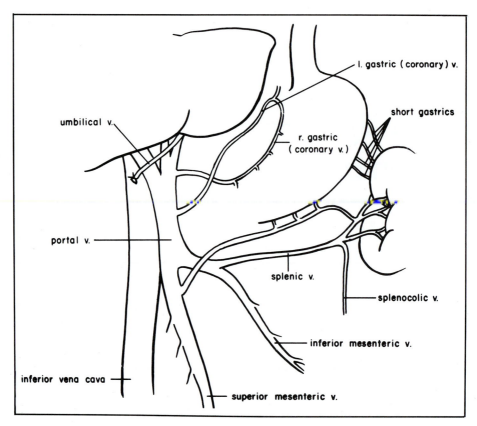

Figure 58-1. Anatomy of portal venous system. (*Adapted from Henderson and Warren*[3] *and from Way.*[4])

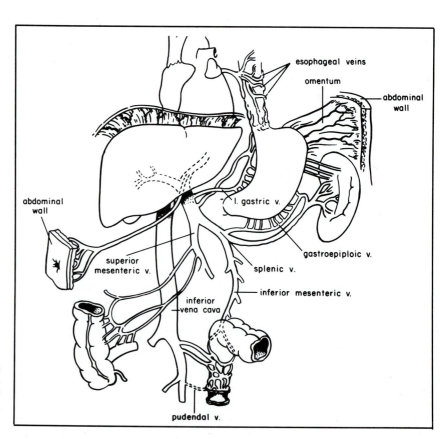

Figure 58-2. Collateral venous pathways and sites of splanchnic systemic communication. (*Adapted from McIndoe*[5] *in Sherlock,*[6] *Orloff*[7] *in Orloff,*[8] *and Sedgwick*[9] *in Brown and Busuttil.*[10])

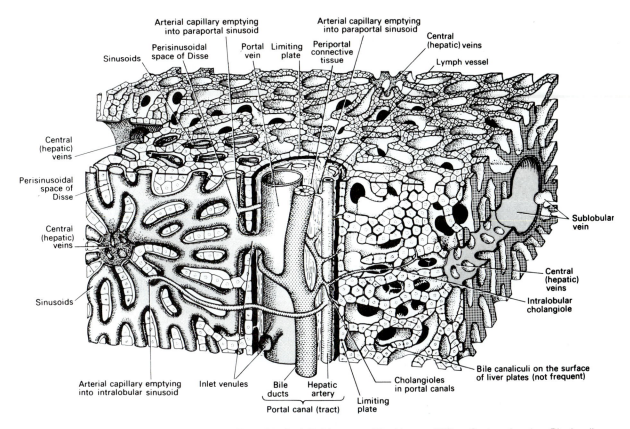

Figure 58-3. Circulation of hepatic lobule. (*From Sherlock S: Diseases of the Liver and Biliary System. London, Blackwell Scientific Publications, 1981.*)

the location of the increased resistance to portal flow[3] (Fig. 58-4). There may be substantial overlap between the presinusoidal and sinusoidal components in different types of cirrhosis. Presinusoidal block is usually associated with normal hepatic function, as opposed to the damaged hepatocyte in intrahepatic or sinusoidal obstruction. The simpler clinical classification of cirrhotic and noncirrhotic portal hyperten-

sion within its prognostic indications is, however, incomplete. The intrahepatic block of cirrhosis has a higher incidence of variceal bleeding than does extrahepatic obstruction such as portal vein thrombosis. A third classification simply identifies prehepatic, intrahepatic, and suprahepatic causes. Extrahepatic portal hypertension is caused by thrombosis of the portal vein or splenic vein or both.

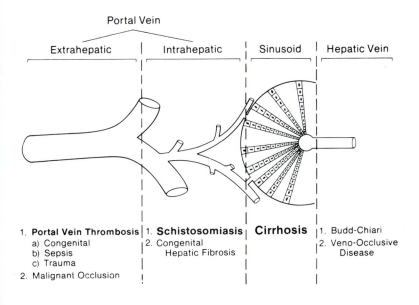

Figure 58-4. Sites of portal and hepatic block. (*From Henderson JM, Warren WD: Surgical complications of cirrhosis and portal hypertension, in Sabiston DC (ed): Textbook of Surgery: The Biological Basis of Modern Surgical Practice, 13th ed. Philadelphia, WB Saunders Co., 1986.*)

It may be of congenital origin, resulting from infection such as pylephlebitis or from trauma or malignancy.

Portal hypertension is most often due to an intrahepatic cause. Cirrhosis is the most frequent. Others are congenital hepatic fibrosis, various types of hepatitis, myeloproliferative disorders, and schistosomiasis.[11] The terminal portions of the portal vein radicals in the liver suffer fibrosis in these latter diseases.

The suprahepatic syndrome is based on obstruction of hepatic venous outflow[12] (Fig. 58-5). Various types of veno-occlusive disease, malignancies, right ventricular failure, and constrictive pericarditis may be the cause.

An uncommon cause of portal hypertension is increased blood flow into the hepatic system. This is associated with splenomegaly and, usually, normal liver function. The Cruveilhier-Baumgarten syndrome applies to patients with intrahepatic or parenchymatous disease, portal hypertension, and recanalization of the umbilical vein. Splenomegaly and caput medusae with a venous hum may be present. The syndrome is to be distinguished from the Cruveilhier-Baumgarten anomaly in which patients have not only a caput medusae but also an umbilical vein that is patent throughout its entire course. Portal hypertension is primary, whereas in the syndrome it is due to liver disease.[13]

Cavernous transformation of the portal vein[12,14,15] (Fig. 58-6), probably commoner than has been thought, is most likely a manifestation of portal vein thrombosis or thrombosis with partial recanalization. It may be a consequence of umbilical vein infection in infancy, or it may occur spontaneously because of sluggish flow through the portal vein, with the chance of thrombosis. In rare instances the portal vein may actually serve as an outflow tract.[4] *Hepatopetal* refers to the direction of flow into the liver in extrahepatic portal vein thrombosis (in the absence of liver disease).

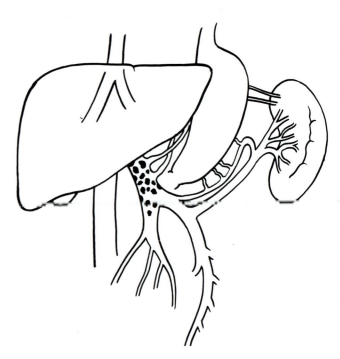

Figure 58-6. Infrahepatic (cavernomatous transformation) obstruction. (*Adapted from Fonkalsrud.*[12,14])

The flow proceeds around the point of occlusion through collateral vessels in the diaphragm and the hepatocolic and hepatogastric ligaments. *Hepatofugal* is the term applied to flow around the liver and into the systemic circulation in the presence of such intrahepatic disease as cirrhosis or portal vein thrombosis. It is the hepatofugal circulation that leads to excessive dilation of other collateral vessels, which results in esophagogastric varices.

Rarely, splenic vein thrombosis causes increased flow from the spleen to the stomach, resulting in gastric varices alone.

NATURAL HISTORY

Hepatitis

Most recent understanding of hepatitis[16] and its consequences stems from two studies. The first study documented the transmission of hepatitis to human volunteers,[17,18] which distinguished hepatitis A, the epidemic form of hepatitis, from hepatitis B, or homologous serum jaundice, and the second documented the transmission of hepatitis A to nonhuman primates,[19] with the consequent recognition of an antigen of hepatitis B virus (HBV) in human blood.[20] Viral hepatitis is important because it is the second commonest cause of intrahepatic cirrhosis and portal hypertension. Four forms are recognized: hepatitis A (HA), hepatitis B (HB), hepatitis non-A, non-B (HNANB), and those hepatitides of other microbial diseases. Synonyms for hepatitis A include infectious hepatitis, epidemic hepatitis, and short-incubation hepatitis. Hepatitis B is identified variously as serum hepatitis, homologous serum jaundice,

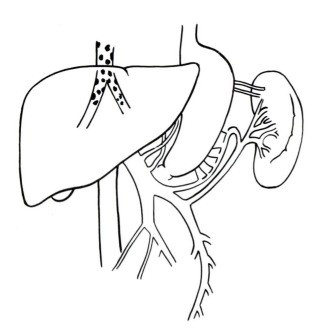

Figure 58-5. Suprahepatic obstruction. (*Adapted from Fonkalsrud.*[12])

transfusion hepatitis, the jaundice of heavy metal injections, and long incubation hepatitis. Hepatitis A never becomes chronic, whereas both hepatitis B and hepatitis non-A, non-B exist in carrier states. Chronic hepatitis B is the commoner cause of cirrhosis, which may include hepatocellular necrosis, fibrosis, and micronodular and macronodular regeneration. Alcoholic cirrhosis has been considered a form of "chronic active" hepatitis[21,22] and, as such, an irreversible progressive condition. Chronic hepatitis describes a process rather than a single disease entity. It may lead to cirrhosis and portal hypertension.[23] Primary biliary cirrhosis, of unknown cause and usually affecting middle-aged women, is characterized by slowly progressing cholestasis, increasing jaundice, and often death from hepatic failure.[24,25] Secondary biliary cirrhosis may be due to sclerosing cholangitis. Both types develop potentially fatal complications: hepatic failure, bleeding varices, fluid retention, and the hepatorenal syndrome. The duration of life from the time of diagnosis is approximately 3 to 5 years. Many patients recover from the acute phase only to suffer the chronic complications of cirrhosis and portal hypertension. For such a patient, a portal decompressive operation may be of value. Careful selection is necessary because sclerosing cholangitis, primary biliary cirrhosis, and hepatolenticular degeneration—Wilson's disease—are usually fatal.[26–30]

Wilson's disease[31–35] is characterized by accumulation of copper in the liver, brain, and kidney, with acute and chronic degenerative organ changes. Although the initial episode may suggest self-limiting viral hepatitis, months to years later the liver and spleen are found to be enlarged. Liver function tests are relatively normal. Hemorrhage from unsuspected varices may herald the disease. Chronic hepatic encephalopathy may be due to large portal systemic shunts. The classic sign is a brown or gray smudge in Descemet's membrane known as the Kayser-Fleischer corneal ring. If Wilson's disease is untreated, it is invariably fatal. Penicillamine forms a soluble chelate with copper, which is then excreted by the kidneys.[36,37] Treatment of the parenchymatous liver disease and its consequences, portal hypertension, hypersplenism, and bleeding varices, is no different from the management of these same complications of other hepatic disorders.

Much of the natural history of cirrhosis remains unknown. The autoimmune response[22] of the alcoholic liver requires further investigation. Possibly only 10 to 15% of alcoholics develop cirrhosis. Many alcoholics do not develop portal hypertension, and of those who do, many do not bleed from varices. Among those who do bleed, however, the mortality rate is high. As many as 66% may be dead 1 year from diagnosis, and 80% may die with the first hemorrhage. Although esophagogastric varices are present in about 70% of patients with cirrhosis, they are responsible for gastrointestinal bleeding in only 30%.[38] Women are more susceptible to the development of alcoholic cirrhosis than men, they acquire it at a younger age, with a shorter history of drinking, and most of them die of hepatocellular failure. By contrast, the predominant causes of death in men are variceal bleeding, intractable ascites, and encephalopathy.[39,40]

Established cirrhosis is characterized by extensive fibrous tissue scarring. It is an end stage of the disease and

is beyond treatment. Five-year survival rates are comparable to those of various malignancies: 16% survival at 3 years and 8% at 5 years.[16,41,42] From the onset of ascites, jaundice, or bleeding, the 5-year survival rate is approximately 5%. By contrast, among 348 patients, most of whom were in Child's group B, who underwent a therapeutic selective distal splenorenal shunt, the 5-year survival rate was 59%.[43]

There is little difference in the survival rates of patients with alcoholic or nonalcoholic cirrhosis who are treated with a nonselective shunt. A difference does become apparent, however, with the distal splenorenal shunt. Here, the median survival rate of the alcoholic patient with cirrhosis is 57 months. More than 50% of nonalcoholic cirrhosis patients who survived the selective shunt were still alive 8 to 9 years later.[43–46]

Hemorrhage

Variceal bleeding is a frequent cause of death.[16,42] In the Boston Inter-Hospital Liver Group Study, esophageal hemorrhage was responsible for one third of the deaths, hepatic failure for a second third, renal failure for 11%, infection for 9%, and miscellaneous causes for the remainder. Although survival with bleeding is more dependent on the severity of the liver disease than on any other single factor, there is little information that a patient with more severe liver disease bleeds more frequently than do others with less severe disease. Among the Child's group A, B, and C patients, the frequencies of rebleeding in groups A and B were similar. Patients with grade C disease had more bleeding episodes than did those with grade A or B disease, but the difference was without statistical significance.

There is little more than anecdotal information as to why some varices bleed and others do not. It is most common at the esophagogastric junction. Here, connective tissue support is less, the varices are more superficial than in the upper part of the esophagus and in the stomach, there may be pressure differences to which the varix is exposed as one moves from the abdomen to the thoracic cavity, and there may be an erosive effect because of gastric reflux.[47–49] Cimetidine should be beneficial, but this has not been established in control series.[50]

The beta blocker propranolol has produced confusing and sometimes conflicting results with a substantial reduction in rebleeding episodes in two studies and no benefit in a third.[51–53] Child's group A patients seemed to be helped more than groups B and C. Beta-receptor blockers should not be used, for fear of producing severe hypotension in the patient with decompensated liver disease.[54]

Ascites

Ascites signals increasing liver failure and limited life expectancy, with bacterial peritonitis, renal failure, and the hepatorenal syndrome resulting ultimately in death. Ascites is frequent in sinusoidal obstruction because of an increase in sinusoidal and intrahepatic pressure and an increase in pressure in the portal and splanchnic veins. Movement of fluid occurs from the intravascular to the extravascular spaces in the entire gastrointestinal tract, and the mesentery may shed water into the peritoneal cavity. There may be an increase of hepatic lymph. Hypoalbuminemia with decreased plasma oncotic pressure may contribute to the development of ascites because a low concentration of plasma albumin impairs resorption of fluid from the extravascular compartment. Decreased glomerular filtration and an alteration in the levels of circulating plasma renin, angiotensin, and aldosterone contribute to sodium retention. Low urinary volume and low urinary sodium are characteristic. Combined hepatic and renal failure is characterized by increasing salt and water retention, oliguria, rising levels of blood urea nitrogen and creatinine, and an elevated bilirubin level. This hepatorenal syndrome is often intractable and ultimately fatal. The survival rate in patients with chronic ascites is as poor as in those with esophageal bleeding.

Other causes of ascites include constrictive pericarditis, tricuspid valve incompetence, peritoneal carcinomatosis, pseudocyst of the pancreas, chylous ascites, and tuberculous peritonitis.

Medical Treatment of Cirrhosis

Modifying the alterations in sodium and water metabolism and correcting the malnutrition usually present in cirrhosis are the objectives. Frequent measurement of urinary sodium, volume, and body weight are necessary if sodium balance is to be achieved, because in the patient with ascites, virtually all ingested sodium ends up in the ascitic fluid. There will be 1 kg of edema fluid for each 120 mEq of ingested sodium.[55] A concentration of 5 mEq/L is evidence of severe sodium retention. Single abdominal taps in which several liters of ascitic fluid are removed, although providing patient comfort, may result in severe hypotension. Serum sodium and albumin levels fall with hemorrhage, and ascitic fluid rapidly reaccumulates.[56,57] Spironolactone and triamterene are helpful but relatively ineffective in refractory ascites.[58] Impaired renal function restricts the use of potassium supplements.

Ascites refractory to good in-hospital therapy is best treated with a peritoneovenous shunt.[59,60] Shunt complications include disseminated intravascular coagulopathy, bacterial peritonitis, variceal bleeding, and congestive heart failure. Rarely, side-to-side portacaval shunt may be needed. The end-to-side shunt may increase sinusoidal pressure in patients with spontaneous reversal of portal flow. The preferred side-to-side anastomosis diverts splanchnic blood away from the liver, may improve hepatic outlow via the portal vein into the vena cava, and substantially reduces sinusoidal pressure.[61,62] It is particularly indicated in the patient with intractable ascites and variceal bleeding.[63-67]

Encephalopathy

Chronic hepatic encephalopathy, as distinguished from the transient episode occurring with any physiologic stress such as variceal hemorrhage, ranks with refractory ascites and fixed elevation of the serum bilirubin level as a predictor of limited survival. Encephalopathy may be of mild degree, with apathy, changes in affect, and inappropriate behavior, including, in the more severe cases, involuntary flapping of the fingers and wrists, so-called asterixis,[68] episodic confusion, disorientation, and drowsiness. Light coma may develop, with fetor hepaticus, hyperreflexia, grimacing, trismus, and sucking reflexes. In deep coma, there is no response to external stimuli, the limbs are flaccid, and the reflexes are depressed. The electroencephalogram shows reduction of the normal dominant alpha rhythm of 8 to 13 cps and high-voltage paroxysmal theta or slow waves. These changes may also be seen in other metabolic derangements, particularly uremia and hypoglycemia.

The pathogenesis is clearly multifactorial, involving shunting of portal venous blood into the systemic circulation and the combined and cumulative effects of a number of metabolic and physiologic impairments in the susceptible brain of the cirrhotic patient.

Although encephalopathy may be spontaneous, the most frequent precipitating cause is gastrointestinal hemorrhage. Infection, often occult in the immunosuppressed cirrhotic patient, and constipation, a root cause of absorption of protein breakdown products, are common offenders. Nitrogenous by-products within the systemic and the splanchnic circulations should be reduced. The colon should be cleared by repeated enemas. Bacterial content should be reduced by administration of neomycin or metronidazole. Lactulose has gained favor as a replacement for neomycin and is administered in doses of 20 to 30 g three or four times daily.[69] Dietary intake of protein should be severely curtailed to less than 20 g per day. Reversal of the encephalopathy occurring as a complication of an end-to-side portacaval shunt, by operative obliteration of the shunt, has been reported. The risk/benefit ratio of reducing encephalopathy by a surgical maneuver that increases the risk of variceal bleeding, is difficult to balance.[70] Conflicting results are reported with the use of L-dopa, a dopamine precursor, and bromocriptine, a dopamine agonist.[71-76] Various forms of colon bypass[77] with or without partial colectomy have been abandoned. There was no significant difference in long-term survival rates between surgically and medically managed groups in the Boston Inter-Hospital trials of 1968, although patients in the surgical group were able to enjoy a higher intake of protein than those treated medically.[78,79]

Encephalopathy is a far more frequent complication of portacaval shunt, whether end-to-side or side-to-side, than of distal splenorenal shunt. The more severe the liver disease, the greater is the likelihood encephalopathy will occur. The elderly patient is so frequently incapacitated by encephalopathy after a portacaval shunt that it should be performed only in exceptional circumstances, such as truly uncontrollable hemorrhage.[77]

PATIENT EVALUATION

The degree of hepatic functional reserve in Laennec's cirrhosis determines survival not only in the natural course of the disease but also after variceal hemorrhage and surgical intervention. Only a few tests are needed. The correlation

TABLE 58-1. CLINICAL CLASSIFICATION OF CIRRHOTIC PATIENTS AS CANDIDATES FOR PORTOSYSTEMIC SHUNT

	Risk		
Criterion	Good (A)	Moderate (B)	Poor (C)
Serum bilirubin (mg/dl)	<2.0	2.0–3.0	>3.0
Serum albumin (g/dl)	>3.5	3.0–3.5	<3.0
Ascites	None	Easily controlled	Poorly controlled
Encephalopathy	None	Minimal	Advanced, "coma"
Nutrition	Excellent	Good	Poor, "wasting"

From Child CG III: The Liver and Portal Hypertension. Philadelphia, WB Saunders Co., 1964.

between reduction of the serum albumin level and the severity of disease is high, because albumin is produced only by the liver. The serum alanine aminotransferase (ALT) level is elevated in the presence of hepatic damage and is more reliable for diagnosis than the serum aspartate aminotransferase (AST) level, because ALT, unlike AST, is much more concentrated in the liver than in skeletal muscle, kidney, pancreas, and myocardium.

Chronic elevation of the serum bilirubin level is a sign of advanced disease. The serum bilirubin and albumin levels, plus the presence of ascites and encephalopathy and the patient's nutritional status, are the items used in Child's evaluation[80] (Table 58-1).

There is confusion concerning the influence of active cellular necrosis on the surgical mortality rate, especially when the necrosis is the result of acute alcoholic hepatitis or chronic active hepatitis, as evidenced by the presence of hyaline in the liver biopsy specimen.[81–84] Needle biopsy of the liver and measurement of portal blood flow have not been as useful in predicting survival, whether after operation or in the natural course of the disease, as have Child's criteria. Adding the serum transaminase determination strengthens Child's classification by providing some indication of active liver cell necrosis.[85,86] (Table 58-2).

Assessment of the hemodynamics of portal flow is of questionable usefulness because preoperative estimation is difficult and there has been little correlation with postoperative encephalopathy and long-term survival.[87–89] Wedged and free hepatic venography, splenoportography (by injection directly into the splenic pulp), celiac and mesenteric angiography, and transhepatic portal venography have all been developed to evaluate hepatic hemodynamics. Although information is gained about portal pressure, direction of flow, spontaneous portal systemic shunts, and anatomic relationships for shunt surgery, most of these tests are not worth the expense and effort when used on a routine basis. They are of greater investigative than clinical value. The wedged hepatic venogram provides a measurement of venous pressure,[90] which correlates well with portal pressure, but, as with free hepatic venography, which reveals how many hepatic veins can be filled and thus the degree of cirrhosis, there is little correlation with operative mortality rate and duration of life. Other causes of portal hypertension can usually be excluded by less invasive and less costly procedures than selective celiac, superior mesenteric, and hepatic angiography. Splanchnic angiography is of value when endoscopic findings are uncertain. In the venous phase, it is useful in determining whether or not there is extrahepatic portal or splenic vein thrombosis.

Transhepatic portography, in which a catheter is passed by means of a guidewire through the portal vein into the splenic or superior mesenteric veins, permits portal vein pressure measurements, indicates the direction of flow and the important contributions of the coronary and short gastric veins, and may also provide an opportunity to occlude, by the use of sclerosing agents or embolization, the coronary and short gastric veins in the patient with a bleeding varix.[91–94] In one series, 71% of most class C patients with bleeding varices who failed to respond to vasopressin had their bleeding controlled by occlusion of these veins; the survival rate was 50% at 1 month. Sclerosing and embolization procedures allow time for the patient to be given supportive therapy, recover from the hepatic failure associated with variceal hemorrhage, and be better prepared for decompressive shunt surgery. Thrombosis may, however, extend into the portal vein, thus precluding creation of a surgical shunt.[95]

Hypersplenism or congestive splenomegaly, once regarded as a distinct entity known as Banti's disease, and probably due to an autoimmune mechanism, is indicated by leukopenia, with a leukocyte count of less than 2,000/mm^3, and thrombocytopenia, with a platelet count of 50,000 or less. Anemia may be present but may have any of several causes. There is sequestration and destruction of platelets, leukocytes, and to some extent erythrocytes. The diagnosis of hypersplenism should not be discarded merely because the spleen is not substantially enlarged.[96]

TABLE 58-2. RESULTS OF 81 PORTOSYSTEMIC SHUNTS BY CLINICAL RISK GROUPS

Group	Operative Mortality Rate (%)	Survival Rate (%) >3 yr	Survival Rate (%) >5 yr	Total No. of Patients
A	15	62	47	34
B	43	20	11	35
C	58	8	8	12

From Smith GW: Evaluation of patients with portal hypertension, in Rutherford RB (ed): Vascular Surgery, 2nd ed. Philadelphia, WB Saunders Co., 1984.

Approximately half of the patients with parenchymatous cirrhosis will have coexisting gastritis and peptic ulcer disease.[97] Thus esophageal varices may not be the source of bleeding, and careful endoscopic examination is essential. Twenty percent of bleeding varices may be gastric.[98] Barium swallow is probably the least reliable test, because it does not localize the active bleeding point.

There are two additional considerations in the selection of patients for operative intervention. There is an increased risk of rupture with a large varix,[47] and surgical therapy for variceal bleeding is approximately twice as costly as medical management. Medically treated patients, however, have more hospital readmissions and are less likely to return to gainful employment than patients who survive surgery.[99]

MANAGEMENT OF ESOPHAGEAL VARICES

Variceal Hemorrhage

Time is of the essence in the management of actively bleeding esophageal varices due to cirrhosis, because the immediate mortality rate, usually due to liver failure, is approximately 50%. By contrast, when the varices are due to extrahepatic portal obstruction, death from hemorrhage is uncommon. Bleeding from esophageal varices is usually severe, whereas it is only mild to moderate with gastritis and duodenal ulcer. It is a misconception that there is no urgency in establishing a diagnosis because in most patients conservative treatment is sufficient. Were it not for secondary liver failure, this might be so. However, correct diagnosis is critical to the plan of therapy and should be made on an urgent basis. Neither barium swallow with upper gastrointestinal tract radiography nor various types of visceral angiography are as useful as expert endoscopy.[100] Selective angiography can identify an active arterial bleeding site. Two thirds of patients will have another hemorrhage within 24 hours of the first variceal hemorrhage, which underscores the need for early management decisions. Intravascular volume replacement with crystalloid and whole blood should commence immediately. Fresh blood is superior to bank blood because fresh blood supplies some still unidentified coagulation factors and does not have the ammonia and potassium that accumulate in stored blood. Blood within the gastrointestinal tract should be removed by gastric lavage and enemas. The administration of a rapid-acting laxative such as magnesium citrate and the administration of neomycin or lactulose or both by nasogastric tube and by enema may also further retard ammonia production. Hypertonic glucose with vitamins C and B complex should be given intravenously. Careful and frequent serum electrolyte determinations must be performed to detect and treat the hypokalemic alkalosis that may develop. Sodium-containing intravenous and lavage solutions compound hepatic and renal failure and contribute to ascites and edema. Neither iced water nor saline solution is superior to these fluids given at room-temperature in arresting hemorrhage. After insertion of a nasogastric tube, vasopressin is administered by the intravenous route at a rate of 0.2 units per minute. The dose is doubled if a significant decrease in bleeding does not occur within 30 to 45 minutes. Higher doses and selective mesenteric intraarterial vasopressin are not enough better to outweigh the systemic side effects and other complications. The infusion is continued at the optimal level for 12 hours after cessation of bleeding and then reduced incrementally until discontinued 12 to 24 hours later. About 70% of patients will stop bleeding, but about the same number will bleed again; thus the hospital discharge survival rate is only approximately 50%.[101] The role of other pharmacologic agents such as somatostatin and propranolol[102,103] has not been precisely established, because the initial enthusiastic reports have been followed by more equivocal results.

Pharmacologic failure is an indication for balloon tamponade. Whether only the gastric balloon should be inflated initially and the esophageal balloon inflated later if bleeding does not stop is probably determined by experience. Tamponade is also indicated in the emergency department when the hemorrhage appears to be exsanguinating. With tamponade, there is a risk of pulmonary aspiration.[104] Tracheobronchial catheter aspiration through the opposite nostril provides some control, which is also available with the Edlich and the Linton-Nachlas tubes. For the obtunded patient, endotracheal intubation is necessary. Proper use of balloon tamponade, which means meticulous monitoring throughout the time it is in place, is associated with 75 to 90% control of the acute hemorrhage. As with the pharmacologic agents, however, about 50% of these patients resume bleeding,[105,106] and the discharge survival rate is no better.

Injection sclerotherapy is difficult in the face of active variceal hemorrhage, even for the skilled surgical endoscopist. Although a success rate of up to 93% has been reported, in some series the hospital mortality rate was 22%.[107] With the use of balloon tamponade, followed immediately by injection sclerotherapy, control of variceal bleeding was achieved in 95% in a second series.[108] Most institutions do not achieve this degree of success.

Although an aggressive sclerotherapy program imposes a substantial work load on the hospital staff, two recent reports indicate its effectiveness. Of 81 patients followed up for a mean of 14 months, 48 had 202 further bleeding episodes, which resulted in nine deaths. Surgical intervention was required 21 times but not for the remainder. Thirty-six patients required tamponade in their initial bleeding episodes.[109] In a second prospective, randomized trial of long-term endoscopic therapy versus distal splenorenal shunt, 71 patients with cirrhosis were hospitalized because of acute variceal bleeding. Alcoholic cirrhosis was present in 61% and nonalcoholic in 39%. All patients were stabilized with blood transfusions, vasopressin, or emergency sclerosis. Distal splenorenal shunt was performed in 35 patients, and 36 were treated with sclerosis.[110] Endoscopic therapy is associated with a high incidence of rebleeding, but it does not contribute to hepatic failure. The distal splenorenal shunt controls bleeding exceptionally well, but hepatic function continues to deteriorate, although at a much slower rate than in patients who have the portal systemic or central splenorenal shunt. The 2-year survival rate of patients treated with sclerosis was significantly better than that of patients treated with a distal splenorenal shunt, with 31 of 36 patients treated with sclerosis alive versus 21 of 35 treated by a shunt. There were 4 operative deaths in the shunt group, and of the 10 later deaths, 8 were due to hepatic failure. Sclerotherapy was recommended as initial therapy for variceal bleeding, and selective shunting was reserved for uncontrollable rebleeding.[110,111]

Percutaneous transhepatic embolization of varices, although associated with a considerable degree of early success in expert hands, has largely been abandoned. Catheterization of the portal vein and its identification by direct venography are achieved through transhepatic puncture. The veins feeding the varices, together with the left gastric and the short gastric veins, are selectively catheterized and obliterated, usually with some form of absorbable gelatin sponge and the patient's own clot or human thrombin. Ultrasonography or venography is required to be certain that the portal vein is patent.[112,113] Limiting features are a rebleeding rate of about 70% and possible thrombosis of the portal vein, rendering it unfit for a subsequent shunt.[95] It is further limited in the presence of ascites. Creation of a distal splenorenal shunt is also precluded should the short gastric veins deliberately or inadvertently be thrombosed.

If all of these measures fail to control bleeding for the class A or B patient, an emergency portacaval or mesocaval shunt should be performed. The extremely high operative mortality rate in Child's group C patients limits emergency surgery to class A and B patients.

Transesophageal ligation of bleeding varices usually gives satisfactory acute control, but the incidence of rebleeding is high. Superimposed on this are the morbidity and mortality rates associated with a major surgical procedure in high-risk patients.[114,115] In the only available control study,[115] emergency variceal ligation consistently controlled hemorrhage, and the survival rate was 54%. Medically treated patients in the same randomized study had a survival rate of only 14%. It is a misconception that surgical variceal ligation has a lower morbidity rate than emergency shunt operations have.

Although bleeding was promptly controlled in 95% of patients undergoing emergency portacaval anastomosis and only 2% had subsequent bleeding, the operative mortality rate of 42% in this series[116] has not been matched by others. In a later experience with 84 patients, the same investigators obtained an operative survival of 83% and a 5-year survival rate of 72%.[8] The following were statistically significant negative risk factors:

1. Ascites on admission
2. ALT of 100 units or higher
3. Sulfobromophthalein sodium (BSP) retention >50% in 45 minutes
4. Hypokalemic alkalosis with an arterial blood pH of 7.5 or greater and a serum potassium level <3.5 mEq/L
5. Requirement of 5 L or more of blood transfusion before and during operation
6. Consumption of alcohol within 7 days before admission.

The operative survival rate of these 17 patients, with this advanced stage of alcoholic cirrhosis, was 47%; however, at 1 year only 18% were alive.

Because of metabolic derangement of multiple organ systems, the postoperative emergency portacaval shunt patient is usually desperately ill. Constant meticulous monitoring of fluid balance and blood gas values, blood and serum

protein levels, pulmonary function, and the need for tracheostomy is required. A hyperdynamic cardiovascular state and severe cardiac output failure often occur. Delerium tremens must be distinguished from hepatic encephalopathy. Intravenously administered alcohol or parenterally administered paraldehyde is contraindicated and is ineffective. Central nervous system depressants such as intramuscular magnesium sulfate or chlordiazepoxide hydrochloride (Librium) are preferable.

There is no specific therapy for progressive liver failure. Only parenteral nutritional support can be offered. Acute tubular necrosis is common. The patient will have oliguria, azotemia, hyperkalemia, a low urine specific gravity and osmolality, and casts and erythrocytes in the urine sediment. Stringent fluid restriction and hemodialysis may help. Less easily recognized and usually fatal is the hepatorenal syndrome.[117–119] The urine is nearly void of sodium, the osmolality is high, there is normal sediment, and the urine specific gravity is widely variable. No therapeutic modality, including the use of diuretics or vasoactive agents to improve flow or the use of hemodialysis, has substantially altered mortality rates.

Elective Nonoperative Therapy and Long Term Management

The natural history of esophageal varices correlates strongly with the degree of hepatic deterioration and the number and severity of repeated variceal hemorrhages. In the alcoholic cirrhotic patient, particularly with continuing use of alcohol, recurrent bleeding 3 or 4 years after the first hemorrhage is in excess of 70%.

Conservative medical management consists of frequent follow-up visits in an effort to provide reinforcement for continuing abstinence from alcohol, avoidance of infections, and improved nutrition. That liver function can be improved by meticulous adherence to such a regimen is demonstrated by a study in which 50% of class C patients had improved sufficiently to be reclassified in group B. Ascites, present in 82% on entry, fell to 30%. Of 14 patients with admission encephalopathy, the abnormality continued in only one. This program of abstinence and nutritional support could be provided only in a hospital setting in these socially deprived patients.[120]

In experienced hands, repeated sclerotherapy gives satisfactory to excellent results. The recommended regimen after emergency sclerotherapy or other nonsurgical means of controlling bleeding is a second injection within 1 week and at 1- to 2-week intervals thereafter until "the varices have been eradicated."[121] Complete endoscopy should be done each time, not only to assess the number and presence of varices, but also to look for ulceration of the esophageal and gastric mucosa, each of which precludes reinjection in the underlying varix. If the varices have been eradicated, outpatient endoscopy at 6 months or yearly intervals is recommended. Lifelong follow-up is required. Effective sclerotherapy over the life of the patient is very successful in preventing recurrent bleeding and does not impair liver function. Inadvertent thrombosis of portal and splenic veins may occur because of "leakage" of sclerosing agents into these vessels with repeated injections over the life of the patient. Details of the techniques and the instrumentation are the subject of numerous reports.[108,112,122-125]

The prophylactic shunt has no place in long-term management of portal hypertension except possibly for veno-occlusive disease, because only one fourth to one third of patients with demonstrated varices will bleed if their history does not include one episode of bleeding. Thus prophylactic shunt subjects some two thirds to three fourths of patients to an operation they may never need. There is no improvement in survival rates between patients with and those without prophylactic shunt.[120,126-128] The same observation, that only one fourth to one third of patients with varices will bleed, applies to prophylactic sclerotherapy, although two series have shown good results.[129,130]

Elective Operative Therapy

Devascularization and Ablative Procedures

The history of ablative gastroesophageal transection and reanastomosis and of devascularization procedures is extensive and mostly of historical interest.[131,132] Except in a few centers, the operative mortality rate and the incidence of recurrent bleeding have made these operations unattractive both for long-term management and for emergency treatment of hemorrhage. Of the many operations, total gastrectomy, esophagogastrectomy, portoazygos disconnection, and various ablative and devascularization procedures are essentially the same in terms of objectives. With rare excep-

tions, all are associated with high mortality and rebleeding rates. They do permit continuing perfusion of the liver, however, and there are fewer cases of encephalopathy than are seen after the standard portacaval and central splenorenal shunt procedures. Three operations deserve more detailed discussion: the Hassab, Sugiura, and ablative operations.

The Hassab Operation. The upper half of the stomach is devascularized in an attempt to disconnect the esophagogastric varices and preserve a portion of portal venous flow. The operation is combined with splenectomy. In some series the mortality rate has been high[108,133-135] (Fig. 58-7)

The Sugiura Operation. A great deal of attention has centered around the very extensive operation developed by Sugiura in Japan.[136,137] Through thoracic and abdominal incisions in one or two stages, transection and devascularization of the esophagus and esophagogastric junction are performed, together with splenectomy and pyloromyotomy.[136] As many as 30 to 50 periesophageal veins may have to be divided. The vagus nerve is preserved. The esophagus is partially transected at the level of the diaphragm, leaving the posterior wall intact. Varices in the region are oversewn, and the anterior wall of the esophagus is closed without suturing the mucosa. Sugiura's operative mortality rate of 4.6% in elective cases and 20% in urgent cases has rarely been achieved by surgeons in the West[133,136-139] (Fig. 58-8).

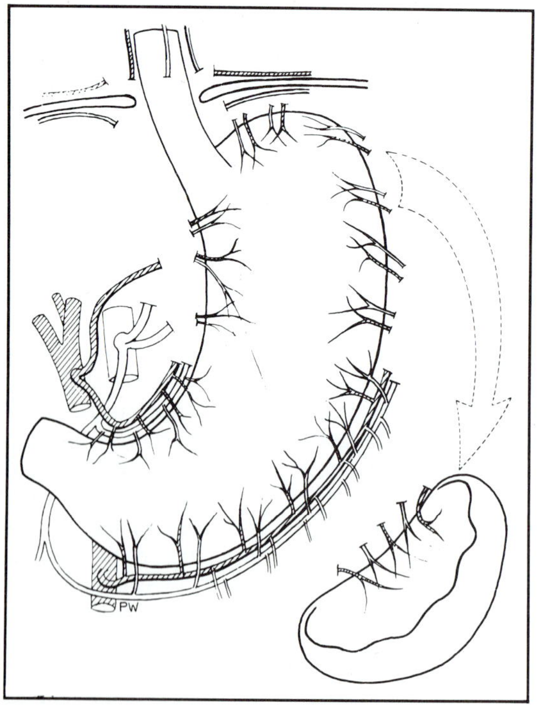

Figure 58-7. Upper gastric devascularization and splenectomy, as performed by Hassab. (*Adapted from Terblanche.*[133])

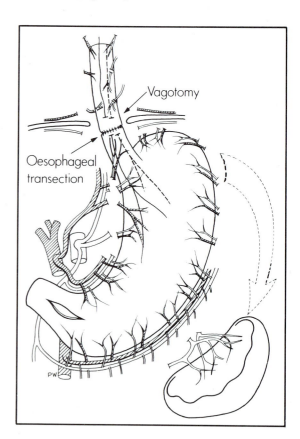

Figure 58-8. The Sugiura operation. (*Adapted from Terblanche.*[133])

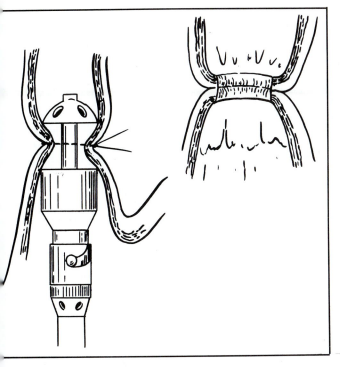

Figure 58-9. Esophageal transection with EEA stapling via gastrotomy and completion anastomosis. (*Adapted from Terblanche.*[133])

Ablative Operations. Experience in this country suggests that ablative operations without simultaneous complete disconnection of the mucosal, submucosal, and extrinsic venous systems of the esophagus will not prevent recurrent variceal bleeding.[140] The EEA stapler has revived interest in the transection procedure, which disconnects varices in the lower part of the esophagus and in the collateral channels[133,141–144] (Fig. 58-9).

For class C patients and emergency control of hemorrhage, esophageal transection and ablative operations with or without transection are of little or no benefit. Operative morbidity and mortality rates are substantial. There is no improvement over sclerotherapy alone. However, for the patient with satisfactory liver function and with no veins appropriate for shunting, and in whom sclerotherapy has failed, ablative operations with esophageal transection may be acceptable.[135,136,145–153] "Shunts control bleeding; ablative procedures buy time."[3]

Shunting Procedures

End-to-Side Portacaval Shunt. This modification of the Eck fistula of 1877 is probably the simplest of all shunts to construct. With the patient in the lateral decubitus position and the right arm elevated and supported over the head, a long right subcostal incision is made from the lateral border of the rectus to the latissimus muscle. The hepatoduodenal ligament is palpated to identify the hepatic artery and the underlying portal vein, which because of high pressure is readily compressible between the index finger in the foramen of Winslow and the overlying thumb. The portal vein is encircled and dissected free from where it bifurcates in the porta hepatis to the point where it issues from behind the head of the pancreas. The right colon is packed away inferiorly. The retroperitoneal space is entered opposite the lateral aspect of the duodenum, which is reflected medially, and the filmy areolar tissue overlying the inferior vena cava is exposed. The portal vein is suture ligated at its bifurcation. The splanchnic end of the vein is anastomosed in end-to-side fashion to the anteromedial aspect of the inferior vena cava after excision of a small elipse of 2 to 4 cm of the anterior vena cava wall. An everting running mattress suture with 6–0 synthetic suture material is used for the posterior wall and tied at each end to prevent a purse-string effect. The anterior row consists of carefully placed everting mattress or interrupted sutures[3] (Fig. 58-10). The splanchnic and splenic beds are decompressed, but sinusoidal pressure within the liver remains high.[154,155]

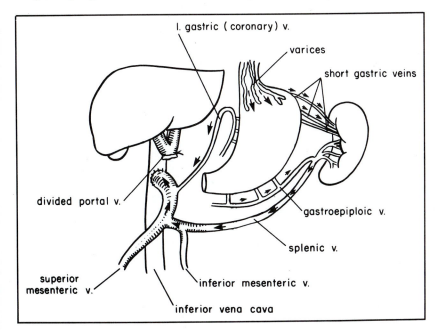

Figure 58-10. End-to-side portacaval shunt. (*Adapted from Henderson and Warren.*[3])

Side-to-Side Portacaval Anastomosis. Although the side-to-side shunt is technically somewhat more difficult than the end-to-side, it is rare that it cannot be constructed except when the liver is huge. The approach and exposure remain the same as in the portacaval shunt, except that the vena cava should be exposed circumferentially and one or two pairs of high lumbar veins should be divided and ligated to lift the vena cava from its bed and bring it closer to the portal vein. The vena cava then becomes more mobile than the portal vein. A 2.5 by 1 cm elipse should be removed from the anteromedial wall of the vena cava and the portal vein. Appropriate "atraumatic" vascular clamps are applied to isolate a generous length of portal vein, and a side-to-side partially occluding clamp is placed on the vena cava. The cava clamp is placed oblique to the long axis to avoid angulation. Before the last few stitches of the anastomosis are placed, as in the performance of an end-to-side portacaval shunt, the portal vein should be flushed to remove any thrombus behind the clamps. Vena cava flow is restored, followed by opening of the portal vein[156] (Fig. 58-11). A side-to-side shunt is preferable to an end-to-side shunt in the presence of ascites. Only with failure of medical management, together with failed peritoneovenous shunts, is ascites an indication for this shunt. The side-to-side, mesocaval, mesorenal, and mesosplenorenal shunts are all distinguished from the end-to-side portacaval shunt by the conversion of the portal vein to an outflow tract of the liver. The side-to-side shunt provides intrahepatic decompression but also serves as an arteriovenous fistula diverting hepatic artery inflow away from the hepatocyte. Neither the end-to-side nor the side-to-side shunt maintains prograde portal perfusion. Both shunts are associated with an appreciably high incidence of postoperative encephalopathy. In the modern management of portal hypertension in the adult alcoholic cirrhotic patient, they have little if any place.[157]

Mesocaval and Mesorenal Shunt. This operation was introduced by Marion[158] and by Clatworthy et al.[159] in the early 1950s for children in whom the splenic vein was too small for construction of a satisfactory anastomosis. Probably the best results have been obtained by Drapanas[160] and associates.

Although direct anastomosis between the superior mesenteric vein and the vena cava is possible, the operation is facilitated by an interposition prosthetic graft, usually made of Dacron or expanded polytetrafluoroethylene, with a diameter of 10 to 20 mm. Too small a diameter may provide insufficient decompression of the varices despite the effort to maintain prograde portal flow. A C-shaped graft was devised[161] on the basis of the observation that the superior mesenteric vein commonly branches at the level of the third portion of the duodenum, leaving a relatively small vessel for anastomosis. The H graft, the C graft, and the mesorenal shunt, as with the side-to-side portacaval shunt, assist in the management of ascites, promptly decompress the portal system and varices, and permit the option of surgical removal should postoperative encephalopathy be impossible to manage medically.[43,162] Mesocaval shunts probably have their best place in the relief of esophageal variceal hemorrhage in children, but they have little to offer over the standard portacaval shunt in terms of survival, recurrence of bleeding, hepatic encephalopathy, and accelerated hepatic failure in the adult. Its usefulness in children is because of the greater frequency of extrahepatic portal hypertension due to occlusion of the portal vein. In this situation, it is very effective. It is not a first choice in the treatment of the adult cirrhotic patient, however, because of the high incidence of thrombosis of synthetic grafts in the venous system. The contention that the mesocaval graft is a technically easier procedure than a conventional end-to-side or side-to-side portacaval shunt is probably based on limited experience with the latter.[163]

Interpositional Mesocaval H Graft. Through a midline incision, the transverse mesocolon is elevated superiorly and the small bowel packed aside below. Superior mesenteric vessels are approached through the peritoneum at the root of the small intestine mesentery. Small venous collateral branches to the mesenteric vein must be carefully ligated and divided. The superior mesenteric vein is anterior and to the right of its accompanying artery. A large intestinal lymphatic trunk is often found to the right of the superior mesenteric vein, from which troublesome leaks may occur if it is not ligated. The anterior surface of the vena cava is approached through the right transverse mesocolon, rather than through mobilization of the right colon. Only partial exposure of the vena cava is required before a partially occluding clamp can be used. The duodenum is mobilized medially to lessen the chance of compressing the graft. It is technically easier to perform the vena cava anastomosis

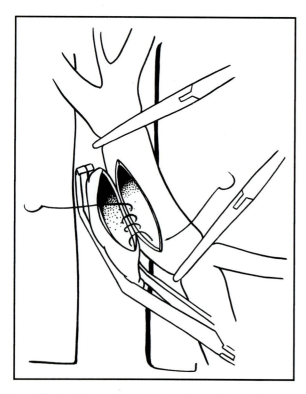

Figure 58-11. Side-to-side portacaval shunt with everting running mattress sutures on posterior wall. *(Adapted from Turcotte.[156])*

first, by means of a continuous 5–0 or 6–0 synthetic suture. Then, if the type of graft used requires it, the graft is preclotted by allowing vena cava blood to enter it momentarily.

Because of the 20- to 30-degree counterclockwise angulation of the superior mesenteric vein in relation to the vena cava, the graft is rotated some 20 to 30 degrees clockwise, and a short length of graft, 3 to 5 cm, is then anastomosed to the posterior surface of the mesenteric vein, with completion of the posterior row of sutures from within the anastomosis[160,161,164–166] (Fig. 58-12).

The more proximal superior mesenteric vein, because of its larger diameter, can be used if a longer C-shaped graft is created.[161,167] These grafts are now favored over the end-to-side caval or iliac superior mesenteric anastomoses, which required division of the inferior vena cava or iliac branch.[158] All of these grafts function as side-to-side or nonselective shunts. Although the meoscaval H-shaped graft was once recommended for emergency control of hemorrhage, the small size of the superior mesenteric vein limits the effectiveness of the shunt. Previous right upper quadrant surgery, infection, a large liver, or a fibrotic portal vein may be indications for these shunts. Operative mortality and long-term survival rates are nearly identical to those associated with the standard portacaval shunt. The incidence of postoperative thrombosis is probably higher than with portacaval shunts.

Despite anatomic and technical variations, the physiologic characteristic of all types of portacaval decompressions is total or partial diversion of splanchnic flow through the hepatic vein to the hepatocyte. The reduction of variceal hemorrhage is countered by acceleration of hepatic failure.

Proximal or Central Splenorenal Shunt. Functioning as a side-to-side splanchnic systemic shunt, the central splenorenal shunt provides no advantage over the portacaval or mesocaval varieties. Two claims have been made in its behalf: that it was associated with a lower incidence of postoperative encephalopathy, and that it maintained prograde hepatic flow.[168,169] Later angiographic follow-up studies failed to demonstrate continuing hepatopetal flow[169–171] (Fig. 58-13).

Arterialization of Liver. Imaginative and innovative attempts to improve hepatic blood flow in the face of total portal vein diversion by arterialization of the distal portal vein stump have been disappointing.

Maillard et al.,[172,173] in 1968, offered the combination of a portacaval shunt and arterialization of the hepatic stump of the portal vein. The splenic artery was anastomosed to the hepatic stump of the portal vein. When the procedure was performed in class A and B patients, the operative mortality rate was 17%. At 1 month, one third of these arteriovenous anastomoses had thrombosed. Adamsons,[174] on the basis of this experience and animal experimentation, recommended this procedure, stating that it has distinct advantages over conventional operations of total portal systemic diversion because of the alleged improved protein tolerance and a diminished incidence of postshunt hepatic

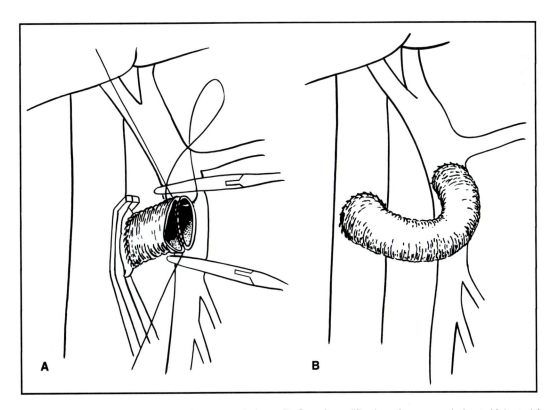

Figure 58-12. A. H graft modification of mesocaval shunt. **B.** C graft modification of mesocaval shunt. (*Adapted from Cameron*[161] *and from Drapanas*[165] *in Sanfey.*[166])

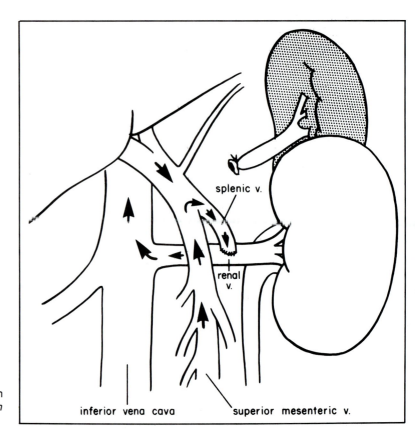

Figure 58-13. Diagrammatic representation of central splenorenal shunt. (*Adapted from Linton*[170] *in Malt.*[171])

encephalopathy. In Maillard's experience, thrombosis developed in the majority of patients appropriately studied, either in the anastomosis or in intrahepatic branches of the portal vein; the incidence of encephalopathy in patients with a patent anastomosis was 17%.

A wide variety of technical maneuvers have been proposed, briefly tried, and largely discarded. The common maneuvers include introduction of arterial blood to the intrahepatic circulation, the use of interpositional saphenous vein grafts between the right gastroepiploic artery and the hepatic stump of the portal vein, end-to-side splenic artery and restored umbilical vein anastomosis, the use of aortoportal vein prosthetic shunt, and the simpler end-to-end splenic artery portal vein anastomosis. These maneuvers have all been combined with conventional portal decompressive shunts.[173,175,176]

Because of these findings and the introduction of the distal splenorenal shunt, these operations have fallen into disfavor.[169,177–184] The incidence of encephalopathy has been disappointingly high. Most of the shunts have been followed by thrombosis because of the limited flow through the cirrhotic liver, and in some instances, there has been acceleration of liver failure, presumably because of excess arterial inflow to the hepatocyte. Therefore, the hepatic arterialization operations have largely been abandoned.

Distal Splenorenal Shunt. Recognition that diversion of portal blood by portacaval shunts accelerated liver failure and increased both the incidence and severity of hepatic encephalopathy as the price for control of variceal bleeding led to the development of selective decompression by Warren et al.[153] in 1966.

Because of compartmentalization of the portal venous system between the territory drained by the splenic vein and that drained by the superior mesenteric vein, only the variceal bed is decompressed and splanchnic flow continues to the liver. The objective of the operation is to separate these two compartments as completely as possible. The splenic end of the divided splenic vein is anastomosed in end-to-side fashion to the left renal vein. Venous return from the esophagus and stomach traverses the short gastric and left gastroepiploic veins and, by way of the spleen and splenic vein, enters the caval circulation. No significant reduction in superior mesenteric or portal venous flow or in pressure occurs[10,185] (Fig. 58-14).

TECHNIQUE. No better description of the details of construction of the distal splenorenal shunt can be provided than that by Warren et al.[3,110,153,186–188] Highlights are depicted in Fig. 58-15. The abdomen is opened through a generous bilateral subcostal incision with division of the falciform ligament to facilitate exposure and begin the portoazygos disconnection. Dividing the gastrocolic omentum begins the approach to the splenic vein and pancreas. Dissection of the splenic vein should be done on the vein, and a sufficient length should be isolated to avoid kinking of the anastomosis. The pancreas should be rotated anteriorly and the fine splenic pancreatic venous branches individually isolated and ligated or clipped in continuity. Division of the ligament of Treitz facilitates exposure of the left renal

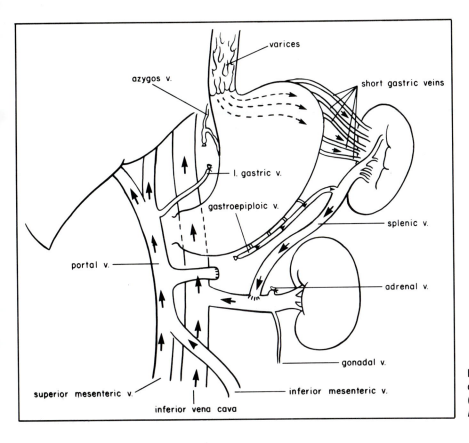

Figure 58-14. Schematic representation of selective (distal) splenorenal shunt. (*Adapted from Salam*[185] *and Brown and Busuttil.*[10])

vein just above the fourth portion of the duodenum. Adrenal vein division improves mobilization. The splenic renal vein anastomosis should avoid both redundancy and buckling. A continuous posterior and an interrupted anterior row of sutures will avoid a purse-string effect.

The development of a "pancreatic siphon" a year or two after operation led to the creation of splenopancreatic disconnection.[189] Large portal-splenic collateral venous pathways may develop 1 to 2 years after operation, with consequent loss of portal and splanchnic venous perfusion. There is also the loss of "pancreatic hepatotropic" factors.[190] There is slow reduction in liver mass[3,191] (Figs. 58-16 and 58-17).

The distal splenorenal shunt accomplishes selective decompression of the gastroesophageal varices, preserves prograde portal flow to the liver, and reduces the incidence of recurrent variceal hemorrhage. It is alleged that hepatotrophic substances from the gut continue to nourish the liver, that potential toxic substances from the gut are harmlessly metabolized, and that by the continuance of the high portal perfusion pressure in the intestinal venous bed, there is decrease in the potential absorption of "toxic substances."[187]

The creation of a distal splenorenal shunt is an operation that requires meticulous attention to operative detail and a degree of skill not often attained by the occasional surgeon.

On the basis of present understanding, variceal decompression is best achieved by selective or distal splenorenal shunt.[2,15,192,193] Nevertheless, from multiple nonrandomized and several randomized studies, overall results, although distinctly better than those of all other types of shunt, are not up to the high theoretic expectations.[43,191,194,195] In mixed groups of alcoholic and nonalcoholic cirrhotic patients, the distal splenorenal shunt, when performed electively, is associated with an operative mortality rate of 7%, an early patency rate of 90%, and control of variceal bleeding in about 90%. Alcoholic cirrhotic patients have a 5-year survival rate of about 45% and the nonalcoholic of 70%.[195] On the basis of the patient's ability to return to work and a reasonably normal life-style, distal splenorenal shunt is clearly superior to the total diversion shunts. Presumably because adequate portal perfusion was continued, and despite the development of collateral venous pathways, encephalopathy was present in only 5% of survivors. There is, however, no statistically significant difference in 10-year survival rates between total portal systemic diverting shunts and distal splenorenal shunts[3] (Fig. 58-18).

In most series the distal splenorenal operation has been used in low-risk patients with mild to moderate liver disease and good blood flow. Ascites, if it responds to diuretics, is not a contraindication. Although insufficient time and numbers of patients have accumulated to permit thoroughly reliable conclusions, the distal splenorenal operation does prevent variceal bleeding in the great majority of patients. In two studies, rebleeding occurred in 29% and 26%, respectively.[196,197] Thus the selectivity of the distal shunt may be lost in time. Portal perfusion may diminish.[198,199]

In a recent report of a randomized study, Warren and his group[110] discussed preliminary results of a prospective randomized trial comparing endoscopic variceal sclerosis

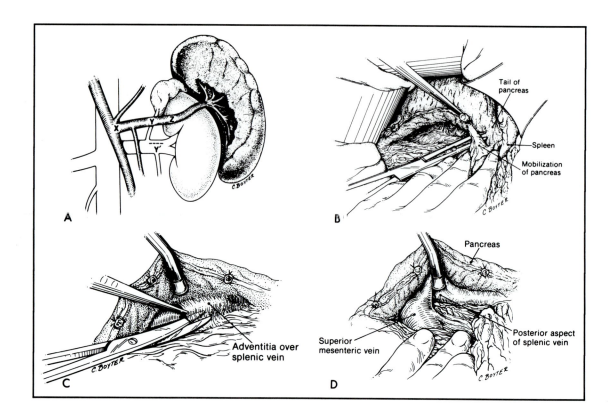

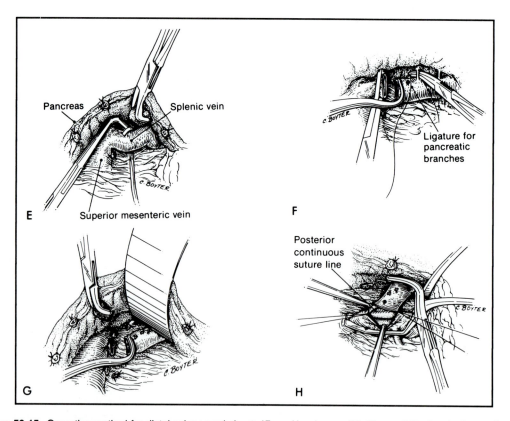

Figure 58-15. Operative method for distal splenorenal shunt. (*From Henderson JM, Warren WD: Surgical complications of cirrhosis and portal hypertension, in Sabiston DC (ed): Textbook of Surgery: The Biological Basis of Modern Surgical Practice, 13th ed. Philadelphia, WB Saunders Co., 1986.*)

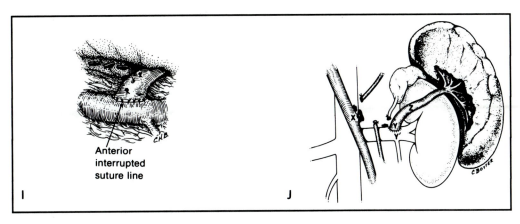

Figure 58-15, cont'd.

therapy with distal splenorenal shunt in patients with cirrhosis and variceal bleeding. Fifty-six percent of patients were in Child's class A or B and 44% were in class C. Cirrhosis was caused by alcoholism in 61% and had other causes in 39%. Median follow-up was 26 months. Provided that surgical backup is available for uncontrolled bleeding, the early survival rate in patients with cirrhosis of mixed causes and severity, with recurrent variceal bleeding, is significantly improved. After sclerotherapy, the rate of rebleeding was 53% and the failure rate 31%, in comparison with a rebleeding rate of 3% after a distal shunt. As measured by galactose elimination capacity, hepatic function was significantly better in the sclerotherapy patients, in comparison with the shunt patients, at a 1-year follow-up test. The authors recommend that, at this time, initial therapy for variceal bleeding and cirrhosis should be sclerosis; the selective shunt should be reserved for patients in whom uncontrollable rebleeding occurs. It is of further interest

that the condition of sclerotherapy patients improved "between the time of randomization and the need for crossover to surgery."[110] As an illustration of the need for prospective controlled randomized trials, in contrast to previous experiences, the alcoholic and the nonalcoholic patients did not differ in their general response and preoperative portal perfusion was basically equal in both. Inasmuch as sclerotherapy does not control the bleeding of gastric varices or "gastritis," these abnormalities are a major indication for crossover from sclerotherapy to the shunt.

SPECIAL SITUATIONS

Portal Hypertension in Children

There are few if any more emotion-packed experiences for the pediatrician, surgeon, and fear-ridden parents than that

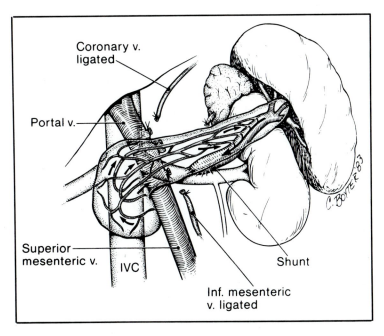

Figure 58-16. "Pancreatic" siphon. These collateral venous pathways from portal vein to intrapancreatic splenic vein have been demonstrated to develop 1 to 2 years after distal splenorenal shunt. (*From Henderson JM, Warren WD: Surgical complications of cirrhosis and portal hypertension, in Sabiston DC (ed): Textbook of Surgery: The Biological Basis of Modern Surgical Practice, 13th ed. Philadelphia, WB Saunders Co., 1986.*)

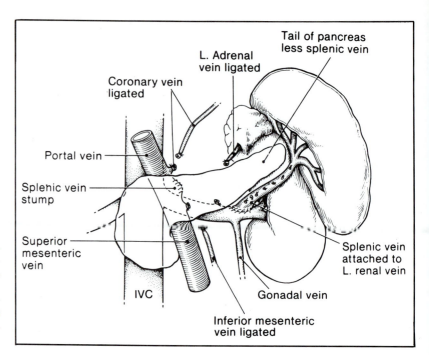

Figure 58-17. Diagram of details of spleno-pancreatic disconnection. (*From Henderson JM, Warren WD: Surgical complications of cirrhosis and portal hypertension, in Sabiston DC (ed): Textbook of Surgery: The Biological Basis of Modern Surgical Practice, 13th ed. Philadelphia, WB Saunders Co., 1986.*)

presented by the frightened child who has suffered a massive esophageal hemorrhage. Fortunately, the child with portal hypertension due to extrahepatic obstruction rarely has impairment of liver function. Children tolerate hemorrhage far better than do adults with cirrhosis. Upper gastrointestinal tract hemorrhage among children is most commonly due to portal hypertension, which is almost always due to portal vein thrombosis. The superior mesenteric and splenic veins may be involved. The usual explanation for portal vein thrombosis is neonatal omphalitis and intraabdominal infection. In about another 50% of children, portal hypertension develops because of congenital or acquired intrahepatic disease, of which cirrhosis is the most common cause in Western countries. The cirrhosis may be due to

hepatitis, extrahepatic biliary atresia, and unknown causes. Although congenital "hepatic fibrosis" is a not uncommon cause of portal hypertension, liver function is usually normal, and the disorder may therefore be confused with the extrahepatic type of portal hypertension.

Intrahepatic causes also include schistosomiasis, "chronic" hepatitis, and the Budd-Chiari syndrome. Many of these disorders are progressive and ultimately fatal. Liver transplantation may be preferable to some type of portosystemic shunt. For the child with extrahepatic portal hypertension, and for whom transplantation need not be considered, one of the questions to be asked is whether the child will "outgrow" the bleeding tendency.[200,201] Reports are anecdotal. A few children do outgrow it, but most do not. Should

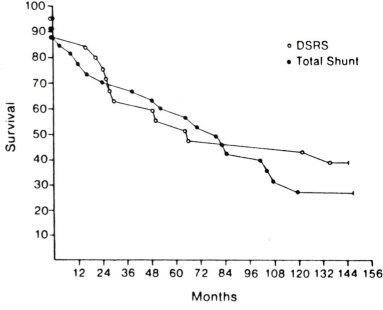

Figure 58-18. Survival rates up to 10 years do not differ significantly between total (central) and distal splenorenal shunts. Incidence of encephalopathy is lower in group that underwent distal splenorenal shunt. (*From Henderson JM, Warren WD: Surgical complications of cirrhosis and portal hypertension, in Sabiston DC (ed): Textbook of Surgery: The Biological Basis of Modern Surgical Practice, 13th ed. Philadelphia, WB Saunders Co., 1986.*)

the child therefore be given multiple blood transfusions, which are necessary to allow him or her to grow to an age where vessel size is sufficient to permit a successful portosystemic decompressive shunt? The extensive experience of the Biçetre Hospital, in France, indicates that 80% of children with portal obstruction experience at least one episode of bleeding and that approximately 40% of these episodes occur before the age of 3 years. In the Biçetre Hospital experience, the endoscopic signs of an increase in the risk of bleeding are (1) "tense" esophageal varices, (2) severe congestion of the esophageal mucosa, and (3) gastric varices.[202] The risk that accompanies multiple bleeding episodes and multiple transfusions must be balanced against the risk of decompressive shunt surgery or sclerotherapy.[12] Portal vein thrombosis is usually diagnosed on the basis of hemorrhage or splenomegaly before 6 years of age.[12] The majority of these patients suffer more than one hemorrhage per year, and the peculiar and unexplained factor is the relationship between hemorrhage and upper respiratory tract infections. In a series of 253 patients, no child died during the first variceal hemorrhage,[12] thus reinforcing the opinion that exsanguinating hemorrhage is uncommon.

Splenomegaly and ascites are the second and third, respectively, most frequent findings suggesting portal vein thrombosis.

Most patients should be managed with temporizing supportive therapy until they reach an age when the splanchnic vessels are large enough to permit construction of a satisfactory shunt.[203] Treatment requires hospitalization with absolute bed rest, antacids, intravenous rather than oral feedings, and administration of vitamin K if appropriate. Only infrequently are systemic vasopressin and sclerotherapy needed.[108,203] Parents should be advised against aspirin.

Recanalization of thrombus within the portal vein is never complete. Thus cavernomatous transformation usually precludes surgical decompression by portal-systemic shunt, and on the rare occasion that flow is achieved, it is so limited that postoperative thrombosis is frequent. Gastroesophageal devascularization, the Sugiura operation,[136] surgical ligation of the bleeding varices, partial esophagogastrectomy, and colon interposition operations have been devised and have had reasonable success.[14,15,204,205] Splenectomy is ill advised because of the increased frequency and severity of infection in later years. It also limits choice of a decompressive surgical procedure. There is a high incidence of rebleeding with splenectomy alone.

Thorough visualization of the portal and splenic venous anatomy is mandatory in planning surgical intervention. Division of the inferior vena cava at the level of the iliac bifurcation or division of the proximal iliac vein for additional length permits anastomosis of the proximal end of the vena cava or iliac vein to the side of the superior mesenteric vein (Marion-Clatworthy shunt).[158,159] Chronic venous insufficiency in the lower extremities usually occurs with time. The mesocaval shunt with an internal jugular vein H graft is the shunt of choice at the Biçetre Hospital in France. Primary hepatic disease suggested by a history of jaundice and, in addition, hepatomegaly, splenomegaly, ascites, and laboratory evidence of impaired liver function

are indications for a liver biopsy to establish the diagnosis of intrahepatic portal obstruction.[8]

Management of portal hypertension is largely determined by the prognosis attached to the underlying liver disease. In contrast to extrahepatic block, the first variceal hemorrhage in children with intrahepatic disease carries a mortality rate of approximately 40%.[12] Survival for many years after decompressive operations has been reported despite the progressive intrahepatic obstruction of posthepatic cirrhosis and liver failure. Provided that the vessels are large enough to permit a satisfactory shunt, successful results have been reported with end-to-side, side-to-side,[206] and mesocaval H shunts and by the distal splenorenal shunt.[199,202,207,208] The devascularization and transection procedures have largely been abandoned, partly because of the greater recent success of shunt surgery and the high incidence of recurrence of varices in the transection procedure.[202] Sclerotherapy is recommended by some as a preferred treatment in children not only when a shunt is not possible but as the initial treatment of a bleeding varix. Serial sclerotherapy, successful in over 90% of patients, does have the complications of hemorrhage, ulceration, and stricture. For the child with good liver function and a nonprogressive form of liver disease, an appropriate shunt is preferred as the initial therapy.[202]

Budd-Chiari Syndrome

Hepatic vein thrombosis with obstruction of hepatic venous outflow is a complication of a number of intraabdominal and systemic disorders.[209,210] These include the endophlebitis originally described by Chiari, obstruction of the inferior vena cava, thrombosis of hepatic veins due to congenital lesions such as atresia, web or membrane formation,[211] neoplasms originating near or metastasizing to the hepatic veins or inferior vena cava, and a variety of infections including schistosomiasis and amebic abscess. Hepatic vein thrombosis has been reported in association with blood dyscrasias, such as polycythemia rubra vera and paroxysmal nocturnal hemoglobinurea, and as a rare complication of pregnancy after the prolonged use of oral contraceptives.[38,212–214] Obstruction of the hepatic venous outflow from whatever cause results in intrahepatic, portal, and splanchnic hypertension with dilation of the sinusoids of the liver, congestion, ischemia, and atrophy of a centrilobular type. Persistence of postsinusoidal pressure leads to irreversible parenchymatous damage with fibrosis and cirrhosis. In many cases the syndrome develops acutely, reaching an irreversible stage within a few weeks to months with a fatal outcome. Possibly in one half to two thirds of patients the syndrome follows a more insidious course, and the diagnosis cannot be established without inferior vena caval and hepatic phlebography. Abdominal pain, ascites, hepatomegaly, anorexia, and wasting are the usual manifestations. In approximately half the cases, no underlying cause can be found. In the acute form, the patient may complain of abdominal pain and severe anorexia; the rapid onset of ascites and rapid demise may ensue. In the chronic form, the patient may survive as long as a few years. In the patient with postsinusoidal obstruction due to suprahepatic ob-

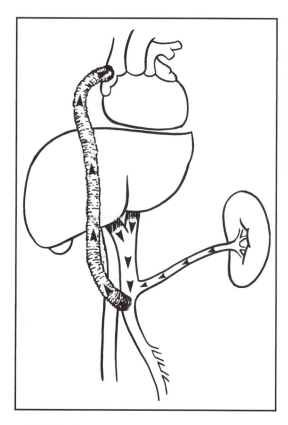

Figure 58-19. In the presence of intrahepatic inferior vena cava obstruction, a mesoatrial bypass graft relieves intrahepatic pressure by means of reversed flow through the portal vein. (*Adapted from Henderson and Warren.*[3])

struction resulting from constrictive pericarditis or prolonged congestive cardiac failure, medical therapy is ineffective. For the few patients who may survive and whose condition is the result of thrombosis of the hepatic veins, a side-to-side portacaval shunt through which the obstructed hepatic venous bed can be decompressed may be effective.[215] A severely obstructed liver, with biopsy evidence of parenchymatous necrosis, requires urgent surgical decompression. Either the side-to-side or the mesocaval shunt is satisfactory. In the presence of an occluded inferior vena cava, in which case portacaval decompression becomes impossible, some success has been reported with a meso-atrial shunt[3,216] (Fig. 58-19). This requires the use of a long bypass graft. For the patient with progressive liver failure in whom a decompressive shunt is unsuccessful or impossible, and in whom the underlying cause is controllable, hepatic transplantation should be considered.[217,218] Percutaneous transluminal dilation has had some limited recent success in patients with stenosis but not occlusion.

Veno-Occlusive Disease

The common feature of a rare group of disorders is outflow obstruction of the hepatic venous system as a result of subendothelial sclerosis of sublobular veins and terminal hepatic venules.[219–221] It was first described in Jamaica, West Indies, among persons who brewed a tea from the leaves

of alkaloid-containing plants. This form of subendothelial sclerosis has also been associated with the administration of antineoplastic drugs and with irradiation therapy in and around the liver. The occlusion of the hepatic venules results in necrosis of liver parenchyma progressing to cirrhosis. The mortality rate in the acute stage is about 20%. Patients who survive do so with all of the complications of hepatic cirrhosis. The discovery of widespread hepatic venular occlusion and centrilobular hemorrhagic necrosis by percutaneous liver biopsy establishes the diagnosis. Decompressive shunts, of which side-to-side portacaval shunt is preferred, are indicated if bleeding esophageal varices develop. Because the mortality rate from chronic veno-occlusive disease is so high, and because the overwhelming cause of death is bleeding from esophageal varices, this may be the one clinical condition in which prophylactic portacaval shunt may have a place.

REFERENCES

1. Graham DY, Smith JL: The course of patients after variceal hemorrhage. Gastroenterology 80:800, 1981.
2. Whipple AO: The problem of hypertension in relation to the hepatosplenopathies. Ann Surg 122:449, 1945.
3. Henderson JM, Warren WD: Surgical complications of cirrhosis and portal hypertension, in Sabiston DC (ed): Textbook of Surgery: The Biological Basis of Modern Surgical Practice, 13th ed. Philadelphia, WB Saunders Co., 1986, pp 1095–1116.
4. Way LW: Portal hypertension, in Way LW (ed): Current Surgical Diagnosis and Treatment, 8th ed. Los Altos, Calif., Lange Medical Publications, 1988.
5. McIndoe AH: Vascular lesions of portal cirrhosis. Arch Pathol 5:23, 1928.
6. Sherlock S: Diseases of the Liver and Biliary System. London, Blackwell Scientific Publications, 1981.
7. Orloff MJ: The liver, in Sabiston DC (ed): Davis-Christopher Textbook of Surgery, 12th ed. Philadelphia, WB Saunders Co., 1981.
8. Orloff MJ: Portal venous hypertension, in Wilson SE, Veith FJ, et al. (eds): Vascular Surgery: Principles and Practice. New York, McGraw-Hill Book Co., 1987, pp 768–800.
9. Sedgwick CE, et al.: Portal Hypertension. Boston, Little, Brown, 1967.
10. Brown SL, Busuttil RW: Portal hypertension, in Moore WS (ed): Vascular Surgery: A Comprehensive Review, 2nd ed. Orlando, Fla., Grune & Stratton, 1986, pp 999–1042.
11. Dunn MA, Kamel R: Hepatic schistosomiasis. Hepatology 1:653, 1981.
12. Fonkalsrud EW: Portal hypertension in children, in Rutherford RB (ed): Vascular Surgery. Philadelphia, WB Saunders Co., 1984, pp 1078–1083.
13. Bolt RJ: Diseases of the hepatic blood vessels, in Bockus HL, Berk JE (eds): Gastroenterology, 4th ed. Philadelphia, WB Saunders Co., 1985, pp 3259–3277.
14. Fonkalsrud EW: Surgical management of portal hypertension in childhood: Long-term results. Arch Surg 115:1042, 1980.
15. Clatworthy HW Jr, Boles ET Jr: Extrahapatic portal bed block in children: Pathogenesis and treatment. Ann Surg 150:371, 1959.
16. Garceau AJ, Chalmers TC, Boston Hospital Liver Group: The natural history of cirrhosis. I. Survival with esophageal varices. N Engl J Med 268:469, 1963.
17. Krugman S, Friedman H, Lattimer C: Hepatitis A and B: Serologic survey of various population groups. Am J Med Sci 275:249, 1978.

18. Decker RH, Overby LR, et al.: Serologic studies of transmission of hepatitis A in humans. J Infect Dis 139:74, 1979.

19. Coursaget P, Lesage G, et al.: Frequency of inapparent hepatitis A infection. Biomedicine 33:246, 1980.

20. Maynard JE, Bradley DW, et al.: Preliminary serologic studies of antibody to hepatitis A virus in populations in the United States. J Infect Dis 134:528, 1976.

21. Hodges JR, Millward-Sader GH, Wright R: Chronic active hepatitis: The spectrum of disease. Lancet 1:550, 1982.

22. Zetterman RK, Sorrell MF: Immunologic aspects of alcoholic liver disease. Gastroenterology 81:616, 1981.

23. Sherlock S: Chronic hepatitis, in Bockus HL, Berk JE (eds): Gastroenterology, 4th ed. Philadelphia, WB Saunders Co., 1985, pp 2902–2921.

24. Shaffner F: Primary biliary cirrhosis, in Bockus HL, Berk JE (eds): Gastroenterology, 4th ed. Philadelphia, WB Saunders Co., 1985, pp 3150–3176.

25. Schaffner F: Sclerosing cholangitis, in Bockus HL, Berk JE (eds): Gastroenterology, 4th ed. Philadelphia, WB Saunders Co., 1985, pp 3177–3188.

26. Leevy CM, Popper H, Sherlock S: Diseases of the Liver and Biliary Tract. Standardization of Nomenclature, Diagnostic Criteria and Diagnostic Methodology. Fogarty International Center Proceedings No. 22, DHEW Publication No. (NIH) 76–725, Washington, DC, 1976.

27. LaRusso NF, Wiesner RH, et al.: Current concepts: Primary sclerosing cholangitis. N Engl J Med 310:899, 1984.

28. Lefkowitch JH: Primary sclerosing cholangitis. Arch Intern Med 142:1157, 1982.

29. Castleman B, Towne VW: Case records of the Massachusetts General Hospital. Case 40041. N Engl J Med 150:169, 1954.

30. Wiesner RH, Larusso NF: Clinicopathologic features of the syndrome of primary sclerosing cholangitis. Gastroenterology 79:200, 1980.

31. Walshe JM: Wilson's disease (hepatolenticular degeneration), in Bockus HL, Berk JE (eds): Gastroenterology, 4th ed. Philadelphia, WB Saunders Co., 1985, pp 3222–3235.

32. Walshe JM: Wilson's disease, hepatolenticular degeneration, in Vinken PJ, Bruyn GW, Klawans HL (eds): Handbook of Clinical Neurology; vol 27: Metabolic and Deficiency Disease of the Nervous System. New York, Elsevier, 1976, pp 379–414.

33. Uzman LL, Iber FL, et al.: The mechanism of copper deposition in the liver in hepatolenticular degeneration (Wilson's disease). Am J Med Sci 231:511, 1956.

34. Schaffner F, Sternlieb I, et al.: Hepatocellular changes in Wilson's disease: Histochemical and electron microscopic studies. Am J Pathol 41:315, 1962.

35. Williams FJB, Walshe JM: Wilson's disease: An analysis of the cranial computerized tomographic appearances found in 60 patients and the changes in response to treatment with chelating agents. Brain 104:735, 1981.

36. Walshe JM: Copper chelation in patients with Wilson's disease. Q J Med 42:441, 1973.

37. Walshe JM: Treatment of Wilson's disease with trientine (triethylene tetramine) dihydrochloride. Lancet 1:643, 1982.

38. Westaby D, Williams R: Portal hypertension, in Bockus HL, Berk JE (eds): Gastroenterology, 4th ed. Philadelphia, WB Saunders Co., 1984, pp 3062–3082.

39. Spain DM: Portal cirrhosis of the liver: A review of two hundred fifty necropsies with references to sex differences. Am J Clin Pathol 15:215, 1945.

40. Galambos JT: Alcoholic liver disease: Fatty liver, hepatitis, and cirrhosis, in Bockus HL, Berk JE (eds): Gastroenterology, 4th ed. Philadelphia, WB Saunders Co., 1985, pp 2985–3048.

41. Creutzfeldt W, Beck K: Cirrhosis of the liver: On the aetiology, pathogenesis, results of treatment and period of survival in an unselected series of 560 patients. Ger Med Month 11:259, 1966.

42. Ratnoff OD, Patek AJ Jr: Natural history of Laennec's cirrhosis of liver: An analysis of 386 cases. Medicine 21:207, 1942.

43. Warren WD, Millikan WJ Jr, et al.: Ten years portal hypertensive surgery at Emory: Results and new perspectives. Ann Surg 195:530, 1982.

44. Zeppa R, Hensley GT, et al.: The comparative survival of alcoholics versus nonalcoholics after distal splenorenal shunt. Ann Surg 187:510, 1978.

45. Bleeding oesophageal varices [Editorial]. Lancet 1:139, 1984.

46. Reynolds TB: Portal-systemic shunt: Finally, some good news (editorial). N Engl J Med 295:1131, 1976.

47. Lebrec D, DeFleury P, et al.: Portal hypertension, size of esophageal varices and risk of gastrointestinal bleeding in alcoholic cirrhosis. Gastroenterology 79:1139, 1980.

48. Adamsons RJ, Butt K, et al.: Prognostic significance of portal pressure in patients with bleeding esophageal varices. Surg Gynecol Obstet 145:353, 1977.

49. Palmer ED, Brick, IB: Correlation between the severity of esophageal varices in portal cirrhosis and their propensity toward hemorrhage. Gastroenterology 30:85, 1956.

50. Macdougall BRD, Williams R: A controlled trial of cimetidine in the recurrence of variceal haemorrhage: Implications about the pathogenesis of haemorrhage. Hepatology 3:69, 1983.

51. Lebrec D, Poynard T, Hillon P: Propranolol for prevention of recurrent gastrointestinal bleeding in patients with cirrhosis. N Engl J Med 305:1371, 1981.

52. Sogaard PE: Propranolol in portal hypertension. Lancet 1:1204, 1981.

53. Burroughs AK, Jenkins WJ, et al.: Controlled trial of propranolol for the prevention of recurrent variceal hemorrhage in patients with cirrhosis. N Engl J Med 309:1539, 1983.

54. Wilkinson SP: Propranolol and portal hypertension in cirrhosis. Lancet 2:429, 1980.

55. Reynolds TB, Campra JL: Ascites in liver disease, in Bockus HL, Berk JE (eds): Gastroenterology, 4th ed. Philadelphia, WB Saunders Co., 1985, pp 3121–3137.

56. Gabuzda GJ, Traeger HS, Davidson CS: Hepatic cirrhosis: Effects of sodium chloride administration and restriction and of abdominal paracentesis on electrolyte and water balance. J Clin Invest 33:780, 1954.

57. Kao HW, Rakov NE, Reynolds TB: Large volume paracentesis: Does it cause hypovolemia? Clin Res 31:32A, 1983.

58. Campra JL, Reynolds TB: Effectiveness of high-dose spironolactone therapy in patients with chronic liver disease and relatively refractory ascites. Dig Dis Sci 23:1025, 1978.

59. LeVeen HH, Christoudias G, et al.: Peritoneovenous shunting for ascites. Ann Surg 180:580, 1974.

60. Lund RH, Newkirk JB: Peritoneovenous shunting system for surgical management of ascites. Contemp Surg 14:31, 1979.

61. Sampliner SE, Iber FL: High-protein ascites in patients with uncomplicated hepatic cirrhosis. Am J Med Sci 267:275, 1974.

62. Hoefs JC: Increase in ascites white blood cell and protein concentrations during diuresis in patients with chronic liver disease. Hepatology 1:249, 1981.

63. Blendis LM, Greig PD, et al.: The renal and hemodynamic effects of the peritoneovenous shunt for intractable hepatic ascites. Gastroenterology 77:250, 1979.

64. Bernhoft A, Pellegrini CA, Way LW: Peritoneovenous shunt for refractory ascites. Arch Surg 117:631, 1982.

65. LeVeen HH, Wapnick S, et al.: Further experience with peritoneovenous shunt for ascites. Ann Surg 184:574, 1976.

66. Turner WW, Pate RM: The Denver peritoneovenous shunt: Relationship between hepatic reserve and successful treatment of ascites. Am J Surg 144:619, 1982.

67. Orloff MJ: Pathogenesis and surgical treatment of intractable

ascites associated with alcoholic cirrhosis. Ann NY Acad Sci 170:213, 1970.

68. Adams RD, Foley JM: The neurological changes in the more common type of severe liver disease. Trans Am Neurol Assoc 74:217, 1949.

69. Mezey E, Smith GW: Management of ascites and hepatic encephalopathy, in Rutherford RB (ed): Vascular Surgery, 2nd ed. Philadelphia, WB Saunders Co., 1984, pp 1084–1094.

70. Hanna SS, Smith RS, et al.: Reversal of hepatic encephalopathy after occlusion of total portasystemic shunts. Am J Surg 142:285, 1981.

71. Parkes JD, Sharpstone P, Williams R: Levodopa in hepatic coma. Lancet 1:1341, 1970.

72. Fischer JE, Funovics JM, et al.: L-Dopa in hepatic coma. Ann Surg 183:386, 1976.

73. Kurtz RC, Sherlock P, et al.: Levodopa: A study of its efficacy in the management of hepatic coma. Gastroenterology 64:758, 1973.

74. Morgan MY, Jacobovits AW, et al.: Successful use of bromocriptine in the treatment of a patient with chronic portal-systemic encephalopathy. N Engl J Med 196:793, 1977.

75. Morgan MY, Jakobovits AW, et al.: Successful use of bromocriptine in the treatment of chronic hepatic encephalopathy. Gastroenterology 78:663, 1980.

76. Schenker S, Desmond PV, et al.: Cryptic nature of bromocriptine therapy in portal-systemic encephalopathy [Editorial]. Gastroenterology 78:1094, 1980.

77. Picone SB Jr, Donovan AJ, Yellin AE: Abdominal colectomy for chronic encephalopathy due to portal-systemic shunt. Arch Surg 118:33, 1983.

78. Resnick RH, Ishihara A, et al.: Boston Inter-Hospital Liver Group: A controlled trial of colon bypass in chronic hepatic encephalopathy. Gastroenterology 54:1057, 1968.

79. Walker JG, Emlyn-Williams A, Craigie A: Treatment of chronic portal-systemic encephalopathy by surgical exclusion of the colon. Lancet 2:861, 1965.

80. Child CG III: The Liver and Portal Hypertension. Philadelphia, WB Saunders Co., 1964.

81. Eckhauser FE, Appleman HD, et al.: Hepatic pathology as a determinant of prognosis after portal decompression. Am J Surg 139:105, 1980.

82. Mikkelsen WP: Therapeutic portacaval shunt: Preliminary data on controlled trial and morbid effects of acute hyaline necrosis. Arch Surg 108:302, 1974.

83. Mikkelsen WP, Turrill FL, Kerr WH: Acute hyaline necrosis of the liver: A surgical trap. Am J Surg 116:266, 1968.

84. Kanel GC, Kaplan MM, et al.: Survival in patients with postnecrotic cirrhosis and Laennec's cirrhosis undergoing therapeutic portacaval shunt. Gastroenterology 73:679, 1977.

85. Simert G, Persson T, Vang J: Factors predicting survival after portacaval shunt: A multiple linear regression analysis. Ann Surg 187:174, 1978.

86. Smith GW: Evaluation of patients with portal hypertension, in Rutherford RB (ed): Vascular Surgery, 2nd ed. Philadelphia, WB Saunders Co., 1984, pp 985–989.

87. Burchell AR, Moreno AH, et al.: Hemodynamic variables and prognosis following portacaval shunts. Surg Gynecol Obstet 138:359, 1974.

88. Charters AC III, Brown NB, et al.: The influence of portal perfusion on the response to portacaval shunt. Am J Surg 130:226, 1975.

89. Smith GW: Use of hemodynamic selection criteria in the management of cirrhotic patients with portal hypertension. Ann Surg 179:782, 1974.

90. Reynolds TB, Ito S, Iwatsuki S: Measurement of portal pressure and its clinical application. Am J Med 49:649, 1970.

91. Bengmark S, Borjesson B, et al.: Obliteration of esophageal

varices by PTP: A follow-up of 43 patients. Ann Surg 190:549, 1979.

92. Smith GW, Westgaard T, Bjorn-Hansen R: Hepatic venous angiography in the evaluation of cirrhosis of the liver. Ann Surg 173:469, 1971.

93. Smith-Laing G, Camilo ME, et al.: Percutaneous transhepatic portography in the assessment of portal hypertension. Gastroenterology 78:197, 1980.

94. Widrich WC, Robbins AH, Nabseth DC: Transhepatic embolization of varices. Cardiovasc Intervent Radiol 3:198, 1980.

95. Gembarowicz RM, Kelly JJ, et al.: Management of variceal hemorrhage: Results of a standardized protocol using vasopressin and transhepatic embolization. Arch Surg 115:1160, 1980.

96. Rikkers LF: Operations for management of esophageal variceal hemorrhage. West J Med 136:107, 1982.

97. Resnick RH: Portal hypertension. Med Clin North Am 59(4):945, 1975.

98. Phemister DB, Humphreys EM: Gastroesophageal resection and total gastrectomy in the treatment of bleeding varicose veins in Banti's syndrome. Ann Surg 125:397, 1947.

99. O'Donnell TF Jr, Gembarowicz RM, et al.: The economic impact of acute variceal bleeding: Cost-effectiveness implications for medical and surgical therapy. Surgery 88:693, 1980.

100. Mitchell KJ, Macdougall BRD, et al.: A prospective reappraisal of emergency endoscopy in patients with portal hypertension. Scand J Gastroenterol 17:965, 1982.

101. Smith GW: Balloon tamponade, pharmacologic intervention, and catheter embolization for variceal hemorrhage, in Ernst CB, Stanley JC (eds): Current Therapy in Vascular Surgery. Toronto, BC Decker, 1987, pp 330–333.

102. Conn HO: Propranolol in portal hypertension: Problems in paradise? Hepatology 4:560, 1984.

103. Burroughs AK, Jenkins WJ, et al.: Controlled trial of propranolol for the prevention of recurrent variceal hemorrhage in patients with cirrhosis. N Engl J Med 309:1539, 1983.

104. Sengstaken RW, Blakemore AH: Balloon tamponade for the control of hemorrhage from esophageal varices. Ann Surg 131:781, 1950.

105. Conn HO: A plethora of therapies, in Westaby D, Macdougall BRD, Williams R (eds): Variceal Bleeding. London, Pitman Medical, 1982, pp 221–251.

106. Conn HO: Hazards attending the use of esophageal tamponade. N Engl J Med 259:701, 1958.

107. Paquet KJ, Oberhammer E: Sclerotherapy of bleeding oesophageal varices by means of endoscopy. Endoscopy 10:7, 1978.

108. Terblanche J, Yakoob HI, et al.: Acute bleeding varices: A five-year prospective evaluation of tamponade and sclerotherapy. Ann Surg 194:521, 1981.

109. McCormack TT, Kennedy HJ, et al.: Implications of a sclerotherapy program for the medical and surgical care of bleeding in portal hypertension. Surg Gynecol Obstet 161:557, 1985.

110. Warren WD, Henderson JM, et al.: Distal splenorenal shunt versus endoscopic sclerotherapy for long-term management of variceal bleeding: Preliminary report of a prospective, randomized trial. Ann Surg 203:454, 1986.

111. Grace ND: Is sclerotherapy the treatment of choice for bleeding esophageal varices [Editorial]? Mayo Clin Proc 60:207, 1985.

112. Lunderqvist A, Vang J: Transhepatic catheterization and obliteration of the coronary vein in patients with portal hypertension and esophageal varices. N Engl J Med 291:646, 1974.

113. Smith-Laing G, Scott J, et al.: Role of percutaneous transhepatic obliteration of varices in the management of hemorrhage from gastroesophageal varices. Gastroenterology 80:1031, 1981.

114. Wirthlin LS, Linton RR, Ellis DS: Transthoracoesophageal ligation of bleeding esophageal varices: A reappraisal. Arch Surg 109:688, 1974.

115. Orloff MJ: A comparative study of emergency transesophageal ligation and nonsurgical treatment of bleeding esophageal varices in unselected patients with cirrhosis. Surgery 52:103, 1962.

116. Orloff MJ, Bell RH, et al.: Long-term results of emergency portacaval shunt for bleeding esophageal varices in unselected patients with alcoholic cirrhosis. Ann Surg 192:325, 1980.

117. Paper S: Renal failure in cirrhosis (the hepatorenal syndrome), in Epstein M (ed): The Kidney in Liver Disease. New York, Elsevier, 1976, pp 91–112.

118. Wilkinson SP, Williams R: Renal failure in cirrhosis: Current views and speculations. Adv Nephrol 7:15, 1977.

119. Wong PY, McCoy GC, et al.: The hepatorenal syndrome. Gastroenterology 77:1326, 1979.

120. Callow AD, Lloyd JB, et al.: Interim experience with a controlled study of prophylactic portacaval shunt. Surgery 57(1):123, 1965.

121. Terblanche J: Sclerotherapy for variceal hemorrhage, in Ernst CB, Stanley JC (eds): Current Therapy in Vascular Surgery. Toronto, BC Decker, 1987, pp 333–336.

122. Terblanche J: Treatment of esophageal varices by injection sclerotherapy, in MacLean LD (ed): Advances in Surgery. Chicago, Year Book Medical Publishers, 1981, p 257.

123. Crafoord C, Frenckner P: New surgical treatment of varicose veins of the esophagus. Acta Otolaryngol (Stockh) 27:422, 1939.

124. Moersch HJ: Treatment of esophageal varices by injection. Proc Staff Meet Mayo Clinic 15:177, 1940.

125. Macdougall BRD, Westaby D, et al.: Increased long-term survival in variceal hemorrhage using injection sclerotherapy. Lancet 1:124, 1982.

126. Conn PO: Prophylactic portacaval shunts. Ann Intern Med 70:859, 1969.

127. Jackson FC, Perrin EB, et al.: A clinical investigation of the portacaval shunt. II. Survival analysis of the prophylactic operation. Am J Surg 115:22, 1967.

128. Resnick RH, Chalmers TC, et al.: Boston Inter-Hospital Liver Group: A controlled study of the prophylactic portacaval shunt—a final report. Ann Intern Med 701:675, 1969.

129. Koch H, Hennin H, et al.: Prophylactic sclerosing of esophageal varices: Results of a prospective controlled study. Endoscopy 18:40, 1986.

130. Paquet KJ, Koussouris P: Is there an indication for prophylactic endoscopic paravariceal injection sclerotherapy in patients with liver cirrhosis and portal hypertension. Endoscopy 18:32, 1986.

131. Johnson G Jr: Nonshunt operations, in Rutherford RB (ed): Vascular Surgery, 2nd ed. Philadelphia, WB Saunders Co., 1984, pp 1048–1051.

132. Habif DV: Treatment of esophageal varices by partial esophago-gastrectomy and interposed jejunal segment. Surgery 46:212, 1959.

133. Terblanche J: Emergency management of variceal hemorrhage, in Rutherford RB (ed): Vascular Surgery, 2nd ed. Philadelphia, WB Saunders Co., 1984, pp 1003–1012.

134. Hassab MA: Nonshunt operations in portal hypertension without cirrhosis. Surg Gynecol Obstet 131:648, 1970.

135. Hassab MA: Gastroesophageal decongestion and splenectomy in the treatment of esophageal varices in bilharzial cirrhosis: Further studies with a report on 355 operations. Surgery 61:169, 1967.

136. Sugiura M, Futagawa S: Further evaluation of the Sugiura procedure in the treatment of esophageal varices. Arch Surg 112:1317, 1977.

137. Sugiura M, Futagawa S: A new technique for treating esophageal varices. J Thorac Cardiovasc Surg 66:677, 1973.

138. Superina RA, Weber JL, Shandling B: A modified Sugiura operation for bleeding varices in children. J Pediatr Surg 18:794, 1983.

139. Wexler MJ: Esophageal procedures to control bleeding from varices. Surg Clin North Am 63:903, 1983.

140. Terblanche J, Northover JMA, et al.: A prospective evaluation of injection sclerotherapy in the treatment of acute bleeding esophageal varices. Surgery 85:239, 1979.

141. Johnson G Jr, Keagy BA: Variceal ligation and gastroesophageal devascularization for variceal hemorrhage, in Ernst CB, Stanley JC (eds): Current Therapy in Vascular Surgery. Toronto, BC Decker, 1987, pp 341–345.

142. Johnston GW: Simplified oesophageal transection for bleeding varices. Br Med J 1:1388, 1979.

143. Johnston GW: Bleeding oesophageal varices: The management of shunt rejects. Ann R Coll Surg Engl 63:3, 1981.

144. Wexler MJ: Treatment of bleeding esophageal varices by transabdominal esophageal transection with the EEA stapling instrument. Surgery 88:406, 1980.

145. Boerema I: Bleeding varices of the esophagus in cirrhosis of the liver and Banti's disease. Arch Chir Neurol 1:253, 1949.

146. Crile GS: Transesophageal ligation of bleeding esophageal varices: A preliminary report of seven cases. Arch Surg 61:654, 1950.

147. Futagawa S, Sugiura M, et al.: Emergency esophageal transection with paraesophagogastric devascularization for variceal bleeding. World J Surg 3:229, 1979.

148. Johnson GW: Six years' experience of oesophageal transection for oesophageal varices using a circular stapling gun. Gut 23:770, 1982.

149. George P, Brown G, et al.: Emergency oesophageal transection in uncontrolled variceal haemorrhage. Br J Surg 60:635, 1973.

150. Wanamaker SR, Cooperman M, Carey LC: Use of the EEA stapling instrument for control of bleeding esophageal varices. Surgery 94:620, 1983.

151. Umeyama K, Yoshikawa K, et al.: Transabdominal oesophageal transection for oesophageal varices: Experience in 101 patients. Br J Surg 70:419, 1983.

152. Van Beek DF, Gleysteen JJ, et al.: Mortality and rebleeding after hypertensive variceal disconnections. Arch Surg 119:446, 1984.

153. Warren WD, Zeppa R, Foman JJ: Selective transsplenic decompression of gastroesophageal varices by distal splenorenal shunt. Ann Surg 166:437, 1967.

154. Reuter SR, Orloff MJ: Wedged hepatic venography in patients with end-to-side portacaval shunts. Radiology 111:563, 1974.

155. Redman HC, Reuter SR: Angiographic demonstration of portacaval and other decompression liver shunts. Radiology 92:788, 1969.

156. Turcotte JG, Erlandson EE: Portacaval shunt, in Rutherford RB (ed): Vascular Surgery, 2nd ed. Philadelphia, WB Saunders Co., 1984, pp 1013–1020.

157. Reuter SR, Berk RH, Orloff MJ: An angiographic study of the pre- and postoperative hemodynamics in patients with side-to-side portacaval shunts. Radiology 116:33, 1975.

158. Marion PO: Traitement chirurgical de l'hypertension portale. Helv Med Acta 21:375, 1954.

159. Clatworthy HW Jr, Wall T, Watman RN: A new type of portal-to-systemic venous shunt for portal hypertension. Arch Surg 71:588, 1955.

160. Drapanas T: Interposition mesocaval shunt for treatment of portal hypertension. Ann Surg 176:435, 1972.

161. Cameron JL, Harrington DP, Maddrey WC: The mesocaval "C" shunt. Surg Gynecol Obstet 150:401, 1980.

162. Reynolds TB, Donovan AJ, et al.: Results of a 12-year random-

ized trial of portacaval shunt in patients with alcoholic liver disease and bleeding varices. Gastroenterology 80:1005, 1981.

163. Cope C: Balloon dilatation of closed mesocaval shunts. AJR 135:989, 1980.

164. Drapanas T, LoCiciero J, Dowling JB: Hemodynamics of the interposition mesocaval shunt. Ann Surg 181:523, 1975.

165. Drapanas T, Akdamar K: Interposition mesocaval shunt for portal hypertension. Hosp Pract, Sept 1984.

166. Sanfey H, Cameron JL: Mesocaval shunts, in Rutherford RB (ed): Vascular Surgery, 2nd ed. Philadelphia, WB Saunders Co., 1984, pp 1029–1047.

167. Cameron JL, Zuidema GD, et al.: Mesocaval shunts for the control of bleeding esophageal varices. Surgery 85:257, 1979.

168. Pliam MB, Adson MA, Foulk WT: Conventional splenorenal shunts. Arch Surg 110:588, 1975.

169. Linton RR, Ellis DS, Geary JE: Critical comparative analysis of early and late results of splenorenal and direct portacaval shunts performed in 169 patients with portal cirrhosis. Ann Surg 154:446, 1961.

170. Linton RR: Atlas of Vascular Surgery. Philadelphia, WB Saunders Co., 1973.

171. Malt RA: Proximal splenorenal venous shunts, in Rutherford RB (ed): Vascular Surgery, 2nd ed. Philadelphia, WB Saunders Co., 1984, pp 1021–1028.

172. Maillard JN, Benhamou JP, Rueff B: Arterialization of the liver with portacaval shunt in the treatment of portal hypertension due to intrahepatic block. Surgery 67:883, 1970.

173. Maillard JN, Rueff B, et al.: Hepatic arterialization and portacaval shunt in hepatic cirrhosis: An assessment. Arch Surg 108:315, 1974.

174. Adamsons RJ: Arterialization of the portal vein, in Rutherford RB (ed): Vascular Surgery, 2nd ed. Philadelphia, WB Saunders Co., 1984, pp 1061–1070.

175. Adamsons RJ, Butt K, et al.: Portacaval shunt with arterialization of the portal vein by means of a low flow arteriovenous fistula in patients with cirrhosis of the liver. Surg Gynecol Obstet 146:869, 1978.

176. Otte JB, Reynaent M, et al.: Arterialization of the portal vein in conjunction with a therapeutic portacaval shunt. Ann Surg 196:656, 1982.

177. Fischer JE, Bauer R, et al.: Comparison of distal and proximal splenorenal shunts: A randomized prospective trial. Ann Surg 194:531, 1981.

178. Barnes BA, Ackroyd FW, et al.: Elective portosystemic shunts: Morbidity and survival data. Ann Surg 174:76, 1971.

179. McDermott WV, Pallazzi H, et al.: Elective portal systemic shunt. N Engl J Med 264:419, 1961.

180. Mikkelson WP, Turrill FR, Pattison AC: Portacaval shunt in cirrhosis of the liver: Clinical and hemodynamic aspects. Am J Surg 104:204, 1962.

181. Voorhees AB Jr, Price JB Jr, Britton RC: Porta-systemic shunting procedures for portal hypertension: Twenty-six year experience in adults with cirrhosis of the liver. Ann Surg 119:501, 1970.

182. Walker RM, Shaldon C, Vowles KD: Late results of portacaval anastomosis. Lancet 2:727, 1961.

183. Ottinger LW: The Linton splenorenal shunt in the management of the bleeding complications of portal hypertension. Ann Surg 196:664, 1982.

184. Resnick RH, Sher FL, et al.: The Boston Inter-Hospital Liver Group: A controlled study of the therapeutic portacaval shunt. Gastroenterology 67:843, 1974.

185. Salam AA: Selective shunts, in Rutherford RB (ed): Vascular Surgery, 2nd ed. Philadelphia, WB Saunders Co., 1984, pp 1052–1060.

186. Warren WD, Millikan WJ Jr: Selective transsplenic decompres-

sion procedure: Changes in technique after 300 cases. Contemp Surg 18:11, 1981.

187. Warren WD: Control of variceal bleeding: Reassessment of rationale: Founder's Lecture SSAT. Am J Surg 148:8, 1983.

188. Warren WD, Millikan WJ Jr, et al.: Selective variceal decompression after splenectomy or splenic vein thrombosis—with a note on splenopancreatic disconnection. Ann Surg 199:694, 1984.

189. Inokuchi K, Beppu K, et al.: Exclusion of nonisolated splenic vein in distal splenorenal shunt for prevention of portal malcirculation. Ann Surg 200:711, 1984.

190. Starzl TE, Porter KA: A hundred years of the hepatotropic controversy: Hepatotropic Factors. Ciba Foundation Symposium. Amsterdam, Elsevier/Excerpta Medica/North Holland Publishing Co., 1978, pp 111–138.

191. Henderson JM, Millikan WJ Jr, et al.: Hemodynamic difference between alcoholic and nonalcoholic cirrhotics following distal splenorenal shunt: Effect on survival? Ann Surg 198:325, 1983.

192. Tylen V, Simert G, Vand J: Hemodynamic changes after distal splenorenal shunt studied by sequential angiography. Radiology 121:585, 1976.

193. Widrich WC, Robbins AH, et al.: Long-term follow-up of distal splenorenal shunts. Radiology 134:341, 1980.

194. Henderson JM, Warren WD: Current status of the distal splenorenal shunt. Semin Liver Dis 3:251, 1983.

195. Zeppa R, Hensley GT, et al.: The comparative survival of alcoholics versus nonalcoholics after distal splenorenal shunt. Ann Surg 187:510, 1978.

196. Martin EW Jr, Molnar J, et al.: Observations on fifty distal splenorenal shunts. Surgery 84:379, 1978.

197. Vang J, Simert G, et al.: Results of a modified distal splenorenal shunt for portal hypertension. Ann Surg 184:224, 1976.

198. Henderson M, Millikan WJ Jr, et al.: The incidence and natural history of thrombus in the portal vein following distal splenorenal shunt. Ann Surg 126:1, 1982.

199. Belghiti J, Grenier P, et al.: Long-term loss of Warren's shunt selectivity: Angiographic demonstration. Arch Surg 116:1121, 1981.

200. Fonkalsrud EW, Longmire WP Jr: Reassessment of operative procedures for portal hypertension in infants and children. Am J Surg 118:148, 1969.

201. Fonkalsrud EW, Myers NA, Robinson MJ: Management of extrahepatic portal hypertension in children. Ann Surg 80:487, 1974.

202. Turcotte JG, Rosenberg L, et al.: Portal hypertension in children, in Ernst CB, Stanley JC (eds): Current Therapy in Vascular Surgery. Toronto, BC Decker, 1987, pp 342–345.

203. Fonkalsrud EW, Boles ET Jr: Choledochal cysts in infancy and childhood. Surg Gynecol Obstet 121:733, 1965.

204. Clatworthy HW Jr, de Lorimier AA: Portal decompression procedures in children. Am J Surg 107:447, 1964.

205. Koop CE, Roddy SR: Colonic replacement of distal esophagus and proximal stomach in the management of bleeding varices in children. Ann Surg 147:17, 1958.

206. Longmire WP Jr, Fonkalsrud EW: Portal hypertension in early childhood. Presented at International Conference on Liver Disease in Infancy and Childhood, Paris, France, June 1985.

207. Boles ET Jr: Discussion of paper: Martin LW: Changing concepts of management of portal hypertension in children. J Pediatr Surg 7:559, 1972.

208. Boles ET, Wise WE, Birken G: Extrahepatic portal hypertension in children: Long-term evaluation. Am J Surg 151:734, 1986.

209. Budd G: Disease of the Liver. Philadelphia, Lea and Blanchard, 1846.

210. Chiari H: Uber die selbstandige Phlebitis obliterans der Haup-

stamme der Venae hepaticae als Todesurache. Beitr Pathol Anat 26:1, 1899.

211. Okuda K: Membranous obstruction of the interior vena cava: Etiology and relation to hepatocellular carcinoma. Gastroenterology 82:376, 1982.

212. Remigo P: Budd-Chiari syndrome in a patient with amebic abscess of the liver. Lab Invest 20:600, 1969.

213. Hoyumpa AM Jr, Schiff L, Helfman L: Budd-Chiari syndrome in women taking oral contraceptives. Am J Med 50:137, 1971.

214. LaLonde G, Theoret G, et al.: Inferior vena cava stenosis and Budd-Chiari syndrome in a woman taking oral contraceptives. Gastroenterology. 82:1452, 1982.

215. Orloff MJ, Johansen KH: Treatment of Budd-Chiari syndrome by side-to-side portacaval shunt: Experimental and clinical results. Ann Surg 188:494, 1978.

216. Cameron JL, Herlong HF, et al.: The Budd-Chiari syndrome: Treatment by mesenteric-systemic venous shunts. Ann Surg 198:335, 1983.

217. Starzl TE, Iwatsuki S, et al.: Analysis of liver transplantation. Hepatology 4:47S, 1984.

218. Schenker S: Medical treatment vs. transplantation in liver disorders. Hepatology 4:102S, 1984.

219. Bras G, Jelliffe DB, Stuart KL: Veno-occlusive disease of the liver with non-portal type of cirrhosis occurring in Jamaica. Arch Pathol 57:285, 1954.

220. Bras G, McLean E: Toxic factors in veno-occlusive disease. Ann NY Acad Sci 111:392, 1963.

221. Stuart KL, Bras G: Veno-occlusive disease of the liver. Q J Med 26:291, 1957.

CHAPTER 59
Vascular Access

Vivian A. Tellis and Frank J. Veith

The enormous strides made in science and technology in the last decade have greatly influenced the practice of medicine and created new needs. One of these is the necessity for access to the circulation, which is needed in diverse groups of patients. On the one hand are patients with multiple organ failure, whose care requires monitoring of vital functions and body chemistry. At the other end of the spectrum are those receiving hemodialysis therapy or home parenteral nutrition, who lead normal lives in spite of the total failure of an essential organ system. In short, countless lives depend on temporary or permanent access to the circulation. To make an appropriate choice for each patient's needs, the surgeon undertaking the responsibility of providing such access must be familiar with the many options and the complications of each.

HISTORICAL ASPECTS

The history of vascular surgery is considered elsewhere in this volume; vascular access surgery could not exist without the development of vascular suturing technique, anticoagulation, and graft materials, as well as the other aspects that have been discussed previously. The description by Seldinger,[1] in 1953, of the technique for percutaneous cannulation of vessels was the essential prelude to most present-day acute monitoring catheters. However, the major factor in creating a need for vascular access was the development of a practical artificial kidney by Wilhelm Kolff in 1943 (cited by Graham[2]). With the artificial kidney, life in patients requiring dialysis could last only as long as the patients could be connected to the machine. This was achieved initially by *external* direct cannulation of vessels for each dialysis until exhaustion of potential sites led to the patient's death. Long-term maintenance dialysis did not therefore become truly practical until the development of Teflon-Silastic external arteriovenous shunts by Quinton et al.[3] in 1960. However, external shunts invariably failed because of infection or occlusion after several months. Specialized external shunts such as the Thomas femoral shunt,

although providing excellent long-term function, posed serious hazards to life and limb in the event of infectious complications.[4] The introduction of the *internal* arteriovenous fistula (AVF) by Brescia et al.[5] was therefore a major advance. In persons with normal blood vessels, cannulas were avoided and a single procedure could provide lifetime access. Creation of the side-to-side AVF therefore continues to be the procedure of choice for long-term vascular access. As older and sicker patients are accepted for dialysis, increasing numbers of patients are encountered in whom an AVF cannot be created by direct arteriovenous anastomosis. In such patients the gap has been bridged by autogenous vein or prosthetic grafts.[6-9] In these individuals, dialysis is performed by direct graft puncture. Although no ideal material exists, expanded polytetrafluoroethylene (PTFE) grafts have been used most extensively, with the lowest rate of complications. Finally, permanent indwelling venous catheters, introduced by Broviac and Hickman,[10,11] have proved invaluable in the management of many diseases and conditions: one such catheter has been modified to provide vascular access.

INDICATIONS: TYPES OF ACCESS

The necessity for vascular access first arose because of the possibility of treating patients with end-stage renal disease. As knowledge and skill have grown, so too have the applications of vascular access procedures, which may be external or internal. An *external* device is one in which a synthetic tube or cannula traverses the skin so that one end is within the lumen of a blood vessel while the other rests on the skin externally. Circulatory access is readily obtained by connection to the external portals, which are heparinized and capped when not in use. With *internal* access methods, intact skin is present over an arteriovenous fistula or graft, or synthetic reservoir. Access to the circulation is obtained by the temporary insertion of a needle through the skin into the device for each use. Short-term access may be required for monitoring vital signs in intensive care situations. It may also be necessary in acute renal failure and apheresis and for parenteral alimentation, chemotherapy, and the frequent administration of blood products (as in hemophilia).[12-15] In some of these situations, access may be required permanently, although the most common indication for permanent access remains end-stage renal disease.

Temporary access, required for a few hours or days, usually involves the use of a semirigid catheter, made of Teflon or a similar material, that is passed into the appropriate vessel over a guide wire by the Seldinger technique.[1] This is the standard method for central venous and pulmonary artery pressure measurements. Intermittent femoral venipuncture can be used for maintenance hemodialysis until acute renal failure resolves or until permanent access is created. The need for repeated punctures can be avoided by special central venous catheters, which can be left in place for several days[16] (Fig. 59-1C). These are heparinized and capped between treatments. However, semirigid catheters are prone to infection along the tract.[17] Sheath formation, erosion of the vessel wall and subclavian vein thrombosis can also occur.[18] If a treatment period of several weeks rather than days is anticipated, a cuffed silicone "permanent" catheter is preferable. Although the external shunt was an essential step in making hemodialysis practical, in our opinion it has no place in the modern management of renal failure. The placement of a shunt mandates the ligation of an artery and vein and is an unnecessary sacrifice of blood vessels, which may complicate the future provision of access.

Permanent access may be internal or external and may require the insertion of synthetic materials. The simple side-to-side AVF remains the ideal. When an AVF is created with good technique in an adequately hydrated host whose vessels are not diseased, that access procedure may be the only one required during a patient's lifetime. When, as a result of occlusion or disease, adequate segments of artery and vein are not in proximity with each other, the gap between the two must be bridged by a graft. All prosthetic grafts are subject to outflow stenosis, occlusion, and infection. They should therefore be avoided if any possibility exists that a direct arteriovenous anastomosis can arterialize accessible veins for puncture. However, when there is no possibility, PTFE appears to be the graft material of choice, inasmuch as thrombectomy is easy, intimal proliferation is often minimal, and infection can frequently be managed while the access route is preserved.[19-21] For these reasons, it enjoys wide popularity as a graft substance. The saphenous vein is undesirable for a "bridge" graft because repeated puncture of the vein leads ultimately to its occlusion.[22] Bovine carotid heterografts, although widely used for several years, have been found by numerous workers to have unacceptably high long-term complication rates[19-22] (Fig. 59-2). Thrombosis and infection are difficult to treat, and dissolution of actual graft substance leads to aneurysm formation, serious hemorrhage, and occasionally death. Tanned human umbilical vein grafts and Dacron velour grafts have been used in a few centers but have not found wide application.[7,8]

Permanent external devices have a role in specific circumstances. Percutaneous long-term cannulation of the central venous system, with the use of a soft silicone catheter to which a Dacron cuff has been fused, is now common[12,23] (Fig. 59-1B). The silicone material resists thrombosis, and fibrous ingrowth into the cuff, which is buried in a subcutaneous tunnel, prevents infection along the tract. Such catheters are used mainly for patients receiving parenteral nutrition, as portals for blood sampling in patients whose peripheral veins are exhausted, and for the administration of chemotherapeutic drugs. Percutaneous catheterization

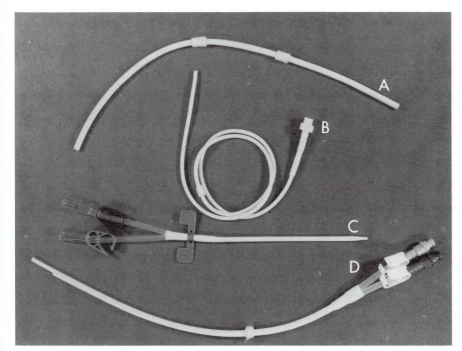

Figure 59-1. Selected external prostheses. **A.** Tenckhoff peritoneal dialysis catheter. **B,C,D.** Central venous catheters. Temporary double-lumen dialysis catheter **(C)** is rigid and has no cuff. Hickman catheter **(B)** is soft, has a cuff for tissue ingrowth, and can be cut to size. Permanent double-lumen cuffed dialysis catheter **(D)** has larger diameter and firmer consistency than Hickman catheter; openings of the two lumina are separated to minimize recirculation.

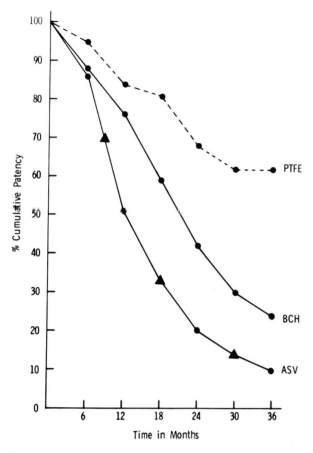

Figure 59-2. Comparison of graft materials for AVF (Haimov et al.).[22] ASV, saphenous vein; BCH, Bovine graft; Superior patency of PTFE. (*From Haimov M, Burrows L, et al.: J Cardiovasc Surg 21:150, 1980.*)

infection, extrusion, and hemorrhage can occur.[29] There seems to be little to justify the expense of this type of device at the present time.

Finally, a review of types of access cannot be considered complete without mention of the permanent peritoneal dialysis catheter[30] (Fig. 59-1A). Although not a vascular device, it is invaluable in the management of acute renal failure, especially in the postoperative period. Unlike hemodialysis, peritoneal dialysis is unaffected by fluctuating blood pressures, and, in addition, the hazards of heparinization can be avoided. There are several types of peritoneal catheters, all of which consist of silicone tubing with an attached Dacron cuff to prevent infection from tracking along the tube. The catheter may also be used for permanent access if peritoneal dialysis is selected as the long-term method of treatment.

SELECTION OF OPTIMUM METHOD

The selection of the best access method depends on both the indication for access and the patient. For short-term purposes, such as monitoring vital signs, performing apheresis, or giving dialysis treatment for acute tubular necrosis that is expected to resolve, a percutaneously inserted semirigid intravascular catheter is used.[13,16] For long-term chemotherapy, parenteral alimentation, and the treatment of blood disorders that do not require rapid aspiration of large volumes of blood, a permanent soft catheter is ideal. The advantage of these methods lies in the fact that vessels are preserved to be reused repeatedly. The disadvantages are those of a blind puncture; occasional hemorrhage and hematomas may occur, and the surrounding vessels and nerves may occasionally be injured. In the case of the subclavian vein, the possibility of pneumothorax and hemothorax exists. However, with experienced personnel, such problems can be minimized. Chemotherapy and parenteral alimentation can also be administered into veins arterialized by an AVF, although this method is used with diminishing frequency because of the convenience and safety of permanent central venous catheters. The fistula must also be created before the beginning of therapy. Internal access through an AVF performed for chemotherapy after superficial veins are sclerosed requires a graft that must be attached to a large vein, such as the femoral vein, because the highly irritating solutions will inevitably cause occlusion of smaller veins.

The provision of access for dialysis requires special consideration. It involves cooperation among the nephrologist, dialysis technician, patient, and surgeon. Inasmuch as these patients can survive more than 20 years, the emphasis should be on preservation of blood vessels. In all hospitalized patients in whom any possibility of renal failure exists, one upper extremity should be preserved from arterial and venous puncture.[31] Creation of an AVF weeks or months before the anticipated need for dialysis is often possible (e.g., in cases of diabetes mellitus or polycystic disease), if the patient's peripheral blood vessels have not been destroyed by repeated puncture of arteries and veins. In such circumstances, the surgical procedure is easy and the first dialysis can be accomplished on an ambulatory

of an occluded superior vena cava has been described.[24] For drug administration, a version of the catheter can be attached to a subcutaneous reservoir. Because there is no external component, the risk of infection is further reduced. Drugs are administered through special needles that puncture the skin and the self-sealing silicone rubber diaphragm of the device, which is heparinized between uses.[25] A single-lumen version of the external cuffed catheter has been used to maintain patients on dialysis therapy for up to 1 year.[26] Permanent double-lumen catheters (PermCath) (Fig. 59-1D) are now available; they are useful in many difficult circumstances and have the added advantage of obviating needle punctures.[23] Another choice for "no needle" dialysis is available in two commercial versions (Bentley Diatap button, and Hemasite).[27,28] Briefly, the device consists of a rigid T tube that is lined with material of low thrombogenicity and is attached to a PTFE graft that is then anastomosed to an artery and a vein. A Dacron cuff, for fibrous ingrowth, is fused around the neck of the T. The lip of the device protrudes through the skin, and dialysis is performed by inserting special cannulas through the self-sealing skin portal. Special equipment and training at the dialysis center are required. The device is subject to the disadvantages of grafts and to those of external devices. Thus occlusion, basis by simple venipuncture. When a patient comes to the physician for the first time and is in acute renal failure without access, hemodialysis is accomplished by intermittent femoral venipuncture or by an indwelling central venous catheter, or peritoneal dialysis can be carried out. (We have not found it necessary to implant an external shunt at Montefiore Medical Center, New York, since 1976.) Permanent access should be created as soon as possible.

The purpose of permanent access is to permit easy and rapid cannulation of two portals so as to obtain blood flows of 200 ml or more per minute, three times weekly for a lifetime. Thus a surgical anastomosis between an artery and a deep vein should not be considered a success just because of a palpable thrill. If the resulting arterialized veins cannot be punctured easily, the procedure is considered to be a failure. The side-to-side AVF at the wrist or antecubital fossa fulfills many objectives. If created distally in the forearm, it provides an abundance of accessible superficial veins. If either vessel at the preferred location just proximal to the crease of the wrist is unsuitable, the radial artery is anastomosed at the most distal point to which an appropriate vein can be approximated (Fig. 59-3). If available, the radial artery should always be used because if it becomes occluded, the ulnar artery can almost still supply blood flow to the hand. Several modifiations of the side-to-side fistula have been described.[32,33] Of special interest is the AVF created in the anatomic "snuffbox," which allows easy approximation of artery and vein. Its use has been reported without major problems, but its prominent location may be cosmetically unappealing to some patients. It also has the potential of creating ischemia of the thumb, which may not be easily correctable. In the absence of a patent radial artery, the use of the ulnar artery to basilic vein fistula has been reported. However, we believe this practice should be avoided, for two reasons: First, it increases the risk of ischemia to the forearm and hand; second, it is difficult to puncture the resultant arterialized basilic vein and to stabilize a needle within it. Moreover, it requires that the patient's arm be placed in awkward and impractical positions for dialysis. If the radial artery cannot be used in either arm, the brachial artery must then be considered for an antecubital AVF. A vein can almost always be located in proximity to the brachial artery for the creation of a patent fistula, especially in thin individuals.[34,35] Limitation of the size of the brachial arteriotomy will minimize the risks of limb ischemia and congestive heart failure. In obese individuals, a brachial AVF may be a poor choice because the resulting veins may be inaccessible. In such patients, Dagher[36] suggested a method in which the basilic vein is mobilized completely, transected distally, redirected through a superficial tunnel on the upper part of the arm, and then anastomosed to the brachial artery. This method has the advantage of avoiding synthetic substances, and Dagher reports 70% patency at 8 years. However, it is a complicated procedure that requires a prolonged period for maturation and then ultimately provides only a short segment of usable arterialized vein.

When an AVF is not feasible, the gap between a suitable artery and vein must be bridged by a graft. In addition, a graft may also be used in obese patients in whom a direct AVF is technically possible but in whom the veins would

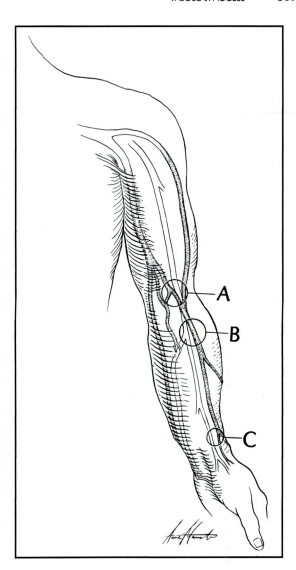

Figure 59-3. Sites for AVF. **A.** Brachial artery used when entire radial artery is occluded. **B.** Midforearm location. **C.** Preferred location at wrist.

be at too great a depth for easy puncture. As has already been pointed out, PTFE grafts are at present generally agreed to be the most suitable prosthetic material for this purpose. It must clearly be understood that the relative ease of graft insertion and of its initial use for dialysis does not justify its insertion when a wholly autogenous AVF is possible. Unlike human tissue, a graft cannot regenerate, and it is only a matter of time before repeated needle punctures lead to ostruction, occlusion, infection, bleeding, or a combination of these. In fact, it is the ease of treating these common complications when they occur that has led to the popularity of PTFE as a graft material for access.

When possible, the site of the graft should be in the *upper extremity*. The distal radial artery should be used as the arterial source, because it can be ligated in case of infection and because proximal vessels are thereby preserved for possible future use. The brachial artery is used when the radial is occluded up to its origin. The graft diameter should not exceed 6 mm to reduce the risk of ischemia. Anastomosis of the venous end into the basilic vein above the elbow permits easy bypass to a proximal site in the event of future occlusion (Fig. 59-4; see also Fig. 59-7). A graft should be easy to puncture and should provide as much length as possible, so that the sites of graft puncture can be varied. The short, deeply placed upper arm graft between the brachial artery and axillary vein is therefore undesirable and contributes to the creation of future "access problems." An infection or a venous outflow stenosis of such a graft poses serious problems in management and may require a major, dangerous operation[37] or lead to loss of access. A graft placed in a loop configuration is preferred by some surgeons to the straight forearm graft because of a supposedly superior patency rate. This approach bears further scrutiny. Numerous variables, such as surgical technique, size and character of blood vessel, frequency of use for dialysis, and technique of dialysis puncture, affect graft patency. Therefore graft patency is of limited value in assessing the adequacy of a particular type of dialysis access.

Many straight grafts remain patent for years. When occlusion occurs, revision of the graft can be simple if the basilic vein has been used. If, at the time of the initial operation, the artery is unsuitable or the distal artery becomes occluded after functioning for awhile, a loop graft can still be placed. By means of occasional reoperation, the life of the initial graft can be prolonged for years. On the other hand, the placement of a loop in the forearm between the brachial artery and antecubital vein as the initial procedure unnecessarily limits and complicates future options. If the venous end of the graft is in the antecubital fossa, revision is often impossible and the graft may have to be abandoned.

The use of *axilloaxillary* grafts has little appeal. By using the roots of both upper extremities, the future use of both upper limbs is compromised. Graft occlusion is inevitable during the patient's life, and this approach makes subsequent procedures difficult or impossible. Furthermore, because dialysis is conducted in an open outpatient setting, the requirement that the patient's chest be bared is eminently impractical, especially for women. Arterioarterial

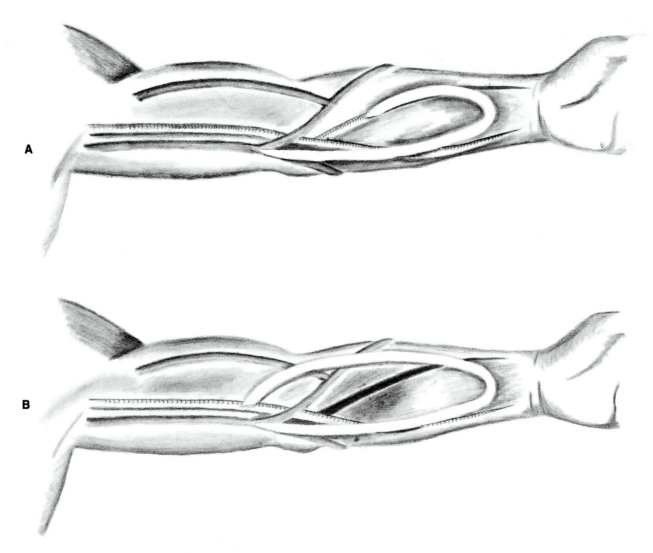

Figure 59-4. Arterial end of graft from **(A)** proximal radial artery when distal radial artery is occluded and from **(B)** brachial artery when entire radial is occluded. Note grafts cross joint at ends of crease. See Fig. 59-7 for preferred configuration.

grafts occasionally have been used,[38] with brief follow-up periods.

The *lower extremity* is less desirable for access. Leg AVF are impractical because venipuncture is very difficult and made even worse by edema of the extremity. The saphenous vein itself can be used in a manner similar to Dagher's procedure using the arm; here again, the vein should be of considerable length so that a sufficiently long segment is available for puncture. To avoid extensive dissection, one can use a PTFE graft for such patients. The graft originates at the proximal superficial artery, is looped into the distal portion of the thigh, and is anastomosed to the saphenous vein near its termination. The common femoral and popliteal arteries should be avoided because a graft complication requiring arterial ligation would create an unacceptably high risk of limb loss in a patient without major vascular disease. Moreover, virtually all prosthetic graft fistulas sooner or later occlude. The risks and problems of reoperating on femoral vessels are greater than those of reoperating on vessels in the upper extremity. Because of proximity to the groin, the hazards of infection and its consequences are also greater. Rather than subject patients to these risks, we now prefer to use a permanent venous catheter (Perm-Cath) in patients who cannot have any upper limb access procedure. This group includes patients with vascular disease, those with exhaustion of usable sites from previous access attempts, and patients with hemodynamic instability, low cardiac output, or disorders of coagulation that result in repeated occlusion of grafts that seem technically and mechanically sound. The catheter is inserted under direct vision into the internal jugular vein and is tunneled subcutaneously to exit on the chest wall, where it can be concealed under clothing. Like all cuffed silicone catheters, it is tolerated for long periods and has a low infection rate. The ends of its two lumina are separated from each other to minimize recirculation, and the walls of the catheter are stiffer than those of other venous catheters so that negative pressure does not cause collapse (Fig. 59-1D). Because blood is drawn from a venous reservoir, unstable blood pressure does not affect the catheter's function. Catheter occlusion can sometimes be corrected by streptokinase infusion; if unsuccessful, replacement of the catheter may be required. Such replacement is often a simple matter of surgically exposing the catheter tract and using a guide wire to facilitate sliding the new catheter into the tract of the old one.

For patients in whom none of these alternatives is possible, peritoneal dialysis should be considered. It may be the method of choice for those with severe vascular or cardiac problems. If this, too, is impossible, one must accept the fact that some circumstances are beyond our present capacity to correct; these should be rare indeed.

PREOPERATIVE EVALUATION

Evaluation of the Patient

A general assessment of the patient is essential. Operative risk factors should be sought. Bleeding and clotting parameters should be normal; there should be no major source of sepsis that might cause endocarditis. The patient's hemo-

dynamic status should be adequate. Patients with renal disease may have been treated with fluid restriction and aggressive diuresis, resulting in dehydration and hypovolemia, both of which should be corrected before operation. Cardiac decompensation, if present, should be treated. A patient with low blood pressure may not be able to maintain patency of a fistula. If these factors are not amenable to correction, consideration should be given to a central venous or peritoneal catheter as the definitive access route.

Evaluation of the Extremity

In patients whose arms have been spared arterial and venous punctures, the nondominant arm is preferred, because it allows the patient the freedom to read or eat while receiving dialysis therapy. The venous system is evaluated for patency. For discrimination between a recently thrombosed vein and an engorged patent one, the veins should collapse after the release of tourniquet compression. The presence of cutdown scars or of many tortuous collateral veins should alter the examiner to the possibility that the main cephalic vein is occluded. Superficial collateral veins are poorly suited to the creation of fistulas, because they are fragile and too convoluted for cannulation with any degree of consistency.

The pulses in the extremity should be palpated. If there is doubt about the adequacy of the arteries or veins in one extremity, the other should be used. A severely edematous arm should be elevated and wrapped with an elastic bandage for a few hours so that the veins can be assessed. When distal forearm veins are occluded, a proximal radial AVF can frequently be created in the mid forearm; this is useful only if the patient has prominent antecubital or upper arm cephalic and basilic veins. When prolonged illness or drug abuse has resulted in obliteration of superficial veins, a graft may be required as the primary procedure. In the majority of instances, careful clinical examination (occasionally reinforced by pulse volume recordings) provides the same information as do cumbersome and expensive contrast studies, which should be reserved for patients with multiple previous procedures or serious vascular problems.

OPERATIVE TECHNIQUES

General Principles

Most AVF procedures can be done on an outpatient basis with the patient under local infiltration anesthesia. Graft insertions and some reoperative or complicated procedures may require axillary or supraclavicular nerve block; epidural anesthesia may be required for femoral operations. Only occasionally should a brief hospitalization be necessary. The hazards of general anesthesia in these patients do not justify its use except in extraordinary circumstances. Antibiotics are unnecessary for routine creation of an AVF. However, all graft insertions and reoperative surgery should be performed under the protection of perioperative antibiotics. A single preoperative intravenous dose of a broad-spectrum cephalosporin provides adequate protection against common pathogens. In patients receiving regular dialysis therapy, the operation should be done on the day of, or the day following, dialysis to ensure optimum electrolyte balance.

Upper limb procedures are done with the patient supine and the arm draped free and extended at right angles on a hand table; the surgeon and assistant are seated, facing each other across the table. Incisions should be as small as commensurate with safety and should be placed away from vascular anastomoses. Systemic heparin is avoided; heparinized saline solution is instilled into the blind segments of all vessels before they are occluded for anastomosis. Vascular occlusion should be by silicone tapes, rather than clamps. Subcutaneous tunnels for grafts should be created by gentle dissection and should not exceed the

diameter of the graft. Grafts that cross the antecubital crease should be led across either end, rather than the middle, to avoid acute angulation (Fig. 59-4).

Arteriovenous Fistula

To create an arteriovenous fistula (Fig. 59-5), the surgeon makes a transverse incision 2 cm proximal to the flexion crease of the wrist. (If a more proximal fistula is to be created, a longitudinal incision affords better exposure.) The incision is carried through the superficial fascia, and the cephalic vein is identified and bluntly mobilized on silicone rubber vessel tapes to the limits of the incision (Fig. 59-5B). All overlying soft tissue is divided longitudi-

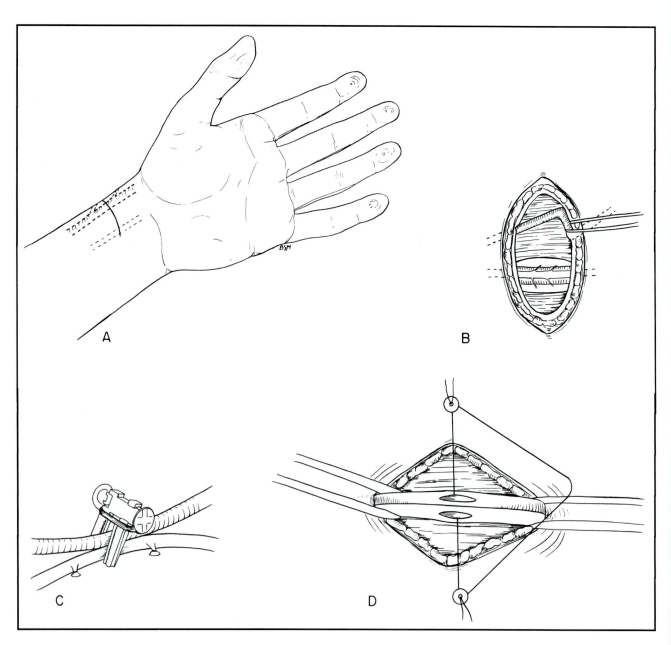

Figure 59-5. Operative technique for creation of AVF. Details in text.

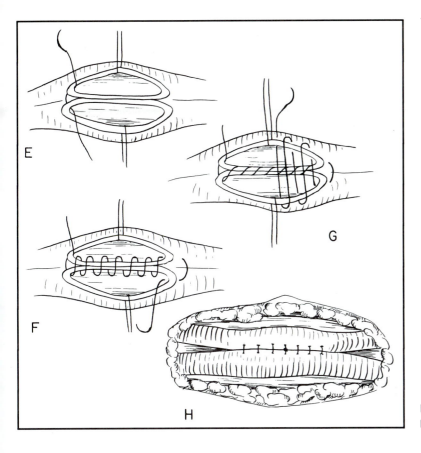

Figure 59-5, cont'd. For legend see opposite page.

nally, layer by layer. Major tributaries are preserved, although smaller ones may be divided. Next, with fine ophthalmologic forceps and blunt-nosed tenotomy scissors, the adventitial areolar tissue coverings of the vein itself are dissected away. The vein is then released from traction and allowed to return to its resting place. The deep fascia is infiltrated with lidocaine and then opened longitudinally on the ulnar side of the brachioradialis tendon. The vascular bundle is revealed. The investing fascia is opened (Fig. 59-5B), and a vessel tape is passed around the artery, which is mobilized by sharp dissection, division of overlying areolar tissue, and ligation and division of several paired muscular branches. It should now be possible to approximate the mobilized artery and vein without tension or distortion. A lightweight disposable plastic bulldog clamp is now placed across both vessels at the proposed fistula site while in the relaxed position (Fig. 59-5C). This maintains proper alignment of the vessels while vessel tapes are passed around the vessels, proximally and distally, and clamped to the drapes with just enough tension to occlude blood flow. The clamp is removed and a 6 mm venotomy made at the predetermined site, facing the artery. The vein is irrigated with heparinized saline solution. Tension on both tapes is then released and the bulldog clamp reapplied to ensure that the relative position of the vessels has not been altered by the manipulations. The tapes are then reapplied. An arteriotomy is made facing the venotomy and both incisions are equalized; the final size should not exceed 8 mm. Vascular dilators up to 3 mm in size are progressively introduced cephalad, each passage being permitted by momen-

tary relaxation of the tapes. Dilatation is not done toward the hand. Finally, heparinized saline solution is instilled into all four vascular limbs to prevent clotting in any potential dead space.

A stay suture of 6–0 silk is now placed at the midpoint of the outer edges of artery and vein, and attached to a vascular anastomosis bow.[39] This lightweight device allows tension on the sutures to be adjusted as desired and retracts the edges apart for good visibility (Fig. 59-5D). One end of a double-armed, 6–0 polypropylene suture is tagged. The other needle is passed from within the lumen, out of the cephalad venous apex. This needle is now passed from outside into the arterial lumen, near the apex (Fig. 59-5E); the posterior wall is then completed from within, in an over-and-over manner (Fig. 59-5F). The suture is continued around the caudal apex and on to the anterior wall, until the stay suture is approached (Fig. 59-5G). This end, with the suture on the outside, is now tagged, and the other end is released and passed from within and then out the cephalad arterial apex. The anterior wall is completed in an over-and-over fashion. The irrigating cannula is now introduced through the anastomosis, first into the artery and then into vein, while tapes are momentarily released for each passage. Each vessel is aspirated and irrigated with heparinized saline solution. The cannula is withdrawn, the stays are removed, the suture is tied, and the vascular occlusion is released (Fig. 59-5H). Compression is applied for several minutes to ensure hemostasis. Uremia may cause prolonged bleeding, and patience is essential. Additional sutures should not be required in a well-performed anasto-

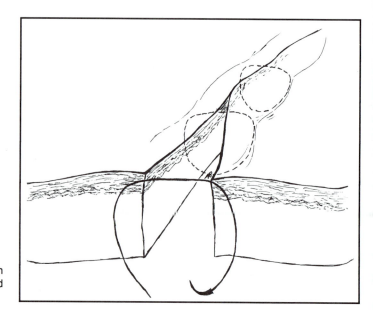

Figure 59-6. Diagrammatic representation of skin and subcutaneous closure with buried interrupted vertical sutures.

mosis, although the application of topical agents (thrombin, bovine collagen) to promote clotting may occasionally be necessary. A thrill should be palpable in most instances. The fistula should now be inspected. Further division of deep fascia may be required, as well as the gentle teasing away of residual adventitial bands. When bleeding has subsided, the incision is closed with a few interrupted sutures of 4–0 polyglactin (Fig. 59-6). These are placed from the deep surface, incorporating superficial fascia and dermis on one side and dermis and superficial fascia on the other. The knot is thus buried, and the resultant closure approximates both subcutaneous tissue and skin, allows for serous drainage, is cosmetically atttractive, and obviates the fear that a skin suture infection might contaminate the vascular anastomosis. A light dressing is applied, and after brief observation, the patient is discharged with a prescription for analgesics.

Polytetrafluoroethylene Graft Fistula

If local anesthesia is to be used to create a PTFE graft fistula (Fig. 59-7), a mixture of lidocaine and bupivacaine (Marcaine) is employed to obtain prolonged analgesia without toxic effects. An oblique incision is made proximal to the antecubital crease, on the medial aspect of the upper arm, directed toward the medial condyle of the humerus. The superficial fascia is opened, and the basilic vein is identified and mobilized on tapes at a point proximal to the confluence of the medial cubital vein. If superficial vessels are occluded, the venae comitantes of the brachial artery will have undergone compensatory enlargement and can be mobilized by means of the same incision. The selected vein is now allowed to return to its resting position, and a transverse incision is made over the distal radial artery, as for an AVF fistula. The deep fascia is opened longitudinally and the artery mobilized by division of paired branches. (If the artery is occluded or unsuitable at this level, a third incision is made longitudinally in the midline of the forearm distal to the

antecubital crease; the radial artery is then mobilized at its origin from the brachial. If this, too, is impossible, the brachial artery itself can be mobilized [Fig. 59-8].) A size 20 French trocar chest catheter is placed on the forearm distal to the venous incision, parallel to the ulnar border of the forearm, but sufficiently anterior so that the forearm will not rest on it (Fig. 59-7A). A marking pencil is used to outline its location on the skin. The lines are curved to meet the edge of the arterial incision in a gentle J shape. The area under the outlined skin is infiltrated with local anesthesia, unless a regional block has been used. The trocar catheter is now introduced into the venous incision and pushed distally under the outlined skin to create a subcutaneous tunnel (Fig. 59-7B). In most patients, the tunnel lies deep to the superficial fascia; in obese patients, the tunnel lies superficial to the fascia. The tunnel created by a 20 French catheter will accommodate a 6 mm graft exactly. When the tip of the catheter is palpated to be opposite the arterial incision, the trocar is removed. A clamp is introduced into the arterial incision, and the end of the catheter is drawn out, leaving most of it within the tunnel to provide hemostasis (Fig. 59-7C). A 6 mm graft is brought into the field and obliquely transected at one end. The vein is atraumatically occluded by vessel loops on traction, and a 1 cm venotomy is created. Patency is confirmed by the passage of dilators and by irrigation with heparinized solution. From within outward, a double-armed 6–0 polypropylene suture is passed through the apex of the graft and of the cephalic end of the venotomy; it is then tied. A second suture is passed through the heel of the graft and the other end of the venotomy, which is first lengthened if necessary. This suture is not tied (Fig. 59-7D). The posterior graft-to-vein suture line is run from the apex downward. The lower suture is tied to itself and the posterior suture; the anterior wall is completed from below upward (Fig. 59-7E). Before the suture is tied, the vein is flushed with heparinized solution. A vascular clamp is placed across the graft, traction released, and the vein allowed to assume its natural resting position. Hemostasis is obtained by compression with a sponge. At this point, one end of a disposable plastic vein stripper is introduced into the distal end of the previously placed catheter, to emerge at the proximal end (Fig. 59-7F). The catheter is withdrawn, leaving the stripper in the tunnel. The proximal end of the stripper is introduced into the free end of the graft and securely tied (Fig. 59-7G). Traction is applied to the distal end of the stripper, and the graft is drawn through the tunnel until it emerges from the distal incision. Care is taken to avoid twisting or kinking the graft. For J-shaped grafts, the graft is now divided precisely where it overlies the artery while both are in the resting position; the arterial anastomosis is then begun (Fig. 59-7H).

The U-shaped grafts require a different approach (Fig. 59-8). We prefer to use a PTFE graft with the middle 5 cm segment supported by polystyrene rings around the external surface to prevent kinking. After the chest tube is inserted as described above (Fig. 59-7C), the stripper is inserted immediately and one end of the graft is attached to it at the distal end after the tube is removed (Fig. 59-8A). Traction is applied from above, until the polystyrene rings enter the distal incision. The graft is divided and the venous anastomosis completed as previously described. The chest tube is now reintroduced from the proximal arterial incision, to emerge at the distal loop incision (Fig. 59-8B). The trocar is removed. The free end of the stripper is passed into the tube to emerge at the arterial end. The tube is removed. The free end of the graft is secured to the other end of the stripper and drawn through the other

limb of the tunnel until the ringed segment is seated snugly in the middle of the loop. The graft is cut to size (Fig. 59-8C). For both J-shaped and U-shaped grafts, the artery is now placed under traction and an arteriotomy made at a site determined before the traction was applied. Patency is confirmed by irrigation and dilators. An end-to-side anastomosis is performed with a suture of 6–0 polypropylene. Before this suture is tied, an irrigating cannula is introduced through the suture line—first into the artery and then into the graft, while occlusion is momentarily released. The suture is tied, all occlusion released, and compression applied for hemostasis. A thrill is usually palpated throughout the graft. The incisions are closed as for AVF, and light dressings are applied.

POSTOPERATIVE CARE

Surgical Aspects

Uncomplicated AVFs require minimal care. After a brief period of observation, the patient is discharged with instruction to avoid wetting the incision until healing has occurred. Analgesics are prescribed for pain. If edema occurs, elevation is necessary; this is more common when a graft has been inserted and may take several days to subside. Severe edema is more commonly associated with the use of the brachial artery as inflow, the axillary vein as outflow, and a large-diameter graft as the conduit. This is an additional

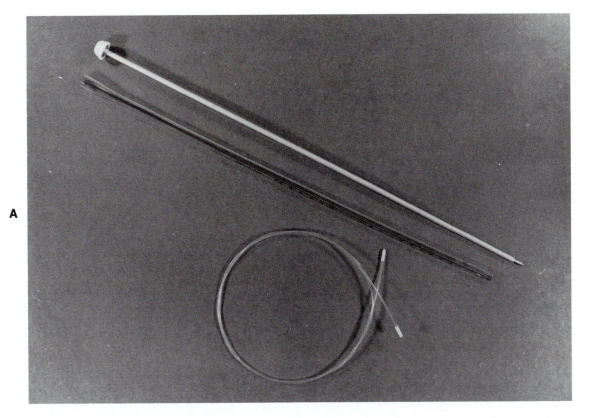

Figure 59-7. Operative technique for creation of PTFE graft fistula. **A.** (*Top*) Chest tube with its trocar alongside, used for making tunnel. (*Bottom*) Vein stripper used to draw graft through tunnel. *Continued.*

816

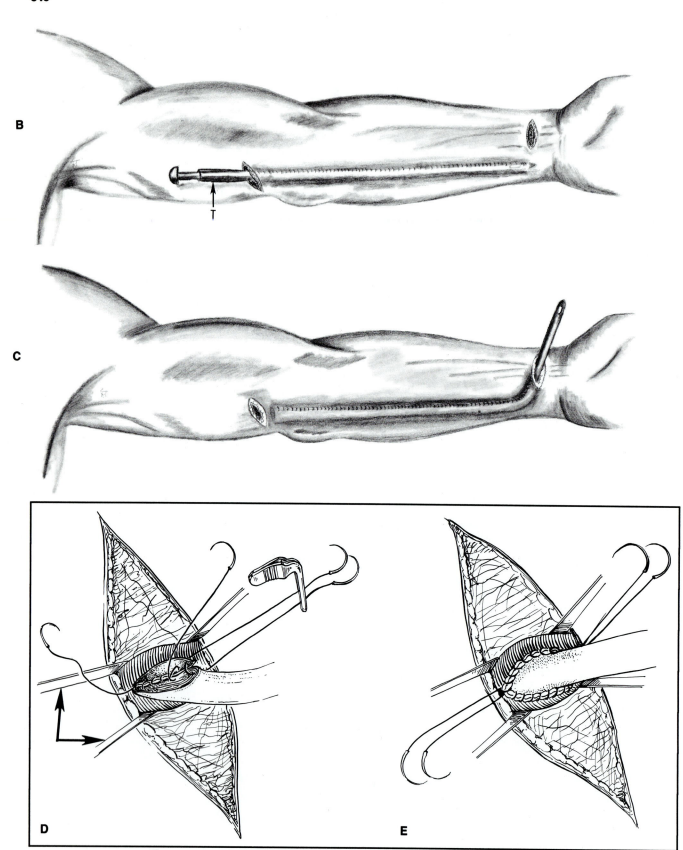

Figure 59-7, cont'd. B. Trocar chest tube (*T*) has been inserted under skin of forearm from upper (venous) incision. **C.** Trocar has been removed. Distal end of catheter has been drawn out through distal (arterial) incision. **D.** Detail of anastomosis. Vein occluded by silicone loops (*L*) on traction. Apical suture between graft and vein has been tied. Posterior wall of anastomosis in progress from above downward. Heel suture placed, tagged, but not tied until posterior wall is completed. **E.** Anastomosis completed from below upward.

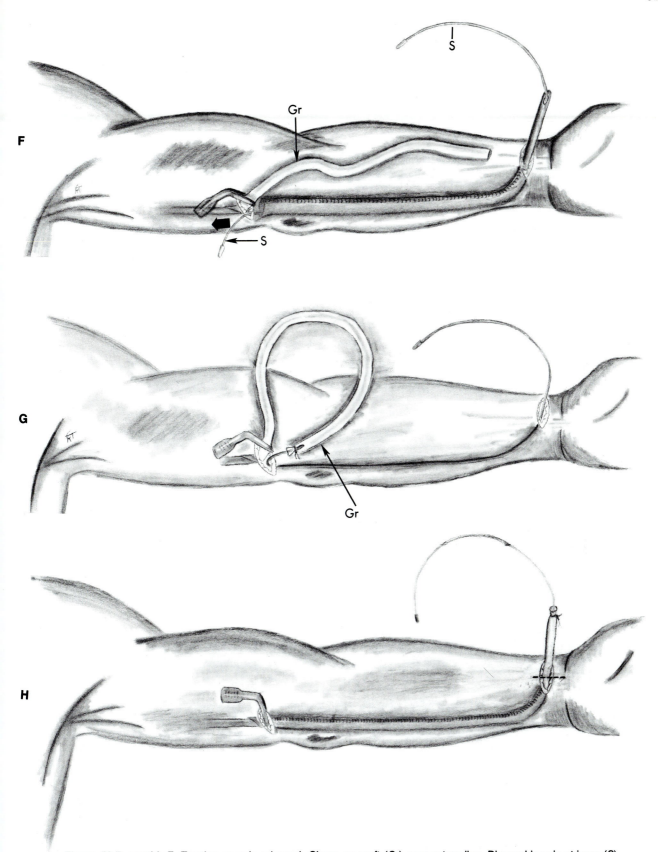

Figure 59-7, cont'd. F. Traction on vein released. Clamp on graft (*Gr*) near suture line. Disposable vein stripper (*S*) passed through distal end of tube, to emerge from incision at proximal end. Tube removed in direction of arrow, leaving stripper in tunnel. **G.** Proximal end of stripper introduced into free end of graft (*Gr*) and securely tied. Traction applied on distal end of stripper to draw graft into tunnel. **H.** Graft in tunnel. Excess graft divided (*dotted line*) where it overlies artery.

Continued.

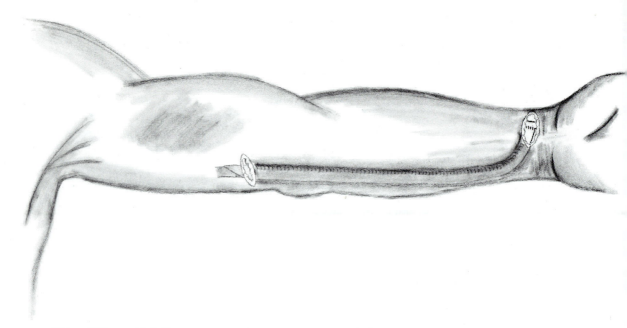

Figure 59-7, cont'd. I. All anastomoses completed. Clamp removed from vein. Incisions to be closed.

reason to use the radial artery and to avoid graft diameters over 6 mm. As a general rule, the arm should not be used for blood pressure measurement, intravenous therapy, or venipuncture other than for dialysis.

Dialysis Aspects

Problems associated with the use of the access for dialysis can be minimized by adherence to a few basic principles. Skin preparation before puncture should be scrupulous, as in a surgical scrub, with the use of povidone-iodine or an equivalent. Large superficial veins resulting from an AVF may be used within 24 hours; however, if veins are small or if local factors such as edema make puncture difficult, use of the fistula should be postponed for fear of damaging the main outflow. PTFE grafts can also be used within 24 hours; however, the insertion or withdrawal of a needle may result in a massive hematoma in the tunnel, jeopardizing or occluding the graft. It is therefore preferable to wait two weeks or more for better adherence of the graft to surrounding tissue. The needles, which should have a short bevel and not exceed 15 gauge, should never be inserted in the vicinity of a surgical scar to avoid disruption of an anastomosis; the corollary is that scars should not be excessive in length, creating a dilemma for the dialysis technician. Proper training is essential so that needles are properly inserted and positioned and damage to the back wall of the vein or graft is avoided. Needle puncture sites should be varied because repeated assault with a needle at the same location will inevitably destroy vessel or graft and cause occlusion or bleeding. If tourniquets must be used, they should be left on for the minimum possible time. On withdrawal of the needle after dialysis, firm pressure should be applied to the puncture site in the vessel, rather than at the skin puncture site, which may not be

directly over the needle hole in the vessel. The pressure should be sufficient to stop bleeding but not flow; it is best applied with a gloved fingertip, rather than a wad of gauze, which may obscure underlying bleeding or hematoma.

COMPLICATIONS

Occlusion

Occlusion is the commonest complication with all types of access. It can occur early, within hours after access has been created, or late, after prolonged use of the access route. Early occlusion is usually caused by a simple thrombus, resulting from poor inflow, poor outflow, or a surgical infection. Occlusion that occurs later often has a more complex origin. The management depends on the type of access and the duration of function. If a side-to-side AVF becomes occluded *intraoperatively* shortly after the anastomosis has been completed, an arteriotomy is made distal to the fistula, through which embolectomy catheters, dilators, and heparinized solution are introduced into the artery and through the fistula into the vein. After restoration of flow, the artery is ligated distal to the anastomosis, effectively converting it to an end-to-side anastomosis. If occlusion has occurred *postoperatively* in a fistula between suboptimal vessels, with a low expectation of success and with the hope of avoiding more intricate procedures, new access must be planned. If, however, such occlusion is unexpected, contributory factors must be sought and corrected. These may include systemic or local causes. Rather than attempt to reopen the old anastomosis, with its now traumatized and occluded vessels, it is expedient to create a new fistula immediately proximal to the old one, with the use of a fresh site in the vessel that may be adjacent to that used previously.

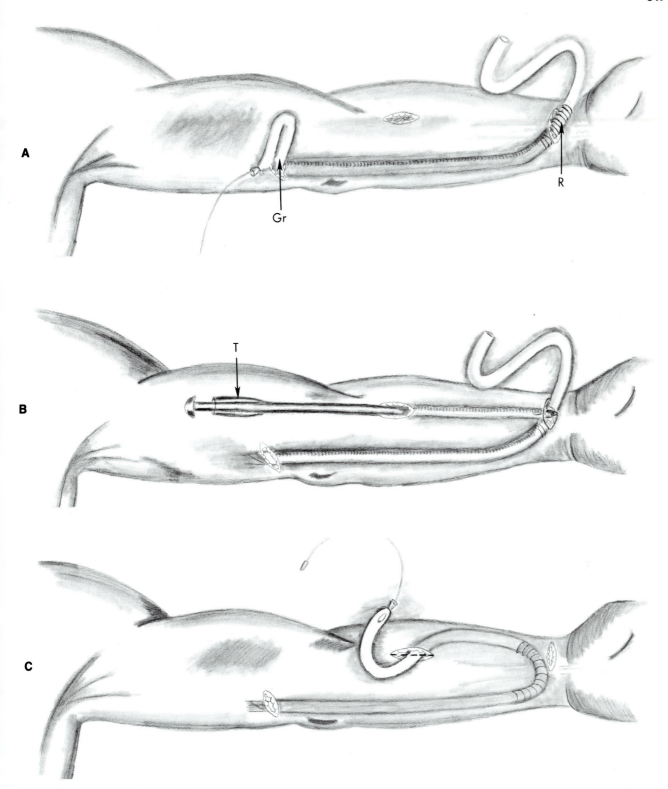

Figure 59-8. PTFE graft fistula. Variation of technique when distal artery is occluded. **A.** Tube inserted as in Figure 59-7B and C. Stripper passed through as in Figure 59-7F and G, and tube removed. Graft (*Gr*) secured to *distal* end of stripper, and drawn through tunnel to emerge at *proximal* end, until ringed segment (*R*) enters distal incision. Excess graft removed at venous end, and anastomosis completed as in Figure 59-7D and E. **B.** Chest tube (*T*) reinserted from proximal forearm arterial incision, to emerge at distal incision. Trocar removed, stripper introduced, and tube withdrawn from above. **C.** Free end of graft attached to stripper and drawn through other limb of tunnel. Graft divided (*dotted line*) over artery, and anastomosis completed. Note ringed segment supporting loop of graft, and seated in tunnel, away from incision.

The same objectives are thus achieved, with increased expectation of success.

When an access route has been functioning for *weeks or months*, its occlusion requires a search for a cause. With AVF, an autologous arteriosclerotic occlusion of the artery or neointimal hyperplasia of the fistula opening may have caused inflow occlusion; the outflow may be blocked by scarring due to repeated punctures at the same site. When a graft fistula is occluded, a common finding is stenosis of the lumen by intimal hyperplasia at the venous anastomosis or in the vein just distal to the graft. The causes of hyperplasia are debated, but turbulent blood flow may play a role. With all types of access, prolonged hypotension, or compression such as by tight garments or sleeping on the arm, may also result in occlusion.

A nonoperative approach to the correction of occlusion has been described by some authors.[40,41] The technique requires the insertion of a catheter through the occluded access route so that the end, guided fluoroscopically, lies near the arterial opening. Streptokinase solution is then infused by a pump or injected directly into the clot. After several hours, clot lysis takes place and the fistula or graft again begins to function. At that time, contrast material is injected to determine the presence of a cause of the occlusion. A stenotic lesion may be corrected by transluminal angioplasty or by subsequent surgical operation. The method must be used with caution. The patient must be hospitalized. Alternative means of dialysis must be arranged while attempts are made to restore permanent access. Since serious bleeding can occur, administration of streptokinase is contraindicated in postoperative patients and those in whom gastrointestinal or intracranial bleeding is present or suspected. Streptokinase can also cause bleeding from dialysis puncture sites. Hypersensitivity reactions can also occur, especially if the patient has previously received the drug. Advocates of this approach, however, report success in a high percentage of cases and suggest that the use of low doses of streptokinase (10,000 units/hour) given directly into the clot results in very few adverse reactions.

Another alternative is the operative approach, which may be simpler and safer under most circumstances. In occlusion of a longstanding AVF in the distal forearm, when a dilated patent artery and vein are present beyond the point of occlusion, a new fistula can be created proximal to the old one, with the previous venous network rearterialized. If the entire radial artery has been occluded, a brachial artery anastomosis may be required. This can be done on an outpatient basis, and the patient can return immediately to his previous dialysis schedule.

After a prosthetic graft has functioned for several months, arterial and venous dilation may have occurred, so that an autologous AVF, previously impossible, can now be created. This is the ideal solution to an occluded graft and should always be considered as the first option. Thrombectomy of an occluded graft is attempted through the original venous skin incision. An oblique incision is made into the graft near the venous suture line, and thrombectomy is carried out with balloon embolectomy catheters. The venous anastomosis should freely accept the largest (5 mm) Garrett dilators. Resistance encountered at or beyond the suture line suggests the presence of intimal hyperplasia

as a cause of occlusion. This must be corrected by patch angioplasty or by extending the graft to a new proximal vein by the addition of an extra PFTE segment (Fig. 59-9). This is easily done if the original venous outflow was to the basilic vein (Fig. 59-7) rather than to the deep antecubital veins, which do not easily permit this option.

Arterial flow can usually be reestablished by the retrograde passage of balloon catheters through the graft and past the arterial anastomosis. If this procedure is easily done and the venous end is also free of impediments, an arteriogram is essential to seek a cause for the occlusion. In the absence of a mechanical cause, occlusion may be explained by hypotension, which should be corrected to prevent recurrence of the problem. Aspirin and dipyridamole have been used for such patients, but these drugs increase the possibility of internal bleeding. PTFE grafts may be repeatedly thrombectomized through the same incision in those patients with recurrent uncorrectable hypotensive episodes; other alternatives for such patients are central venous catheters and peritoneal dialysis. Finally, an arterial cause may be suspected if a graft feels flaccid and there is no palpable pulse in the artery of origin. This type of occlusion may respond to arterial thrombectomy but is likely to require a segmental extension to provide new inflow from a proximal, patent artery (Fig. 59-4).

All graft reoperations are preceded by intravenous administration of antibiotics. For prevention of clotting while a segment of graft is clamped near the venous end during closure of the graft incision, heparin should be instilled into the graft before it is clamped. When new segments of graft are added, the old segments may be used immediately for dialysis.

Occlusion of an AVF or graft can be simple or complicated, and so can its management. Clinical evaluation, angiography, operation, angioplasty, and streptokinase infusion all have a role in management. They are not mutually exclusive, and, in fact, many patients will require more than one of these modalities. Selection of the appropriate course of action will depend on the nature of the problem, the availability of resources, and the judgment and expertise of the surgeons managing the problem. If all reasonable efforts to salvage a failed access have been exhausted, access must be created at a new site.

Infection

Infection at the surgical site of an AVF is a rare occurrence that should usually be assumed to occur from a breach of a technique. Infection through dialysis puncture sites, however, is more common. In patients with good hygiene and with careful puncture techniques—as in patients receiving home dialysis therapy, it rarely occurs. However, careless technique—including multiple punctures at the same site, double puncture, and puncture resulting in hematoma formation—invites infection from the host of skin organisms.[42] When such infection occurs, it is treated like an endocarditis, with prolonged antibiotic therapy. Surgical drainage may be necessary, and sometimes a segment of vein must be excised. If other arterialized channels exist, the access can be preserved, but if the infection involves the main vein,

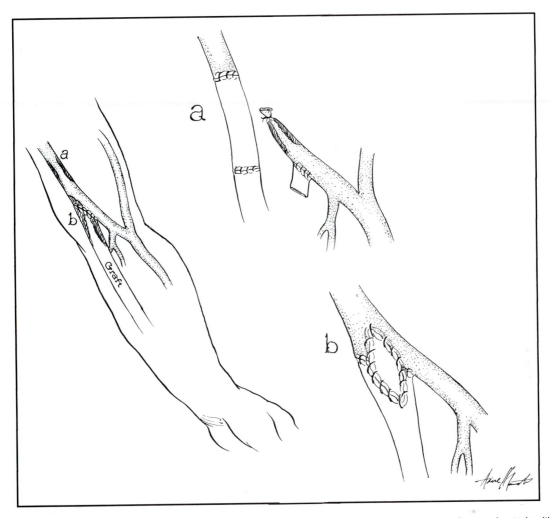

Figure 59-9. Treatment of outflow stenosis. **a.** Long segment beyond anastomosis treated by graft extension to healthy vein. **b.** Stenosis confined to anastomotic area treated by patch angioplasty.

there is no alternative to sacrificing the fistula. New access is created when the systemic threat is over.

Postoperative graft infection is also a rarity that must be differentiated from the mechanical sequelae of dissection in the subcutaneous plane. Erythema, edema, ecchymoses, and mild tenderness are common findings along the graft for several days after operation. If the patient appears to have toxic effects or is febrile, blood cultures are obtained, as well as a grain-stained smear and culture of any exudate from the incisions. A graft must be removed if there is a serious possibility that it may be infected. A graft that has been in use may become infected for reasons that are similar to those related to AVF infection, but with greater frequency because of the presence of a foreign body. Management depends on the circumstances. The patient may be febrile, with an obvious abscess localized to one area of a functioning graft that has undergone soft tissue fixation. The patient is placed on a regimen of antibiotic therapy, and the area is widely drained. As such infections arise at puncture sites, bleeding may occur during the drainage procedure. Larger lacerations in the graft may have to be repaired with No.

6–0 polypropylene suture material. The wound is packed with povidone-iodine and allowed to heal by secondary intention.[21] If defervescence occurs, graft use is continued and the access route is salvaged. During healing, the exposed graft may be displaced above skin level. It may then be necessary to rotate skin flaps to cover the site, after the acute process has subsided.[43] If the infection is extensive or is at or near a suture line in the blood vessel, or if the patient continues to be febrile, the access route should be sacrificed. Nonfunctioning grafts that have been left in situ may occasionally become infected, and draining sinuses or localized abscesses may appear. Since the vascular connections are occluded, the grafts may be removed by simple traction, the site being left open to provide drainage.

It must be reemphasized that the management outlined here for graft infection refers specifically to PTFE grafts. The only other prosthetic graft with which experience has been gained is bovine heterograft. This material undergoes dissolution when infected, and it cannot be sutured. Attempts should never be made to salvage these grafts because serious bleeding may occur.

Ischemia

A functioning radial-cephalic AVF may occasionally result in ischemia of the hand. This is caused by diversion of blood from the palmar arch into the low-resistance venous system. The patient complains of coldness, numbness, and cramps that worsen during dialysis. Manual compression of the fistula results in perceptible improvement of the distal pulses. This confirms the diagnosis and the adequacy of the circulation. Ligation of the radial artery distal to the fistula resolves the problem and preserves access. Ischemia resulting from brachial artery anastomoses requires more careful assessment. Ischemia resulting from fistulas or grafts with too great a flow may be resolved by narrowing of a fistula or banding of a graft. The incidence of this complication will be minimized if the brachial artery is avoided when possible, and by limiting the unavoidable anastomoses to 5 mm. Finally, some patients may have diffuse arterial disease, and arteriography may occasionally be justified if inflow problems are suspected. In such patients, any diversion of blood flow into the low-resistance venous system may cause ischemia. Such fistulas must be closed.

Other Complications

Venous Hypertension

Venous hypertension is manifested by severe edema of the hand, pain, and, if the condition is allowed to progress, ulceration of the digits. It may result when the proximal venous limb of a functioning fistula or graft is occluded and arterialized blood is pumped into a hand with inadequate venous drainage (Fig. 59-10). Ligation of the distal venous limb relieves the hypertension. If this represented the only outflow of the fistula, a proximal fistula must also be created to a patent vein. Lesser degrees of venous compromise may first occur as outflow resistance during dialysis. Angiography may reveal a stenosis that may be amenable to transluminal dilatation, which could prevent a later occlusion (Fig. 59-11). If venous hypertension results from brachial artery inflow into the axillary vein of an extremity that has had a considerable amount of venous compromise, the only treatment alternatives may be banding of the graft or closure of the access.

Nerve Complications

Nerve complications may occasionally occur.[44] Notable among these are nerve entrapment syndromes, which cause sensory and motor changes in the hand. Nerve conduction studies are useful in differentiating this problem from peripheral neuropathy and from ischemia due to a steal syndrome, which may also be manifested as numbness and weakness. The treatment is release of the median nerve at the wrist.

Aneurysm Formation

If confined to arterialized veins, aneurysm formation does not require treatment. Aneurysm formation at the site of repeated needle punctures of PTFE grafts is inevitable after a period of years. The offending area is repaired by suture, patch, or segmental replacement, as indicated, permitting continued use of the rest of the graft. Pseudoaneurysms

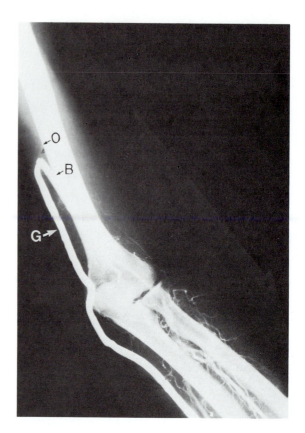

Figure 59-10. Graft angiogram in venous hypertension. Proximal outflow (*O*) occluded. Total flow from graft (*G*) is retrograde into basilic vein (*B*). Treated by graft extension to proximal vein, as in Figure 59-9A.

at suture lines represent anastomotic dehiscences that must be repaired. If infection is the cause, the fistula must be closed.

Congestive Heart Failure

Congestive heart failure may occur with large left-to-right shunts. It is rarely seen with peripheral AVF. However, it occurs more commonly if the brachial or femoral artery is used, especially if the arteriotomy or graft diameter exceeds 6 mm. Excessive flow may be corrected by banding. The technique requires the use of a strip of Teflon felt, which is wrapped around the graft near the arterial end (or the venous outflow of an autologous AVF). Constriction is adjusted until the flow is reduced adequately and the band sutured to itself in the appropriate position. Adequacy of the reduction in flow may be gauged by palpation or more accurately measured by means of electromagnetic flow probes.

Graft angiography[45] can play an important role in the evaluation of problem fistulas and in the identification of defects before they cause occlusion. The arterialized vein or graft is punctured directly, and multiple rapid-sequence x-ray films are obtained during dye injection. The first few films are obtained during tourniquet compression, thus revealing the arterial inflow. The rest are taken after release, to reveal the outflow. All grafts that undergo occlusion should be studied after correction; occasional stenoses may be encountered that can be dilated transluminally (Fig. 59-

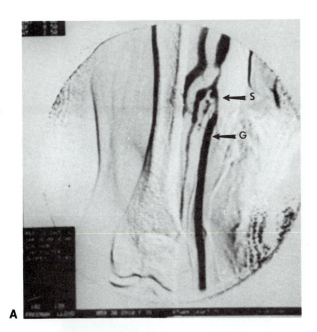

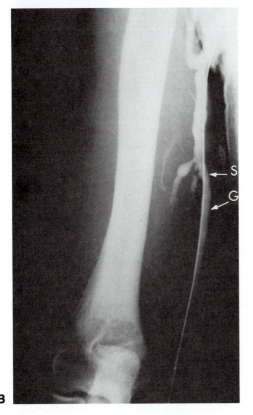

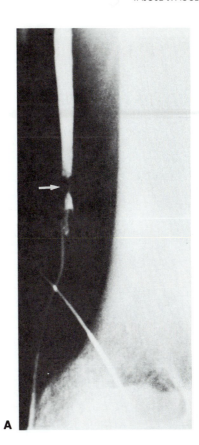

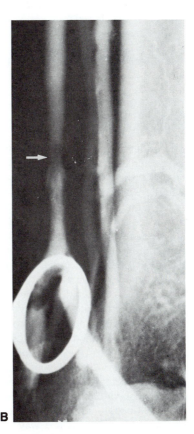

Figure 59-11. Venous hypertension. **A.** Digital intravenous angiogram showing long segment stenosis of vein (*S*), beyond insertion of graft (*G*). **B.** Contrast study after transluminal dilatation of narrowed segment. Guide wire has not yet been withdrawn.

12), or information may be obtained that will be useful in future surgery (Fig. 59-13). Angiography is especially useful when high venous resistance is noted during dialysis, the appearance of or increase in size of needle-site aneurysms is noted, or prolonged bleeding occurs after removal of needles. These suggest outflow obstruction, which can be

Figure 59-12. Postoperative graft angiogram showing stenotic segment in vein (*arrows*) before **(A)** and after **(B)** transluminal dilatation.

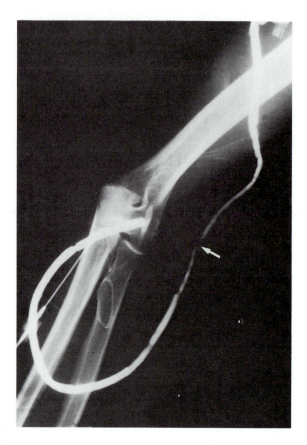

Figure 59-13. Graft angiogram after successful thrombectomy shows long, narrowed segment with severe stenosis at midpoint (*arrow*). Treated by replacement of segment.

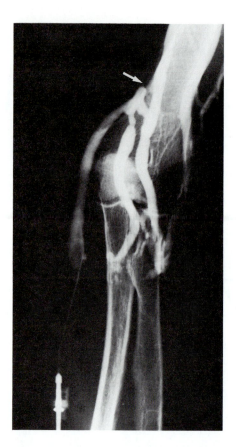

Figure 59-14. Graft angiogram for increased venous pressure on dialysis: complete occlusion of main outflow (*arrow*). Venous hypertension prevented by multiple collateral vessels.

corrected, preventing almost certain occlusion (Figs. 59-12 to Fig. 59-14).

CONCLUSIONS

The surgeon who undertakes the provision of vascular access must have a thorough understanding of the many available options, and the advantages and disadvantages of each. The selection of a particular method should be dictated by the needs and limitations posed by the disease process and the patient. With regard to dialysis access, the surgeon should have an understanding of the procedures involved, and there should be a cooperative arrangement with the dialysis personnel and the nephrologists, as well as with the patient. Every attempt must be made to conserve blood vessels, to avoid prosthetic materials, and to preserve or restore access sites once they are functioning. Because the procedures are not performed for the treatment of vascular disease, they should be designed to avoid placing life and limb in jeopardy except under the most extraordinary circumstances. If at all possible, investigations, evaluations, and operations should be scheduled so as not to disrupt established dialysis routines. In this way, the existence of 70,000 people in the United States alone, as well as others for whom dialysis is a way of life, may be made more tolerable.

REFERENCES

1. Seldinger SI: Catheter replacement of a needle in percutaneous arteriography: A new technique. Acta Radiol 39:368, 1953.
2. Graham WB: Historical aspects of hemodialysis. Trans Proc 9:xlix, 1977.
3. Quinton WE, Dillard D, et al.: Cannulation of blood vessels for prolonged hemodialysis. Trans Am Soc Artif Intern Organs 6:104, 1960.
4. Thomas TI: Large vessel applique arteriovenous shunt for hemodialysis: A new concept. Am J Surg 120:244, 1970.
5. Brescia MJ, Cimino JE, et al.: Chronic hemodialysis using venepuncture and a surgically created arteriovenous fistula. N Engl J Med 275:1089, 1966.
6. Chinitz JL, Yokoyama T, et al.: Self-sealing prosthesis for arteriovenous fistula in man. Trans Am Soc Artif Intern Organs 18:452, 1972.
7. Rubio PA, Farrell EM: Modified human umbilical vein arteriovenous fistula for maintenance hemodialysis. Arch Surg 117:943, 1982.
8. Burdick JF, Scott W, et al.: Experience with Dacron graft arteriovenous fistulas for dialysis access. Ann Surg 187:262, 1978.
9. Soyer T, Lempineu M, et al.: A new venous prosthesis. Surgery 72:864, 1972.
10. Broviac JW, Cole JJ, et al.: A silicone rubber arterial catheter for prolonged parenteral alimentation. Surg Gynecol Obstet 136:602, 1973.
11. Hickman RO, Buckner D, et al.: A modified right artrial catheter for access to the venous system in marrow transplant recipients. Surg Gynecol Obstet 148:871, 1979.

12. Goldenberg HS, Goldberg EM, et al.: The arteriovenous fistula: Its construction in the management of hemophilia. Arch Surg 115:857, 1980.

13. Spindler JS: Subclavian vein catheterization for apheresis access. J Clin Apheresis 1:202, 1983.

14. Raaf JM: Vascular access grafts for chemotherapy. Ann Surg 190:614, 1979.

15. Wade JC, Newman KA, et al.: Two methods for improved venous access in acute leukemia patients. JAMA 246:140, 1981.

16. Tapson JS, Hoenich NA, et al.: Evaluation of the Shiley dual lumen subclavian hemodialysis catheter. Trans Am Soc Artif Intern Organs 31:140, 1985.

17. Dahlberg PJ, Yutuc WR, Newcomer KL: Subclavian hemodialysis catheter infections. Am J Kidney Dis 6:421, 1986.

18. Cheung AK, Gregory MC: Subclavian vein thrombosis in hemodialysis patients. Trans Am Soc Artif Intern Organs 31:131, 1985.

19. Tellis VA, Kohlberg WI, et al.: Expanded polytetrafluoroethylene graft for chronic hemodialysis. Ann Surg 189:101, 1979.

20. Lilly L, Nghiem D, et al.: Comparison between bovine heterograft and expanded PTFE grafts for dialysis access. Amer Surg 46:694, 1980.

21. Bhat DJ, Tellis VA, et al.: Management of sepsis involving expanded polytetrafluoroethylene grafts for hemodialysis access. Surgery 87:445, 1980.

22. Haimov M, Burrows L, et al.: Experience with arterial substitutes in the construction of vascular access for hemodialysis. J Cardiovasc Surg 21:150, 1980.

23. Francis DMA, Hoernich NA, et al.: An indwelling right atrial catheter for long-term hemodialysis. Trans Am Soc Artif Intern Organs 29:348, 1983.

24. Torosian MH, Meranze S, Mullen J: Central venous access with occlusive superior central venous thrombosis. Ann Surg 203:30, 1986.

25. Bothe A, Piccione W, et al.: Implantable central venous access system. Am J Surg 147:565, 1984.

26. McGonigle DJ, Schrock L, et al.: Experience using central venous access for long-term hemodialysis: A new concept. Am J Surg 145:571, 1983.

27. Lipsig LJ, Hedger RW, et al.: Clinical experience with transcutaneous vascular access. Dialysis Transplantation 13(12):786, 1984.

28. Kaplan AA, Grant J, et al.: Regional experience with the Hemasite no-needle access device. Trans Am Soc Artif Intern Organs 29:369, 1983.

29. Barth RH, Schwartz S, Lynn RI: High incidence of infectious complications with the Hemasite® vascular access device. Trans Am Soc Artif Intern Organs 30:450, 1984.

30. Tenckhoff H, Schecter H: A bacteriologically safe peritoneal access device. Trans Am Soc Artif Intern Organs 14:181, 1968.

31. Kaufman JL: Planning and protecting vascular access sites in the future hemodialysis patient. Arch Intern Med 145:1384, 1985.

32. Patrick W, May J: Basilic vein transposition. Am J Surg 143:254, 1982.

33. Mehigan JT, McAlexander RA, et al.: Snuff box arteriovenous fistula for hemodialysis. Am J Surg 143:252, 1982.

34. Cantelmo NL, Logerfo FW, et al.: Brachiobasilic and brachiocephalic fistulas as secondary angioaccess routes. Surg Gynecol Obstet 155:545, 1982.

35. Tellis VA, Veith FJ, et al.: Internal arteriovenous fistula for dialysis. Surg Gynecol Obstet 132:866, 1971.

36. Dagher FJ: The upper arm AV hemoaccess: Long-term follow-up. J Cardiovasc Surg 27:447, 1986.

37. Haimov M: Vascular access for hemodialysis: New modifications for the difficult patient. Surgery 92:109, 1982.

38. Giacchino JL, Geis WP, et al.: Vascular access: Long-term results, new techniques. Arch Surg 114:403, 1979.

39. Sako Y: Vascular anastomosis bow: An aid for coronary artery bypass and other vascular operations. Arch Surg 108:380, 1974.

40. Klimas VA, Denny KM, et al.: Low-dose streptokinase therapy for thrombosed arteriovenous fistulas. Trans Am Soc Artif Intern Organs 30:511, 1984.

41. Zeit RM: Arterial and venous embolization: Declotting of dialysis shunts by direct injection of streptokinase. Radiology 159:639, 1986.

42. Appel GB: Vascular access infections with long-term hemodialysis. Arch Intern Med 138:1610, 1978.

43. Tellis VA, Weiss P, et al.: Skin-flap coverage of polytetrafluoroethylene vascular access graft exposed by previous infection. Surgery 103:118, 1988.

44. Bradish CF: Carpal tunnel syndrome in patients on hemodialysis. J Bone Joint Surg 8:130, 1985.

45. Hughes K, Adams FG, et al.: The radiology of local complications of hemodialysis access devices. Clin Radiol 31:489, 1980.

PART VI
Thoracic Outlet Syndromes and Sympathectomies

CHAPTER 60
Thoracic Outlet Compression Syndromes

J. Manly Stallworth

While the thoracic outlet syndrome (TOS) has been recognized as a clinical entity for more than a century and a half, controversies related to theories of the compression process, methods of diagnosis, and choices of treatment continue unabated. Opinions vary as to classification methods and anatomic features involved in the compressive processes on the arteries, veins, and nerve components comprising the elemental features of the clinical syndrome. The three simple, original methods used to delineate the various causes of TOS have been altered to the point of confusing not only the diagnosis but also operative approaches and interpretive criteria.

Treatment varies from nonsurgical to radical excision methods above and below the clavicle. Some surgeons excise the first rib in all circumstances. Others make the operative exposure above or below the clavicle, depending on the clinical level of nerve or vessel compression symptoms. While some initially expose the first rib posteriorly, others reserve this approach for patients with recurrent symptoms. The trend is toward a direct approach to the area where the compression point clinically exists, a thorough search for abnormally functioning soft tissues or bones, and excision of the offending structure.

Historically, Sir Astley Cooper first described the symptoms of thoracic outlet syndrome in 1821.[1] In 1861 Coote[2] reported the excision of a cervical rib as the first operative treatment for TOS. Subsequently, Bramwell[3] in 1903 suggested the relationship of possible brachial plexus compression and a normal first rib. Five years later, Roberts[4] emphasized the relationship of symptoms to variation in the configuration of the cervical rib.

While many papers have been written to describe the mixture of neurologic, arterial, and venous symptoms, the phrase "thoracic outlet syndrome" was first used by Peet[5] in 1956 in a summary article. Later, Lord and Rosati[6] published an excellent review of the clinical picture, diagnostic methods, and anatomic descriptions.

Operative measures designed to relieve the compression syndromes included scalenotomy as recommended by Adson and Coffey in 1927,[7] removal of cervical ribs, initially by Coote[2] and later by Rob,[8] resection of clavicle by Lord[9] in 1971, and resection of the normal first rib by Murphy[10] in 1910. In 1962 Clagett[11] reviewed the posterior approach as a method of relief in all variations of TOS. The transaxillary approach was described by Roos and Owens[12,13] as a means of resection of the first rib, along with anterior and medial scalene muscle division. Later in 1971 Roos[14] advocated excision of the second rib, if it were found to be involved in the compression of the neurovascular bundle. Excision of the pectoralis minor tendon, along with the first rib, was proposed by Silver[15] in 1972. Lord[9] in 1971 proposed division of the costocoracoid tendon and the scalenus medius muscles, and at about the same time Johnson[16] suggested the appropriateness of a posterior approach in wide exploration and excision of abnormal tendinous bands.

In the late 1960s and 1970s the dominant operative trend centered around the transaxillary resection of the first rib and was advocated more or less empirically to relieve TOS by Roos,[12] Sanders et al.[17] Urschel and Razzuk,[18] and many others. In recent years, however, the tendency has been toward seeking a more precise localization of the mechanical fault during both the preoperative and intraoperative evaluations, to explicitly eliminate the pressure at operation by dividing the offending structure rather than routinely excising the first rib.[9,19,20]

ANATOMY

Basic understanding of the anatomy is absolutely vital in all diagnostic and operative considerations in TOS (Fig. 60-1). Following the course of the subclavian artery from its origin in the superior thoracic outlet, through its passage via the scalene triangle to its costoclavicular exit and its continuation as the axillary artery through the axilla, reveals any possible point of compression. The thoracic outlet difficulties begin in the scalene hiatus, made up of the scalene anterior muscle frontally, the scalene medius posteriorly, and the first rib inferiorly. In this area accessory cervical ribs, taut or anomalous scalene muscles, and aberrant bands

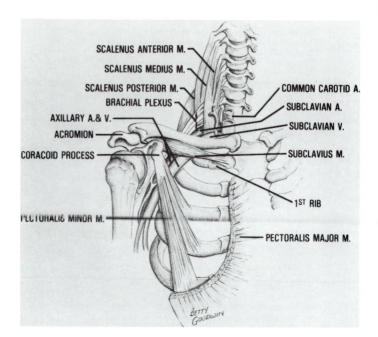

Figure 60-1. Basic anatomy involved in the thoracic outlet syndrome.

may individually or collectively be involved with compressive processes. These structures encircle not only the artery but also the contiguous brachial plexus, constituting the neurovascular bundle, which continues as a unit through the axilla. The subclavian vein, which usually lies anterior to the scalene anterior muscle, also joins the nerve-artery combination forming a unit that proceeds together peripher-

ally to pass between the clavicle and first rib into the axilla. At this junction the subclavius muscle, costocoracoid tendon, and possibly aberrant tissue cross over the neurovascular bundle, which then proceeds superiorly over the pectoralis minor muscle and inferiorly beneath the pectoralis major muscle. All of these structures become involved in the motions of the shoulder, the only human "universal

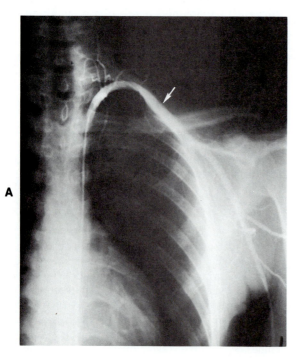

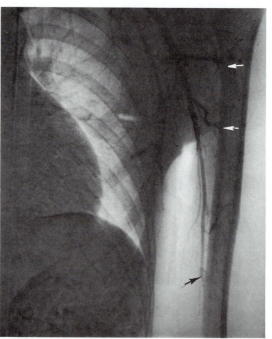

Figure 60-2. A. Arteriogram shows flattening of subclavian artery (*arrow*), apparently the source of emboli seen in **B. B.** Embolic occlusion of the brachial artery (*top arrow*) and its branches (*second arrow*), resulting in amputation of the hand in this 18-year-old patient. (*From Stallworth JM, Quinn GJ, Aiken AF: Ann Surg 185:581, 1977.*)

joint," which is ordinarily maintained in motor balance by the attachment of 24 muscles and 18 ligaments. Anatomic details and variations have been superbly described by Pollak.[21]

CLINICAL PICTURE

The clinical manifestations of TOS vary according to the nerves and vessels compressed and the site of the pressure point. Neurologic symptoms are the result of brachial plexus compression and generally may be classified in two major groups. The upper plexus consisting of C-4 to C-7, is correlated with symptoms involving the head, neck, and upper back; the lower plexus (C-8 and T-1) is usually related anatomically to the arm and hand. Early symptoms of intermittent paresthesia, pain, and numbness may progress with time to include muscle weakness and atrophy if compression is unrelieved. These neurologic manifestations often simulate those resulting from abnormal cervical discs, cord tumor or injury, spondylitis, spondylolisthesis, and carpal tunnel sydrome.

Arterial symptoms vary from digital vasospasm to gangrene depending upon the degree of compression and irritation. Irritation of the vessel wall by bony pressure may lead to damage to the intima—thrombosis and embolization—(Fig. 60-2) or to the media, resulting in aneurysm formation.[22] Adventitial scarring and palpable callouslike formation, caused by tendinous irritation, are often present. This scar formation can be helpful in localizing the exact point of compression during operative exploration. Arterial insufficiency caused by embolization, arteriosclerosis, vasospasm associated with Raynaud's disease, and reflex vasomotor dystrophy must be considered in the differential diagnosis.

Venous symptoms, consisting of tingling, aching, tired, painful limbs associated at times with cyanosis, swelling, and distended distal veins, are the result of obstruction of the axillary-subclavian venous system (Fig. 60-3). Other venous disorders, including "effort" thrombosis,[23] thrombophlebitis, heart failure, tumors and aneurysms of the mediastinum and thoracic outlet canal, arteriovenous fistulas, and chronic or acute lymphangiitis, must be differentiated. Because of the anatomically close relationships of these vessels and the brachial plexus, any combination of neurovascular symptoms may be present.

The clinical diagnosis is usually established during the patient's interview and detailed physical examination. When taking the patient's history, it is most important to elicit and closely evaluate the exact positional attitudes

A

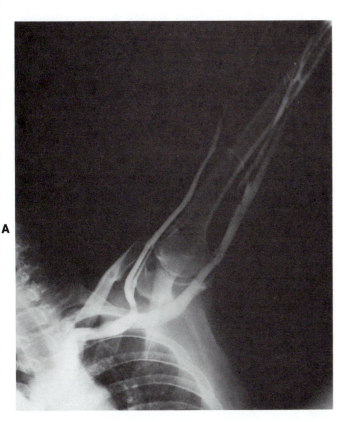

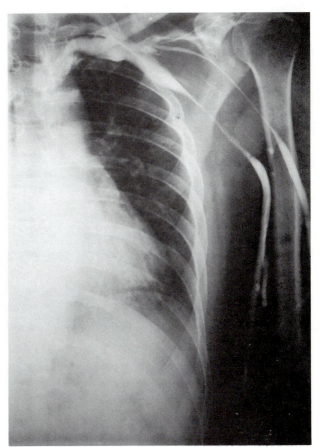

B

Figure 60-3. A. Normal phlebogram with arm abducted. **B.** Marked symptomatic compression of brachial and cephalic veins by pectoralis major muscle with arm adducted. (*From Stallworth JM, Quinn GJ, Aiken AF: Ann Surg 185:581, 1977.*)

adopted during work or play that provoke the symptoms, for example, athletic practices such as swimming, volleyball, baseball, and hiking (wearing a backpack); work habits involved in painting, carpentry, paperhanging, hairdressing, transporting heavy objects by hand, and so forth; and routine household duties like hanging clothes and washing windows. Historically, it is important to question sleeping habits, especially when related to hyperabduction of the arms. Likewise, possible relationships to trauma, operations, malignancies, and unusual systemic diseases should be vigorously investigated.

It is necessary to carry out a thorough, general physical examination with emphasis on posture, anatomic faults in the neck or arms, localized swelling and tenderness, deficiency in brachial blood pressure or pulses of the arms, venous cyanosis or distension, bruit of the neck and shoulder, and skin temperature change in hands and to include a neurologic evaluation of the brachial plexus distribution. Finally, the three classic thoracic outlet maneuvers must be carried out precisely. Since these maneuvers are often misinterpreted after being inaccurately performed, the original descriptions and photographs are presented once more for purposes of clarification.

Adson Maneuver

In 1927 Adson and Coffey wrote: "Clinically we were able to demonstrate the influence of the scalenus anticus muscle by having the patient elevate the chin and extend the neck or rotate the head *to the affected side* while taking a deep inspiration, this produces paresthesia over the distribution of the brachial plexus and, frequently, obliteration of the pulse at the wrist of the affected side."[7] [italics added] (Figs. 60-4 and 60-5).

Costoclavicular Maneuver

In 1943, Falconer and Weddell[24] published diagrams "illustrating the mechanism of costoclavicular compression of the subclavian artery on backward and downward bracing of the shoulders" (Figs. 60-6 and 60-7). In addition, these authors wrote that "this [position] may be occasioned by carrying heavy weights or in the services by marching with full pack."[24] Some authors have stated that hyperabduction of the arm and external rotation of the hand are the appropriate test for the costoclavicular syndrome, while others have advocated exercises of the arm muscles during hyperabduction. As can be seen, the costoclavicular maneuver is an opposite mechanism from hyperabduction, and failure to recognize this fact may lead not only to inaccurate diagnoses but to incorrect operative approaches.

Hyperabduction Maneuver

The hyperabduction maneuver was originally described in 1945 by Wright[25] and illustrated by photographs (Figs. 60-8 and 60-9). "The term 'hyperabduction' is used . . . to mean that phase of circumduction which brings the arms together above the head."[25] Despite the clarity of this description and the fact that the clavicle can be seen to be elevated away from the first rib during the maneuver, some surgeons continue to use the hyperabduction maneuver as a test for costoclavicular compression syndrome. When abduction of the arm is practiced during surgical exposure of the first rib, it becomes obvious that hyperabduction mechanically produces the *opposite* effect from that of the costoclavicular maneuver (Fig. 60-10). This is important to recognize. The anatomic relationships in all thoracic outlet compression syndromes have been accurately described by Lord and Rosati and superbly illustrated by Frank Netter.[6]

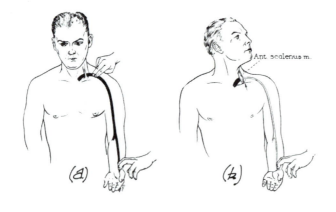

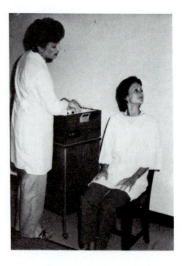

Figure 60-4. Original description by Adson.[7] "The vascular test: (a) the subclavian and radial arteries identified, (b) pulsations of arteries obliterated by inspiration; elevation of patient's chest and rotation of his·head to the affected side, in this case the left." (*From Surg Gynecol Obstet 85:688, 1947.*)

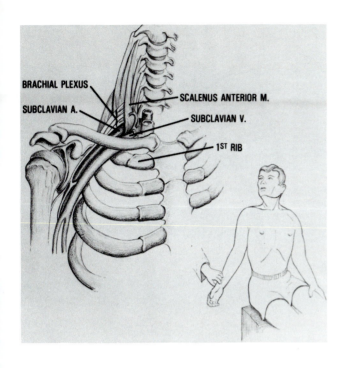

Figure 60-5. Anatomic features seen during an Adson maneuver.

ANCILLARY EXAMINATIONS

Radiologic Examination

X-ray films, including oblique projections of the cervical spine, are routinely made in the search for malformations in associated cervical ribs, vertebrae, and other bones. Chest radiographs are made in each patient to look for structural deformities and at the same time for tumors or other factors that could produce pressure symptoms in the thoracic outlet.

Arteriograms of the subclavian-axillary distribution are indicated when there is evidence of partial or complete arterial obstruction, suspected aneurysm, or peripheral emboli (Fig. 60-2). Intermittent arterial stenosis can usually be localized by noninvasive techniques using Doppler, B-mode ultrasound, or plethysmography.

Phlebograms (Fig. 60-3) are necessary in patients who show signs of venous obstruction at any of the outlet areas determined clinically or by noninvasive methods.

Computed tomography scans are ordinarily recommended when the differential diagnosis includes cervical cord compressive lesions such as discs, cord tumors, and spinal stenosis.

Noninvasive Vascular Examination

Plethysmographic studies at wrist level, bilaterally, are carried out before, during, and after the Adson, costoclavicular,

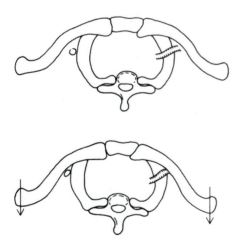

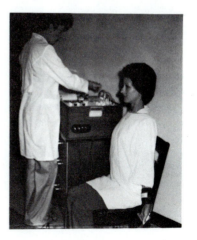

Figure 60-6. Mechanism of costoclavicular compression of subclavian artery on backward and downward bracing of shoulders. (*From Falconer MA, Weddell G: Lancet 2:542, 1943.*)

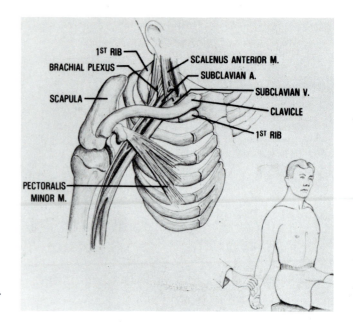

Figure 60-7. Anatomic relationships during costoclavicular maneuver.

and hyperabduction maneuvers. If the patient's symptoms are reproduced simultaneously with diminished arterial flow during the maneuver, a diagnosis of the anatomic level of compression can be readily ascertained and recorded (Fig. 60-11). Diminished arm arterial flow during outlet studies, when not associated with ischemia or neurologic symptoms, is common and requires no treatment.[26]

Doppler and duplex ultrasound examinations may be of value in patients with diminution or obstruction of blood flow in both large vein and artery of the arms and low axillae. At higher anatomic levels, in the axilla or low neck areas, these studies may be technically difficult but are worthwhile when the appropriate equipment and qualified technicians are available.

Skin temperature, digital plethysmography, and sweat studies are indicated in those patients who manifest ischemic symptoms of the fingers. It is important to differentiate digital spasm of Raynaud's type from embolic digital artery obstruction, since the treatment for the two types of ischemic processes is significantly different.

Neurologic Examination

While nerve conduction studies have been strongly advocated by many authors,[27] some have found them of little or no value in the differential diagnosis.[15,19,28] This author has found nerve conduction studies and electromyograms impressively accurate in distinguishing carpal tunnel syndrome but not useful otherwise in TOS.

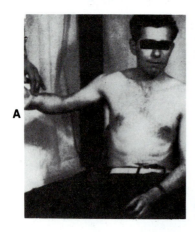
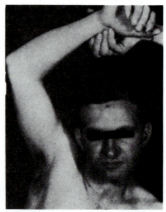
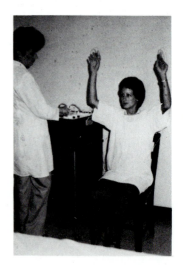

Figure 60-8. Original Description by Wright. **A.** "Patient in position of the test. Arm abducted anteriorly and laterally." **B.** "Second position for test. In many instances the pulse is completely obliterated." (*From Wright IS: Am Heart J 29:1, 1945.*)

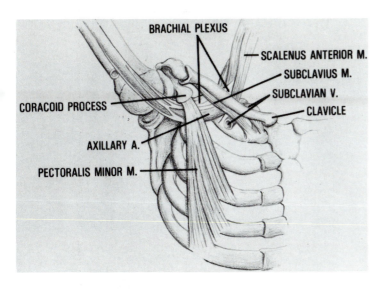

Figure 60-9. Anatomic changes during hyperabduction maneuver.

CONSERVATIVE TREATMENT

Following a definitive diagnosis of thoracic outlet syndrome utilizing detailed clinical evaluation and appropriate ancillary examinations, treatment is planned according to the severity and type of symptoms and precise localization of the compression site in its relationship to the clavicle. If the syndrome involves injury to the vessels, immediate treatment is indicated; however, if the clinical picture is dominantly neurogenic or is mixed with intermittent neurovascular disorder, operation can usually be deferred until nonoperative treatment methods have been tried. Physical therapy under supervision is recommended if there are postural faults; otherwise, the exercises designed by Peet[5] to promote muscle function necessary to maintain mechanical balance in the entire shoulder-neck unit are carried out at home for at least 6 weeks. Female patients with pendulous breasts supported by narrow cloth straps over the midclavicle level often complain of costoclavicular compression symptoms. Simple widening and padding of these straps can relieve this localized pressure point and alleviate symptoms. In the obese patient rolls of fatty tissue may produce localized axillary pressure when the arm is maintained in adduction, which is intensified by carrying objects at the side, such as suitcases. Effective management for such patients is weight reduction. Cervical traction may be tried when there are symptoms suggestive of cervical disc pressure versus TOS. The same is true in the trial use of a cervical collar. During the period of nonoperative treatment, the patient is reminded to record the position of

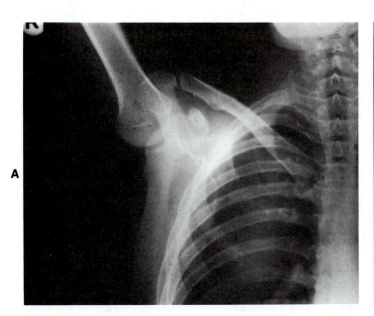

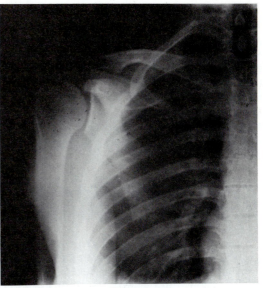

Figure 60-10. A. Radiographic evidence of clavicle elevated away from the rib cage during hyperabduction maneuver. **B.** Note compressive effect of clavicle on first rib during costoclavicular maneuver.

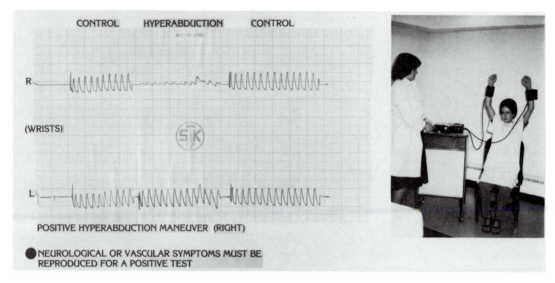

CONTROL   HYPERABDUCTION   CONTROL

R

(WRISTS)

L

POSITIVE HYPERABDUCTION MANEUVER (RIGHT)

● NEUROLOGICAL OR VASCULAR SYMPTOMS MUST BE
REPRODUCED FOR A POSITIVE TEST

Figure 60-11. Noninvasive plethysmographic diagnostic test.

the body at the onset of symptoms, that is, what motion causes or aggravates symptoms and what offers relief. Should there be a question of hyperabduction symptoms in arms during sleep, the arms may be secured loosely to a waist belt at night as a therapeutic trial. When the patient's occupation, such as driving a motor vehicle or typing, causes symptoms, change in jobs may be considered. Analgesics and muscle relaxants are often helpful during the nonoperative trial period.

OPERATIVE CONSIDERATIONS

Only a small percentage of patients having a diagnosis of TOS require operative treatment[19]—in our series, only 143 (12%) of 1,140 patients examined. Generally time is sufficient to totally evaluate the patient's status and apply appropriate nonsurgical techniques; however, when acute vascular symptoms are present, urgent evaluation and treatment is usually indicated. Such patients often present with thrombosis of the artery or vein in the low neck or axillary area, producing symptoms of ischemia or venostasis distally in the arms. Aneurysms may occur at the site of mechanical compression and are often associated with embolic changes in the distal tissues. In all events, acute arterial symptoms, with the exception of intermittent vasospasm, require urgent evaluation. After every clinical effort is made to localize the mechanical compressive problem, arteriograms correlated with the appropriate TOS maneuver may be obtained. Operative plans are formulated not only to relieve the mechanical compressive object but simultaneously to expose the damaged artery segment, which may require thrombectomy or segment replacement, depending upon the presenting pathologic findings. If intermittent vasospasm of the Raynaud's type is the presenting picture, an extensive general evaluation including noninvasive extremity flow studies must be sought, since appropriate treatment for varying vasospastic disorders may be strikingly different. Plans for possible operative exposure must include not only the site

of the compressive tissue but also available visualization and, when indicated, excision of the upper dorsal sympathetic ganglia.

Since the venous occlusive symptom may be acute, intermittent (Fig. 60-3), or chronic, the exact point of pressure on the vein wall must be localized. While appropriate Doppler and imaging diagnostic methods may be helpful, phlebography is usually necessary for accurate diagnosis. Treatment varies according to the location and nature of the mechanical obstruction. When the obstruction is intermittent, the anatomic cause for compression dictates the type of operative approach and the results are usually excellent. On the other hand, if the vein is acutely obstructed, thrombectomy via the cervical or axillary approach is recommended. When the clot has been present for several days, enzyme digestion should be considered.[29] Should there be chronic or long-standing venostasis symptoms, a period of observation is recommended, with treatment directed toward prevention of swelling. Venous replacement is controversial and seldom necessary; its use depends entirely upon the severity of venostatic disabling effects to the patient.

OPERATIVE APPROACHES

Should conservative measures fail, or if the symptoms are aggravated by treatment and worsen, surgical intervention should be offered.

Supraclavicular Approach

When the dominant symptom involves the upper roots of the brachial plexus, thought should be directed toward exploration of the neck through a supraclavicular approach,[17,30,31] which affords exposure of the scalene muscles, the upper brachial plexus, the great vessels, accessory ribs, and related congenital anomalies, along with access

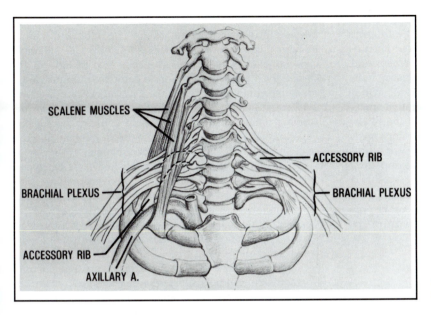

Figure 60-12. Anatomic relationships of neck structures to accessory ribs.

to the first rib and clavicle (Fig. 60-12). If the anterior scalene muscle requires decompression, it must be excised (Fig. 60-13) rather than simply divided because of possible adhesive reformation or perforation of the muscle with lower plexus nerve roots. In such case, the original symptoms would be aggravated by retraction of the divided muscle fibers against the imbedded nerves.[20]

Transaxillary Approach

When the clinical picture suggests costoclavicular or hyperabductor symptom, surgical exploration through a transaxillary incision described by Roos and Owens[13] is usually preferred, except in secondary operations, when the posterior approach may be selected. Some of the advantages of the axillary approach include excellent cosmesis and readily palpable and visual access to traversing axillary muscles, ligaments, and bony structures which may be involved in the compression of the neurovascular bundle. At the same time, it allows access for dorsal sympathectomy when indicated.

We believe that sufficient compression of the brachial plexus to produce symptoms simultaneously causes measurable compression of the incorporated vasculature even in the absence of vascular symptoms. At operation, if the patient has been prepared so that the axilla, shoulder, and lower neck are exposed with the arm draped in a sterile

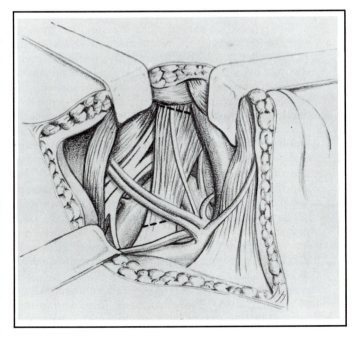

Figure 60-13. Exposure of scalene anterior muscle in preparation for its wide resection. Brachial nerves or subclavian artery which sometimes perforate this muscle must be sought out and avoided.

field, it is possible to perform the hyperabduction and costo-clavicular maneuvers under anesthesia with the thoracic outlet structures directly exposed. Under these circumstances, the physiology of the compressive process and the *offending structure*, whether bony or soft tissue, can be identified and divided or excised as indicated. In our series using this method in 194 consecutive operative procedures, 92% of patients had excellent results. Of the 14 patients who required bone resection, only six were improved. In the remaining 180 operations, soft tissue alone was found to cause the neurovascular bundle compression symptoms, and simple division or excision of these tissues resulted in a 96% success rate.[20] In each instance, the point of anatomic compression was identified during the operative procedure simultaneously with mechanical performance of appropriate thoracic outlet maneuver.

Subclavicular Approach

Among other operative approaches we used the subclavicular incision only when the patient's neurovascular symptoms occurred bilaterally during the hyperabduction studies. Under these instances, the operative exposure was similar to that used in the axillo-axillary bypass procedure, thus permitting ready access to the underlying, compressive soft tissues and a positive correlation to the appropriate arm-shoulder diagnostic maneuvers. Good functional results followed in the few patients treated in this way, but cosmetic results were less favorable than in the other approaches.

Posterior Approach

The posterior thoracic exposure has been used successfully by some surgeons[16,32] as a primary procedure, but in our experience, both in thoracic outlet as well as thoracoplasty operations, it often offers relatively difficult exposure and requires excessive muscle division. However, when used as a secondary procedure following failure of an initial thoracic outlet operation, it permits a fresh operative field, free of dangerous adhesions.

In repair of the great vessels, it matters little whether the specific localizing diagnosis originates above or below the clavicle, since a combination of supraclavicular and transaxillary surgical approaches[33] is most often indicated as the safest and most efficient operation for the patient.

COMMENT

Safeguards in the treatment of thoracic outlet diagnoses are varied and complicated. First, the anatomy is basically complex and spliced with multitudes of anomalies, all of which must be thoroughly understood before any operative procedure is carried out. Second, the nerve dysfunction and bizarre ramifications commonly seen require detailed neurologic consultation regarding specific nerve patterns, possible nerve conduction, and electromyographic studies. Also to be evaluated are possible underlying CNS problems

or a combination of thoracic outlet syndrome and unsuspected allied neurologic disorders. The difficult questions of returning to work, the work load, physical limitation, and monetary liability must be answered in light of the clinical evaluation. In addition to compensation problems, many patients with TOS may be psychoneurotic. The term *crock* suggested by Dale[19] would seem appropriate for describing them. Whether one should consider neurosis in equating therapeutic results is a matter for debate. No one seems to have the solution to this dilemma.

In the more than 225 articles published on TOS between 1980 and 1986 there is much disagreement about its management. For example, a typical patient is the young, nonathletic, uninjured adult, free of bony abnormalities, who has TOS-like symptoms and comes for treatment. It is our view that the removal of soft tissue is less hazardous and more beneficial than automatic removal of the first rib. Often it is thought that since the first rib, being an anatomic boundary for the three outlets, must in some way act as a "common denominator," and its excision will meet operative criteria for cure. However, the question arises, why or how does a normal rib in its stable anatomic position become misaligned? Its dense fixation to the second rib allows little motion during respiration. If motion is due to tension of the superior elevators, such as the scalene muscles, that could readily be demonstrated by fluoroscopy. Likewise, its relationship to the clavicle during all of the thoracic outlet maneuvers can also be recorded radiologically. Elevation of the clavicle by abduction of the arm does not cause compression between the rib and clavicle (see Fig. 60-10). Also, rotation of the hand in any direction when the arm is abducted causes little or no pressure effect of the clavicle on the rib. Yet abduction with external rotation of the hand (A.E.R.) is perhaps the most frequent diagnostic criterion used as indication for first rib resection. This maneuver actually causes reduction of compression between the two bony structures, relieving costoclavicular syndrome!

The dominant cause of thoracic outlet symptoms is neurologic, not vascular compression. Intermittent pressure on nerves causes pain while equal pressure on an associated vessel may have no clinical effect. Keeping in mind the composite relationship of the nerves and vessels in the thoracic outlet, would not the pressure needed to cause nerve root symptoms simultaneously constrict the associated vessels sufficiently to affect volume measurements but not necessarily sufficiently to produce ischemic symptoms? If this theory is correct, would it not be simple anatomically to locate the pressure point by accurately measuring the distal artery flow at the moment the patient becomes symptomatic during the course of the thoracic outlet examination? Would it not be reasonable to look for this point of arterial compression concomitantly with performance of thoracic outlet maneuvers during operative exposure? As explained, costoclavicular and hyperabduction maneuvers can be easily accomplished under operative conditions. The Adson maneuver is not readily reproduced in the anesthetized patient, but as in other operative exposures, points of chronic irritation on the artery wall may be observed, such as early aneurysmal dilatation or chafing of the adventitial structures that produces callous formation. Some palpable or visible arterial injury or abnormality was observed at operation in 51 of the 194 consecutive thoracic outlet operative procedures in our series. There was physical evidence of vessel wall compression in all patients with costoclavicular or hyperabduction complaints.

CONCLUSIONS

Acknowledging the problems of diagnosis and management of TOS, it appears reasonable to return to the basic anatomic and physiologic processes as they relate to the compressive "trigger" site. These specific pressure points, having been generally located by clinical evaluation, can be further localized by pulse volume plethysmographic tracings performed during all of the thoracic outlet maneuvers. With this information, a direct anatomic operative approach affords palpable and visible access to the compression site and is advantageous to the patient, since in this instance there is minimal disruption and less likelihood of secondary complication.

In essence, when the patient voices the chief complaint during one of the diagnostic maneuvers and *at the same time* there is a stenotic vascular effect on the recorded waveform (Fig. 60-11), a precise diagnosis can be obtained and proper treatment instituted.

REFERENCES

1. Cooper AP: On exostosis, in Cooper, Cooper As Travers B: Surgical Essays, 3rd ed., Philadelphia, Webster, 1821, p 128.
2. Coote H: Exostosis of the left transverse process of the seventh cervical vertebra surrounded by blood vessels and nerves: Successful removal. Lancet 1:360, 1861.
3. Bramwell F: Lesion of the first dorsal nerve root. Rev Neurol Psychiat 1:236, 1903.
4. Roberts JB: The surgical importance of cervical ribs to the general practitioner. JAMA 51:1126, 1908.
5. Peet RM, Hendricksen JD, et al.: Thoracic outlet syndrome: Evaluation of a therapeutic exercise program. Proc Mayo Clin 31:281, 1956.
6. Lord JW Jr, Rosati LM: Thoracic outlet syndromes. Clinical Symposia, Ciba 23:3, 1971.
7. Adson AW, Coffey JR: Cervical rib: A method of anterior approach for relief of symptoms by division of the scalenus anticus. Ann Surg 85:839, 1927.
8. Rob CG, Standeven A: Arterial occlusion complicating thoracic outlet compression syndrome, Br Med J 2:709, 1958.
9. Lord JW Jr: Thoracic outlet syndromes: Current management. Ann Surg 173:700, 1971.
10. Murphy T: Brachial neuritis caused by pressure of first rib. Aust Med J 15:582, 1910.
11. Clagett OT: Presidential Address: Research and prosearch. J Thorac Cardiovasc Surg 44:153, 1962.
12. Roos DB: Transaxillary approach for first rib resection to relieve thoracic outlet syndrome. Ann Surg 163:354, 1966.
13. Roos DB, Owens JC: Thoracic outlet syndrome. Arch Surg 93:71, 1966.
14. Roos DB: Experience with first rib resection for thoracic outlet syndrome. Arch Surg 173:429–442, 1971.
15. Silver, D: Thoracic outlet syndrome, in Sabiston DC Jr (ed): Christopher's Textbook of Surgery, 10th ed. Philadelphia, WB Sanders Co., 1972, p 1858.
16. Johnson CR: Treatment of thoracic outlet syndrome by removal of first rib and related entrapments through posterolateral approach. J Thorac Cardiovasc Surg 68:536, 1974.
17. Sanders RJ, Monsour JW, Baer SB: Transaxillary first rib resection for the thoracic outlet syndrome. Arch Surg 97:1014, 1968.
18. Urschel HC Jr, Razzuk MA: Management of the thoracic outlet syndrome. N Engl J Med 286:1140, 1972.
19. Dale WA: Thoracic outlet compression syndrome: Critique in 1982. Arch Surg 117:1437, 1982.
20. Stallworth JM, Quinn GJ, Aiken AF: Is rib resection necessary for relief of thoracic outlet syndrome? Ann Surg 185:581, 1977.
21. Pollak EW: Thoracic Outlet Syndrome: Diagnosis and Treatment. Mount Kisco, N.Y., Futura Publishing Co., 1986, p 3.
22. Haimovici H: Arterial thromboembolism of the upper extremity associated with the thoracic outlet syndrome. J Cardiovasc Surg 23:214, 1982.
23. Adams J, DeWees J: Effort thrombosis of axillary and subclavian veins. J Trauma 11:923, 1971.
24. Falconer MA, Weddell G: Costoclavicular compression of the subclavian artery and vein. Lancet 2:539, 1943.
25. Wright IS: The neurovascular syndrome produced by hyperabduction of the arms. Am Heart J 29:1, 1945.
26. Gerdoodis R, Barnes WR: Thoracic outlet arterial compression: Prevalence in normal persons. Angiology 31:538, 1980.
27. Glover JL, Worth RM, et al.: Evoked responses in the diagnosis of thoracic outlet syndrome. Surgery 89:86, 1981.
28. Roos DB in Machleder H (ed): Vascular disorders of the Upper Extremity. Mount Kisco, NY, Futura Publishing Co., 1983, p 91.
29. Marden UJ: The use of thrombolytic agents: Choice of patient, drug administration, laboratory monitoring. Ann Intern Med 90:802, 1979.
30. Qvarfordt G, Ehrenfeld W, Stoney R: Supraclavicular radical scalenectomy and transaxillary first rib resection for thoracic outlet syndrome. Surgery 148:111, 1984.
31. Sanders RJ, Ramer S: The supraclavicular approach to scalenectomy and first rib resection: Description of technique. J Vasc Surg 2:75L, 1985.
32. Marinez NS: Posterior first rib resection for total thoracic outlet syndrome decompression. Contemp Surg 15:13, 1979.
33. Roos DB: The place for scalenectomy and first rib resection in thoracic outlet syndrome. Surgery 92:1077, 1982.

CHAPTER 61
Arterial Thromboembolism Due to Thoracic Outlet Complications

Henry Haimovici

Acute arterial thromboembolism of the upper extremity associated with the thoracic outlet syndrome differs in many ways from a cardiogenic embolism, particularly in its pathophysiology and management. Indeed, the thromboembolic process originates in a damaged subclavian artery as a result of its prolonged compression by congenital or acquired anomalous anatomic structures at the thoracic outlet.

Although rare, these vascular complications were first reported long ago; nonetheless, their potential threat to the viability of the limb is still not widely recognized. This point is reflected in most reviews of large series of cases of thoracic outlet syndrome, which dealt almost exclusively with the neurologic manifestations and rarely, if at all, with vascular complications.[1-3]

Traditionally, the neurovascular manifestations have been attributed to a number of separate entities, the main ones being the cervical rib, scalenus anticus, costoclavicular, and hyperabduction syndromes. These entities, either alone or in combination, have been held responsible for vascular complications.

However, it is now well recognized that of these entities, the major anatomic abnormalities associated with these complications are mainly cervical ribs, rarely anomalous first and second thoracic ribs and only occasionally a callus of malunion of a fractured clavicle. In contrast to the skeletal abnormalities, the muscular and ligamentous elements are usually secondary factors in the overall entrapment process.

The term "thoracic outlet syndrome," introduced by Peet et al. in 1956 and popularized in 1958 by Rob and Standeven as "thoracic outlet *compression* syndrome," helped provide a unifying concept of the underlying pathogenesis of the various separate entities.[4,5]

The important role which the first rib seems to play in the costoclavicular vise has led in recent years to its routine removal in the management of the thoracic outlet syndrome with neurologic complications.[6] However, contrary to some early expectations, these same operative principles are not usually suitable in the presence of arterial lesions.

The increasing interest in this condition justifies a more detailed description of its various aspects. This chapter will therefore give a broader view of vascular complications and their management and will also briefly include a critical review of the pertinent literature.

HISTORICAL BACKGROUND

While cervical ribs and other anatomic abnormalities have been reported for over a century as anatomic curiosities, it was not until 1861 that Coote removed a cervical rib which caused pressure on the subclavian and axillary vessels with resulting ischemia of the arm.[7] Then, in 1863, Hilton reported a case of thrombosis of the subclavian artery resulting from the artery's compression by an exostosis of the first thoracic rib.[8] The patient had no radial pulse and two gangrenous fingers. Other publications appeared subsequently which confirmed the significance of the osseous compression of the subclavian vessels.[9-11] It was only after the development of roentgenologic identification that cervical ribs and other osseous anomalies were more frequently noted. Thus Halsted was able in 1916 to collect from the literature 716 cases of cervical ribs.[12] Of these, 525 were clinical cases and the rest were represented by autopsy and museum specimens. Some 360 cases presented symptoms of compression; of these, 125 cases presented with vascular symptoms. In 27 of the 125 cases (21.6%), there were subclavian aneurysms. This review led Halsted to reinvestigate the causes of subclavian aneurysm formation and of poststenotic dilatation.[12] On the basis of his experiments, he attributed poststenotic dilatation to two chief factors: (1) to "a whirlpool-like play of the blood below the site of the constriction and (2) to the lowered blood pressure." Holman later essentially confirmed the mechanism of the poststenotic dilatation by attributing it to mural structural fatigue secondary to the turbulent flow which induces vibrations leading to the histologic changes of the artery.[13]

The nature of the vascular complications of the thoracic outlet compression syndrome remained unsettled for some time. Thus Todd advanced the theory in 1912 "that vascular symptoms occurring in association with cervical ribs are not mechanical in origin but are trophic in character caused by paralysis of the periarterial sympathetic fibers."[14]

Subsequent carefully observed anatomopathologic findings failed to agree with this theory. Thus Lewis and Pickering postulated in 1934 that the vascular changes in the upper extremity were due to traumatic compression of the subclavian artery by the cervical rib, followed by mural thrombosis and the embolic manifestations.[15] Later, Lewis clearly summarized this concept as follows[16]:

Such compression, oft repeated, is calculated to damage the artery and to promote clotting within it; actually its walls have been found greatly thickened and adherent to surrounding structures, or the vessel dilated or aneurysmal and partly or completely filled with clot. All the vascular symptoms displayed could not arise, however, directly out of compression or out of permanent obstruction of the subclavian artery, but they could arise out of thrombosis with embolism. The thrombi form where the wall is damaged by compression; these, so it is supposed, become detached by repeated movement and from time to time, causing embolism of smaller or larger branches in the arterial tree.

The correctness of this description has since then been abundantly demonstrated by arteriographic and operative findings. While vascular manifestations may range from minor to major symptoms of arterial ischemia, it is mostly the thromboembolic episodes that represent the real threat to the viability of the limb.

Brief Review of the Literature

One of the earliest reviews on this subject appeared in 1916 in Halsted's classic paper on the experimentally induced poststenotic arterial dilatation.[12] This paper included a tabulation of 21 clinical cases presenting a subclavian aneurysm in association with a cervical rib. In the 1930s, such related vascular complications were being reported with greater frequency, as reflected in Eden's review of 48 cases.[17] In our own 1956 review of the literature, special focus was placed on the evaluation of the thromboembolic manifestations on the basis of anatomopathologic criteria in a selected group of 29 cases.[18] In 1958, Rob and Standeven reported ten cases of arterial occlusion of the upper extremity associated with the thoracic outlet compression syndrome.[5] Subsequent papers continued to report an increasing number of vascular complications due to cervical ribs.[19-31] In these papers, great emphasis was placed on the early recognition and treatment of these complications. More recently, the need for first rib resection in the management of the vascular lesions was brought into question by a number of vascular surgeons.[32,33] A better understanding of the surgical management of the compressing structures of the thoracic outlet has thus been evolved, as reflected in several recent papers.[25,27,29] The increasing number of cases being reported suggests that vascular complications are likely less infrequent than they seemed to be from the earlier literature.

CLINICAL PATHOLOGIC BACKGROUND

The majority of patients fall into the 21- to 50-year-old age group, with a range between 16 and 66 years of age in our series.[18] Eden mentioned in his review the uncommon occurrences of this condition in a 5-year-old child and in a 75-year-old woman.[17] The vast majority of cases occur in young or middle-aged adults. In our review, 18 were men and 12 were women. Eden noted a reversed ratio of 20 males to 26 females, which may have been due to a possible preponderance of neurologic complications. Most reports indicate that vascular symptoms are more common in the right arm, which corresponds to the greater number of right-handed individuals; however, in Eden's series, 24 cases occurred in the left arm, as opposed to 20 in the right. In 70 percent of the cases, the condition is bilateral.

The incidence of cervical ribs encountered in routine chest films has been estimated as between 0.5 and 0.7 percent.[18] The vast majority of these patients are asymptomatic. The largest group of symptomatic patients comprises those with impingement upon the brachial plexus by an incomplete cervical rib. Ischemic symptoms are rare. Adson reported vascular symptomatology in 5.6% of his patients.[34] These symptoms were manifested as Raynaud's phenomenon with signs referable to partial intermittent subclavian artery occlusion.

The type of cervical rib is of great significance in vascular complications. It has been well established since Gruber's study[35] that short (type I) and incomplete (type II) ribs produce neurologic complications, while only long or complete ones (type III) are associated with arterial complications. In our review, every case except one had a complete cervical rib.[18] This was also true in the asymptomatic contralateral side.

The Subclavian Artery

In the presence of a complete cervical rib, the supraclavicular course of the subclavian artery is displaced. There is an upward extension of the thorax so that the subclavian artery passes high in the neck; as it emerges from the lateral border of the anterior scalene muscle it is elevated and usually readily palpable well above the clavicle. Indeed, in all these patients there is a supraclavicular mass represented by the cervical rib at its articulating site with the first rib. The artery at this level is occasionally tender. Short described two variants of the course of the subclavian artery in relation to the cervical rib articulating exostosis with the first rib. In type A, the subclavian artery crosses the first rib medially to its exostosis. Short found that in this type all patients had major vascular symptoms. In type B, the subclavian artery crosses the first rib lateral to the exostosis and the symptoms are neurologic rather than vascular. Short further pointed out that the two groups can be distinguished clinically and that each type has a different prognostic value.

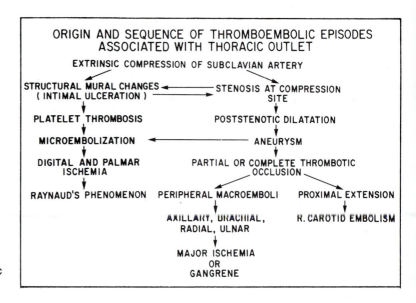

Figure 61-1. Origin and sequence of clinicopathologic events associated with the thoracic outlet.

The prolonged compression of the subclavian artery may lead to (1) structural changes of the arterial wall, consisting often of a greatly thickened vessel adherent to the surrounding structures, (2) stenosis at the site of the extravascular compression, and (3) often a poststenotic dilatation (Fig. 61-1). If the entrapment of the artery is of short duration, the caliber of the vessel may return to normal following surgical correction of the compression.[19]

Subclavian Aneurysms

Following Halsted's report in 1916[12] of a group of 27 cases of cervical rib associated with subclavian artery aneurysm, a small number of reports dealing with thoracic outlet syndrome confirmed the relationship to vascular complications, but only rarely did those reports note the presence of aneurysm. Instead, most reports dealt primarily with thrombosis of the subclavian artery associated with peripheral embolic manifestations. In 1962 Wellington and Martin[22] could find only 57 such cases. Since that time, however, many more cases of this entity have been reported.

Many papers dealing with the thoracic outlet syndrome and circulatory complications fail to specifically identify the presence of aneurysm, probably because they are silent and because diagnosticians are unaware that these aneurysms occur. On the other hand, a number of observations of poststenotic dilatation have been interpreted as a simple dilatation and not aneurysm. Of course, depending on the size of the dilatation relative to that of the subclavian artery, it may be difficult to differentiate between the two, especially when the dilated poststenotic lesion is thrombosed.

Based on a personal series of observations, Short stated that "a large number of crippling cases of ischemia of the arm or hand which are due to thromboembolic propagation originate from silent subclavian aneurysms."[36] He believed that aneurysms are sufficiently common to give concern and that complications would be best prevented by attempting to understand more fully those factors, congenital or acquired, which predispose to aneurysm formation. Fur-

thermore, in his series of 16 patients with complete cervical ribs, Short found that in a group of eight female patients with a mean age of 24, those without thromboembolic manifestations had no aneurysm or dilatation, while in a group of six females and two males with a mean age of 44, thromboembolic manifestations originated from a subclavian aneurysm.

Reports before the 1960s failed to mention aneurysm formation of the poststenotic area of the subclavian artery. Later, observations became more frequent, either of so-called simple dilatation of the subclavian artery or actual aneurysmal appearance of that dilatation.

Thus in Bertelsen et al's report[23] of six cases, two had aneurysmal lesions and two simple dilatations of the subclavian artery. On the other hand, Judy and Heyman in 1972 stated that in seven cases no aneurysm or dilatation was noted on the arteriographic studies.[25] The features in those cases were overwhelmingly thromboembolic manifestations. The thrombosis in the sac likely obscured the aneurysms in the angiograms. With the newer techniques of CT scans and B-mode ultrasonography the aneurysmal presence may be revealed more often, because of the technical superiority of these noninvasive procedures over simple arteriography.

In the late 1960s a number of papers dealt specifically with arterial aneurysms distal to points of subclavian constriction.[22,23] Since this artery passes through a narrow, rigid confine of the thoracic outlet, this vessel is particularly prone to excessive compression and aneurysm formation, even when muscular or ligament variations of the normal anatomy are not present. Thus, Wellington and Martin[22] reported eight cases of subclavian aneurysms which led them to believe, like Short,[36] that all patients with symptoms of arterial insufficiency due to predisposing anatomical abnormality at the thoracic outlet, such as cervical rib in particular, should be explored surgically when other causes of ischemia have been excluded.

Wellington and Martin's experience included eight patients between 18 and 50 years of age, average age 36. They reported five patients with bilateral ribs; one patient had a right-sided lesion only. The five patients with bilateral ribs were righthanded and had only unilateral symptoms at the time of first admission to the hospital, but all eight patients had digital symptoms of pain, paresthesia, coldness, numbness, or blueness, and two had frank digital ulceration. Aortic arch angiography was performed in five of the eight patients before operation. A definite subclavian aneurysm was demonstrated in only one. In the other four patients, the third part of the subclavian artery was completely thrombosed in two, narrowed at the point of compression in one, and appeared completely normal in one. Distal vessels were obstructed at varying sites of the arterial tree of the upper extremity.

In conclusion, postcompression occlusion of the third portion of the subclavian artery may present aneurysmal formation more often than has been reported in the literature. This would confirm what Halsted produced experimentally and Holman demonstrated later, namely, that compression in one area of the arterial tree due to hemodynamic factors results in variable degrees of lesions from simple dilatation to aneurysmal formation in the majority of cases. Although some reports in the past failed to mention the diagnosis of aneurysmal dilatations, based on the analysis of the above cases, one may conclude that the thromboembolic complications must be anticipated as part of the aneurysmal lesion. The thrombotic manifestations originate in the aneurysmal sac and embolize into the distal portion of the upper extremity and hand, as demonstrated by the statistical observations of Short and others.[36]

Subclavian Thrombosis

Further in the sequence of events, long-standing compression of the artery may result in an ulceration of the intimal layer (Fig. 61-2). During its initial stage, local thrombi often arise from this lesion. This may eventually lead to a completely occluding thrombosis of the arterial lumen. Partial or complete thrombosis of the subclavian artery without distal embolization may remain silent because of the extensive collateral circulation available at this level. However,

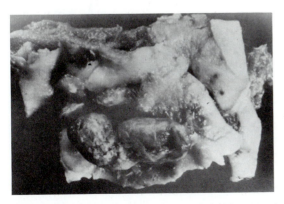

Figure 61-2. Specimen of an open, excised subclavian artery showing an ulcerated plaque with a firmly attached thrombus, taken from a 32-year-old woman with cervical rib and arterial thrombosis. (*From Schein, Haimovici, et al: Surgery 40:428, 1956*)

there is commonly an increasing danger of embolization of the distal arterial tree. These emboli may be small or large. Small emboli may lodge in the digital and palmar arteries, producing a picture of unilateral Raynaud's phenomenon. Larger emboli blocking the brachial bifurcation at the antecubital fossa may result in major ischemia or gangrene of the hand and fingers. A more rare complication is extension of subclavian artery thrombosis proximally to involve the vertebral or carotid artery, with consequent contralateral hemiplegia. About 12 such cases have been mentioned in the literature through 1974.[27]

CLINICAL MANIFESTATIONS

Most vascular complications associated with the thoracic outlet take months or years to become apparent or significant. However, when first seen by the physician, patients with these complications *usually* present with an acute stage of the process. Generally, the clinical picture has three phases: the prodromal, the advanced ischemic, and the severe ischemic.

Prodromal Phase. The most common symptoms at *onset* are largely confined to the fingers and hand and consist of attacks of coldness, numbness, cyanosis or pallor, and pain, especially on exposure to cold. Often these attacks resemble a typical Raynaud's phenomenon. Sometimes associated neurologic involvement is evidenced by symptoms which are not always easy to distinguish accurately from symptoms of ischemic origin, such as numbness, wasting, and pain.

The initial manifestations are usually attributed to occlusion of digital or palmar arterioles. The color and temperature changes and response to cold are confined to the acral parts of the limb and often show temporary regression.

The natural course of this process, however, consists of episodic and repetitive peripheral microemboli which impart a progressive ischemia to the hand or forearm. Depending on the degree of ischemia, the clinical course may assume either of the following forms.

Advanced Ischemic Phase. The color changes of Raynaud's phenomenon on exposure to cold become more severe and are usually confined to the involved hand only and sometimes to one finger—most commonly the index. Pulsations present in the previous phase disappear first in the digital arterioles and later at the radial and ulnar or even brachial artery. Pain experienced in the arm becomes more pronounced, especially during exercise.

Severe Ischemic Phase. Since this process sometimes progresses at a rapid pace, the ischemia may become severe enough to prevent the patient from sleeping at night, especially if the collateral circulation has decreased. Sometimes this phase may be preceded by some episode of trauma, which obviously is only an incidental event, not uncommonly with medicolegal implications.

The usual duration of the entire spectrum of the ischemic manifestations ranges from a few weeks to a few months or longer before the condition becomes critical.

When the symptoms worsen, the pain becomes acutely intolerable, and the patient presents himself or herself to the physician at this point.

Physical examination usually turns up evidence of a cervical rib in the supraclavicular region. A thrill is palpable and a systolic bruit is audible in most instances. The hand and arm may show evidence of vascular compromise. Blood pressure may be decreased or absent; wrist and brachial pulses may be unobtainable. Muscle atrophy may be present not only in the intrinsic muscles of the hand, but also in the thenar or hypothenar regions. In advanced cases, the forearm and the arm musculatures may show similar changes. Ulcerations or gangrene of the tips of the fingers, either focal or extensive, may be noted in these advanced cases. In a previously reported review of 29 patients, 11 (36.7%) sustained a loss of a phalanx or a digit, and 2 (6.7%) required major upper extremity amputations.[18]

DIAGNOSIS

Differential Diagnosis

Many of the symptoms described in the *early stages* of the thromboembolic complications associated with the thoracic outlet syndrome may mimic symptoms of other lesions, requiring careful differentiation. Of these, carpal tunnel syndrome, cervical root entrapment, cervical arthritis, and a protruded cervical disk (most of which produce severe pain) are often more typical of neurologic than of vascular complications. In the presence of unilateral vascular symptoms, it is necessary to rule out collagen vascular disease, vasospastic syndromes, autoimmune vasculitis, traumatic thrombosis of hand vessels, and actual cardiogenic embolic disease. Unfortunately, quite often identification of the source of microemboli is not directed toward the possible thoracic outlet origin.

At the *stage of acute vascular manifestations*, differential diagnosis should pose less of a problem. Awareness of the potential presence of cervical ribs or anomalies of the osseous structures of the thorax aperture is essential in recognizing the nature of the disease and in deciding the management of these complications at an earlier stage.

Diagnostic Tests

Routine Roentgenograms. These should obviously be obtained for determining the presence of cervical ribs, abnormal transverse process of C7, anomalous first rib, clavicular exostosis or callus of malunited fracture, or vertebral abnormalities.

Shoulder Girdle Classical Maneuvers. These maneuvers for detecting vascular, neurologic, or neurovascular manifestations of the thoracic outlet syndrome may be helpful but are not of critical significance. The costoclavicular,[37] hyperabduction,[39] and Adson maneuvers,[34] the most commonly used clinical tests, may only help to alert one to the existence of compressing anatomic structures in this region.

Noninvasive Tests. Pulse volume recording at digital, wrist, forearm, and arm levels may indicate relative arterial patency and pulsatility or their absence. The pulse volume index at various levels may also be of help in assessing the results of treatment and the overall prognosis. Unless associated neurologic signs are present, electrodiagnostic tests are of limited or no value in the diagnostic evaluation of the arterial complications.

Arteriography. In the presence of arterial manifestations, arteriography of the entire arterial tree is mandatory, including views of the aortic arch, the subclavian, the axillary, the brachial, the ulnar, the radial, and the hand arterial systems. This can best be achieved through a transfemoral arch aortogram study.[25,39] Evaluation of the runoff into the brachial, forearm, and hand arterial network is essential for assessment of the extent of the occlusions. Because of the multiple arterial lesions, especially in cases of advanced ischemia, the arteriographic findings are not always easy to fit into simple patterns. As a rule, a combination of two or more segmental occlusions may be present at various levels of the upper extremity vasculature.

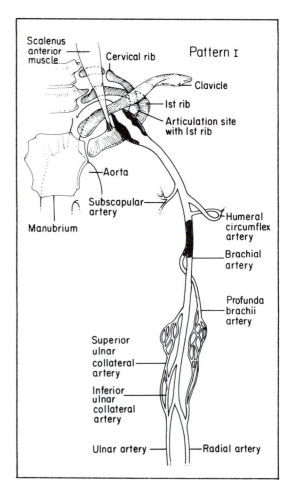

Figure 61-3. *Pattern I* of arterial lesions involving (1) the subclavian and (2) the proximal brachial. These lesions are amenable to complete restoration of arterial patency (see text), although prior microemboli of the hand arterioles may be present.

On the basis of our arteriographic findings and those in the literature it is possible to discern the following four major patterns.

PATTERN I.   This involves poststenotic aneurysmal dilatation of the third part of the subclavian artery with occlusion of the proximal or distal brachial artery with an apparently normal distal arterial tree (Fig. 61-3). A frequent shortcoming in this pattern is the underestimation of the presence of mural thrombi of the subclavian.[25] Furthermore, mild poststenotic dilatation may go undiagnosed, especially if collaterals are minimal around the shoulder. In such cases, the brachial occlusion may remain unrelated to the subclavian lesion.[5]

PATTERN II.   This involves poststenotic aneurysmal dilatation with (1) obvious subclavian mural thrombi, (2) brachial occlusions, (3) radial/ulnar embolic occlusions, and (4) patent interosseous arteries (Fig. 61-4). In mild to moderate subclavian artery changes seen on the arteriogram, there is usually a discrepancy between the aforementioned problems and the operative findings, which are generally more severe. Judy and Heyman found mural thrombosis and ulcerated intimal plaques to be far more pronounced than suggested by the arteriogram in three of seven cases.[25]

PATTERN III.   This involves complete thrombosis of the third part of the subclavian artery with acute multiple segmental embolic occlusion of the axillary-brachial, radial, or ulnar artery. Prior microemboli to the hand vasculature are often also found (Fig. 61-5). A typical example can be seen in the personal case report described later in this chapter. The severity of such cases requires good arteriographic techniques and multiple operative explorations of the major arteries of the extremity for disobstructing as many as is feasible.

PATTERN IV.   This involves complete thrombosis of the third part of the subclavian artery with no significant reentry into the axillary-brachial segment, with collateral circulation inadequately perfusing the forearm and hand. The vasculature of the hand may have already been impaired by prior

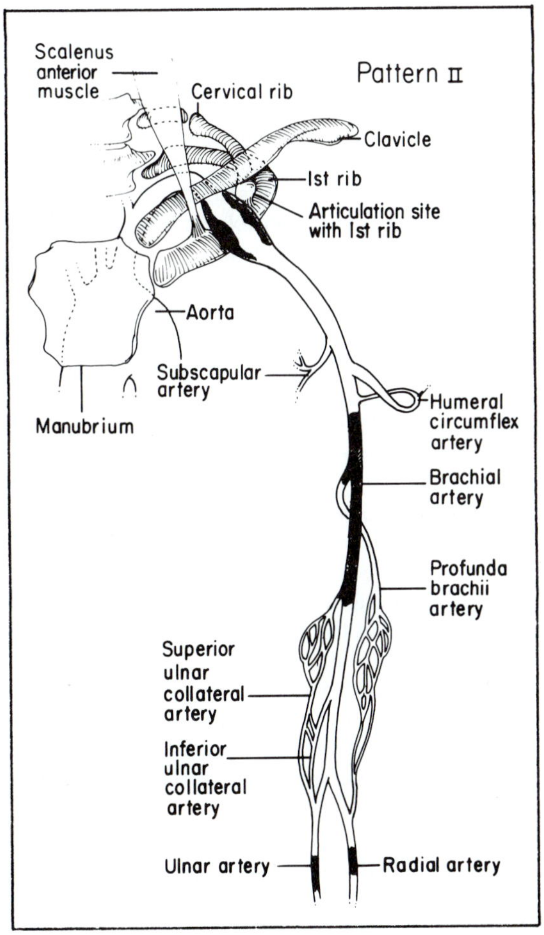

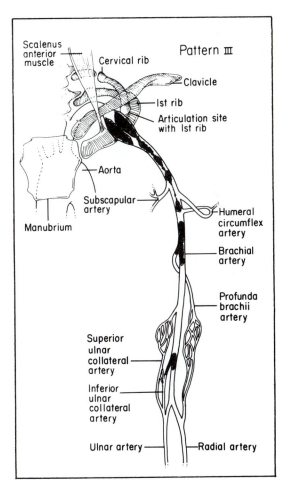

Figure 61-4. *Pattern II* of arterial lesions involving (1) the subclavian; (2) the proximal half of the brachial, with blockage of bifurcations at the profunda and superior ulnar levels; and (3) the radial and ulnar. These lesions are still amenable to restoration of direct arterial flow to the elbow and, through collaterals, to the forearm and hand, although microemboli may occur prior to major arterial emboli in the larger vessels.

Figure 61-5. *Pattern III* of arterial lesions involving (1) the subclavian, (2) the axillary, (3) the proximal bifurcation of the brachial, (4) the distal brachial at the inferior ulnar, and (5) possible digital microemboli (not shown in the diagram). Reconstructive procedures of the proximal arterial tree and a thoracic sympathectomy are indicated here.

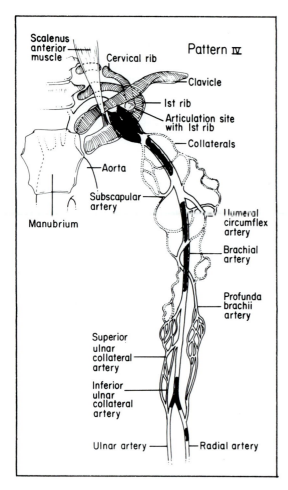

Figure 61-6. *Pattern IV* of arterial lesions involving (1) the subclavian; (2) nearly total thrombosis of the axillary, brachial, and radial-ulnar; and (3) collaterals of varying degrees of efficacy. An aggressive approach is indicated: one should thrombectomize or bypass the occlusive process, if possible, and perform a thoracic sympathectomy in an attempt to salvage the hand.

microemboli (Fig. 61-6.). If the proximal lesions involve the brachial bifurcation at the elbow, the sudden ischemia may result in gangrene of the hand.[18,25] The only way this will not occur is if the proximal thromboembolic process develops gradually and concurrently with the formation of a collateral circulation (Figs. 61-7 and 61-8).

Obviously, these four arteriographic patterns offer only a framework for other combinations of arterial lesions, some of which may defy the description of a specific pattern. Notwithstanding the patterns specified above, careful identification of the lesions preoperatively and, if necessary, by intraoperative arteriograms is essential for proper planning of the operation.

TREATMENT

The vascular complications associated with the thoracic outlet assume by far a greater urgency than do purely neurologic manifestations. Presence of threatening ischemia of

the upper extremity should receive prompt attention in every case, whether moderate or severe. Lack of awareness of its serious prognostic significance may lead to irreversible ischemic changes with tissue loss.

Surgical treatment of the thromboembolic manifestations arising from entrapment of the subclavian artery by the abnormal structures of the thoracic outlet is as follows: (1) decompression of the subclavian artery, (2) repair of the arterial lesions, and (3) management of the associated ischemia of the hand, unrelieved by arterial reconstruction.

Surgical Exposure for Subclavian Artery Decompression

Surgical Approach. The surgical approach for exposure of the thoracic outlet structures depends on the type of the neurologic or vascular lesions and to some extent on the preference of the individual surgeon.

The posterior approach described by Clagett in 1962 is suitable for patients with a primarily neurologic symptomatology.[40] However, Clagett and others have recognized that if arterial complications are present, it is necessary to use an anterior approach for dealing separately and adequately with them.[41]

The transaxillary approach advocated by both Roos and Owens in 1966 gained wide acceptance because of the easy exposure and the cosmetic results.[6,42] As with the posterior approach, this approach is satisfactory in patients having mostly, if not exclusively, neurologic complications.[2] Neither of these two procedures, however, facilitates concomitant vascular repair of the subclavian artery.

The supraclavicular approach, used originally in 1910 by Murphy,[10] is still favored by most vascular surgeons. It provides access not only to the subclavian vessels but also to the cervical rib and almost all of the other structures of the thoracic outlet. However, if the axillary-brachial vessels and the first thoracic rib are to be exposed, this approach is not adequate.

The infraclavicular or anterior approach will then offer good access to the first rib and to the distal portion of the subclavian and axillary vessels. This exposure also affords easy evaluation of the potential compressive effects of the pectoralis minor tendon in the hyperabduction syndrome.

Combined supra- and infraclavicular approaches may offer a logical solution to the exposure of the many structural elements.[29]

A *claviculectomy*, either partial or total, provides exposure for both the supra- and the infraclavicular areas. Lord and Rosati found the claviculectomy to offer easy access with favorable results.[43] Our experience and that of others supports their viewpoint.

Removal of Compressive Structures. These structures include the first thoracic rib, the cervical rib, the anterior scalene muscle, the clavicle, and the pectoralis minor tendon.

Routine removal of the first *thoracic rib* through the posterior or especially the transaxillary approach, as favored by Roos and most cardiothoracic surgeons, is being challenged as a "cure-all" by those dealing primarily with the

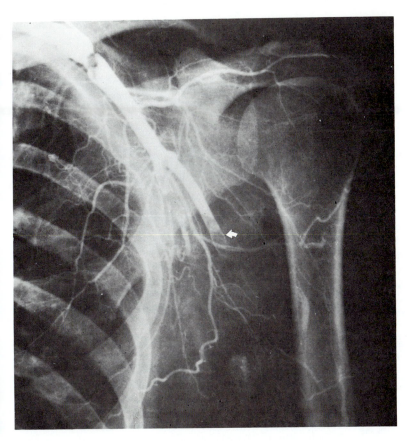

Figure 61-7. Left percutaneous subclavian arteriogram showing an occlusion of the proximal brachial and subscapular arteries due to thrombi, displaying oval filling defects within the vascular lumen, which suggest its embolic nature. Eighteen months before, the patient had had intermittent ischemic manifestations of the hand, with all pulses palpable. A cervical rib was not demonstrated. A scalenotomy and pectoralis minor tenotomy were performed, with resolution of symptoms. Sudden onset of pain in the arm extending to the fingertips 18 months later led to this arteriogram. An upper thoracic sympathectomy was then performed, with good functional results.

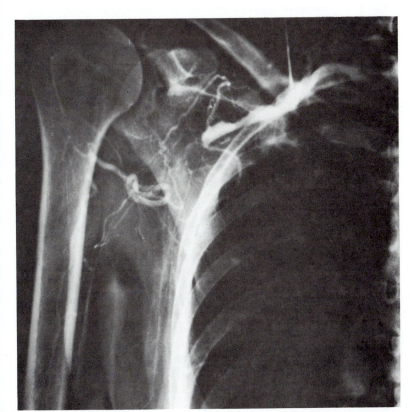

Figure 61-8. Right percutaneous subclavian arteriogram showing mural thrombi in the dilated third part of the subclavian with abrupt occlusion of the midportion of the axillary. The brachial artery is not visualized. Bilateral cervical ribs are present. Excision of the right cervical rib and scalenotomy resulted in increased warmth of the hand and healing of digital ulcers.

arterial complications. Stallworth et al. reported only nine first rib resections in 146 procedures for thoracic outlet syndrome.[32] On the basis of current experience, excision of the first rib should be reserved for patients with proven compression of the subclavian artery directly related to it. In these cases with clear indications, its resection is carried out through the anterior approach concomitantly with the other procedures (cervical rib, scalene division, arterial repair).

Satisfactory decompression of the subclavian artery can be achieved in the majority of cases only by removal of the cervical rib, scalenotomy, and occasionally pectoralis minor tenotomy.

The excision of the *cervical rib* is in most cases the first and most important step. It should be done "together with the resection of the bony prominence on the first rib which forms part of the joint between cervical rib and first rib."[19] Ross emphasized this technical point, since this bony prominence is a primary cause of impingement upon and indentation of the subclavian artery. In the absence of definite compression, resection of the cervical rib has been omitted by some, including this author.

Scalenotomy is mandatory whenever the subclavian artery is exposed. It is automatically severed when the first rib is resected. Simple scalenotomy does not always provide long-term subclavian decompression. A rate of recurrence of symptoms after first rib resection of over 15% was recently reported by Sanders et al.[33] The reason for recurrence was scalene muscle reattachment to the bed of the first rib. As a result, scalenectomy is recommended instead. Its good to excellent long-term results appear to support its routine use instead of the simple severance of the muscle.

Pectoralis minor tenotomy, although rarely indicated, may be useful when there is clear evidence of axillary artery compression by the hyperabduction of the arm. Lord and Rosati[43] some time ago and Stallworth et al.[32] later pointed out the usefulness of this procedure in selected cases. Removal of the costocoracoid ligament and of the subclavius muscle may be of additional value in the decompressive process.[37]

Claviculectomy, as mentioned above, may be indicated when the clavicle plays a significant compressive role in the costoclavicular syndrome and when necessary to achieve a wider access to the various vascular and bony structures of the thoracic outlet.

Arterial Repair

The reconstructive arterial procedures obviously must be tailored to each individual patient, depending on the nature, location, and extent of the occlusive process.

Direct surgical approach to the subclavian, axillary, and brachial arteries, as the case may indicate, is necessary and often feasible.

Thrombectomy or thromboendarterectomy of the subclavian-axillary arteries, excision of these arteries with graft interposition, and bypass graft to the distal arm may be used either alone or in combination. Before we review the merits of these procedures, the following case report will illustrate the diagnostic findings and some of the problems in management.

CASE REPORT

The patient (MP), a 45-year-old white woman, was admitted to Montefiore Hospital on April 20, 1965, with a 6 month history of pain, paresthesias, motor weakness, and coldness of the right-upper extremity. In October 1964 she had a sudden onset of pain in this extremity extending from the elbow to the fingertips.

Physical examination revealed marked rubor on dependency and blanching on elevation of the hand. Superficial ulcers on the fingertips failed to heal. Atrophy of the thenar, hypothenar, and small muscles of the hand was quite pronounced.

The subclavian artery pulse was palpable only in the supraclavicular fossa, but no thrill or bruit was detectable. No other pulses were felt distally. Blood pressure and oscillometric readings of the right arm were unobtainable, but these readings were normal in the left arm. Roentgenograms of the chest and cervical spine demonstrated the presence of bilateral cervical ribs.

A retrograde aortic arch aortogram obtained through the percutaneous transfemoral Seldinger technique showed (1) complete occlusion of the third part of the right subclavian artery, (2) thrombosis of the axillary-brachial artery, (3) poor runoff into the collaterals supplying the upper arm, and (4) poststenotic dilatation of the left distal subclavian and the initial part of the axillary (Figs. 61-9 and 61-10).

Exposure of the subclavian and axillary arteries was easily achieved following a scalenotomy and resection of the middle third of the clavicle. The third part of the subclavian and the first part of the axillary arteries were dilated and nonpulsating. The poststenotic right subclavian artery was not visible on the arteriogram but was seen on the left side. An arteriotomy of the subclavian-axillary artery disclosed the presence of a thrombus attached firmly to a thickened atherosclerotic intima. A thromboendarterectomy was easily performed after developing a cleavage plane. The entire thickened intima was removed, along with a well-organized thrombus (Fig. 61-11).

The upper brachial artery was then exposed through the medial upper third of the arm. Through an arteriotomy at this level, organized thrombi were extracted. Excellent pulses were obtained in the subclavian, axillary, and brachial arteries down to the elbow. At the completion of the operation, a weak ulnar pulse was also palpable. Postoperatively, the ischemic changes improved and the patient could resume her work 3 weeks later. The patient was seen periodically. When last examined 11 years postoperatively, her blood pressure and pulse volume recordings disclosed nearly normal findings in the arm and forearm. Pulsatile flow was obtained in the fingers as well (Figs. 61-12 and 61-13).

A 15 year follow-up showed the patient doing quite well. The left side, in spite of the poststenotic dilatation, remained asymptomatic.

Methods of Arterial Reconstruction

The subclavian artery, site of origin of the thromboembolic process, becomes accessible after its decompression to direct repair. If by history and arteriographic findings there is even minimal evidence of mural lesions, an arteriotomy of the subclavian is indicated. Mere decompression of the artery may not be advisable, even when combined with a sympathectomy, since it leaves behind a damaged, ulcerated, and thrombus-covered intima, a likely source of later embolism.

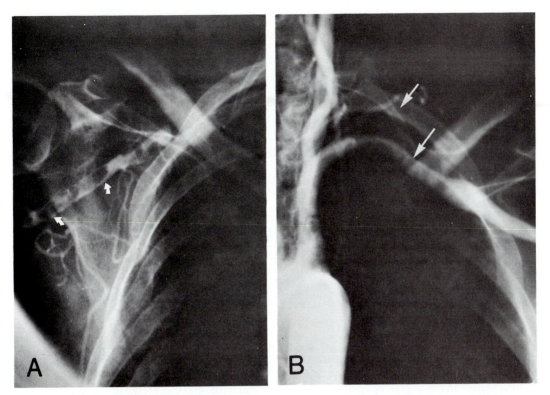

Figure 61-9. A. Right subclavian arteriogram via transfemoral retrograde thoracic aortogram 5 seconds after contrast injection. There is collateral filling of the axillary artery, which contains numerous defects characteristic of incompletely obstructing thrombi. **B.** Left subclavian arteriogram from the same retrograde thoracic aortogram as seen in **A.** Note narrowing on the subclavian as it passes over the cervical rib (*arrows*) and the poststenotic dilatation of the axillary.

Simple thrombectomy under these conditions is rarely sufficient. A thromboendarterectomy at the level of the compression of the artery, consisting of excision of both the ulcerated intima and the thrombus, is the more appropriate procedure.

However, if the arterial wall is too thin or friable due to degenerative changes, if a cleavage plane cannot be easily developed, or if the subclavian is actually aneurysmal, a

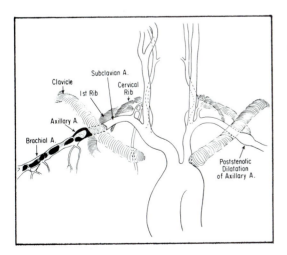

Figure 61-10. Diagram representing the arteriographic findings in Figure 61-9 A and B.

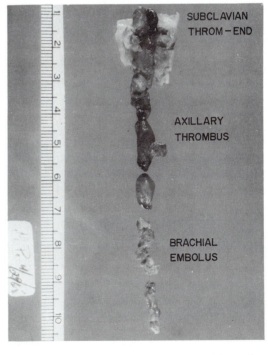

Figure 61-11. Operative specimen consisting of (1) an atherosclerotic intima and thrombus removed from the third part of the subclavian during the thromboendarterectomy; (2) an organized thrombus of recent date, extending from the subclavian into the axillary; and (3) old organized thrombi representing emboli of the brachial.

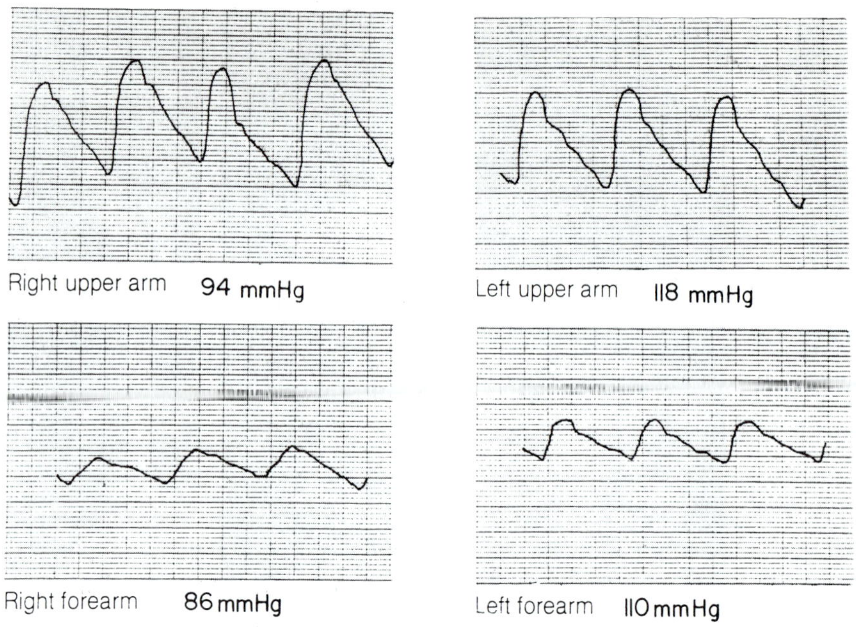

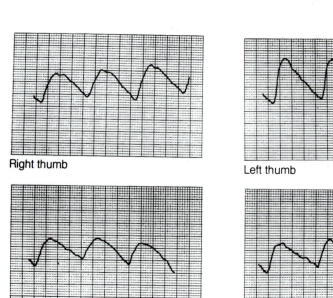

Figure 61-12. Bilateral upper extremity pulse volume recordings (PVRs) and Doppler blood pressure determinations 11 years postoperatively. Note that the routine blood pressure taken with a mercury sphygmomanometer was equal in both arms (R = 120/78, L = 118/78). The upper arm pulse waves are nearly identical on both sides, while the pulse waves of the forearm on the right display sawtooth contours characteristic of decreased systolic pressure (R = 86, L = 110).

Right upper arm   94 mmHg

Left upper arm   118 mmHg

Right forearm   86 mmHg

Left forearm   110 mmHg

thromboendarterectomy is contraindicated. Instead, it is best to excise the involved segment and reestablish arterial continuity by direct anastomosis or preferably by interposition of a graft (autogenous vein or plastic tube).

Axillary and brachial thromboembolic occlusions, if long-standing, may be difficult to impossible to disobstruct with an embolectomy catheter. A direct approach through a separate exposure is then necessary, especially for the brachial. An intraoperative arteriogram may be useful in localizing the extent of the occlusion and delineating the outflow below the brachial. It is important to distinguish between the brachial occlusion at its origin just proximal to the profunda brachii and the occlusion at the elbow, where it divides into radial and ulnar. Prognosis appears better with a proximal than with a distal occlusion, because

disobstruction is easier. Thromboembolectomy of the proximal brachial may provide adequate flow to the forearm and hand, especially if the distal brachial is patent. Reestablishing patency of the deep brachial artery in the event that the distal brachial thrombus cannot be dislodged is somewhat equivalent to profunda femoris revascularization in the thigh when the superficial femoral is occluded. Should the thromboembolectomy fail, an autogenous vein or Gore-Tex graft bypass from the subclavian or axillary to the brachial should be considered if a runoff is available.[27]

Direct repair of the forearm or hand is most often not feasible because of the chronic multiple repetitive embolic episodes affecting these distal vessels. These episodes often account for failure to restore normal wrist pulses.

Indications for cervicothoracic sympathectomy are dic-

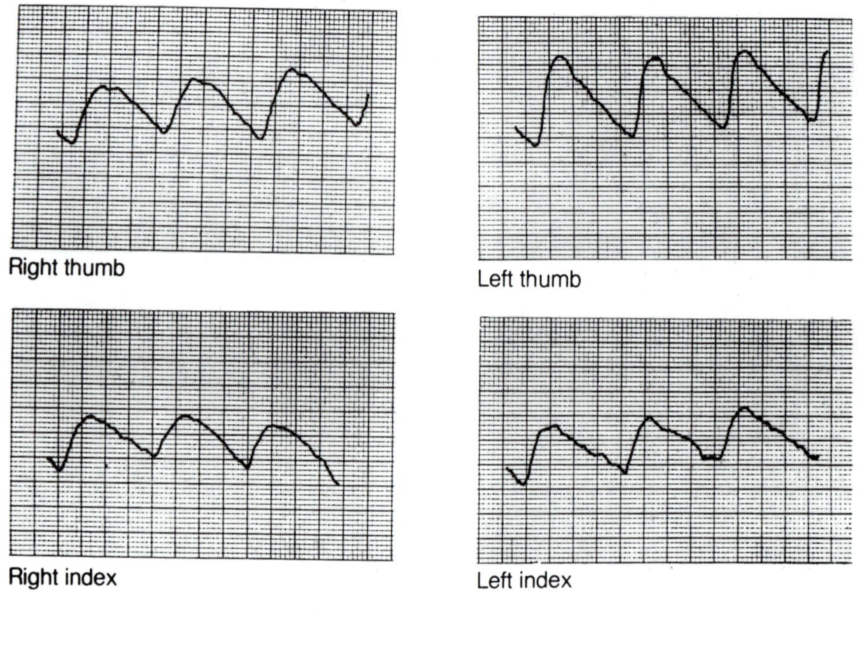

Right thumb

Left thumb

Right index

Left index

Figure 61-13. Pulse waves of the thumbs and index fingers of both hands indicate pulsatile flow. The pressures were not recorded for technical reasons.

tated essentially by the frequent difficulty or inability to restore arterial patency below the elbow for the reasons stated above. This procedure is particularly appropriate when there is evidence of hand ischemia of a threatening nature (patterns III and IV). The procedure is carried out through the supraclavicular exposure used for dealing with the decompressive maneuvers, which adds little time to the operation. The actual sympathectomy consists of removal of the distal half of the stellate ganglion and the second and third thoracic ganglia. This provides sympathetic denervation of the forearm and hand with corresponding revascularization of the latter.[44] Most vascular surgeons have found the cervicothoracic sympathectomy to be an important additional step in the overall management of this syndrome.[5,11,19,20,22,23,25,27,31]

The results of management of these arterial lesions have improved since 1966 because of greater awareness of their presence and a more prompt combined use of the various methods of decompression and revascularization. Tables 61.1, 61.2, and 61.3 reflect the changing concepts of these lesions and their management.

Table 61.1, in which 29 cases were evaluated during the period up to 1955, indicates that most decompressive procedures were cervical rib resection and scalenotomies and were performed in 58% and 42% of the cases, respectively. Arterial repair consisting of arteriotomy for thrombectomy was rarely performed except in combination with a few other procedures.

Table 61.2, which includes 50 cases during the period between 1956 and 1965, shows greater use of cervical rib resection than that of the first thoracic rib. Scalenotomy alone, excluding its mandatory use with the first thoracic rib resection, was done in 23% of the cases. Arterial repair used in only 14 cases included thrombectomy, thromboembolectomy, and excision of subclavian artery with graft interposition, while the remaining cases were treated by thoracic sympathectomy either alone or in conjunction with arterial repair.

Table 61.3, which includes 49 cases treated between 1966 and 1978, indicates a more aggressive approach to these lesions. It consists of wider application of decompressive procedures associated with more advanced techniques of arterial repair. The results obtained were more gratifying,

TABLE 61-1. MANAGEMENT OF CERVICAL RIB WITH ARTERIAL COMPLICATIONS (1815–1955)

	No.	%
1. Decompressive procedures		
Cervical rib resection	17	58
Scalenotomy	12	42
Total	29	
2. Arterial repair and/or thoracic sympathectomy		
Arteriotomy	7	63.6
Periarterial stripping	1	9.1
Dorsal sympathectomy	1	9.1
Thrombectomy	1	9.1
Resection with graft replacement	1	9.1
Total	11	

Based on data from ref. Schein et al.[18]

TABLE 61-2. MANAGEMENT OF CERVICAL RIB WITH ARTERIAL COMPLICATIONS (1956–1965)

	No.	%
1. Decompressive procedures		
Cervical rib resection	15	57.7
First thoracic rib resection	5	19.2
Scalenotomy	6	23.1
2. Arterial repair and/or thoracic sympathectomy		
Arterial repair (thrombectomy, thromboembolectomy, excision of SCA with graft replacement)	14	51.8
Thoracic sympathectomy	13	48.2

Based on data from Judy and Heyman.[25]

TABLE 61-3. MANAGEMENT OF CERVICAL RIB WITH ARTERIAL COMPLICATIONS (1966–1978)

	No.	%
1. Decompressive procedures		
Cervical rib resection	26	44.0
First thoracic rib resection	14	23.7
Claviculectomy	10	17.0
Scalenotomy	8	13.5
Exostosis of first rib	1	1.8
2. Arterial Repair and/or Thoracic Sympathectomy		
Thrombectomy	4	
Thromboendarterectomy	7	52.7
Excision of SCA with graft interposition	11	
Aneurysmectomy with anastomosis or graft	8	
Embolectomy	7	12.3
Sympathectomy	13	22.7
Miscellaneous	7	12.3

Based on data from Williams and Carpenter[3] Peet et al.[4] Bertelsen et al.[23] Mathes and Salam[26] and Banes et al.[31]

although a perfect revascularization of the limb is always difficult to achieve because of the multiple microembolic and repetitive lesions present distally.

The results of the combined arterial repair and cervicothoracic sympathectomy obviously depend on the collateral network available at the hand and finger levels. If gangrene is present, either of the digits or of the hand, every effort should be made to delay amputation in order to provide time for development of the collateral circulation. Obviously, loss of a hand carries a greater disability, especially in the right-handed individual, than does loss of a foot.

A greater awareness of this unusual thromboembolic process associated with the thoracic outlet may lead to an earlier diagnosis with a better outlook for more complete limb salvage.[45]

CONCLUSIONS

The relatively rare vascular complications resulting from abnormal structures of the thoracic outlet with a potential threat to the viability of the upper limb are still not widely appreciated. Early recognition of the underlying thromboembolic process—the cause of the clinical manifestation—

is the key to prevention and appropriate management of these complications.

REFERENCES

1. Nelson RM, Davis RW: Collective review: Thoracic outlet compression syndrome. Ann Thorac Surg 8:437, 1969.
2. Roos DB: Experience with first rib resection for thoracic outlet syndrome. Ann Surg 173:429, 1971.
3. Williams HT, Carpenter NH: Surgical treatment of the thoracic outlet compression syndrome. Arch Surg 113:850, 1978.
4. Peet RM, Hendricksen JD, et al.: Thoracic outlet syndrome: Evaluation of a therapeutic exercise program. Proc Mayo Clin 31:281, 1956.
5. Rob CG, Standeven A: Arterial occlusion complicating thoracic outlet compression syndrome. Br Med J 2:709, 1958.
6. Roos DB, Owens JC: Thoracic outlet syndrome. Arch Surg 93:71, 1966.
7. Coote H: Exostosis of the left transverse process of the seventh cervical vertebra surrounded by blood vessels and nerves: Successful removal. Lancet 1:360, 1861.
8. Hilton J: Lectures on Rest and Pain. London, 1863, p. 179.
9. Murphy JB: Case of cervical rib with symptoms resembling subclavian aneurysm. Ann Surg 41:399, 1905.
10. Murphy T: Brachial neuritis from pressure of the first rib. Aust Med J 15:582, 1910.
11. Telford ED, Stopford JSB: The vascular complications of the cervical rib. Br J Surg 18:577, 1931.
12. Halsted WS: An experimental study of circumscribed dilatation of an artery immediately distal to a partially occluding band, and its bearing on the dilatation of the subclavian artery observed in certain cases of cervical rib. J Exp Med 24:271, 1916.
13. Holman EF: The obscure physiology of poststenotic dilatation: Its relation to the development of aneurysms. J Thorac Cardiovasc Surg 28:109, 1954.
14. Todd TW: The vascular symptoms in "cervical" rib. Lancet 2:362, 1912.
15. Lewis T, Pickering GW: Observations upon maladies in which the blood supply to digits ceases intermittently or permanently, and upon bilateral gangrene of digits: Observations relevant to so-called "Raynaud's disease." Clin Sci 1:327, 1934.
16. Lewis R: Vascular Disorders of the Limbs. London, Macmillan, 1946, p 86.
17. Eden KC: The vascular complications of cervical ribs and first rib abnormalities. Br J Surg 27:111, 1939–1940.
18. Schein CJ, Haimovici H, Young H: Arterial thrombosis associated with cervical ribs: Surgical considerations. Report of a case and review of the literature. Surgery 40:428, 1956.
19. Ross JP: Vascular complications of cervical rib. Ann Surg 150:340, 1959.
20. Eastcott HHG: Reconstruction of the subclavian artery for complications of cervical-rib and thoracic-outlet syndrome. Lancet 2:1243, 1962.
21. Gunning AJ, Pickering GW, et al.: Mural thrombosis of the subclavian artery and subsequent embolism in cervical rib. Q J Med 33:133, 1964.
22. Wellington JL, Martin P: Post-stenotic subclavian aneurysms. Angiology 16:566, 1965.
23. Bertelsen S, Mathiesen FR, Phlenschlaeger HH: Vascular complications of cervical rib. Scand J Thorac Cardiovasc Surg 2:133, 1968.
24. Swinton NW, Hall RJ, et al.: Unilateral Raynaud's phenomenon caused by cervical first rib anomalies. Am J Med 48:404, 1970.
25. Judy KL, Heyman RL: Vascular complications of the thoracic outlet syndrome. Am J Surg 123:521, 1972.
26. Mathes SJ, Salam AA: Subclavian artery aneurysm: Sequela of thoracic outlet syndrome. Surgery 76:506, 1974.
27. Blank RH, Connar RG: Arterial complications associated with thoracic outlet compression syndrome. Ann Thorac Surg 17:315, 1974.
28. Sachatello CR, Ernst CB, Griffen WP: The acutely ischemic upper extremity: Selective management. Surgery 76:1002, 1974.
29. Martin J, Gaspard DJ, Johnston PW, et al.: Vascular manifestations of the thoracic outlet syndrome. Arch Surg 111:779, 1976.
30. Kim GE, Imparato AM, et al.: Arterial embolization of the upper extremity associated with thoracic outlet syndrome. Vasc Surg 12:85, 1978.
31. Banis JC, Rich N, Whelan TJ: Ischemia of the upper extremity due to noncardiac emboli. Am J Surg 134:131, 1977.
32. Stallworth JM, Quinn GJ, Aiken A: Is rib resection necessary for relief of thoracic outlet syndrome? Ann Surg 185:581, 1977.
33. Sanders RJ, Monsour JW, Gerber WF, et al.: Scalenectomy versus first rib resection for treatment of the thoracic outlet syndrome. Surgery 85:109, 1979.
34. Adson AW: Surgical treatment for symptoms produced by cervical ribs and the scalenus anticus muscle. Surg Gynecol Obstet 85:687, 1947.
35. Gruber W: Ueber die Halsrippen des Menschen mit vergleichendanatomischen Bemerkungen. Mem Acad Sci (St Petersburg) 7:(2): 1969.
36. Short DW: The subclavian artery in 16 patients with complete cervical ribs. J Cardiovasc Surg 16:135, 1975.
37. Falconer MA, Weddel G: Costoclavicular compression of the subclavian artery and vein. Lancet 2:539, 1943.
38. Wright IS: The neurovascular syndrome produced by hyperabduction of the arms. Am Heart J 29:1, 1945.
39. Haimovici H, Caplan LH: Arterial thrombosis complicating the thoracic outlet syndrome: Arteriographic considerations. Radiology 87:457, 1966.
40. Clagett OT: Research and prosearch. J Thorac Cardiovasc Surg 44:153, 1962.
41. Fairbairn JF, Clagett OT: Neurovascular compression syndromes of the thoracic outlet, in Fairbairn JF, Juergens JL, Spittell JA (eds): Peripheral Vascular Diseases, 4th ed. Philadelphia, Saunders, 1972, p 459.
42. Owens JC: Thoracic outlet compression syndromes, in Haimovici H (ed): Vascular Surgery: Principles and Techniques. New York, McGraw-Hill, 1976, p 733.
43. Lord JW Jr, Rosati LM: Thoracic outlet syndromes: Clinical symposia. Ciba Found Symp 23:3, 1971.
44. Haimovici H: Arterial thromboembolism: Thoracic outlet complications, in Haimovici H (ed): Vascular Emergencies, Appleton-Century-Crofts, NY, 1982, p 190.
45. Scher LA, Veith FJ, Haimovici H, et al.: Staging of arterial complications of cervical rib: Guidelines for surgical management. Surgery 95:644, 1984.

Chapter 62
Arterial Surgery of Upper Extremity

James S. T. Yao

Unlike occlusive disease affecting the lower extremities in which the etiology is either atherosclerotic or embolic, a wide variety of systemic diseases may cause ischemic symptoms of the upper extremity. Because of this, evaluation of upper extremity ischemia and selection of patients for surgery requires a thorough history and a careful physical examination. A good history taking, including occupational, athletic, pharmacologic, and medical history, helps guide the diagnostic workup. For surgical treatment, the type of procedure depends on the location of the disease and the classification into proximal vs. distal lesions. Surgical intervention is often indicated in patients with severe ischemia due to proximal arterial occlusion. Table 62-1 enumerates the causes of upper extremity ischemia.

SYMPTOMS

Presenting symptoms of upper extremity ischemia include Raynaud's phenomenon, pain, evidence of arterial emboli, and easy fatigue of the forearm after exercise. Raynaud's phenomenon, first described in 1862,[1] is episodic digital ischemia provoked by stimuli such as cold or emotion. It is manifested by pallor (white) followed by cyanosis (blue) and then redness. Raynaud's phenomenon must be distinguished from acrocyanosis, which is characterized by persistent, diffuse cyanosis of the fingers and hands. Also, Raynaud's phenomenon is often referred symptoms secondary to underlying disease, which must not be confused with Raynaud's disease. Raynaud's disease is a primary disease without underlying cause, and the diagnosis is made only after exclusion of all etiologic factors listed in Table 62-1. The criteria suggested by Allen and Brown[2] are helpful in establishing the diagnosis:

1. Raynaud's phenomenon excited by cold or emotion
2. Bilaterality of Raynaud's phenomenon
3. Ischemic lesions, when present, limited to small areas of cutaneous gangrene
4. Exclusion of diseases that might be causal (Table 62-1)

5. Symptoms for at least 2 years in the absence of any disease that might be causal.

Adhering to these guidelines helps establish the definitive diagnosis of Raynaud's disease. In general, unilateral Raynaud's phenomenon is due to organic arterial occlusive disease and seldom to primary Raynaud's disease.[3] Arterial emboli can occur as livedo reticularis, petechiae of the skin, or gangrene of the tips of the fingers. Easy fatigue or intolerance to exercise of the forearm is usually due to proximal artery lesions.

CLINICAL EXAMINATION

Examination in patients who present with symptoms of upper extremity ischemia must include the thoracic outlet and the entire upper extremity. Palpation of the supraclavicular region may help detect the presence of a subclavian artery aneurysm or a cervical rib. Auscultation of the subclavian artery and listening for the presence of a bruit during various thoracic outlet maneuvers (see Chapter 60) helps establish the diagnosis of thoracic outlet compression to the artery. Arteries in the upper extremity are accessible to pulse palpation, and a decrease of pulse or absence of a pulse is diagnostic for major artery occlusion. Examination of hand ischemia is not complete unless an Allen test is performed.[4] The test is done as follows: The examiner stands beside or facing the subject. The radial and ulnar arteries of one wrist are compressed by the examiner's fingers. The subject is asked to open and close the hand rapidly for 1 minute in order to squeeze blood out of the hand, then to extend the fingers quickly. The radial or the ulnar artery is released, and the hand is observed for capillary refilling and return of color. The test is judged normal if refilling of the hand is complete within a short period (<6 seconds). Any portion of the hand which does not blush is an indication of incomplete continuity of the arch. Hyperextension of the fingers must be avoided because this will give a false-positive result.

853

TABLE 62-1. ETIOLOGY OF UPPER EXTREMITY AND DIGITAL ISCHEMIA

I. Atherosclerosis
   A. Arteriosclerosis obliterans
   B. Embolization
      1. Cardiac
      2. Atheromatous emboli
II. Arteritis
   A. Collagen disease
      1. Scleroderma
      2. Rheumatoid arteritis
      3. Systemic lupus erythematosus
      4. Polyarteritis
   B. Allergic necrotizing arteritis
   C. Takayasu's disease (autoimmune disorder)
   D. Buerger's syndrome
   E. Giant cell arteritis
III. Blood dyscrasias
   A. Cold agglutinins
   B. Cryoglobulins
   C. Polycythemia
IV. Drug-induced occlusion
   A. Ergot poisoning
   B. Drug abuse
V. Occupational trauma
   A. Vibration syndrome
   B. Hypothenar hammer syndrome
   C. Electrical burns
VI. Thoracic outlet syndrome
VII. Congenital arterial wall defects
VIII. Trauma
   A. Iatrogenic catheter injury
      1. Cardiac catheterization
      2. Arterial blood gas and pressure monitoring
      3. Arteriography
IX. Renal transplantation and related problems
   A. Azotemic arteriopathy
   B. Hemodialysis shunts
X. Aneurysms of the upper extremity

In addition to the Allen test, examination of the hand must include palpation of the palm for pulsatile mass. Assessment of patency of the digital arteries by palpation is often difficult and unreliable.

LABORATORY EXAMINATION

Serologic Tests

In severe bilateral hand ischemia, a systemic cause of the arterial insufficiency should be sought. The major causes of such ischemia can be identified by serologic testing. Although patients harboring these conditions are seldom candidates for surgical intervention, it is important for interested surgeons to establish proper diagnoses.

In detection of scleroderma (systemic sclerosis) and its variant, the CRST syndrome, a battery of tests is used. Because the features of the condition include calcinosis, Raynaud's phenomenon, esophageal dysfunction, and tel-

angiectasia, a combination of physical examination, soft tissue roentgenograms, and esophageal motility studies may be revealing. The immunologic abnormalities are unfortunately nonspecific.

Systemic lupus erythematosus (SLE), another important cause of bilateral hand ischemia, is characterized by multisystem abnormalities caused by a variety of autoantibodies. The characteristic antibody in SLE is directed against native DNA. Low levels of serum complement are found in 70% of patients with SLE, and acute phase reactants, such as C-reactive protein and elevated fibrinogen, may be found also. The ESR is often elevated and remains so, even during disease remission. Even extensive serologic or immunologic testing may not disclose causes of rapid onset of hand ischemia.[5,6]

Noninvasive Tests

Several noninvasive tests, including plethysmography and transcutaneous Doppler ultrasound flow detection, are now available for objective evaluation of hand ischemia. Of these techniques, Doppler flow detection is simplest.

The Doppler examination of the upper extremity consists of both arterial waveform recording and analysis and pressure measurements. Bilateral examinations should be performed because many of the diseases affecting the hand are symmetric,[7] and often the asymptomatic hand will have significant disease.

Since the axillary and brachial arteries are superficially located, they lend themselves to Doppler examination throughout their entire course in the upper arm. Distal to the elbow, however, arterial signals are more difficult to obtain, and it is not until the wrist that both the radial and ulnar arteries become superficially situated once again.

In the hand, the palmar arches are best heard at the midthenar and hypothenar regions. The common digital vessels are heard at the base of the fingers at their division into the proper digital arteries along the shaft of each finger. The waveforms are analyzed for their shape and contour, similar to examination of the lower extremity.

For segmental upper extremity pressures, a pneumatic cuff is placed at the upper arm, as routinely used for blood pressure recording. The arm pressure will represent the brachial pressure, which should be within 10 to 20 mmHg of the opposite extremity. A greater difference signifies innominate, subclavian, axillary, or brachial artery stenosis. If brachial artery occlusion is suspected, a pressure cuff may be applied to the forearm and the pressure recorded in a similar manner using the radial artery for signal detection. If there is a pressure drop of 20 to 30 mm Hg, this signifies an obstruction distal to the brachial artery. For digital pressure measurement, a 2.5 cm cuff is placed at the base of the finger, and the return of Doppler signals following cuff deflation is monitored at the fingertip.

The palmar circulation is assessed by listening over the hypothenar and thenar eminences for the palmar arches. Patency of the palmar arch is assessed by the modified Allen test described by Kamienski and Barnes.[8] The Doppler probe is placed over the radial artery while compressing the ulnar artery. Should the waveform be obliterated, the

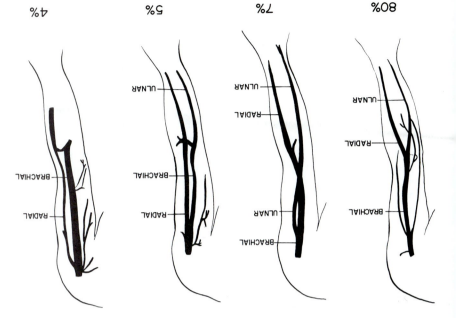

80%

7%

5%

4%

Figure 62-1. Normal variation of the brachial artery and its major branches. (*From Bergan JJ (ed): Arterial Surgery. New York Churchill Livingstone, 1984.*)

---

artery and its branches and in the palmar arch of the hand.

The origin of the radial and ulnar vessels has been noted to be variable by McCormack et al.[11] In 750 upper extremity dissections, 139 specimens had high origin of the radial branch (14%), either from the axillary (2%) or midbrachial (12%) artery (Fig. 62-1). High origin of the ulnar artery was seen less frequently, being present in 2.6% of cases. Rare anomalies, such as an accessory brachial artery or partially duplicated radial artery, were also identified.

Of all arterial patterns of the upper extremity, the palmar arch is subject to most variation (Fig. 62-2). In a study by Coleman and Anson,[12] the superficial arch was found to be complete in 80% of cases. In this group, five subgroups were identified:

Type A   The arch was formed by the ulnar artery and the superficial palmar branch of the radial artery (35.5%).

Type B   The arch was formed entirely by the ulnar artery (37%).

Type C   The arch was formed by an enlarged median artery (3%).

Type D   The arch was formed by the radial, median, and ulnar arteries (1.2%).

Type E   The arch was formed by the ulnar artery joined by vessel from the deep palmar arch at the base of the thenar eminence.

Incomplete arches are present in the remaining 20% of individuals and probably are a major underlying factor in the etiology of digital ischemia (Fig. 62-2). An incomplete arch is defined as one in which the superficial arch does not anastomose with any radial branch and the ulnar branch does not supply the thumb and radial aspects of the index finger. There are four subgroups of incomplete arches:[12]

Type A   The superficial palmar branches of both the radial and ulnar arteries supply the palm and fingers but do not anastomose (3.2%).

---

arch is dependent on the ulnar artery for supply. If the pulse remains present, the arch is complete. The procedure is repeated by listening over the ulnar artery while compressing the radial artery. The Allen test can be repeated while listening at the base of each digit or along the proper digital vessels of each finger. In some cases, even though the arch appears patent, pulsatile flow will be lost to the digits.

The Doppler technique is of particular value to determine palmar arch patency in a patient who is unconscious or uncooperative in performing an Allen test. Arterial obstruction distal to the palmar arch is best detected by digital pressure measurements. An arterial occlusion distal to the palmar arch is defined by a pressure gradient between the fingers of greater than 15 mm Hg or a wrist-to-digit difference of 30 mm Hg. These very distal occlusions are caused by emboli, Buerger's disease, or arteritis. There is good correlation between Doppler criteria and radiographic findings.[9]

Arteriography

Arteriography remains the most conclusive test for diagnosis of upper extremity ischemia, and it must be done if surgery is contemplated. The preferred method for arteriography of the upper extremity, including the hand, is transfemoral catheterization of the subclavian and brachial arteries, with selective contrast injection.[10] The innominate or external rotation with abduction view is obtained to detect the presence of compression. If thoracic outlet syndrome is suspected, a hyperabduction or external rotation with abduction view is obtained to detect the presence of compression.

In addition to establishing a diagnosis, arteriography defines the normal anatomy of the brachial artery and its branches. Such variations are of surgical significance if an operative procedure is contemplated, since normal anatomic variations have been observed in the brachial

DIAGNOSIS

In most instances, the diagnosis of large artery occlusion is not difficult, and a careful pulse examination will establish the diagnosis. In hand and digital ischemia, the use of noninvasive testing to detect digital artery occlusion helps distinguish Raynaud's phenomenon from Raynaud's disease. The diagnosis of Raynaud's disease should not be made until all diagnostic tests are completed and proven negative. The onset of Raynaud's phenomenon may precede other manifestations of underlying collagen disease by many years. Therefore, the diagnosis of Raynaud's disease must not be made until 2 years have elapsed with no systemic disease appearing. If this strict criterion is followed, most patients will be found to have Raynaud's phenomenon, and Raynaud's disease will become a rare clinical entity.

Type B	The ulnar artery forms the entire superficial palmar arch but does not supply the thumb or index finger (13.4%)
Type C	The median artery reaches the hand to supply the digits but does not anastomose with the radial or ulnar arteries, and the median artery supplies a branch to the thumb (3.8%)
Type D	The radial, median, and ulnar arteries all give origin to the superficial vessels but do not anastomose (1.1%)

PROXIMAL ARTERIAL LESIONS

Atherosclerosis

Atherosclerotic stenosis or occlusion is common in the subclavian artery but less so in the axillary, brachial, and distal arteries. Because of the rich collateral networks of the scapular region, occlusion of the subclavian artery seldom causes severe digital ischemia unless there is associated embolization. Atheromatous embolization to the digital arteries may present with Raynaud's phenomenon, and the source may be an ulcerating proximal plaque or aneurysm (Fig. 62-3). Proximal subclavian artery occlusion is often associated with the vertebral steal phenomenon. Occlusion of the subclavian artery in the second or third part is less common. Collateral pathways in such instances depend on the site of the occlusion.

Atherosclerotic occlusion of the axillary artery is uncommon. Instead, most occlusions of the axillary artery are from unrecognized emboli originating from proximal atheromatous plaques or intracardiac thrombi.

Arterial Emboli

The upper limbs are the site of acute arterial occlusion in 10 to 20% of acute embolic events,[13] and the brachial artery is the most common site (65%) for lodgment of emboli in the upper extremity.[14]

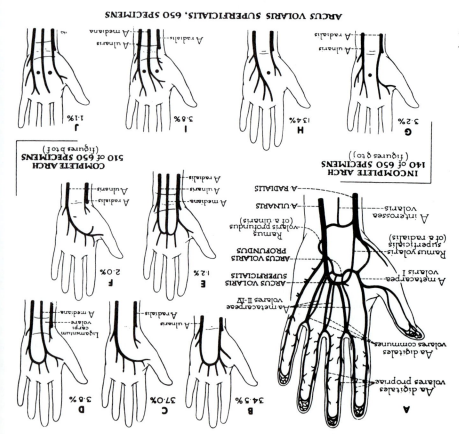

Figure 62-2. Patterns of normal palmar anatomy. (From Coleman SS, Anson BJ: Surg Gynecol Obstet 113:409, 1961.)

first affecting the adventitia and vasa vasorum. Later, the media is affected with a loss of elastic fibers. The intima responds by proliferation, with subsequent thrombosis resulting in stenosis, occlusion, or aneurysm formation. In addition to symptoms referable to the arterial lesions, acute or chronic systemic illness occurs which mimics countless other conditions. The etiology remains obscure, but the current consensus favors a hypersensitivity or autoimmune reaction.

Arteriography provides definitive diagnosis. Because of the widespread involvement of various arteries, total aortography has been advocated.[17,18] In its most familiar form, the aortic arch and the main trunks are affected (Fig. 62-4), but as indicated above, lesions are also common in the descending thoracic and abdominal aorta. The pulmonary artery was affected in 45% of patients reported by Nasu.[19]

One of the distinct features of Takayasu's arteritis is the presence of abundant collateral vessels (see Fig. 62-4). This finding is probably due to the chronicity of the disease. Unlike atherosclerosis, subclavian occlusion proximal to the vertebral artery is rare. Rich collateral pathways from the subclavian, axillary, and proximal brachial arteries participate in the network.

Giant Cell Arteritis

The most frequently recognized clinical features of giant cell arteritis (cranial, temporal, and granulomatous arteritis) result from involvement of cranial arteries. Systemic symp-

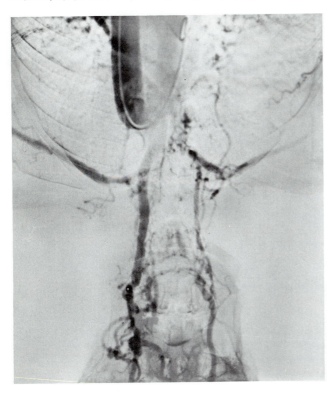

Figure 62-4. Occlusion of innominate artery at left subclavian artery in a patient with Takayasu's arteritis.

Diagnosis of embolism of the brachial artery is not difficult. A careful pulse examination, with history and symptoms, usually establishes the diagnosis. Because of this, arteriography in a clear-cut case is seldom needed. A cardiac origin of emboli of the upper limb accounts for over 90% of these cases.[14] Myxoma is one possible source of the emboli.[15] Occasionally, arterial emboli may go unnoticed, and the patient will present with recurrent symptoms. In this circumstance, arteriography is helpful in establishing the diagnosis.

Takayasu's Arteritis

Takayasu's arteritis is a nonspecific inflammatory process of unknown etiology affecting segmentally the aorta and its main branches. Since Takayasu's description of this disease in 1908,[16] it has been known by many names: pulseless disease, aortic arch syndrome, young female arteritis, and Martorell's syndrome. In 1977, Ishikawa et al.[17] referred to Takayasu's disease as occlusive thromboaortopathy to denote the widespread disease process which affects carotid, subclavian, axillary, and pulmonary arteries and the thoracic and abdominal aorta. Because the subclavian-axillary arteries are often involved, it is not unusual for patients to present with upper extremity ischemia.

Classically, the disease affects young women between 10 and 30 years of age, the sex ratio being at least 7 to 1. Though the bulk of cases have been reported in Japan, Takayasu's arteritis is also seen in other parts of Asia and in Mexico. Reports from the Western world, however, have been sparse.

The basic pathologic process is panarteritis, probably

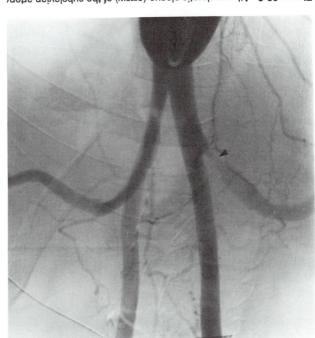

Figure 62-3. Atherosclerotic plaque (arrow) of the subclavian artery in a patient with embolization to fingers.

toms, such as malaise and fever, are common in these patients. Although involvement of large arteries by giant cell arteritis is uncommon, it has received some attention.[20] Of 248 patients with giant cell arteritis reported by Klein et al.,[20] 15 were found to have ischemic symptoms of the upper extremity. Of these 15 patients, five had Raynaud's phenomenon. Characteristic arteriographic findings in these patients included long segments of smooth arterial stenosis alternating with areas of normal or increased caliber; smooth, tapered occlusions; and absence of irregular plaques and ulcerations (Fig. 62-5).

Ergot Poisoning

With the introduction of ergotamine tartrate for the treatment of migraine, vascular complications as a result of overdosage have become a diagnostic problem for those who are not familiar with ergot poisoning. The affected arteries may be in the upper extremities or the lower extremities.[21,22] Most arterial occlusions may be reversed, if prompt diagnosis of ergot poisoning is made and the medication is discontinued instantly.[23] In prolonged ischemia due to ergot poisoning, thrombosis with tissue necrosis may occur.

Pharmacologically, the ergot compounds produce intense vasoconstriction because of direct stimulation of the alpha receptors in the vessel wall. The characteristic finding on the arteriogram is intense spasm seen as long, smooth areas of narrowing. This is often bilateral and tends to be symmetric. Occasionally, focal spasm is seen. Other prominent features are the presence of abundant collateral vessels. Although rare, thrombi may be present and are seen as

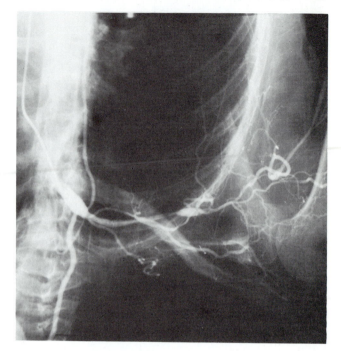

Figure 62-5. Arteriogram in a patient with proven giant-cell arteritis. Note the typical tapering appearance of the subclavian artery.

filling defects on the arteriogram. Spasm and narrowing of the affected artery often reverse to normal when ergot drugs are completely withdrawn (Figs. 62-6, 62-7). Treatment of ergot poisoning may occasionally benefit from the administration of sodium nitroprusside.

Thoracic Outlet Syndrome

Thoracic outlet syndrome consists of neurologic and vascular manifestations. The anatomic boundaries of the thoracic outlet generally correspond to the area traversed by the subclavian artery and vein and the brachial plexus. These structures pass through the interscalene triangle (anterior and medial), with the exception that the subclavian vein lies anterior to the scalene muscle. They then lie in the retroclavicular fossa, pass beneath the clavicle, and enter the upper extremity. The subclavian vessels and brachial plexus can be compressed extrinsically in three sites: (1) the costoclavicular space, (2) the interscalene triangle, or (3) the angle between the insertion of the pectoralis minor

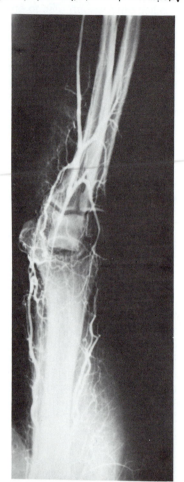

Figure 62-6. Arteriogram demonstrating occlusion of the brachial artery in a young woman with ergot poisoning. Note extensive spasm of the brachial artery. (From Neiman HL, Yao JST (eds): Angiography of Vascular Disease. New York, Churchill Livingstone, 1985.)

Radiation Injury

Irradiation may cause damage not only to small vessels but also to large arteries such as the subclavian.[24] Morphologic changes in small arteries have been described by several investigators.[25,26] These changes include endothelial proliferation, degeneration of the cells of the media with subsequent cystic medial necrosis, and fibrosis. Most injuries to the arteries present with late manifestations, and for the most part injury to the vasa vasorum is present. Fonkalsrud et al.[26] documented these changes by light electron microscopy. Fibrosis of the arterial wall as a result of damage to the vasa vasorum leads to narrowing of the vessel lumen.

As stated by Butler et al.,[24] there are three stages following irradiation. The first is at 5 years following radiation, when most patients present with mural thrombosis. These patients are also found to have multiple digital artery occlusions, presumably due to embolization from the injured subclavian artery (Fig. 62-10). The second stage occurs 10 years after irradiation, when patients present with symptoms caused by fibrotic occlusion of the irradiated vessel. The third stage is much later (20 to 25 years or more following irradiation), when the lesion involves periarterial fibrosis together with accelerated atherosclerosis.

DISTAL ARTERIAL LESIONS

Collagen Disease

Collagen diseases are a broad category of disorders having in common the finding of generalized connective tissue damage with an increase in the amount of collagen in skin, muscle, tendons, fascia, and viscera. Each of the different types of disease classified under this grouping has prominent, nonspecific, constitutional manifestations, along with varying patterns of organ involvement. When the characteristic histologic changes of fibrinoid degeneration and intimal thickening occur in the blood vessels, signs of ischemia can occur. In addition, the added insult of vasospasm may adversely contribute to the clinical picture. Collagen disease includes scleroderma, rheumatoid arthritis, systemic lupus erythematosus, polyarteritis nodosa, and dermatomyositis. All these diseases have systemic symptoms, and the diagnosis is made by elevation of ESR and positive serologic tests.

Buerger's Disease (Thromboangiitis Obliterans)

Raynaud's disease and Buerger's disease have met with similar controversy in regard to their being distinct clinical entities. Buerger's disease was first described by von Winiwarter in 1879. In 1908, Buerger[27] described the disease in Jewish patients who presented with digital gangrene without occlusion of the larger arteries. Today it is noted that such patients are heavy smokers. While the disease, if it exists, is more common in the lower extremity, it may occur in the upper extremity. As arteriography became more frequent, patients suspected of having Buerger's disease were

muscle and the coracoid process in the axilla. Of these three sites, the costoclavicular space, formed by the first thoracic rib and clavicle, is the most common site of compression.

Any structure that encroaches upon the thoracic outlet or any process that functionally reduces its dimensions can produce compression of the brachial plexus and underlying vascular structures. Thoracic outlet syndrome may be due to cervical rib, abnormalities of the scalenus anticus muscle, or bony abnormalities of the cervical vertebrae, clavicle, or first rib. Although between 0.5 and 1% of the population have a cervical rib, 10% of fewer of such persons have symptoms of neurovascular compression. The majority of patients with thoracic outlet syndrome present with neurologic rather than ischemic symptoms. Pain is usual and involves the C8 and T1 dermatome. Vascular abnormalities in thoracic outlet syndrome include direct compression of the artery or poststenotic dilatation or aneurysm formation with thrombus formation and distal embolization (Figs. 62-8, 62-9). Raynaud's phenomenon is not uncommon as an initial complaint, and it is often unilateral.

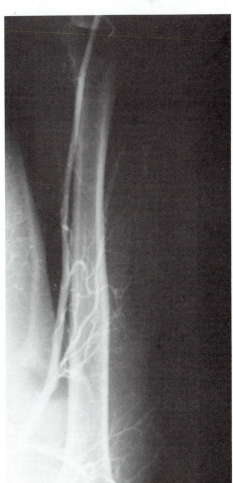

Figure 62-7. Repeat arteriogram in the same patient 10 days after cessation of drug. The brachial artery has returned to normal appearance. (From Neiman HL, Yao JST (eds): Angiography of Vascular Disease. New York, Churchill Livingstone, 1985.)

Blood Dyscrasias

Cold agglutinins, cryoglobulin, and polycythemia vera are the most common forms of blood dyscrasias which may be associated with occlusion of the arteries of the legs or hands. In 1903, William Osler first drew attention to vascular complications of polycythemia. Norman and Allen[29] reported their experience with polycythemia in the Mayo Clinic and found that a third of these patients had vascular complications. Of 200 patients with polycythemia vera, the arterial complications ranged from cerebrovascular accident to peripheral artery occlusion and included venous thrombosis in 34%.[30] The cause of small artery occlusion is generally thought to be local thrombosis or embolism. Regardless of the cause, acute digital ischemia may occur.

found to have atherosclerosis rather than thromboangiitis obliterans. Similarly, modern investigation in suspected patients often uncovers a collagen disease. At present, the diagnosis of Buerger's disease depends on histologic examination with involvement not only of arteries but of veins as well. This is manifested clinically as migrating phlebitis.

Characteristic arteriographic findings are occlusion of small arteries of the digits, with abundant collaterals (Fig. 62-11). A characteristic corrugated appearance of the artery proximal to an occlusion is often seen, and this finding has been cited as one of the diagnostic findings in Buerger's disease. However, the corrugated artery may also be seen in other conditions. Not only does the symptomatic hand demonstrate digital artery occlusion, but the asymptomatic hand may show it as well.[28]

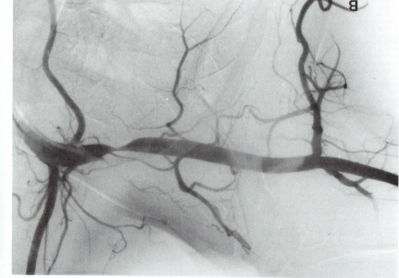
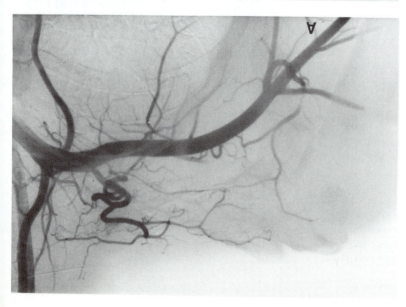

Figure 62-8. Arteriogram of a patient with thoracic outlet compression syndrome. **A.** Neutral position. **B.** Hyperabduction. The subclavian artery became stenotic.

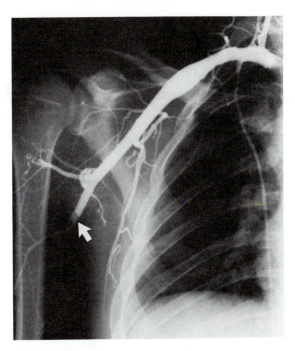

Figure 62-9. Arteriogram in a patient with cervical rib and hand ischemia, showing aneurysm dilatation of the subclavian artery. A filling defect (arrow) is seen in the brachial artery, indicating embolization.

Drug Abuse

Drug abuse presents social problems and also a new, wide variety of medical problems. Vascular complications due to drug abuse may be related to local damage to the artery by unsterile needles leading to infection, false aneurysm formation, or arteriovenous fistula. Apart from the systemic effect of various drugs on the arterial system itself, the inadvertent injection of hypertonic solution or powder into

the arterial system often causes multiple digital arterial occlusions. Raynaud's phenomenon following this form of obstruction is not uncommon.

Catheter Injury

With increasing use of diagnostic and therapeutic procedures involving catheterization, damage to the radial or brachial artery has become more common, especially when an incomplete palmar arch is not recognized prior to placement of a catheter in the radial artery.[30] Catheterization of the heart or arteriographic examination of the extremities and trunk may result in damage to the brachial artery, which causes thrombosis, embolization, or dissection. Failure to recognize normal anatomic variation of the brachial and hand arterial anatomy may cause puzzling problems. Further, unrecognized injury to the brachial artery following cardiac catheterization may cause exercise pain in the forearm or cold sensitivity of the involved extremity. Arteriographic examination is often needed to clarify the situation. The arteriographic finding is often occlusion of the brachial artery with irregularity of the arterial wall. When there is associated embolization, multiple occlusions of the digital arteries may be seen.

Injuries to the radial artery from blood gas monitoring are not uncommon. Severe ischemia may result if there is incompleteness of the superficial and deep volar arches, and gangrene of the hand has been reported. Arteriography is seldom needed when acute thrombus is recognized and promptly treated. In chronic ischemia, arteriography may be necessary to define the anatomy of the hand, thus allowing consideration of microvascular repair of the artery.

Vibration Syndrome

Blanching and numbness of the hands after using pneumatic drills is now a recognized clinical entity of hand isch-

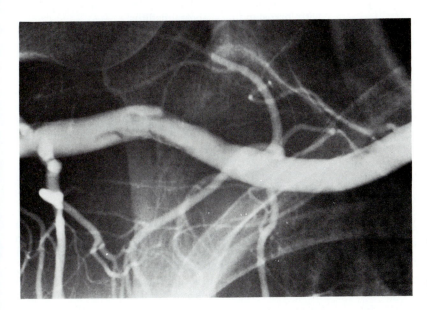

Figure 62-10. Arteriogram in a patient with a history of irradiation of the shoulder region. Note the linear weblike defect in the artery. (*From Neiman HL, Yao JST (eds): Angiography of Vascular Disease. New York, Churchill Livingstone, 1985.*)

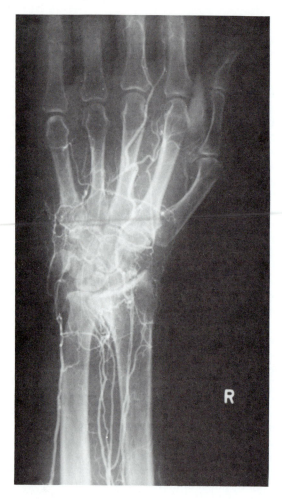

Figure 62-11. Arteriographic appearance of the hand vasculature in a patient with a history of heavy smoking without collagen disease.

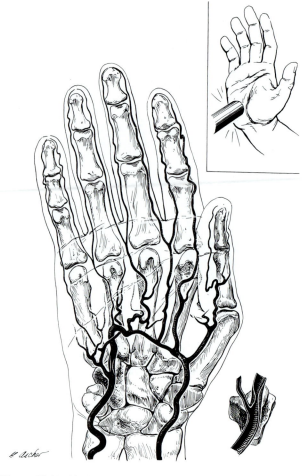

Figure 62-12. Mechanism of injury to the ulnar artery in hypothenar hammer syndrome. (See text for explanation)

emia. The vibratory white-finger is a form of occupational trauma. Repetitive trauma to the digital arteries is the primary responsible factor.

Hypothenar Hammer Syndrome

The predisposing factor in the development of hypothenar hammer syndrome is the repetitive use of the palm of the hand in activities which involve pushing, pounding, or twisting (Fig. 62-12). The anatomic location of the ulnar artery in the area of the hypothenar eminence places it in a vulnerable position. When this area is repeatedly traumatized, ulnar or digital artery occlusion or aneurysm formation can result.[31]

Azotemic Arteriopathy

In chronic renal failure, calcification, such as is seen in Monckeberg's arteriosclerosis of the lower extremity, may affect the digital arteries of the hand, causing gangrene of the digits. The so-called azotemic arteriopathy[32] is character-

ized by calcification of the media of the digital arteries, resulting in a pipestem pattern on plain x-ray film (Fig. 62-13). A similar condition may be observed in patients with long-standing diabetes mellitus.

ANEURYSMS OF UPPER EXTREMITY ARTERIES

Common sites for aneurysm formation in the upper extremity are the subclavian artery and the hand. False aneurysm due to trauma, however, may occur along the course of the arterial system in the upper extremity. Innominate artery aneurysm may cause hand ischemia, but this is rare.

Subclavian Artery Aneurysm

Aneurysms of the subclavian artery are rare in comparison with other peripheral aneurysms, and most subclavian aneurysms are caused by blunt or penetrating trauma or by the thoracic outlet syndrome. In the latter condition, poststenotic dilatation is often observed in patients with cervical rib. The incidence of arteriosclerotic aneurysm of the subclavian artery is unknown, but the condition is rare,

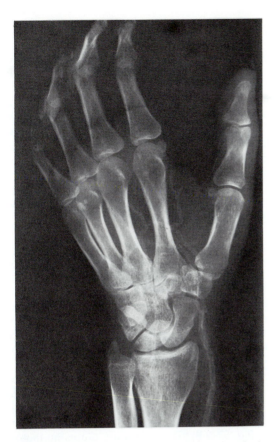

Figure 62-13. Typical appearance of azotemic arteriopathy in a diabetic patient with renal transplant. All digital arteries are distinctly seen on plain x-ray film. The radial artery also shows heavy calcification. Arteriogram in this patient shows multiple digital artery occlusions.

Arteriography allows examination of the integrity of the volar arch and the collateral pathways. With the development of microvascular surgery, most aneurysms are now being treated with vein graft interposition or simply by end-to-end anastomosis.

TREATMENT

Treatment of upper extremity ischemia is strictly according to the etiology. Withdrawal of drugs such as ergot derivatives, dopamine, or chemotherapeutic agents will help reverse ischemia. For patients with collagen disease, treatment must be directed toward the underlying cause and steroid or immunosuppressive treatment may be necessary. Patients with digital artery occlusion without proximal artery lesions are not candidates for surgical intervention. The severity of Raynaud's phenomenon in these patients may require a course of pharmacologic treatment. At present, the use of calcium channel blocker (nifedipine, 10 mg every 8 hours) appears to be the drug of choice. Both clinical and hemodynamic assessment have demonstrated nifedipine as effective in the treatment of Raynaud's phenomenon.[38]

Severe hand ischemia associated with major arterial lesions is the prime indication for arterial reconstructive surgery in the upper extremity. In patients with associated arteritis or autoimmune disease with a high ESR, the use

even in patients with multiple aneurysms. Several authors, however, have reported series of arteriosclerotic subclavian artery aneurysms,[33,34] and aneurysm of the anomalous subclavian artery has received attention.[35] Other, less common causes of subclavian artery aneurysm are syphilis,[36] cystic medial necrosis, congenital defects, and invasion from tuberculous lymphadenitis. Subclavian artery aneurysm may present as a late complication or Blalock-Taussig anastomosis and may also be a part of an arteriovenous malformation.

Subclavian artery aneurysm may cause digital artery occlusion because of embolization from debris or thrombi within the aneurysm.

Aneurysms of the Hand

False aneurysms due to penetrating trauma or needle puncture are the most common forms of aneurysm of the hand. Other aneurysms of the hand arteries may be due to occupational trauma with injury to the ulnar artery where it passes across the hook of the hamate bone (Fig. 62-14). Arteriosclerotic aneurysms of the hand are rare and have been reported sporadically.[37] The lesions are usually associated with significant arteriosclerotic disease involving other vessels. Either the radial or the ulnar artery may be involved.

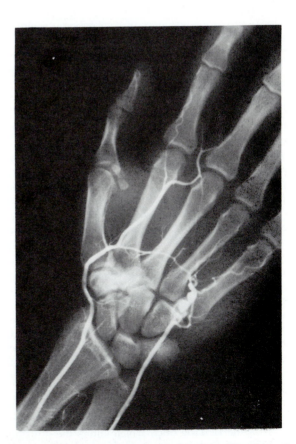

Figure 62-14. Aneurysm of the terminal branch of the ulnar artery in a carpenter with hypothenar hammer syndrome.

of a steroid preparation may be necessary. The type of procedure employed varies according to the location of the lesion.

Proximal Artery Occlusion

Lesions involving the innominate, subclavian, or axillary artery are best treated by bypass grafting. In selected cases in which the atherosclerotic process, such as ulcerating plaque, is localized, a short segment endarterectomy with patch may be used. An intrathoracic approach using the thoracic aorta as the origin of the graft is needed if the innominate or proximal subclavian artery is occluded. Long segment occlusion of the axillary or brachial artery is also best treated by bypass grafting. Once again, the use of autogenous vein (saphenous or cephalic) is preferred to prosthetic materials. Short segmental stenosis or occlusion of the brachial artery (<2 cm) is amenable to endarterectomy with vein patch. In extensive occlusion of the forearm arteries, bypass to the ulnar, radial, or interosseous artery using autogenous vein is indicated to relieve severe ischemia.

Management of vascular complications of the thoracic outlet syndrome depends on the extent of injury and the mechanism of compression. Damage to the artery such as mural thrombosis, poststenotic dilatation, or aneurysm formation must be dealt with by replacement of the injured segment with a short bypass graft. At the same time, the responsible compression structure (cervical rib, anterior scalene muscle) must be removed. If there is no arterial damage but there is evidence of compression, removal of the cervical rib or offending muscle is needed to prevent future assault on the artery. Distal embolization as a result of mural thrombus or thrombosed aneurysm may require distal bypass to relieve severe ischemia.

Exposure of Subclavian Artery
The skin incision is made 1 cm above and parallel to the clavicle, beginning medially at the sternal head of the sternocleidomastoid muscle and extending laterally to the midpoint of the clavicle (Fig. 62-15A). The incision is carried through the subcutaneous tissue and platysma muscle to expose the clavicular head of the sternocleidomastoid muscle (Fig. 62-15B). The muscle is then divided parallel to the clavicle using the coagulation mode of the electrocautery, exposing the scalene fat pad. Dissection medially in the scalene fat should identify the anterior scalene muscle and its attachment to the first rib (Fig. 62-15C). Particular care must be given to this dissection, because the phrenic nerve courses along the anterior border of the anterior scalene muscle and must be preserved. The phrenic nerve is mobilized from the anterior scalene muscle and retracted gently with a silastic sling. The anterior scalene muscle may then be divided close to its junction with the first rib, thus exposing the more proximal portion of the subclavian artery (Fig. 62-15D). It must be remembered that the subclavian vein lies just anterior to the anterior scalene muscle and should be protected during division of the muscle. Also, the thoracic duct, which enters the junction of the left internal jugular vein and the left subclavian vein,

can easily be injured inadvertently at this point in the dissection.

At this time, the subclavian artery is skeletonized. Remember that the pleura lies just deep to the vessel. The vertebral artery should be preserved unless it is occluded by atherosclerotic disease. The internal mammary artery and thyrocervical trunk should be preserved, but division of the internal mammary artery increases mobility of the subclavian artery. Vascular control is obtained through the use of silastic slings on the proximal and distal extent of the subclavian artery, proximal control being obtained as early as possible during the dissection. Branch vessels are controlled by the double-looping of silastic slings that are placed on mild tension prior to arteriotomy.

Exposure of Axillary Artery
A horizontal incision is made approximately 6 to 8 cm in length, about two finger-breadths below the clavicle (Fig. 62-16A). This is similar to exposure of the axillary artery for axillary-femoral bypass. The pectoralis major muscle fibers between the clavicular and sternocostal heads are split horizontally, parallel to the skin incision. After division of the pectoralis minor close to its insertion, the axillary artery is exposed easily. Great care must be taken to avoid injury to the surrounding structure, such as the axillary vein, which lies inferiorly, and the lateral cord of the brachial plexus, which is located above the artery. Exposure of the axillary artery may be facilitated by dividing the pectoralis nerve (Fig. 62-16B). This procedure causes no motor loss. The lateral thoracic artery must be identified and looped with a silastic tape for control of bleeding during the arteriotomy. After exposure of the axillary artery proximally and distally for about 4 cm, the artery is ready for the bypass procedure.

Exposure of Brachial Artery
The arm is placed in abduction with the forearm and hand in supination. An incision of 6 to 8 cm is made medially along the posterior border of the biceps muscle (Fig. 62-17A). After medial and lateral retraction of muscle, the brachial artery is identifiable. The sheath of the neurovascular bundle is entered through an avascular area. The artery is normally surrounded by the median nerve and medial cutaneous nerve of the forearm. A 4 cm segment of brachial artery is exposed (Fig. 62-17B), which can be used either to accept a vein graft from the axillary artery or as the proximal supply of a brachial to radial or brachial to ulnar artery bypass.

Exposure of Radial, Ulnar, or Interosseous Artery
Depending on the nature of the occlusion, the radial or ulnar artery can be exposed and used for bypass at either the elbow or the wrist. At the elbow, the radial or ulnar artery is exposed simply by extending the incision across the elbow joint as depicted in Figure 62-18A. The lacertus fibrosus (bicipital aponeurosis) of the biceps muscle can be retracted laterally to facilitate the exposure of these two major branches. If necessary, the bicipital aponeurosis may be divided. The brachial vein is seen between the artery and the median nerve. The recurrent radial artery, a small

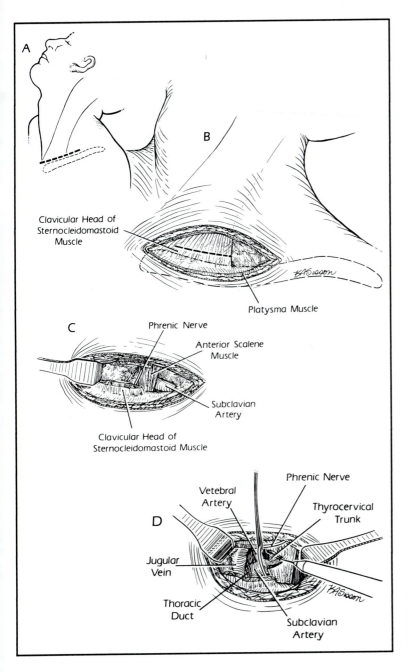

Clavicular Head of
Sternocleidomastoid
Muscle

Platysma Muscle

Phrenic Nerve

Anterior Scalene
Muscle

Subclavian
Artery

Clavicular Head of
Sternocleidomastoid Muscle

Phrenic Nerve

Vetebral
Artery

Thyrocervical
Trunk

Jugular
Vein

Thoracic
Duct

Subclavian
Artery

Figure 62-15. Exposure of the subclavian artery. (See text for explanation). (*From Bergan JJ, Yao JST (eds): Cerebrovascular Insufficiency. New York, Grune & Stratton, 1983.*)

branch, may be seen and must be identified for control of back-bleeding. Either the ulnar or radial artery may be used as the recipient for the bypass. If both the ulnar and radial arteries are occluded, the interosseous artery may be used. The common interosseous artery originates from the dorsal lateral surface of the ulnar artery about 2 to 3 cm distal to the brachial bifurcation (Fig. 62-18B). The size of this artery is close to the size of the proximal ulnar artery, and it divides into posterior and anterior branches just proximal to the interosseous membrane (Fig. 62-19). Exposure of the anterior interosseous artery follows the anatomic landmark of the ulnar artery. The anterior interosseous artery is found between the flexor digitorum profundus muscle and the flexor pollicis longus (Fig. 62-20) and is accompanied by the anterior interosseous branch of the median nerve. The latter provides motor regulation to the flexor digitorum profunda and the flexor pollicis longus. The posterior interosseous artery is located on the dorsal aspect of the forearm, and a separate skin incision on the dorsum of the forearm is needed to expose this artery.

Surgical Procedure

The patient is placed in supine position with the hand and upper arm positioned at 90 degrees abduction and resting on an arm board. The arm must be draped free in sterile fashion using a stockinette so that an incision on the inner aspect of the upper arm can be made easily, if necessary. This position allows palpation of distal pulses

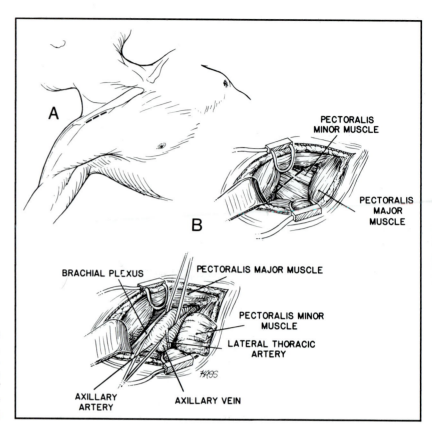

Figure 62-16. A. Skin incision for axillary to brachial, ulnar, radial artery bypass. **B.** Exposure of the axillary artery is greatly facilitated by dividing the pectoris minor muscle at its insertion. (*From Bergan JJ, Yao JST (eds): Operative Techniques in Vascular Surgery. New York, Grune & Stratton, 1980.*)

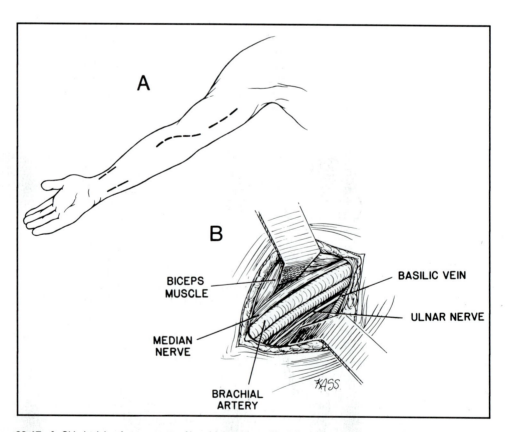

Figure 62-17. A. Skin incision for exposure of brachial artery and its trifurcation. **B.** The brachial artery is readily identifiable after the sheath of the neurovascular bundle is entered. (*From Bergan JJ, Yao JST (eds): Operative Techniques in Vascular Surgery. New York, Grune & Stratton, 1980.*)

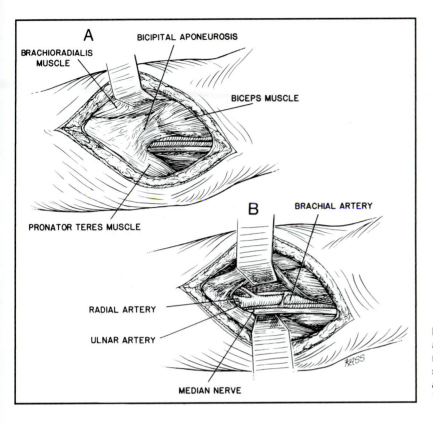

Figure 62-18. The radial and ulnar arteries are often seen beneath the bicipital aponeurosis, which may be divided to facilitate exposure. (*From Bergan JJ, Yao JST (eds): Operative Techniques in Vascular Surgery. New York, Grune & Stratton, 1980.*)

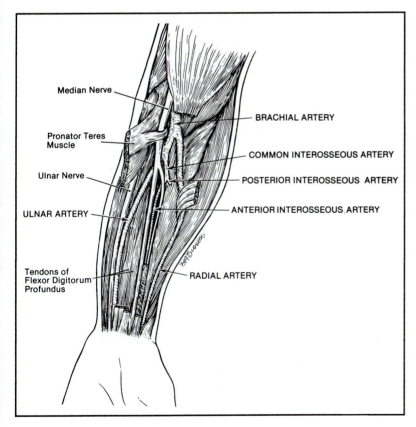

Figure 62-19. Anatomy of left forearm. Note relationship between the median nerve and the anterior interosseous artery. (*From McCarthy WJ, Flinn WR, et al.: J Vasc Surg vol 3, 1986.*)

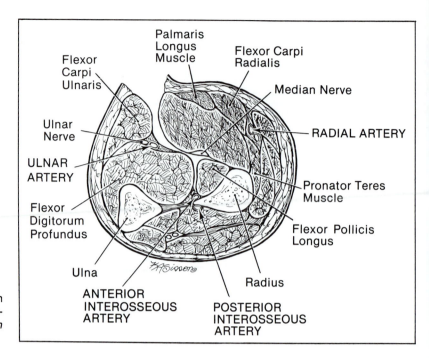

Figure 62-20. Cross section of forearm shows exposure of the interosseous digitorum profundus. (*From McCarthy WJ, Flinn WR, et al.: J Vasc Surg vol. 3, 1986.*)

(radial, ulnar, and brachial) to ascertain the success of the operation.

Bypass procedures in the upper extremity are normally done with autogenous vein harvested from the lower limb. Therefore, one of the lower extremities, including the groin, must be prepared and draped during the procedure. If saphenous vein is not available, the cephalic vein from the contralateral arm may be used. Expanding polytetrafluoroethylene (PTFE) is used only when no autogenous vein is available.

Once the sites for inflow and distal anastomoses are determined, the exposure described above is executed on the appropriate artery. Following this, the saphenous vein is harvested and prepared. The vein is distended with normal saline, and all leaking branches are ligated with 4–0 sutures. The vein is then ready for anastomosis.

Tunneling of the bypass graft follows the normal pathway of the artery using a long DeBakey clamp placed subfascially. If necessary, a separate jump incision is made to facilitate passing of the graft. The vein graft is placed in reverse position and passed through the subfascial tunnel. At this point, 5000 units of heparin are given.

Anasotomosis of vein to artery is often done in end-to-side manner using 6–0 Prolene sutures. At the completion of the anastomoses, an electromagnetic flowmeter is used to ascertain the flow value, followed by an intraoperative arteriogram to evaluate the integrity of the distal anastomosis. The latter procedure is done by placing a 20-gauge intraarterial shunt catheter into the graft. Injection of 20 ml of contrast media is often sufficient to visualize the distal arm and the hand. The hand must be included to allow detailed study of the palmar arch anatomy.

Distal Arterial Lesions

This refers to stenosis, occlusion, or aneurysm at the wrist level or in the hand. A short segmental occlusion of either the radial or ulnar artery is best treated by thrombectomy or endarterectomy with vein patch. Aneurysm in the hand is not uncommonly associated with hypothenar hammer syndrome, and the aneurysm can be resected and replaced with either primary end-to-end anastomosis or an interposed vein graft. Occlusion distal to the proximal palmar crease is not ordinarily amenable to surgery, but perhaps microvascular repair should be considered.

Results

Garrett et al.[39] were the first to report use of an autogenous vein bypass for upper extremity ischemia. Subsequently, others have also reported good results with bypass grafting.[40–45] In our recent analysis of bypass grafting for upper limb ischemia,[46] we found the result to be similar to lower extremity revascularization, that is, proximal grafts fared better than distal grafts. The 2-year patency was 83% for grafts at or above the brachial artery but only 53% for grafts distal to the brachial bifurcation (Fig. 62-21). Unlike lower extremity surgery, major amputation was not required in any case even after graft occlusion.

Cervical Sympathectomy

Like lumbar sympathectomy, cervical sympathectomy is done less and less frequently. This is because of the better understanding of episodic vasospasm and, in particular, an improvement in diagnostic techniques. Many patients thought to have Raynaud's disease have been found to have secondary disease, and sympathectomy is not helpful in patients with collagen disease. As a result, cervical sympathectomy is done only in selected instances. Sympathectomy is indicated in hyperhidrosis and causalgia.

Cervical sympathectomy is performed through the transaxillary approach. A small incision is made in the axilla between the second and third intercostal spaces. The sympathetic chain is identified after the pleural cavity is entered, and the sympathetic ganglia from the lower third of the stellate ganglion, including T2 through T4, are removed.

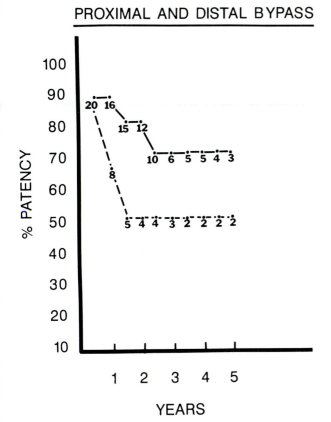

Figure 62-21. Life table analysis of primary patency rates (2 years) of upper extremity bypass grafts. Top: Distal anastomosis above brachial artery trifurcation. Bottom: Distal anastomosis below the brachial artery trifurcation. (*From McCarthy WJ, Flinn WR, et al.: J Vasc Surg vol. 3, 1986.*)

REFERENCES

1. Raynaud M: De l'Asphyxe Locale et de la Gangrene Symetrique des Extremities. Paris, Rignoux, 1862.
2. Allen EV, Brown GE: Raynaud's disease affecting men. Ann Intern Med 5:1384, 1932.
3. Bouhoutsos J, Morris T, Martin P: Unilateral Raynaud's phenomenon in the hand and its significance. Surgery 82:547, 1977.
4. Allen EV: Thromboangiitis obliterans: Methods of diagnosis of chronic occlusive arterial lesions distal to the wrist with illustrative cases. Am J Med 178:237, 1929.
5. Baur GM, Porter JM, et al.: Rapid onset of hand ischemia of unknown etiology: Clinical evaluation and follow-up of ten patients. Ann Surg 186:184, 1977.
6. Porter JM, Taylor LM: Limb ischemia caused by small artery disease. World J Surg 7:326, 1983.
7. Erlandson EE, Forrest ME, et al.: Discriminant arteriographic criteria in the management of forearm and hand ischemia. Surgery 90:1025, 1981.
8. Kamienski RW, Barnes RW: Critique of the Allen test for continuity of the palmar arch assessed by Doppler ultrasound. Surg Gynecol Obstet 142:861, 1976.
9. Yao JST, Gourmos C, Irvine WT: A method for assessing ischemia of the hand and fingers. Surgery 135:373, 1972.
10. Yao JST, Bergan JJ, Neiman HL: Arteriography for upper extremity and digital ischemia, in Neiman HL, Yao JST, (eds): Angiography of Vascular Disease. New York, Churchill Livingstone, 1985, pp 353–419.
11. McCormack LJ, Cauldwell EW, Anson BJ: Brachial and antebrachial arterial patterns: A study of 750 extremities. Surg Gynecol Obstet 96:43, 1953.
12. Coleman SS, Anson BJ: Arterial patterns in the hand based upon a study of 650 specimens. Surg Gynecol Obstet 113:409, 1961.
13. Metz P, Sager P: Acute arterial occlusion of the upper limbs. A follow-up study of 31 extremities. Acta Chir Scand 140:195, 1974.
14. Savelyev JS, Zatevakhin II, Stepanov NV: Arterial embolism of the upper limbs. Surgery 81:367, 1977.
15. Thompson JR, Simmons CR: Arterial embolus. Manifestation of unsuspected myxoma. JAMA 228:864, 1974.
16. Takayasu M: A case with peculiar changes of the central retinal vessels. Acta Soc Ophthal Japan 12:554, 1908.
17. Ishikawa K, Serin Y, et al.: Occlusive thromboaortopathy (Takayasu's disease) and allied diseases. Proceedings 34th Asian-Pacific Congress Cardiology 1:43, 1964.
18. Lande A, Rosse P: The value of total aortography in the diagnosis of Takayasu's arteritis. Radiology 114:287, 1975.
19. Nasu T: Pathology of pulseless disease. A systematic study and critical review of twenty-one autopsy cases reported in Japan. Angiology 14:225, 1963.
20. Klein RG, Hunder GG, et al.: Large artery involvement in giant cell (temporal) arteritis. Ann Intern Med 83:806, 1975.
21. Kempczinski RF, Buckley CJ, Darling RC: Vascular insufficiency secondary to ergotism. Surgery 79:597, 1976.
22. Yao JST, Goodwin DP, Kenyon JR: Case of ergot poisoning. Br Med J 3:86, 1970.
23. Fielding JWL, Donovan RM, et al.: Reversible arteriopathy following an ergotamine overdose in a heavy smoker. Br J Surg 67:247, 1980.
24. Butler MJ, Lane RHS, Webster JHH: Irradiation injury to large arteries. Br J Surg 67:341, 1980.
25. Moss WT, Brand WN, Battifora H: The heart and blood vessels, in *Radiation Oncology, Rationale, Technique, Results*. St. Louis, C. V. Mosby Co., 1973, p 248.
26. Fonkalsrud EW, Sanchez M, et al.: Serial changes in arterial structure following radiation therapy. Surg Gynecol Obstet 145:395, 1977.
27. Buerger L: Thrombo-angiitis obliterans. A study of the vascular lesions leading to presenile spontaneous gangrene. Am J Med Sci 136:567, 1908.
28. Hirai M, Shionoya S: Arterial obstruction of the upper limb in Buerger's disease: Its incidence and primary lesion. Br J Surg 66:124, 1979.
29. Norman IL, Allen EV: The Vascular Complications of Polycythemia. Am Heart J 13:257, 1937.
30. Rich NM, Hobson RW II, Fedde CW: Vascular trauma secondary to diagnostic and therapeutic procedures. Am J Surg 128:715, 1974.
31. Conn J, Bergan JJ, Bell JL: Hypothenar hammer syndrome: Posttraumatic digital ischemia. Surgery 68:1122, 1970.
32. Conn J, Krumlovsky FA, et al.: Calciphylaxis. Etiology of progressive vascular calcification and gangrene? Ann Surg 177:206, 1973.
33. Hobson RW II, Sarkaria J, et al.: Atherosclerotic aneurysms of the subclavian artery. Surgery 85:368, 1979.
34. Pairolero PC, Walls JT, et al.: Subclavian-axillary artery aneurysms. Surgery 90:757, 1981.
35. Rodgers BM, Talbert JL, Holenbeck JI: Aneurysm of anomalous subclavian artery: An unusual cause of dysphagia lusoria in childhood. Ann Surg 187:158, 1978.
36. Bjork VO: Aneurysm and occlusion of the right subclavian artery. Acta Chir Scand Suppl 356:103, 1965.
37. Thorrens S, Trippel OH, Bergan JJ: Arteriosclerotic aneurysms

of the hand. Excision and restoration of continuity. Arch Surg 92:937, 1966.

38. Aldoori M, Campbell WB, Dieppe PA: Nifedipine in the treatment of Raynaud's syndrome. Cardiovasc Res 20:466, 1986.

39. Garrett HE, Morris GC, et al.: Revascularization of upper extremity with autogenous vein bypass graft. Arch Surg 91:751, 1965.

40. Wood PB: Vein-graft bypass in axillary and brachial artery occlusions causing claudication. Br J Surg 60:29, 1973.

41. Holleman JH Jr, Hardy JD, et al: Arterial surgery for arm ischemia. A survey of 136 patients. Ann Surg 191:727, 1980.

42. Gross WS, Flanigan DP et al.: Chronic upper extremity arterial insufficency. Etiology, manifestations, and operative management. Arch Surg 113:419, 1978.

43. Bergqvist D, Ericsson BF, et al.: Arterial surgery of the upper extremity. World J Surg 7:786, 1983.

44. McNamara MF, Takaki HS, et al.: A systematic approach to sever hand ischemia. Surgery 83:1, 1978.

45. Welling RE, Cranley JJ, et al.: Obliterative arterial disease of the upper extremity. Arch Surg 116:1593, 1981.

46. McCarthy WJ, Flinn WR, et al.: Result of bypass grafting for upper limb ischemia. J Vasc Surg 3:741, 1986.

CHAPTER 63
Cervicothoracic and Upper Thoracic Sympathectomy

Henry Haimovici

Sympathetic denervation of the upper extremity may be achieved by various techniques. In spite of technical improvements, it is well recognized that a lasting denervation of the upper extremity has remained a goal that is sometimes difficult to achieve. A review of the neuroanatomy of the sympathetic chain[1,2] providing the innervation to the upper extremity and a discussion of the criteria for completeness of sympathetic denervation should provide a basis for understanding some of the technical difficulties and the unpredictable clinical results observed in some cases.

NEUROANATOMY OF CERVICOTHORACIC SYMPATHETIC CHAIN

The inferior cervical ganglion, the lowest structure of the cervical sympathetic trunk, is commonly fused with the first thoracic ganglion. These two constitute the stellate ganglion and are situated anterior to the head of the first rib and behind the pleura. Sometimes, but rarely, they appear as separate structures.

The thoracic or dorsal sympathetic trunk includes 10 or 11 ganglia joined together by longitudinal fibers. In most instances the first thoracic ganglion and only rarely the second are fused with the inferior cervical to form the stellate ganglion.

Each thoracic ganglion is connected with a corresponding spinal nerve by a white and a gray ramus. In a large percentage of cases, an intrathoracic ramus arising from the second thoracic nerve joins the first, usually proximal to the origin of the first intercostal nerve.

To achieve an adequate sympathetic denervation of the upper extremity, removal of the inferior cervical and upper three or four thoracic segments of the sympathetic trunk is essential. In performing a denervation of the upper extremity, two different pathways are encountered: the oculopupillary and upper-extremity fibers.

The preganglionic fibers supplying the oculopupillary apparatus arise in the lateral horn of the spinal cord, emerge with the anterior root of T-1 and C-8, and traverse the stellate ganglion. The preganglionic outflow to the upper extremity usually emerges from T-2 to T-9. These pathways and their variables are of interest to the surgeon. The preganglionic fibers accompany the anterior spinal roots and ascend uninterrupted into the paravertebral chain until they synapse with postganglionic fibers in the first, second, and possibly third ganglia. The postganglionic fibers to the upper extremity are supplied by the brachial plexus. The median nerve carries the most important sympathetic supply; the ulnar and radial have a lesser number of fibers.

To achieve complete denervation of the upper extremity the first thoracic or dorsal ganglion must be removed. In addition, it is desirable to remove partially the lower cervical ganglion. As a result of its ablation, however, a Horner's syndrome may be produced. To avoid this in most patients, sectioning of the sympathetic chain below the preganglionic fibers emerging from the first thoracic segment of the cord may be necessary.

The difficulty of identifying the proper fibers is often the cause of the significant incidence of failure of sympathectomy of the upper limb.

INDICATIONS

Indications for sympathectomy of the upper extremity are relatively less frequent than for similar conditions of the lower extremity. The most common indications are as follows:

- *Vasospastic syndromes:* Raynaud's disease with disabling symptoms and signs, unyielding to medical management and lasting over 1 to 2 years; Raynaud's phenomenon secondary to scleroderma, one of the most common of the collagen diseases; lupus erythematosus; periarteritis nodosa; and rheumatoid arthritis. The vasospastic changes of the digits associated with the latter three conditions are less amenable to this type of surgery. In hyperhidrosis, when severe enough and disabling, an upper thoracic sympathectomy will provide excellent results.

- *Organic diseases:* Thromboangiitis obliterans, arteriosclerosis obliterans, affecting mostly the lower extremities, may also involve the upper. In advanced cases with ischemic lesions and vasomotor changes in the absence of reconstructive arterial surgery, an upper thoracic sympathectomy may sometimes yield gratifying results.
- *Thoracic outlet syndromes* with involvement of the subclavian or axillary arteries, resulting in peripheral emboli, may occasionally be managed by a combined first rib resection and an upper thoracic sympathectomy.[3,4] This is also applicable in cases of severe ischemia in embolic occlusions of cardiac origin in which the distal arterial patency could not be achieved by a thromboembolectomy.
- *Causalgia* or causalgia-like syndromes may occasionally benefit from an upper thoracic sympathectomy.
- *Posttraumatic sympathetic dystrophy* (Sudeck's atrophy) with marked osteoporosis, swelling, coldness, sweating, and pain of the hands has been successfully controlled by this procedure. (See Chapter 60).

OPERATIVE TECHNIQUES

The choice of one of the several approaches available depends essentially on which one offers the easiest exposure of the sympathetic trunk and carries the least operative risk. The following three approaches, having somewhat different indications, will be described: (1) the supraclavicular, (2) the anterior transthoracic, and (3) the axillary transthoracic.

Suffice it to only mention a fourth operative approach hardly used today, except by some neurosurgeons, known as the posterior transthoracic procedure, originally described by Adson,[5] later modified by Telford,[6] and popularized by Smithwick.[7] This technique offers limited visualization of the structures and has a high incidence of inadequate results. It is carried out by a paraspinal incision with resection of the third rib and an extrapleural approach.[7-9]

Supraclavicular Approach

One of the earliest approaches was the supraclavicular. Leriche and Fontaine[10] and Gask and Ross[11] were among its advocates.

Right Cervicothoracic Sympathectomy
Position of Patient. The patient is placed in the supine position with the head turned away from the side of the incision and the neck somewhat hyperextended. The shoulders are elevated by a bolster (Fig. 63-1A)

Anesthesia. Intratracheal general anesthesia is safest, as the potential risks of a pneumothorax secondary to a pleural tear are eliminated. Local anesthesia has been used, but its risks appear unwarranted.

Incision. The skin incision is horizontal, just above the clavicle, and extends from the medial border of the sternocleidomastoid for 2 to 3 inches medial to the anterior border of the trapezius. The skin incision extends through the platysma, the superficial cervical fascia, and the descending supraclavicular nerves. The external jugular vein is divided and ligated.

Division of Muscles. The clavicular head of or the entire sternocleidomastoid muscle may be sectioned and later resutured. The omohyoid muscle, which runs obliquely across the field, is cut across and the deep cervical fascia is opened (Fig. 63-1B). At this point the carotid and internal jugular vein sheath lie on the medial side of the incision; the floor is formed by the anterior scalene muscle. The scalene adipose pad lying in front of this muscle is carefully dissected, and the vessels within it are divided and ligated. The adipose pad is retracted, and the scalene muscle is then easily identified.

The phrenic nerve crosses the anterior surface of the muscle from the posterior to the medial side. It is carefully mobilized, and a Vesseloop is placed about it and retracted medially (Fig. 63-1C). The scalene muscle is then divided slightly above its insertion, care being taken not to injure the phrenic nerve and the underlying subclavian vessels.

Medial to the scalene is the internal jugular vein which should be retracted and not severed. Care should be taken to avoid the thoracic duct on the left side. (One should bear in mind that a branch of the thoracic duct may also be present on the right.)

The brachial plexus is identified laterally; its injury can be avoided, facilitated by retracting the supraclavicular structures to the medial side of the operative area. At the lower part of the field are the subclavian vessels which partially cover the pleural dome.

After the scalene muscle is mobilized and transected, the subclavian artery comes into view and is separated from the internal jugular vein under which lies the vertebral artery, a branch of the subclavian just opposite to the internal mammary artery. The thyrocervical trunk coming off the subclavian, distal to the vertebral artery, should be carefully ligated to avoid injury and hazardous bleeding.

The vertebral artery, the first anatomic target before reaching the sympathetic trunk, usually covers the lower cervical ganglion (Fig. 63-1D). The subclavian artery is then retracted downward, a maneuver that is the key to obtaining sufficient exposure of the upper two to three thoracic ganglia. (The subclavian vein lies behind the clavicle and is not usually in the operative field.) After ligation and section of the thyrocervical axis have been achieved, the proximal end of the subclavian is freed by blunt dissection to allow good exposure of the vertebral artery which is behind these tissues.

By deepening the dissection behind the subclavian artery, the seventh cervical transverse process is exposed along with the pleural dome and suprapleural membrane (Sibson's fascia). The fascia is dissected bluntly from the rib to the retropleural space. The stellate ganglion and the upper thoracic chain emerge into view in front of the neck of the first and the second ribs. After the apical pleura is freed, the inferior cervical and the first and sometimes the second thoracic ganglia are easily visualized.

Excision of Cervicothoracic Sympathetic Ganglia. The first structure visualized is the stellate ganglion, a dumbbell-

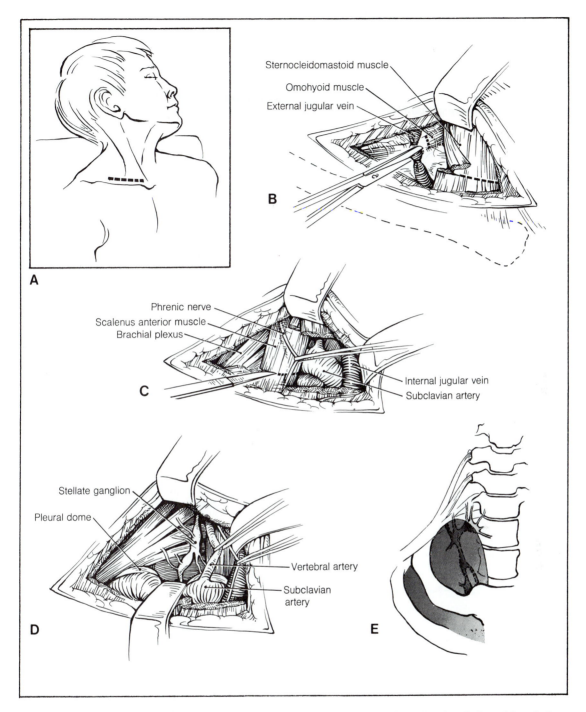

Figure 63-1. Right supraclavicular approach. **A.** Position of the patient and line of skin incision. **B.** Dotted lines indicate the site of sectioning of the sternocleidomastoid and omohyoid muscles. The external jugular vein is being divided. **C.** Anterior scalene muscle is divided along dotted line, care being taken to retract the phrenic nerve medially. **D.** Retraction of the subclavian artery downward and the vertebral artery and phrenic nerve medially helps to expose the stellate ganglion. Note the brachial plexus laterally and the pleural dome behind the subclavian artery. **E.** Cervicothoracic sympathetic ganglia in their retropleural relationship.

shaped structure, 1.5 to 2.5 cm in length, which is usually a fused single mass of the two ganglia. Its lower portion lies in front of the first thoracic nerve and against the head of the first rib. Its upper pole has a number of fine rami which connect it with the lower trunks of the brachial plexus (Fig. 63-1E). Other fibers surround the vertebral artery and

the subclavian by the annulus of Vieussens, connecting the inferior cervical with the small intermediate and middle cervical ganglia above. These star-shaped rami have given to the structure the name of stellate ganglion and make its identification an easy matter. When this structure has been freed from its bed, the chain can often be followed down as far as the third ganglion with minimal difficulty. However, care should be taken not to injure the intercostal arteries, the highest being a branch of the costocervical trunk of the subclavian.

After the lower cervical to the third dorsal ganglia have been freed, the handling of the stellate ganglion, its rami, and adjacent nerves may pose some problems. To achieve adequate denervation of the upper extremity, the lower half of the stellate ganglion and the second, third, and possibly the fourth dorsal ganglia together with the rami should be removed in all cases. The question revolves only about the upper part of the stellate, which may contain some of the postganglionic fibers to the upper extremity. Their removal may therefore be necessary for completeness of denervation, although a Horner's syndrome is usually anticipated. Should the procedure be bilateral, the latter inconvenience may be acceptable, especially in the presence of severe vasospastic or ischemic changes of the hand. For hyperhidrosis the sympathectomy entending from T-1 to T-3 may be adequate.

Closure of Incision. After closure in layers without drainage, a No. 20 catheter should be placed in the extrapleural space along the spine until the closure of the skin is airtight. The platysma edges are approximated with fine suture material. At this point the catheter left in the extrapleural space is aspirated and then withdrawn.

Left Cervicothoracic Sympathectomy

The procedure on the left side is, of course, identical to that on the right, except that the thoracic duct must be identified and retracted out of the field with a thin ribbon retractor. It should be borne in mind that the thoracic duct emerges forward out of the depth of the mediastinum from behind the jugular vein and enters the subclavian just lateral to its junction with the jugular (Fig. 63-2). At this stage of the procedure, a bloodless field is essential; the procedure should be aided by a good light provided by a lighted retractor or a headlight necessary to identify the duct. It goes without saying that considerable care must be exercised not to injure the pleural dome or the thoracic duct or one of the large blood vessels.

Pitfalls and Complications

Two important pitfalls are most often connected with this approach: (1) limited exposure of the dorsal sympathetic nerve, thus allowing only a partial sympathectomy, and (2) difficulties in controlling serious hemorrhage if a large vessel is injured, which may lead in some instances to ischemia of the limb.[12]

Complications include injuries to the subclavian artery, thoracic duct, brachial plexus, phrenic nerve, and the pleura. A thoracic duct injury must be carefully ligated to prevent lymphorrhea. Pneumothorax may be easily treated by insertion of a chest tube in some cases. If a Horner's syndrome occurs, anhidrosis of the affected side of the face and neck will be present in addition to that of the upper extremity, including the upper chest and part of the axilla.

Anterior Transthoracic Upper Dorsal Sympathectomy

In contrast to the supraclavicular technique, the anterior transthoracic approach provides direct and easy exposure of the sympathetic chain.[13]

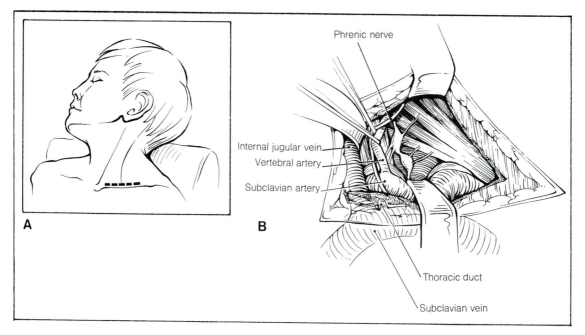

Figure 63-2. A. Position of the patient and line of skin incision in the left supraclavicular area. **B.** Exposure of the left stellate ganglion, using an approach similar to that shown in Fig. 63-1D. Note position of the thoracic duct.

Position of Patient

The patient is placed in the supine position with the side of the thorax to be operated upon elevated about 15 degrees by a bolster under the scapula. The upper extremity is abducted to 90 degrees with the forearm anchored to a crossbar. An endotracheal anesthesia is used.

Procedure

The skin incision extends anteriorly from the parasternal line to the anterior or midaxillary line over the third intercostal space (Fig. 63-3A).

The pectoralis major and intercostal muscles are divided, and the pleura is opened (Fig. 63-3B). The costal cartilage of the third rib is divided with a scalpel to facilitate retraction toward the upper thoracic cage. The lung is then deflated and depressed downward to permit exposure of the upper posterior aspect of the thoracic wall (Fig. 63-3C and D).

The parietal pleura overlying the angles of the ribs posteriorly is incised from below the fifth rib to the apex of the thoracic cage (Fig. 63-4A). The sympathetic chain is then dissected free from the chest wall, particular care being taken at each intercostal space to avoid injury to the intercostal vessels. The rami and the lower part of the chain below the fourth or fifth dorsal ganglia are clipped and divided. The chain is then dissected cephalad toward the upper border of the first rib.

As in the previous procedure, handling of the stellate ganglion may raise some difficulty concerning the number of fibers to be divided for achieving total denervation of the upper extremity. In order to prevent Horner's syndrome, partial freeing of the stellate ganglion is advisable.

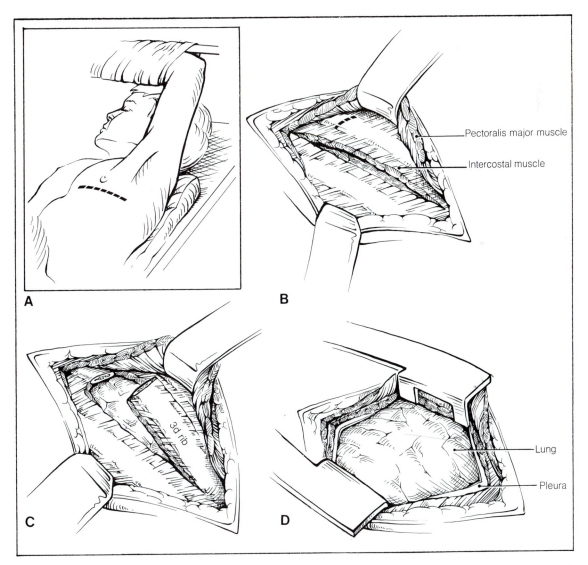

Figure 63-3. Anterior transthoracic approach. **A.** Position of the patient, showing the line of incision in the third intercostal space. Left upper extremity is in marked abduction with the forearm supported by a crossbar in a sling. **B.** Transection of the pectoralis major and intercostal muscles. **C.** Detachment of the third rib after dividing of the costochondral junction. **D.** Retraction of the third interspace and exposure of the lung.

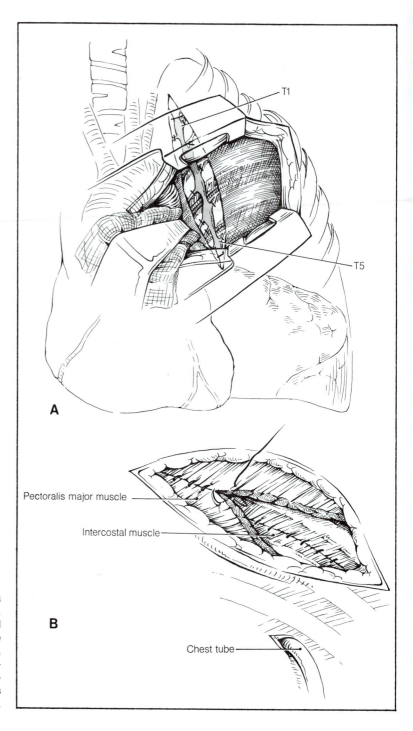

Figure 63-4. A. Posterior parietal pleura overlying the sympathetic chain is opened. The shaded segment of the ganglionated chain and the position of the clips indicate the segment to be removed (T-1 to T-5), excluding the lower cervical ganglion. **B.** Closure of the chest. Note the chest tube emerging through a stab wound two interspaces below the third in the anterior axillary line.

The dissection of the first thoracic nerve should be done just cephalad to the rami going to this nerve, and only the lower half of the stellate ganglion should be removed.

Closure of Chest
After the chain has been resected and hemostasis carefully obtained, the lung is reexpanded under direct vision. The chest wound is closed in layers, using interrupted nonabsorbable sutures. A small intercostal chest tube is inserted through a small stab wound in the anterior axillary line about two interspaces below the intercostal incision. This is connected to an underwater-seal suction-type apparatus. The chest tube is usually removed in 24 to 48 hours (Fig. 63-4B).

This procedure provides excellent access to the sympathetic chain except that, in some instances, the upper part of the stellate ganglion may be difficult to expose. Whether one can achieve in each case a complete denervation of the upper extremity by this procedure depends largely upon proper identification of the first thoracic and lower cervical ganglion. Complication and mortality rates are reported to be low with this approach.[13]

Transaxillary Approach

Atkins, in 1949,[14] was the first to publish the transaxillary technique. The operation consists of a transaxillary and transpleural approach to the upper thoracic sympathetic nerve, a procedure that seems to have gained great favor with vascular surgeons.

Right Transaxillary Sympathectomy

An endotracheal anesthesia is used. The patient is placed in the left lateral prone position, which is crucial for adequate exposure. The upper arm is abducted to approximately 100 degrees, is drawn slightly forward with the

elbow at 90 degrees, and is supported on an arm rest. The arm should be wrapped loosely and secured in place on the arm rest with a bandage (Fig. 63-5A).

The skin incision is carried out over the third intercostal space and extends from the lateral border of the pectoralis major muscle to the anterior border of the latissimus dorsi muscle. The incision is deepened through the subcutaneous fatty tissue layer to expose the line of incision in the axillary fascia.

The pectoralis major and latissimus dorsi muscles are retracted, care being taken to protect the long thoracic and thoracodorsal nerves which lie at the edge of the latissimus dorsi (Fig. 63-5B). The long thoracic nerve supplies the

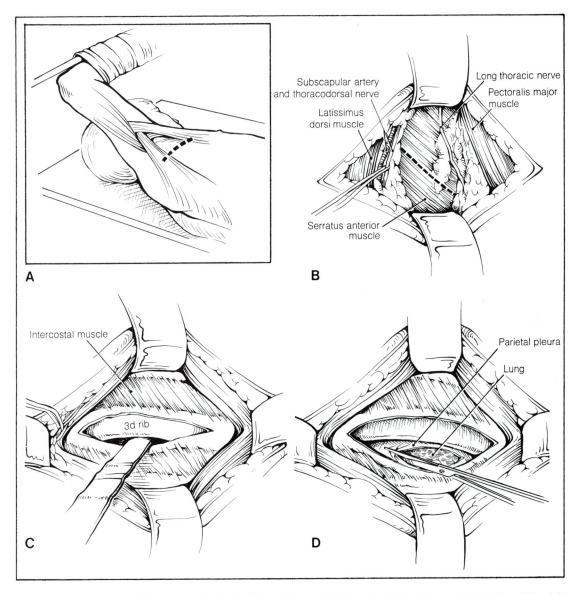

Figure 63-5. Right transaxillary approach. **A.** Position of the patient, line of skin incision, and abduction of the right upper extremity with the forearm supported by a crossbar. **B.** Exposure of the serratus anterior muscle and line of incision overlying the third rib. Note the long thoracic and thoradorsal nerves, the latter along the latissimus dorsi muscle and the former overlying the serratus, posteriorly to the pectoralis major muscle. **C.** Retraction of the edges of the divided serratus muscle, and the extraperiosteal mobilization of the third rib. **D.** Incision of the anterior parietal pleura and exposure of the lung.

serratus anterior and rests on the outer surface of this muscle. The thoracodorsal nerve follows the course of the subscapular artery, along the posterior wall of the axilla to the latissimus dorsi in which it may be traced as far as the lower border of the muscle. The long thoracic nerve is retracted anteriorly, and the fatty areolar tissue is cleared, together with the lymph nodes. The anterior serratus muscle is freed and is then divided along the broken line indicated in Figure 63-5B. The cut margins of the muscle are retracted,

uncovering the third rib. Its periosteum is incised, the lower half of it is separated from the third rib, and a periosteal elevator is inserted between the periosteum and the rib to mobilize it by blunt dissection from the underlying endothoracic fascia and parietal pleura (Fig. 63-5C).

The pleura is incised, and the opening of the pleural cavity is extended by scissors (Fig. 63-5D). The incision is then expanded with a small Finochietto rib retractor (Fig. 63-6A).

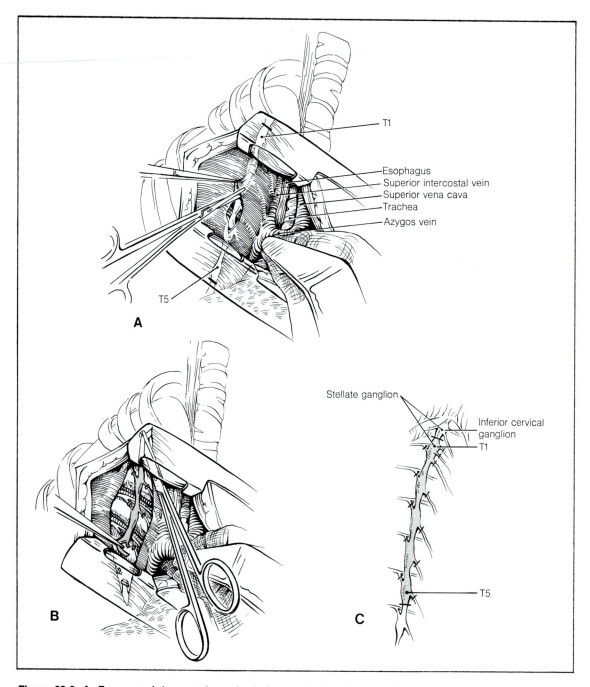

Figure 63-6. A. Exposure of the posterior parietal pleura and its incision over the underlying sympathetic chain. **B.** Excision of the upper thoracic sympathetic ganglionated chain below the inferior cervical ganglion. Note the clips on the rami connecting the chain to the intercostal nerves and other plexuses not shown in the drawing. **C.** Details of the upper thoracic sympathetic chain and inferior cervical ganglion.

The thoracic sympathetic chain becomes readily apparent beneath the posterior parietal pleura. The latter is incised along the chain, which is lifted up with a hook. The rami are divided after tantalum or silver clips are applied. Care must be taken to avoid injury to the intercostal vessels. The sympathetic chain is freed all the way up to the stellate ganglion. The chain is then divided below the fourth or fifth ganglion and is then mobilized cephalad by sharp dissection, using curved blunt-tipped scissors (Fig. 63-6B).

Near the location of the stellate ganglion, the intercostal vessels are frequently closely adherent to the chain, requiring careful handling to avoid injuring them. The inferior half of the stellate ganglion should be included in the ganglionectomy. The fibers that pass superiorly to the ganglion should be preserved in order to prevent a Horner's syndrome that accompanies its total excision (Fig. 63-6C).

Closure of the thoracotomy is carried out in the usual fashion. The rib cage is approximated with two pericostal double-strength sutures of chromic catgut (Fig. 63-7A). A catheter is placed in the pleural cavity for temporary water-seal drainage of the pleural cavity (Fig. 63-7B).

The anterior serratus muscle and axillary fascia are closed with interrupted nonabsorbable suture material. The catheter is aspirated while the anesthetist maintains positive pressure; it is withdrawn after the skin is closed.

Left Transaxillary Sympathectomy

The patient's position for a left transaxillary sympathectomy (Fig. 63-7C) is similar to that for the right.

After the left pleural cavity is entered and the lung is deflated and retracted gently inferiorly and medially, the sympathetic chain comes into view behind the parietal pleura. On the medial side of the exposure the arch of the aorta is visible. The parietal pleura is incised along the sympathetic chain, which is mobilized down the fourth or fifth thoracic ganglion. Proximally the dissection is carried to the stellate ganglion of which the first thoracic ganglion is excised. Among the structures to be watched carefully

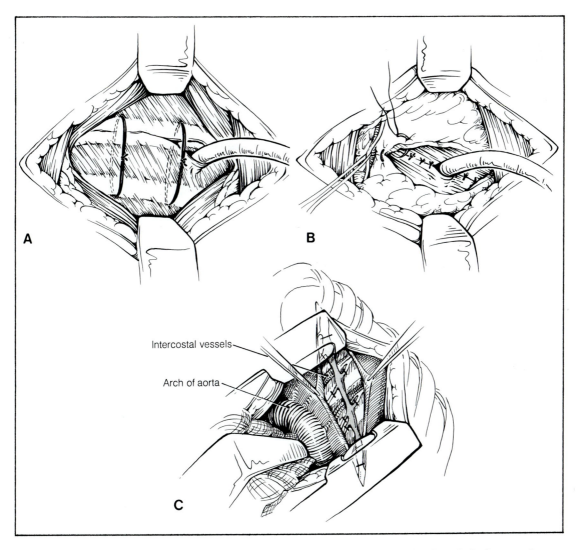

A

B

Intercostal vessels

Arch of aorta

C

Figure 63-7. A. Closure of the thoracotomy with pericostal sutures. Note the chest tube through the intercostal space. **B.** Closure of the muscle layers. **C.** Drawing of the left transaxillary upper thoracic sympathectomy.

to avoid inflicting any injury are the intercostal vessels and the thoracic duct, the latter close to the upper end of the sympathetic chain. Closure is carried out in layers as indicated for the right side.

Simultaneous bilateral transthoracic sympathectomy is inadvisable. In patients with hyperhidrosis involving both hands and feet, it is best to carry out the procedure in three operative sessions, one for the bilateral lumbar sympathectomies and one for each of the upper thoracic procedures.

Advantages and Disadvantages

Advantages of the transaxillary approach are several: relatively rapid performance, avoidance of large muscle or motor nerve division, good visualization of the chain, good cosmetic result, and usually minor postoperative disability and pain. The overall success rate is interpreted as 77% in one statistical report.[15]

Disadvantages are primarily related to the relatively small incision, which in certain individuals limits the exposure and renders difficult the access to the stellate ganglion, especially in the presence of adhesions at the apical portion of the pleural cavity.

Approach to the second intercostal space should be avoided because of the difficulty in spreading it with retractors. As a result of a narrower access than through the third, there is danger of injuring the long thoracic nerve, which may lead to palsy of the serratus muscle.

Postoperative Care

After a successful upper thoracic sympathectomy with any of the above approaches, the skin of the denervated extremity, as a rule, will become warm and dry almost immediately. In the presence of a Horner's syndrome, one finds typical signs of myosis, ptosis of the upper eyelid, slight elevation of the lower lid, and anhidrosis of the face and neck on the side of the sympathetic denervation.

The patient may be out of bed the day after the operation. Routine chest films for the presence of pleural effusion or pneumothorax are taken. Intercostal pain is usually present postoperatively. This is controlled by analgesics or mild narcotics. The arm may be protected in a sling if pain is due to pulling on the suture line.

PITFALLS AND COMPLICATIONS

Operative Pitfalls

Injury to intercostal vessels or the azygos vein or the thoracic duct has been dealt with above.

Complications

Postsympathectomy Neuralgia

This postoperative pain varies from patient to patient. Two types of pain are generally observed: one due to the operative exposure and manipulation of the intercostal nerves,

and the other more deep-seated, disappearing or becoming much less pronounced within a few weeks. Gentle handling of the intercostal nerves during the operation will minimize to a great extent this postoperative pain. Occasional procaine block of intercostal nerves at the posterior origin may control the pain if the usual analgesics fail to do so.

Sudomotor Changes

Compensatory body sweating may be a complication of sympathetic denervation of the large surface area of the body. This occurs most often in a four-extremity sympathectomy for hyperhidrosis. Usually, after several months, readjustment of the sudomotor activity occurs, consisting of lessening of this hyperhidrosis in the nondenervated skin.

Gustatory sweating on half of the face is a common occurrence, especially after bilateral operations. It is associated with eating and is accompanied by tingling and flushing as well as pilomotor changes in the skin. The use of spicy or acid foods or sweets may initiate the complaint. It is more frequently noted whenever a cervicodorsal sympathectomy is performed for hyperhidrosis or Raynaud's disease. This phenomenon may be delayed, although most often it appears in the first 12 months postoperatively.

Treatment of this complication includes the use of ganglionic blocking drugs and, in some cases, excision of any residual stellate ganglion tissue.

Return of Sympathetic Activity

It is well known that a cervicothoracic sympathectomy may sometimes fail to offer permanent denervation to the upper extremity. In the immediate postoperative period, a residual vasospasm is attributable to a hypersensitivity of the denervated arteriolar smooth muscle to epinephrine. This interpretation is based on Cannon's law of denervation,[16] which states that interruption of the postganglionic fibers results in an increased sensitivity of the neuroeffector cells to circulating epinephrine. Although this phenomenon was clearly demonstrated in animal experiments, the physiologic importance in humans appears undoubtedly overstated.[17] The return of vasomotor tone, particularly in cases of Raynaud's disease, may rather be related to inadequate denervation or local digital arteriolar sensitivity to cold, or a combination of the two.

Regeneration of the Sympathetic

In a preganglionic denervation by the Telford[6] technique, regeneration of these fibers was incriminated as a factor responsible for the return of the vasomotor tone. However, if this were possible, the reconnection of the preganglionic fibers with the postganglionic neuron still remains difficult to understand, although regeneration of preganglionic fibers does take place in accordance with Waller's law.

In experimental animals there is indeed evidence for regeneration of preganglionic fibers. Haimovici and Hodes[18] presented evidence for regeneration of certain fibers (adrenal, pupillary) even after removal of the entire sympathetic chain on both sides. Similar findings were reported by other investigators.[19] Whether an identical regeneration occurs in humans in the upper extremity and by what mechanism is still a moot question.

Among other likely possibilities to account for return

of sympathetic activity is the presence of accessory ganglia described by Wrete[20] and Skoog.[21] These findings would account for the fact that some degree of residual sweating is always present over some areas.

The inescapable fact remains, however, that in a certain number of cases a lasting denervation of the upper extremity is difficult to achieve, for reasons that are equally difficult to interpret. The recurrence may be related to a return of some vascular tone as well as to some technical problems responsible for incompleteness of denervation. The more complex neuroanatomy of the autonomic nervous system at this level may account, at least partially, for the latter fact.

REFERENCES

1. Kuntz A: Distribution of the sympathetic rami to the brachial plexus. Arch Surg 15:871, 1927.
2. White JC, Smithwick RM, et al.: The Autonomic Nervous System: Anatomy, Physiology and Surgical Application, 3 edt. New York: Macmillan, 1941.
3. Schein CJ, Haimovici H, et al.: Arterial thrombosis associated with cervical ribs: Surgical considerations. Report of a case and review of the literature. Surgery 40:428, 1956.
4. Roos DB: Transaxillary approach for first rib resection to relieve thoracic outlet syndrome. Ann Surg 163:354, 1966.
5. Adson AW, Brown GE: The treatment of Raynaud's disease by resection of the upper thoracic and lumbar sympathetic ganglia and trunks. Surg Gynecol Obstet 48:577, 1929.
6. Telford ED: The technique of sympathectomy. Br J Surg 23:448, 1935.
7. Smithwick RH: Modified dorsal sympathectomy for vascular spasm (Raynaud's disease) of the upper extremity. A preliminary report. Ann Surg 104:339, 1936.
8. Mackay HJ: Improved approach for posterior upper thoracic sympathectomy. JAMA 159:1261, 1955.
9. Cloward RB: Upper thoracic sympathectomy: Surgical technique. Surgery 66:1120, 1969.
10. Leriche R, Fontaine R: Technique de l'ablation du ganglion étoilé. J Chir 41:353, 1933.
11. Gask GE, Ross JP: The Surgery of the Sympathetic Nervous System, 2nd ed. Baltimore, William Wood & Co, 1937.
12. Lord JW: Post-traumatic vascular disorders and upper extremity sympathectomy. Orthop Clin North Am 1:393, 1970.
13. Palumbo LT, Lulu DJ: Anterior transthoracic upper dorsal sympathectomy. Arch Surg 92:247, 1966.
14. Atkins HJB: Peraxillary approach to the stellate and upper thoracic sympathetic ganglia. Lancet 2:1152, 1949.
15. Berguer R, Smit R: Transaxillary sympathectomy (T2-T4) for relief of vasospastic/sympathetic pain of upper extremities. Surgery 89:764, 1981.
16. Cannon WB: A law of denervation. Am J Med Sci 198:737, 1939.
17. Simeone FA, Felder DA: Observations upon the supersensitivity of denervated digital blood vessels in man. Surgery 30:218, 1951.
18. Haimovici H, Hodes R: Preganglionic nerve regeneration in completely sympathectomized cats. Am J Physiol 128:463, 1940.
19. Hinsey JC, Phillips RA, et al.: Observations on cats following pre- and postganglionic sympathectomies. Am J Physiol 126:534, 1939.
20. Wrete M: Die Entwicklung der intermediären Ganglien béim Menschen. Gegenbauers Morphol Jahrb 75:229, 1935.
21. Skoog T: Ganglia in the communicating rami of the cervical sympathetic trunk. Lancet 253:457, 1947.

CHAPTER 64
Lumbar Sympathectomy

Henry Haimovici

Although lumbar sympathectomy was introduced many decades ago as a method of treatment for ischemic and painful disorders of the lower extremity, much controversy still persists over its physiologic effects, clinical indications, and long-term results.

Previously the operation called "periarterial sympathectomy" by Leriche, was advocated for a great variety of circulatory and painful disorders of the extremities.[1] However, its physiologic effects were fleeting. Another procedure, devised by Royle of Australia in 1924, used sympathetic ramisection in the treatment of spastic paralysis.[2] Royle noted improved circulation in the legs of the patients, but the procedure offered little lasting effect.

The first actual lumbar sympathectomy for arterial occlusive disease of the lower extremity was performed in 1924 by Julio Diez of Buenos Aires.[3] From this point on, the history of lumbar sympathectomy has been one of mixed fortunes. Its place in the management of vascular disorders underwent periodic reappraisals because of uneven clinical results. This became especially relevant after the advent of reconstructive arterial surgery. However, when reconstructive arterial procedures were contraindicated, lumbar sympathectomy reassumed a second place, since its objective usually is to promote development of collateral circulation. Thus lumbar sympathectomy has limited indications in the management of peripheral vasospastic and occlusive arterial disease.

NEUROANATOMY OF THE LUMBAR SYMPATHETIC TRUNK

The standard anatomy textbooks indicate that, as a rule, the lumbar sympathetic trunk[4-6] contains four to five ganglia. These ganglia are usually found in the lumbar chain, but the number may vary between two and eight, and, rarely, only one continuous ganglion is found.

Ganglion L1 is described as lying anterior to the body of vertebra L1, over the second lumbar vertebra or anterior to the intervertebral disk. The second ganglion (L2) has been described as lying anterior to the body of the second lumbar vertebra. Specific positions have also been assigned to ganglia below the second.

Although the variations in position of the ganglia are common, the second and the fourth lumbar ganglia are the more constant ones. The latter is usually located behind the origin of the iliac vessels.

The number of rami of any ganglion vary from two to seven. In general, there are more rami between the first and second lumbar spinal nerves and the sympathetic trunk than between the third, fourth, or fifth lumbar spinal nerves and the sympathetic trunk. The rami of the first ganglion have a cephalic direction, the second has a cephalic or transverse direction, and the third and fourth ganglia have a transverse or caudal direction.

Cross communications between the right and left sympathetic trunks are also variable.[7] Some investigators have found up to 80% of such communications in their dissections, whereas others have failed to encounter any in their anatomic studies. Because of the intermediate ganglia sometimes encountered on the rami communicantes, division of all the rami in the course of the sympathectomy is important. The genitofemoral nerve supplies branches to the external iliac and femoral arteries and seems to be intimately connected with the lumbar sympathetic trunk via rami and collaterals. Knowledge of these variations in the anatomic structures may be helpful in performing correctly a lumbar sympathectomy.

Distribution of Sympathetic Innervation of the Lower Extremity

Completeness of anatomic denervation is important for achieving adequate sympathectomy of a given segment of an extremity. Excision of the chain from L2 to L4, sometimes including L1, offers satisfactory results. Removal of a lesser portion of the sympathetic chain may, however, prove to be inadequate. The source of sympathetic fibers as related to the lumbar ganglia may be helpful in determining the extent of the sympathectomy. Thus, the first lumbar ganglion supplies the femoral and obturator nerves, which in turn provide the sympathetic innervation of the thigh and parts of the leg. The ablation of the second and third lumbar ganglia denervates the posterior aspect of the thigh, the leg, and the foot. To obtain denervation of the anterior surface of the thigh and of the medial aspect of the leg, the first lumbar ganglion must also be removed.

Criteria for Completeness of Sympathetic Denervation

Evaluation of the degree of denervation following a lumbar sympathectomy relies upon two main physiologic effects: (1) vasomotor responses as determined by skin thermometry and (2) cessation of the secretory activity of the sweat glands.[8,9] Electrical skin resistance is convenient and simple for routine clinical testing of changes in sweat function.

INDICATIONS

Indications for lumbar sympathectomy are limited essentially to patients with nonreconstructible arterial disease or vasospastic conditions of the leg and foot. In such cases, to be successful a lumbar sympathectomy depends on: (1) proper selection of the patients, (2) adequate denervation, and (3) meticulous postoperative care of the lesions. Predicting the effects of a sympathectomy upon the circulation of the lower extremity, especially the foot and toes, is essential for determining the operative indications. The degree of accuracy that any one of the available methods offers in forecasting the results has been the subject of much debate, especially regarding diabetics.[10] The poor results of the procedure are often due to lack of a uniform method of selecting patients for the operation. Essentially, one has to evaluate properly (1) the collateral circulation or its potential availability, (2) the vasomotor activity of the extremity, and (3) clinical findings, all of which may provide in most instances a fairly accurate prediction of the operative results.[11]

The physiologic effects of a lumbar sympathectomy, despite its long clinical use, still remain ill defined, as attested by a number of reports. Interpretation of blood flow increase effect has been called into question. Indeed, recent investigations of arteriovenous (AV) shunting following lumbar sympathectomy have raised the question of the therapeutic value of its nutritive blood flow to the denervated tissues, especially to the skin. It should be noted that such data were obtained primarily in acute animal experiments, which disclosed that after sympathectomy there is an increased AV flow with no change in total capillary nutritive flow, both to skin and muscle.[12] Other investigations, however, are at variance with these results. One of the reasons invoked is the experimental model, and the other is the possible lack of correlation with the arteriosclerotic human extremity. Thus, while in the above-mentioned experimental model the arterial tree was undisturbed, by contrast, when the femoral arteries were ligated so as to mimic ischemic clinical conditions, significant increase in

tissue blood flow was obtained following sympathectomy.[13]

Furthermore, Moore and Hall,[14] utilizing xenon-133 clearance before and after lumbar sympathectomy in patients with rest pain or minimal gangrene, were able to show an increase of capillary skin blood flow by a factor of 10%. There is also clinical evidence of enhanced blood flow in cases of bypass grafts with poor runoff in which concomitant lumbar sympathectomy was carried out.[15,16]

Therefore, interpretation of the relative significance of AV anastomoses and capillary flows following lumbar sympathectomy in patients must be cautiously viewed. Its effects on the vascular bed of the skin are shared by both the AV channels and the capillary circulation. In contrast to the skin, the effect on the skeletal muscle blood vessels has remained controversial.

The failure of sympathectomy to relieve intermittent claudication in the majority of cases has been interpreted as a lack of sympathetic innervation of those vessels. Confusion surrounding this problem may be considerably dispelled by bearing in mind that local metabolic factors inherent in muscular activity are more important in the control of blood flow in skeletal muscle than is the sympathetic innervation. Furthermore, in the absence of patency of the major limb artery, whether or not the collateral network in the muscles will be adequate to relieve intermittent claudication is, in our opinion, determined by the mathematical relationship of the squared cross section of collaterals correlated with that of the occluded major artery, as expressed by Poiseuille's law. These considerations, rather than the vasomotor factors, explain the low percentage of improvement in intermittent claudication as noted by most observers.[11]

Vasospasm, hyperhidrosis, causalgia, or causalgic-type pain may occur as isolated manifestations but are more often associated with occlusive arterial disease. Their relief or elimination in the context of the latter is one of the important indications for a lumbar sympathectomy. In the presence of advanced arterial disease due to diffuse lesions not lending themselves to reconstructive vascular surgery, sympathectomy may be the only measure of limb revascularization. In these cases, its role and greatest effectiveness reside in the physiologic ability to increase the collateral system for improving and preserving the viability of the skin.

Use of distal thigh to arm or ankle perfusion pressure as a criterion for predicting response to lumbar sympathectomy is fraught with a number of flaws.[12] The bottom line is what happens to the collateral flow of the foot. Arterography and noninvasive modalities may be more useful.

Based on our experience and that of others, relief of rest pain and prevention of major amputations in a significant percentage of patients attest to the effectiveness of this procedure, even in patients with advanced ischemic changes.[11,13,17,18] It should be pointed out that, during the critical postoperative period, meticulous care of the foot lesions, cessation of smoking, and avoidance of any other vasoconstrictor influence may greatly enhance the effectiveness of the sympathectomy.

The role of diabetes mellitus is generally recognized as an accelerating and aggravating factor in limb and life prognosis. Indications of lumbar sympathectomy in diabetes are questionable, because of the frequency of "autosympathectomy" in such patients. The diffuse nature of the arteriosclerotic process may account primarily for the greater severity of ischemic changes in diabetics as compared with nondiabetics. This is substantiated by arteriographic studies of the lower extremity.[19] As shown by our own findings, occlusion of the distal arterial tree (popliteal, tibials), poor or absent runoff, and inefficient collaterals are more prevalent among diabetic patients.[12,20]

The long-range effectiveness of lumbar sympathectomy on limb survival is difficult to assess. Progression of the disease may be one of the important factors for late amputations. In a number of reports and in our own study, it is apparent that sympathectomy in a certain number of cases may have only a delaying action, since it does not arrest the downgrade progression of the atherosclerotic process.

Contraindications to lumbar sympathectomy are rapidly progressing ischemic lesions and poor general condition of the patient. Unsatisfactory results may be avoided by adhering to the criteria for selection of patients as outlined above.

Lumbar sympathectomy alone or in combination with reconstructive arterial surgery, however, may be a valuable procedure in patients with advanced arterial insufficiency.[12]

OPERATIVE TECHNIQUES

The method of choice for either unilateral or bilateral lumbar sympathectomy is by the extraperitoneal exposure. Two approaches are most convenient and simple: (1) anterior transverse and (2) anterolateral. The former is the most commonly used. The latter is employed in conjunction with exposure of an iliac vessel.

Anterior Transverse Exposure

Right Lumbar Sympathectomy
General endotracheal anesthesia is preferred, although epidural or spinal anesthesia is often used in certain patients.

Position. Proper positioning of the patient on the operating table is important for adequate exposure of the sympathetic chain. A bolster is placed under the lower ribs and the iliac crest so as to achieve an elevation of the right side of about a 20 to 30 degree angle to the table (Fig. 64-1A). If necessary, the table may be tilted further by another 10 degrees. Rarely do we use a kidney break except in obese individuals. The thigh is flexed at 45 degrees to provide relaxation of the psoas muscle by means of a pillow placed between two extremities.

Procedure. A transverse skin incision is carried out at the level of the umbilicus, starting at the lateral border of the rectus abdominis and extending laterally toward the tip of the 12th rib (Fig. 64-1A).

A muscle-splitting technique is used,[21] involving the external oblique fascia, the internal oblique muscle and the transversus abdominus muscle. Blunt digital dissection in the retroperitoneal space is used to separate the abdominal contents, which are retracted medially from the lumbar

adipose tissue. In continuing the retraction of the peritoneum, the psoas major muscle comes into view. It is located more anteriorly than one generally assumes. One should avoid dissecting between the psoas and the quadratus lumborum, which is more posterior and lateral.

Before retracting the abdominal contents, it is important first to identify the ureter so that it may be properly protected from any injury (Fig. 64-2A). Retraction of the peritoneal sac combined with blunt dissection, using a long tissue forceps, facilitates exposure to the lumbar sympathetic trunk (Fig. 64-2B). The ganglionated chain lies on the anterolateral surface of the vertebral column. Its identification is usually first made by digital palpation against the sides of the vertebrae.

The ilioinguinal and genitofemoral nerves, especially the latter, not to be mistaken for the sympathetic trunk, course downward and lateralward along the medial aspect of the psoas muscle (Fig. 64-2A). These have neither ganglionated structures nor rami. In addition, they are easy to mobilize and are not attached to the vertebral bodies. Such anatomic characteristics should differentiate them, especially the genitofemoral nerve, from the sympathetic trunk.

Adequate retraction is obtained to allow exposure of the proximal segment of the lumbar sympathetic trunk, namely, L1 and L2. The crus of the diaphragm may sometimes overlap and hide the origin of the lumbar sympathetic trunk.

Mobilization of the sympathetic trunk is accomplished from the proximal end downward. The distal portion of the sympathetic to be dissected lies under the iliac vessels, which should be carefully retracted. The rami are divided after lifting the sympathetic chain. Usually the latter lies in front of the lumbar vessels, which must be avoided when dividing the rami. If the lumbar vessels (artery and vein) pass in front of the chain, the latter is divided proximally and then is slipped behind the vessels downward. If this is not feasible, the lumbar vessels may be divided to facilitate this maneuver, although this has never been necessary in our experience.

The sympathetic trunk may not always be a single nerve but may include two or three branches, as well as crossover fibers. All the rami and fibers must be divided in the area between L2 and L4. If a bilateral lumbar sympathectomy is carried out, only one L1 ganglion is removed (Fig. 64-3), the other one being left in place, especially in males. Silver or tantalum clips are placed at both remaining ends above and below the severed sympathetic chain (Fig. 64-2D).

Closure of the abdominal incision is carried out in layers, using interrupted sutures of absorbable material (Fig. 64-4A, B, C). The skin is closed with simple or mattress sutures of silk or synthetic material (Fig. 64-4D).

Left Lumbar Sympathectomy
The skin incision, the muscle-splitting technique and the exposure of the sympathetic trunk are similar to the maneuvers used for the right side (Fig. 64-5A).

The left lumbar sympathetic trunk is more easily accessible, since it is located posterior and lateral to the abdominal aorta and left iliac artery. Care should be taken to avoid

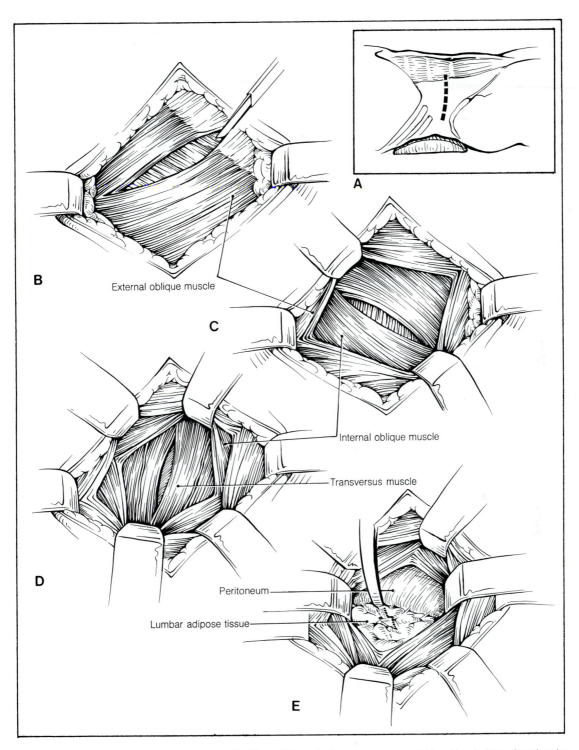

Figure 64-1. Right lumbar sympathectomy. **A.** Position of the patient on the operating table with a bolster placed under the thoracolumbar region. Heavy, broken line indicates the site of the skin incision. **B.** Incision of the external oblique muscle and of its aponeurosis along their fibers. **C.** Retraction of the external oblique muscle and divided internal oblique muscle along its fibers. **D.** Transversus muscle divided along its fibers, exposing the retroperitoneal space. **E.** Retroperitoneal space enlarged, showing the peritoneum and lumbar adipose tissue.

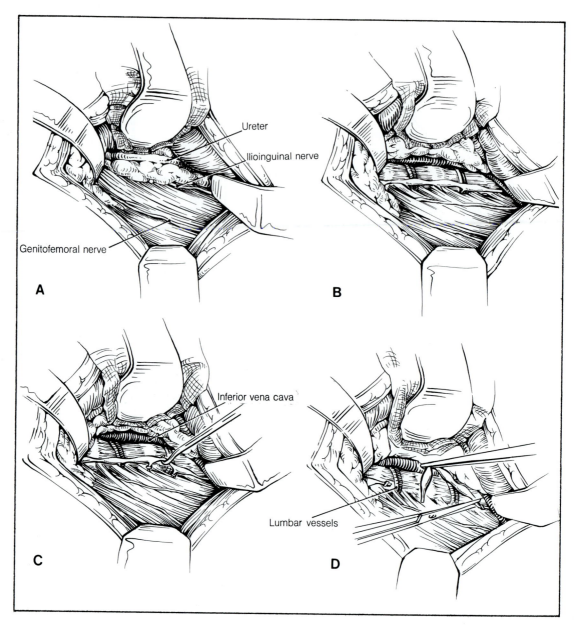

Figure 64-2. A. Abdominal contents retracted medially, thus exposing the ureter. Note the ilioinguinal and genitofemoral nerves lying on the psoas. **B.** Further retraction of the abdominal contents, exposing the inferior vena cava and right iliac vein, lumbar sympathetic trunk, and lumbar vessels. **C.** Mobilization of the sympathetic trunk lifted by a nerve hook. **D.** Excision of the sympathetic trunk.

injuring the latter with the retractor, especially in those cases in which these vessels are calcified, for fear of causing thrombosis.

The sympathetic trunk is mobilized and then lifted away from the vertebrae with a Smithwick or any other type of dissector-hook. Clips are placed on the rami, as well as on the chain above and below its excision (Fig. 64-4B). Figure 64-5B also shows that the sympathetic trunk passes behind the lumbar vessels. In mobilizing the lower portion of the trunk, one should avoid avulsing it, which might lead to injury of the vessels. The chain should therefore be carefully mobilized before slipping it behind the latter.

Comment

As already mentioned, the number and location of the ganglia are variable. From a practical point of view, the chain should be removed between a point of emergence near the diaphragmatic crura and the point of disappearance beneath the common iliac vessels. This segment usually comprises the essential L2, L3, and L4 ganglia. For denervation of the anterior surface of the thigh, L1 should also be included. In some instances, the crus of the diaphragm may have to be divided in order to reach L1.

In some patients, the sympathetic trunk may be obscured by overlying fibrous bands. When invisible, the trunk may be located by digital palpation over the vertebrae.

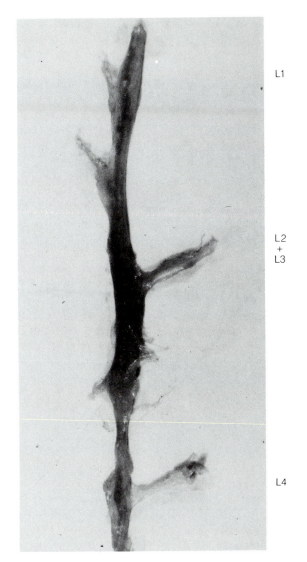

L1

L2
+
L3

L4

Figure 64-3. Specimen of sympathetic trunk removed between L1 and L4.

tures are easily demonstrable and should not be confused with the lumbar sympathetic chain.

Anterolateral Exposure

The patient is placed in the supine position similar to the previous exposure, with the operating table being rotated about 30 degrees away from the surgeon.

The *skin incision* (Fig. 64-6A) begins at the tip of the 11th rib and extends inferiorly parallel to the inguinal ligament about $\frac{1}{2}$ to 2 inches medial to the iliac crest and terminates at the lateral border of the rectus abdominis.

The external oblique and its aponeurosis are incised in the direction of the fibers from one end to the other along the skin incision (Fig. 64-6).

The internal oblique and the transversus abdominis muscles are transected in the same direction as the external oblique. Care should be taken to transect these two muscles about $1\frac{1}{2}$ to 2 inches from the inguinal ligament and the iliac crest in order to avoid entering the peritoneum.

The transversalis fascia is opened and, by using blunt manual dissection, the peritoneal sac is retracted medially. Its separation is continued beyond the medial border of the psoas muscle up to the midline. The ureter and the genital vessels and the genitofemoral nerve are identified. Then a moist lap is placed over the peritoneum, and Deaver retractors are used for enlarging and maintaining the opening.

Exposure of the sympathetic chain is carried out in a fashion similar to the previously described procedure. Usually this approach to the sympathetic is carried out for a double purpose: the sympathectomy and exposure of the iliac vessels for a reconstructive procedure.

In the event that the sympathectomy requires excision of L1, it may sometimes be necessary to enlarge its proximal exposure by resecting the distal portion of the rib. The latter is removed subperiosteally (Fig. 64-6C).

Closure of the incision is carried out in a fashion similar to the previous approach, using a muscle layer approximation by means of interrupted sutures.

Incision of the fibrous layer is then necessary before the chain is exposed and isolated.

On the right side, the inferior vena cava covers the sympathetic trunk and hides it completely from view before its retraction. The left sympathetic chain is always more readily exposed when the adipose and lymphatic tissue masses are reflected medially toward the aorta.

The transversalis fascia and the peritoneum are often inseparably adherent anteriorly and separated laterally by the properitoneal fat. If inadvertently incised or opened during the separation, the peritoneal rent should be promptly closed. The peritoneum should be reflected toward the midline before reaching the anterior surface of the psoas. Otherwise, the dissecting fingers may stray into the gutter between the quadratus lumborum and psoas muscles.

The ureter with the genital vessels is incorporated in and retracted with the parietal peritoneal leaf. These struc-

Operative Pitfalls

Injury to the structures adjacent to the sympathetic chain, if minor and consisting of bleeding from lumbar vessels, should be treated by temporary compression with gentle packing, to be followed immediately by the use of clips. Inadvertent rupture of a lumbar artery may be more difficult to control and may necessitate temporary occlusion of the aorta in order to secure the stump of the ruptured lumbar vessel. A tear in the inferior vena cava or abdominal aorta or iliac vessels is by far a more serious complication because of potentially significant loss of blood. Compression or clamping of the aorta or compression of the inferior vena cava is necessary for control of bleeding before repair of the vessels is carried out. Likewise, injury to the ureter should be recognized promptly in order to repair any rent.

Removal of the genitofemoral nerve or iliolumbar nerve, mistaken for the sympathetic trunk, may cause less

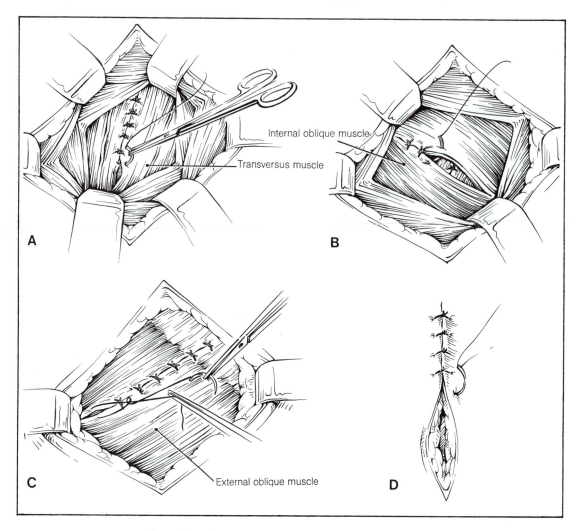

Figure 64-4. Steps of layer closure of the abdominal incision.

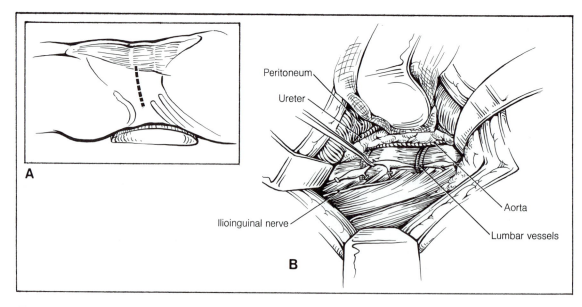

Figure 64-5. Left lumbar sympathectomy. **A.** Position of the patient on the operating table and the line of the skin incision. **B.** Exposure of the lumbar sympathetic trunk and application of clips on the chain and its rami. Note the presence of lumbar vessels anterior to the sympathetic trunk.

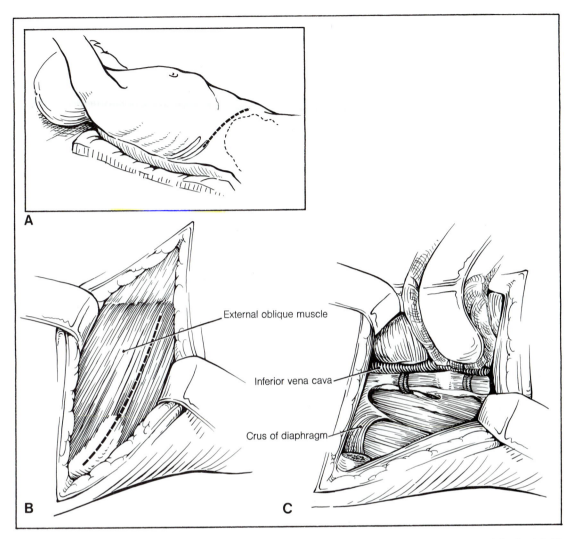

Figure 64-6. Anterolateral exposure of the right lumbar sympathetic trunk. **A.** Position of the patient and the line of skin incision extending from the 11th rib to the lateral border of the rectus abdominis muscle. Note the skin incision is oblique. **B.** Line of incision of the external oblique muscle extending proximally to the tip of the 11th rib. Except for the latter muscle, the internal oblique and transversus muscles are transected along the oblique incision of the skin. **C.** Exposure of the sympathetic trunk, inferior vena cava, and right iliac vein. Note also exposure of the crus of the diaphragm. (See text for further details.)

tragic consequences but may be responsible for some neuritic pain and, obviously, results in failure of the desired sympathetic denervation.

Postoperative Care

As a rule, after a successful sympathectomy, the extremity becomes warm and dry within a matter of hours. Painful ulcers or rest pain usually subside in the majority of cases.

Postoperative abdominal distention due to a paralytic ileus may be a source of discomfort to the patient for 2 to 3 days. In such instances, administration of 250 or 500 μg of neostigmine (Prostigmin) every 6 hours, combined with intermittent use of a rectal tube, may promptly alleviate the discomfort.

COMPLICATIONS

Postsympathectomy Neuralgia

A frequent, if not common, complication following sympathectomy is postsympathectomy neuralgia, the nature of which is not entirely elucidated. It may occur suddenly after a latent period of 10 to 17 days. The pain is severe, unremitting, and worse at night. Fortunately, it is a self-limiting process, with spontaneous remission common after periods of several weeks.[22–24]

This neuralgia usually occurs after the abdominal incision is completely healed, and the patient has usually been discharged from the hospital. It consists of severe, deep aching or burning and as a rule is exacerbated at rest.

Distribution of the pain is over the cutaneous segments

of L1, L2, L3, and occasionally T12. Essentially, the distribution is along the anterior femoral cutaneous, lateral femoral cutaneous, genitofemoral, and ilioinguinal nerves. Hyperesthesia may often be noted over the anterolateral thigh and in the groin, and there may be limitation of straight leg raising.

The etiology of postsympathectomy neuralgia is obscure. Several mechanisms have been postulated, but none has been entirely documented.[23]

Neuromas of severed sympathetic fibers, manifestation of ischemic neuritis, and traumatic neuritis of sensory nerves adjacent to the excised sympathetic chain are some of the mechanisms invoked to account for this postoperative complication.

Treatment of postsympathectomy neuralgia is symptomatic and consists of doses of strong narcotics frequently required for pain relief, especially at night. The patient is more comfortable during the daytime and requires much less or no analgesia.

In any event, it is important to reassure the patient that this postsympathectomy neuralgia does not reflect aggravation of the disease and that the process is self-limited and will subside within a reasonable period of time.

Postsympathectomy Causalgia

The complication of postsympathectomy causalgia is extremely rare and occurs at the operative site, sometimes weeks or months after surgery. Infiltration of the area with procaine may be helpful in relieving the pain. Several injections may be necessary before the causalgia is brought under control.

Paradoxical Gangrene

The mechanism invoked, so-called paradoxical gangrene, is not entirely clear. Very likely it is due to a local vascular

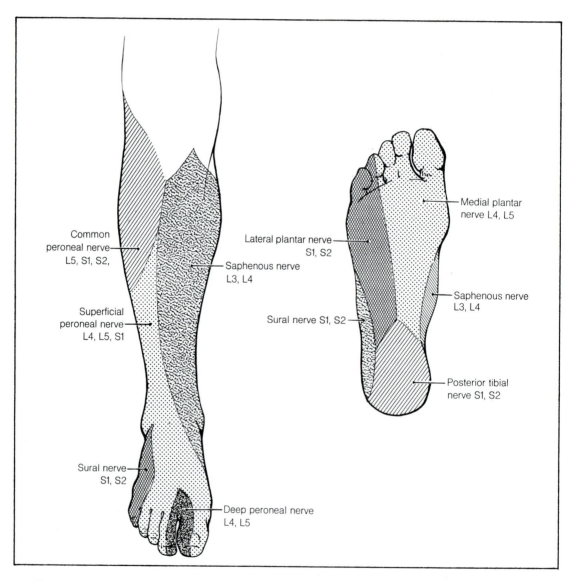

Figure 64-7. Diagrams of the distribution of the five sensory nerves and their dermatomes in the leg and foot.

complication related to intraoperative trauma of the aorta or iliac artery, or of spontaneous thrombosis as a result of prolonged hypotension during surgery or during the postoperative period. In other instances, a latent progressive ischemia, combined with a minor intraoperative trauma, may precipitate paradoxical gangrene.

Prophylactic measures against postoperative ischemia, including gangrene, should always be taken during and after surgery. They consist of avoiding (1) compression of the involved limb during surgery, (2) any direct retraction of the aorta or iliac arteries, and (3) hypotension during or after the procedure by alerting the anesthetist about maintaining the arterial pressure at a preoperative level.

If such a complication occurs in spite of these measures, arteriography should be done to detect any acute thrombosis, and it should be dealt with accordingly.

In rare cases not yielding to conventional analgesic methods, sensory nerve interruption in the leg may be necessary, provided that adequate skin circulation is present (Figs. 64-7 to 64-9).

Disturbances of Sexual Function

There is general agreement that bilateral removal of L1 in male patients may result in loss of libido, failure of ejaculation, and even sterility. If bilateral lumbar sympathectomy is performed, it is recommended that only one side should include L1. Whitelaw and Smithwick[25] showed that bilateral lumbar sympathectomy below L2 offers complete assurance that sexual function will not be altered in any respect, contrary to what happened in those individuals in whom the

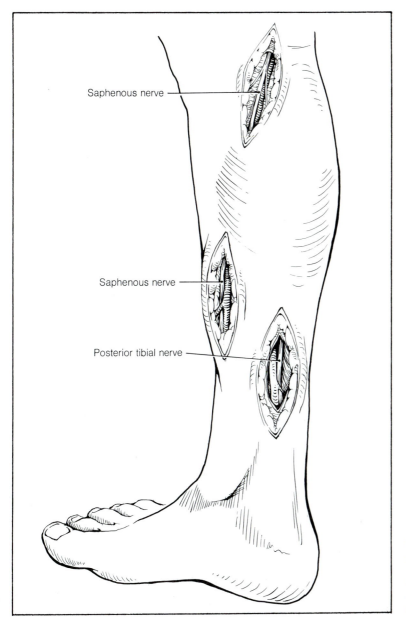

Figure 64-8. Diagram of exposures of the posterior tibial nerve at the lower third, the saphenous nerve at the middle third, and the same nerve at the upper third at its emergence from underneath the deep fascia near the knee.

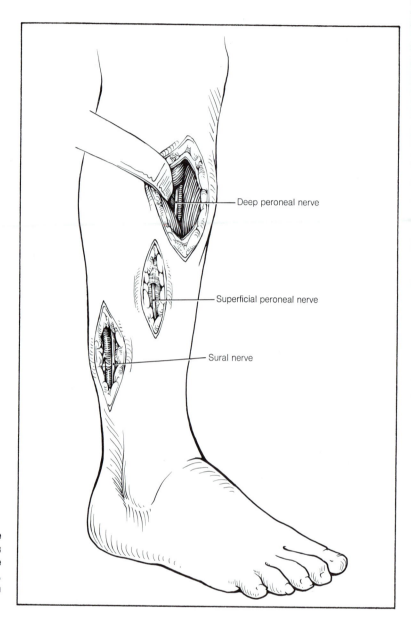

Figure 64-9. Diagram of exposures of the sural nerve adjacent to the short saphenous vein, the superficial peroneal nerve at the site of its emergence from the deep fascia, and the deep peroneal nerve in the depth of the anterior tibial compartment.

sympathectomy included L1 to L3, and in 63% of whom significant changes in sexual function occurred. Apparently, sympathectomy has no adverse effect on the female genital tract when L1 is included in the procedure bilaterally. Another observation made by the same investigators indicated that, by contrast, 7% of the male patients reported that sexual function had increased following sympathectomy. In diabetic patients, sexual impotence following bilateral lumbar sympathectomy should be cautiously interpreted, since in diabetics, disturbances of sexual function may exist independently in a certain percentage of cases.

Sudomotor Changes

Loss of sweating is a physiologic response of any extremity following sympathectomy. However, compensatory body sweating may be a complication of sympathetic denervation of a large surface area of the body and may alter its heat control. This occurs most often in bilateral high lumbar sympathectomy or in a four-extremity sympathectomy. Patients exhibit excessive sweating in nondenervated areas, as a rule, only immediately after surgery. Although the patient may be disabled for a few months postoperatively, usually readjustment of the sudomotor activity appears within 3 months, consisting of lessening of this hyperhidrosis in the nondenervated skin.

Return of Sympathetic Activity

Lasting physiologic results of a lumbar sympathectomy may not always be achieved, for a variety of reasons. Of these the main are (1) inadequate removal of the sympathetic trunk, (2) variations in the number of ganglia and the pattern of distribution of the rami, (3) the presence of intermediate ganglia, (4) the crossover fibers from the contralateral side, (5) sensitization phenomenon of the blood vessels, and (6) regeneration of the sympathetic.

Removal of the sympathetic trunk between L2 and L4 inclusive should, as a rule, provide adequate denervation of the leg and foot except for the area of the medial aspect of the leg, which depends on the innervation from L1.

An occasional sensitization phenomenon, consisting of exaggerated response of smooth muscle to catecholamines may be present. The physiologic parameters of the sensitization phenomenon were formulated by Cannon under the law of denervation.

Sympathetic Regeneration

The concept of sympathetic regeneration to account for a return of sympathetic activity in man may have been overstated. To prevent regeneration, a considerable length of the sympathetic trunk must be removed and this may not always be certain, since we have presented evidence for regeneration even after removal of the entire sympathetic chain on both sides.[26]

Another possibility is progression of the disease, which may at a later stage nullify partially or completely the beneficial effects of a sympathectomy. Reevaluation of the arterial process should be carried out to ascertain the cause of sympathectomy failure.

SUMMARY AND CONCLUSIONS

Lumbar sympathectomy is an important adjunct in the management of occlusive arterial disease provided that (1) patients are properly selected, (2) removal of the sympathetic trunk is adequate, (3) postoperative care of the foot lesions is meticulous, and (4) use of tobacco is rigorously eliminated.

Knowledge and understanding of the therapeutic limitations of the sympathectomy may help to dispel much of the controversy regarding its effectiveness. The procedure neither alters the basic arterial lesion nor prevents its progression.

The operative technique is usually simple and safe, with a low mortality rate. Although varied, the postoperative complications are mostly sympathetic denervation-related. Understanding of their mechanisms will facilitate both prevention and subsequent management.

REFERENCES

1. Leriche R: De l'élongation et de la section des nerfs perivasculaires dans certains syndromes douloureux d'origine artérielle et dans quelques troubles trophiques. Lyon Chir 10:378, 1913.
2. Royle ND: A new operative procedure in the treatment of spastic paralysis and its experimental basis. Med J Aust 1:77, 1924.
3. Diez J: Un nuevo metodo de simpatectomia periferica para el tratamiento de los afecciones troficas y gangrenosas de los miembros: La disociacion fascicular. Bol Soc Cir B Aires 8:792, 1924.
4. Yeager GH, Cowley RA: Anatomical observations on the lumbar sympathetics with evaluation of sympathectomies in organic peripheral vascular disease. Ann Surg 127:953, 1948.
5. Lowenberg RI, Morton DE: The anatomic and surgical significance of the lumbar sympathetic nervous system. Ann Surg 133:525, 1951.
6. Edwards EA: Operative anatomy of the lumbar sympathetic chain. Angiology 2:184, 1951.
7. Webber RH: An analysis of the sympathetic trunk, communicating rami, sympathetic roots and visceral rami in the lumbar region in man. Ann Surg 141:398, 1955.
8. Haimovici H: Criteria for completeness of sympathetic denervation (Editorial). Angiology 2:423, 1951.
9. Haimovici H: Evidence for adrenergic sweating in man. J Appl Physiol 2:512, 1950.
10. Da Valle MJ, Baumann FG, et al: Limited success of lumbar sympathectomy in the prevention of ischemic limb loss in diabetic patients. Surg Gynecol Obstet 152:784, 1981.
11. Haimovici H, Steinman C, Karson IH: Evaluation of lumbar sympathectomy. Advanced occlusive arterial disease. Arch Surg 89:1089, 1964.
12. Terry HJ, Allan JS, Taylor GW: The effect of adding lumbar sympathectomy to reconstructive arterial surgery in the lower limb. Br J Surg 57:51, 1970.
13. Smithwick RH: Lumbar sympathectomy in treatment of obliterative vascular disease of lower extremities. Surgery 42:415, 567, 1957.
14. Moore WS, Hall AD: Effects of lumbar sympathectomy on skin capillary blood flow in arterial occlusive disease. J Surg Res 14:151, 1973.
15. Delaney J, Scarpino J: Limb arteriovenous shunting following sympathetic denervation. Surgery 73:202, 1973.
16. Cronenwett JL, Lindenauer SM: Direct measurement of arteriovenous anastomotic blood flow after lumbar sympathectomy. Surgery 82:82, 1977.
17. De Takats G: Place of sympathectomy in treatment of occlusive arterial disease. Arch Surg 77:655, 1958.
18. Gillespie JA: Future place of lumbar sympathectomy in obliterative vascular disease of lower limbs. Br Med J 2:1640, 1964.
19. Haimovici H: Patterns of arteriosclerotic lesions of the lower extremity. Arch Surg 95:918, 1967.
20. Haimovici H: Peripheral arterial disease in diabetes. NY State J Med 61:2988, 1961; in Ellenberg M, Rifkin H (eds): Diabetes Mellitus: Theory and Practice. New York, McGraw-Hill, 1970, Chap 42, p 890.
21. Pearl F: Muscle-splitting extraperitoneal lumbar ganglionectomy. Surg Gynecol Obstet 65:107, 1937.
22. Tracy CD, Crockett FB: Pain in the lower limb after sympathectomy. Lancet 1:12, 1957.
23. Litwin MS: Postsympathectomy neuralgia. Arch Surg 84:121, 1962.
24. Owens JC: Postsympathectomy pain syndromes. Bull Soc Int Chir 23:500, 1964.
25. Whitelaw GP, Smithwick RH: Some secondary effects of sympathectomy, with particular reference to disturbance of sexual function. N Engl J Med 245:121, 1951.
26. Haimovici H, Hodes R: Preganglionic nerve regeneration in completely sympathectomized cats. Am J Physiol 128:463, 1940.

PART VII
Venous and Lymphatic Surgery

CHAPTER 65
Noninvasive Evaluation of Venous Disease

Robert W. Barnes

The six common clinical syndromes of venous disease are acute deep vein thrombosis, recurrent deep vein thrombosis, postthrombotic (stasis) syndrome, varicose veins, superficial thrombophlebitis, and pulmonary embolism. The clinical diagnosis of these syndromes is frequently in error, being both falsely positive and falsely negative in up to 50% of patients.[1] Contrast phlebography (venography) is the standard for diagnosis, but the technique is expensive, painful, and time consuming, which limits its application as a routine screening and follow-up procedure. For the past 20 years, several noninvasive diagnostic techniques have been developed to assess venous disease. These techniques can be classified into three broad categories: studies that evaluate venous obstruction and thrombosis, tests of venous valvular incompetence, and procedures designed to assess the activity of venous thrombosis. This chapter reviews the basic principles and techniques of these diagnostic methods, including their interpretation and accuracy as well as their advantages and limitations. The application of the methods to the six clinical syndromes is discussed, using diagnostic algorithms, and their cost-effectiveness is documented.

DOPPLER ULTRASOUND

Principle

The Doppler ultrasonic velocity detector evaluates arterial or venous blood flow by a frequency shift in ultrasound reflected from moving blood cells. The instrument provides an audible sound signal or recordable waveform. Arterial signals are distinguished by their multiphasicity, with frequency changes with each heartbeat. Venous flow velocity is cyclic with respiration and can be augmented by limb compression maneuvers.[2] The Doppler detector permits assessment of both venous obstruction and valvular incompetence. The deep, communicating, and superficial veins of the upper and lower extremities may be evaluated, and the major veins, including the iliac and vena cava, indirectly assessed with the instrument.

Technique[3]

Lower Extremity Deep Veins
The patient is evaluated in the supine position with the head of the bed elevated and the lower extremity in a slightly flexed position at the hip and knees (Fig. 65-1). The Doppler probe is coupled to the skin with acoustic gel. Venous flow signals are elicited sequentially at the posterior tibial vein at the ankle, the common femoral vein in the groin, the superficial femoral vein in the thigh, and the popliteal vein behind the knee. At each location, the venous flow characteristics are elicited, including spontaneity, phasicity with respiration, augmentation during distal limb compression, and competence with cessation of flow during proximal limb compression. In addition, the venous flow signal should be nonpulsatile; that is, it should not be cyclic with each heart beat. The venous flow signals should be elicited adjacent to the named arteries at each of the aforementioned locations.

Superficial Veins
The greater (or lesser) saphenous vein can be assessed with the Doppler probe positioned lightly over the skin along the course of the superficial veins. Spontaneous flow may not be heard in cool extremities, but venous flow velocity should be elicited by distal compression. The vein should be competent during proximal limb compression or the Valsalva maneuver.

Perforating Veins
The perforating veins of the lower leg may be incompetent in patients with postthrombotic chronic venous insufficiency. The veins can be located by the Doppler probe at sites of incompetent flow signals during manual compression of the calf above a rubber tourniquet, which prevents

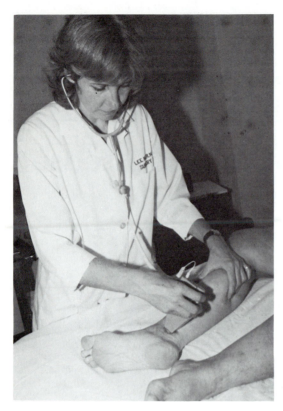

Figure 65-1. Doppler ultrasonic evaluation of the posterior tibial vein.

reflux flow down incompetent superficial veins. The location of incompetent perforators can be marked for subsequent injection sclerotherapy or surgical ligation.

Upper Extremity

The Doppler probe can be positioned over the brachial, axillary, and subclavian veins as well as the superficial veins of the upper extremity. In the neck the internal jugular vein can also be assessed. The flow characteristics in the upper extremity and neck may differ somewhat from those in the lower extremity. In the legs, venous flow is usually attenuated during inspiration, as the diaphragm descends and intraabdominal pressure increases. Conversely, in the upper extremity, flow may increase during inspiration unless thoracic outlet compression of the subclavian vein exists. In the jugular vein, flow velocity may be more continuous and relatively high-pitched, particularly with the patient in the upright position.

Interpretation

Normal venous flow is audible with the Doppler probe at all locations except in superficial veins and occasionally in the posterior tibial vein at the ankle, particularly in cool, vasoconstricted extremities. In the presence of venous thrombosis, flow velocity may not be elicited at the expected location. Alternatively, continuous high-pitched flow velocity may be associated with collateral circulation or a recanalized vein. In venous thrombosis, the flow velocity in distal

veins is more continuous, and augmentation may be attenuated or absent. Venous valvular incompetence occurs several weeks or months after the thrombotic episode. Venous valvular incompetence is typical of varicose veins.

Accuracy

The accuracy of Doppler ultrasound is proportional to the experience of the examiner. The technique is subjective and requires several months of regular application of the instrument in patients with suspected venous disease in order to achieve maximal diagnostic accuracy. With experience, a physician or technologist can correctly identify over 95% of patients with acute deep vein thrombosis. The accuracy is somewhat less in isolated calf vein disease, although the technique still permits detection of over 90% of patients with major calf thrombi.[4] Small thrombi in muscular calf veins are not detected by the instrument.

Advantages

Doppler ultrasound is the least expensive and most portable method of evaluating venous disease. The technique is versatile, inasmuch as both venous obstruction and valvular incompetence can be assessed in both deep and superficial veins of the lower and upper extremities as well as in communicating (perforating) veins. A modification of the examination can be employed in patients in orthopedic traction devices or plaster casts.

Limitations

Doppler ultrasound is a subjective technique in which much time is required for the examiner to gain facility and accuracy. Although hard-copy recordings can be made with the instrument, the accuracy is not improved over audible interpretation by an experienced examiner. The technique is insensitive to isolated small calf vein thrombi. It also will not detect partial thrombi in major veins if the thrombus does not involve more than 50% of the cross-sectional area of the vessel. The technique is insensitive to disease in internal iliac or profunda femoris veins.

VENOUS OUTFLOW PLETHYSMOGRAPHY

Principle

Plethysmography is the recording of changes in volume or other dimension of the body in response to each heartbeat or temporary occlusion of venous return (venous occlusion plethysmography). The plethysmograph includes a transducer to sense the change in body dimension, an amplifier to magnify this change, and a recorder to permit a hard-copy tracing of the dimensional change. In venous outflow plethysmography, the detection of deep vein obstruction is reflected in an attenuation of the decrease in limb volume after deflation of a pneumatic cuff that temporarily occludes

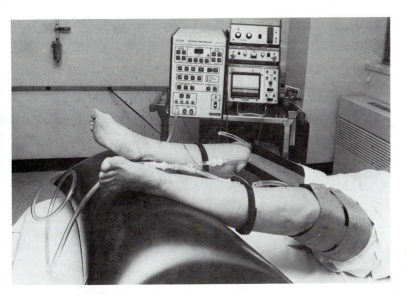

Figure 65-2. Technique of determining maximum venous outflow with a strain-gauge plethysmograph (SPG).

venous return on the proximal limb. Several transducers are available, the most common being strain-gauge plethysmograph (SPG), impedance plethysmograph (IPG), and air (volume pulse recorder).

Technique[5,6]

The patient is evaluated in the supine position with the lower extremities elevated and placed in a relaxed position with slight flexion of the hip and knee. A pneumatic cuff is applied to the thigh, and the transducer is applied to the calf (Fig. 65-2). After calibrating and balancing the transducer, the pneumatic thigh cuff is inflated (30 to 55 mm Hg) to temporarily occlude venous return. The transducer on the calf records the increase in calf volume or circumfer-

ence. After stabilization of calf size, usually in about 2 minutes, the thigh cuff is rapidly deflated, and the decrease in calf volume or circumference is recorded (Fig. 65-3). The procedure is repeated several times until consistent outflow tracings are obtained.

Interpretation

Several types of interpretation of venous outflow tracings are possible, depending upon the type of transducer employed on the calf. Most techniques involve plotting or analyzing both the incremental volume (capacitance) of calf change during the period of venous occlusion as well as the rate of decrease in calf volume or circumference after cuff deflation (outflow). The outflow rate can be calculated instantaneously at the beginning of outflow (maximum venous outflow), or the rate of outflow over a period of time (up to 3 seconds) may be noted. With the SPG, the venous outflow can be calculated in millimeters per minute per 100 g of tissue. Normal values for outflow depend upon the instrument employed and the rapidity of cuff deflation. The position of the leg, the amount of calf circumference subtended by the gauge, and the relaxation of the leg all contribute to the venous outflow. The impedance technique usually is interpreted by plotting the incremental volume (capacitance) on one axis of the chart paper and the outflow in 3 seconds on the other axis.[7]

Accuracy

Venous outflow plethysmography detects 85 to 95% of deep vein thrombi at or above the level of the popliteal vein. The specificity exceeds 90% in most reported series.[8] The technique is insensitive to isolated calf vein thrombi, although if massive, such calf vein thrombosis may result in attenuated capacitance during the period of thigh cuff inflation.

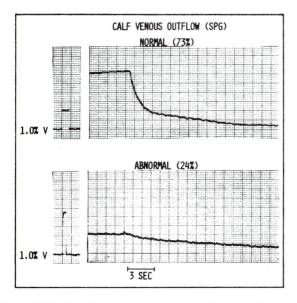

Figure 65-3. Recordings of normal (*top*) and abnormal (*bottom*) venous outflow using a strain-gauge plethysmograph (SPG).

Advantages

Venous outflow plethysmography is objective and relatively simple to perform. Most instruments are portable. A hardcopy tracing is obtained that simplifies diagnostic interpretation. Such objective recordings permit longitudinal followup of patients to detect improvement in venous outflow during the postthrombotic period of recanalization or collateral development.

Limitations

Venous outflow plethysmography is more expensive than Doppler ultrasound, with instruments costing between $2000 and $10,000. The technique is insensitive to isolated calf vein thrombi and thrombi in the profunda femoris or internal iliac veins. The method may be falsely negative in patients with chronic venous disease and recanalization or large collateral development. The technique may be influenced by positional factors and may be impossible in patients who are uncooperative or who are in orthopedic traction appliances or plaster casts.

PHLEBORHEOGRAPHY

Principle

The phleborheograph is an air plethysmograph that employs pneumatic cuffs to sense volume fluctuations in the lower extremity during respiration as well as pneumatic compression maneuvers.[9] The normal cyclic fluctuations in limb volume are attenuated in the presence of venous thrombosis, which also result in abnormal increases in limb volume during distal limb compression maneuvers. The technique detects deep venous obstruction as well as gross valvular incompetence of the deep veins.

Technique

The patient is studied in the supine position with the head of the bed elevated and the lower extremities in a slightly dependent position to permit filling of the veins of the extremity. The patient must be positioned so that the leg is relaxed and in a slightly flexed position at the hip and knee. Pneumatic cuffs are placed on the foot, calf, and thigh, as well as the chest (to record respiratory movement). The initial recording is taken to identify cyclic changes in lower extremity volume associated with respiration. Subsequent stages of the procedure involve recording changes in thigh, calf, and foot volume during sequential maneuvers of repetitive rapid inflations of either the foot or calf cuffs.

Interpretation

Normally, the lower extremity should have recordable changes in volume during respiration, as venous flow is cyclically attenuated by descent of the diaphragm and increased intraabdominal pressure. This cyclic volume change is analogous to the change in flow velocity that is audible by Doppler ultrasound. In the presence of venous thrombosis, there will be attenuation or absence of respiratory wave change in limb volume distal to the occlusive thrombus. Normally, rapid compression of the foot or calf should not lead to increase in extremity volume if the major veins are patent. In the presence of venous thrombosis, such distal limb compression maneuvers result in a temporary increase in limb volume distal to the obstructing thrombosis. Finally, compression of the calf should result in a decrease in foot volume as blood is emptied from the foot into the compressed calf veins. In the presence of calf vein thrombosis, such diminution in foot volume during calf compression may be attenuated or absent. In the presence of chronic venous insufficiency, the foot volume may return to the baseline more rapidly than normal.

Accuracy

The phleborheograph is the most accurate plethysmographic technique to detect deep vein thrombosis. Most reports suggest an accuracy exceeding 95% in detection of major leg vein thrombi. In addition, the method is sensitive to major calf vein thrombi.

Advantages

The phleborheograph provides objective hard-copy recordings of venous pathophysiology, including both the venous outflow obstruction as well as gross venous valvular incompetence. The technique is the most accurate of the plethysmographic methods to evaluate venous disease. The method permits objective recording of changes associated with recanalization of venous thrombi or development of prominent collaterals. The multiple recording channels of the device also permit evaluation of arterial disease, with the ability to record hemodynamic events from a variety of other transducers.

Limitations

The phleborheograph is the most expensive diagnostic instrument for venous disease, with the cost exceeding $10,000. The examination is time consuming, and the instrument, while portable, is bulky. The technique requires considerable patient cooperation. The method is insensitive to minor calf thrombi and obstruction of the profunda femoris and internal iliac veins.

VENOUS REFLUX PLETHYSMOGRAPHY

Principle

Several plethysmographic transducers permit assessment of limb volume or skin blood content changes associated with chronic venous insufficiency. The most useful devices are the SPG and the photoplethysmograph (PPG). The transducers record abnormal changes in calf volume or skin blood content in response to proximal pneumatic compression on the thigh or after muscular exercise in the erect position.

Technique

The SPG records calf volume changes with the patient in the supine position.[10] A proximal thigh tourniquet is inflated above the arterial systolic pressure to temporarily isolate the limb from the circulation. A distal thigh cuff is then inflated up to 50 mm Hg, which may displace underlying thigh venous blood in a distal direction through incompetent veins. The strain-gauge on the calf records the abnormal increase in calf circumference during the period of thigh cuff inflation.

A more suitable method for assessing altered calf venous dynamics in chronic venous insufficiency is to record changes in calf volume with the patient sitting or standing during calf muscle exercise[11] (Fig. 65-4). The strain-gauge is placed on the calf, and the transducer is calibrated and balanced. The patient then contracts the calf muscle while sitting, or the calf volume can be recorded while the patient walks on a treadmill. The calf volume changes recorded with the strain-gauge are a reflection on deep venous capacity and function.

In order to record abnormalities of communicating (perforating) or superficial veins, the PPG[12] is taped to the skin on the medial aspect of the lower leg, using two-faced clear plastic tape (Fig. 65-5). The PPG transducer is connected to the recorder via an amplifier set in the DC (venous) mode. Changes in skin blood content result in a change in the reflection of the light-emitting infrared diode in the transducer. The patient can exercise in the sitting or standing position, and changes in skin blood content are recorded during and after the exercise.

Interpretation

Normally, the calf volume decreases by at least 2% during active contraction of the calf in the sitting or standing position. In the presence of chronic deep venous insufficiency, the decrease in calf volume may be attenuated or absent, and the return to baseline may be accelerated. The skin blood content recorded with the PPG transducer should normally decrease during erect exercise and gradually return to baseline in 20 to 60 seconds after cessation of exercise (Fig. 65-6). In patients with incompetent communicating (perforating) or superficial veins, the decrement in skin blood content is attenuated, and the recovery time to baseline is accelerated. Differentiation of superficial from deep venous incompetence can be assessed by applying rubber tourniquets to the leg above the transducer. The tourniquets

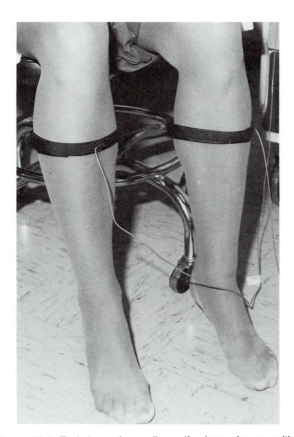

Figure 65-4. Technique of recording calf volume changes with a strain-gauge plethysmograph (SPG) during calf muscle exercise while sitting.

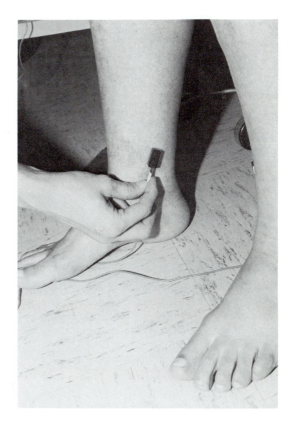

Figure 65-5. Method of attaching photoplethysmograph (PPG) transducer to skin using two-faced plastic tape to measure skin blood content changes during calf contraction.

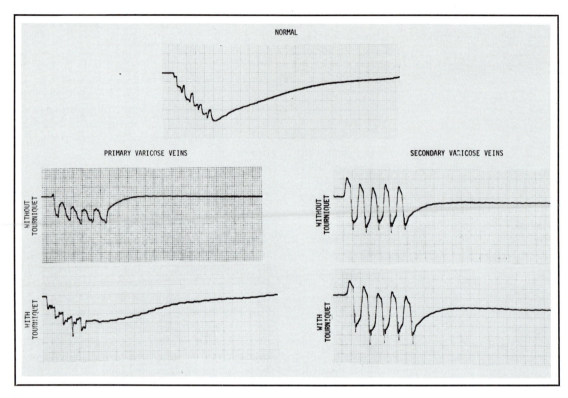

Figure 65-6. Normal (*top*) and abnormal (*bottom*) ankle skin blood content changes in response to calf muscle exercise.

should normalize the PPG tracing if the valvular incompetence is limited to the superficial veins, whereas if deep and perforating venous incompetence exists, the tracing may remain abnormal.

Accuracy

Venous reflux plethysmography correlates well with clinical syndromes and venographic evidence of chronic venous insufficiency. The tracings recorded by the PPG on the lower leg correlate closely with simultaneous tracings of superficial venous pressure in patients with chronic venous insufficiency.

Advantages

Venous reflux plethysmography offers objective confirmation of the extent and localization of superficial and deep venous incompetence. The techniques are simple to perform and can document changes in patients during maneuvers that mimic normal upright muscular exercise.

Limitations

Venous reflux plethysmography is influenced by lack of patient cooperation and by local inflammatory changes in the leg. Insufficient calf muscle exercise may result in false-positive recordings. Likewise, local inflammation associated

with ulceration may result in rapid recovery times in patients undergoing venous reflux photoplethysmography.

FIBRINOGEN ^{125}I LEG SCANNING

Principle

When injected intravenously, human fibrinogen labeled with iodine 125 becomes incorporated into actively forming thrombi. The localized radioactivity at such sites can be detected by an external scintillation counter[13] (Fig. 65-7).

Technique

The thyroid should be blocked with oral potassium iodide or intravenous sodium iodide. Fibrinogen ^{125}I, 100 μCi, is injected intravenously. The fibrinogen should be prepared from hepatitis-free donors. The radioactive count in the lower extremities is made with an external portable scintillation detector at intervals along the course of the major deep veins in the thigh and the calf. The counts at each location are compared to the cardiac background activity. Leg scanning is performed approximately 1 hour after injection of the labeled fibrinogen and then daily.

Interpretation

Normally, the leg counts at any location should not exceed 15 to 20% of cardiac background activity. Likewise, counts

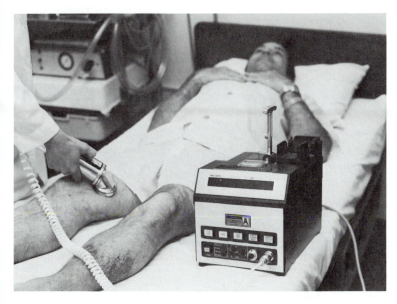

Figure 65-7. Technique of using portable scintillation probe to detect sites of increased radioactivity during fibrinogen ^{125}I leg scanning.

should not differ between adjacent locations or similar sites on the opposite extremity by more than 15 to 20%. Localized increased radioactivity is indicative of active thrombosis at that location.

Accuracy

Fibrinogen ^{125}I leg scanning is sensitive to 85 to 90% of thrombi proved by contrast phlebography. The technique is most sensitive to active thrombi in the calf, popliteal, or distal thigh veins. The technique is insensitive to thrombi that are not actively forming. The method may not detect proximal thrombi in the iliofemoral segment because of the high background activity associated with the large muscle mass in these areas and radioactivity accumulating in the urinary bladder. The test may be falsely positive at sites of trauma, operative wounds, hemorrhage, or inflammation.

Advantages

Fibrinogen ^{125}I scanning is the most sensitive technique for detecting calf vein thrombi. The method is fairly specific for active venous thrombosis, making it useful in evaluating patients with suspected recurrent venous thrombosis. The technique has had its greatest application in prospective screening of high-risk patients, such as those undergoing major operation or with serious underlying medical illnesses.

Limitations

The fibrinogen I^{125} commercially available is expensive, costing more than $60 per dose. This, coupled with the length of time necessary to make an accurate diagnosis, makes the method expensive. The required wait of 24 to 72 hours

before confirming a diagnosis makes the test of limited application in suspected acute deep vein thrombosis unless used with another technique.[14] The technique is insensitive to inactive disease and will not detect proximal venous thrombi. The method carries a theoretic risk of transmission of hepatitis.

RADIONUCLIDE PHLEBOGRAPHY

Principle

Radionuclide phlebography (venography) involves the visualization of isotope during its passage through the major veins from a distal intravenous injection on the extremity.[15] The technique is in essence a dynamic venous scan and can be performed at the time of perfusion lung scanning.[16]

Technique

Approximately 6 to 7 mCi of sodium pertechnetate (technetium ^{99m}Tc) is divided between two syringes and injected intravenously in a vein on the dorsum of each foot. With ankle tourniquets in place, the isotope ascends the deep venous system and is imaged with a gamma (Anger) camera. The resultant images provide a dynamic view of the popliteal, femoral, and iliac veins and the inferior vena cava. If necessary, visualization of the upper extremity veins can be performed with isotope injection into the veins of the arms.

Interpretation

Normally, the major venous channels are visualized as a single venous trunk extending from the knee to the inferior vena cava (Fig. 65-8). Isolated calf veins cannot be resolved with the technique. In the presence of venous thrombosis,

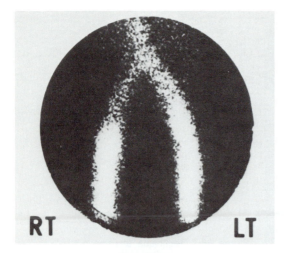

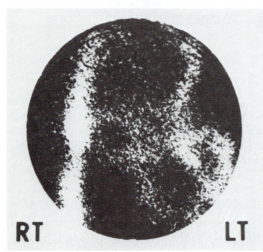

Figure 65-8. Normal (*top*) and abnormal (*bottom*) radionuclide phlebogram of iliac veins and inferior vena cava.

there may be interruption of the normal venous channel and the development of multiple collateral veins. Venous thrombosis may also delay the ascent of the isotope, which normally should reach the inferior vena cava within 10 to 15 seconds. Release of the superficial tourniquets at the ankle may permit filling of the superficial (saphenous) vein. Application of a patch of radioactive marker at each knee and on the pubis may help localization of the venous images.

Accuracy

The sensitivity of radionuclide phlebography is about 95% compared with contrast phlebography. The technique is insensitive to nonocclusive thrombi, and the method is not sensitive to isolated calf vein thrombi.

Advantages

The injectate is painless, making the technique particularly useful in patients who require repeat or follow-up studies.

The method is more rapid than conventional contrast phlebography and can be performed at the time of perfusion lung scanning. The dynamic flow characteristics make radionuclide phlebography particularly useful for evaluating collateral venous circulation. The method provides better visualization of the intraabdominal veins than contrast phlebography from peripheral injections.

Limitations

Radionuclide phlebography has poorer resolution of the venous system than contrast phlebography. This factor makes the method of little value in detecting isolated calf vein thrombi or small nonocclusive thrombi in the proximal veins. The method exposes the patient to a low dose of radioactivity. The technique is not portable and is relatively expensive.

VENOUS IMAGING

Principle

Ultrasonic imaging of the venous system involves high-resolution ultrasound to screen for the following:

1. The presence or absence of an intraluminal soft-tissue mass
2. Compressibility of the vein (ability to coapt the vessel walls)
3. Response to performance of the Valsalva maneuver
4. The structure and function of vein valves

Recently, real-time B-mode imaging has been coupled with pulsed Doppler capabilities to allow for concomitant assessment of anatomic structure and venous flow characteristics. This system, referred to as duplex scanning, combines two testing modalities into one efficient diagnostic technique.

Technique

The patient is first evaluated in the supine position with the head of the bed elevated and the lower extremities in a slightly flexed position at the hips and knees (Fig. 65-9). The scanner is coupled to the skin with acoustic gel, and the common femoral artery is identified. Medially the common femoral vein is visualized and confirmed with the Doppler. The superficial femoral, deep femoral, greater saphenous, anterior tibial, and posterior tibial veins are also examined. The popliteal vein is approached in an identical fashion but with the patient either in the prone or decubitus position. Many laboratories are presently scanning iliac veins with deep Doppler instrumentation. Longitudinal and transverse views are routinely obtained on all veins. Each vein is examined for intraluminal soft-tissue masses. The transducer probe is used to gently compress each vein while observing the video monitor for changes in vein caliber. Femoral vein diameter is observed during the Valsalva maneuver and during distal vein compression. Venous valve structure and function are visualized.

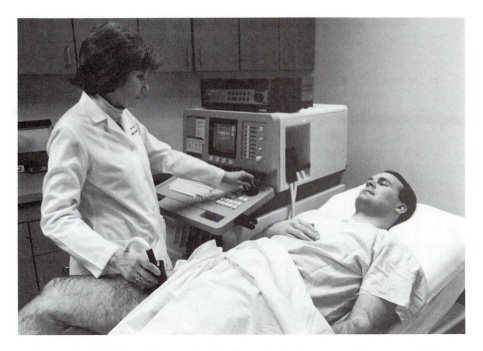

Figure 65-9. Technique of venous imaging for evaluating lower extremity venous pathology.

Interpretation

Doppler flow velocity is interpreted as described earlier in this chapter. Normal veins, both noncompressed and compressed, and veins with thrombus can be identified (Fig. 65-10). Real-time imaging for the identification of deep venous obstruction has frequently shown the obstructed vein to be larger and filled with a speckled mass.[17] Deep venous thrombosis causes the vein to be noncompressible with the transducer probe and to show no change in diameter with the Valsalva maneuver.[18] Likewise, veins well proximal to areas of deep vein thrombosis retain their compressibility and normal response to the Valsalva maneuver. Valve structure and function are observed and correlated with the patients' clinical presentation. Nonfunctional valves without intraluminal thrombus suggest old deep vein thrombosis with recanalization.

Accuracy

The accuracy of venous imaging is proportional to the experience of the examiner and to the training of the interpreting physician. The echogenicity of chronic vs. acute thrombus is variably reported[19–21]; thus interpreting thrombus age remains fertile ground for investigation. Comparing B-mode ultrasound with venography shows the former to have an overall specificity of 92 to 100% and sensitivity of 94 to 100%.[22–24]

Advantages

Venous imaging affords an anatomic assessment of the vein and its contents (thrombus, valves, and communicating

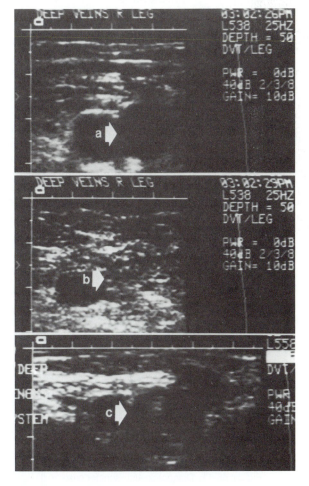

Figure 65-10. Normal noncompressed (*a*) and normal compressed (*b*) femoral veins. Thrombus in femoral vein (*c*).

veins). It is advantageous for patients with extrinsic venous compression, amputations, contrast allergies, renal compromise, and chronic venous insufficiency.

Limitations

The deep femoral vein, the superficial femoral vein at the adductor canal region, and the iliac veins are difficult to examine. The equipment is expensive compared to that required for other noninvasive tests but is the same equipment used by most large laboratories for B-mode carotid scans. An experienced examiner and interpreting physician are required for excellent results.

CLINICAL APPLICATIONS

Acute Deep Vein Thrombosis

A diagnostic algorithm for the evaluation of patients with suspected acute deep vein thrombosis is shown in Figure 65-11. Such patients should receive intravenous heparin until the diagnosis is confirmed. Initial screening may involve Doppler ultrasound, venous imaging, venous outflow plethysmography, phleborheography, or radionuclide phlebography. If the noninvasive study is unequivocally positive, the patient may be treated for deep vein thrombosis unless some predisposing factor exists that might result in a false-positive noninvasive study. Patients with such conditions as trauma, possible ruptured Baker's cyst, or malignancy may have extrinsic compression of the venous system, which will result in an abnormal screening study. Such patients deserve contrast phlebography for clarification of the diagnosis. If the noninvasive study is unequivocally normal and no isolated calf vein thrombosis is suspected (frequently overlooked by noninvasive techniques), the heparin therapy may be discontinued. Such patients may require contrast phlebography to clarify the diagnosis. Contrast phlebography is also indicated in patients in whom the noninvasive study is equivocal or who are uncooperative, making the examination difficult.

Recurrent Deep Vein Thrombosis

A diagnostic algorithm for the evaluation of patients with suspected recurrent deep vein thrombosis is shown in Figure 65-12. Such patients are usually treated with repeat hospitalization and anticoagulation. However, many patients have recurrent symptoms on the basis of chronic, inactive postthrombotic disease. Furthermore, some patients with recurrent symptoms have a condition other than venous disease and have been previously misdiagnosed and iatrogenically mistreated. Noninvasive screening by Doppler ultrasound, venous imaging, and venous outflow and reflux plethysmography or phleborheography is useful to determine whether the venous system is normal, obstructed, or incompetent. Patients with normal results on noninvasive studies should be thoroughly investigated for other problems to clarify their underlying symptoms. Contrast phlebography may be useful to convince referring physicians that the condition is not due to venous disease.

Patients with predominant venous outflow obstruction are particularly prone to develop recurrent leg pain with exercise, so-called venous claudication. Such patients can usually be managed with supportive measures but occasionally require venous reconstruction procedures such as crossover venous bypass. If recurrent active thrombosis is present, the patient requires anticoagulation. Such patients may be identified by contrast phlebography with the visualization of fresh clot outlined by contrast material. Alternatively, such patients may be studied by fibrinogen ^{125}I leg scanning to identify active thrombi. If noninvasive studies show only chronic venous valvular incompetence without outflow obstruction, such patients may develop recurrent leg swelling and pain on the basis of chronic venous insufficiency. These patients are best managed with elastic support stockings and leg elevation, although some patients may benefit from venous valvular reconstruction procedures.

Postthrombotic (Stasis) Syndrome

An algorithm for the evaluation and management of patients with suspected postthrombotic chronic venous insuf-

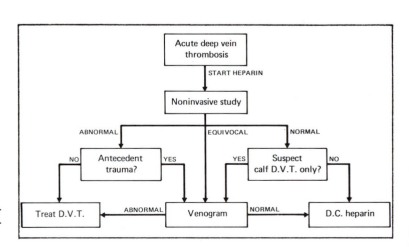

Figure 65-11. Diagnostic algorithm for evaluation of suspected acute deep vein thrombosis.

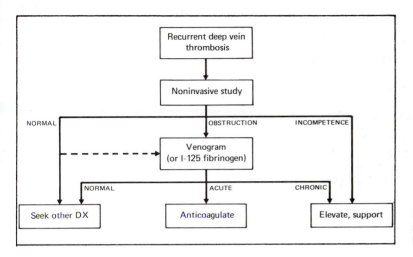

Figure 65-12. Diagnostic algorithm for evaluation of suspected recurrent venous thrombosis.

ficiency is shown in Figure 65-13. Patients with leg pain, stasis, dermatitis, and ulceration are usually diagnosed by a bedside examination. However, some patients may have stasis-like signs due to other conditions such as contact dermatitis, rheumatoid vasculitis, or chronic traumatic ulceration. These patients may be evaluated by Doppler ultrasound, venous imaging, and venous outflow and reflux plethysmography to clarify their underlying pathophysiologic sequelae. Most patients have deep and perforating incompetence without associated deep venous obstruction. Patients with extensive deep venous outflow obstruction may require venous reconstruction or bypass procedures. More commonly, patients have venous incompetence of the deep and perforating veins, with or without superficial venous incompetence. Such patients are best managed by elastic support. Patients with chronic stasis ulcers usually benefit from application of a medicated bandage (Unna's boot). Doppler ultrasound may document sites of incompetent perforating veins, which may be ligated to improve the chronic venous insufficiency. Venous imaging can confirm valvular incompetence and identify patients who may be considered for vein valve reconstruction. Venous reflux photoplethysmography can document occasional patients with ambulatory venous hypertension who also benefit from ligation of perforating veins.

Varicose Veins

An algorithm to evaluate patients with varicose veins is depicted in Figure 65-14. The basic clinical objective is to differentiate patients with isolated superficial venous incompetence (primary varicose veins) from those individuals with underlying deep venous disease (secondary varicose veins). Doppler ultrasound and venous outflow and reflux plethysmography are helpful in evaluating such patients. If venous abnormalities are limited to the superficial system, the patient may be reassured that chronic stasis ulceration and the risk of major venous thrombosis or pulmonary embolism are unlikely. Patients with primary varicose veins can be treated conservatively with elastic support, by injection therapy, or by stripping for control of the cosmetic problem. However, if underlying deep venous disease is documented, stripping of the varicose veins is not advised, and the prognosis is that of the postthrombotic syndrome.

Superficial Thrombophlebitis

The patient with an inflammatory streak along the course of the greater saphenous vein may have superficial thrombophlebitis or lymphangiitis. If an obvious varicose vein

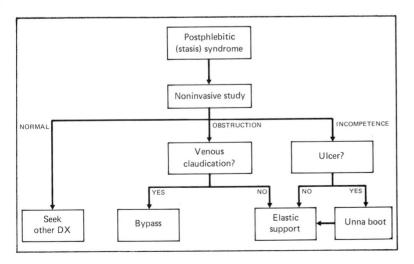

Figure 65-13. Diagnostic-therapeutic algorithm for management of suspected postthrombotic chronic venous insufficiency.

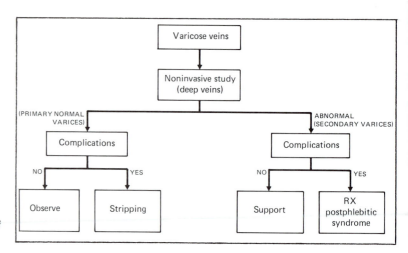

Figure 65-14. Algorithm for management of patients with varicose veins.

is thrombosed, the clinical diagnosis is simple. However, if predisposing varicose veins are not present, the patient is best evaluated by Doppler ultrasound (Fig. 65-15). If the superficial vein is patent, lymphangiitis is probable, and the patient should respond to antibiotic therapy. If the superficial vein is thrombosed, a Doppler examination of the deep veins may establish the presence of associated deep vein thrombosis. In the latter condition, anticoagulants are the treatment of choice. If thrombosis is limited to the superficial veins, the saphenofemoral junction can be ligated if the process extends near that point. For more distal superficial thrombophlebitis, nonsteroidal antiinflammatory drugs provide the best therapy.

Pulmonary Embolism

The clinical diagnosis of pulmonary embolism is falsely positive and falsely negative in about 50% of patients. A diagnostic algorithm for the evaluation of such patients is shown in Figure 65-16. After initiating heparin therapy,

screening perfusion and ventilation lung scanning is performed. If the lung scan is normal, a significant pulmonary embolus can be ruled out. If the scan is positive, noninvasive evaluation of the lower extremities may be helpful in order to improve the specificity of the lung scan. If the noninvasive study reveals leg vein thrombosis, the patient may be safely treated for pulmonary embolus. If the noninvasive study is normal, pulmonary arteriography should be considered unless the ventilation-perfusion scan is highly diagnostic. In our experience, ventilation-perfusion lung scans are frequently falsely positive, and pulmonary arteriography becomes an important diagnostic modality to correctly manage the patient.

COST-EFFECTIVENESS

The noninvasive diagnostic techniques discussed in this chapter have proven to be both cost beneficial[25] and cost effective.[26] The clinical diagnosis is not cost effective. Contrast phlebography is cost effective and is even more so

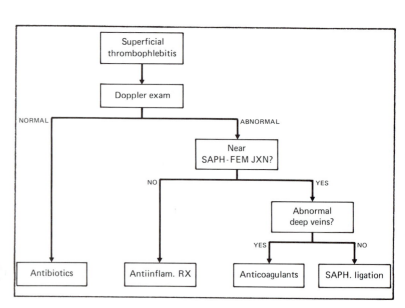

Figure 65-15. Algorithm for evaluation and management of patients with suspected superficial thrombophlebitis.

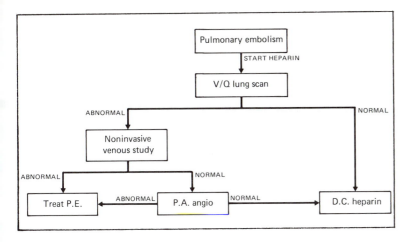

Figure 65-16. Diagnostic algorithm for evaluation of suspected pulmonary embolism.

when applied as an outpatient investigation. Noninvasive studies, likewise, compare favorably with contrast phlebography on a cost-benefit or cost-effective analysis. The major cost of evaluation of venous thrombosis is hospitalization. It is thus apparent that judicious use of noninvasive techniques with documented accuracy on an outpatient basis may greatly reduce total expenditure in assessing patients with clinical venous syndromes.

REFERENCES

1. Barnes RW, Wu KK, et al.: Fallibility of the clinical diagnosis of venous thrombosis. JAMA 234:605, 1975.
2. Strandness DE, Sumner DS: Ultrasonic velocity detector in the diagnosis of thrombophlebitis. Arch Surg 104:180, 1972.
3. Barnes RW, Russell HE, et al.: Doppler Ultrasonic Evaluation of Venous Disease: A Programmed Audiovisual Instruction, 2nd ed. Iowa City, University of Iowa Press, 1975, p 251.
4. Barnes RW, Russell HE, et al.: Accuracy of Doppler ultrasound in clinically suspected venous thrombosis of the calf. Surg Gynecol Obstet 143:425, 1976.
5. Barnes RW, Collicott PE, et al.: Noninvasive quantitation of maximum venous outflow in acute thrombophlebitis. Surgery 72:971, 1972.
6. Wheeler HB, O'Donnell JA, et al.: Bedside screening for venous thrombosis using occlusive impedance phlebography. Angiology 26:199, 1975.
7. Hull R, van Aken WG, et al.: Impedance plethysmography using the occlusive cuff technique in the diagnosis of venous thrombosis. Circulation 53:696, 1976.
8. Wheeler HB: Diagnosis of deep vein thrombosis; review of clinical evaluation and impedance plethysmography. Am J Surg 150(4A):7, 1985.
9. Cranley JJ, Gay AY, et al.: A plethysmographic technique for the diagnosis of deep venous thrombosis of the lower extremities. Surg Gynecol Obstet 136:385, 1973.
10. Barnes RW, Collicott PE, et al.: Noninvasive quantitation of venous reflux in the postphlebitic syndrome. Surg Gynecol Obstet 136:769, 1973.
11. Holm JSE: A simple plethysmographic method for differentiating primary from secondary varicose veins. Surg Gynecol Obstet 143:609, 1976.
12. Barnes RW, Yao JS: Photoplethysmography in chronic venous insufficiency, in Bernstein EF (ed): Noninvasive Diagnostic Techniques in Vascular Disease. St. Louis, C. V. Mosby, 1982, p 514.
13. Hirsh J, Gallus AS: ^{125}I-labeled fibrinogen scanning. JAMA 233:970, 1975.
14. Hull R, Hirsh J, et al.: Combined use of leg scanning and impedance plethysmography in suspected venous thrombosis: An alternative to venography. N Engl J Med 296:1497, 1977.
15. Barnes RW, McDonald GB, et al.: Radionuclide venography for rapid dynamic evaluation of venous disease. Surgery 73:706, 1973.
16. Yao JST, Henkin RE, et al.: Combined isotope venography and lung scanning. Arch Surg 107:146, 1973.
17. Talbot SR: Use of real-time imaging in identifying deep venous obstruction; a preliminary report. Bruit 6:41, 1982.
18. Raghavendra BN, Rosen RJ, et al.: Deep venous thrombosis: Detection by high-resolution real-time ultrasonography. Radiology 152(3):789, 1984.
19. Coelho JCU, Sigel B: B-mode sonography of blood clots. J Clin Ultrasound 10:323, 1982.
20. Alanen A, Kormano M: Correlation of the echogenicity and structure of clotted blood. J Ultrasound Med 4:421, 1985.
21. Shung KK, Fei DY, et al.: Ultrasonic characterization of blood during coagulation. J Clin Ultrasound 12:147, 1984.
22. Sandler DA, Duncan JS, et al.: Diagnosis of deep-vein thrombosis: Comparison of clinical evaluation, ultrasound, plethysmography, and venoscan with x-ray venogram. Lancet, Sept 29, 1984, p 716.
23. Dauzat MM, Laroche JP, et al.: Real-time B-mode ultrasonography for better specificity in the noninvasive diagnosis of deep venous thrombosis. J Ultrasound Med 5:625, 1986.
24. Sullivan ED, Peter DJ, et al.: Real-time B-mode venous ultrasound. J Vasc Surg 1:465, 1984.
25. Barnes RW: Cost/benefit analysis of noninvasive testing for venous thromboembolism, in Bernstein EF (ed): Noninvasive Diagnostic Techniques in Vascular Disease. St. Louis, C. V. Mosby, 1982, p 570.
26. Hull R, Hirsh J, et al.: Cost effectiveness of clinical diagnosis, venography, and noninvasive testing in patients with symptomatic deep-vein thrombosis. N Engl J Med 304:1561, 1981.

CHAPTER 66

Venous Imaging: Contrast Phlebography and Duplex Ultrasonography

Seymour Sprayregen, Cheryl Montefusco, and Henry Haimovici

CONTRAST PHLEBOGRAPHY

Lower Extremity Venous Thrombosis

Clinical diagnosis of deep venous thrombosis (DVT) is well known to be often deceptive or misleading.[1-3] Although massive deep venous thrombosis or phlegmasia cerulea dolens are generally easily detectable on the basis of clinical evaluation the diagnosis of the common form of DVT, which involves the small-, medium-, or even large-sized veins, has an accuracy of less than 50%.[4] Because of the ever-present potential complication of pulmonary embolism, objective methods for establishing an accurate diagnosis of DVT are therefore essential.

Contrast phlebography previously was accepted as the most dependable modality for establishing an accurate diagnosis of DVT. Recently, however, duplex ultrasonography has been shown to have an accuracy rivaling that of contrast studies in the extremities.[5-8] The evidence suggests that duplex ultrasonography will also be extremely accurate in the diagnosis of pelvic and caval thrombosis. In our institution duplex ultrasonography is the preferred diagnostic modality for establishing the diagnosis of DVT and for venous mapping prior to bypass surgery. Only when duplex studies are inadequate, which is quite infrequent, are contrast examinations performed.

Historical Background

The early attempts of phlebography in the 1920s were hampered by the chemical nature of the contrast media and the inadequate techniques. It was not until 1938 that phlebography became more standardized, when dos Santos introduced the ascending method for outlining the deep and superficial veins by injecting the contrast material into a superficial vein of the foot.[9] Serial films were taken as the contrast medium ascended in the leg and thigh. In 1941 Luke introduced descending phlebography, in which the contrast material is injected into the femoral vein at the groin with the patient in the upright position.[10] Its main objective was to show whether the valves in the thigh and calf veins were intact or incompetent. It was subsequently shown, however, that contrast material may descend in the absence of pathologic valves, therefore severely limiting the value of this technique.

At present, ascending phlebography with various modifications since its introduction is the standard procedure most commonly used.[11,12] Concurrent with improvement of the phlebographic technique, better understanding of the dynamics of venous and contrast material flow led to more accurate interpretation of the phlebographic findings in normal and pathologic states.

Anatomy of Venous System of Lower Extremity
The radiologic visualization and interpretation of venous disorders, especially those of DVT, are more difficult than those of arterial disorders. Four major problems must be adequately analyzed in most cases of venous occlusion or insufficiency:

1. Anatomic integrity of the superficial and deep veins
2. Level and extent of partial or complete thrombotic occlusion
3. Competency of the venous valves
4. Presence of artifacts or variants.

Knowledge of the normal anatomy and pathologic features of the veins of the lower extremity is essential for proper phlebographic interpretation.

The superficial and deep veins of the foot are drained by the great and small saphenous veins and their tributaries.

The *superficial veins* are located on the dorsal and plantar surfaces of the foot. On the dorsum the digital veins join the plantar branches to form a dorsal venous arch. Proximal to this arch are irregular venous networks, which form medial and lateral marginal veins.

The superficial plantar veins form an arch that extends across the roots of the toes and leads into the medial and lateral marginal veins. These superficial veins of the foot communicate with deep veins that drain into the great and small saphenous veins as well as into the deep veins of the leg.

The great saphenous vein, the longest vein in the body,

begins in the medial marginal vein of the dorsum of the foot and ends in the femoral vein below the inguinal ligament. The number of its valves varies from 10 to 20, and the valves are more numerous in the lower leg than in the thigh. The small saphenous vein begins behind the lateral malleolus as a continuation of the lateral marginal vein. Running directly upward, it perforates the deep fascia in the lower part of the popliteal fossa and ends in the popliteal vein between the heads of the gastrocnemius. It also communicates with the deep veins on the dorsum of the foot and receives numerous large tributaries from the back of the leg. Before piercing the deep fascia, it gives off a branch that runs upward and forward to join the great saphenous vein. The small saphenous vein possesses from 9 to 12 valves, one of which is always found near the termination in the popliteal vein.

The *deep veins* of the foot are represented by the deep plantar venous arch, which lies alongside the plantar arterial arch. These veins communicate with the great and small saphenous veins and unite behind the medial malleolus to form the posterior tibial and the peroneal veins. The anterior tibial veins are the upward continuation of the venae comitantes of the dorsalis pedis artery, and unite with the posterior tibial to form the popliteal vein. Of the deep calf veins, those draining the gastrocnemius and soleus muscles appear to play a significant role as an early site of acute thrombosis. The gastrocnemius veins drain into the popliteal vein, whereas those of the soleus empty into the posterior tibial and peroneal veins.

The popliteal vein ascends through the popliteal fossa to the aperture of the adductor magnus, where it becomes the femoral vein. There are usually four valves in the popliteal vein.

The femoral vein accompanies the femoral artery through the upper two thirds of the thigh. It receives numerous muscular tributaries and about 4 cm below the inguinal ligament is joined by the profunda femoris vein. Near its termination it receives the great saphenous vein. There are three valves in the femoral vein.

The deep femoral vein receives the medial and lateral femoral circumflex veins and tributaries corresponding to the arterial perforating branches, and through these establishes communications with the popliteal vein below and the inferior gluteal vein above.

Perforating or *communicating* veins connect the superficial with the deep veins by passing through the deep fascia. They are found mostly in the foot and lower half of the leg and are less frequent in the thigh. The valves in these communicating veins are designed to allow flow from the superficial to the deep system. In postphlebitic cases following destruction and incompetence of valves, the flow is reversed from the deep to the superficial veins.

Technique of Phlebography

Unlike the technique of arteriography, that of phlebography is far from standardized. The technique used by us is that of ascending phlebography. The patient is placed in the semiupright position (40° to 60° from the horizontal). This allows the superficial veins to become well distended and the valves to be well visualized. This position is well tolerated by most patients. The extremity being examined does

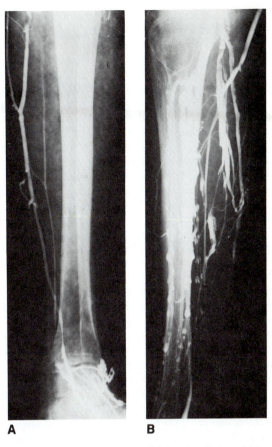

A   **B**

Figure 66-1. A. Leg phlebogram, weightbearing. **B.** Leg phlebogram of the same patient, nonweightbearing. Note the striking difference between the two methods: in **A,** only superficial veins are visualized; in **B,** both deep and superficial veins are opacified.

not bear weight, a fact accomplished by placing a box under the opposite foot and having the patient support his weight on that side. This allows the deep leg veins of the examined side, as a result of the non-weight-bearing position, not to be compressed by the calf muscles (Fig. 66-1). It also permits the examined side to be freely rotated for proper filming.

An exception to the upright position is in the evaluation of the saphenous veins for bypasses. This examination is performed with the patient supine (on the long leg changer) and without tourniquets. The contrast medium is injected into a superficial vein in the dorsum of the foot. A No. 21 or 23 butterfly needle is used and is connected with a three-way stopcock to a heparinized saline solution (5000 units of heparin in 500 ml of normal saline solution). At times, the large vein draining the great toe may be the only vein available. If no vein is distended after placement of a tourniquet, the leg is placed in a dependent position, with the patient sitting or standing. If distended veins are still not evident, the foot is soaked in warm water for 10 minutes. This usually induces distension of the veins. The presence of edema usually makes identification of veins extremely difficult. Even in the presence of edema, however, local finger compression with a tourniquet applied to the ankle usually allows at least one vein to be visualized.

The injection is usually made antegrade. Some authors, however, prefer a retrograde injection (needle pointing to the toes) claiming that this type of injection will ensure more complete opacification of the superficial and deep veins of the foot and leg. With injection of the dorsal superficial arch, contrast material passes directly to the anterior tibial veins and the deep plantar arch, which in turn empty into the posterior tibial and peroneal veins. A tourniquet is applied above the ankle to direct the contrast into the deep veins. A tourniquet is not used when the saphenous veins are being studied[13] for bypass surgery.

A 45% contrast solution is used. This contrast results in adequate opacification of the veins and in a lesser incidence of postphlebography thrombophlebitis and pain than a 60% contrast solution[14,15] does.

It is extremely important that the injection site be closely monitored so that extravasation of contrast, which can lead to skin sloughing, does not occur. The tip of the needle should be inspected visually and palpated during the injection to make certain that extravasation does not occur. Periodically throughout the injection an attempt is made to aspirate blood into the tubing. Blood return is a helpful (but not totally reliable) sign that the needle is in the correct position. Fluoroscopy and plain film examination of the puncture site can also be performed to further exclude the possibility of extravasation.

The initial film is taken after injection of 60 ml of contrast medium; additional increments of 10 ml are then given for the subsequent three films. Anteroposterior, lateral, and oblique films of the foot and leg are obtained. These views allow differentiation of the deep and superficial veins and separation of the many deep veins from each other. Occasionally a small thrombus will be demonstrated on only one of the four views. Anteroposterior views of the thigh and pelvis are then taken, with the pelvic film obtained immediately after the patient is placed in the horizontal

supine position. A single anteroposterior view is all that is necessary for visualization of the popliteal, femoral, and iliac veins.

Upon completion of the examination the patient is returned to the horizontal position, and the examined leg is elevated for 10 to 15 minutes. Approximately 200 ml of the heparinized solution is rapidly infused. These steps are performed to clear the venous system of contrast medium because the incidence of contrast-induced phlebitis is related to its contact time with the venous endothelium.

Indications for phlebography are

1. Diagnosis and evaluation of the extent of DVT
2. Evaluation of the saphenous veins prior to bypass surgery
3. Postphlebitic syndrome
4. Varicose veins
5. The rare congenital malformations

This chapter is primarily concerned with acute venous thrombosis.

The main phlebographic criterion of acute venous thrombosis is the presence of a filling defect within an opacified vein, with a sharply delineated thrombus demonstrated on at least two films. Nonfilling of the deep veins (when strict criteria for the performance of the phlebogram have been fulfilled) usually indicates venous thrombosis.

Nonfilling of the entire deep system with proper technique is due to the inability of the contrast medium to enter the occluded veins. Localized nonfilling of veins with bypassing collaterals indicates venous obstruction (recent or long standing).

Phlebographic Patterns of Acute Deep Venous Thrombosis of Lower Extremity

While past phlebographic exploration focused primarily on the leg and thigh veins, recent findings have emphasized

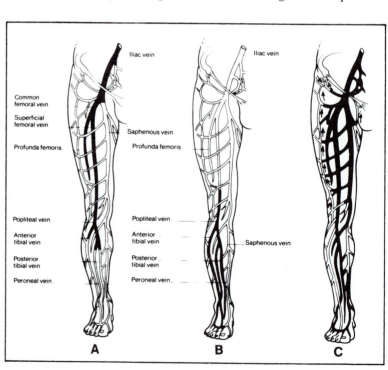

Figure 66-2. Diagrams of three patterns of lower extremity venous thrombosis: **A.** Pattern of an iliofemoral venous thrombosis. **B.** Pattern of calf vein thrombosis extending into the popliteal vein. **C.** Pattern of massive vein thrombosis involving both deep and superficial channels characteristic of phlegmasia cerulea dolens.

the necessity of examining all segments of the venous tree. Phlebographic patterns of venous thrombosis are diagrammed in Figure 66-2.

Venous Thrombosis in the Foot

Acute venous thrombosis in the foot has rarely been mentioned or reported in the literature. However, it has been shown that not infrequently venous thrombosis of the leg originates in the foot veins. Thomas and O'Dwyer[16] in a study of 188 legs found thrombosis in 106 cases, distributed as follows: veins above and below the ankle were affected in 46%; above the ankle in 44%; and in the foot alone in only 10%. The age of the thrombi in the foot and leg often differed: in certain cases the plantar thrombus was more recent, whereas in other cases the thrombi appeared to be of similar ages at both sites. The most commonly involved veins were the lateral plantar and, much less commonly, the medial ones. It is of interest that a number of these thromboses in the foot were accompanied by pulmonary emboli. If the examination were confined to the leg and thigh veins alone, the source of emboli would have remained undetected. The recent literature on the subject suggests that foot vein thrombosis is less infrequent than previously believed, and it is therefore recommended that at the time of the leg phlebogram, a view of the foot also be incorporated in the study.

Lower Leg Thrombosis

Thrombosis confined to the leg veins may affect one, two, or all three major trunks (Figs. 66-3 to 66-6). In our experience isolated involvement of the anterior tibial veins is rare. As they are paired, only one of the two venae comitantes of the leg arteries may be involved, thereby allowing the venous flow return to be relatively normal. In the latter instance the clinical symptoms may not be pronounced. Thrombi may be completely or only partially obstructive. In the latter case the thrombus is separated from the wall of the vein by a stream of contrast material. Visualization of the soleal sinuses, which may be the origin of the deep vein thrombosis, is best demonstrated on the lateral view. In a series of 100 phlebograms of the lower extremity, De-Weese and Rogoff found thrombotic lesions in 43% confined to the tibial-peroneal veins.[17]

Femoropopliteal Vein Thrombosis

Femoropopliteal venous thrombosis may be localized to this segment, or associated with calf vein thrombi (Fig. 66-5 and 66-7). Thus, of 23 extremities with femoral vein involvement, DeWeese and Rogoff found 13 to be associated with thrombosis of calf veins.[17] Usually the occlusion of the superficial femoral vein extends from the adductor ten-

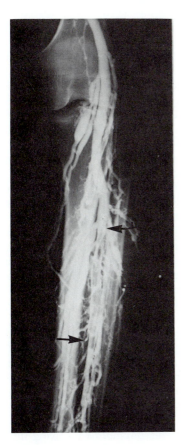

Figure 66-3. Tibial vein thrombosis incompletely occluding the lumen.

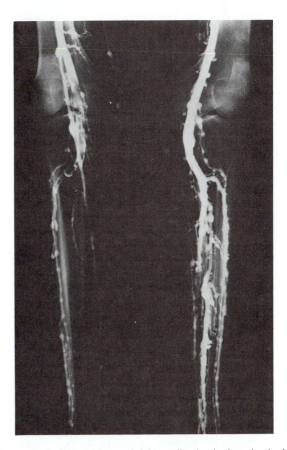

Figure 66-4. Bilateral leg and right popliteal vein thrombosis. Note absence of right peroneal and posterior tibial vein opacification, suggesting their complete thrombotic occlusion. *Right:* Anterior tibial and popliteal veins show thrombotic material in continuity, with free-floating clots within the veins. *Left:* Leg presents thrombosis of posterior tibial veins at the midcalf level.

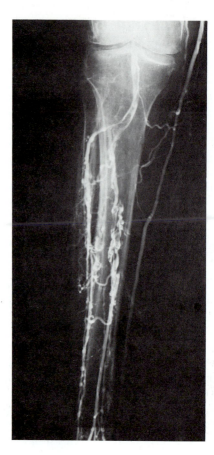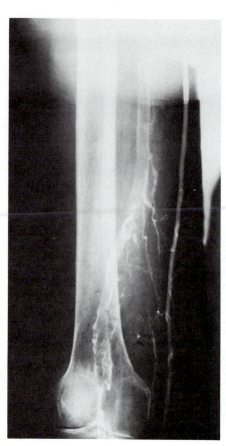

Figure 66-5. Extensive venous thrombosis involving the leg and thigh. *Leg:* Tibial and popliteal vein thrombosis. Note thrombi in peroneal and posterior tibial vein, extending into the popliteal at the confluence of these veins and into the proximal segment (*arrows*). *Thigh:* Popliteal and superficial femoral thrombotic occlusion. The two veins are completely blocked by massive thrombosis. The greater saphenous vein is opacified.

don level and includes the common femoral vein. It appears that the initial location of the venous thrombosis is often similar to that of the femoral artery, as a result of mechanical trauma at the adductor canal level. Occlusion of the superficial femoral vein is shown on the venogram by nonfilling of this vein and by extensive collateral branches in the thigh. The saphenous and the profunda femoris veins serve as collaterals. In the presence of extensive femoropopliteal occlusion associated with calf vein thrombosis, clinical manifestations are quite evident (edema, tenderness, and cyanotic discoloration of the skin). Occasionally, the condition may assume the more dramatic form of phlegmasia cerulea dolens (Fig. 66-6).

Iliofemoral Venous Thrombosis

This pattern of venous thrombosis may be confined to the iliac veins or may be associated with involvement of the common femoral and possibly the superficial femoral vein and even with the lower leg veins. The origin of the thrombosis is often difficult to determine. In the combined iliofemoral and lower leg venous thrombosis, it is likely that the initial lesion is usually in the proximal tree. The age of the thrombi may provide a clue as to the sequence of the lesions. Thus, the thrombi removed from the older occlusions are more adherent and histologically more organized.

The relative incidence of iliofemoral thrombosis varies. It is reported as 12 to 14% by Mayor et al.[18] and as 34% by DeWeese and Rogoff.[17] In the latter authors' study of 100 phlebograms, there were 34 iliofemoral venous throm-

boses, of which ten had additional extensive obstruction of the lower leg and femoral veins. It is difficult to determine whether the thrombosis originated distally and subsequently had ascended towards the iliac or, conversely, had extended distally.[19,20] The clinical sequence of events or examination of the age of the venous clots may offer some help. If the latter are more adherent in the proximal venous segment, it is likely that the thrombotic process originated in the iliac veins (Fig. 66-8).

In the phlebographic interpretation of this pattern, the extent of collaterals may be indicative of the degree of deep vein occlusions. The great saphenous vein is usually patent to the groin level. The tributaries of the common and deep femoral veins, if opacified, communicate with the pelvic veins of the ipsilateral and contralateral iliac systems.

An interesting aspect of iliac vein thrombosis is the far more frequent involvement of the left common iliac vein than of the right. This is explained by the anatomic relationship of the right common iliac artery, which passes anterior to the left common iliac vein and thus results in compression of the vein against the spine.[21] This venous compression may induce decreased venous flow, which in some cases leads eventually to iliac vein thrombosis.

Clinically, the typical iliofemoral venous thrombosis may present as the classic phlegmasia alba dolens or "milk leg," well described during the last century.[22] In combined extensive venous thrombosis involving the distal venous tree, the clinical picture potentially may assume that of phlegmasia cerulea dolens, an ischemic form that is poten-

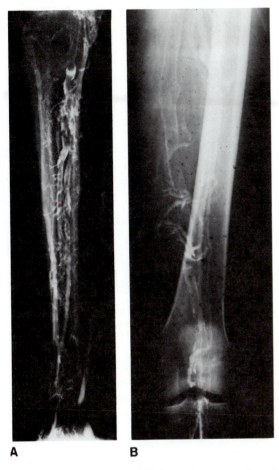

A **B**

Figure 66-6. A, B. Acute leg and thigh massive venous thrombosis of the phlegmasia cerulea dolens type. Note involvement of all leg veins, with thrombosis extending into the popliteal and femoral veins.

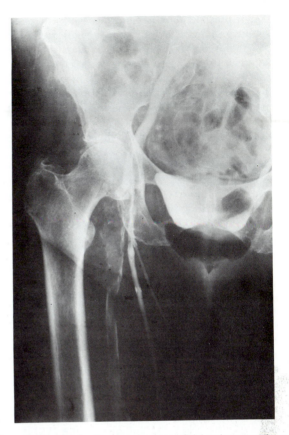

Figure 66-7. Massive thrombosis of superficial and common femoral veins associated with ipsilateral pelvic compression of iliac vein.

tially reversible but that if untreated may lead to gangrene.[23–25]

External and common iliac vein thrombosis may be demonstrated by ascending phlebography. If their visualization is inadequate, the involved side may be safely used for a percutaneous femoral vein injection of contrast medium. Alternatively the opposite iliac vein may be catheterized and the catheter advanced into the involved side through the inferior vena cava.

Internal Iliac and Pelvic Veins Thrombosis

Phlebography of the internal iliac vein (hypogastric) and its pelvic tributaries is technically more difficult than the previous phlebographic studies.[26] Internal iliac phlebography is rarely performed. The relative incidence of thrombosis of the pelvic veins is rather infrequent, as compared with that of the common and external iliac veins. Also, pulmonary embolism from these veins is equally rare. The pelvic veins are represented by a network around the bladder, rectum, and vagina. They are not easily demonstrable by phlebography unless they act as collaterals to an occlusion of the iliac veins and inferior vena cava.

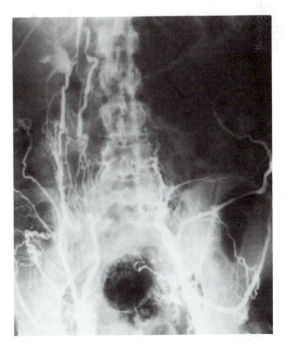

Figure 66-8. Complete thrombosis of the inferior vena cava and of both common iliac veins. Note marked collateral circulation attempting to compensate for the venous blockage.

Pelvic phlebography is performed with the patient in the supine position. The Valsalva maneuver with a percutaneous femoral contrast medium injection may demonstrate the internal iliac as far as the first competent valve. This may be followed by selective hypogastric phlebography, during which its tributaries may be enhanced by having the patient perform a Valsalva maneuver. In the past, intraosseous phlebography with a direct injection into the greater trochanter was used to opacify the hypogastric tributaries. This is rarely if ever used today.

A common problem, especially in patients with a pelvic tumor, is whether iliac vein obstruction is due to extrinsic compression, primary thrombosis, or a combination of the two. This diagnostic problem can usually be resolved by combined use of phlebography and CT, sonography, or MRI.

Inferior Vena Cavography

Occlusion of the inferior vena cava (IVC) may be congenital or acquired. The most common congenital obstructing lesion of the IVC is azygos continuation of the IVC in which the infrahepatic vena cava does not develop. Lower extremity drainage is then through the IVC and the ascending lumbar-azygos system. These patients may or may not have lower extremity edema. A rare congenital lesion (with most of the cases reported from Japan) is a bandlike obstruction of the IVC just below the entrance of the IVC into the right atrium.

Primary thrombosis of the IVC is rare. Thrombosis is usually due to extension of an iliofemoral thrombosis (Fig. 66-9) or to progression of a renal vein tumor-thrombus with carcinoma of the kidney. Tumor can also produce extrinsic

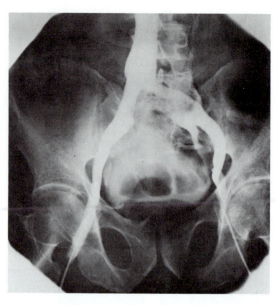

Figure 66-10. Iliocaval phlebogram showing partial occlusion of left common iliac vein due to compression by right iliac artery.

narrowing of the IVC (Fig. 66-10), as well as of the iliac veins (as mentioned above), with thrombosis occasionally superimposed upon the narrowing. When thrombosis of the IVC is secondary to that of the iliofemoral veins, venous thrombosis of the lower extremities may also be present. In a series of 178 combined lower extremity and IVC phlebographies, Ranniger[27] found an overall involvement of the IVC in 35%. Of this group, isolated IVC involvement occurred in 12%; there was associated involvement of one iliac vein in 11%, and lower leg involvement in 12%.

As the above findings demonstrate, in the presence of bilateral lower extremity edema, inferior vena cavography should be performed because it may reveal congenital or acquired obstruction of the IVC.

Inferior vena cavography is usually performed by unilateral percutaneous femoral vein catheterization. The IVC should be studied up to its entrance into the right atrium. Biplane examination is important for proper identification of the normal and pathologic features.

IVC thrombus, if an extension from an iliac lesion, may occlude the IVC only partially and thus may be floating in the caval lumen. If detached, such a thrombus is a grave potential hazard of a fatal pulmonary embolism.

Complications

Systemic

Contrast media produce various types of adverse reactions. Idiosyncratic "allergic-type" reactions may result in hives, itching, layngeal edema, bronchospasm, and circulatory collapse. Nonidiosyncratic reactions due to direct toxic effects of the contrast medium may result in nausea, vomiting, cardiac arrhythmias, pulmonary edema, and cardiovascular collapse. It is sometimes difficult to differentiate between these two types of reactions. In addition, contrast media

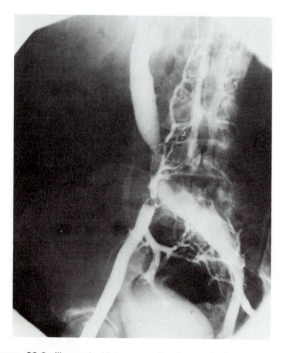

Figure 66-9. Iliocaval phlebogram showing extrinsic narrowing at the iliocaval junction due to tumor.

are known to cause nephrotoxicity, especially in patients with impaired renal function. A good review of the adverse reactions to contrast media was written by Cohan and Dunnick.[28]

Before phlebography is performed, an allergy history is taken. Minor allergic reactions such as urticaria may occur in 5% of patients. With a history of allergies, the incidence is 10%; if the patient has had a previous reaction to contrast media, the incidence is 15%.[29] There is evidence which indicates that premedication with steroids will lower the incidence of these reactions.[30] Because of this we place patients who have had contrast reactions or who have a history of other allergies or hay fever on steroids for 1 day prior to the examination. In addition, an antihistaminic is given immediately preceding the phlebogram. There is evidence that allergic-type reactions are less frequent with low-osmolarity agents, so these agents are given to patients who have had reactions in the past or who have a history of other allergies.

Most phlebographic techniques require the use of at least 100 ml of contrast medium. Contrast-induced nephropathy may occur in patients given contrast media. Contrast-induced nephropathy may occur in patients with normal renal function, but it is much more likely to occur in patients with impaired renal function. Recent evidence seems to indicate that the incidence of contrast nephropathy is lessened when the low-osmolarity agents are used.

Local

Extravasation of contrast medium at the site of the injection is avoidable in most instances, provided great care is taken to assure the proper position of the needle or catheter in the vein.[31] Injection should be done slowly if there is any evidence of the slightest leakage through the needle puncture of the vein. In a normally vascularized foot, extravasation of small amounts of contrast medium may resolve itself with local applications of moist heat, elevation of the limb, and anti-inflammatory agents. However, in a foot in which there is arterial insufficiency superimposed on the venous problem, one has to be extremely cautious to avoid the extravasation of contrast medium that may result in a necrotic lesion of the overlying skin. However, such an event should be treated promptly as mentioned above.

Morphologic changes in vessel endothelium caused by contrast media are well known.[32] The harmful effects are translated clinically as pain, local redness, swelling, and ultimately, thrombosis. Thrombotic side effects of lower limb phlebography have been reported, but the incidence is rather small.[33]

Increased uptake of fibrinogen ^{125}I occurs with venous thrombosis but also occurs with phlebitis without thrombosis. Increased uptake of fibrinogen ^{125}I was encountered in 30 of 55 patients after normal ascending phlebography. However, only three patients had symptoms develop and were treated for thrombophlebitis. In another study, two thirds of patients with abnormal fibrinogen ^{125}I scans after phlebography had thrombus demonstrated on repeated phlebography. This report also showed that by using dilute contrast medium the incidence of deep vein thrombosis after phlebography was 26% when ionic contrast medium

was used; the incidence was reduced to 2% by the use of nonionic contrast medium. In addition, superficial thrombophlebitis was observed in 14% of patients after phlebography with ionic contrast agent but in no patients studied with nonionic contrast medium. Anticoagulation therapy was also shown to be effective in preventing contrast medium–induced thrombophlebitis.

Phlebography often produces discomfort and pain (often considerable) during the procedure. Occasionally it produces a postphlebography syndrome of pain, swelling, heat, and erythema beginning 12 to 36 hours after the study. As noted in the section on techniques, pain is considerably increased when tourniquets are used. One report demonstrated that the use of dilute contrast medium reduced the incidence of pain during the procedure from 59 to 30% and reduced the incidence of the postphlebography syndrome from 24 to 7.5%. Pain during the procedure can also be reduced by the use of nonionic contrast medium. In addition, the postphlebography syndrome likely can be eliminated by techniques that minimize the contact time between the contrast agent and the venous endothelium, as described above.

Presumptive diagnosis of pulmonary embolization has been reported by some observers. Usually these instances are related to small pulmonary emboli, and if the emboli are treated promptly with intravenous heparin, the condition resolves within 10 to 14 days.

Cases of extensive thrombosis have been reported exceptionally.[34] Even more exceptionally reported were cases of phlegmasia cerulea dolens and gangrene following peripheral phlebography.[35,36]

In general, phlebography in the hands of experienced angiographers has proved safe and useful in the diagnosis and management of patients with deep venous thrombosis. Knowledge of potential hazards should guide the angiographer or vascular surgeon to prevent any serious after effects.

Upper Extremity Venous Thrombosis

Acute DVT of the upper extremity (Fig. 66-11) is uncommon, formerly accounting for only 1 to 2% of the total incidence of all DVT.[37] The relative and absolute incidences have increased in recent years because of the frequent use of transvenous pacemakers and indwelling catheters (Swan-Ganz, dialysis, hyperalimentation). Studies have shown an incidence of DVT in at least 25% in this pacemaker-catheter group of patients. In other cases the DVT may result following fracture or dislocation of the clavicle or more commonly may not be related to any known injury. This latter form of DVT is usually known as the Paget-Schroetter syndrome.[38] The Paget-Schroetter syndrome is attributed to compression of the subclavian vein between the first rib and clavicle. Some authors emphasize the primary or unknown aspect, and others emphasize the traumatic or stress aspect of Paget-Schroetter syndrome. Hughes, in a comprehensive review in 1949, concluded that most such cases bear some relationship to the thoracic outlet compression syndrome.[38] This opinion was subsequently documented by many others. Although in these cases the clinical manifestations are mostly due to subclavian

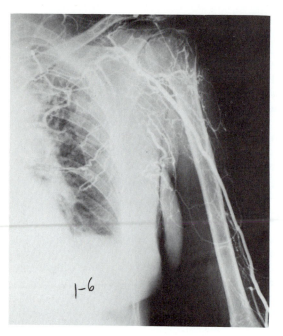

Figure 66-11. Subclavian-axillary vein thrombisis of undetermined etiology. Note extensive collateral channels around the shoulder and the chest.

venous thrombosis, Adams et al. reported an entity of intermittent subclavian vein obstruction without thrombosis. All these cases occur predominantly in the right arm.[39]

Other causes of acute thrombosis of the upper extremity are congestive heart failure, cor pulmonale, coagulation abnormalities, lymphoma, polycythemia, and thrombocytosis.[37] Of these factors, congestive heart failure was reported by Loring as the most frequent. It occurs most commonly in women (male:female ratio, 1:25). The vein most frequently involved was the subclavian, often combined with the lower jugular vein.[40]

A few other rare etiologic factors include metastases to the axillary lymph nodes (especially from carcinoma of the breast) and intravenous injections of chemicals, antibiotics, etc. known to injure the venous endothelium.

Phlebography of Upper Extremity

Phlebography of the upper extremity is best obtained by injecting the contrast medium into the basilic vein. If injected into the cephalic vein or one of its tributaries, the contrast medium may bypass a thrombus in the axillary vein. In cases with intermittent subclavian-axillary compression, phlebographic study combined with venous pressure determinations extending from the superior vena cava to the axillary vein or more distally may help in establishing the correct diagnosis (Fig. 66-11).

Swinton et al., in a series of phlebographies performed on 20 of 23 patients with venous thrombosis, found two more common patterns: (1) localized plugs in the subclavian-axillary junction and (2) long blocks of the entire axillary vein.[41] Brachial and cephalic venous thrombosis were not noted in this series. Campbell et al., in a series of 25 patients in whom 22 phlebograms were carried out, found that they

all confirmed the diagnosis but often failed to define the proximal extent of the obstruction.[42]

In the majority of cases phlebography is important for establishing the diagnosis of DVT and also for planning the method of treatment.

Management

The still prevailing opinion that nonoperative treatment of major venous thrombosis of the upper extremity carries little residual disability is at variance with the results of its natural course. Tilney et al.,[43] based on a study of 48 patients, have found that 16 of 34 with residual symptoms, or 48%, had resulting long-term disability. In support of this finding, DeWeese et al.[44] have shown that in 6 of 23 patients, or 25%, subclavian thrombectomy was necessary and resulted in complete relief of symptoms. While conservative management is adequate in many patients, some patients probably require more aggressive therapy. In this regard a recent study of 41 patients[45] showed that thrombosis due to intrinsic damage (venous lines, drug abuse, hypercoagulable states) responded well to anticoagulation and rarely caused persistent symptoms. Conversely, when thrombosis was due to extrinsic narrowing (effort-induced, trauma, neoplastic disease), only 50% of patients were free of symptoms at long-term follow-up. Since this latter group of patients does poorly with anticoagulation alone, additional treatments with fibrinolytic agents or operation should be considered.

DUPLEX ULTRASONOGRAPHY

The recent application of duplex ultrasonography to the problems inherent in the diagnosis of venous diseases has attracted widespread interest.[5–8] Because of its noninvasive character, duplex ultrasonography is painless and has no associated morbidity or mortality. For these and other reasons, duplex techniques enjoy a high level of patient acceptance, and for the physician who suspects the presence of venous thrombosis, duplex ultrasonography provides a quick, comfortable, and inexpensive method for differential diagnosis.

Technique for Detection of Venous Thrombi

Lower Extremity

A systematic approach to the named veins of the lower extremity begins by applying the duplex probe to the femoral triangle in a manner that provides a longitudinal image of the common femoral vein just below the inguinal ligament. The Doppler gate is adjusted to lie in the center of the venous channel, and the Doppler angle is set parallel to the direction of blood flow. To test for the presence of blood clots within the vein, the examiner applies probe pressure while watching the vein walls approach each other and meet.

By rotating the probe so that it is perpendicular to the long axis of the vein, a transverse image is obtained. Repetition of the compression maneuver must result in complete collapse of the vessel for normalcy to be deter-

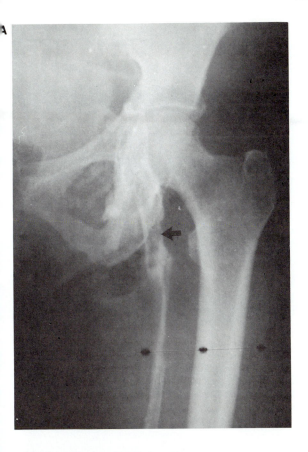

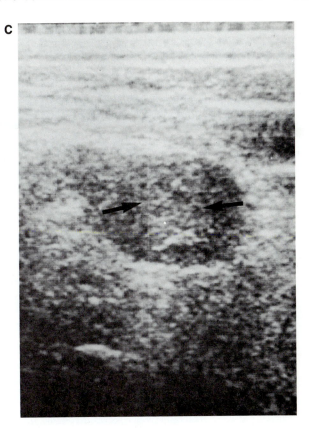

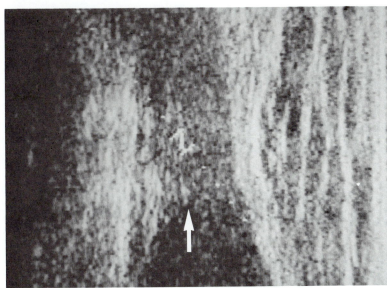

Figure 66–12. A large thrombus in the common femoral vein is indicated on contrast venography **(A)** by the *black arrow*. The same thrombus is visualized on duplex ultrasonography in the longitudinal projection **(B)** by the *white arrow* and in the transverse projection **(C)** by the *black arrows*.

mined. Partial compressibility or incompressibility in both the longitudinal and transverse projections is considered an indication of the possible presence of thrombus. Incompressibility in both projections, coupled with the absence of Doppler evidence of blood flow, even with augmentation maneuvers, is strong evidence of the presence of occlusive thrombus. Partial compressibility in both projections with accompanying weak Doppler signals indicates the presence of nonocclusive thrombus, partial recanalization, or chronic thrombosis.

In each lower extremity tested, the entire length of the common femoral, superficial femoral, greater saphenous, popliteal, peroneal, and anterior and posterior tibial veins must be visualized, insonated, and compressed as described.

Upper Extremity
As with the lower extremity, the entire length of the cephalic, basilic, brachial, axillary, and subclavian veins must be visualized, insonated, and compressed to rule out the

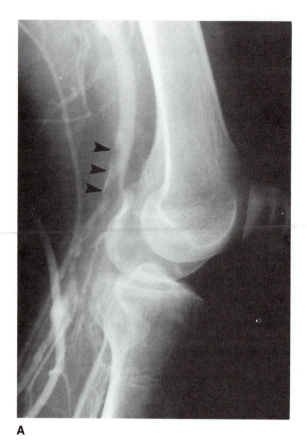

A

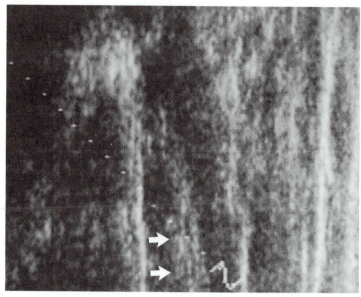

B

Figure 66-13. Contrast venogram **(A)** reveals the presence of a large, tongue-shaped thrombus (*black arrows*) in the popliteal vein. Duplex ultrasonography **(B)** visualizes the same thrombus (*white arrows*) with similar detail and definition.

presence of thrombus. In some patients the curvature of the clavicle may prevent compression of the subclavian vein. The vein walls can be made to approximate by instructing the patient to inhale sharply through the nose or to "sniff." This maneuver exaggerates negative intrathoracic pressure enough to collapse the normal subclavian vein.

Comparison of Duplex Ultrasonography and Ascending Contrast Venography in Diagnosis of Venous Thrombosis

Several such comparisons have been reported and all of them utilize the results of contrast venography as the standard against which duplex ultrasonographic results are compared. In this setting, reported sensitivities range from 90 to 100%; specificities range from 89 to 99%; positive predictive values range from 93 to 100%, and overall accuracies range from 93 to 100%. By their nature, these types of statistics are based on the presumption that contrast venography is 100% accurate all of the time. However, experienced radiologists acknowledge that although diagnostic errors are infrequent, they do occcur. When coming from an experienced and skilled laboratory, duplex results are as reliable as those of contrast venography and can be used confidently as the basis for treatment decisions in cases of venous thrombosis (Figs. 66-12 and 66-13).

REFERENCES

1. Kakkar VV: Deep vein thrombosis: Detection and prevention. Circulation 51:8, 1975.
2. Cranley JJ, Canos AJ, et al: The diagnosis of deep venous thrombosis. Arch Surg 111:34, 1976.
3. Moser KM, Brach BB, et al.: Clinically suspected deep venous thrombosis of the lower extremities. JAMA 237:2195, 1977.
4. Barnes RW, Collicott PE, et al.: Noninvasive quantification of maximum venous outflow in acute thrombophlebitis. Surgery 72:971, 1972.
5. Montefusco CM, Bakal CB, Sprayregen S, Veith FJ: Comparison of duplex ultrasonography and ascending contrast venography in the diagnosis of deep vein thrombosis. J Vasc Surg (accepted for publication).
6. Sullivan ED, Peter DJ, Cranley JJ: Real-time B-mode venous ultrasound. J Vasc Surg 1:465–471, 1984.
7. Oliver MA: Duplex scanning in venous disease. Bruit 9:206–209, 1985.
8. Hannan LJ, Stedje KJ, et al.: Venous imaging of the extremities. Bruit 10:29, 1986.
9. dos Santos JC: La Phlébographie directe: Conception, technique, premiers resultats. J Intern Chir 3:625, 1938.
10. Luke JC: Diagnosis of chronic enlargement of leg, with description of new syndrome. Surg Gynecol Obstet 73:472, 1941.
11. Rabinov K, Paulin S: Roentgen diagnosis of venous thrombosis in the leg. Arch Surg 104:134, 1972.
12. Thomas ML: Phlebography. Arch Surg 104:145, 1972.
13. Veith FJ, Moss CM, Sprayregen S, Montefusco CM: Preopera-

tive saphenous venography in arterial reconstructive surgery of the lower extremity. Surgery 85:253, 1979.

14. Bettman MA, Paulin S: Leg phlebography: The incidence, nature and modification of undesirable side effects. Radiology 122:101, 1977.

15. Bettman MA, Salzman EW, Rosenthal D, Clagett P, et al.: Reduction of venous thrombosis complicating phlebography. AJR 134:1169–1172, 1980.

16. Thomas ML, O'Dwyer JA: A phlebographic study of the incidence and significance of venous thrombosis in the foot. AJR 130:751, 1978.

17. DeWeese JA, Rogoff SM: Phlebographic patterns of acute deep venous thrombosis of the leg. Surgery 53:99, 1963.

18. Mavor EE, Galloway JMD, et al.: Venography in iliofemoral venous thromboembolism. Surg Gynecol Obstet 129:57, 1969.

19. Thomas ML, McAllister V: The radiological progression of deep venous thrombus. Radiology 99:37, 1971.

20. Warren R: Behavior of venous thrombi. Arch Surg 115:1151, 1980.

21. May R, Thurner J: The cause of predominantly sinistral occurrence of thrombosis of the pelvic veins. Angiology 8:419, 1957.

22. Trousseau R: Clinique Médicale de l'Hotel Dieu de Paris, Vol III. Paris: Bailliere, 1868.

23. Haimovici H, Suffness G: Gangrene of the extremities of venous origin: Case report. Am J Med Sci 215:278, 1948.

24. Haimovici H: Gangrene of the extremities of venous origin: Review of literature with case reports. Circulation 1:225, 1950.

25. Haimovici H: Ischemic Forms of Venous Thrombosis: Phlegmasia Cerulea Dolens, Venous Gangrene. Springfield, Ill: Charles C. Thomas, 1971.

26. Thomas ML, Browse NL: Internal iliac vein thrombosis.

27. Ranniger K: Obstruction of the inferior vena cava with edema or thrombophlebitis of the lower extremities. AJR 109:563, 1970.

28. Cohan RH, Dunnick NR: Intravascular contrast media: Adverse reactions. AJR 149:665–670, 1987.

29. Shehadi WH: Contrast media adverse reactions: Occurrence, recurrence and distribution patterns. Radiology 143:11–17, 1982.

30. Lasser EC, Berry CC, et al.: Pretreatment with corticosteroids to alleviate reactions to intravenous contrast material. N Engl J Med 317:845–849, 1987.

31. Spigos DG, Thane TT, et al.: Skin necrosis following extravasation during peripheral phlebography. Radiology 123:605, 1977.

32. Zinner G, Gottlob R: Morphologic changes in vessel endothelia caused by contrast media. Angiology 10:207, 1959.

33. Albrechtsson U, Olsson CG: Thrombosis following phlebography with ionic and non-ionic contrast media. Acta Radiologica 20:46, 1979.

34. Albrechtsson U, Olsson CG: Thrombotic side-effects of lower-limb phlebography. Lancet 1:723, 1976.

35. Thomas ML: Gangrene following peripheral phlebography of the legs. Br J Radiol 43:528, 1970.

36. Lipchik EO, Altman DP: Phlegmasia cerulea dolens. Radiology 133:81, 1979.

37. Prescott SM, Tikoff G: Deep venous thrombosis of the upper extremity: A reappraisal. Circulation 59:350, 1979.

38. Hughes ESR: Venous obstruction in upper extremity (Paget-Schroetter's syndrome). Surg Gynecol Obstet 88:89, 1949.

39. Adams JT, DeWeese JA, et al.: Intermittent subclavian vein obstruction without thrombosis. Surgery 63:147, 1968.

40. Loring WE: Venous thrombosis in the upper extremities as a complication of myocardial failure. Am J Med 12:397, 1952.

41. Swinton NW, Edgett JW, et al.: Primary subclavian-axillary vein thrombosis. Circulation 38:737, 1968.

42. Campbell CB, Chandler JG, et al.: Axillary, subclavian, and brachiocephalic vein obstruction. Surgery 82:816, 1977.

43. Tilney NL, Griffiths HJG, et al.: Natural history of major venous thrombosis of the upper extremity. Arch Surg 101:792, 1970.

44. DeWeese JA, Adams JT, et al.: Subclavian venous thrombectomy. Circulation (suppl II) 41:158, 1970.

45. Donayre CE, White GH, Mehringer SM, et al.: Pathogenesis determines late morbidity of axillosubclavian vein thrombosis. Am J Surg 152:179–184, 1986.

CHAPTER 67
Varicose Veins

Kenneth J. Cherry, Jr., and Larry H. Hollier

Varicose veins are a problem throughout the world. Prevalence rates vary from 0.1 to 50% in adult populations, with striking geographic disparities.[1-4] Coon and colleagues in 1973 estimated that 12% of the U.S. adult population, or 24 million persons at that time, had varicose veins.[5] Western industrialized nations have much higher prevalence rates than traditional nonindustrialized countries,[6] and one study of South Pacific peoples showed a marked disparity between those living traditionally and those adopting Western lifestyles.[7]

The etiology of varicose veins remains unknown. Diet, activity, female sex, race, weight, pregnancy, age, and hereditary predisposition have all been implicated. At the Mayo Clinic, over half the patients seen for varicose veins have family members with varicosities. Reagan and Folse reported that femoral vein reflux was twice as common in the children of parents with varicose veins.[8] Adults with positive family histories and normal limbs have a greater incidence of incompetent iliofemoral valves.[9] Occupations requiring prolonged sitting or standing are thought to exacerbate the problem.[1] Pregnancy, if not a cause of varicosities, is certainly an aggravating factor, with many patients dating the onset of varicosities to a specific pregnancy. Women are afflicted more often than men; Coon et al. reported a 36% prevalence in women and a 19% prevalence in men.[5] Older persons are more commonly affected, with a reported prevalence in the United States of less than 1% in persons 20 to 29 years old, and greater than 50% in persons over 70 years old. The female to male ratio decreases as age increases.[5]

PHYSIOLOGY AND PATHOPHYSIOLOGY

The deep veins normally return 85 to 90% of the venous blood to the heart, with the superficial veins transporting the remainder. It is thought that the saphenous systems contribute to thermal regulatory functions of the body by expanding or contracting in response to nerve stimuli or temperature changes without alterations in pressure.[10] The superficial system also seems to function as an accessory venous system, becoming clinically important in the presence of acute deep venous disease.

Primary varicosities of both the greater and lesser saphenous systems are the result of incompetent valves. McIrvine et al. found saphenofemoral junction incompetence in 82% of patients with primary varicosities studied by Doppler ultrasound.[11] Sequential retrograde valvular incompetence arises from the saphenofemoral junction or, less commonly, from incompetent perforator valves. Whether the incompetence is the result of inherently weak valves or of weak walls with secondary weakening of the valves is a subject of much debate.[4,5,8,9] The superficial veins are poorly supported by surrounding tissues and inherently lacking in strength. Whatever the cause of valvular incompetence, the resulting relative venous hypertension gives rise to symptoms of heaviness and aching over the varicosities and localized swelling. Complications include thrombophlebitis, dermatitis, variceal hemorrhage, and less commonly, ulceration. The greater saphenous system is involved five to six times more frequently than the lesser saphenous system.

Arteriovenous shunts in patients with varicose veins have been documented by several authors.[12-14] Whether they cause or result from the varicosities is unknown, as is the role they play in pathophysiology.

ANATOMY

The venous system of the lower extremities is essentially made up of three elements: the deep system, the perforating or communicating system, and the superficial system. All these systems have valves designed to drive blood flow into the deep system and thence to the heart. The greater saphenous vein begins in the medial foot at the confluence of the dorsal venous arch, digital veins from the toes, and the perforating tributary vein from the medial aspect of the foot (Fig. 67-1). It receives tributaries from the deep foot veins up to the level of the malleolus. Above this level

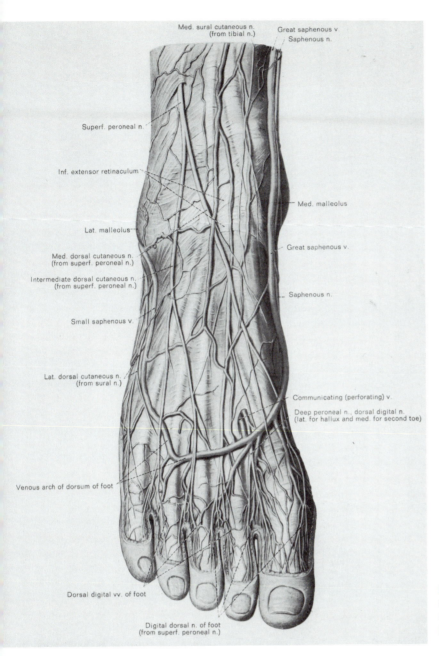

Med. sural cutaneous n. (from tibial n.)

Great saphenous v.
Saphenous n.

Superf. peroneal n.

Inf. extensor retinaculum

Med. malleolus

Lat. malleolus

Great saphenous v.

Med. dorsal cutaneous n. (from superf. peroneal n.)

Intermediate dorsal cutaneous n. (from superf. peroneal n.)

Saphenous n.

Small saphenous v.

Lat. dorsal cutaneous n. (from sural n.)

Communicating (perforating) v.

Deep peroneal n., dorsal digital n. (lat. for hallux and med. for second toe)

Venous arch of dorsum of foot

Dorsal digital vv. of foot

Digital dorsal n. of foot (from superf. peroneal n.)

Figure 67-1. Cutaneous nerves and veins of dorsum of right foot. (From Sobotta and Figge: *Atlas of Human Anatomy*, vol. 3, 9th English ed., Baltimore-Munich, Urban & Schwarzenberg, 1977.)

the valve system directs flow inward toward the deep system. The vein passes anterior to the medial malleolus, along the anteromedial border of the leg (Figs. 67-2 and 67-3). It runs posterior to the medial condyles of the tibia and femur and along the medial side of the thigh toward the fossa ovalis, where it joins the femoral vein. Along its course it is joined by perforating veins; the most common sites are along the distal third of the leg. The perforating veins in the distal third of the leg join the posterior venous arch, which rejoins the saphenous vein at or above the knee level. Between the greater and lesser saphenous systems are freely communicating veins. A persistent perforating vein is found near the junction of the middle and distal thirds of the thigh (Fig. 67-4). At the saphenofemoral junction are many named tributaries, including the lateral and medial femoral cutaneous veins, the external circumflex

iliac vein, the superficial epigastric vein, and the external pudendal veins. The saphenous nerve is in intimate contact with the greater saphenous vein from the medial malleolus to just above knee level. At this level it pierces the deep fascia and joins the superficial femoral artery just above the adductor hiatus.

The lesser saphenous system begins posterior to the lateral malleolus. It is a continuation of the lateral marginal vein of the foot. It receives tributaries from the medial and lateral aspects of the leg and communicates with the deep system through perforating veins. Many of these deep perforating veins are continuous with the deep venous sinusoids of the soleus muscle. Avulsion of these may give rise to major hemorrhage at operation. The lesser saphenous vein courses posteriorly along the leg; unlike the greater saphenous it pierces the fascia, so at the popliteal level

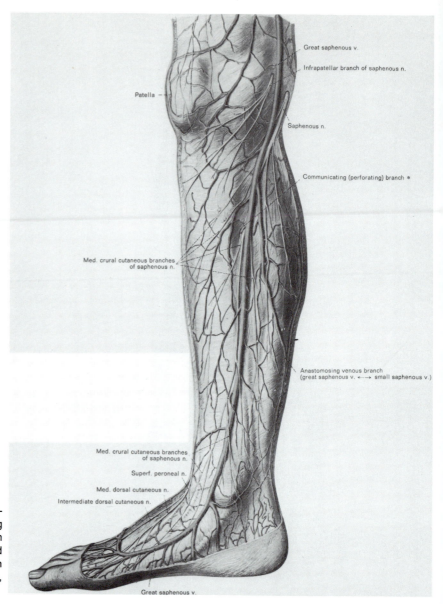

Figure 67-2. Cutaneous nerves and veins of medial side of right leg and foot. The communicating (perforating) veins connect the subcutaneous with the deep muscular veins. (From Sobotta and Figge: *Atlas of Human Anatomy*, vol. 3, 9th English ed., Baltimore-Munich, Urban & Schwarzenberg, 1977.)

the vein is deep to the fascia and is technically a part of the deep venous system. The lesser saphenous vein normally terminates in the popliteal vein, but it may continue up the posterior aspect of the thigh to join the deep muscular veins or indeed to join the medial femoral cutaneous branch of the greater saphenous system. The lesser saphenous vein is accompanied in its distal two thirds by the sural nerve.

DIAGNOSIS

Patients usually come to the physician with complaints of unsightliness, aching, heaviness, fatigue, or burning, which are aggravated by standing or sitting and which seem to worsen as the day progresses. The symptoms are relieved by elevation of the extremities. The varicosities may be easily seen in most patients. In markedly obese patients, varicosities that are not visible can be palpated.

Classically the competence of valves is determined by clinical tests, such as the Trendelenburg or retrograde filling test. In this test the extremity is elevated, thereby emptying the superficial veins, and a tourniquet applied at the mid-thigh level. The patient then stands up. If the superficial veins do not refill until the tourniquet is released, saphenous incompetence and primary varicosities are diagnosed. The lesser saphenous system is examined in a similar manner but with digital compression of the popliteal space. When the patient stands, if the veins fill before release of the tourniquet, the perforating veins are incompetent. These two entities can exist separately or in combination.

Ascending phlebography, descending phlebography, and varicography have been advocated as tests to assess and document incompetence of the superficial system.[15–18] Doppler examination and duplex scanning (Fig. 67-5) of the superficial system are now performed, and documentation of incompetence is easily obtained.[11,19–21] Normally in the management of varicose veins, more formal testing

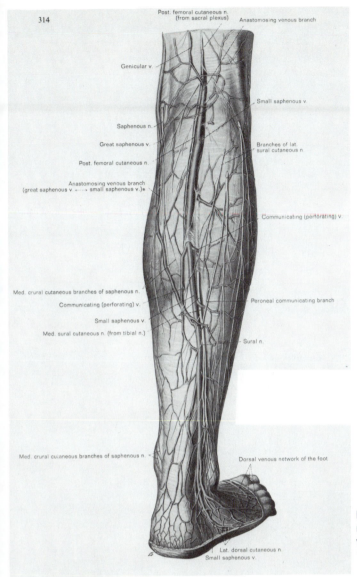

314

Post. femoral cutaneous n.
(from sacral plexus)

Anastomosing venous branch

Genicular v.

Small saphenous v.

Saphenous n.

Great saphenous v.

Branches of lat.
sural cutaneous n.

Post. femoral cutaneous n.

Anastomosing venous branch
(great saphenous v. ←· · · · → small saphenous v.)·

Communicating (perforating) v.

Med. crural cutaneous branches of saphenous n.

Communicating (perforating) v.

Peroneal communicating branch

Small saphenous v.

Med. sural cutaneous n. (from tibial n.)

Sural n.

Med. crural cutaneous branches of saphenous n.

Dorsal venous network of the foot

Lat. dorsal cutaneous n.
Small saphenous v.

Figure 67-3. Cutaneous nerves and veins of the dorsal aspect of right leg and foot. (From Sobotta and Figge: *Atlas of Human Anatomy*, vol. 3, 9th English ed., Baltimore-Munich, Urban & Schwarzenberg, 1977.)

than clinical testing is not necessary unless one suspects chronic venous insufficiency. Phlebography is not indicated unless chronic venous insufficiency with deep venous obstruction is suspected or unless the patient has unusual varicosities, for example, reminiscent of a Klippel-Trenaunay syndrome.

INDICATIONS

Patients whose varicosities have been complicated by phlebitis, skin changes, hemorrhage, or ulceration should be considered candidates for stripping of the appropriate superficial system and excision of varicosities, especially if the episodes have been multiple. Those patients whose varicosities are without complications but who are symptomatic with localized heaviness or aching are also considered suitable candidates for operation. Those patients whose varicosities are of cosmetic concern only are not so clearcut. It is the general practice at the Mayo Clinic to excise

these varicosities if the patient is young, rather than prescribe lifelong elastic support. Elderly patients who are more amenable to wearing elastic stockings are often treated nonoperatively. Debate continues about the preservation of the saphenous veins for coronary artery bypass. If the saphenous vein is massively dilated with varicosities in its own course as well as those of its tributaries, it would seem a poor conduit for coronary blood flow. If varicosities are present, but the saphenous itself is neither dilated nor incompetent, it can be preserved.

Of more concern is the treatment of secondary varicose veins. Varicosities may be excised in the face of an incompetent deep venous system, but excision is contraindicated when chronic venous insufficiency is on the basis of deep venous obstruction. Patients with varicose veins and chronic venous insufficiency whose varicosities are symptomatic and warrant excision should be studied by reliable noninvasive methods or by phlebography to determine whether obstruction or valvular incompetence is the cause of their deep venous disease. Patients with obstruction usually are

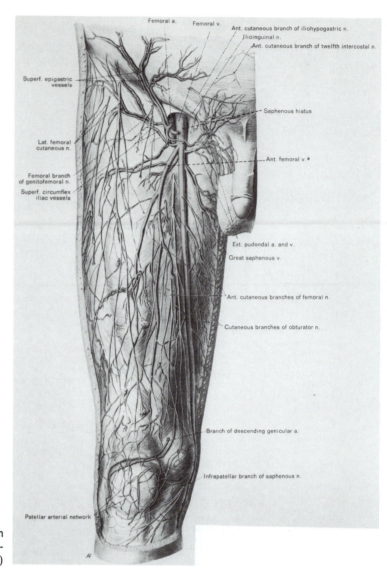

Figure 67-4. Cutaneous nerves and veins of thigh. (From Sobotta and Figge: *Atlas of Human Anatomy*, vol. 3, 9th English ed., Baltimore-Munich, Urban & Schwarzenberg, 1977.)

not candidates for excision of varicosities. Patients who have deep valvular incompetence and who undergo excision of symptomatic varicosities must still be treated with lifelong elastic support for the underlying chronic venous insufficiency.

SURGICAL TECHNIQUES

The necessity of stripping the saphenous system in addition to the excision of varicosities is undergoing continued and renewed questioning.[22–25] Currently at the Mayo Clinic, formal stripping of the appropriate saphenous system and individual excision of varicosities is the operative procedure of choice for most patients with primary varicose veins. Patients with localized varicosities and without demonstrable saphenous incompetence or dilation undergo excision of the varicosities without a formal stripping. Ligation of the saphenous at the saphenofemoral junction and excision of varicosities without formal stripping is not currently performed at the Mayo Clinic; review of the experience here makes us consider this a less than adequate operation.

Prior to operation the varicosities are marked with the patient standing. General anesthesia is employed in most instances. The patient is placed in the head-down position with the foot of the table elevated 15 to 30 degrees to minimize bleeding. An oblique incision is made in the groin, two finger-breadths lateral and two finger-breadths inferior to the pubic tubercle. The saphenofemoral junction is dissected free. The various tributaries are divided and ligated. In the ankle, the saphenous vein is dissected free just anterior to the medial malleolus. Disposable strippers are passed from distal to proximal, and the vein stripped. The distal stump is ligated, and the proximal stump, flush with the femoral vein, is both ligated and suture ligated.

Small incisions are then made over the varicosities, which are excised by the avulsion technique, generally without ligation. Perforating veins are ligated, if necessary, at the fascial level. The groin wounds are closed with subcutaneous and subcuticular Vicryl. The other wounds are closed with subcutaneous Vicryl and Steri-strips. The extremities are dressed with sterile gauze dressings, padding, Kerlex, and Ace wraps.

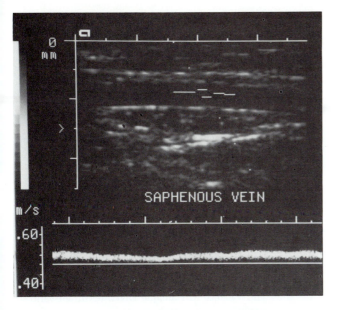

Figure 67-5. Duplex scan showing normal saphenous vein.

POSTOPERATIVE MANAGEMENT

On the night after operation, the patient's extremities are elevated in bed. On the first postoperative day, dressings are changed and elastic wraps reapplied. Patients are allowed to walk or to lie in bed. Standing or sitting is not allowed. Most patients are discharged on the second postoperative day with instructions to wrap their extremities to knee level for 1 month. Patients with chronic venous insufficiency are instructed to wrap their legs for 2 months, after which they are asked to return to the use of elastic stockings. The use of absorbable sutures obviates the need for suture removal. No complications from early mobilization and early discharge from the hospital have been encountered. Many patients are now admitted on the morning of surgery. It is anticipated that in the future some patients may be offered this operation on an outpatient basis.

RECURRENT VARICOSE VEINS

Recurrent varicose veins develop in 3 to 65% of patients after operation, depending on length of follow-up and modality of study.[26–28] The use of Doppler assessment may well increase the reported incidence of recurrence of varicosities. At the Mayo Clinic, 20% of patients return with recurrences, both minor and major. It is felt that the causes of recurrences are incomplete surgical removal or subsequent development of varicosities because of inherent weakness of the veins. Despite these reports attributing some recurrences to the presence of tributaries at the saphenofemoral junction, groin incisions are not reentered currently in our practice unless varicosities are demonstrated in that area. Small recurrences are treated by sclerotherapy, whereas generalized recurrences are best treated by excision of the varicosities.

COMPLICATIONS

Complications after vein stripping are infrequent. Residual and recurrent varices are the most troublesome; the most common is probably ecchymosis, which resolves in all patients. Dysesthesias because of injury to the saphenous or sural nerves occur in a variable number of patients. Decrease in the incidence of this has been reported by surgeons advocating stripping from the groin distally as opposed from the ankle upwards.[29] Infection is also a rare complication.

Deep vein thrombosis, though it might be thought to be a frequent complication of these operations, is rarely encountered. Keith and Smead reported a 0.6% incidence.[30]

LONG-TERM RESULTS

The Mayo Clinic reported good to excellent results in 85% of patients followed for 10 or more years[31] and in 68% of patients followed for 20 or more years.[32]

SCLEROTHERAPY

Sclerotherapy has been advocated as treatment for varicose veins, having been practiced extensively in Europe for decades. Incompetent greater and lesser saphenous veins must be excised prior to sclerotherapy, since these long-incompetent channels cannot be satisfactorily compressed. Hobbs showed that sclerosant therapy is not satisfactory treatment when follow-up time is longer than 1 year.[33] It is our feeling that this form of therapy is best reserved for small recurrences or for venous stars. Many different solutions are used, the most common now being sodium tetradecyl sulfate. The varicosities are injected with a sclerosant in a 25- to 30-gauge needle. Compression of the varix is applied immediately. Generally, compression is maintained for periods ranging from 3 hours to 1 week, depending on physician practice and extent of varicosities.

LASER THERAPY

Laser therapy is being tried as treatment for venous varicosities, particularly cutaneous scars. It is a new modality of therapy, the early results of which have been only modestly successful.[33,34] It is anticipated that the coming years will see more promising reports as this technology is developed and refined.

REFERENCES

1. Beaglehole R: Epidemiology of varicose veins. World J Surg 10:898, 1986.
2. Madar G, Widmer LK, et al.: Varicose veins and chronic venous insufficiency: Disorder or disease? A critical epidemiological review. VASA (Bern) 15(2):126, 1966.
3. Maffei FHA, Magaldi C, et al.: Varicose veins and chronic venous insufficiency in Brazil: Prevalence among 1755 inhabitants of a country town. Int J Epidemiol 15:210, 1986.

4. Rose SS, Ahmed A: Some thoughts on the aetiology of varicose veins. J Cardiovasc Surg 27:534, 1986.

5. Coon WW, Willis PW III, Keller JB: Venous thromboembolism and other venous disease in the Tecumseh Community Health Study. Circulation 48:839, 1973.

6. Ludbrook J: Primary great saphenous varicose veins revisited. World J Surg 10:954, 1986.

7. Beaglehole R, Prior IAM, Salmond CE, Davidson F: Varicose veins in the South Pacific. Int J Epidemiol 4:295, 1975.

8. Reagan B, Folse R: Lower limb venous dynamics in normal persons and children of patients with varicose veins. Surg Gynecol Obstet 132:15, 1971.

9. Ludbrook J, Beale G: Femoral venous valves in relation to varicose veins. Lancet 1:79, 1962.

10. Shepherd JT: Role of the veins in the circulation. Circulation 33:484, 1966.

11. McIrvine AJ, Corbett CRR, et al.: The demonstration of saphenofemoral incompetence; Doppler ultrasound compared with standard clinical tests. Br J Surg 71:509, 1984.

12. Baron HC, Cassaro S: The role of arteriovenous shunts in the pathogenesis of varicose veins. J Vasc Surg 4:124, 1986.

13. Haimovici H: Arteriovenous shunting in varicose veins. Its diagnosis by Doppler ultrasound flow detector. J Vasc Surg 2:684, 1985.

14. Reikeras O, Sorlie D: The significance of arteriovenous shunting for the development of varicose veins. Acta Chir Scand 149:479, 1983.

15. Corbett CR, McIrvine AJ, et al.: The use of varicography to identify the sources of incompetence in recurrent varicose veins. Ann R Coll Surg Engl 66:412, 1984.

16. Sutton R, Darke SG: Stripping the long saphenous vein: Preoperative retrograde saphenography in patients with and without venous ulceration. Br J Surg 73:305, 1986.

17. Thomas ML, Bowles JN: Incompetent perforating veins: Comparison of varicography and ascending phlebography. Radiology 154:619, 1985.

18. Thomas ML, Bowles JN: Descending phlebography in the assessment of long saphenous vein incompetence. AJR 145:1255, 1985.

19. Hoare MC, Royle JP: Doppler ultrasound detection of saphenofemoral and saphenopopliteal incompetence and operative venography to ensure precise saphenopopliteal ligation. Aust NZ J Surg 54:49, 1984.

20. Large J: Doppler testing as an important conservation measure in the treatment of varicose veins. Aust NZ J Surg 54:357, 1984.

21. Wales LR, Azose AA: Saphenous varix: Ultrasonic diagnosis (case reports). J Ultrasound Med 4:143, 1985.

22. Kistner RL, Ferris EB III, Randhawa G, Kalauokalani DA: The evolving management of varicose veins. Straub Clinic experience. Postgrad Med 80:51, 1986.

23. Large J: Surgical treatment of saphenous varices, with preservation of the main great saphenous trunk. J Vasc Surg 2:886, 1985.

24. Schobinger RA: Conservative varicose vein surgery—a modern necessity. Helv Chir Acta 52:7, 1985.

25. Tremblay J, Lewis EW, Allen PT: Selecting a treatment for primary varicose veins. Can Med Assoc J 133:20, 1985.

26. Lofgren EP, Lofgren KA: Recurrence of varicose veins after the stripping operation. Arch Surg 102:111, 1971.

27. Royle JP: Recurrent varicose veins. World J Surg 10:944, 1986.

28. Starnes HF, Vallance R, Hamilton DNH: Recurrent varicose veins: A radiological approach to investigation. Clin Radiol 35:95, 1984.

29. Cox SJ, Wellwood JM, Martin A: Saphenous nerve injury caused by stripping of the long saphenous vein. Br Med J 1:415, 1974.

30. Keith LM Jr, Smead WL: Saphenous vein stripping and its complications. Surg Clin North Am 63:1303, 1983.

31. Larson RH, Lofgren EP, et al.: Long-term results after vein surgery. Study of 1,000 cases after 10 years. Mayo Clin Proc 49:114, 1974.

32. Lofgren KA: Unpublished data.

33. Hobbs JT: The ten-year results of the random trial at St. Mary's Hospital, London. Presented at Sixth World Congress of Phlebologists, Buenos Aires, Argentina, 1977.

34. Lofgren EP: Varicose Veins, in Haimovici H: Vascular Surgery: Principles and Techniques, 2nd ed. Norwalk, Conn., Appleton-Century-Crofts, 1984.

CHAPTER 68

Venous Interruption

Lazar J. Greenfield and Barbara A. Michna

HISTORICAL BACKGROUND

Virchow developed his theory of the pathogenesis of thromboembolism between 1846 and 1856.[1-3] Several years later Spencer, Wells, and Hegan[4] reported the first cases of fatal postoperative pulmonary embolism (PE). In 1883 and 1885 Kocher and Billroth ligated the inferior vena cava (IVC) for control of bleeding in trauma, but the patients did not survive. Bottini[5] in 1893 performed the first successful IVC interruption, and in 1906 Trendelenburg ligated the infrarenal vena cava to prevent septic thromboembolism from pelvic and ovarian veins.

When autopsy studies related pulmonary embolism to peripheral vein thrombi, Homans[6] in 1934 recommended femoral vein ligation to prevent embolism. Four years later, Läwen[7] performed the first iliofemoral venous thrombectomy with restoration of patency as a means of removing potentially embolic thrombi. High failure rates with femoral vein ligation and recognition of more proximal embolic sources led Homans to recommend IVC ligation as the preferred treatment for proximal thrombosis.[8] Although venous ligation was effective in preventing pulmonary embolism, it became apparent that the procedure was associated with significant early and late morbidity.

As a means of reducing postoperative sequelae, Dale[5] in 1958 suggested using absorbable suture for vena caval ligation in the hope that recanalization would occur after the risk of acute embolism passed. This idea subsequently led to the concept of filtration of the IVC rather than ligation, prompting the development of numerous thrombi trapping devices. Late mortality was reduced, but the procedure still required general anesthesia and transabdominal or retroperitoneal dissection, often in critically ill patients. Intraluminal devices inserted through femoral or jugular veins with the patient under local anesthesia were introduced in the 1960s. The initial devices were removable, but it was quickly recognized that permanent devices were not associated with an increase in morbidity. Intraluminal filters have since become the treatment of choice in virtually all patients requiring mechanical protection against pulmonary embolism.

COMPLICATIONS OF VENOUS THROMBOSIS

Pulmonary Embolism

The most serious complication of venous thrombosis is pulmonary embolism (PE). An estimated 200,000 deaths per year[9] are due to embolism, and despite an increased awareness of the significance of the problem, the mortality rate has not significantly declined. In one large autopsy series of over 5,000 cases 55% showed evidence of gross PE, and an additional 14% had microscopic emboli only. The cause of death was felt to be directly related to embolism in 18% of patients autopsied.[10]

Of all patients who develop pulmonary embolism, 11% die within the hour, obviating the opportunity for diagnosis or treatment. Of untreated patients, 24% die of the embolism, with roughly 13% surviving longer than 1 hour but dying prior to treatment, presumably because of delay in diagnosis. The incidence of missed diagnosis is thought to be as high as 70%. In addition, the recurrent embolism rate of untreated patients surviving their first event is 30%, with 18% of the recurrent events fatal. As few as 30% of affected patients are diagnosed and treated.[11]

The major source of PE is the lower extremity, with 90 to 95% of emboli originating there; in the remaining 5 to 10% of patients, cardiac or upper extremity thrombosis is the source. Although it was once thought that all significant PE came from above the calf level, with more peripheral thrombosis representing minimal embolic risk, it is now recognized that 50 to 65% of PE originate below the inguinal ligament, many in the calf and soleal veins.

Factors contributing to formation of peripheral deep venous thrombosis (DVT) include trauma, the postoperative state, malignancy, pregnancy, cardiac failure, and a sedentary life-style, among others. All these conditions contribute to the stasis component of Virchow's triad of thromboembolism pathogenesis. Malignancy is associated with changes in blood favorable to DVT formation in addition to causing stasis from mechanical tumor bulk compression. In Havig's series of 5,000 autopsy cases,[10] the most significant risk factor for PE, not venous thrombosis, was the bedridden state.

Prior to consideration of major vein interruption for PE, the diagnosis must be firmly established. The most commonly seen signs and symptoms are nonspecific. In one series of 43 cases of embolism,[12] chest pain was the first symptom in 92%, with hemoptysis present half the time. Results of the Urokinase Pulmonary Embolism Trial (UPET)[13] showed dypsnea and pleuritic chest pain to be the most frequent symptoms while tachypnea, rales, and accentuated P_2 were the most frequently encountered signs (Table 68-1). Goodall and Greenfield in 1980[14] reviewed 73 patients with a clinical suspicion of PE who underwent pulmonary angiography. Twenty-nine percent had positive findings, and the remainder had no evidence of embolism on angiography. Comparing the two groups (PE vs. no PE), there was no difference in the incidence of chest pain, dyspnea, hemoptysis, collapse, sweats, or levels of pH, Pa_{O_2}, or blood pressure. It was found that a pulse rate greater than 100 per minute and a respiratory rate greater than 30 per minute were significantly more common in embolism patients, as was a Pa_{CO_2} value less than 30 mm Hg. The combination of hypoxemia and hypocarbia strongly suggested PE, especially if the pH were normal or alkaline. In any case, any of the signs mentioned above, with or without evidence of peripheral DVT, should alert the clinician to the need for further workup.

In addition to levels of arterial gases, other laboratory parameters have been examined for correlation with PE, all with nonspecific findings. No consistent association was found between serum lactic dehydrogenase (LDH), alanine amino transferase (ALT), aspartate aminotransferase (AST), or bilirubin levels. Examination of breakdown products of fibrinogen-fibrin in patients with thromboembolism failed to show a significant increase. Quantitation of factors thought to reflect active thrombosis, including fibrinopeptide A, have been encouraging, but the assays are as yet too sophisticated to be completed rapidly enough to aid

in diagnosis. Again, arterial blood gas measurements are the most useful laboratory diagnostic tool. The finding of a normal Pa_{O_2} in a postoperative patient in respiratory distress virtually excludes the diagnosis of PE, while hypoxemia associated with hypocarbia is more suggestive of embolism.

Electrocardiographic changes are likewise nonspecific. The classic findings reflecting acute right heart strain, P pulmonale, right-axis deviation, and right bundle-branch block or the $S_1Q_3T_3$ pattern, are seen only in 25% of patients with PE. The most common changes seen are nonspecific ST segment and T-wave abnormalities. In most instances the electrocardiograph is more helpful in ruling out a primary cardiac diagnosis.

Similarly, the major importance of the plain radiograph is to rule out other disorders causing respiratory distress such as pneumothorax, aspiration, congestive heart failure, or pneumonia. In Hendricks and Barnes' study of 43 cases,[12] the chest radiograph was found to be helpful in 92% of cases. Goodall and Greenfield[14] in comparing chest x-ray films in patients undergoing angiography for clinical suspicion of PE, found that overall 85% of radiographs were abnormal, but there were no differences between chest radiographs in the group with positive angiography and the group with negative angiography. Westermark's sign of segmental or lobar perfusion loss, considered one of the hallmark signs of PE, is seen infrequently (Table 68-2). Pleural effusion, pulmonary infiltrate, atelectasis, and elevated hemidiaphragm are seen commonly but are not specific for PE.

In a patient without underlying pulmonary disease and a nearly normal chest radiograph, the lung perfusion scan to detect regional alterations in pulmonary blood flow may be valuable. The lung scan has an overall accuracy rate of 73%,[14] with few false negatives but a specificity of only 61%. A previously healthy individual with a normal chest radiograph and a high probability lung scan could reasonably begin treatment without a further diagnostic workup, although there is prognostic value in the finding of proximal DVT by noninvasive tests. The less underlying pulmonary or cardiac disease a patient has, the more reliable the lung scan will be. In other patients, the diagnosis of PE requires angiographic confirmation. An added benefit of angiogra-

TABLE 68-1. PRESENTING SIGNS AND SYMPTOMS IN DOCUMENTED MAJOR PULMONARY EMBOLISM (UPET)[13]

Symptoms	Incidence (%)	Signs	Incidence (%)
Dyspnea	81	Tachypnea	88
Pleural pain	72	Rales	53
Apprehension	59	Increased P_2	53
Cough	54	Tachycardia	43
Hemoptysis	34	Fever	42
Sweats	26	S_3, S_4	34
Syncope	14	Sweating	34
		Phlebitis	33
		Cyanosis	18
		Hypotension	6

TABLE 68-2. CHEST RADIOGRAPHIC FINDINGS IN PATIENTS WITH NEGATIVE (GROUP A) AND POSITIVE (GROUP B) PULMONARY ARTERIOGRAMS

Finding	Group A (n = 51)	Group B (n = 20)
Infiltrate	17	4
Effusion	12	2
Elevated diaphragm	2	1
Atelectasis	8	1
Westermark's sign	1	1
Cardiomegaly	7	6
Normal	7	4
Pulmonary edema	4	3
Other	11	2

phy is the opportunity to measure pulmonary artery systolic pressures via right heart catheterization at the time of the study. The arteriographic diagnosis is established when a filling defect is seen in the pulmonary arteries or obstruction is seen with an area of decreased distal pulmonary vascular perfusion.

Once the diagnosis of PE is established, the treatment of choice is intravenous heparin. At the time of diagnosis an effort should also be made to identify the source of embolism via venography. A venogram demonstrating a free-floating thrombus in the iliofemoral system or the inferior vena cava (IVC) suggests the patient is a candidate for mechanical vena caval interruption, particularly if a significant embolic event has already been sustained. Although heparin is the mainstay of therapy, its action is to prevent further thrombosis peripherally and in the pulmonary circuit without actually causing clot lysis. A superior pharmacologic therapy has not yet been discovered; the UPET study[13] showed an 18% recurrent embolism rate, which was fatal in 9% of patients adequately anticoagulated. More recently, tissue plasminogen activator has shown promise in the management of PE in terms of its thrombolytic properties, but the complication rate was significant in one reported study.[15]

Recurrent Venous Thrombosis

The incidence of recurrent venous thrombosis is difficult to determine. One possibility is the rate of recurrent PE after an appropriate period of treatment, but recurrent embolism could be attributable to preexisting thrombus as well as recurrent disease. Another indicator of recurrent thrombosis is the incidence of recurrent phlebitis following appropriate initial management. In a recent review of patients receiving intraluminal IVC filtration devices,[16] often in association with anticoagulant therapy, patients were followed annually for symptomatic changes as well as undergoing Doppler and plethysmographic examinations. Of 106 Doppler examinations a new abnormality was detected in 5%; venography and plethysmography demonstrated new defects in 8% and 9%, respectively. Considering that these were routine follow-up visits, many without associated symptom changes, the incidence of asymptomatic and therefore overall DVT may be higher than reported.

INDICATIONS

Most patients with PE receive adequate therapy with anticoagulation alone. But in patients with a contraindication to or failure of anticoagulant therapy, venous interruption is indicated. The most frequent indications for caval interruption are contraindication to anticoagulation (38%), recurrent PE (27%), complication of anticoagulation (17%), and prophylaxis (17%).[16]

Ligation was the first method of interruption to become popular, and the surgical indications include those listed above. Prophylactic ligation was acceptable in instances of thrombus above the superficial femoral vein with associated PE. In addition, pelvic phlebitis with septic thrombo-

embolism was felt to require ligation. When partial vein interruption replaced ligation as the primary mechanical protection therapy, ligation was still the preferred management for septic embolism since embolism of small thrombi (<3 mm) was felt to be unacceptable. However, both clinical and experimental studies show that the Greenfield filter is preferable to ligation for septic embolism provided that the patient is receiving appropriate antibiotics.[17] The increased popularity of partial interruption over ligation led many to expand their indications for vena cava plication. It was felt by some surgeons[18] that high-risk patients—over 65 years old, overweight, hypertensive, or with a cardiac history—undergoing a major intraabdominal procedure were candidates for caval interruption. Consequently, patients undergoing abdominal surgery with any of the factors mentioned above had vena caval interruption recommended as a prophylactic measure against recurrent embolism. Generally today, the indications for prophylaxis are more stringent and include the following:

1. Chronic pulmonary hypertension
2. DVT with severe respiratory impairment
3. Free-floating thrombus in the iliofemoral system or vena cava
4. Significant hip or pelvic fractures
5. A prior history of DVT in patients undergoing surgical procedures at high risk for PE

A significant number of patients may be unable to take anticoagulants because of increased bleeding risks from recent surgery, trauma, ulcer disease, or stroke. Others may have a drug sensitivity, heparin-induced thrombocytopenia being seen most commonly. Other indications include recurrent embolism while receiving adequate anticoagulation and following pulmonary embolectomy.

PREOPERATIVE ASSESSMENT

For the patient who presents with PE and who may require venous interruption, it is helpful to identify the source of thrombosis. Five to ten percent of pulmonary emboli originate from sources other than the lower extremity, and interruption is not indicated if the embolus originated from an upper extremity or cardiac source. It is also important to know whether thrombus is present in the vena cava in order to provide appropriate filter positioning in the case of an intraluminal device and, during surgical placement of an extraluminal device, to prevent thrombus dislodgement and embolism during manipulation of the vena cava. The most accurate method of assessing the lower extremity venous system remains the venogram. Criteria that confirm venous thrombosis include the following:

1. Visualization of thrombus with sharp margins in a heavily opacified vein
2. Thrombus present within a vein on at least two radiographs
3. Nonvisualization of a long segment of vein
4. Demonstration of enlarged collateral vessels.

If venography through a dorsal foot vein does not identify the most proximal extent of thrombus, injection through the ipsilateral groin is performed. In certain cases in which thrombus involves the femoral system, injection through the contralateral groin may be necessary to determine the patency of the IVC.

Many patients with PE have severe underlying disease, and every effort should be made prior to surgery to optimize the patient's condition. Swan-Ganz and Foley catheter monitoring may be necessary to improve management of fluid balance and cardiac function. Legs should be elevated to provide for maximal venous return. All procedures for caval interruption except insertion of intraluminal devices should be performed in patients with normal clotting times, so vitamin K and protamine may be required to reverse the effects of heparin, and anticoagulation should be withheld postoperatively for at least 12 hours.

VENA CAVA LIGATION

The procedure of vena cava ligation was developed in response to a high recurrent PE rate following superficial femoral vein ligation.[19] Although the procedure is associated with a high morbidity rate, the patients who underwent the operation were at such high risk for recurrent PE that the morbidity was felt to be justified. With the discovery of heparin, ligation was used for patients in whom anticoagulation was unsuccessful or contraindicated.

Ligation of the IVC is accomplished through a transabdominal or right retroperitoneal approach. In the retroperitoneal approach, a transverse muscle-splitting incision is used, and the extraperitoneal space is entered by displacing the peritoneal sac medially. Following exposure of the IVC, the caval ligation is performed using a heavy, nonabsorbable, 2.0 double-silk ligature just below the renal veins. Cases of septic thrombophlebitis with embolism should be managed with a transabdominal approach so that the ovarian veins can also be ligated. Generally, whenever possible the retroperitoneal approach should be used, since it is associated with less early postoperative morbidity.

In patients undergoing IVC ligation, recurrent embolism has occurred in 0 to 50%.[20,21] A review of results of several authors who performed caval ligation on a total of 1,358 patients found the overall rate of recurrent PE to be 6.4%.[22] Sources of recurrent embolism were primarily from thrombus extending above the level of ligature or from large (<3 mm), tortuous collateral vessels that invariably develop following complete caval occlusion. Only in rare instances were upper extremity or cardiac sources of recurrent embolism suspected. The consistent development of large collateral vessels as potential embolic sources was felt by many to obviate the theoretical advantage of complete occlusion of the cava.

Significant morbidity and mortality occurred in patients who had caval ligation. Operative mortality rates ranged from 0 to 40%,[20,23] with an average of 15% in 1,358 patients.[22] Many authors[24,25] noted a high correlation between operative mortality and underlying cardiac disease, with mortality rates of 40 to 60% in cardiac patients compared with 12 to 32% in patients without cardiac disease undergoing IVC ligation. The decreased venous return resulting from ligation was often poorly tolerated in patients with cardiac dysfunction, who could not compensate for decreased flow with increased cardiac output.

Acute and chronic morbidity rates also remained high. In the series of 71 patients with surgical caval occlusion reported by Gazzaniga and co-workers,[26] 34% developed a syndrome of hypotension and oliguria within 24 hours after surgery. Lower extremity edema was seen in the majority of patients in the immediate postoperative period, with many resolving their edema over subsequent months and years. Postthrombotic syndrome rates ranged from 10 to 90% and appeared to a certain extent dependent on patient cooperation and motivation. With ligation the uninvolved limb also became subject to the same stasis sequelae as the limb with thrombosis, leading to symptoms in the previously healthy contralateral limb in up to 70% of cases in one series.[21] In addition to edema, other stasis sequelae developed, including ulceration, gangrene, phlebitis, and disabling pain.

Vena caval ligation provides acceptable protection against recurrent PE. However, the procedure requires an abdominal or retroperitoneal incision under general anesthesia in an often unstable patient who is compromised either from the embolic event or underlying disease. Mortality rates are therefore high, and acute caval occlusion may contribute significantly to cardiac decompensation in patients with preexisting disease. Long-term morbidity, although common, is generally nondisabling and may be influenced by patient compliance. For these reasons there are few if any indications for the procedure.

EXTRALUMINAL INTERRUPTION

The concept of partial venous interruption was developed out of concern for a high incidence of venous stasis sequelae following total caval occlusion. It was felt that a venous channel not larger than 3 mm would trap any clinically significant thrombus while preserving venous return and preventing venous stasis. The earliest method developed was a suture grid[27] which filtered out large thrombi, followed by suture plication[28] and then stapling of the cava (Fig. 68-1). Later, smooth and serrated Teflon and non-Teflon clips which did not violate the intima were developed to partially occlude the vena cava lumen (Fig. 68-2).

Operative Technique

Partial venous interruption can be performed under general anesthesia through a retroperitoneal or transabdominal incision similar to that used for ligation. Because of exposure variance, when a transabdominal route is used, the procedure is generally done just distal to the renal veins while a retroperitoneal approach provides the best exposure of the IVC a few centimeters proximal to the caval bifurcation. The technique of suture filtration described by DeWeese and Hunter[27] uses a transabdominal route, and the infrarenal IVC must be mobilized over a distance of 8 cm. Using Dacron continuous mattress sutures, a grid is constructed by positioning sutures 2 to 3 mm apart without narrowing the caval lumen. For plication, the vena cava is mobilized

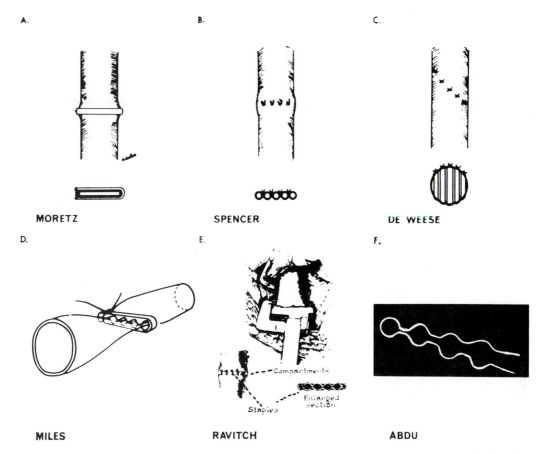

Figure 68-1. Methods of partial occlusion of the inferior vena cava. **A.** Moretz smooth plastic clip. **B.** Plication (Spencer). **C.** Filter (DeWeese). **D.** Serrated clip (Miles). **E.** Stapling technique (Ravitch). **F.** ABDU clip. (From Hendricks GL, Barnes WT: Am Surg 37:558, 1971.)

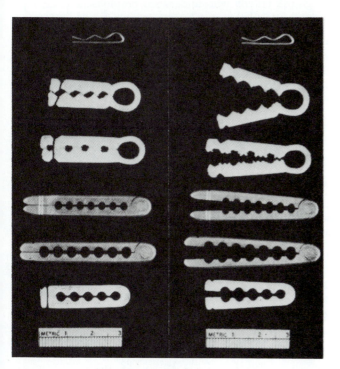

Figure 68-2. Stages of development of serrated Teflon and non-Teflon partially occluding vena caval clips. (From Miles RM, Chappell F, Renner O: Am Surg 30(1), 1964.)

2 to 3 cm, and interrupted mattress sutures are placed 5 mm apart, constructing channels that divide the cava into compartments each measuring 3 mm in diameter. To reduce dissection of the vena cava, Ravitch et al.[29] proposed using a stapling device similar to that for bronchial stump closure but leaving a 5 mm gap between staples to ensure adequate flow and reduce distal IVC thrombosis.

Although the devices vary in configuration, vena caval clips are all applied the same way. The infrarenal IVC is exposed, and an area large enough to pass a clip under is mobilized. The clip is placed preferably below a sizeable lumbar vein to prevent the formation of a cul-de-sac. Clips are adjusted so that apertures range between 3.0 and 3.5 mm in diameter; since they are extraluminal, they have the theoretical advantage of being less likely to induce caval thrombosis (Fig. 68-3). Generally, anticoagulation is withheld in the immediate perioperative period. As with ligation, postoperatively the legs are elevated and wrapped in Ace bandages to facilitate venous return.

Complications and Results

Not surprisingly, each caval filtration device is felt by its designer to be superior to others. Animal studies comparing ligation and plication with caval clipping in terms of patency, ability to trap thrombus, recurrent embolism, and

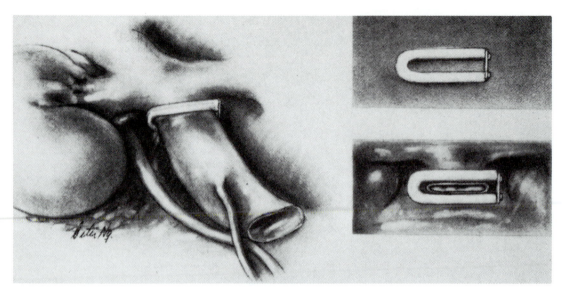

Figure 68-3. Application of smooth-edged clip. (From Adams JT, DeWeese JA: Surgery 57(1):82, 1965.)

venous pressure gradients above and below the site of interruption showed no difference between the three groups.[30] It was felt that plication and grid filter construction were technically more difficult to perform, and therefore aperture size was more likely to be variable.

Operative mortality rates for caval interruption range from 6 to 10%, primarily from underlying disease. There is generally only a minimal venous pressure gradient above and below the site of clipping, and hypotension secondary to delayed venous return is rarely a problem. Patency of the vena cava confirmed by cavogram or autopsy ranges from 23 to 100%, for an overall average patency of 74% (Table 68-3).[27,28,31-36] The incidence of recurrent PE ranges from 0 to 18%, with an average of 6%.

Postoperative morbidity includes early complications of bleeding, wound infection, hematoma, and lower extremity edema. Late morbidity is primarily in terms of development of venous stasis sequelae. Edema is present in 48 to 86% of patients but is permanent in only 10 to 40%. New onset of phlebitis is noted in 27% of patients after caval interruption, and 10% and 37% develop ulceration and varicosities, respectively.

A factor to consider in reviewing results of extraluminal interruption devices is the indication for placement. As the procedure became more popular and increased use of clips made application easier, the percentage of patients receiving prophylactic interruption increased dramatically in some series. A study of 120 patients[18] with two or more high-risk criteria who underwent prophylactic caval clipping revealed that in 97 cases age greater than 65 years and in 118 cases abdominal surgery more complicated than cholecystectomy constituted the indication for operation. Thus most patients had clipping performed because of their age and the fact they were having abdominal surgery, without any prior history of DVT or PE. A prospective study[37] of epidemiologically similar patients, 101 of whom had abdominal surgery and 51 of whom had vena caval clips placed prophylactically at operation, found no significant differ-

TABLE 68-3. VENA CAVAL PATENCY PROVEN BY CAVOGRAM OR AUTOPSY

Author	Type of Interruption	No. Patients	Postoperative Follow-up (mo)	No. Examined by Autopsy or Cavogram	No. Patent	Patent (%)
DeMeester[31]	Plication	56	<36	35	21	60
DeWeese[27]	Filter	17	6-55	6	6	100
Spencer[28]	Plication	39	<36	19	16	84
Moretz[32]	Clip	44	?	27	23	85
Miles[33]	Clip	11	<4	5	2	40
Taber[34]	Clip	42	4-6	4	4	100
Bergan[32]	Mixed	33	<6	13	3	23
Burget[35]	Plication	24	30	17	14	82
Leather[36]	Clip	62	59	43	36	84
		328		169	125	74%

ence in deaths from PE. Interpretation of any study in which a sizeable number of patients had similar operative indications must take this into account. Once the patients without prior history of deep venous thrombosis or PE are excluded, the recurrent embolism rate may be higher than 6% and the adjusted patency rate lower than 74%.

INTRALUMINAL INTERRUPTION

The concern for the morbidity and potential mortality of subjecting seriously ill patients to general anesthesia and abdominal surgery for placement of an extraluminal filtration device prompted the development of intraluminal vena caval filtration devices that were inserted through peripheral veins with the patient under local anesthesia. Early devices were designed to totally occlude the IVC as in ligation but that could be removed after recovery from the acute event. Soon after, nonremovable intraluminal filters were developed. Initially, the procedure was performed on moribund patients felt to be too compromised to withstand laparotomy. Intraluminal filters were used only in extreme situations because of concern for possible filter migration. Over time, there proved to be a low incidence of migration of intraluminal devices with adequate embolism protection and lower morbidity. Therefore, these devices have replaced

ligation and extraluminal interruption as the preferred method of PE prevention in patients who require mechanical protection.

Early Intraluminal Devices

In 1968, Eichelter and Schenk[38] reported the development of the first intraluminal vena caval filtration device, which could be inserted with the patient under local anesthesia. The Eichelter catheter was a plastic umbrella-sieve that could be placed in the infrarenal IVC through the saphenous vein and removed after several weeks when the greatest risk of embolism had passed (Fig. 68-4). The catheter was inserted in 10 patients, all of whom were too unstable to tolerate a more invasive procedure. The mortality rate was 80%, with the longest duration of catheter placement 49 days. There were two cases of recurrent embolism, one wound hematoma, one case of phlegmasia cerulea dolens from pericatheter thrombosis, and an episode of temporary venous congestion.

Concern over the potential for trapped or attached thrombi to embolize at the time of catheter removal led Pate to design the first permanent caval narrowing device.[39] His model was a single piece of thin spring steel wire, bent to form a loop in the center, with each arm bent back

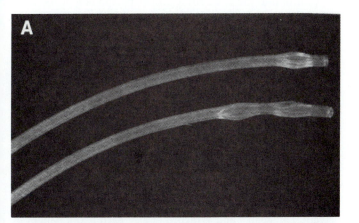

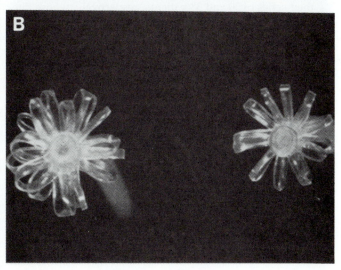

Figure 68-4. Eichelter catheter in closed position **(A)** and open position **(B)** with double sieve on bottom and left, respectively. (From Eichelter P, Schenk WG: Arch Surg 97:348, 1968.)

acutely under itself and the entire wire wrapped in unspun Dacron yarn (Fig. 68-5). After successful animal studies, the filter was inserted in two moribund patients, both of whom died without evidence of local trauma from the clip or recurrent embolism.

The Hunter balloon[40] was developed in 1970 to provide a permanent, minimally invasive means of complete IVC occlusion. It is a 75 cm long, 6.3 mm wide double catheter device with a detachable balloon at one end and ports for intravenous infusion, venography, and balloon inflation. Insertion is via an internal jugular vein exposed between the heads of the sternocleidomastoid. The catheter is passed into the infrarenal cava and confirmed by venography through the instrument. The balloon is inflated and tested for fixation by providing firm upward traction on the inserting catheter. Prior to release a configuration of well-developed elongation is confirmed. Over time, the balloon slowly collapses, with scarring and fibrosis of that segment of vena cava.

In 96 cases of balloon insertion, there was no operative mortality, and two cases of hypotension with balloon inflation that responded to volume expansion. There were no confirmed instances of recurrent embolism or of balloon migration. In terms of morbidity, 15% of patients on anti-coagulants had worsened venous stasis compared to 36% not receiving anticoagulation. Approximately half the patients had permanent lower extremity edema similar to the incidence of postthrombotic syndrome in caval ligation patients.[41] Enlargement of collateral vessels was similar to that seen in ligation of the IVC.

The results of patients having intraluminal interruption in the late 1960s and early 1970s cannot be compared to that group receiving extraluminal interruption since the patient populations are dissimilar. Initially, intraluminal devices were utilized only in those patients too ill to tolerate an abdominal procedure, so higher morbidity and mortality rates are to be expected.

Mobin-Uddin Umbrella

The Mobin-Uddin umbrella was the first intraluminal caval filtration device to gain widespread application. The design consists of six spokes of stainless steel Silastic-coated alloy radiating from a central hub with spokes extending 2 mm beyond the Silastic body for caval wall fixation. Eighteen fenestrations 3 mm in diameter allow continued venous flow (Fig. 68-6).

Umbrella insertion is via the internal jugular vein only. The application capsule containing the collapsed umbrella is inserted via a venotomy and advanced under fluoroscopic control into the IVC. After proper positioning at the level of the third lumbar vertebra and with the guide wire in position, the filter is ejected with fixation provided by firm upward traction on the guide wire. The catheter is withdrawn, and venotomy and skin incisions are closed.

The operative mortality rate for the Mobin-Uddin umbrella has ranged from 0 to 8%, with a collective mortality rate of 0.6%.[22] Most of the deaths have been from proximal filter migration, which is the most serious immediate complication of filter insertion. The initial umbrella design utilized a 23 mm diameter filter, but after 20 instances of proximal migration with a 63% mortality rate the 28 mm umbrella was introduced which reduced but did not eliminate the migration problem. Mobin-Uddin et al.[42] reported proximal migration of two of the 28 mm filters. Santos and Lansman[43] and Wingerd et al.[44] each had a patient in their series of 30 and 38 patients, respectively, whose filter migrated to the right heart or pulmonary artery, resulting in death in one case.

In addition, complications from filter perforation have been reported,[42,45–47] including one fatality from a retroperitoneal bleed, retroperitoneal hematomas (5), duodenal perforation (1), and ureter perforation (1). Right recurrent laryngeal nerve damage and acute renal failure have been reported rarely.

The incidence of recurrent PE is variable among series and ranges from 0 to 34%.[22] In Mobin-Uddin's collective review of 2,215 patients[42] who had umbrellas inserted, an overall recurrent embolism rate of 3% was found, which was fatal in 0.8% of the cases.

The design of the Mobin-Uddin umbrella allows for slow occlusion resulting in a vena cava patency rate of 15 to 40% with an average patency of 33% over time. Not surprisingly, there is a higher incidence of postoperative

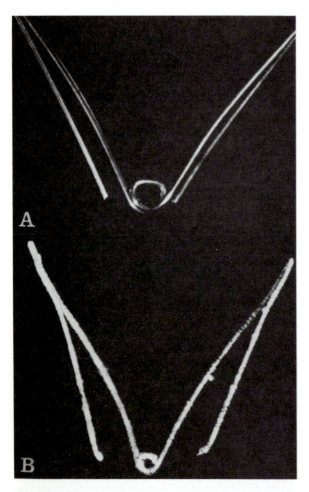

Figure 68-5. Pate clip before **(A)** and after **(B)** Dacron wrapping. (From Pate JW, Melvin D, Cheek RC: Ann Surg 169(6):873, 1969.)

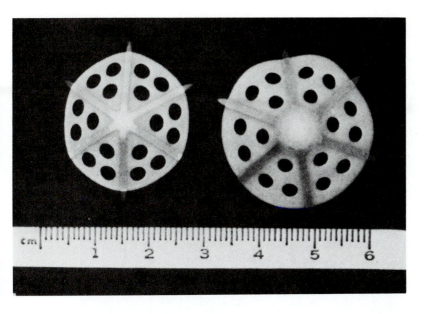

Figure 68-6. Mobin-Uddin umbrella. *Left,* 23 mm filter. *Right,* 28 mm filter. (From Mobin-Uddin K, Utley JR, Bryant LR: Prog Cardiovasc Dis 17(5):391, 1975.)

edema in patients with occluded umbrellas. Stasis problems are seen in 16 to 75% of patients with umbrellas, which is also correlated to some degree with the preoperative status, although it is not uncommon to develop postoperative edema in the contralateral limb. Because of the high incidence of IVC occlusions following filter insertion, it is recommended that patients with umbrellas misplaced in the suprarenal vena cava undergo surgical removal with simultaneous placement of a clip infrarenally.

Greenfield Vena Cava Filter

The Mobin-Uddin umbrella became more widely used as its low recurrent embolism rates became established, but concern remained about the 66% occlusion rate. The next major design was the Greenfield filter, in which a cone shape was selected to provide a maximal entrapment area while preserving blood flow. The geometry of the cone permits filling to 80% of its depth before the cross-sectional area is reduced by 64%. Spacing between the six stainless steel wires ensures trapping of all emboli greater than 3 mm (Fig. 68-7).

The filter can be inserted by a femoral or internal jugular approach, but the jugular route is used more commonly. Through a venotomy, the catheter carrier is passed with the aid of a guide wire into the IVC. Following fluoroscopic positioning at the level of the third lumbar vertebra, the filter is discharged, the guide wire and catheter withdrawn, and the venotomy repaired. Final positioning is confirmed by plain abdominal radiograph.

No deaths have been reported resulting from Green-

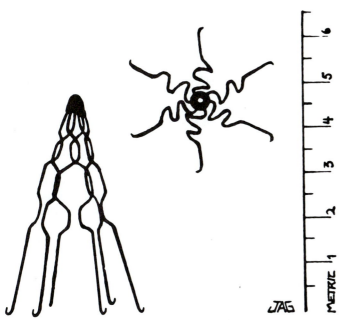

Figure 68-7. Greenfield filter. *Left,* Side view with recurved hooks at the end of each limb for secure fixation to the vena cava wall. *Right,* End-on view showing axial filtering pattern. (From Stewart JR, Greenfield LJ: Surg Clin North Am 62(3), 1982.)

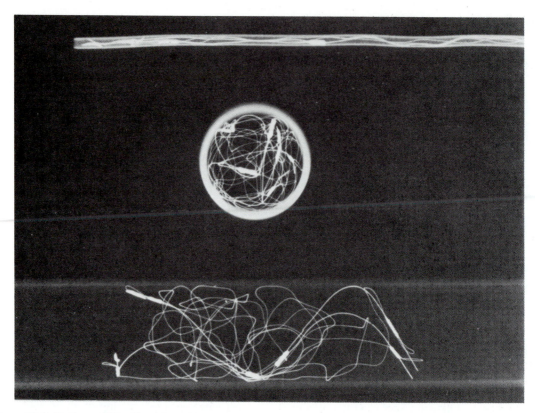

Figure 68-8. Bird's nest filter. *Top,* Filter within catheter. Axial (*middle*) and lateral (*bottom*) projections of filter in plastic tube. (From Roehm JOF Jr: J Vasc Surg 1:498, 1984.)

field filter insertion. Because of the construction of the steel hooks and fixation within the caval wall, migration has not occurred, although it is not uncommon to note a gradual 0 to 18 mm distal change in filter position relative to underlying bony structures, thought to be due to fibrosis around the struts. Perforation of the struts through the vena caval wall has been reported[48] in several cases but without associated morbidity except one instance of hematuria, which resolved when warfarin was discontinued, and one case of a filter misplaced in the iliac vein that had a strut embedded in the obturator nerve, causing symptoms and necessitating filter removal. Other complications have included rare instances of air embolism when the jugular vein was open during insertion.

Filter misplacement has occurred in 4% of patients, but because of a documented long-term patency rate of 96%,[16] filters mistakenly placed in the renal vein or suprarenal IVC generally contribute no morbidity. In fact, in renal transplant patients or patients with malignant tumors or thrombus within the IVC or renal vein, use of suprarenally positioned Greenfield filters has become accepted.[49–52] Venous stasis sequelae are seen in 44% of patients receiving Greenfield filters, with the majority having edema prior to filter insertion. Roughly 15% of venous sequelae which develop over long-term follow-up are new or are more severe but can be attributed to recurrent DVT and are not correlated with filter patency.

The long-term recurrent PE rate is 3.8% over a 12-year follow-up period, with a 1.9% fatal embolism incidence.[16]

At present, the Greenfield filter is the only FDA-approved intraluminal device being marketed.

Bird's Nest Filter

One of the most recent developments in the design of intraluminal vena cava filtration devices is the filter constructed for percutaneous insertion, eliminating the need for a neck incision and potentially difficult dissection in obese patients. The bird's nest filter consists of four thin strands of stainless steel wire, each 25 cm long, attached to a pair of short-angled hooks at each end for fixation to the wall of the inferior vena cava (Fig. 68-8). The stainless steel wire is thought to be nonthrombogenic, although a similar technique has been used to induce thrombosis. A side arm of the catheter allows injection of radiopaque medium for proper localization.

Following percutaneous access through the femoral, internal jugular, or subclavian vein, the sheath is positioned just proximal to the renal veins for a femoral vein approach, and at the inferior border of the third lumbar vertebrae if a jugular or subclavian vein route is used. The hooks are then exposed until they contact the caval wall, and the filter is pushed into place, engaging the hooks within the wall. The preformed curved wires produce a fine criss-crossing network similar in appearance to a bird's nest. Theoretically, the procedure could be performed at the same time as pulmonary angiography if results showed that filter placement was indicated, thus eliminating the need for a second procedure either in the operating room or in the radiology suite under fluoroscopic guidance.

After initial filter placement work in animals produced no complications, the filter was inserted in 28 patients in a 1-year period. During the short follow-up period no patient developed symptoms of recurrent emboli or vena cava thrombosis, and cavograms performed in two patients demonstrated patency, although an additional two patients moribund at the time of insertion were found to have occluded filters at autopsy 24 to 48 hours following filter placement.[53]

In another experimental model,[54] the bird's nest filter was found to allow an 83% incidence of clot lysis over a 1-week period with increasing thrombus size in one animal. However, difficulty in affixing the hooks of the filter into the vein wall resulted in abandonment of the procedure in two instances and placement of the device too proximally in another two cases. In one other instance, a set of hooked wires migrated to the right atrium despite correct insertion. The issues of proximal migration and possible thrombogenic properties of the bird's nest filter require further study before any conclusions can be drawn.

Comparison of Intraluminal Devices

Except in rare instances, intraluminal vena cava filter devices have replaced extraluminal devices since they provide the same effective protection against recurrent PE without the added morbidity and mortality rates associated with general anesthesia and an abdominal or retroperitoneal procedure. Among the intraluminal devices the Greenfield filter is the most widely used today and is the only device marketed that is approved by the FDA. The high patency rate of the Greenfield filter permits intentional suprarenal filter placement in selected cases without added morbidity.

The percutaneous insertion of the bird's nest filter is advantageous, but questions regarding the potential for migration and misplacement must be answered prior to its availability for widespread use.

REFERENCES

1. Virchow R: Uber die Vertpfung der Lungenarterie. Neue Notizen und Geb d Natur Heilk 36:26, 1846.
2. Virchow R: Die cellular Pathologie in ihrer Begrundung auf physiologische und pathologische Gewebelehre. Berlin, A. Hirschwald, 1858.
3. Welch WH: Papers and Addresses. Baltimore, Johns Hopkins Press, 1920, pp 66–258.
4. Matas R: Postoperative thrombosis and pulmonary embolism before and after Lister. A retrospect and prospect. Univ Toronto Med Bull 10:1, 1932.
5. Dale WA: Ligation of the inferior vena cava for thromboembolism. Surgery 43:22, 1958.
6. Homans J: Thrombosis of the deep veins of the lower leg causing pulmonary embolism. N Engl J Med 221:993, 1934.
7. Läwen A: Weitere Erfahrungen über operative Thrombenentfernung bei Venenthrombose. Arch Klin Chir 193:723, 1938.
8. Homans J: Deep venous thrombosis in the lower limb. Surg Gynecol Obstet 79:70, 1944.
9. Dalen JE, Alpert JS: Natural history of pulmonary embolism. Prog Cardiovasc Dis 17:257, 1975.
10. Havig O: Deep vein thrombosis and pulmonary embolism. An autopsy study with multiple regression analysis of possible risk factors. Acta Chir Scand 478 (suppl 1):120, 1977.
11. Coon WW, Coller FA: Clinicopathologic correlation in thromboembolism. Surg Gynecol Obstet 109:259, 1959.
12. Hendricks GL Jr, Barnes WT: Experiences with the Moretz clip: 100 cases. Am Surg 37:558, 1971.
13. Urokinase Pulmonary Embolism Trial: A national cooperative study. Circulation 48(suppl 2), 1973.
14. Goodall RJR, Greenfield LJ: Clinical correlations in the diagnosis of pulmonary embolism. Ann Surg 191:219, 1980.
15. Goldhaber SZ, et al.: Acute pulmonary embolism treated with tissue plasminogen activator. Lancet 2(8512):886–889, 1986.
16. Greenfield LJ, Peyton R, et al.: Greenfield vena caval filter experience. Late results in 156 patients. Arch Surg 116:1451, 1981.
17. Peyton JWR, Hylemon MB, et al.: Comparison of Greenfield filter and vena caval ligation for experimental septic thromboembolism. Surgery 93:533, 1983.
18. Rahma AFA, Boland J, et al.: Long-term follow-up of prophylactic caval clipping. J Cardiovasc Surg 22:550, 1981.
19. Mozes M, Adar R, et al.: Vein ligation in the treatment of pulmonary embolism. Surgery 55:621, 1964.
20. Krause RJ, Cranley JJ, et al.: Caval ligation in thromboembolic disease. Arch Surg 87:184, 1963.
21. Piccone VA, Vidal E, et al.: The late results of caval ligation. Surgery 68:980, 1970.
22. Bomalaski JS, Martin GJ, et al.: Inferior vena cava interruption in the management of pulmonary embolism. Chest 82:767, 1982.
23. Amador E, Li TK, Crane U: Ligation of inferior vena cava for thromboembolism. Clinical and autopsy correlations in 119 cases. JAMA 206:1758, 1968.
24. Schowengerdt CG, Schreiber JT: Interruption of the vena cava in the treatment of pulmonary embolism. Surg Gynecol Obstet 132:645, 1971.
25. Lepore AA, Bottino CG: Transvenous filter for pulmonary embolism. N Y State J Med p. 1645, October 1981.
26. Gazzaniga AB, Cahill JL, et al.: Changes in blood volume and renal function following ligation of the inferior vena cava. Surgery 62:417, 1967.
27. DeWeese MS, Hunter DC: A vena cava filter for the prevention of pulmonary embolism. A five-year clinical experience. Arch Surg 86:852, 1963.
28. Spencer FC: Plication of the vena cava for pulmonary embolism. Surgery 62:388, 1967.
29. Ravitch MM, Snodgrass E, et al.: Compartmentation of the vena cava with the mechanical stapler. Surg Gynecol Obstet 122:561, 1966.
30. Adams JT, DeWeese JA: Experimental and clinical evaluation of partial vein interruption in the prevention of pulmonary emboli. Surgery 57:82, 1965.
31. DeMeester TR, et al.: Plication of the inferior vena cava for thromboembolism. Surgery 62:56, 1967.
32. Moretz WH, Bergan JJ, et al.: Prevention of pulmonary embolism: Comparison of vena caval ligation, plication, and filter operations in prevention of pulmonary emboli. Arch Surg 92:605, 1966.
33. Miles RM: Prevention of pulmonary embolism by the use of a plastic vena caval clip. Ann Surg 163:192, 1966.
34. Taber RE, et al.: Prevention of pulmonary emboli with a vena caval clip. JAMA 195:889, 1966.
35. Burget DE Jr, et al.: Inferior vena cava plication for prevention of pulmonary embolism: Results in 24 cases. Ann Surg 165:437, 1967.

36. Leather RP, Clark WR, et al.: Five-year experience with the Moretz vena caval clip in 62 patients. Arch Surg 97:357, 1968.

37. Gardner AMN, Askew AR, et al.: Partial occlusion of the IVC in the prevention of fatal pulmonary embolus. Surg Gynecol Obstet 138:17, 1974.

38. Eichelter P, Schenk WG Jr: Prophylaxis of pulmonary embolism. A new experimental approach with initial results. Arch Surg 97:348, 1968.

39. Pate JW, Melvin D, Cheek RC: A new form of vena caval interruption. Ann Surg 69:873, 1969.

40. Hunter JA, Sessions R, Buenger R: Experimental balloon obstruction of the inferior vena cava. Ann Surg 171:315, 1970.

41. Hunter JA, DeLaria GA, et al.: Requirements for a method of transvenous inferior vena cava interruption. Arch Surg 115:1324, 1980.

42. Mobin-Uddin K, Utley JR, Bryant LR: The inferior vena cava umbrella filter. Prog Cardiovasc Dis 17:391, 1975.

43. Santos GH, Lansman S: Prevention of pulmonary embolism with use of Mobin-Uddin filter. N Y State J Med p. 185, February 1982.

44. Wingerd M, Bernhard VM, et al.: Comparison of caval filters in the management of venous thromboembolism. Arch Surg 113:1264, 1978.

45. Mobin-Uddin K, Callard GM, et al.: Transvenous caval interruption with an umbrella filter. N Engl J Med 286:55, 1972.

46. Mobin-Uddin K: Vena cava umbrella filter. Edwards Laboratories Clinical Report, September 1972.

47. Praiss DE, Marmar JL, et al.: Letters to the editor: Is the umbrella filter safe? N Engl J Med 286:1006, 1972.

48. Greenfield LJ, Zocco J, et al.: Clinical experience with the Kim-Ray Greenfield vena cava filter. Ann Surg 185:692, 1977.

49. Stewart JR, Peyton JWR, et al.: Clinical results of suprarenal placement of the Greenfield vena cava filter. Surgery 92:1, 1982.

50. Rosenthal D, Gershon CR, Rudderman R: Renal cell carcinoma invading the inferior vena cava: The use of the Greenfield filter to prevent tumor emboli during nephrectomy. J Urol 134:126, 1985.

51. Orsini RA, Jarrell BE: Suprarenal placement of vena caval filters: Indications, techniques, and results. J Vasc Surg 1:124, 1984.

52. Jarrell BE, Szentpetery S, et al.: Greenfield filter in renal transplant patients. Arch Surg 116:930, 1981.

53. Roehm JOF Jr: The bird's nest filter: A new percutaneous transcatheter inferior vena cava filter. J Vasc Surg 1:498, 1984.

54. Burke PE, Michna BA, et al.: Experimental comparison of percutaneous vena caval devices: Titanium Greenfield filter versus bird's nest filter. J Vasc Surg (Accepted but not published)

CHAPTER 69
Iliofemoral Venous Thrombectomy

Lazar J. Greenfield and Barbara A. Michna

HISTORICAL BACKGROUND

In 1937 Läwen first described femoral venous thrombectomy with restoration of the venous circulation.[1] Although thrombectomy had been performed previously, Läwen was first to repair the venotomy following thrombectomy, thereby restoring venous patency. It was thought that chronic venous obstruction was responsible for the postthrombotic syndrome and that reestablishing continuous flow would prevent late stasis changes. Prior to this, common femoral vein ligation was advocated by Homans to prevent pulmonary embolism (PE).[2] Not only did this produce lower extremity stasis changes, but significant recurrent embolism rates suggested that pelvic and iliac veins served as potential embolic sources. In his 1953 report, Allen noted that patients who had thrombectomy prior to vein ligation had less postthrombotic edema.[3] Later in that decade, Fontaine described three surgical procedures for treatment of patients with recurrent PE or phlegmasia alba dolens not responsive to anticoagulant therapy: inferior vena cava (IVC) ligation, phlebectomy, and thrombectomy.[4] Lumbar sympathectomy had been used earlier but was found to be ineffective. Mahorner in 1957 was among the first in North America to advocate thrombectomy for iliofemoral thrombosis,[5] and with the introduction of the Fogarty balloon catheter in 1966, the procedure gained more popularity[6] and proved more effective than with previously used suction catheters.

Following several reports of success in the late 1950s and early 1960s, the procedure fell into disfavor when a report by Lansing and Davis in 1968 described poor long-term results despite initial success, with a 61% 5-year follow-up of surviving patients.[7] Since that time, results have been varied. Use of an arteriovenous fistula for both acute and chronic venous occlusion and improvements in venous reconstructive techniques have expanded the surgical options available for management of iliofemoral thrombosis.

PATHOPHYSIOLOGY

The natural history of untreated iliofemoral thrombosis is a 60 to 70% incidence of PE with a mortality rate of 18%.[8,9] The mortality rate for untreated venous gangrene, the most severe clinical presentation of iliofemoral thrombosis, is 83%.[10] Late morbidity as expressed in the postthrombotic syndrome is seen in 90%.[11] When peripheral venous thrombosis extends into the IVC, a 35% embolism rate is seen, even with adequate anticoagulation.[12,13] Heparinization for treatment of deep venous thrombosis (DVT) reduces the incidence of PE to 12% with a mortality rate less than 1%, but the postthrombotic syndrome is still seen in 50 to 80%.[14–16]

To address the issue of frequency of iliofemoral thrombosis, McLachlin and Paterson prospectively autopsied 100 unselected male patients over 40 years of age with particular attention to the lungs and peripheral leg veins, which were removed in continuity.[17] They found 76 individual thrombi in 34 positive cases, 37 of which arose above the level of the superficial femoral vein. This was in contradiction to early investigators' conclusions that all DVT originated in the calf veins and that femoral and iliac vein thrombi were extensions from thrombus in the posterior tibial veins. Mavor and Galloway also disputed this when examination of 252 instances of iliofemoral thrombosis in 228 patients showed only 24 cases in which the distribution of clot suggested a peripheral to proximal propagation.[18] Studies by Fontaine[4] and DeWeese et al.[19] supported this theory when they found a 60% incidence of DVT localized to the femoral, iliac, or pelvic veins on phlebography.

The pathogenesis of iliofemoral thrombosis is multifactorial. The classic work of Virchow on the three causative factors of venous thrombosis still holds credence today, although the issue is recognized as much more complex than originally described. Fontaine felt that the balance between vein wall change, stasis, and blood composition determined whether a thrombus was adhesive with significant inflammatory response, in which case it was unlikely to embolize, or embologenic with minimal inflammation, resulting in a loosely adherent clot which could easily dislodge and migrate proximally.[4] Sevitt localized the initial site of thrombus formation to valve cusps and vein bifurcations with clot extending into the vein wall from the primary site of adherence.[20] McLachlin and Paterson questioned the theory of vein injury when serial sections of thrombosed veins failed to reveal a lesion, although one third of thrombi originated in relation to a valve pocket.[17]

In iliofemoral thrombosis, arteriospasm appears to be an injury response association rather than an inciting factor. Diminished arterial flow is often clinically evident following massive thrombosis with elevated venous pressures. Efforts to relieve arteriospasm pharmacologically or via sympathetic blockade have not alleviated clinical DVT symptoms, whereas medical or surgical relief of venous obstruction usually improves arterial insufficiency.

Thrombus formation within the iliofemoral system has been related to a multitude of factors, including extension of pelvic vein thrombosis secondary to inflammatory processes or direct venous compression from tumor bulk, pregnancy, hematoma, and so forth. Direct venous compression, from the right iliac artery crossing the left iliac vein, the internal iliac artery crossing the iliac vein, or from the left inguinal ligament impinging on the femoral vein, has played a significant role in thrombus formation as evidenced by the left-sided predominance of thrombosis seen consistently in published reports (Table 69-1). Cockett and Thomas described an apparently distinct obstruction etiology, the iliac compression syndrome, in a select group of generally young patients who developed acute iliofemoral thrombosis following a period of bed rest.[21] Six of these patients underwent vena caval bifurcation exploration, and all were found to have a localized fibrous stricture in the vein which was the initiating source of occlusion and unrelated to extrinsic compression.

TABLE 69-1. LEFT- vs. RIGHT-SIDED ILIOFEMORAL THROMBOSIS

Study		Left	Right	Bilateral
DeWeese[37]	(1964)	22	9	
Smith[30]	(1965)	15	3	
Fogarty[6]	(1966)	24	9	2
Haimovici[10]	(1966)	175	80	44
Barner[31]	(1969)	49	24	
Mavor[18]	(1969)	182	70	
Edwards[32]	(1970)	44	17	
Johansson[25]	(1973)	12	11	
Lindhagen[35]	(1978)	24	4	
Goto[39]	(1980)	66	21	1
Matsubara[56]	(1982)	165	46	11
Horsch[34]	(1983)	109	52	
Röder[40]	(1983)	31	15	
Plate[53]	(1984)	44	14	
Stirneman[36]	(1984)	31	6	
		993	381	58

Defects in the coagulation system can predispose to venous thrombosis. Fontaine, in 1957, attempted without success to correlate thromboplastic activity and prothrombin and fibrinogen levels in patients with iliofemoral thrombosis.[4] He concluded that hypercoagulability of blood was not uncommon and could be triggered by nonspecific mediators such as stress. With more refined diagnostic techniques, Gaston described a case of hereditary factor V level elevation in a 6-year-old girl with spontaneous iliofemoral thrombosis.[22] Also, isolated instances of antithrombin III deficiency have been found to cause hypercoagulability, and Egeberg reported a family pedigree with decreased levels of antithrombin III transmitted in an autosomal dominant manner with a strong tendency to venous thrombosis.[23] Though certainly not commonplace, congenital coagulation disorders may be more prevalent than reported. Technical inability to reliably measure many of the factors involved in coagulation has precluded a clearer understanding of their importance in thrombogenesis.

Certain conditions or disorders are known to be associated with iliofemoral thrombosis. The association of the prepartum or postpartum state with mechanical compression of pelvic veins is clearly recognized. Major pelvic or lower extremity fractures, trauma, and the postoperative state frequently precede thrombus formation. Other conditions which play an etiologic role are malignancy, use of oral contraceptives, the bedridden state, cardiac failure, postthrombotic syndrome, and infection. Unfortunately, the cause of most cases of thrombosis remains unknown.

CLINICAL DATA

The clinical presentation of iliofemoral thrombosis is varied and may be silent, as in partial thrombotic occlusion in which the extremity appears normal and the diagnosis is made by venography after PE occurs. In symptomatic cases, proximal venous occlusion develops, and distal venous pressure may increase as much as 10 times normal. Virtually all these patients demonstrate uniform limb swelling and have tenderness over the femoral vein at the level of the inguinal ligament. Depending on the extent of the occlusion and the availability of collateral veins, the signs and symptoms vary from phlegmasia alba dolens, with "milk" or "white" leg appearance from edema in subcutaneous tissues, to the ischemic forms of DVT, including phlegmasia cerulea dolens, in which cyanosis is present with signs of arterial insufficiency, and venous gangrene, in which tissue death occurs. These forms represent the spectrum of the same pathologic process, with reversible injury at all stages except with venous gangrene. In addition, many patients with ischemic thrombosis develop hypovolemic shock secondary to massive fluid sequestration. In an experimental model, Vasko and Brockman found that 55% of the blood volume was lost into the interstitial space within 8 hours of massive venous occlusion.[24] Untreated thrombosis may lead to progression, susceptibility to PE, and the postthrombotic syndrome. The latter results from valve incompetence following recanalization and also within large collateral veins, since dilatation of the vein distorts the valves. Therefore, the postthrombotic syndrome as characterized by dependent edema, venous ulceration, brawny induration, and pigmentation does not imply persistent obstruction but usually reflects a patent recanalized or well-collateralized venous system.

In cases of phlegmasia cerulea dolens or venous gangrene, the clinical diagnosis of iliofemoral thrombosis is justified, and venographic confirmation is not mandatory. However, it may be helpful for assessment of the contralateral limb, for identifying the most proximal extent of thrombus, and for comparison with postoperative studies. If thrombosis is present within the vena cava, management is altered. Generally, ascending venography is performed first, with contrast medium injected through any dorsal foot vein. If this technique fails to adequately visualize flow in the iliac vein, an ipsilateral femoral vein contrast study is done. Failure to aspirate blood from the femoral vein is presumptive evidence of thrombosis, and contralateral femoral vein venography is done next to exclude vena caval thrombosis. Cockett and Thomas used the technique of pertrochanteric venography in patients with suspected iliofemoral thrombosis.[21] However, this involves sterile puncture of the outer aspect of the greater trochanter with fluoroscopy under general anesthesia. Others have used noninvasive assessment such as Doppler and plethysmography to correlate with venographic results and to establish a baseline for postoperative follow-up. More recently, real-time B-mode imaging has been added in duplex studies and offers the prospect of direct visualization. These techniques currently lack the specificity and sensitivity to be used as the primary means of diagnosis but will undoubtedly gain in acceptability with further experience.

INDICATIONS

The presumed advantages of iliofemoral venous thrombectomy over standard heparin therapy are immediate relief of compromised venous drainage of the lower extremity, lessened morbidity, venous valve preservation, and prevention of the postthrombotic syndrome.[7] The present controversy over acceptance of these advantages is reflected in the published indications for surgical management of this problem. Johansson et al.,[25] Lansing and Davis,[7] and McLachlin et al.[26] noted long-term results not significantly different than with anticoagulant therapy and felt the procedure was indicated only in the threat of limb loss. Lansing and Davis advocated a 3- to 4-hour trial of heparin and elevation prior to thrombectomy even in cases of impending ischemia. Others who felt thrombectomy to be a superior form of treatment used more liberal indications in assessing possible surgical candidates. Mavor and Galloway[18] and Haller and Abrams[27] advocated thrombectomy for any patient with venous occlusion at the iliofemoral level, partial or complete, excluding those unable to tolerate the procedure. Based on clinical results, Harris and Brown felt patients with venous thrombosis proximal to the popliteal tributaries should undergo thrombectomy.[28] Fogarty et al.[6] and DeWeese et al.[29] believed duration of clinical symptoms to be related to prognosis and objected to performing thrombectomy after a 7- to 10-day preoperative clinical course, whereas Andriopoulos et al. advocated iliac vein thrombec-

tomy within 21 days of the onset of symptoms.[16] It is generally believed that patients with iliofemoral occlusion who fail medical therapy in terms of relief of acute symptoms should undergo thrombectomy or IVC interruption or both to protect against embolism. One exception, septic thrombosis, particularly originating from a pelvic source, is believed to be best managed conservatively or with IVC interruption without thrombectomy if recurrent embolism occurs on anticoagulant therapy. Evidence of major PE prior to therapy is felt by most to justify more aggressive management, either thrombectomy or vena caval interruption or both.

OPERATIVE TECHNIQUE

Adequate patient resuscitation must be undertaken before surgery. Specifically, patients are usually hypovolemic secondary to fluid sequestration in the obstructed, swollen limb. Since these patients commonly have significant underlying disorders, a Swan-Ganz catheter is often indicated to facilitate volume repletion. A urinary catheter should be inserted for additional fluid status monitoring, and at least two units of packed red cells should be available in the operating room.

The operation can be performed under general or local anesthesia, with the latter preferred. The entire involved leg, lower abdomen, and opposite groin are prepared, with a sterile stockinette placed on the involved leg to facilitate intraoperative manipulation.

A longitudinal incision (Fig. 69-1) is made over the

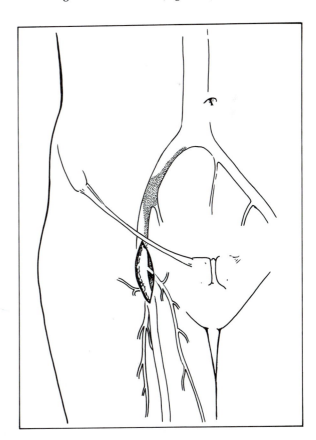

Figure 69-1. Incision.

femoral vein. The common femoral vein is mobilized (Fig. 69-2) from the inguinal ligament to the profunda branch, and the profunda, superficial femoral, and saphenous veins are isolated. If the patient was not heparinized earlier and there is no contraindication to heparin, a dose of 100 U/kg should be administered. A transverse venotomy (Fig. 69-3) is made in the common femoral vein, and a No. 12 Fogarty venous catheter is passed proximally (Fig. 69-4). Fogarty's initial description of venous thrombectomy called for placement of a second Fogarty catheter through the contralateral limb into the IVC to prevent migration of any major thrombi dislodged while the first catheter was being passed through the area of proximal thrombosis.[6] Generation of positive intrathoracic pressure by the Valsalva maneuver, if the patient is awake during embolectomy, has proved equally effective in prevention of PE without the morbidity of an additional incision and venotomy.

The Fogarty catheter is passed into the vena cava and the balloon inflated. Slow withdrawal of the catheter (Fig. 69-5) with extrusion of thrombus is usually followed by brisk retrograde bleeding. The procedure is performed several times until no further proximal clot is extracted. After clearance proximally, thrombus distal to the common femoral vein is removed by milking the distal clot out with an Esmarch bandage (Fig. 69-6) applied from the foot proximally. Again, brisk bleeding should be seen, and if retained thrombus is seen, a small Fogarty catheter can be passed distally (Fig. 69-7) through thrombus to the popliteal vein. Gentle passage should minimize damage to valves.

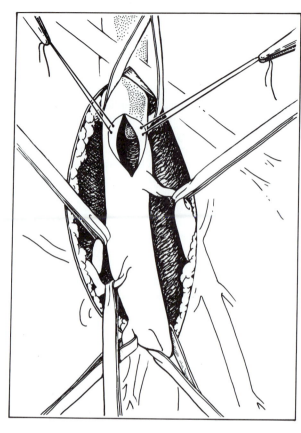

Figure 69-3. Venotomy.

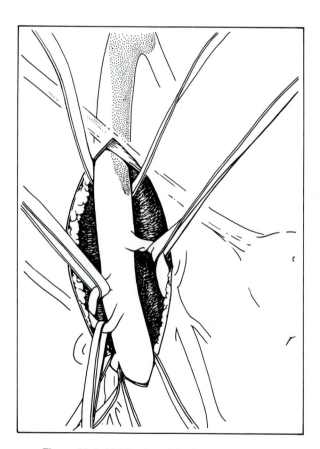

Figure 69-2. Mobilization of the femoral vein.

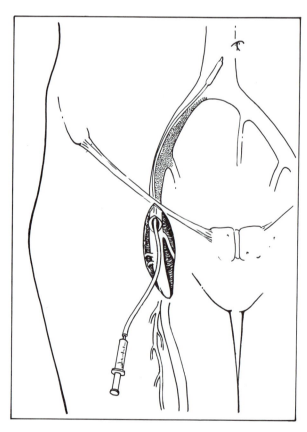

Figure 69-4. Passage of a Fogarty catheter.

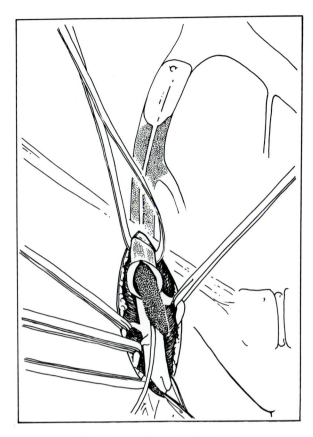

Figure 69-5. Catheter withdrawal.

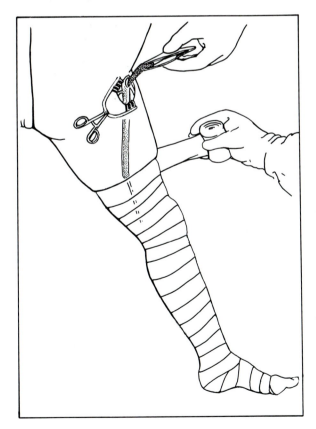

Figure 69-6. Distal compression with Esmarch bandage to extrude thrombus.

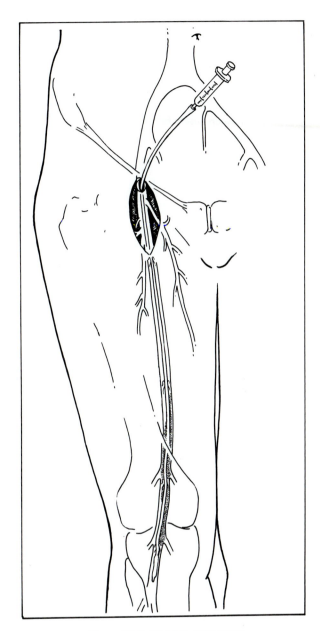

Figure 69-7. Distal thrombectomy.

Retrograde flow is often not an accurate assessment of vein clearance. An occluded common iliac vein will still bleed briskly if the internal iliac vein is patent. Conversely, poor retrograde flow may be seen when the iliac vein valve is intact, despite removal of all proximal thrombus. Therefore, intraoperative venography should be performed by injecting 20 ml of contrast medium into the femoral vein. If clot remains, thrombectomy should be repeated. Following completion of thrombectomy, a small catheter is placed through a tributary of the greater saphenous vein into the femoral vein for postoperative regional heparin administration and for postoperative venography. The venotomy closure (Fig. 69-8) is then completed with fine running suture and the skin closed. Generally, there is no indication for wound drainage.

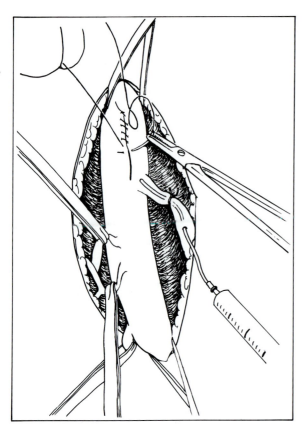

Figure 69-8. Closure of venotomy with placement of catheter in saphenous vein for postoperative heparin infusion.

Postoperatively, heparin is continued for 5 to 7 days, and venography via the saphenous vein catheter is performed prior to discontinuance of heparin. Warfarin (Coumadin) should be started early to allow 4 days minimal overlap with heparin, adjusting levels to maintain the prothrombin time 1.4 times normal. Warfarin is generally continued for 3 to 4 months postoperatively. Calf-length elastic stockings or pneumatic compression devices are worn in the early postoperative period and the legs are elevated. Although agreement does not exist on when to ambulate patients, the trend has been toward earlier mobilization. Smith has all patients ambulatory by the first postoperative day,[30] and many others begin active leg exercises soon after surgery. Harris and Brown found that the patient's ability to walk postoperatively was the most important factor in maintaining patency, to the extent that they consider thrombectomy contraindicated in patients with hemiparesis or those unable to walk because of other injury.[28]

Complications

The most dreaded complication of iliofemoral thrombectomy is PE resulting from dislodgement of thrombus while manipulating the Fogarty catheter or other suction device. For this reason Fogarty proposed placing an occluding catheter in the IVC through a contralateral groin incision. Using this technique he had no instances of intraoperative PE in 43 patients, although one patient who was inadequately anticoagulated developed PE 3 weeks postoperatively. By and large, this method of embolism prevention has never been used widely because of reluctance on the part of surgeons to incise and manipulate the contralateral femoral vein. Most surgeons prefer increased intraabdominal pressure during Fogarty passage to prevent proximal migration of any thrombus dislodged. Of 165 thrombectomies, Andriopoulos and coworkers[16] reported two fatal intraoperative and four nonfatal cases of PE. Barner et al.,[31] Edwards et al.,[32] and Bertelsen[33] had no cases of PE in 70, 69, and 15 patients, respectively, using increased intraabdominal pressure during thrombectomy. Mavor and Galloway's series[18] of 228 cases reported seven fatalities from PE, two of which were intraoperative. Of the five postoperative deaths, two patients had IVC ligation following PE, which was felt to have contributed to their deaths. All five instances of postoperative embolism were associated with incomplete thrombectomies. However, the issue of bilaterality must be considered. In this and other series,[25,34] it is assumed that the embolus originates from the involved side despite a known significant incidence of bilateral vein involvement. Although less likely, thrombus may embolize from the contralateral side, which again argues the need for preoperative venography or noninvasive duplex examination.

DeWeese and colleagues[19] examined the complication rates between 11 thrombectomy patients and 12 patients treated conservatively. In the medically treated group, there were five deaths, the ultimate cause of which was related in all cases to venous thrombosis or its complications. Six patients developed venous gangrene, and four of them died. Another became uremic because of renal tubular necrosis possibly secondary to phlegmasia cerulea dolens. All five had signs and symptoms of PE, which was demonstrated at autopsy in four cases. In the surgery group three patients died: one of aspiration pneumonia postoperatively; one, with severe hypertension, from a cerebrovascular accident; and one from carcinomatosis on day 8. There were no documented cases of PE. Wound complications secondary to bleeding and hematoma and delayed wound healing, including one case of abdominal wound dehiscence, were also seen. Smith[30] noted one fatality from PE in his group of 16 patients treated by anticoagulation alone and one surgical death from multiple PE in a patient moribund prior to thrombectomy.

The remainder of the thrombectomy-associated complications have been wound problems, usually hematoma with or without superimposed infection. Lindhagen and coworkers[35] had 16 complications in 14 patients for a 50% complication rate, including six wound infections, four cases of bleeding, one slipped heparin catheter, and five cases of rethrombosis, three of which required reoperation. Smith[30] described a one-third incidence of delayed wound healing from prolonged lymphatic drainage. In many of these series, bleeding problems were controlled with more careful attention to heparin and warfarin regulation. Among other complications, postthrombectomy progression of thrombus leading to ischemia and amputation was seen rarely,[16,30] and even less frequently reported were femoral, iliac, or IVC perforation from Fogarty or other catheters.[34,36]

The majority of the above complications can be avoided with meticulous technique and hemostasis, close monitoring of heparin administration, and careful manipulation of catheters.

Perhaps the most frequent complication but the hardest to assess is prevalence of rethrombosis. Without preoperative and intraoperative venography it is difficult to distinguish thrombus never cleared from new thrombus formed after patency is reestablished. Clearance, of course, is dependent upon many variables. Operator technique, duration of symptoms, clot adherence, isolated proximal vs. extensive thrombus, and mechanical obstruction each affects to a greater or lesser degree the patency achieved and therefore the rethrombosis rate.

RESULTS

Early reports of thrombectomy were encouraging. One of the earliest series was by Mahorner et al. in 1957[5] who described results of 16 thrombectomies in 15 patients with phlegmasia alba or phlegmasia cerulea dolens using increased abdominal pressure, common duct stone forceps, and suction catheters to extrude the clot. Excellent results were obtained in 12 patients, good results in two patients, and poor results in two patients. Postoperative venograms showed patency of the iliofemoral system in 3 of 4 patients. In 1963, Haller and Abrams reported on 45 patients with iliofemoral thrombosis and concluded that duration of symptoms preoperatively determined postoperative results.[27] Of 34 patients with a history of less than 10 days, 26 had normal limbs postoperatively with an 84% normal limb rate at 6 months, and the remaining 16% had slight to moderate disability. In contrast, of 11 patients with symptoms present 14 or more days, only one had a normal leg after 6 months, two required amputation from progression of disease, and two died from extension of the thrombus into the vena cava.

DeWeese reported on 31 thrombectomy patients in 1964, six of whom had femoral vein ligation and five of whom had femoral vein suture grid interruption performed after thrombectomy when it was felt that residual clot remained.[37] Twenty-one had good or excellent results, with the best results seen in patients with segmental iliac and proximal femoral vein involvement with distal segments clear. No patient with excellent results had femoral vein

ligation or plication, and better results were seen following filter procedures than ligations. Follow-up of 16 patients from 1 to 5 years found only one patient with uncontrollable edema.

Table 69-2 shows the results of a comparison of medical and surgical therapy conducted by Smith in 1965.[30] Of patients in the thrombectomy group, 78% had an excellent or satisfactory result, whereas only 50% of the medically treated group had similar clinical results. Smith also found the mean duration of hospitalization to be 6 days shorter for the surgical patients, including the surgical failures. Interestingly, there was little correlation between postoperative venography and clinical result, although this may be explained by operative assessment of patency being made by back-bleeding and not intraoperative venography.

Following development of the Fogarty balloon catheter to extrude clots, Fogarty reported on short-term and 22-month follow-up results in 43 patients.[6] Twenty-one patients had thrombectomy with a 90% excellent short-term result and an 82% excellent long-term result. Ten patients had IVC plication at the time of therapy with good results initially in 7 of 12 and mixed results at late follow-up.

In the large series of 228 patients reported by Mavor and Galloway in 1969, 67% had phlegmasia cerulea dolens and two had venous gangrene[18]; PE was the initial diagnosis in 38 patients. Total clearance of the venous system was achieved in 78 patients, all of whom had good clinical results. Another 126 patients had partial clearance with satisfactory clinical findings. Table 69-3 demonstrates the correlation of PE to degree of clearance. This high rate of PE following thrombectomy was not seen in any other series and occurred despite postoperative urokinase and local heparin therapy.

Overall, initial reports were good, and thrombectomy appeared a superior treatment to conventional medical therapy until it fell into disfavor with the 1968 report by Lansing and Davis[7] on the 5-year follow-up of 45 patients initially reported by Haller and Abrams.[27] Of the 17 initial 45 patients (38%) who were alive and available for follow-up, Lansing and Davis found only one without significant edema. Venograms done in 15 of 17 patients showed all with an incompetent deep venous system without functioning valves. Encouraging reports such as those of Harris and Brown in 1968 who reported good clinical results with venographic patency and normal valves in 15 of 17 patients[28] were overshadowed by the discouraging results of Lansing and Davis.

TABLE 69-2. COMPARISON OF MEDICAL AND SURGICAL THERAPY

Treatment	Clinical Result			
	Excellent	Satisfactory	Failure	Death
Iliofemoral thrombectomy 18 patients (mean follow-up 17 mo)	39%	39%	17%	5%*
Heparin and warfarin 16 patients (mean follow-up 16 mo)	12%	38%	44%	6%†

* Patient moribund prior to surgery with multiple PE.
† Fatal PE during therapy.
From Smith GW. Surg Gynecol Obstet 121:1298, 1965.

TABLE 69-3. CONTROL OF EMBOLISM BY ILIOFEMORAL VENOUS THROMBECTOMY

	Complete Clearance	Partial Clearance	Failure
Total	38	52	23
Further embolism	5 (13%)	12 (23%)	8 (35%)
Fatal embolism	0	4 (8%)	3 (13%)

One year later, Barner and coworkers[31] described good clinical results in 42 of 70 patients who underwent iliofemoral venous thrombectomy despite almost universal evidence of thrombosis or recanalization on venograms done several weeks postoperatively, calling into question the true efficacy of thrombectomy in cases of late morbidity. Additional poor results—a postthrombotic syndrome rate of 74%—reported by Johanssen and coworkers in 1972[25] further questioned the effectiveness of the procedure. A comparison of surgical and medical treatment was conducted by Young et al. in 1974[14] who concluded that the incidence of postthrombotic syndrome was no different in the two groups. However, their surgical group consisted of patients with IVC and superficial femoral vein ligation with and without thrombectomy, and only three patients underwent thrombectomy alone.

After an almost 10-year period of negativism, proponents of the procedure began publishing favorable results. Lindhagen and colleagues in 1978[35] published a series of 28 patients undergoing thrombectomy, 18 with phlegmasia alba dolens and five with phlegmasia cerulea dolens. Intraoperative venography was performed to confirm clearance in all patients. Early results showed 86% excellent clinical results and 56% incidence of complete clearance on venography, with excellent clinical results in 82% of patients at 6-month follow-up. Provan and Rumble[38] operated on 12 patients with duration of symptoms less than 48 hours and found eight patients had normal limbs postoperatively which remained asymptomatic over time. The four remaining patients in the series had minor symptoms which did not progress, and three of them were found to have the iliac vein compression syndrome described earlier by Cockett and Thomas.[21]

Over the next few years, several papers were published showing superiority of thrombectomy over conservative treatment for iliofemoral thrombosis.[16,32,39] The study by Röder et al. in 1985[40] in which 46 thrombectomies were performed, 21 for phlegmasia cerulea dolens and 10 with preoperative PE, reported good results. At 5-month follow-up, 44% of the patients were asymptomatic, which decreased only to 40% after 10 years. Minor edema was seen in 27% of patients, with 33% showing significant edema or ulceration at 10 years. Horsch and Pichlmaier[34] found 75% good or excellent results with a mean follow-up of 26 months in their study of 161 patients.

Several conclusions can be reached on the basis of the published results of various authors. Success of thrombectomy is dependent upon the ability to completely clear the proximal thrombus. Many of the earlier studies used the degree of back bleeding as a measure of clearance, which is unreliable since bleeding may occur from a patent internal iliac vein despite a thrombosed proximal common iliac vein. Before development of the Fogarty catheter, most of the suction devices could not be passed proximal to the level of the pelvic brim because of anatomic constraints. It is likely that thrombectomy was perceived as complete when resistance was met, when in fact an obstructing clot remained proximal to the catheter. It was not until intraoperative venography was instituted on a routine basis that more accurate assessment of clearance was obtained, and therefore a more valid assessment of the efficacy of thrombectomy was possible.

The longer a thrombus is present the more adherent to the vein wall it becomes and the less likely that it can be cleared at thrombectomy. Goto et al.[39] and Provan and Rumble[38] found their best results when thrombectomy was done within 48 hours after the onset of symptoms. Lindhagen et al.[35] reported 91% excellent results if thrombectomy was performed within 7 days, which decreased to 60% at 7 to 14 days; the procedure was impossible when symptoms were present over 2 weeks. Edwards and coworkers[32] noted similar findings at 10 days. According to Andriopoulos et al.[16] patency of femoral and pelvic veins following thrombectomy declined from 29/41 at less than 4 days to 8/41 at 5 to 8 days and 4/41 at more than 8 days. Röder and colleagues[40] showed no correlation between preoperative duration of symptoms and postoperative patency. Patency rates of 54% were seen when the symptoms had been present less than a week and 64% when symptoms were more prolonged.

Correlation between venographic and clinical results is usually good when patients have a normal limb. That is, venography consistently demonstrates patency and competent valves when the clinical result is excellent. In cases of only partial clearance, rethrombosis, or recanalization, with or without competent valves, clinical results vary from excellent to poor.[31,35] There is no linear relationship between the degree of residual disease on venographic studies and symptoms. Early ambulation, venous intermittent compression boots, and active and passive leg exercises have all contributed to improved recovery and a better clinical result. Edwards and colleagues[32] were so convinced of the importance of early ambulation that they revised their indications for surgery to exclude hemiplegics, pelvic fracture patients, and others unable to ambulate within the first 1 to 2 postoperative days.

Finally, careful operative technique is essential. Complete extrusion of clot proximally and distally while maintaining valve integrity is important. Failure of absolute hemostasis with resultant hematoma may contribute to early rethrombosis. Since patients as a general rule receive either local or systemic heparin followed by warfarin treatment postoperatively to minimize rethrombosis, they are at an increased risk of bleeding and hematoma formation.

ADJUNCTIVE MEASURES

Anticoagulation

The role of anticoagulation in the treatment of iliofemoral thrombosis is well established and was discussed previously, with a PE rate of 1 to 12% and a mortality rate of 1% in patients treated with anticoagulant therapy alone. Postthrombotic syndrome occurs in 50 to 80% of patients, and it is in this area of late morbidity that thrombectomy can provide a superior result by restoring patency and preserving valve function.

Heparin has been used in the perioperative and postoperative period to maintain patency, particularly in those instances of partial clearance by thrombectomy. There is some doubt as to the benefit of postoperative heparin in cases of isolated proximal thrombosis, but in the cases of extensive disease, particularly with calf thrombosis not readily cleared with Fogarty catheters, it helps prevent proximal clot propagation. The current trend in heparin therapy has been toward local infusion into a branch of the saphenous vein to provide anticoagulant therapy locally at a lower overall dosage and thereby reduce systemic complications. Whether this will prove to be more efficacious remains to be established. The maximal anticoagulation benefit is derived within the first 2 to 3 months, at which time the endothelialization of damaged intima has been completed and the majority of thrombogenic sources are no longer present.

One question that remains is whether other thrombolytic drugs such as streptokinase and urokinase may prove more effective than heparin in clot dissolution and restoration of normal venous anatomy. In 1978, Dhall and coworkers[41] reported on 39 patients who underwent streptokinase therapy for venous thrombosis, 37 of which were at the iliofemoral level. They found 9 of 39 patients with complete clearance on final venogram, generally 7 to 9 days after start of treatment. Incomplete clearance was seen in 30 patients, with five patients demonstrating complete reocclusion after an initial lysis period. Dhall et al. found the maximum lysis period to be the first 36 to 48 hours of therapy, and it was associated with lower fibrinogen and plasminogen levels. Heparin therapy at 625 USP units per hour to maintain saphenofemoral cannula patency was given to 15 patients, while 24 received additional heparin therapy, and 16 of them were given warfarin. Interestingly, therapeutic heparin dosages did not influence rethrombosis rates in either the partial or complete clearance group, calling into question the value of continuing anticoagulant therapy after the rethrombosis period begins at 24 to 48 hours following treatment. Since the total clearance rate was only 23% with a 13% incidence of total reocclusion, it seems unlikely that streptokinase would be any more effective in preventing the postthrombotic syndrome than heparin therapy. In support of this, Seaman and colleagues[42] compared the effects of streptokinase (24 patients) with heparin therapy (26 patients) in patients who had DVT at any level, confirmed by venography, with symptoms of 5 days or less duration. They found more rapid lysis with streptokinase at 3 days, but after 10 days of therapy there was no difference in the two groups. Furthermore, bleeding complications caused interruption of therapy in 29% of the group treated with streptokinase and 19% of the group treated with heparin.

In a prospective study of 29 patients with major DVT (thrombosis involving the popliteal or proximal veins or both, with or without calf DVT), Kakkar and Lawrence[43] compared hemodynamic and clinical results in patients receiving 5-day treatment with heparin or streptokinase, followed by a 6-month course of warfarin. Overall, at 2-year follow-up they found over half of the limbs with evidence of severe hemodynamic changes equivalent to those seen in established postthrombotic changes. Clinically, 14% of patients had no symptoms, 20% had severe symptoms, and the remainder demonstrated mild to moderate changes. No difference was seen between patients receiving heparin and streptokinase. It appears, then, that the hope of developing a drug to restore venous patency and preserve valve function as thrombectomy proposes to do has not yet materialized. Other thrombolytic drugs such as tissue plasminogen activator are currently under investigation. If these demonstrate efficacy in lysis of thrombosis in the deep venous system, they may provide new alternatives in treatment.

Vena Cava Interruption

Inferior vena cava or superficial femoral vein ligation was used long before thrombectomy in management of patients with PE and proximal DVT, but it had an unacceptably high incidence of severe postthrombotic syndrome. Therefore, it seemed logical to perform thrombectomy at the same time as venous interruption to reestablish patency of major veins and reduce postoperative edema and ulceration while providing protection against embolism in high-risk patients. In his 1964 article, DeWeese[37] found that plication or filter placement caused less morbidity and was as effective as femoral vein or IVC ligation in preventing PE in patients with incomplete clearance following thrombectomy. Brockman and Vasko in their 1965 article[44] on the pathophysiology and treatment of phlegmasia cerulea dolens advocated IVC plication with thrombectomy for iliofemoral thrombosis with preoperative PE or "impending embolism." Clearly, the patients who had plication with thrombectomy had more severe sequelae than those with thrombectomy alone, but whether this was caused by more severe disease in the patients requiring plication or by the operative procedure itself was not established. In 1967, DeWeese et al.[29] reported on 21 patients with partial femoral vein interruption and six patients with IVC plication. Of the patients with femoral vein interruption, 10 had clinical evidence of distal thrombus progression confirmed by venography in seven cases. Of those with IVC interruption, half had further distal progression, suggesting that the plication procedure itself leads to further thrombus production by causing increased stasis. Two years later, Edwards and coworkers[32] described 3 of 58 patients who had IVC interruption at the time of iliofemoral thrombectomy. All had further thrombosis, and two had contralateral occlusion 11 and 10 months postoperatively while taking oral anticoagulants.

Currently, indications for vena cava interruption at the time of thrombectomy are recurrent PE or unsuccessful or incomplete thrombectomy in a high-risk patient. The issue of increased morbidity following IVC filtration today is less important since the Greenfield vena cava filter has a documented long-term patency rate of 95%[45] and has not been shown to be associated with an increase in the postthrombotic syndrome in patients treated with the filter alone or the filter and anticoagulants.

VENOUS BYPASS AND GRAFT REPLACEMENT

The role of venous bypass or graft replacement surgery in the management of iliofemoral venous thrombosis has traditionally been one of ameliorating symptoms in the patient with chronic pain or ulceration. One of the earlier techniques was replacement of part of a diseased vein with autogenous vein graft with intact valves, the concept being to control edema caused by valve incompetence or obstruction. The results showed high patency rates but with recanalization rates of 30 to 40% with functionless valves.[46,47] Palma and Esperon developed the crossover saphenous vein graft in 1959, tunneling the saphenous vein across the pubis to the involved femoral vein below the point of obstruction while leaving the proximal saphenous vein intact[48] (Figs. 69-9 to 69-12). Initial reports claimed a success rate of greater than 60%, but subsequent reports suggested that clinical status of the limb often had little correlation to bypass graft patency.[36]

Taking into account all venous bypass procedures, clinical improvement is seen in 75% of selected patients.[49] Again, these procedures have been used in patients who have already developed the postthrombotic syndrome.

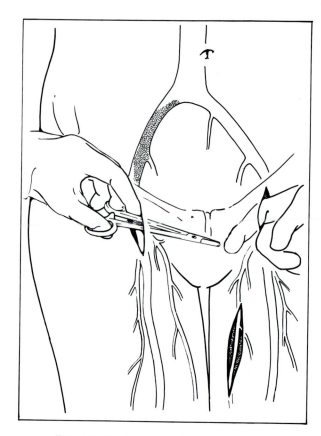

Figure 69-10. Formation of cross pubis tunnel.

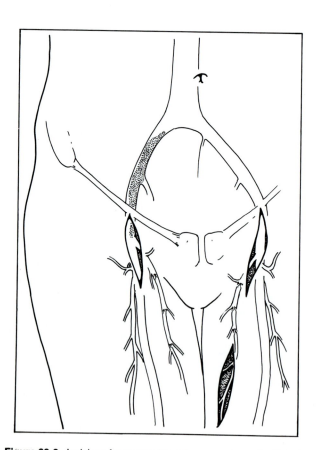

Figure 69-9. Incisions for crossover saphenous vein graft with isolation of the contralateral saphenous vein.

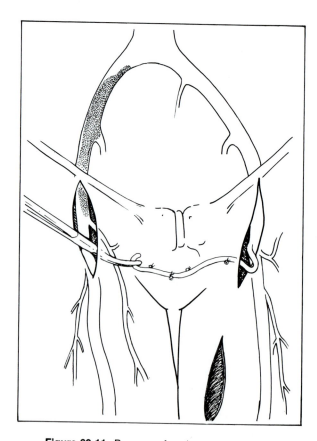

Figure 69-11. Passage of saphenous vein graft.

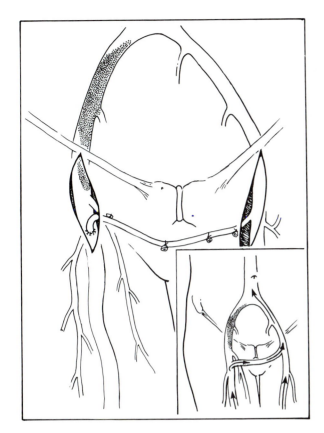

Figure 69-12. Venous outflow restored through contralateral limb.

An application of the Palma procedure to acute management of proximal venous occlusion was reported by McNeil and Sorour in 1980.[50] They described two cases of phlegmasia cerulea dolens that failed thrombectomy as documented by operative venography. Greater saphenous vein crossover bypass graft to the femoral vein of the affected side was performed under the same anesthesia, with excellent results in both cases and normal limbs at 30- and 48-month follow-up. This result suggests that the procedure may be an effective approach for patients who fail thrombectomy despite relative acuteness of symptoms or for those in whom a poor result is anticipated based on residual thrombus present at venography.

Role of AV Fistula in Post-Thrombectomy Patency

Just as the initial work with venous bypass techniques was conducted in patients with late morbidity following acute occlusion, initial work with arteriovenous (AV) fistulas was in conjunction with venous reconstruction in the patient with chronic venous changes. The theory behind creation of an AV fistula was to increase venous flow in the bypass segment, thereby maintaining patency. It soon followed that this concept could be used in the acute setting to prevent the newly thrombectomized segment from reoccluding.

Levin et al., in 1971,[51] created either side-to-side or H-type AV fistulas in dogs, using autogenous external jugular vein to replace femoral vein bilaterally. The contralateral

side was replaced without fistula for control in each dog. The H-type fistula (Fig. 69-13) was found to be superior to the side-to-side fistula with a 90% 6-week patency and no late reocclusion following fistula closure. Interestingly, in the side-to-side fistula group four dogs occluded their grafts and never regained patency, while in the control group, 6 of 10 dogs thrombosed their grafts early, but all were recanalized by 6 weeks. This led Levin and coworkers to conclude that venous blood contains more fibrinolytic activity than arterial blood and that the dilution effect of the arterial blood from the AV fistula prevented recanalization.

Delin and colleagues[52] reported in 1982 their clinical experience using postthrombectomy AV fistula in 13 women with acute iliofemoral thrombosis. Fistulas were created between the saphenous vein and femoral artery at thrombectomy and were closed at 3 months. At follow-up venography, early patency of the iliofemoral segment was 85%, and plethysmographic values reverted to normal in 8 of 11 patients. Prior to treatment the level of plasminogen activator in the thrombosis group was lower than in the control group without thrombosis, suggesting a deficiency in release of plasminogen activators as a thrombosis etiology.

In 1984, Plate et al.[53] published results comparing 32 patients with iliofemoral thrombosis treated with anticoagulation alone and 31 patients with proximal occlusion treated by thrombectomy, temporary AV fistula, and anticoagulation. At 6-month follow-up, only 7% of the medically treated group were symptom free compared to 42% of the surgically treated group, in which there was a 13% reocclusion rate. Clinical, venographic, Doppler, and venous exercise pressure measurements in both groups showed nine patients with all measurements normal; all were from the surgically treated group. No patient in the medically treated group had all normal findings. In a recent large study Einarsson and colleagues[54] performed iliofemoral venous thrombectomy and temporary AV fistula in 57 patients with acute thrombosis. They found 75% with good and 20% with fair clinical results and a venographic iliofemoral patency rate of 61%. Eighty-two percent had normal femoral venous pressures. However, follow-up was less than a year, and long-term effects of AV fistula combined with thrombectomy are not yet well established. Also, no author has published a series comparing thrombectomy results with those of thrombectomy and AV fistula.

Arteriovenous fistula with venous bypass for acute occlusion was recently carried out by Ijima and coworkers[55] using an EPTFE (expanded polytetrafluroethylene) synthetic graft instead of a crossover saphenous vein graft. All patients had failed attempt at thrombectomy. The bypass graft remained patent in 3 of 4 cases, and although some edema was present when the fistula was open, symptoms disappeared following fistula closure.

Arteriovenous fistula with thrombectomy or in conjunction with venous bypass following failed thrombectomy appears to yield consistently higher short-term patency rates. However, the key to success of any surgical procedure for proximal venous thrombosis is in reduction of postthrombotic sequelae, for which further follow-up study is needed.

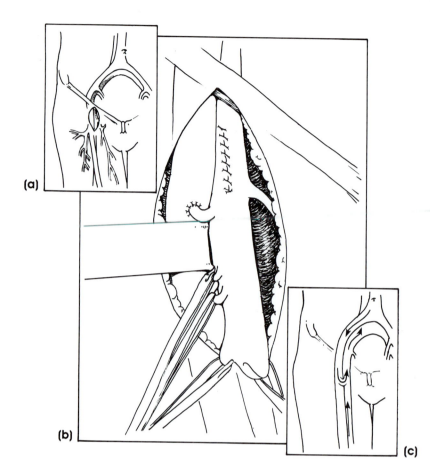

Figure 69-13. Construction of H-type fistula. **(a)** Incision. **(b)** Fistula formation and venotomy closure following thrombectomy. **(c)** Restoration of blood flow through fistula and previously occluded segment.

REFERENCES

1. Läwen VA: Über Thrombektomie bei Venenthrombose und Arteriospasmus. Zentralbl Chir 17:961, 1937.
2. Homans J: Thrombosis of the deep veins of the lower leg causing pulmonary embolism. N Engl J Med 211:993, 1934.
3. Allen AW: Management of thromboembolic disease in surgical patients. Surg Gynecol Obstet 96:107, 1953.
4. Fontaine R: Remarks concerning venous thrombosis and its sequelae. Surgery 41:6, 1957.
5. Mahorner H, Castlebury JW, Coleman WO: Attempts to restore function in major veins which are the site of massive thrombosis. Ann Surg 146:510, 1957.
6. Fogarty TJ, Dennis D, Krippaehne WW: Surgical management of iliofemoral venous thrombosis. Am J Surg 112:211, 1966.
7. Lansing AM, Davis WM: Five-year follow-up study of iliofemoral venous thrombectomy. Ann Surg 168:620, 1968.
8. Browse NL, Clemenson G, Croft DN: Fibrinogen-detectable thrombosis in the legs and pulmonary embolism. Br Med J 1:603, 1974.
9. Havig O: Deep vein thrombosis and pulmonary embolism. An autopsy study with multiple regression analysis of possible risk factors. Acta Chir Scand 478:1, 1977.
10. Haimovici H: The ischemic forms of venous thrombosis. 1. Phlegmasia cerulea dolens. 2. Venous gangrene. J Cardiovasc Surg 7(suppl):164, 1966.
11. Bauer G: Thrombosis. Early diagnosis and abortive treatment with heparin. Lancet 1:447, 1945.
12. Orsini RA, Jarrell BE: Suprarenal placement of vena caval filters: Indications, techniques, and results. J Vasc Surg 1:124, 1984.
13. Bauer G: Clinical experiences of a surgeon in the use of heparin. Am J Cardiol 14:29, 1964.
14. Young AE, Thomas ML, Browse NL: Comparison between sequelae of surgical and medical treatment of venous thromboembolism. Br Med J 4:127, 1974.
15. Bauer GT: Roentgenologic and clinical study of the sequels of thrombosis. Acta Chir Scand 86(suppl 74):5, 1942.
16. Andriopoulos A, Wirsing P, Botticher R: Results of iliofemoral venous thrombectomy after acute thrombosis. Report on 165 cases. J Cardiovasc Surg 23:123, 1982.
17. McLachlin J, Paterson JC: Some basic observations on venous thrombosis and pulmonary embolism. Surg Gynecol Obstet 93:1, 1951.
18. Mavor GE, Galloway JMD: Iliofemoral venous thrombosis. Pathological considerations and surgical management. Br J Surg 56:45, 1969.
19. DeWeese JA, Jones TI, et al.: Evaluation of thrombectomy in the management of iliofemoral venous thrombosis. Surgery 47:140, 1960.
20. Sevitt S: The acutely swollen leg and deep vein thrombosis. Br J Surg 54:886, 1967.
21. Cockett FB, Thomas ML: The iliac compression syndrome. Br J Surg 52:816, 1965.
22. Gaston LW: Studies on a family with an elevated plasma level of factor V (proaccelerin) and a tendency to thrombosis. J Pediatr 68:367, 1966.
23. Egeberg O: Inherited antithrombin deficiency causing thrombophilia. Thromb Diath Haemorrh 13:516, 1965.
24. Vasko JS, Brockman SK: Massive venous occlusion of the lower extremity: An experimental study. Surg Forum 13:233, 1964.

25. Johansson E, Nordlander S, Zetterquist S: Venous thrombectomy in the lower extremity—clinical, phlebographic and plethysmographic evaluation of early and late results. Acta Chir Scand 139:511, 1973.

26. McLachlin AD, Carroll SE, et al.: Experimental venous thrombectomy. Ann Surg 171:956, 1970.

27. Haller AJ, Abrams BL: Use of thrombectomy in the treatment of acute iliofemoral venous thrombosis in forty-five patients. Ann Surg 158:561, 1963.

28. Harris EJ, Brown WH: Patency after thrombectomy for iliofemoral thrombosis. Ann Surg 167:91, 1968.

29. DeWeese JA, Adams JT, Rogoff SM: Restoration and maintenance of venous patency in venous thrombosis: Anticoagulation, thrombectomy and partial venous interruption. Pac Med Surg 75:77, 1967.

30. Smith GW: Therapy of iliofemoral venous thrombosis. Surg Gynecol Obstet 121:1298, 1965.

31. Barner HB, Willman VL, et al.: Thrombectomy for iliofemoral venous thrombosis. JAMA 208:2442, 1969.

32. Edwards WH, Sawyers JL, Foster JH: Iliofemoral venous thrombosis: Reappraisal of thrombectomy. Ann Surg 171:961, 1970.

33. Bertelsen S: Surgical management of iliofemoral thrombophlebitis. Acta Chir Scand 135:149, 1969.

34. Horsch S, Pichlmaier H: Surgery of the venous system—present state of the art. Thorac Cardiovasc Surg 31:8, 1983.

35. Lindhagen J, Haglund M, et al.: Iliofemoral venous thrombectomy. J Cardiovasc Surg 19:319, 1978.

36. Stirnemann P, Althaus U, et al.: Early phlebographic results after iliofemoral venous thrombectomy. Thorac Cardiovasc Surg 32:299, 1984.

37. DeWeese JA: Thrombectomy for acute iliofemoral venous thrombosis. J Cardiovasc Surg 5:703, 1964.

38. Provan JL, Rumble EJ: Re-evaluation of thrombectomy in the management of iliofemoral venous thrombosis. Can J Surg 22:378, 1979.

39. Goto H, Wada T: Iliofemoral venous thrombectomy. Follow-up studies of 88 patients. J Cardiovasc Surg 21:341, 1980.

40. Röder OC, Lorentzen JE, Hansen HJB: Venous thrombectomy for iliofemoral thrombosis. Early and long-term results in 46 consecutive cases. Acta Chir Scand 150:31, 1984.

41. Dhall DP, Dawson AA, Mavor GE: Problems of resistant thrombolysis and early recurrent thrombosis in streptokinase therapy. Surg Gynecol Obstet 146:15, 1978.

42. Seaman AJ, Common HH, et al.: Deep vein thrombosis treated with streptokinase or heparin. Angiology 27:549, 1976.

43. Kakkar VV, Lawrence D: Hemodynamic and clinical assessment after therapy for acute deep vein thrombosis. A prospective study. Am J Surg 150:54, 1985.

44. Brockman SK, Vasko JS: Observation on the pathophysiology and treatment of phlegmasia cerulea dolens with special reference to thrombectomy. Am J Surg 109:485, 1965.

45. Greenfield LJ, Peyton R, et al.: Greenfield vena cava filter experience: Late results in 156 patients. Arch Surg 116:1451, 1981.

46. DeWeese JA, Niguidula F: The replacement of short segments of veins with functional autogenous venous grafts. Surg Gynecol Obstet 110:303, 1960.

47. Dale WA: Thrombosis and recannulization of veins used as venous grafts. Angiology 12:603, 1961.

48. Palma EC, Esperon R: Vein transplants and grafts in the surgical treatment of the postphlebitic syndrome. J Cardiovasc Surg 1:94, 1960.

49. Dale WA: Venous bypass surgery. Surg Clin North Am 62:391, 1982.

50. McNeil AD, Sorour NN: Veno-venous internal saphenous crossover graft for phlegmasia cerulea dolens. Br J Surg 67:877, 1980.

51. Levin PM, Rich NM, et al.: Role of arteriovenous shunts in venous reconstruction. Am J Surg 122:183, 1971.

52. Delin A, Swedenberg J, et al.: Thrombectomy and arteriovenous fistula for iliofemoral venous thrombosis in fertile women. Surg Gynecol Obstet 154:69, 1982.

53. Plate G, Einarsson E, et al.: Thrombectomy with temporary arteriovenous fistula: The treatment of choice in acute iliofemoral venous thrombosis. J Vasc Surg 1:867, 1984.

54. Einarsson E, Albrechtsson U, et al.: Follow-up evaluation of venous morphologic factors and function after thrombectomy and temporary arteriovenous fistula in thrombosis of iliofemoral vein. Surg Gynecol Obstet 163:111, 1986.

55. Ijima H, Kodama M, Hori M: Temporary arteriovenous fistula for venous reconstruction using synthetic graft: A clinical and experimental investigation. J Cardiovasc Surg 26:131, 1985.

56. Matsubara J, Hirai M, et al.: Treatment of ilio-femoral venous occlusion. J Cardiovasc Surg 23(3):256, 1982.

CHAPTER 70

Ischemic Venous Thrombosis: Phlegmasia Cerulea Dolens and Venous Gangrene

Henry Haimovici

One of the outstanding features of acute venous thrombosis of the extremities is absence of any appreciable anoxemia of the tissues. In contrast to this classic form, characterized primarily by manifestations of acute venous insufficiency, there are instances of thrombophlebitis exhibiting truly dramatic and often catastrophic circulatory disturbances. These may range from transient severe ischemic changes to actual gangrene.[1,2]

Historically, ischemic manifestations of vascular disturbances were thought to have an arterial origin. Acceptance of the idea that such manifestations could be induced by acute venous thrombosis alone without arterial participation was slow in coming (Fig. 70-1). Venous-induced, tissue-threatening ischemia in the presence of persistent patency of the arterial tree at times poses difficult diagnostic and therapeutic questions.

Definition of Terms

Earlier terms used to define this condition were often inadequate and at times misleading, such as pseudoembolic phlebitis,[3] acute massive venous occlusion,[4] and thrombophlebitis with spasm and gangrene.[5] Currently, phlegmasia cerulea dolens (blue thrombophlebitis)[6] and gangrene of venous origin[7-9] have gained wide acceptance. However, used interchangeably, these terms, although conveying some of the highlights of the syndrome, have also often led to some confusion. The multiplicity of terms primarily is due to uncertainty as to the exact pathogeneis of this entity.

The ischemia of the tissues appeared the outstanding common denominator as conveyed by the various terms for this type of acute venous thrombosis. For the sake of emphasizing the true ischemic nature of the clinicopathologic manifestations, in the early 1960s I proposed for this entity the comprehensive term *ischemic venous thrombosis*[1] (IVT) and subdivided it into two distinct clinical stages for which two of the widely used terms were retained and redefined: (1) *phlegmasia cerulea dolens* (PCD), a reversible stage, and (2) *venous gangrene*, an irreversible stage of the process associated with varying degrees of tissue loss.

It should be pointed out that although these two stages or forms are part of the same overall clinicopathologic entity, the difference between them not only is a matter of degree of the underlying venous occlusion but also of their course and ultimate prognosis. Early recognition and treatment of PCD is of the utmost importance if gangrene is to be prevented. Herein lies the significance of this classification into two stages.

Historical Background

Historically, the notion of causal relationship between acute venous occlusion and gangrene of the extremities is not new. As early as 1593, Fabricius Hildanus[10] recognized the possibility of gangrene associated with venous thrombosis. Subsequently, particularly during the eighteenth and nineteenth centuries, this condition was the subject of sporadic case reports. From findings made primarily at autopsy, several pathogenic mechanisms were proposed. Thus, Godin, in 1836, explained this condition by stating, "the edema associated with gangrene is of venous etiology, and venous occlusion causes the gangrene because once the blood reaches the distal parts, it can no longer return" (because of the blockage of the veins). Subsequent case reports and reviews reinforced this notion of venous gangrene in the latter part of the nineteenth century. Despite a number of subsequent contributions, the idea that ischemia can be induced only by acute venous thrombosis has not been readily accepted.

Experimental reproduction of this condition in the 1930s, solely by extensive occlusion of the venous channels, attempted to provide a pathogenic basis for this entity.[11,12] Consequently, this condition gained greater clinical significance and attention. It was in 1938 that the term *phlegmasia cerulea dolens* was introduced[6] and that attention was drawn to the association of venous gangrene with deep venous thrombosis.[7]

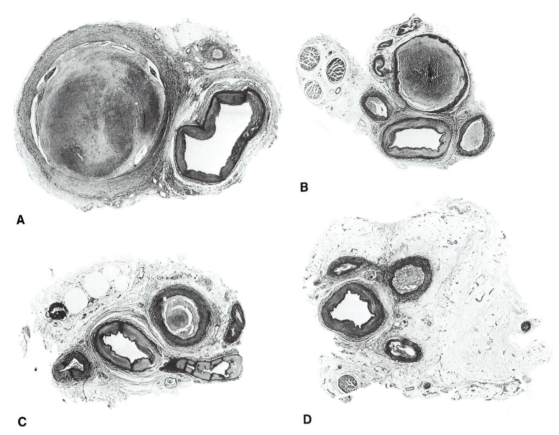

Figure 70-1. Cross sections of the blood vessels in the case of venous gangrene shown in Figure 70-4. The cross sections are through the following vessels: popliteal **(A)**, posterior **(B)**, anterior tibial **(C)**, and dorsalis pedis **(D)**. The veins are all thrombosed, whereas the arteries are all patent.

After that time a steadily increasing number of reports on IVC showed that it was more prevalent than was previously believed.

Despite accumulating information, however, the severe form of venous thrombosis was often poorly or incorrectly differentiated from the common form and moreover was often mistaken for other vascular disorders (see Differential Diagnosis).

Incidence

Ischemic forms of venous thrombosis are rarely reported or emphasized. One of the reasons is lack of correlation to the overall problem of deep venous thrombosis. Only a few statistical studies indicate such a correlation; see Table 70-1. Our own experience of over 60 cases was based on more than 600 patients.[2,13]

Greater awareness of this clinical entity is important if it is to have wider recognition. Based on the data presented in Table 70-1, it appears that IVT is probably more common than is generally believed. It is also important to emphasize that 82% of cases were due to PCD and only 18% to venous gangrene. Prompt and appropriate treatment of the PCD could have prevented the gangrene.

Etiology

The etiologic factors of IVC I described in 1971 were based on a study of 175 patients with 189 extremities involved with PCD and of 158 patients with 199 extremities involved with venous gangrene.[2] Subsequent experience has not disproved these factors. The etiology of IVT is not much different from that of common DVT except that DVT occurs more frequently. The most common etiologic factors in both groups are a postoperative state and neoplastic disease.

A postoperative state was noted in 24.8% of PCD cases and in only 13.30% of venous gangrene cases. In contrast, neoplastic disease was associated with PCD in 14.6% and with venous gangrene in 24.8% of cases. It appears, therefore, that about 1 out of 7 patients with PCD and 1 out of 4 patients with venous gangrene had an underlying visceral malignancy. The slightly higher incidence of neoplastic diseases associated with this group of cases of venous thrombosis has led a few authors to overemphasize this relationship and thus to give the erroneous impression that venous gangrene in particular is always associated with terminal illness.[21] This is fortunately not the case, unless the report is based on a small selected group of patients.

In PCD the lower extremities were involved in 95.4% of cases and the upper extremities in only 4.6% (Fig.

TABLE 70-1. INCIDENCE OF ISCHEMIC VENOUS THROMBOSIS RELATIVE TO OVERALL DEEP VENOUS TROMBOSIS

Author (year)	# of DVT	IVT		PCD		VG	
		#	%	#	%	#	%
Anlyan[14] (1957)	453	19	4.2	17	89.4	2	10.6
Devambez[15] (1953)	589	31	5.2	29	93.5	2	6.5
Fogarty[16] (1963)	655	11	1.7	8	72.9	3	27.1
Fontaine[17] (1965)	300	32	10.7	32	100	—	—
Natali[18] (1982)	117	5	4.3	5	100	—	—
Gouiran[19] (1983)	185	35	18.9	29	82.9	6	17.1
Haimovici[20] (1983)	610	62	10.1	40	64.5	22	35.5
Totals	2,909	195	6.9	160	82.0	35	18.0

DVT, deep venous trombosis; IVT, ischemic venous thrombosis; PCD, phlegmasia cerulea dolens; VG, venous gangrene.

70-2, Table 70-2). In unilateral cases the left lower extremity was affected four times as often as the right. Bilateral involvement occurred in only 6.2% of cases.

In venous gangrene, by contrast, the left lower extremity was affected only slightly more often than the right (left 56%, right 46%). In addition, there were more bilateral cases of venous gangrene than PCD. Analysis of the data shows that venous thrombosis is more extensive in venous gangrene than in PCD, indicating the highest index of thrombogenicity in this type of venous disease.

TABLE 70-2. PATHOGENESIS OF ISCHEMIC VENOUS THROMBOSIS

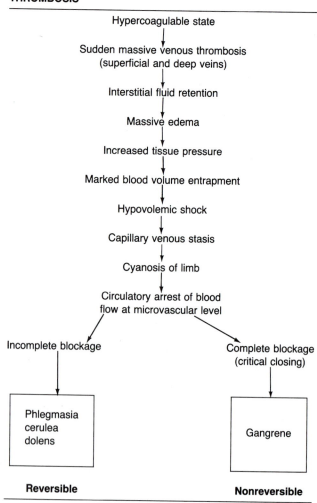

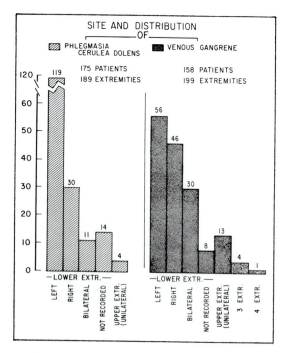

Figure 70-2. Etiology. Site and distribution of phlegmasia cerulea dolens in 175 patients with 189 extremities involved (*left*) and of venous gangrene in 158 patients with 199 extremities involved (*right*).

CLINICAL MANIFESTATIONS

Phlegmasia Cerulea Dolens

The syndrome of this form of acute circulatory disturbance (often preceded by a typical phlegmasia alba dolens) includes the classic triad of edema, cyanosis, and pain, hence the term *phlegmasia cerulea dolens*. Pain is usually severe and always present. Cyanosis is pathognomonic and is as striking as the severity of the pain. The edema, occasionally absent at the inception of PCD, is generally characteristic, having a hard, woody or rubbery consistency. After a few days, cutaneous blebs or bullae may appear.

Peripheral arterial pulses, pedal or wrist, at the initial stage may be felt in only one half the cases. Arteriography and noninvasive tests are helpful in disclosing patency of the arterial tree. Phlebography, on the other hand, will disclose extensive venous thrombosis, often up to and including the iliac veins and inferior vena cava. Circulatory collapse or hypovolemic shock from excessive fluid loss occurs in most cases because of entrapment in the involved extremity of from 3 to 5 liters of fluid. Pulmonary embolism is a frequent complication of PCD, seen in approximately 14.9% of the nonfatal cases and 3.4% of fatal cases (Fig. 70-3). This is in contrast to its greater frequency in cases of venous gangrene. Immediate recognition and treatment of PCD are essential for preventing progression to gangrene.

Venous Gangrene

The clinical picture of an IVT resulting in gangrene may go through three different phases: (1) phlegmasia alba dolens, (2) phlegmasia cerulea dolens, and (3) gangrene (Fig. 70-4).

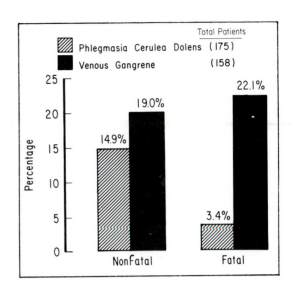

Figure 70-3. Incidence of pulmonary embolism in ischemic venous thrombosis.

Phlegmasia alba dolens will often precede by a few days the blue thrombophlebitis and venous gangrene, although in a certain number of cases it may fail to appear or may pass unnoticed.

Phlegmasia cerulea dolens is present in all instances. All peripheral pulses at the initial stage are palpable in more than half the cases. As in simple PCD, circulatory collapse is noted in many instances (21.5%) of IVT. Multiple venous occlusions involving two or more extremities are most characteristic. In addition, about 1 out of 4 patients also has uncomplicated venous thrombosis, either as phlegmasia

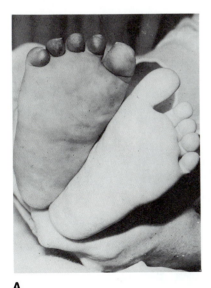
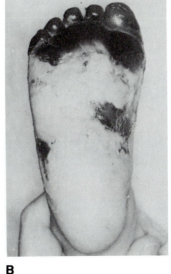
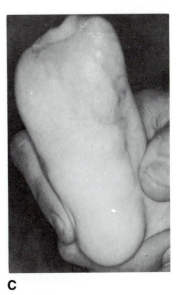

A   **B**   **C**

Figure 70-4. A. Incipient gangrene of the toes with marked cyanosis of the right foot. **B.** Extent of gangrenous lesions of the plantar surface, sites of skin incisions for the fasciotomies performed earlier for decompression of a swollen foot. **C.** Healing of the foot after self-amputation of toes and spontaneous separation of the adjacent necrotic skin 3 months after onset of the gangrene.

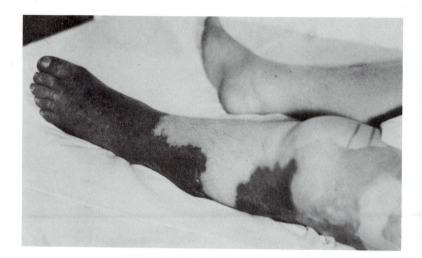

Figure 70-5. Gangrene of the left foot and the lateral aspect of the leg up to the knee, with a patchy area of discoloration above the knee. The entire extremity is massively swollen.

alba dolens or as phlegmasia cerulea dolens, affecting other extremities.

Gangrene usually develops within 4 to 8 days after the onset of the ischemic signs (Fig. 70-5). This gap between the two phases affords early recognition of the symptoms and treatment to prevent gangrene. The extent of the gangrene varies. In most patients the gangrenous lesions are limited to the toes or foot (Fig. 70-6). Rarely, they affect the leg or even the thigh, in which case the incidence of pulmonary embolism is greater, ranging from 19.0% in the nonfatal cases of venous gangrene to 22.1% in the fatal cases.

CLINICOPATHOLOGIC PATTERNS OF ISCHEMIC THROMBOSIS

Patterns of Lower Extremity

Clinical, phlebographic, and operative findings, as well as post-mortem examination, indicate that several patterns are associated with the two types of IVT of the lower extremities.

In PCD there are essentially three patterns: (1) iliofemoral, (2) femoropopliteotibial, and (3) a combined form (Fig. 70-7). Characteristic in each of the three types is patency of a number of major and collateral veins at the *root* of

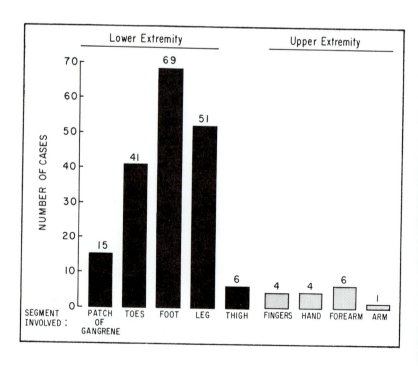

Figure 70-6. Distribution and extent of gangrene involving the lower and upper extremities. Note the relatively high incidence of distal and localized gangrene of the toes and fingers.

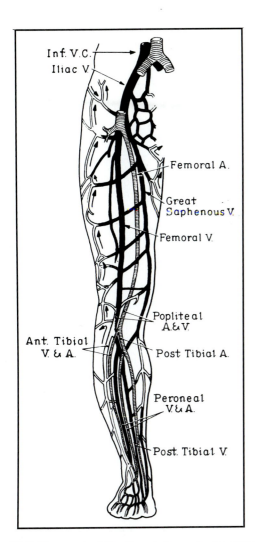

Figure 70-7. Diagram depicting the arteries and veins of the lower extremity in which venous occlusion is associated with phlegmasia cerulea dolens. Note the presence of venous collaterals at the root of the extremity where patent veins provide venous outflow and account for the reversibility of the ischemic syndrome.

the extremity, thus providing escape pathways for venous return and potential reversibility of the ischemic syndrome.

In venous gangrene there are essentially two patterns: (1) complete occlusion of the femoroiliocaval axis but with patency of the popliteotibial veins (Fig. 70-8A) and (2) complete or nearly complete occlusion of the entire venous system of the extremity, including both superficial and deep channels (Fig. 70-8B). Figure 70-8 depicts the patterns of venous occlusion leading to venous gangrene.

Patterns of Upper Extremity[2]

The anatomicopathologic patterns in the upper extremity are not so well defined as those in the lower extremity. The clinical findings and the severity of the venous thrombosis do not always correlate with the extent of gangrene. Two patterns based on the presence of (1) phlegmasia ceru-

lea dolens and (2) gangrenous lesions best express this correlation of the various findings (Table 70-3).

First Group: PCD Only

- Of the 175 patients with 189 PCD cases, only four patients had associated upper extremity involvement.
- One involved the right side, and three the left side.
- The causes varied. No precipitating cause was reported for the PCD of the right extremity. The patient was a 48-year-old man. He was treated by thrombectomy of the subclavian-axillary veins and had a complete recovery.

The causes of the other three cases were as follows:

- Influenza in a 52-year-old man treated with papaverine; he had a complete recovery.
- Hypertensive cardiovascular disease in a 64-year-old man treated with heparin and elevation; recovery was complete.
- Breast carcinoma with metastases in a 67-year-old woman treated with heparin and papaverine. She eventually died from her malignant metastatic disease.

Second Group: Gangrene of Upper Extremity

Of the 158 patients with gangrene of 199 lower extremities, 21 displayed upper-extremity gangrenous lesions, and 5 displayed only simple PCD or phlegmasia alba dolens (PAD).

Following is the extent of upper extremity involvement to be correlated with the extent of venous thrombosis:

1. Discoloration of the skin may involve the hand, the forearm, or the entire arm.
2. The gangrenous lesions may involve the fingers alone, the fingers and hand, the hand and forearm, or the entire arm.

Correlation of the number of thrombosed veins with the upper extremity segment(s) affected is indispensable. However, the most significant correlation was that of venous thrombotic lesions of the subclavian axillary veins with extensive gangrenous lesions of the hand and forearm (Table 70-3).

From an etiologic point of view, most gangrenous lesions of the upper extremity were related to lung, breast, or colon carcinoma with metastatic findings in the lungs.

All the cases of upper extremity gangrene were part of an overall picture of extensive venous thrombosis involving the lower as well as the upper extremities. The hypercoagulability state, mentioned earlier, incites this complex picture in which upper extremity involvement is only one feature of the entire thrombotic disease involving large territories of the body.

Recently, three isolated cases of gangrene of the upper extremity were reported.[22] Their causes were intravenous chemical injury, fracture of the thoracic outlet region, and prolonged bilateral placement of IV catheters. Each of the three patients had superimposed systemic diseases, which precipitated or contributed to the thrombogenic process, thus resulting in gangrene. These cases are somewhat different from the cases analyzed above.

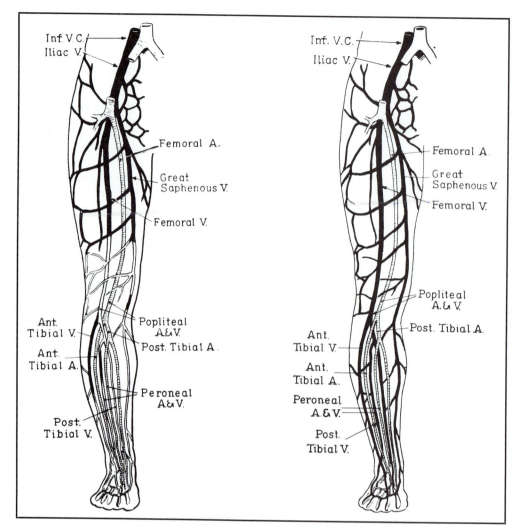

Figure 70-8. Diagram depicting complete occlusion of the entire venous system of both the superficial and deep channels. In contrast to Figure 70-3, there are no patent veins at the root of the extremity to provide venous outflow.

PATHOPHYSIOLOGY

The hypercoagulable state appears to be the initiating factor of IVT, followed by a sequence of pathophysiologic events (see Table 70-2).

A number of hematologic components have been implicated in the pathogenesis of hypercoagulability but are still not well documented. Most of the evidence is based on observations of allied conditions of venous thrombosis.

A defective fibrinolytic system due to low levels of plasminogen activators and to the liberation of thromboplastic substances from an undetectable source, often a tumor, has been postulated as one cause. Additional more specific factors present a series of complex interrelated reactions that involve the plasma coagulation mechanism. Of these, antithrombin deficiency has been suggested as a cause of unexplained thrombosis in vascular surgery. In addition, heparin-induced platelet aggregation may be a cause of unexplained thrombosis in some patients. But the chief contributing factors revealed in a recent study of unexplained thrombosis, primarily venous thrombosis, are re-

lated to the low activity level of antithrombin II (heparin cofactor activity) or antithrombin III or both.

Antithrombin II appears to be controversial. Some investigators feel that antithrombin II, depending on the method used for its determination, is in reality a function of antithrombin III.[23,24] The controversy is due to the variability of laboratory results in which normal antithrombin III and elevated antithrombin II levels are a cause of bleeding and are considered to be two different factors. The biochemical structure of antithrombin II has not been defined, and therefore its existence is speculative.

Antithrombin III deficiency is inherited and rarely causes clinically manifest thrombosis during the second decade of life. The thrombotic episodes related to antithrombin III are initiated by such predisposing factors as surgery, childbirth, and infection. The thrombosis rarely occurs spontaneously as a result of antithrombin III deficiency. Like antithrombin II, it functions as a heparin cofactor necessary for heparin's anticoagulant activity. Radioimmunoassay measures antithrombin III with the greatest accuracy. In this fashion one can estimate the total amount of the

TABLE 70-3. VENOUS GANGRENE OF UPPER EXTREMITY

Case No.*	Etiology	Clinical Manifestations	Extent of Gangrene	Anatomic Findings of Veins
7.	After IV infusion	PCD of hand and forearm	Distal phalanges of last 4 fingers	Not reported
8.	After IV infusion	Cyanosis and motor loss of hand	Hand and lower third of forearm	Thrombosis of cephalic vein
9.	Unknown	PCD	Second finger	Thrombosis of brachial veins
18.	Posttraumatic (wound of axilla)	Discoloration of ulnar aspect; no edema	Hand and forearm	Brachial ulnar and superficial veins thrombosed; radial veins patent
22.	Cancer of left lung	PCD	Hand	Thrombosis of all veins of entire extremity
26.	Posttraumatic	PCD	Hand and lower half of forearm	Thrombosis of all veins of amputated specimen
30.	Polycythemia	a. PCD b. PCD 4 days later	Hand and foot, midforearm (wet gangrene)	Thrombosis of all veins
36.	Metastatic cancer of lungs and abdomen	PCD	Patchy gangrene of right forearm and hand only	Subclavian vein thrombosed; all distal veins thrombosed
53.	Unknown	35 days after RLE	Left hand	Not reported
60.	Right lobar pneumonia	PCD	All right fingers	Clinical evidence of extensive venous thrombosis
61.	Status asthmaticus		Hand and lower third of forearm	Major veins patent (dissection incomplete); occlusion of distal veins?
108.	Heart failure	PCD, gangrene	Hand and lower half of forearm	Thrombosed
137.	Cancer of bladder, hematuria, levophed infusion	PAD, PCD, gangrene	Arm	Thrombosed
149.	Cancer of ovary	PCD	Fingers	Thrombosed
157.	Bronchogenic cancer	Distal cyanosis, edema	Left hand, right hand	Thrombosed

* Case numbers correspond to one of the 158 numbered cases reported in Hacimovici H: Ischemic Forms of Venous Thrombosis: Phlegmasia Cerulea Dolens, Venous Gangrene. Charles C Thomas, Publisher, Springfield, Ill, 1971.

protein available and assay the biologic activity of antithrombin as well. The cause of antithrombin deficiency in patients with hypercoagulability is unknown. It is assumed that these patients probably have an inherited trait. Heparin cofactor II is activated by higher concentrations of heparin and seems to selectively inhibit thrombin. Patients with reduced levels of heparin cofactor II suffer from recurrent venous thrombosis.

Another important aspect of coagulation is the proteins designated C and S.[23] Protein C is a vitamin K–dependent plasma proenzyme produced in the liver. Thrombin is the only known circulating enzyme capable of activating protein C. Activated protein C (APC) inactivates factors Va and VIIIa and thus interferes with the activation of factor X. Protein C deficiency is hereditary and is transmitted as an autosomal dominant trait. Patients with protein C deficiency are at risk for recurring thromboembolism. These patients are usually treated with warfarin. However, they should receive heparin for the first few days of warfarin therapy because protein C levels are depressed more rapidly than are the coagulation factor levels. The full expression of the anticoagulant potential of activated protein C is dependent on the availability of a second glycoprotein known as protein S. Protein S acts as a cofactor protein with APC in the inactivation of Xa. Deficiencies of protein S are also inherited as an autosomal dominant trait.

These factors of coagulation mechanism are mentioned particularly in relation to venous thrombosis leading to PCD and venous gangrene. Venous thrombosis associated with PCD and venous gangrene massively affects the deep as well as the superficial veins. Its link to warfarin in this situation is depletion of protein C and protein S. Their vitamin K–dependent synthesis is blocked, thereby tipping the hematologic coagulation-anticoagulation scale toward thrombosis.

These various factors and their interdependence may play a significant role in the coagulation or hypercoagulable state that initiates the venous thrombosis leading to venous gangrene. So far, few studies have been carried out in which these factors were used as criteria for the development and severity of the thrombogenic factors.

Besides the antithrombin II and III deficiencies and the deficiencies of proteins C and S, heparin-induced thrombocytopenia can be an inciting or complicating factor in IVT. Cryoglobulinemia and polycythemia are also found in patients who present the massive venous thrombosis which occurs in phlegmasia cerulea dolens and venous gangrene. In addition to these hematologic factors, some patients displayed disseminated intravascular coagulation (DIC) based on laboratory findings. Thus, in addition to the preceding factors, there are strictly hematologic aspects of coagulation that complicate the underlying thrombosis in the PCD and venous gangrene. All combined lead to the hypercoagulable state, which has been poorly defined in the past. Recent studies have provided a more coherent understanding of what the hypercoagulable state is: a process in which factors of different natures combine to produce this thrombogenic entity.[24]

It is important to point out that all these factors do not act individually to produce the thrombotic result. Several of these factors act at one time. They are usually associated with precipitating factors such as trauma, infection, intravenous infusion, and especially a number of life-threatening illnesses such as those which constitute low cardiac output, sepsis, congestive heart failure, and many of the other elements enumerated in the etiology of this condition.

If antithrombin deficiencies are recognized early, thrombosis could be prevented by long-term use of warfarin (Coumadin). It is claimed that warfarin or sodium warfarin, if maintained indefinitely, may elevate antithrombin III levels in some patients. This statement is based on preliminary results of a study of arterial lesions. No definite conclusions could be drawn from the laboratory studies, or from the effects of the anticoagulants in the antithrombotic treatment. It is obvious from the uncertainty about some aspects of thrombogenesis and its treatment that further experience is necessary before a definitive understanding of the underlying mechanism of the hypercoagulable state can be achieved.

Hemodynamics of Venous Blockage

The extensive blockage of venous return causes the interstitial or extravascular fluid retention reflected by the massive edema and the marked increase in tissue pressure. After 8 hours of massive venous occlusion, there is a rise in tissue pressure of 38 mm Hg on the affected side as compared to 3 mm Hg on the control side.[25]

The critical closure of arterial flow occurs mostly in complete blockage. It is in these cases that the Burton principle may account for the capillary stasis leading to ischemia.[26] Another consequence of the aforementioned physiopathologic events is a marked entrapment of blood due to excessive fluid loss in the extravascular compartment of the involved extremity. This leads to hypovolemic shock. The quantity of trapped fluid in the swollen limb has been estimated to range from 3 to 5 L. As a corollary, the average control hematocrit rises considerably, increasing by about 53%.

Vasomotor changes affecting the veins and arteries may also play a role, but such changes have been variously interpreted by clinicians and experimentalists alike. The most commonly encountered vasomotor change is a spasm in the major arteries adjacent to the thrombosed veins, primarily seen during their exposure in the femoral vessels. Vasospasm appears more pronounced in PCD than in venous gangrene cases.

Total or near total venous occlusions immediately produce a rise in venous pressure that corresponds to the mean arterial pressure. Concomitantly, the blood flow falls to zero level. Arterial blood pressure and visible arterial pulsations remain normal for a number of hours. Experimentally these changes have been shown to peak in a 6-hour period. After 12 hours of occlusion the pulse and arterial pressure distal to the occlusion usually disappear.[27]

These experimental hemodynamic data confirm the possibility of reversing the ischemic phenomena within the 6- to 12-hour period. In the clinical setting it may take slightly longer for the ischemic changes, depending on their extent, to become irreversible, a factor to bear in mind in the management of some cases.

A clear understanding of the pathophysiology of this form of venous thrombosis and proper assessment of the clinical findings are essential for determining effective management of these patients.

DIAGNOSIS

The clinical picture of both forms of IVT offers, at onset, the characteristic association of venous and arterial manifestations. Therefore a differential diagnosis from other vascular conditions may have to be made in the presence of either PCD or venous gangrene. For example, internal hemorrhage, myocardial infarction, pulmonary embolism, or traumatic injuries can cause acute peripheral circulatory failure, so common in PCD.

To diagnose venous gangrene there must be thrombophlebitis without arterial occlusion. Arteriography is helpful in differentiating venous from arterial gangrene. Other difficult diagnoses are acute infectious diabetic gangrene, gangrene complicating acute prolonged vascular collapse, and embolic gangrene (see Table 70-4). At onset it may be difficult if not impossible to predict whether the ischemic manifestations in a case of PCD would be reversible or would continue to progress toward necrosis of the tissues.

DIFFERENTIAL DIAGNOSIS

As Table 70-4 indicates, the need for differential diagnosis arises from three major clinical findings. Most of the condi-

TABLE 70-4. DIFFERENTIAL DIAGNOSIS

Phelgmasia Cerulea Dolens
  Reflex arteriospasm
  Acute inflammatory lymphedema
  Acute peripheral circulatory failure
  Peripheral arterial embolism
  Concomitant acute arterial and venous occlusion
Venous Gangrene
  Palpable pulses
  —Acute infectious gangrene
  —Gangrene complicating vascular collapse
  —Digital gangrene due to endarteritis
  Nonpalpable pulses
  —Embolic gangrene
  —Gangrene due to actue arterial thrombosis
  —Gangrene due to mixed arterial and venous occlusions
Skin Necrosis Associated with Anticoagulant Therapy

tions mentioned in Table 70-4 are discussed elsewhere in this book and need not be repeated here.

However, in recent years skin necrosis secondary to anticoagulant therapy has raised difficult problems in diagnosis. Because it is secondary to anticoagulants, drugs universally used in the management of vascular diseases, a special discussion of its differential diagnosis is warranted. One of the entities from which it should be differentiated is venous gangrene.

A number of European authors, and in recent years a few American investigators as well as surgeons dealing with these problems, have pointed out this little-known complication. Unawareness of the exact pathogenesis of venous gangrene of the extremities has often led to misdiagnosis.

In 1961, Feder and Auerbach[28] described "purple toes" as an uncommon complication of oral coumarin drug therapy. They presented six cases with a cutaneous vascular lesion occurring 3 to 8 weeks after anticoagulant therapy with coumarin derivatives had been initiated. These were differentiated from other dermatologic effects that have been observed in the course of anticoagulant therapy. The mechanisms ascribed to the production of the cutaneous vascular lesions were direct capillary and cellular damage and vasodilatation. Of course, because these lesions appeared 3 to 8 weeks after initiation of the anticoagulant therapy, doubts arose as to whether this mechanism alone would explain this phenomenon. It is possible that another effect on the blood clotting mechanism is present but has not been isolated.

Nalbandian et al.[29] reviewed the literature and gave an excellent description of these complications. In their experience, this appears to be a rare complication of coumarin-congener anticoagulant therapy characterized by a sequence of skin lesions such as petechiae, ecchymoses, and hemorrhagic infarcts. These lesions occur in random sites and have been well documented for several years in the European literature. The lesions appear between the third and the tenth day of anticoagulant therapy, 90% occurring within the third to the sixth day. These alarming lesions were associated only with the use of coumarin-congeners, dicumarol being involved most frequently. Heparin had never been implicated before 1979. Nalbandian et al.[29] suggested as a possible mechanism a toxic action of the coumarin-congeners, which would occur at the dermovascular loop, precisely at the junction of the capillary and the precapillary arteriole. The stage of hemorrhagic infarct that is actually a gangrenous lesion correlates with the thrombosis of the venules resulting from stasis immediately distal to the dermovascular loop. The authors[29] recognize that many aspects remain unresolved and therefore feel that more pathophysiologic studies are indicated to understand more accurately its mechanism.

Warfarin-induced Skin Necrosis and Venous Gangrene of the Extremities

Warfarin (Coumadin)-induced skin necrosis is rare. Its recognition has emerged slowly in the literature in the past three decades. It is characterized by its unique affinity for skin and subcutaneous tissue. Lesions are found in areas where abundant subcutaneous tissue is present, such as breasts, buttocks, abdominal wall, anterior surface of the thighs, and exceptionally in the legs or arms. Furthermore, characteristically these lesions are localized in small areas. Pathologically, arteries in the skin and subcutaneous tissue are spared, whereas the capillaries and venules, and occasionally the subcutaneous veins, are selectively occluded. Hemorrhage originating from the capillaries leads to necrosis of connective and fatty tissue. In its extreme manifestations the Coumadin-induced lesion is a hemorrhagic infarct of the skin and subcutaneous tissue.

Warfarin-induced skin necrosis may mimic other skin conditions and may be confused with other entities. Thus a few studies have appeared in which the clinical and pathologic features of venous gangrene resulting from PCD were mistaken for warfarin-induced necrosis. Under these circumstances, warfarin may be erroneously implicated as the cause of the skin lesions and of extensive venous gangrene of the extremities. Such lack of precision in diagnosis may have serious therapeutic consequences. Should such a case also involve a medicolegal question, the consequences of mistaken diagnosis could become financially catastrophic.

As is well known, venous gangrene is the result of untreated PCD. It is essential to distinguish between venous gangrene, which results from massive venous occlusion, and skin necrosis induced by warfarin, which involves capillary hemorrhage and thrombosis of localized skin venules. Making a differential diagnosis may be difficult for the uninitiated, since patients treated initially for venous thrombosis may have warfarin-induced necrosis, which can progress to PCD and ultimately to venous gangrene. It is important to strongly emphasize that these two conditions are fundamentally, pathologically, and pathogenetically different. Massive thrombosis of all the veins of the extremity is the key to the differential diagnosis. This can be confirmed by ultrasound scanning in vivo, by examination of the amputated limb, or by autopsy. The presence of thrombosed major and small veins and patency of the arterial system are a *sine qua non* of the diagnosis of venous gangrene (see Fig. 70-1).[30]

Heparin-induced Necrosis and Thrombotic Complications

For many years warfarin was the only anticoagulant thought capable of inducing skin necrosis. As recently as 1968 it was stated that heparin did not cause similar lesions. Since then, however, cases in which heparin induced similar skin complications as well as thrombotic vascular lesions have been reported.

In 1978 Wu reported hyperaggregability of platelets and thrombosis in patients in whom thrombocytopenia was present.[31] The same year Weismann and Robin reported on arterial embolism occurring during systemic heparin therapy.[32] Roberts et al.[33] had questioned this causal relationship in 1964. Rhodes et al.[34] investigated this problem in more detail and in 1973 reported thrombocytopenia with thrombotic and hemorrhagic manifestations associated with the use of heparin. Later in 1977 the same investigators reported on eight cases with thrombotic-hemorrhagic complications associated with heparin-induced thrombocytopenia.[35] As a result, clinical papers on this subject sounded the warning that not only warfarin but also heparin can induce necrotic, as well as hemorrhagic and thrombotic, skin lesions.

White et al.[36] in 1979 reported eight cases of skin necrosis, of which six were heparin-induced and two were due to thrombotic complications. Skin and subcutaneous necrosis developed at the sites of subcutaneous heparin injection in the six patients. Systemic thrombotic events and thrombocytopenia were observed in two of the patients with skin necrosis when they received intravenous heparin and in two other patients receiving heparin who did not have primary skin necrosis. The complications included peripheral ischemia in three patients, two of whom required amputation, myocardial infarction in two, and a cerebral infarction in one. The complications occurred after 6 days of heparin administration. The type of heparin these patients received was of bovine origin.

The heparin-induced lesions are initiated by thrombocytopenia, followed by platelet aggregation, a fact that White et al.[36] found in six of the eight patients in vitro. The same mechanism is assumed to happen in vivo by platelet aggregation, followed by intravascular thrombosis.

Some papers report only heparin necrosis and refer to it as an anticoagulation syndrome. Towne et al.,[24] focus their attention primarily on peripheral vascular complications of heparin therapy. They treated seven patients with thromboses resulting from platelet aggregation induced by heparin. Four of the patients had acute arterial ischemia of the lower extremity; two had venous gangrene, and one had occlusion of an autogenous vein placed as a femoral popliteal bypass. In all these instances, platelet count was noticeably reduced in the affected patients. They considered the thrombus white because it was predominantly composed of fibrin-platelet aggregates with an occasional entrapped WBC and rare RBC. All these patients received heparin therapy and demonstrated thrombocytopenia and platelet aggregation.

As is the case with warfarin, the complications occurring after heparin are paradoxical, since the therapy is indicated to prevent thrombosis.

The mechanism triggering intravascular thrombosis appears to be chemically induced immune thrombocytopenia. As with warfarin, this complication usually arises after several days of exposure to heparin.

Although complications following heparin therapy are rare, it is important to add this potential hazard of the use of heparin to the list of potential dangers if the patient is not evaluated in vitro before treatment for thrombocytopenia and aggregation of platelets. Should such a test be positive prior to surgery, heparin should not be administered. Dextran is preferable. Some reports indicate that warfarin has been used in cases of heparin complications. But heparin is not recommended in cases of warfarin complications. Use of any of these anticoagulants should be based on the immune response of the patient's blood to these agents.

TREATMENT

Although management may vary according to the clinical finding of PCD or venous gangrene, a number of objectives are nevertheless common to both. In order of priority, conditions one must direct immediate attention to are the following:

1. Combatting the venous stasis (edema) by maximum limb elevation
2. Relieving shock by appropriate blood volume replacement
3. Starting intravenous heparin
4. Treating angiospasm
5. Treating concurrently underlying conditions if feasible
6. Assessing the extent of gangrene

Medical Management

Elevation of the Extremity

Medical management should be applied without delay in each case. Elevation of the extremity as the first step is essential for combatting the venous stasis. Although most of the venous bed may be obstructed, there often still remain patent venous channels, especially in the PCD stage. These channels can be made to empty large quantities of blood from the extremity, thus relieving the venous engorgement. To accomplish this, the involved limb is elevated quite high to a 60- or even a 70-degree angle, with the head placed on one pillow only.[4] When the venous engorgement has been reduced, fresh arterial blood may be able to enter the vascular bed and thus reduce the acute symptoms.

Elevation can be continued and maintained until the ischemic and venous stasis subside substantially or completely. The improvement is reflected in gradual disappearance of cyanosis, rapid subsidence of pain, diminished distension of veins, and improvement of skin temperature.

Maximal elevation is applicable not only in PCD but also in patients with venous gangrene. The reduction in edema is greater in the former than in the latter. Returning trapped blood from the limb to the systemic circulation not only decreases the subfascial tension but also relieves extensive pressure on the arterial tree and combats the existing hypovolemic shock. Elevation alone or in conjunction with other measures has resulted, as previously reported by myself and others, in the recovery of about 92% of patients with PCD.[2] While the extremity is elevated, additional exercises, passive or active, of the toes and ankle may be attempted with caution, but one should bear in mind that it may at times result in fragmentation of a floating thrombus with the possibility of pulmonary embolism.

Circulatory Collapse (Shock)

Circulatory collapse or hypovolemic shock, that is, the hypovolemic condition, often presents as a result of excessive entrapment of blood in the involved extremity and may require immediate administration of whole blood or plasma or packed red cells. Fluid and cell replacements are urgently needed for the relief of the existing shock and hemoconcentration. In the absence of whole blood or packed red cells, plasma expanders, such as dextran, can be useful adjuncts for combatting this complication.

Anticoagulants and Plasma Expanders

In PCD, heparin is the optimal anticoagulant for preventing further propagation of thrombosis, especially when it is

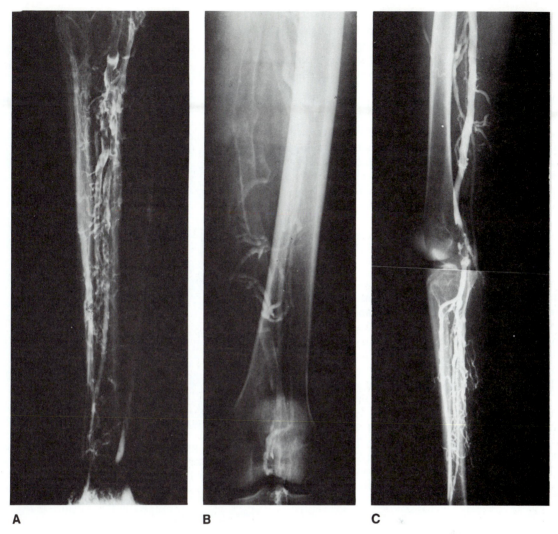

Figure 70-9. A. Venogram of the left leg disclosing multiple areas of thrombosis in the calf veins of a patient with phlegmasia cerulea dolens. **B.** Extension of the calf thrombosis in the popliteal and superficial femoral veins. **C.** Venogram obtained 9 days after onset of the process shows patency of the leg and thigh veins with exception of a small defect in the popliteal area. The patient remained edema-free throughout the 7 year observation.

used concomitantly with elevation of the extremity. Some patients may show complete resolution of the thrombi in the context of this combined treatment. An example is shown in Figure 70-9.

Occasionally the usefulness of heparin is questioned in severe hypercoagulable states when the process involves the totality of the venous tree. In such cases venous thrombectomy or fibrinolytic agents are indicated as alternatives.

Dextran may be used as fluid replacement if whole blood or packed red cells are not immediately available. Dextran 40 (Rheomacrodex [Pharmacia]) is preferable to dextran 70 (Macrodex [Pharmacia]) since it lowers blood viscosity more, has better rheologic properties, and is more rapidly excreted by the kidneys. Although it has been used mostly in the uncomplicated forms of deep venous thrombosis, it is also useful in cases of ischemic venous thrombosis. One of the main hematologic effects on the platelets is to reduce their adhesiveness and aggregation and thus prevent clotting. Because of a few known side effects (overloading,

anaphylaxis, renal damage) one should be cautious when using it as a blood substitute.

Hypertonic mannitol has been used to prevent rethrombosis in the revascularization syndrome after acute arterial embolism.[2] The patients were first given 100 ml of 20% mannitol as an intravenous bolus, followed by an infusion of 10 g/h of mannitol. This was continued for 6 to 24 hours, depending on the degree of the clinical severity.

Fibrinolytics

The two major fibrinolytic agents currently used are streptokinase and urokinase. In a few controlled multicenter clinical trials sponsored in the U.S. by the National Heart, Lung, and Blood Institute, as well as in several clinics in Europe, these agents were found to be effective in the management of deep venous thrombosis and pulmonary embolism.

These agents are not, however, widely used because of side effects such as allergic reactions, pulmonary emboli, fever, general malaise, and potentially lethal hemorrhage, particularly in the brain. Contraindications to their use are fresh surgical wounds, following trauma, during pregnancy or postpartum, arterial hypertension, recent streptococcal infection, and obviously in persons with hemorrhagic conditions.

Fibrinolysis is indicated only for established thrombophlebitis and should not be used for prophylaxis. Best results may be obtained in relatively fresh thrombi of not more than a week's duration. Long-term results are sometimes difficult to determine as reported by Partsch et al.[37] in six cases. Encouraging results of a few isolated cases are being reported such as the use of urokinase in two cases, one of PCD and the other of venous gangrene, with complete resolution of the lesions.[38]

Further experience in IVT is needed before its efficacy is better established.

Vasodilators

With regard to vasodilator procedures, the question of associated vasospasm in PCD or venous gangrene has been the subject of great debate. When present, associated spasm of the major arteries adjacent to the veins may extend to the more peripheral branches and collaterals and thus further compromise limb viability. Although not always documented clinically, experimental data have suggested that spasm of the arterial tree, and possibly of unobstructed venules, may be observed in PCD. Application of hot packs and use of papaverine or sympathetic nerve blocks may relieve angiospasm and venous engorgement. The validity and effectiveness of these procedures are difficult to assess. It should be understood that vasospasm, when present in ischemic venous thrombosis, is only secondary and contributory.

Management of Underlying Diseases

Many patients with ischemic venous thrombosis suffer from serious visceral conditions, such as neoplastic diseases, postoperative situations, and infections or metabolic diseases. Treatment of these conditions must be undertaken concurrently or whenever possible or indicated

Surgical Management

From the preceding review of medical management, especially the use of anticoagulants and fibrinolytic therapy, it is obvious that under certain circumstances the resolution of the venous thrombi is difficult to achieve. Venous thrombectomy is then indicated.

In the 1970s, many surgeons who attempted surgical removal of the thrombi became disappointed because of the frequent rethrombosis of the veins postoperatively. Recently, with improved technique, there has been a renewed interest in this procedure.

Indications for venous thrombectomy upon which there is most general agreement are (1) phlegmasia cerulea dolens, especially if conservative management failed within 24 to 72 hours, (2) recurrent pulmonary embolism, (3) floating thrombi in the iliocaval axis as determined phlebograph-

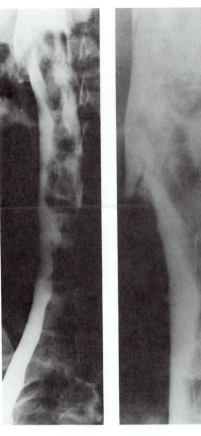

Figure 70-10. Phlegmasia cerulea dolens. Inferior venacavogram showing a floating thrombus. On the *right*, enlargement of the *left* picture, showing greater detail of the thrombus curling up above the renal veins. A transfemoral thrombectomy of the inferior vena cava was carried out in addition to ligation of ovarian veins because of pelvic pathology.

ically (Fig. 70-10), and (4) rapidly progressive thrombosis in any type of acute femoroiliocaval thrombosis.[39,40]

This procedure by removing the thrombus carries a threefold salvage role: (1) it prevents further extension of the thrombosis that could cause gangrene of the limb, (2) it removes the source of pulmonary embolism, frequently fatal in this condition, and (3) it forestalls a serious postthrombotic syndrome with the well-known dreaded sequelae.

Venous Thrombectomy

Comprehensive Thrombectomy of Proximal and Distal Venous Channels: Iliac and Popliteotibial Veins. This is paramount for complete success of the procedure. Fresh thrombi less than 24 to 48 hours old offer the best chance for removal from the venous system. In contrast, thrombi 72 to 96 hours old or more adhere to the venous wall and cannot be pulled out with the balloon catheters. Radiologic control during thrombectomy may be helpful in visualizing the exact position of possible residual thrombi. Use of an intraoperative image intensifier has been advocated by some as a means of simplifying this evaluation.

More recently, Vollmar and Hutschenreiter[41] have recommended routine use of intraoperative vascular endoscopy. Although a relatively simple procedure in the hands of experienced technicians, endoscopy may offer difficulties to the uninitiated. In some cases, endoscopy would seem superior to venous angiography. According to Vollmar, it is helpful in the diagnosis of a venous spur, which is frequently seen in recurrent occlusions.

Distal Tree Clearance. The distal tree may be difficult or impossible to clear in the presence of old organized thrombi. If, on the other hand, the distal thrombi appear of recent date, "milking" of the leg and lower thigh could be achieved by use of an Esmarch rubber elastic bandage wrapped tightly around the limb from foot up to midthigh. By vigorous wrapping and elevation of the leg, the thrombi may be extruded through an open venotomy of the femoral vein.

Prevention of Pulmonary Embolism During Thrombectomy. In some cases, cava temporary obstruction of the vena may be useful for prevention of pulmonary embolism during thrombectomy.

Role of Temporary Arteriovenous Fistula. Concomitant temporary AV fistula is being advocated by a few European surgeons. Vollmar,[41] a strong proponent of this procedure, in a series of 42 cases with AV fistula achieved patency in 83.8% of cases, but without AV fistula in only 61.5% of 13 cases. Delin et al.[42] reported similar success with AV fistula in 85% of their cases.

The AV procedure as an adjunct in arterial or venous diseases for enhancing blood flow is not entirely new. Its protective value in maintaining patency of veins after thrombectomy needs further study to confirm the above successful results.

Regional Fibrinolysis as Adjunct to Surgical Thrombectomy. Streptokinase may be delivered directly to its site of action to avoid systemic side effects. However, successful results could be obtained in certain cases with systemic administration of streptokinase. Control of the results should be obtained by intraoperative phlebography.

Postoperative anticoagulation, in addition to fibrinolysis, is highly recommended in these cases.[43]

Indications
In the nonischemic forms of DVT, with proper selection of patients, DeWeese and Adams[44] pointed out that patency was achieved in as many as 77 to 88% of cases, documented by postoperative venograms, as reported by several U.S. surgeons. During the period from 1978 to the present, further encouraging reports have appeared in European and Japanese literature confirming the efficacy of the procedure. There is often a discrepancy between decreased patency rates postoperatively and successful clinical findings. This is accounted for by decreasing patency rates from iliac to the leg veins. Thus, Minar[45] had found the following decrease in patency rates: iliac 57%, femoral 32%, and the leg veins 26%. Similar rates have been reported by other recent publications.

Comments

While the DeWeese and Minar reports deal mostly with nonischemic forms of deep venous thrombosis, the principles and techniques of venous thrombectomy for managing PCD and venous gangrene are the same.

In the present group of ischemic forms the immediate results of this procedure in preventing the acute complications make its indications for surgery more urgent and valid than in the nonischemic forms.

Inferior Vena Cava Interruption
As an isolated surgical procedure, this is rarely used except to prevent further pulmonary embolism. Following thrombectomy, if in doubt about the possibility of pulmonary embolism from a peripheral venous tree not adequately disobstructed, interruption of the IVC may be necessary. Extraluminal interruption or intraluminal interruption is done depending on circumstances. The former may be carried out either by the extraperitoneal or transperitoneal approach.

Since most venous thrombectomies are done through the femoral area, the extraperitoneal approach using a plastic clip or a stenosing ligation of the IVC is preferable.

The intraluminal method is indicated when the abdominal operation appears contraindicated. Use of the cone filter (Kimray-Greenfield) appears to offer the least immediate and late disadvantages.

One word of caution against complete ligation: interruption of IVC alone without thrombectomy may in itself induce an ischemic syndrome. Our own method of stenosing ligation is by far easier, safer, and more expeditious.[46-49] A few points concerning this technique are illustrated in Figures 70-11 and 70-12.

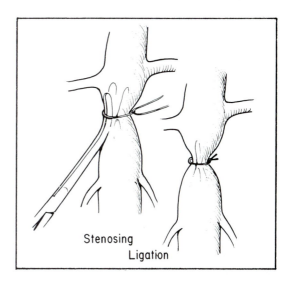

Figure 70-11. Diagram of stenosing ligation of inferior vena cava. Note that the ligation is carried out around the tip of a Kelly clamp, and when it is completed the residual vena cava lumen is slightly more than the thickness of the tip of the clamp.

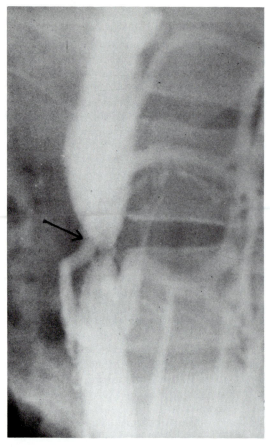

Figure 70-12. An inferior vena cavogram of a case in which a stenosing ligation was carried out in a patient in whom repeated pulmonary emboli could not be controlled by intravenous heparin over a period of several weeks. Note the ligation below a lumbar vein, with development of collateral circulation around the ligation. No further pulmonary emboli were noted after this interruption. The patient died 2 months later, and examination of the specimen showed complete clearance of thrombi in the distal veins. (*From Haimovici H: Vascular Emergencies. New York, Appleton-Century-Crofts, 1982.*)

Fasciotomy

There is little doubt that in the presence of massive venous thrombosis with corresponding increased subcutaneous subfascial edema a fasciotomy is mandatory for relieving the compression of the various structures involved. It usually restores the caliber of major arteries, reestablishes capillary flow, and decompresses the muscles, which may be on the verge of severe ischemia or necrosis. In recent years the therapeutic potential of fasciotomy has been fully appreciated in PCD, as well as in other vascular conditions. The procedure used in such instances results in relief of the ischemic manifestations and therefore should be recommended widely.

In contrast to the technique applied in arterial cases, in PCD the incisions should be wider and carried out not only below but also above the knee, both medially and laterally when necessary. Only in this way can one hope to decompress rapidly the various structures and prevent the impending severe ischemia.

TABLE 70-5. DISTRIBUTION OF CASES OF GANGRENE ACCORDING TO LEVELS OF AMPUTATION

Levels of Amputation	Recovered	Died
Toes	13	0
Transmetatarsal	5	0
Midleg	15	4
Midthigh	19	13
Fingers	2	0
Forearm	1	0
Arm	3	0
Total	58	17

From Haimovici H: Vascular Emergencies. New York, Appleton-Century-Crofts, 1982.

Amputations

It should be pointed out that venous gangrene is usually limited to the distal part of the extremity and mostly to the skin and sometimes the subcutaneous tissue. It rarely extends to the subfascial region and muscle layers, but the possibility that it can should always be considered as well as lymphangitis and cellulitis. With or without superimposed infection, most cases of venous gangrene are of the moist variety because of the presence of edema, although dry necrosis is not incompatible with venous gangrene. The line of demarcation usually takes several weeks. If the infection is prevented or controlled, the necrotic process, which is mostly superficial, appears to be self-limiting. In contrast, spreading of the infection to the deep tissues may lead to loss of the extremity despite patent arteries.

Mortality risks are quite high in this group of patients (22.6%). In a series of 75 patients I reviewed, 17 died after the procedure; most of these deaths occurred in above-knee amputations (13 out of 17) (Table 70-5). It should be pointed out that a large number of these patients had superficial lesions and could be treated conservatively. It is noteworthy that 20 out of the 58 survivors had such lesions and many of these required only local debridement and skin grafting. It should again be underscored that venous gangrene is usually superficial and more limited than arterial gangrene. Prevention of infection is essential to avoid major loss of tissue. Demarcation of the necrotic areas and their spontaneous eliminations may thus occur.

PROGNOSIS

Local and systemic factors, alone or in combination determine the prognosis concerning both the limb and life of the patient. Analysis of the clinicopathologic data has disclosed that the outcome of this disease is vastly different in the two forms of ischemic thrombophlebitis.

Factors that dominate the prognosis are (1) *local:* the presence or absence of gangrene; (2) *systemic:* shock, pulmonary embolism, and the underlying disease; and (3) *therapeutic:* the method of treatment and the speed with which it is applied.

In PCD the overall recovery rate in the entire group

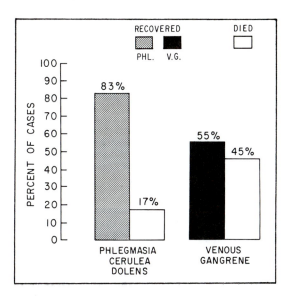

Figure 70-13. Overall prognosis in all cases of ischemic venous thrombosis, both treated and untreated.

of treated and untreated patients reported earlier was 84% (Fig. 70-13). The 16% mortality was related primarily to systemic factors.

Circulatory collapse was present in 28% of the cases, but from the available data it is difficult to determine whether this condition contributed significantly to fatal outcome. It would appear that in most cases, when adequate treatment was applied in time, circulatory collapse could be reversed. By contrast, the fatal pulmonary emboli that occurred in 3.4% of the patients and the underlying disease were by far the two most important causes of immediate death. Although neoplastic lesions associated with PCD were present in 15.4% of the cases, only about a third of these patients died shortly after onset of the acute venous thrombosis. Death occurring sometime after the acute venous thrombosis has subsided is obviously attributable to the underlying disease rather than to the vascular lesion.

Treatment addressed primarily to reversing shock and providing supportive measures is essential at the onset of this condition. Lack of treatment resulted in ten deaths out of 11 patients in this series.

In venous gangrene, in contrast to PCD, the presence of gangrene, especially if it is extensive and associated with infection, represents a serious local factor that may play a significant role in the fatal outcome of the patient. The overall mortality rate associated with venous gangrene was 42%. Patients with bilateral lower extremity gangrene with or without amputation had a 71% mortality rate, associated systemic factors obviously contributing to this high incidence. Circulatory collapse was present in 21.5% of the cases. As in the preceding group, it is difficult to determine from the available data the extent to which the presence of shock could be held responsible for the fatal outcome of these patients. Most significant were two major factors: pulmonary embolism and neoplastic disease.

Fatal pulmonary emboli were reported in 22.1% of patients in the neoplastic disease group. The various conditions—multiple gangrenous lesions, severe shock, pulmo-

nary emboli, and terminal neoplastic diseases—are most often combined in cases with a fatal outcome. The immediate prognosis, however, can be favorably influenced if adequate and prompt treatment is applied. Failure to do so in 18 cases resulted in 15 deaths (83%), as compared to a 36.4% mortality rate for the treated patients. These data clearly indicate that the prognosis in cases of venous gangrene is extremely severe, as opposed to the prognosis with PCD, in which the outcome is more favorable.

Conclusions

From these data it is clear that there is a fundamental difference between PCD and venous gangrene in their respective survival rates. With better understanding of the two clinical forms, of the pathogenesis of this unusual entity, and of its immediate treatment, a substantial improvement can be achieved in the prognosis concerning both limb salvage and survival of the patient.

REFERENCES

1. Haimovici H: The ischemic forms of venous thrombosis. J Cardiovasc Surg (suppl Philadelphia Congress 1965) 7:164, 1966.
2. Haimovici H: Ischemic Forms of Venous Thrombosis: Phlegmasia Cerulea Dolens, Venous Gangrene. Charles C Thomas, Publisher, Springfield, Ill., 1971.
3. Magendie J, Tingaud R: Phlebite a forme pseudoembolique (phlebite bleue de Gregoire). Bordeaux Chir 3(4):112, 1945.
4. Veal JR, Dugan TJ, et al.: Acute massive venous occlusion of the lower extremities. Surgery 29:355, 1951.
5. Decoulx P, Bastien P: Gangrene par spasme arteriel au cours d'une phlebite. Ann Anat Phathol 16:353, 1939.
6. Gregoire R: La phlebite bleue (phlegmatia caerulea dolens). Presse Med 46:1313, 1938.
7. Audier M, Haimovici H: Les Gangrenes des membres d'origine veineuse. Presse Med 46:1403, 1938.
8. Haimovici H: Gangrene of the extremities of venous origin. Review of the literature with case reports. Circulation 1:225, 1950.
9. DeBakey ME, Ochsner A: Phlegmasia cerulea dolens and gangrene associated with thrombophlebitis. Surgery 26:16, 1949.
10. Fabricius Hildanus G: De Gangraena et Sphacelo, Cologne, 1593.
11. Fontaine R, de Sousa Pereira A: Obliterations et resections veineuses experimentales; contribution a l'etude de la circulation collaterale veineuse. Rev Chir (Paris) 75:161, 1937.
12. Perlow S, Killian ST, et al.: Shock following venous occlusions of a leg. Am J Physiol 134:755, 1941.
13. Haimovici H: Ischemic forms of venous thrombosis. Heart Bull 16:101, 1967.
14. Anlyan WG, Hart D: Special problems in venous thromboembolism. Ann Surg 146:499, 1957.
15. Devambez J: Trente et une phlebites bleues; deux amputations pour gangrene. Phlebologie 13:187, 1960.
16. Fogarty TJ, Cranley JJ, et al.: Surgical management of phlegmasia cerulea dolens. Arch Surg 86:256, 1963.
17. Fontaine R, Kieny R, et al.: Contribution a l'etude clinique et therapeutique de la phlegmatia coerulea dolens (phlebite bleue). A propos de 32 observations personneles. Lyon Chir 61:321, 1965.
18. Natali J, Tricot JF: Place de la chirurgie dans le traitement des phlebites aigues des membres inferieurs. Phlebologie 35:187, 1982.

19. Le Bideau-Gouiran G: Etude de 35 cas de phlebites ischemiques operees. Phlebologie 36:101, 1983.

20. Haimovici H: Ischemic venous thrombosis, in Haimovici H (ed): Vascular Emergencies, Appleton-Century-Crofts, Norwalk, Conn., 1982, p 589.

21. Bulow S, Sager P: Venous gangrene. Acta Chir Scand 141:272, 1975.

22. Smith BM, Shield GW, et al.: Venous gangrene of the upper extremity. Ann Surg 201:511, 1985.

23. Towne JB, Bernhard VM, et al.: Antithrombin deficiency—A cause of unexplained thrombosis in vascular surgery. Surgery 89(b):735, 1981.

24. Towne JB, Bernhard VM, et al.: White clot syndrome. Arch Surg 114:372, 1979.

25. Brockman SK, Vasco JS: Observations on the pathophysiology and treatment of phlegmasia cerulea dolens with special reference to thrombectomy. Am J Surg 109:485, 1965.

26. Burton AC: On the physical equilibrium of small blood vessels. Am J Physiol 164:319, 1951.

27. Stallworth JM, Najib A, et al.: Phlegmasia cerulea dolens: An experimental study. Ann Surg 165:860, 1967.

28. Feder W, Auerbach R: "Purple toes": an uncommon sequela of oral Coumadin drug therapy. Ann Intern Med 55:911, 1961.

29. Nalbandian RM, Masler IJ, Barrett JL, Pearce JF, Rupp EC: Petechiae, ecchymoses and necrosis of skin induced by coumarin congeneres. JAMA 192:603, 1965.

30. Haimovici H, Bergan JJ: Coumadin-induced skin necrosis versus venous gangrene of the extremities. Editorial. J Vasc Surg 5(4):655, 1987.

31. Wu KK: Platelet hyperaggregability and thrombosis in patients with thrombocythemia. Ann Intern Med 88:7, 1978.

32. Weismann RE, Robin RW: Arterial embolism occurring during systemic heparin therapy. Arch Surg 76:219, 1958.

33. Roberts B, Rosato FE, Rosato EF: Heparin: a cause of arterial emboli? Surgery 55:803, 1964.

34. Rhodes GR, Dixon RH, Silver D: Heparin induced thrombocytopenia with thrombotic and hemorrhagic manifestations. Surg Gynecol Obstet 136:409, 1973.

35. Rhodes GR, Dixon RH, Silver D: Heparin induced thrombocytopenia: Eight cases with thrombotic-hemorrhagic complications. Ann Surg 186:752, 1977.

36. White PW, Sadd JR, Nensel RE: Thrombotic complications of heparin therapy. Ann Surg 190:595, 1979.

37. Partsch H, Weidinger P, Mostbeck A, et al: Funktionelle Spatergebnisse nach Thrombecktomie, Fibrinolyse und konservativer Therapie von Bein-Beckenvenenthrombosen. VASA 9:53, 1980.

38. Zimmermann R, Morl H, Harenberg J: Urokinase-behandlung der phlegmasia coerulea dolens. Dtsch Med Wochenschr 104:1563, 1979.

39. Moreau P, Chevalier JM, Enon B, et al: Thrombectomie veineuse pour thrombose aigue femoro-ilio-cave. Nouv Presse Med 10:3159, 1981.

40. Valici A, Isman H, Migliori B, et al: Thrombose aigue femoro-ilio-cave en gerontologie, Thrombectomie veineuse avec amplificateur de brillance. Nouv Presse Med 11:1421, 1981.

41. Vollmar JF, Hutschenreiter: Temporary arteriovenous fistulas. In Pelvic and Abdominal Veins: Progress in Diagnostics and Therapy, Excerpta Medica, Princeton, 1980.

42. Delin A, Swedenborg J, Hellgren M, et al: Thrombectomy and arteriovenous fistula for iliofemoral venous thrombosis in fertile women. Surg Gynecol Obstet 154:69, 1982.

43. Nachbur B, Beck EA, Senn A: Can the results of treatment of deep venous thrombosis be improved by combining surgical thrombectomy with regional fibrinolysis? J Cardiovasc Surg 21:347, 1980.

44. DeWeese JA, Adams JT: Iliofemoral venous thrombectomy. In Haimovici H (ed), Vascular Surgery, Appleton-Century-Crofts, Norwalk, CT, 1984, p 1007.

45. Minar E, Ehringer H, Marosi L, et al: Klinische, funktionelle, und morphologische spatergenbnisse nach venoser thrombektomie. VASA 12:346, 1983.

46. Steinman C, Alpert J, Haimovici H: Inferior vena cava bypass grafts: An experimental evaluation of a temporary arteriovenous fistula on their long-term patency. Arch Surg 93:747, 1966.

47. Goto H, Wada T, Matsumoto A, et al: Iliofemoral venous thrombectomy: Follow-up studies of 88 patients. Surgery 21:341, 1980.

48. Raithel D, Sohnlein B: Die venose thrombektomie–Technik und ergebnisse. VASA 10:119, 1981.

49. Andriopoulos A, Wirsing P, Botticher R: Results of iliofemoral venous thrombectomy after acute thrombosis: Report on 165 cases. J Cardiovasc Surg 23:123, 1982.

CHAPTER 71
Pathophysiology of Postphlebitic Syndrome with Leg Ulcer

Henry Haimovici

The pathogenesis of venous stasis leg ulcers is the result of many factors. A clear understanding of the mechanisms leading to these ulcerations of the leg should be based on several parameters: (1) the pathologic valvular destruction of the involved deep and superficial veins, (2) phlebodynamics of the leg, (3) phlebographic findings, and (4) microcirculatory changes. When properly correlated, the various parameters involved may provide a more comprehensive picture of the pathogenesis of this condition.

PATHOLOGIC VALVULAR INCOMPETENCE

Although it has been claimed that the destruction of the valves of the iliac, femoral, and popliteal veins is the main etiologic factor in the ulceration of the leg, findings based on morphologic characteristics and hemodynamics of the venous system have shown that these veins alone could not account for the development of ulceration of the lower leg. This holds true also for primary varicose veins, especially because stasis ulcers are often erroneously associated with the term "varicose ulcers." This terminology implies that the incompetent superficial veins of the leg and thigh are responsible for the immediate mechanism of ulceration. Contrary to this concept, the lesions of an ulceration are due primarily to local valve destruction of the deep veins of the lower leg and ankle. Although the presence of varicose veins in association with a postphlebitic syndrome is common, such veins may be contributing but are not the main factor in the causation of these ulcers. The dysfunction of the deep veins resulting from a postthrombotic disease plays the major role in the initiation of this process. It should be noted that the varicose veins resulting from a postthrombotic syndrome do not exhibit the usual pattern of the primary type of varicose veins, which involves essentially the long or short saphenous systems and their tributaries.

The malfunction of the valves of the deep veins becomes apparent weeks or months after recanalization of the thrombosed veins, which occurs in the majority of cases,

as demonstrated mostly by phlebography and noninvasive hemodynamic evaluation.[1]

The role of ankle-perforating veins is widely recognized in the overall pathogenesis of this syndrome. It is well known that the lower leg and ankle veins are drained by ankle-perforating veins, which empty normally into the posterior tibial veins (Fig. 71-1). When these veins, which are relatively large, become incompetent, they dilate further to a considerable degree. These ankle-perforating veins, like the deep veins of the leg, have their valves destroyed as a result of the postphlebitic process and are responsible, in large part, for venous hypertension at that level.[1] This fact accounts for the significant contribution to the lower leg lesion induced by incompetency of the ankle-perforating veins. Surgery for eradication of venous insufficiency, if confined to the great saphenous system without taking into account the incompetent perforators, may represent a serious cause for recurrence of the ulcer. Indeed, omission of this operative detail may result in perpetuation of the ulcerative process as soon as the patient's activity is resumed.

PHLEBODYNAMICS

Essentially, the pathologic physiology of the postphlebitic syndrome appears to be due to local ambulatory venous hypertension in the area of the ankle, as demonstrated repeatedly by a number of investigators. Deep venous pressure measurements have shown that (1) in *normal* legs, with the patient standing, the venous pressure in the subcutaneous veins of the foot and ankle falls rapidly during exercise to between 0 and 30 mm Hg and then rises slowly on cessation of exercise to a previous height of 90 mm Hg, (2) in patients with primary incompetent superficial *varicose veins*, the pressure falls to a value of 45 to 60 mm Hg, rising rapidly to the initial figure of 90 mm Hg on cessation of exercise, and (3) in *postphlebitic* cases, the pressure fall during exercise is minimal, although there appears to be some variation. Most investigations found that there

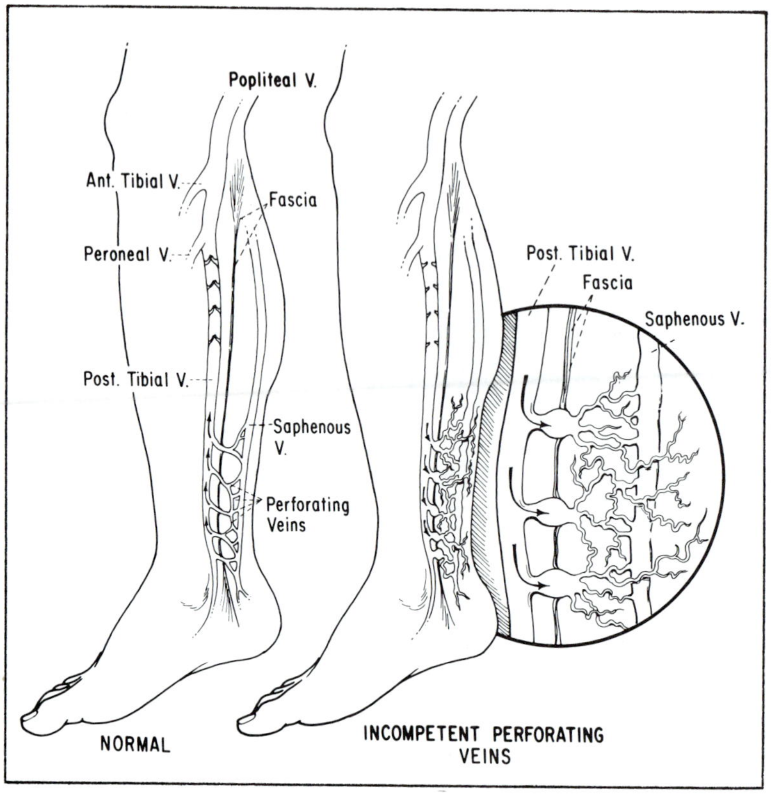

Figure 71-1. Diagram illustrating (*left*) normal valves of the deep venous system of the leg with a normal flow from the superficial to the deep veins and (*right*) incompetent valves involving the deep and perforating veins. The destruction of the valves in the ankle-perforating veins leads to dilatation of these veins, as indicated in this diagram. The resulting increased venous hypertension at the ankle level leads to gradual dilatation of all the small venules in this area, as seen in the blow-up on the right side of the diagram.

is either no fall of pressure during exercise or a slight fall to a value of 75 to 80 mm Hg with an immediate return to the preexercise level on cessation of exercise. DeCamp et al.[2] actually recorded a slight rise in pressure during exercise in a few cases.

PHLEBOGRAPHIC PATTERNS

The scope of venous surgery for this condition is directed toward the eradication of valvular insufficiency of the superficial and communicating veins. Indications for such surgery are based on the return of patency of the previously thrombosed deep veins, thus ruling out their persisting occlusion. Lack of recanalization of the deep veins is a contraindication to surgery of superficial veins, in which instance their role as a collateral venous system must be preserved. Phlebographic demonstration of the anatomic state of the venous system of the entire lower extremity is therefore of great practical value.

The postphlebitic phlebographic findings depend on the location and extent of the involvement of the venous channels. Interpretation of the various phlebographic patterns should also take into account the other parameters mentioned above. (See Chapter 66.)

Pattern 1

In pattern 1 a phlebogram reveals patency of most of the leg veins. It acquires significance only if a clinical history of deep venous thrombosis was present in the past and if

ambulatory venous hypertension at the ankle level is demonstrated and is not relieved by muscular activity (Fig. 71-2).

Pattern 2

In pattern 2, there is a typical history of iliofemoral thrombophlebitis and an ascending phlebogram may reveal only obstruction of leg veins. If varicose veins of the long saphenous tributaries are present, they may play the role of compensating collateral vessels. Continued presence of obstruction of the leg veins contraindicates surgery of the superficial veins (Fig. 71-3).

Pattern 3

In pattern 3, in contrast to the preceding pattern, the indications for surgery differ because the phlebogram of the lower extremity with a previous history of iliofemoral thrombosis reveals patency of both thigh and leg veins. In such a patient with a chronic leg ulcer, edema, and varicose veins, surgery of the superficial veins and excision of the indolent ulcer with skin grafting are properly indicated (Fig. 71-4).

In this connection, it is interesting to point out that in the past, once patients had a deep venous thrombosis, surgery of the superficial incompetent varicose veins was not advised in spite of recanalization of deep veins. Such a notion is totally erroneous, because the known facts based on phlebography, phlebodynamics, and operative findings are at variance with it.

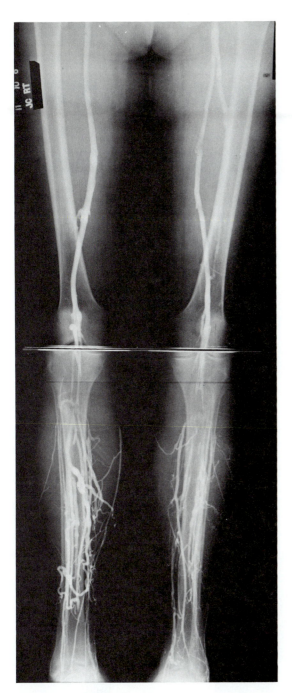

Figure 71-2. Phlebogram of both lower extremities, indicating abnormal venous pattern in the lower leg veins.

In brief, the morphologic state of the veins can be adequately evaluated by phlebography, often in conjunction with duplex ultrasonography, in most cases. The functional state of the veins, however, particularly that of the valves, may require combined phlebographic, noninvasive, and phlebomanometric studies. In this manner, a fair distinction can be established between the normal and the pathologic venous system in most instances.

MICROCIRCULATORY CHANGES

Role of Abnormal Arteriovenous Shunts in Pathogenesis of Chronic Venous Insufficiency

The relationship of the arteriovenous anastomoses (AVAs) to chronic venous insufficiency has received scant attention in the vascular literature. Although AVAs were described over a century ago, their physiologic significance and, in particular, their role in vascular diseases have remained ill defined.[3–7]

The AVAs are normal vascular channels connecting the arterial and venous sides of the circulation. They are much larger than the capillaries and permit arterial blood to pass directly into the veins, thus bypassing the capillary bed (Fig. 71-5). Their physiologic role is largely that of a safety valve for the capillaries. If the shunting of the arterial blood into the venous system is persisting or occurring relatively often, this condition may lead to physiologic disturbances and result in an abnormality.

Identification of arteriovenous communications (AVCs) with varicose veins has been documented by visual observation during surgery and especially by use of high-powered microscopes or magnifying lenses. The AVCs have been found consistently to originate subfascially and to terminate in tributaries extrafascially, thus bypassing the capillary network. By means of serial arteriography, it was shown that in more than 80% of varicose veins there is premature venous opacification. By means of Doppler ultrasonography, it was demonstrated that arteriovenous shunting was present in 80% of the cases. A correlative study of these parameters has shown that the initial significant abnormality in varicose veins is mostly confined to the tributaries, although at an advanced stage the main trunk may also be subsequently affected to a lesser degree.[8,9]

Varicose Veins

Patients with varicose veins of the greater saphenous system have associated lesser saphenous involvement in 20% of the cases. Most of these patients have advanced manifestations of chronic venous stasis, as disclosed by pitting ankle edema, dermatitis, itching, and leg ulcers. In addition, more than 50% complain of coldness of the feet or occasional burning.

Arteriography has disclosed normal arteries in all extremities, in the majority of cases. The following were the characteristics of angiographic events:

1. Arterial phase: The entire arterial tree, including plantar vessels, is visualized within 2 to 5 seconds.
2. Capillary phase: Only minimal or moderate impregnation of the tissues is seen with contrast material.
3. Venous phase: In more than 81% of cases, the pedal veins (plantar and dorsal) are opacified within 5 to 8 seconds.

The veins in the foot and leg appear tortuous and elongated with all the characteristics of varicose disease.

Chronic Venous Stasis Syndrome

In 22 of 25 extremities studied, varicose veins, chronic or recurrent stasis ulcers, and edema, all secondary to deep

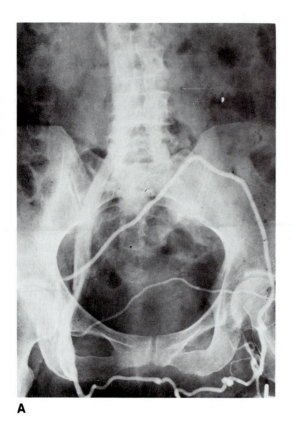

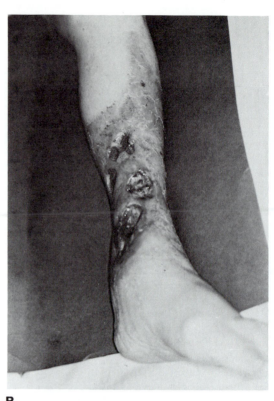

A

B

Figure 71-3. A. Phlebogram of a 60-year-old woman with a pelvic tumor on the left side, with tremendous edema of the left lower extremity. The venogram indicates complete occlusion of the left iliac and femoral veins with crossover collateral circulation from the left to the right side, filling the iliac and inferior vena cava. Obviously, the collateral circulation was insufficient to drain the venous blood from the left lower extremity. **B.** Left leg postthrombotic ulcers in the same patient.

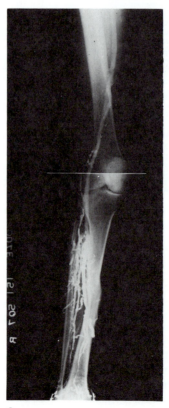

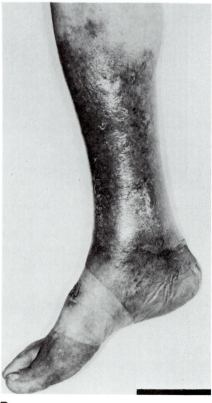

Figure 71-4. A. Phlebogram of a postphlebi-tic case with recanalized leg veins. **B.** Leg of same patient. Note ulcer of medial aspect of the ankle and brownish discoloration of the leg.

A

B

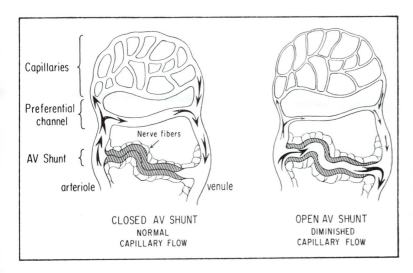

Figure 71-5. Diagram of terminal microvascular bed, including the capillaries, preferential channel, and AVAs with neuromuscular glomus of Masson. On the left is depicted a closed AVA with open normal capillary flow. On the right, there is an open AVA with diminished capillary flow.

venous thrombosis, were present. In two others, only edema of several years' duration was present.

The initial site of venous opacification was at the level of maximum stasis, that is, around the ankle and lower half of the leg (Figs. 71-6 and 71-7). In most instances, the onset of opacification took place within 5 to 8 seconds.

The veins appeared tortuous in the foot and leg area only, the site of predilection of the stasis syndrome.

Varicose Veins and Arteriosclerosis Obliterans
Of 11 patients, 8 had primary varicose veins and 3 had varicosities secondary to a postphlebitic syndrome. The an-

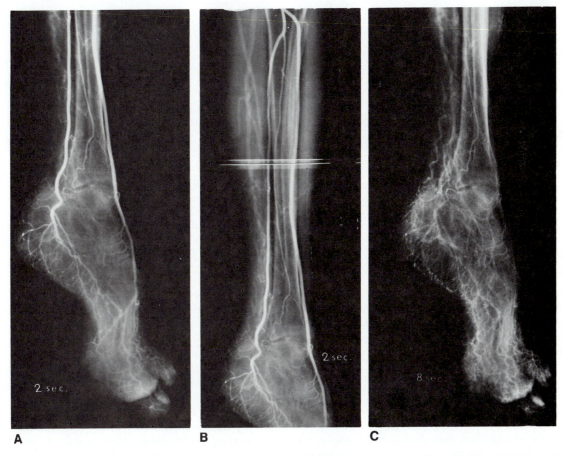

A **B** **C**

Figure 71-6. Serial femoral arteriogram of a patient with postphlebitic syndrome (ankle ulcer and edema). Note, on the first film (2 seconds), the presence of both arterial and venous opacifications. The most pronounced early venous visualization **(A, B)** is around the ankle and leg, sites of the maximum stasis in the patient. At 8 seconds (third film) the angiogram is predominantly composed of both deep and superficial veins. Note the plantar maculas at 8 seconds **(C)**.

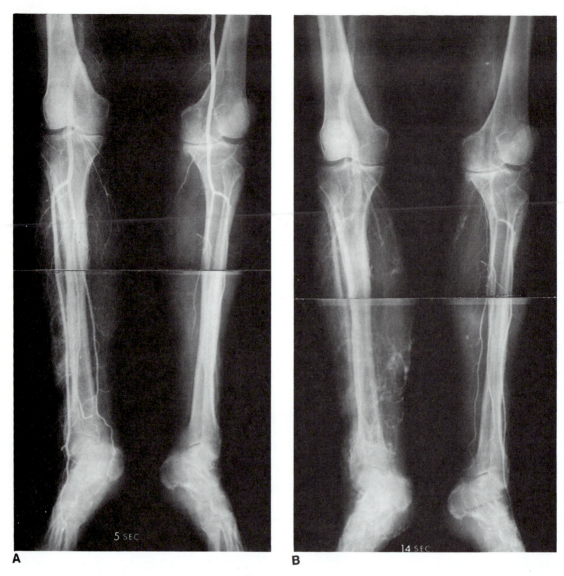

Figure 71-7. Serial femoral arteriogram of a 61-year-old woman with postphlebitic syndrome (extensive leg ulcers) and secondary varicose veins of right lower extremity; the left extremity appears normal. Note the complete arterial visualization within 5 seconds of the involved extremity, whereas the arterial phase on the contralateral side took 14 seconds. In the postphlebitic leg, evidence of AVAs and venous opacification is seen within 5 seconds, and only venous opacification, including of the popliteal-femoral veins, is seen at 14 seconds. In the other leg, there is visualization of the arterial tree only, even at 14 seconds.

giographic findings in this group of patients included arterial lesions and early opacification of the venous channels, which were not very different from those observed in the pure venous cases (varicose veins and chronic venous stasis syndrome.)

DISCUSSION

Rapid venous opacification seen during arteriography for traumatic or congenital arteriovenous fistula is a well-known sign and is easily explained. In chronic venous insufficiency, venous opacification is not as instantaneous as in a large arteriovenous fistula, because of an almost microscopic size (30 to 60 μm) of the AVAs. The question is whether the

AVAs function abnormally. One fact is certain: once a dysfunction of the AVAs is established, shunting of arterial blood directly into the venous system further increases venous dilatation. Thus AVA dysfunction seems to represent an aggravating factor. The abundant venous network opacified mostly at the level of maximum stasis supports this concept. In our study, the dilated veins were opacified prematurely in ulcerated areas and sometimes were diffusely distributed throughout the leg. As a result of AVA shunting, the bypassing of the capillary bed by arterial blood leads to ischemia that is superimposed on the stasis syndrome.

On the basis of the above pathophysiologic findings, the sequence of hemodynamic events leading to a stasis ulcer appears to be as follows: (1) valvular insufficiency

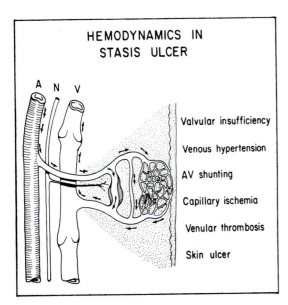

Figure 71-8. Diagram of altered hemodynamics leading to venous stasis ulcer. The usual chronologic order of these changes is indicated on the right side of this diagram. Note the directional flow changes from the arterial through the AVAs instead of through the capillaries.

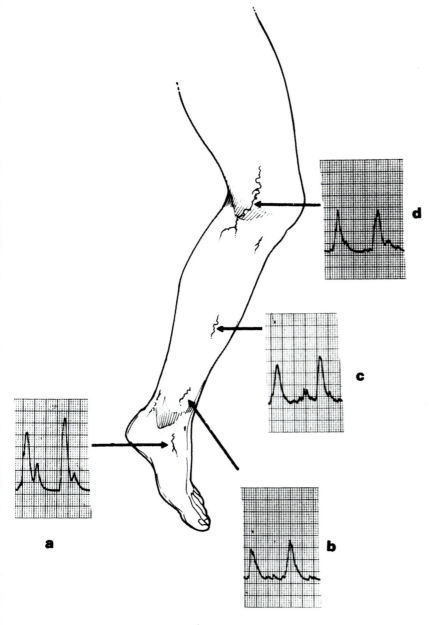

Figure 71-9. Venous flow tracings in recurrent varicose veins with 30-year history in 65-year-old woman associated with healed ulceration of left ankle and chronic dependency-induced edema. Normal dorsalis pedis arterial tracing (a); pulsatile venous tracing in area above ankle at site of previous ulceration (b); pulsatile venous tracings on medial side of and around knee area (c) and (d). Note difference in dorsalis pedis pulse wave characteristics from those in venous tracings. (*From Haimovici H: Vasc Surg 2:687, 1985.*)

occurs first as a result of the venous disease process, (2) insufficiency leads to venous hypertension, (3) arteriovenous shunting results in decreased arterial flow through the capillary system, (4) a decrease in arterial flow leads to a diversion of the oxygenated blood directly from the artery into the veins without going through the capillaries, and (5) superimposed ischemia with tissue anoxia results, contributing ultimately to the skin ulcer (Fig. 71-8).

It appears, therefore, that prolonged and diffuse patency of AVAs results in local venous dilatation and short-circuiting of arterial blood directly into the vein. Bluish discoloration and coldness of the foot and leg are the associated characteristic signs of ischemia.

In patients with varicose veins and postphlebitic syndrome, arteriovenous shunting has been pinpointed with the use of the ultrasonic Doppler flow detector. Pulsatile venous flow was recorded in patients with long-standing typical primary varicose veins without ulcerations and in patients with chronic or recurrent leg ulcers. The significant fact was that the detection of the pulsatile venous flow was obtained at the site of unusually large varicose veins, in the ulcerated areas, or at the site of a healed ulcer (Fig. 71-9). This fact suggests that even though a healed venous ulcer is covered with a new skin, the underlying arteriovenous shunting persists. This further suggests that to eradicate the cause of the ulcer and avoid its possible recurrence, one must excise the arteriovenous shunts.

LUMBAR SYMPATHECTOMY

As a result of local ischemia, manifested clinically by bluish discoloration and coldness of the foot and leg, lumbar sympathectomy has been advocated in some intractable stasis ulcers associated with the postphlebitic syndrome.

In this context, Patman[10] presented clinical evidence of the role of lumbar sympathectomy in the healing of chronic venous leg ulcers.

In a series of 23 patients with a typical history of postphlebitic ulcers, conservative and surgical modalities directed at local care of the ulcer and correction of the underlying venous ulcers remained unsuccessful. In the face of refractory and intractable ulcerations, Patman performed lumbar sympathectomy, with improvement in these patients. He stated that "while sympathectomy may enhance nutrition of the skin, it does not replace the classic methods of therapy for the control of altered fluid dynamics responsible for the ulcerations."[10]

It is widely accepted, and reemphasized by the series discussed above, that lumbar sympathectomy may be helpful *only* in a small intractable group of cases of postphlebitic

ulcers. Furthermore, the indications should be restricted to those patients who display vasomotor changes (coldness, hyperhidrosis) and present evidence of arteriovenous shunting or *associated* arterial insufficiency.

SUMMARY

The lessons derived from this brief review on the pathophysiology of the postphlebitic syndrome with leg ulcers are significant in that they emphasize (1) the role of the valvular incompetence of the deep veins of the leg, with special emphasis on those of the ankle, (2) the role of reverse venous flow through the communicating or ankle-perforating incompetent veins, (3) the resulting venous hypertension at the ankle level, (4) the role of arteriovenous shunting, as yet not well known but significant in reducing the nutritive arterial flow through the capillary bed, and (5) the possible usefulness of lumbar sympathectomy in a small group of patients with postphlebitic ulcers refractory to the classic management of these cases.

REFERENCES

1. Dodd H, Cockett FB: The Pathology and Surgery of the Veins of the Lower Limb. Baltimore, Williams & Wilkins, 1956, Chap 14, p 343.
2. DeCamp PT, Ward JA, Ochsner A: Ambulatory venous pressure studies in postphlebitic and other disease states. Surgery 29:365, 1951.
3. Piulachs P, Vidal-Barraquer F: Pathogenic study of varicose veins. Angiology 4:59, 1953.
4. Malan E: Vascular syndromes from dilatation of arteriovenous communications of the sole of the foot. AMA Arch Surg 77:783, 1958.
5. Gius, JA: Arteriovenous anastomoses and varicose veins. Arch Surg 81:299, 1960.
6. Edwards EA, O'Connor JF: Ordinary varicose veins as an expression of congenital hemangioma. Surg Gynecol Obstet 122:1245, 1966.
7. Haimovici H, Steinman C, Caplan LH: Angiographic evaluation of arteriovenous shunting in peripheral vascular diseases. Radiology 87:696, 1966.
8. Haimovici H: Arteriovenous shunting in varicose veins: Its diagnosis by Doppler ultrasound flow detector. J Vasc Surg 2:684, 1985.
9. Haimovici H: Role of precapillary arteriovenous shunting in the pathogenesis of varicose veins and its therapeutic implications. Surgery 101:515, 1987.
10. Patman RD: Sympathectomy in the treatment of chronic venous leg ulcers. Arch Surg 117:1561, 1982.

CHAPTER 72

Chronic Deep Venous Insufficiency

Kenneth J. Cherry, Jr., and Larry H. Hollier

Chronic venous insufficiency is a widespread and serious, if largely unspectacular, problem. It has been estimated to affect 0.5% of the populations of Great Britain and the United States.[1] Female patients are twice as numerous as male patients. The mean age of presentation for females is 55, and 10% of patients will be hospitalized for recurrent thrombosis, cellulitis, ulceration, or operation.[2] Two million workdays are thought to be lost in the United States each year because of complications associated with this entity.[3] It is believed that the majority of cases represent late sequelae of deep venous thrombosis, hence the term *postphlebitic syndrome*, which is usually used interchangeably, if not entirely correctly, with chronic venous insufficiency. Other disease processes such as congenital absence or incompetence of the valves may give rise to chronic venous insufficiency. Ferris and Kistner[4] have identified a population with primary valvular incompetence, and it may be that some of the patients thought to have silent deep venous thrombosis suffer instead from this malady. The cause of a particular case may not be vitally important when medical management is pursued successfully. Direct operations on the deep venous system, however, discussed in other chapters herein, must be predicated on a firm understanding of the particular disease process and anatomy. The acute onset of chronic venous insufficiency in previously healthy patients, particularly the elderly, mandates a search for extrinsic causes such as pelvic tumors.

PATHOPHYSIOLOGY

The venous system of the lower extremities is divided into three entities or subsystems. The deep system of veins is comprised of those veins lying within the muscular compartments and beneath the deep fascia. This system returns approximately 85% of the blood delivered to the lower extremities. The superficial system is comprised of the greater saphenous and lesser saphenous veins and their tributaries in the subcutaneous tissue, superficial to the deep fascia. The perforating system (communicating system) is comprised of those veins traversing the fascia and connecting the deep and superficial systems. These perforating veins have valves designed normally to direct flow from the superficial to the deep veins in the extremity proximal to the foot level. The valves present in the lower extremity are bicuspid. They are more numerous distally, with many fewer valve stations in the thigh than in the leg. The valves are often absent in the iliac veins.[5]

Iliofemoral venous thrombosis is considered the most common precursor of chronic venous insufficiency, a history of such being elicited in anywhere from 30 to 87% of patients.[6] It has been accepted that the remainder of patients have silent thrombosis (see Fig. 72-3). Nonetheless patients with primary valve agenesis and dysfunction have been identified,[4,7] although the number of such patients is unknown. Conversely, up to 86% of patients with documented deep venous thrombosis may be expected to develop a venous ulcer if followed for 10 years.[8] However, the course of the sequelae of deep venous thrombosis is problematic. Browse and his coworkers pointed out that one fourth of patients with thrombosis extending above the knee level may not develop symptoms in 5 to 10 years.[9] Acutely, the obstruction is complete.

In the months that follow, recanalization of the veins restores patency. However, competency is lost as the thrombotic and healing processes destroy the valves involved. Those valves distal to the thrombotic process are thought to dilate sequentially as the incompetent venous segments cephalad transmit uncorrected hydrostatic pressure to the next distal valve station. This increase in pressure is transmitted to the perforating veins with the same results—loss of competency and reversal of venous flow. It is this combination of deep and perforating venous incompetence that, in most cases, leads to the syndrome of chronic venous insufficiency. Schanzer and Peirce[10] found incompetent perforators to be the pathologic factor in 60% of their patients and incompetent deep veins in 27%. They did not look at the combination. Using different methods, Szendro et al.[11] found deep venous incompetence to correlate best with symptomatic chronic venous insufficiency. Yao et al. believe that deep and perforating valve incompetence together are the most important factors in symptomatic disease. Shull, Nicolaides, and their coworkers[13] have pointed out that popliteal vein incompetence correlates best with symptomatology.

The pathologic process affects the skin and subcutaneous tissues. The hydrostatic pressure transmitted to these tissues causes increased water in the interstitial spaces with resultant edema.[14] Edema is the first manifestation of chronic venous insufficiency. It initially appears at the end of the day, involving the ankle and lower leg, and recedes at night. It may progress with time so that the involved leg does not return to normal size with recumbency. It may progress up into the thigh. Massive swelling of the entire extremity or extremities may be seen with iliac or inferior vena caval occlusion.

The other manifestations of chronic venous insufficiency are dermatitis, induration, pain, and ulceration. Associated with the edema are congestion and cyanosis of the skin, leading to hemosiderin deposition and its resultant brown discoloration (Fig. 72-1). Stasis dermatitis (eczema) is a frequent companion problem. Long-standing edema and dermatitis lead to fibrosis of the tissues and induration of the involved skin and subcutaneous tissues. These changes are usually seen in the malleolar areas, most commonly over the medial malleolus. Ulceration develops in these same areas. Perforating veins here arise directly from the subcutaneous tissues; incompetence of these valves transmits the pressure in the deep veins directly to the subcutaneous tissue.[15] Browse and his coworkers[16] have described an increased escape of fibrin through the microvascular network in these areas. This hyperpermeability

allows for a dense, pericapillary "cuff" of fibrin, which an inadequate fibrinolytic system cannot clear. Patients with chronic venous insufficiency have inadequate fibrinolysis in both blood and the vein wall. This fibrin ring around the capillaries acts as a barrier to gas diffusion, leading to cellular ischemia and ultimately to necrosis. Skin oxygen tensions have been shown by different groups to be decreased in patients with venous stasis disease.[17-19] These ulcers are slow to heal and notoriously recurrent.

Some patients are bothered by pain in the muscles of the leg after standing for some time. Recumbency usually relieves this aching and fatigue. Venous claudication is a severe, bursting pain, usually of the thigh, thought to occur with long-standing iliofemoral occlusion, with a patent system distally. This pain is thought to be the result of venous congestion, made worse with exercise because the increased flow associated with muscle activity cannot be returned to the heart at the same rate delivered. In an interesting study, Qvarfordt et al.[20] have demonstrated increased intramuscular pressure in the anterior and deep posterior compartments and increased water content in the leg muscles ipsilateral to iliac vein occlusion. They and others believe the pain of venous claudication is secondary to this increase in intramuscular pressure.

DIAGNOSIS

The diagnosis of chronic venous insufficiency, with edema, induration, and ulceration, is usually made easily on history and physical examination. The differential diagnoses include congestive heart failure, chronic glomerulonephritis, chronic lymphedema, and lipedema.[14] Probably the most difficult differential diagnosis is between chronic venous insufficiency and chronic lymphedema. The edema of chronic venous insufficiency does not involve the foot, nor do the skin and subcutaneous tissues take on the diffuse thickening of lymphedema, with the latter's firm pitting edema.

Ulceration may result from arterial as well as venous disease. Location of the ulcers in the toes and feet, their pale appearance, and the pain associated with them, as well as the other signs of arterial insufficiency, are useful in distinguishing between the two entities. Combined arterial and venous ulcerations occur, and signs of both arterial and venous disease are present. Edema and chronic skin changes may preclude accurate pulse examination. Vascular laboratory measurements, both arterial and venous, are useful in such situations.

Whereas physical examination may reveal the presence of chronic venous insufficiency, it is not sufficient to elucidate the underlying anatomic and functional defects. Szendro and colleagues[11] and Moore, Himmel, and Sumner[5] have shown that valvular incompetence need not be an all-or-none phenomenon. Femoral veins may reflux separately, as may popliteal veins, or incompetence may be generalized. Popliteal incompetence is believed by many authors to correlate most directly with chronic venous insufficiency,[5,12,13] although Ferris and Kistner[4] make a cogent case for femoral incompetence as a causal factor. Kistner, in his discussion of Moore et al.'s paper, analyzed their data somewhat differently than they did and believed that

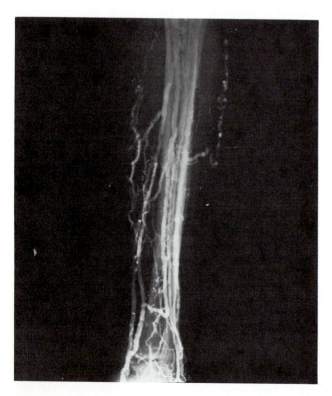

Figure 72-1. Ascending phlebogram demonstrating incompetent perforating vein.

75% of their patients had proximal incompetence, either singly or in conjunction with distal incompetence. At the time of this writing, these differences of viewpoint remain controversial and are undergoing continued investigation.

If there is no history of deep venous thrombosis, other causes of chronic venous insufficiency should be sought. Pelvic tumors, hemangiomas, and arteriovenous fistulas may give rise to venous insufficiency, as may primary valvular agenesis or incompetence.

For years ascending phlebography has been the standard against which new modalities are compared. Deep venous patency and perforator venous patency and competence can be demonstrated (Fig. 72-1). Postphlebitic changes and chronic obstructions are easily seen. Some authorities believe ascending phlebography may be performed in such a way as to define incompetence of valves as well.[21] These studies, however, are probably inadequate if a deep venous reconstruction to restore competency is contemplated. Clear delineation of the state of the venous valves usually requires descending phlebography, although the use of this modality is considered by some authorities to be controversial because of differences in technique and appraisal.[22] Kistner[23] has developed a grading system for evaluating descending phlebography (Table 72-1). Decisions concerning deep venous valvular replacement or reconstruction are dependent on such anatomic and functional assessment (Fig. 72-2). Descending phlebography is a fluoroscopic, hence dynamic, study and as such provides functional as well as anatomic data.

Ambulatory venous pressure is an extremely useful diagnostic measurement and a good method of follow-up for reconstructive procedures, although it is a minimally invasive and moderately cumbersome procedure[24-28] (Fig. 72-2). It is these last two factors that probably have prevented its wider use and acceptance. A small-gauge needle or catheter is placed in a dorsal vein of the foot, and resting supine and standing venous pressures and exercise pressures are obtained. The supine pressures are in the range of less than 10 mm Hg. Assuming an upright position causes the pressure to elevate to the range of about 75 mm Hg, depending on the patient's height. This increase normally takes more than 20 seconds. Exercise causes an initial rise in pressure of small proportions and short duration, followed by a greater than 50% decrease as the muscle pump of the legs comes into play. Ambulatory pressures are normally in the range of 20 mm Hg.

In a patient with chronic venous insufficiency without

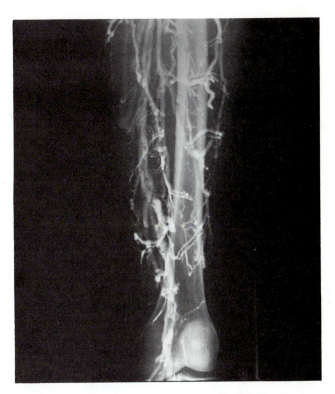

Figure 72-2. Descending phlebogram revealing massive incompetence of deep veins down to infragenicular level.

obstruction, the supine pressure is normal. Upon standing, the rise in venous pressure occurs in less than normal time. The standing resting, or baseline, pressure is usually normal. With exercise the drop in pressure does not achieve the 50% level, and with continued exercise, it may exceed baseline.

With venous obstruction there may be increases in both supine and standing, resting and exercise pressures, depending on collateralization and competency.

Noninvasive laboratory examination of the deep veins has become a mainstay of venous evaluation. Impedance plethysmography (IPG) is useful in the diagnosis of deep venous thrombosis and obstruction but is less helpful in the diagnosis of chronic venous insufficiency. Phleborheography also is of more use in diagnosing deep venous thrombosis. Currently, photoplethysmography (PPG), Doppler venous examination, and duplex scanning are the most useful noninvasive tools available to the surgeon or physician assessing chronic venous insufficiency.

Photoplethysmography measures the cutaneous capillary blood volume through an emitter and detector of backscattered light in these tissues (Figs. 72-3 to 72-5). Cutaneous blood content is an index of venous pressure. When venous valves are competent, capillary refilling is slow, being solely a function of arterial flow. When venous reflux is present, the refilling time is shortened. This test may be used to differentiate between local edema and ulcers due to primary varices and those due to chronic venous insufficiency. When primary varices are present and deep venous insufficiency is absent, application of a tourniquet returns capillary refilling times to normal.[24,29-32]

TABLE 72-1. INTERPRETATION OF DESCENDING PHLEBOGRAPHY

Complete competence
  Does not leak during full Valsalva maneuver

Satisfactory competence
  Mild leakage limited to thigh during Valsalva maneuver

Moderate incompetence
  Prominent leakage into calf during Valsalva maneuver
  Retains prograde flow in iliac vein

Severe incompetence
  Cascading retrograde flow during Valsalva maneuver
  Reflux into calf perforators

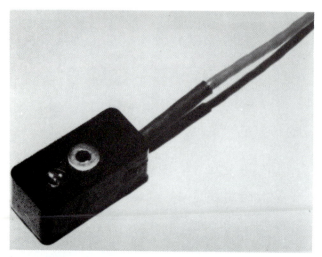

Figure 72-3. Photoplethysmograph consists of two infrared sensors. (*From Kempczinski RF, Yao JST: Practical Noninvasive Vascular Diagnosis, 2nd ed. Chicago, Year Book Medical Publishers, 1987.*)

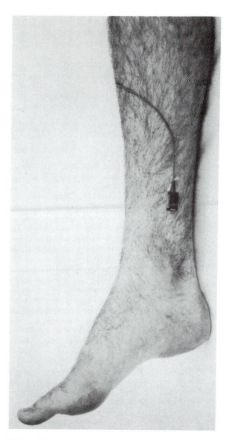

Figure 72-5. Photoplethysmographic transducer, which is attached to the skin. (*From Kempczinski RF, Yao JST: Practical Noninvasive Vascular Diagnosis, 2nd ed. Chicago, Year Book Medical Publishers, 1987.*)

Doppler examination with a directional instrument may reveal forward or reverse flow. Probes of 5, 8, or 10 MHz may be used. The femoral, popliteal, and saphenous veins may be individually studied. Retrograde flow during inspiration occurs when incompetence is present. The presence of attenuated respiratory modulation and an altered response to the Valsalva maneuver are helpful in diagnosing chronic venous insufficiency and obstruction.[24,31-33]

Duplex scanning probably holds more promise for evaluation of the venous system than any other noninvasive mode of examination because it pairs anatomic information (from the B-mode imager) and functional data (from the Doppler). Individual veins in the lower extremity may be individually and accurately evaluated. It is from this tool that our knowledge of segmental reflux has come. In the hands of the St. Mary's group in London, duplex scanning has a sensitivity of 84% and a specificity of 88% when compared to ambulatory venous pressures. Nicolaides and his coworkers[11,13] have shown a high correlation between popliteal vein reflux and symptomatic diseases, that is, ulcers (Fig. 72-6).

NONOPERATIVE TREATMENT

Medical management continues to be the mainstay of treatment for the vast majority of patients with chronic venous insufficiency. Education of patients is a difficult, but neces-

sary, basis of care. Venous disease is insidious, causing its damage over years. Many physicians fail to understand this slow, inexorable course, and it is not surprising that patients do not readily grasp the necessity of protracted care. Graduated elastic support is a lifelong necessity for these patients. Graded compression elastic stockings provide the best support. Strict adherence to the use of these stockings may prevent the consequences of prolonged uncorrected venous hypertension and may also alleviate the pain many patients experience. Knee-length stockings are usually sufficient because thigh-high stockings tend to buckle behind the knees. Some patients with severe disease may benefit from pantyhose stockings. Usually 30 to 40 mm compression weight suffices. Heavier stockings are reserved for patients with associated lymphedema or refractory venous edema.

Figure 72-4. Normalization of venous refilling time after long saphenous vein stripping. The photoplethysmographic tourniquet test accurately predicted response before surgery. (*From Kempczinski RF, Yao JST: Practical Noninvasive Vascular Diagnosis, 2nd ed. Chicago, Year Book Medical Publishers, 1987.*)

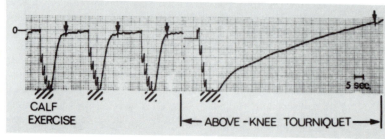

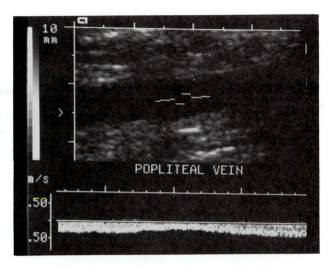

Figure 72-6. Duplex scan showing popliteal vein.

Ulcerations are treated with elevation, medication, and compressive therapy. Small ulcerations may be treated on an outpatient basis. Throughout the United States, Unna's boots are used extensively. They, or variants thereof such as Elastoplast boots, may be used. Antibiotic or antibacterial solutions such as 0.25% aluminum subacetate can be used. If cellulitis intervenes, appropriate antibiotics are used either locally or systemically. Patients' allergies must be noted because local allergic reactions can turn small ulcerations into large defects.

Eczema and dermatitis are treated when appropriate with lanolin solutions, aluminum subacetate, steroid preparations, or antibiotics.

Extensive ulcerations with associated cellulitis may require hospitalization with elevation of the leg. Split-thickness skin grafting may be a necessity for these patients. Large, recurrent ulcerations are an indication for more aggressive management.

SURGICAL MANAGEMENT

Direct surgical correction of chronic venous insufficiency is undergoing evolution and evaluation. A detailed analysis is outside the scope of this chapter and is discussed elsewhere. A few comments nonetheless are in order. Classic operations, such as the Linton procedure, which interrupt or destroy incompetent perforators, have their place when incompetent communicating veins are the major problem. Indeed, the contrasting experiences of Ferris and Kistner[4] and the Northwestern group[34,35] with regard to deep venous reconstruction point out dramatically the necessity of addressing incompetent perforators. Kistner treats both deep and perforator disease. In an early series, the group from Chicago performed deep venous reconstructions but left coexistent incompetent perforators uncorrected. Their reconstructions failed at a later date. The controversies concerning femoral valve reconstructions notwithstanding, it would seem that symptomatic incompetent communicating veins should be corrected whether or not deep venous dis-

ease is to be operated on directly. It is not unusual to find incompetent perforators in the presence of incompetent deep veins, as noted previously. As a consequence, newer procedures have been and are being developed. Kistner, in Honolulu, is responsible in this country for the vigorous reappraisal of venous pathophysiology and the evaluation of reconstructive, rather than extirpative, procedures on the deep veins. There is much controversy about the role of a single, competent valve at the superficial femoral vein level and about the importance of femoral vs. popliteal incompetence. These controversies are far from settled but are representative of the renewed interest, thought, and reappraisal given venous disorders.

The operations for deep venous disease may be classed into two categories: (1) operations to restore venous patency, and (2) operations to restore venous competency.

Patency

At present there are three types of operations performed to restore patency: (1) the Husni operation, (2) the Palma-Dale operation and its variants, and (3) direct reconstructions of the iliac vein and the inferior vena cava.

The Husni operation, or in situ saphenopopliteal venovenous bypass, is designed to relieve obstruction of the femoral and popliteal veins by use of the ipsilateral saphenous vein anastomosed end-to-side to the most proximal patent deep vein, usually the popliteal. Free vein grafts can be used if the ipsilateral saphenous vein is not suitable and if the other extremity is not involved[36] (Fig. 72-7).

In the Palma-Dale operation, iliac obstruction is bypassed by use of the contralateral saphenous vein. Palma and Esperon[37] reported their operation in 1960. Dale[38] has had the most experience in this country. Many of his patients, 43%, had malignancies obstructing the iliac vein, and 65% of the patients over 50 were obstructed by pelvic cancer. It would appear from his experience that the best results occur with extrinsic compression in which the veins themselves are structurally intact (Fig. 72-8). It is imperative that the iliac obstruction be functional as well as anatomic. Ambulatory venous pressures should be consistent with an outflow obstruction. If patency of collaterals is of a degree that distal venous pressures, even after exercise, are only mildly elevated, bypass grafting cannot be expected to be either necessary or successful. In a small experience, surgeons at the Mayo Clinic have had disappointing results with these types of operations. Some surgeons have begun to use externally reinforced polytetrafluroethylene (PTFE) grafts as their crossover component, citing better patency rates.[39] Arteriovenous fistulas are usually created at the time of operation to increase flow rates through the graft. They are usually temporary and are taken down or ligated after 6 to 12 weeks.

Distinct from extraanatomic, or crosspubic, grafting are direct reconstructions of the iliac veins and the superior and inferior vena cavae, which have been performed with spiral vein grafts and with externally supported (ringed) PTFE grafts.[40-42] Results in the early stages are promising, and it may be that direct reconstructions will prove superior to extraanatomic grafts. Gloviczki, Hollier, et al.[43,44] have

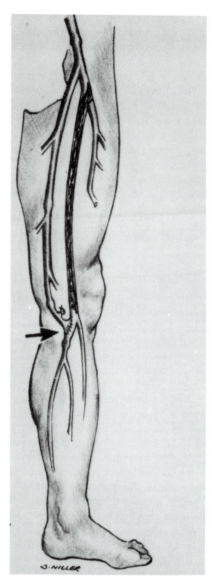

Figure 72-7. Saphenopopliteal anastomosis (*arrow*). (*From Bergan JJ, Yao JST: Venous Problems. Chicago, Year Book Medical Publishers, 1978.*)

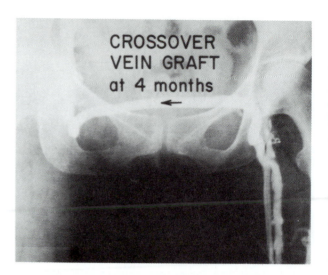

Figure 72-8. Patent crossover vein graft 4 months after surgery. (*From Bergan JJ, Yao JST: Venous Problems. Chicago, Year Book Medical Publishers, 1978.*)

rect through use of a gracilis or silastic band, as described by Psathakis and Psathakis,[45] transplants of valve-containing segments of brachial vein to the femoral and popliteal levels,[4] and vein-segment transpositions, as popularized by Kistner.[4] Early results for highly selective and skilled surgeons such as Kistner, Raju, and Taheri are good.[4,46,47] Patient selection is controversial. The majority of patients probably continue to be treated best at the present time by compressive elastic support. Nonetheless, the 14-year results reported by Ferris and Kistner[4] are encouraging, and surgeons continue to perform these difficult venous reconstructions when medical management proves unsatisfactory for patients.

THE FUTURE

The recognition of regional or segmental reflux by the duplex scan and the advent of direct operations on the venous system offer exciting prospects for the treatment of venous disease. As methods of diagnosis become more precise, diagnosis itself will become more precise, and the term *chronic venous insufficiency* may no longer be an adequate diagnosis. Rather, specific diagnoses such as superficial femoral venous incompetence or popliteal venous incompetence with associated perforator incompetence will be made. Surgeons may expect that, with more precision in diagnostic methods, operations will be tailored for particular and individual disease states just as they currently are for the arterial system. The coming years will witness exciting developments, both promising and disappointing, as chronic venous disease becomes better understood and, it is to be hoped, better managed.

recommended temporary arteriovenous fistulas and anticoagulation as adjuvant therapy. Dale, Harris, and Terry[42] in their clinical placement of grafts did not use arteriovenous fistulas. This is an exciting area, the guiding principles of which have not yet been developed.

Operations to restore patency are applicable to only a small minority of patients with deep venous disease. Schanzer and Peirce[10] found only 7.6% of cases of chronic venous disease to be based on venous obstruction.

Competency

There currently is a multiplicity of operations designed to restore venous competency. They include valvuloplasty, both direct, as performed by Ferris and Kistner,[4] and indi-

REFERENCES

1. Boyd AM, Jepson RP, et al.: The logical management of chronic ulcers of the legs. Angiology 3:207, 1952.
2. Cuthbert Owens, J: The postphlebitic syndrome: Management

by conservative means, in Bergan JJ, Yao JST: Venous Problems. Chicago, Year Book Medical Publishers, Inc, 1978, p 369.

3. Browse NL, Burnand KG: The postphlebitic syndrome: A new look, in Bergan JJ, Yao JST: Chicago, Year Book Medical Publishers, 1978, p 395.

4. Ferris EB, Kistner RL: Femoral vein reconstruction in the management of chronic venous insufficiency. Arch Surg 117:1571, 1982.

5. Moore DJ, Himmel PD, Sumner DS: Distribution of venous valvular incompetence in patients with the postphlebitic syndrome. J Vasc Surg 3:49, 1986.

6. Bauer G: A roentgenological and clinical study of the sequels of thrombosis. Acta Chir Scand 86(suppl 74):1, 1942.

7. Plate G, Brudin L, et al.: Physiologic and therapeutic aspects in congenital vein valve aplasia of the lower limb. Ann Surg 198:229, 1983.

8. O'Donnell TF, Browse NL, et al.: The socioeconomic effects of an iliofemoral venous thrombosis. J Surg Res 22:483, 1977.

9. Browse NL, Clemenson G, et al.: Is the postphlebitic leg always postphlebitic? Relation between phlebographic appearances and deep-vein thrombosis and late sequelae. Br Med J 281:1167, 1980.

10. Schanzer H, Peirce EC II: A rational approach to surgery of the chronic venous stasis syndrome. Ann Surg 195:25, 1982.

11. Szendro G, Nicolaides MS, et al.: Duplex scanning in the assessment of deep venous incompetence. J Vasc Surg 4:237, 1986.

12. Yao JST, Flinn WR, et al.: The role of noninvasive testing in the evaluation of chronic venous problems. World J Surg 10:911, 1986.

13. Shull KC, Nicolaides AN, et al.: Significance of popliteal reflux in relation to ambulatory venous pressure and ulceration. Arch Surg 114:1304, 1979.

14. Juergens JL, Lofgren KA: Chronic venous insufficiency (postphlebitic syndrome, chronic venous stasis), in Juergens JL, Spittell JA Jr, Fairbairn JF II: Peripheral Vascular Diseases, 5th ed. Philadelphia, WB Saunders Co, 1980, p 981.

15. Dodd H, Cockett FB: The Pathology and Surgery of the Veins of the Lower Limb. Edinburgh & London, Churchill Livingstone, 1956.

16. Browse NL, Gray L, et al.: Blood and vein wall fibrinolytic activity in health and vascular disease. Br Med J 1:478, 1977.

17. Dodd HJ, Gaylarde PM, Sarkany I: Skin oxygen tension in venous insufficiency of the lower leg. J R Soc Med 78:373, 1985.

18. Franzeck UK, Bollinger A, et al.: Transcutaneous oxygen tension and capillary morphologic characteristics and density in patients with chronic venous incompetence. Circulation 70:806, 1984.

19. Rooke TW, Hollier LH, et al.: The effect of elastic compression on TcPo$_2$ in limbs with venous stasis. Phlebology 2:23, 1987.

20. Qvarfordt P, Eklöf B, et al.: Intramuscular pressure, blood flow, and skeletal muscle metabolism in patients with venous claudication. Surgery 95:191, 1984.

21. Lundström B, Osterman G: Assessment of deep venous insufficiency by ascending phlebography. Acta Radiol (Diagn) 24:375, 1983.

22. Ackroyd JS, Browse NL: The investigation and surgery of the post-thrombotic syndrome. J Cardiovasc Surg 27:5, 1986.

23. Kistner RL: Diagnosis of chronic venous insufficiency. J Vasc Surg 3:185, 1986.

24. Flanigan DP, Williams LR: Venous insufficiency of the lower extremities: New methods of diagnosis and therapy. Surg Annu 14:359, 1982.

25. Nachbur B: Assessment of venous disorders by venous pressure measurements, in Hobb JT: The Treatment of Venous Disorders. Philadelphia, JB Lippincott Co, 1977.

26. Randhawa GK, Dhillon JS, et al.: Assessment of chronic venous insufficiency using dynamic venous pressure studies. Am J Surg 148:203, 1984.

27. Schanzer H, Peirce EC II: Pathophysiologic evaluation of chronic venous stasis with ambulatory venous pressure studies. Angiology 33:183, 1982.

28. Taheri SA, Pendergast D, et al.: Continuous ambulatory venous pressure for diagnosis of venous insufficiency. Preliminary report. Am J Surg 150:203, 1985.

29. Abramowitz HB, Queral LA, et al.: The use of photoplethysmography in the assessment of venous insufficiency: A comparison to venous pressure measurements. Surgery 86:434, 1979.

30. Flinn WR, O'Mara CS, et al.: The use of photoplethysmography in the assessment of venous insufficiency, in Kempczinski RF, Yao JST: Practical Noninvasive Vascular Diagnosis, 2nd ed. Chicago, Year Book Medical Publishers, 1987, p 486.

31. Kohler TR, Strandness DE Jr: Noninvasive testing for the evaluation of chronic venous disease. World J Surg 10:903, 1986.

32. Barnes RW: Current status of noninvasive tests in the diagnosis of venous disease. Surg Clin North Am 62:489, 1982.

33. Yao JST, Blackburn DR: Doppler venous survey, in Kempczinski RE, Yao JST: Practical Noninvasive Vascular Diagnosis, 2nd ed. Chicago, Year Book Medical Publishers, 1987, p 392.

34. Queral LA, Whitehouse WM Jr, et al.: Surgical correction of chronic deep venous insufficiency by valvular transposition. Surgery 87:688, 1980.

35. Johnson ND, Queral LA, et al.: Late objective assessment of venous valve surgery. Arch Surg 116:1461, 1981.

36. Husni EA: Clinical experience with femoropopliteal venous reconstruction, in Bergan JJ, Yao JST: Venous Problems. Chicago, Year Book Medical Publishers, 1978, p 485.

37. Palma EC, Esperon R: Vein transplants and grafts in the surgical treatment of the postphlebitic syndrome. J Cardiovasc Surg 1:94, 1960.

38. Dale WA: Crossover grafts for iliofemoral venous occlusion, in Bergan JJ, Yao JST: Venous Problems. Chicago, Year Book Medical Publishers, 1978, p 411.

39. Dollmar JF, Hutschenreiter S: Vascular prostheses for the venous system, in May R, Weber J: Pelvic and Abdominal Veins: Progress in Diagnostics and Therapy. Amsterdam, Excerpta Medica, 1981.

40. Chan EL, Bardin JA, Bernstein EF: Inferior vena cava bypass: Experimental evaluation of externally supported grafts and initial clinical application. J Vasc Surg 1:675, 1984.

41. Chiu CJ, Terzis J, MacRae ML: Replacement of superior vena cava with the spiral composite vein graft. Ann Thorac Surg 17:555, 1974.

42. Dale WA, Harris J, Terry RB: Polytetrafluoroethylene reconstruction of the inferior vena cava. Surgery 95:625, 1984.

43. Gloviczki P, Hollier LH, et al.: Experimental replacement of the inferior vena cava: Factors affecting patency. Surgery 6:657, 1984.

44. Gloviczki P, Hollier LH: Remplacement prothétique de la veine inférieure, in Kieffer E: Chirurgie de la Veine Cave Inférieure et de ses Branches. Paris, Expansion Scientifique Francaise, 1985, p 82.

45. Psathakis ND, Psathakis DN: Rationale of the substitute "valve" operation by technique II in the treatment of chronic venous insufficiency. Int Angio 4:397, 1985.

46. Raju S: Venous insufficiency of the lower limb and stasis ulceration: Changing concepts in management. Ann Surg 197:688, 1983.

47. Taheri SA, Pendergast DR, et al.: Vein valve transplantation. Am J Surg 150:201, 1985.

CHAPTER 73

Venous Reconstruction for Treatment of Postphlebitic Syndrome

Henry Haimovici

HISTORICAL BACKGROUND

In contrast to the great strides achieved in arterial reconstructive procedures, venous replacement in the venous tree has not resulted in similar success.[1] However, in recent years, stimulated by the overall progress in vascular techniques, new approaches in the management of venous problems have become available.

It is of interest to note that before the present era, Eck, a Russian surgeon, successfully performed the first anastomosis between the portal vein and the inferior vena cava.[2] This technique of venovenous anastomosis, which enabled primarily physiologists to carry out important laboratory studies, later became the basis for the well-known portacaval shunts, but it remained an essentially isolated historical achievement, without any immediate clinical application, until the modern era.

It was not until the beginning of this century that surgeons began to apply techniques of vascular sutures and anastomoses to the venous system. As an example, Clermont,[3] in 1901, reported experiments in anastomosing a divided inferior vena cava by using a continuous everting mattress suture of fine silk. The follow-up of 1 month was too short to be significant, in spite of the successful result of the procedure.

This isolated experiment was followed by another method devised by Payr[4] in 1904. It consisted of invaginating the ends of divided vessels over cylinders of magnesium, but subsequent attempts at grafting of veins by Payr's method resulted in thrombosis and failure. As a result of a series of unsuccessful attempts, no further experimentation seems to have been carried out for several decades, in spite of Carrel's technique[5] published in 1902, of using circular sutures on the blood vessels. Then later, in 1906, Carrel and Guthrie[6] reported excellent results in the application of their method of arteriovenous anastomoses and transplantation of organs.

In the 1950s, the renewal of interest in implanting grafts in the venous system was stimulated by the renaissance in arterial grafting.

One of the areas that became an early focus of clinical interest was reconstructive surgery to treat postphlebitic syndrome and to provide venous repair by bypass procedures. Thus Kunlin et al.,[7] in 1953, attempted to treat postphlebitic syndrome by inserting 18 cm of a free saphenous segment between the external iliac and long saphenous veins. The bypass graft, however, remained patent for only 3 weeks.

In 1954, Warren and Thayer[8] attempted a similar procedure in another venous area. They transplanted the long saphenous vein in 14 patients to improve postphlebitic stasis of the lower part of the leg. In seven patients the long saphenous vein was transplanted from the subcutaneous area of the groin to the muscular compartment below to increase the blood flow during muscular contraction. This transplantation was carried out in seven other patients, and in addition, the vein was divided at the knee level, where an anastomosis was performed between the proximal segment of the saphenous vein and the distal segment of the divided popliteal vein. Regional heparinization for 24 hours, with a polyethylene catheter tied into the short saphenous vein near the popliteal vein, was carried out in the patients with a saphenopopliteal anastomosis. Postoperative phlebograms revealed patency of all the transplants without the latter type of anastomosis. In the group with popliteal anastomosis, only one transplant was open; the phlebograms were equivocal in the other six.

The first genuinely successful procedure in venous reconstruction that resulted in increased venous flow in postphlebitic syndrome was achieved by Palma and Eperson[9] in 1958. Their procedure was novel and consisted of a crossover graft through the suprapubic region from the normal to the thrombophlebitic limb with the use of the saphenous vein. The great improvement that followed this procedure stimulated great interest in a number of surgeons who applied this principle of the technique to a variety of cases.[10]

INCIDENCE OF POSTTHROMBOTIC VENOUS THROMBOSIS REQUIRING SURGICAL REPAIR

The exact number of patients with previous venous thrombosis of major vessels requiring surgery is not known. One of the major reasons is the pathophysiology of venous thrombosis. A large number of patients with acute thrombosis have recanalization of the thrombus and, instead of having a complete occlusion of a major vein, develop a partial lumen with resulting venous insufficiency. Consequently the patients who require surgical repair do not fall into the category of those with recanalization of the major thrombus but, rather, continue to have venous insufficiency that is manageable by nonsurgical means. Except for the indications mentioned below, the postthrombotic syndrome with incompetent deep veins will develop in most patients who have had lesions of the major veins, but without the need for major surgical replacement of the veins. There have been a few recently published reports of series of patients with clinically suspected venous insufficiency, but only a small percentage of these patients were found to have persistent obstructive disease. Thus, Raju,[11] in a group of 147 patients with *clinically* suspected venous insufficiency, found only 13 (9%) who had signs of occlusion of the main veins. Whether this percentage requires crossover femorofemoral grafting has been questioned by Halliday et al.,[12] who believed that in their own experience thre was probably an even lower proportion of patients suitable for femorofemoral crossover grafting; they found only 47 patients (3%) suitable for this operation in a consecutive series of over 1600 undergoing phlebography so that treatment of their chronic venous disease could be planned. Their finding underscores the fact that this discrepancy is based on phlebography and not on clinical suspicion of venous insufficiency, the clinical accuracy being of course questioned.

EVALUATION FOR VENOUS RECONSTRUCTION

As shown by the studies discussed above, careful preoperative evaluation of suspected venous occlusion by phlebography and noninvasive methods, especially duplex B-mode imaging, is essential.[12–14] Only with these diagnostic methods can one determine the percentage of patients in this category who require either femoropopliteal or femorofemoral crossover bypass.

Indications for Reconstruction

In contrast to indications for reconstructive treatment of arterial occlusive diseases, which appears, in general, much easier to accomplish, those for venous reconstruction are somewhat more difficult to determine.

One of the most common indications is unilateral iliac venous thrombosis with additional evidence of (1) suprapubic collateral veins, (2) limb edema that does not yield to elevation or bandaging, (3) intermittent claudication associated with venous obstruction of the leg veins, and (4) occlusion of the lower segment of the vena cava and the proximal segment of the adjacent iliac vein.

Less common, perhaps, is postthrombotic disease of the femoral vein, for which a saphenopopliteal bypass is indicated.

Contraindications for Reconstruction

Contraindications for venous reconstruction may be (1) chronic venous thrombosis of the lower leg deep veins, in which recanalization of the venous obstruction may not be suitable for such a repair, and (2) the presence of only valvular insufficiency associated with extensive and diffuse postphlebitic changes of the venous tree. An exception may be made for the popliteal vein without obstructive distal venous disease (see below).

GRAFT MATERIALS

Three main types of graft materials are used in venous reconstruction procedures: (1) saphenous vein, (2) synthetic material, and (3) autogenous vein valves.

The saphenous vein is most often the graft material of choice. Two types of methods may be considered: the use of the greater saphenous vein as a crossover and its use as a free vein segment.

Unlike all other types of grafting material, an autogenous vein offers several fundamental advantages: it is, by definition, a live tissue; it is not subject to rejection by the organism, and the endothelial lining, if the vein is properly handled, has a great potential for reducing the chances of thrombosis.

After careful removal of the vein from its location by several small skin incisions or by means of a long thigh approach, dissection is carried out under direct visual control. Some of the adventitia, especially near the section of the vein, is stripped off, according to Palma,[15] although some authors believe that this may not be entirely necessary. The collateral veins of this segment of the saphenous vein are carefully ligated and are divided about 1 to 2 mm away from the junction with the main trunk. This will ensure that the graft will dilate, increasing its lumen by one third, and that it will take on a uniformly cylindrical shape. The use of the autogenous graft avoids the irregular beadlike enlargements of the transplanted graft, which could give rise to turbulence and possible thrombosis.[15]

SAPHENOUS VEIN GRAFTS

Femorofemoral Crossover (Palma Procedure)*

Donor Side. The saphenous vein on the donor side is prepared for the harvest of a length of about 6 to 8 cm of the trunk, with the adventitia stripped off only at the medial third, the free end (Fig. 73-1).

---

* These operative steps are based in part on Palma's description in Chapter 65 of *Vascular Surgery*, second edition.[15]

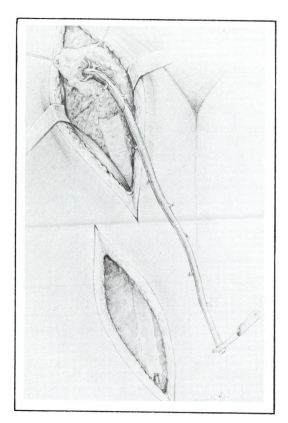

Figure 73-1. Terminal proximal two thirds of saphenous vein divided at above-knee level. Note its junction with femoral vein, which is left intact. (*From Palma EC, Eperson R: J Cardiovasc Surg 1:94, 1960.*)

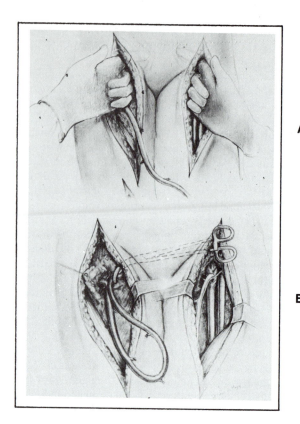

Figure 73-2. A. Construction of suprapubic tunnel by digital dissection. **B.** Note the clamp, which is passed through tunnel from left to right for directing the saphenous graft toward the recipient side. (*From Palma EC, Eperson R: J Cardiovasc Surg 1:94, 1960.*)

Recipient Side. After the donor side has been prepared, the junction of the femoral vein with the saphenous vein in the recipient area is exposed, including the proximal tributaries, namely, the superficial epigastric, the superficial circumflex iliac, and the external pudendal.

Subcutaneous Suprapubic Tunnel. At this point, a deep subcutaneous tunnel is made in the suprapubic region, either by digital dissection if the area is not too long or by using a tunneler (Fig. 73-2).

Passage of Graft Through Tunnel. The saphenous vein is then passed through the suprapubic tunnel to the involved side, with great care being taken to avoid twisting the vessel. The graft is then pulled gently through the tunnel to avoid any kinking.

Once the graft is in the recipient area, a gradual curve is imparted to the graft in the Scarpa triangle of the recipient side. This is necessary to ensure stability by stitching the adventitia to the femoral fascia on the recipient side.

Saphenofemoral Anastomosis. The anastomosis of the free end of the donor saphenous vein to the femoral vein of the postphlebitic side is then carried out. The usual site of the anastomosis is the common femoral vein, but occasionally the superficial femoral or deep femoral vein may be used when the common femoral is unavailable for one

reason or another. An end-to-side technique is used as a method of anastomosis (Fig. 73-3).

Whether an arteriovenous fistula, distal to the anastomosis of the saphenous into the femoral, is also created at the same time will depend on the evaluation of the hemodynamics at the completion of the anastomosis of the saphenous into the femoral vein. This point will be discussed below, because it may be debatable under certain circumstances.

Case Report: Technical Aspects and Follow-up

A 17-year-old patient was referred in July 1977 because of a postphlebitic syndrome of the left lower extremity. A brief medical history before the referral indicated that in July 1972 he underwent a hydrocele operation, after which a deep thrombophlebitis developed in the left lower extremity. Within 3 years, varicose veins developed in the leg and in the suprapubic region, and some of them became thrombosed. On the patient's admission to the hospital, the left lower extremity was considerably larger than the right, as disclosed by measurements of the girth of both lower extremities at various levels. The history was consistent with the findings of deep iliofemoral thrombophlebitis with collateral circulation in the abdominal wall.

The phlebogram disclosed extensive thrombosis involving the left iliac vein with partial recanalization of the left external iliac and common femoral veins. The left superficial vein was partially recanalized, as was the popliteal. The left greater saphenous vein was patent and remarkably enlarged. On the phlebogram, one thrombus was seen in the mid-thigh region. The right iliac vein and the inferior vena cava were normal.

Surgery was performed a few days after the patient's admission to the hospital. The procedure consisted of a contralateral saphenous vein crossover. It is of interest to mention the findings regarding the blood vessels: Numerous veins were encountered by blunt and sharp dissection in the left groin. These veins indicated the presence of collateral vessels of the saphenous vein. The latter was exposed and was traced to its junction with the common femoral vein. All venous tributaries were demonstrated by anatomic dissection. The left saphenous vein was markedly dilated as had been seen on the phlebogram. Likewise, all tributaries were markedly enlarged. In addition to these findings, the left common femoral vein was also markedly dilated with a thrombosed cord along the posterior wall, although the lumen of the common femoral vein was deemed to be patent. This was demonstrated by a longitudinal incision in the anterior wall of the vein, which showed partial patency.

The right saphenous vein was then exposed and harvested in the fashion described above, and then a subcutaneous tunnel was made in the suprapubic area. The saphenous vein from the right side was delivered through the tunnel by maintaining proper orientation for passing it to the left groin. A few adventitial sutures of No. 4-0 silk were tacked between the graft and the pectineus fascia in such a fashion as to prevent angulation or kinking. Longitudinal venotomy was made in the left common femoral and left greater saphenous vein adjacent to its junction. Then the distal end of the donor spahenous vein was appropriately tailored and anastomosed to the left vein venotomy by means of a running suture

of 4-0 Tevdek suture material lubricated with petrolatum. The patient did well postoperatively and was discharged within 2 weeks after surgery.

After surgery and during the postoperative period, serial radioisotope phlebograms showed patency of the crossover graft (Figs. 73-4 and 73-5). They also showed occlusion of the left iliac vessels and patency of the right side up to and including the inferior vena cava. Repeat phlebograms were obtained over a period of several years. When the patient was seen recently, 10 years postoperatively, his left lower extremity was free of varicose veins. Similarly, no varicosities were found in the abdominal wall. Noninvasive tests revealed patency of the crossover graft. This 10-year postoperative follow-up was therefore documented by clinical evaluation and noninvasive imaging.

Contralateral Saphenopopliteal Bypass

In cases of chronic venous occlusion involving not only the iliac but also the common and the superficial femoral veins, a contralateral saphenous vein graft can be extended into the popliteal vein, provided that the latter is adequate. The donor saphenous vein segment must, of course, be longer than that used in the femoral crossover. It is important that the exact length be assessed by measuring the vein before it is harvested along the length of the thigh downward to the popliteal vein on both the recipient side and the donor side. Occasionally, one may have to harvest

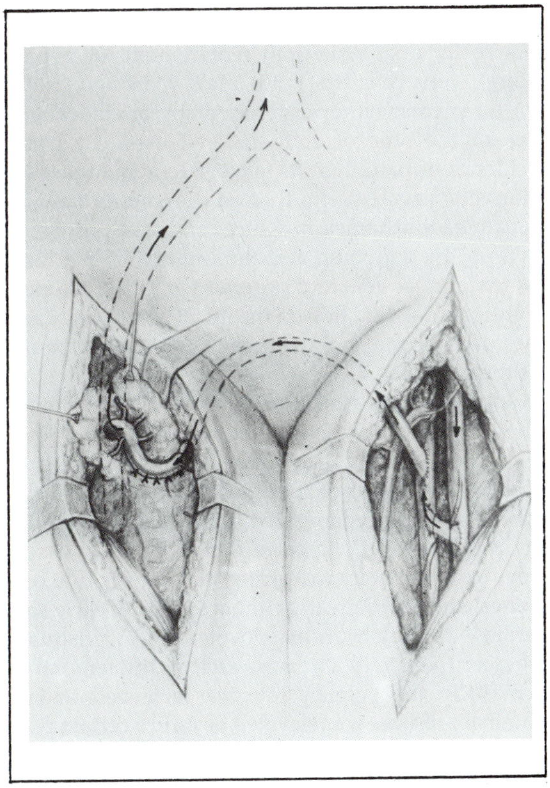

Figure 73-3. Complete position of saphenous graft in its course from right to left and its anastomosis to a branch of left femoral vein. Note arrows indicating direction of blood flow toward donor side. (*From Palma EC, Eperson R: J Cardiovasc Surg 1:94, 1960.*)

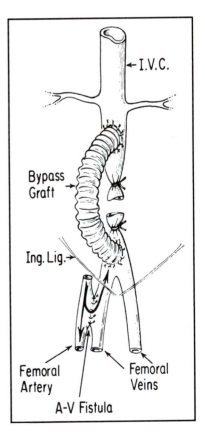

Figure 73-4. Location of constructed arteriovenous fistula, the site of bypass graft, from common femoral vein to inferior vena cava. Latter was divided to simulate occlusion. (*From Steinman C, Alpert J, and Haimovici H: Arch Surg 93:747, 1966.*)

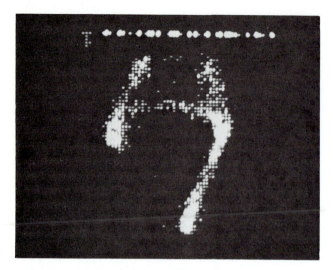

Figure 73-5. Radioisotope phlebogram with technetium (^{99m}Tc) depicting crossover graft connecting left femoral vein with right side and showing flow into right iliac toward inferior vena cava (see case report section in this chapter).

a small segment of vein from another area such as the upper extremity if the length of the segment of the donor side is not sufficient.

Palma[15] suggested for such a case that the vein graft be placed into the subsartorial canal and be opened widely to avoid any possible pressure on the graft or hindrance to the flow in the graft to the popliteal vein. The tendon of the adductor magnus should be divided so as to open the adductor hiatus, thus freeing the vessels. The sartorius muscle may also be divided transversely, its bed serving as a passage through which the saphenous vein is passed until it reaches the popliteal segment to which it is to be anastomosed.

Femoropopliteal Bypass

An in situ saphenopopliteal graft can be used as a transplant on the ipsilateral side in a postphlebitic syndrome affecting the superficial femoral and proximal popliteal veins. In this instance, the bypass would start from the intact common femorosaphenous vein; the sole anastomosis is carried out distally into the popliteal vein. For this purpose, according to Palma,[15] the graft should be placed through the adductor canal after the canal has been divided transversely and opened. The saphenous vein is then anastomosed either to the popliteal vein or to the posterior tibial vein according to the extent of the lesions (Palma[15]). Warren and Thayer,[8] as mentioned earlier, attempted a similar technique in 1954.

Free Saphenous Vein Grafts

The free saphenous vein graft can be used on the ipsilateral side if the external iliac and common femoral veins are occluded, but the common iliac vein must be patent and the ipsilateral saphenous vein normal.

An extraperitoneal approach is used for exposure of the iliac veins. The proximal end of the free graft is anastomosed to the ipsilateral common iliac vein, and the distal anastomosis is carried out in one of the patent veins in the upper part of the thigh or more distally as the case may be (superficial femoral or popliteal).[15]

SYNTHETIC GRAFTS

Expanded polytetrafluoroethylene (PTFE) appears to be the most suitable synthetic alternative to autogenous veins, not only for an arterial graft, but as a venous replacement as well. Historically, as a matter of fact, PTFE was first used experimentally as a venous substitute by Soyer et al.[16] in 1972, and later as an arterial bypass by Matsumoto et al.[17] in 1973. PTFE offers characteristics of strength, durability, proper porosity, and healing properties suitable for venous replacements. Its use is especially indicated when external stenting is part of the graft. This adds to the resistance against the weight caused by the overlying tissues, which tends to collapse the graft.

The use of recently available external stenting eliminates potential compression of the prosthesis. For example, the Gore-Tex vascular graft has rings that encircle the standard PTFE graft. In addition, the thin-walled grafts whose handling and performance surgeons have known for many years are still being used in a large number of implants.[18,19]

Grafts in the Inferior Vena Cava: Role of Temporary Arteriovenous Fistula

The search for a suitable graft replacement for bypassing the inferior vena cava has, until a few years ago, met with little or no success either experimentally or clinically, irrespective of the type of graft material used. By contrast, the incidence of patent grafts is considerably higher in the superior vena caval system than in the inferior vena cava. The negative intrathoracic pressure versus the positive pressure within the abdomen and the isogravitational venous flow in the jugular vein and superior vena cava as opposed to the antigravitational flow in the inferior vena cava appear to play a decisive role in the different outcomes of implantation at the two sites.

In addition to the reasons cited above, internal pressure and the rate of blood flow exert an important influence on the patency of venous grafts, including that of the inferior vena cava. A number of experimental studies have shown that if venous hemodynamics are altered, that is, if a higher venous pressure and a greater intraluminal flow system are provided, the patency of grafts, particularly that of synthetic ones, should be greatly enhanced. In the early studies by Kunlin[20] in which an arteriovenous (AV) fistula was created near the site of a venous graft in the femoral vein, an increase in the patency rate was achieved when the intraluminal pressure was elevated beyond a certain point.[21]

In 1964, my associates and I undertook an experimental study with the objective of evaluating the effect of a temporary fistula on long-term patency of various graft materials in the venous system.[21] For the implantation a bypass procedure was used in the inferior vena cava. In 22 dog experiments, a side-to-side femoral AV fistula was created. The

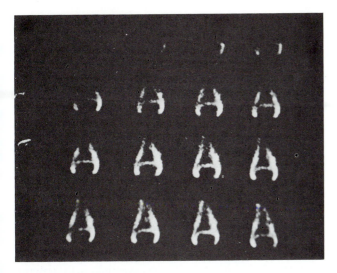

Figure 73-6. Serial phlebogram using same technique as in Figure 73-5 three years after surgery.

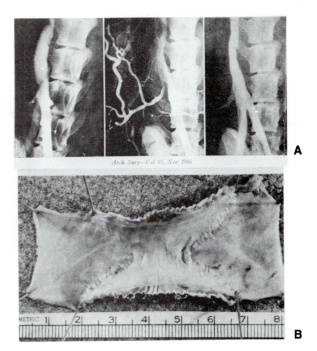

Figure 73-8. A. Dacron graft and adjacent host inferior vena cava after 169 days of implantation. Note smooth neointima of graft and its continuity with intima of inferior vena cava. **B.** Phlebogram of inferior vena cava, showing Dacron bypass graft: (left) immediately after implantation, (center) its appearance 8 days later with partial occlusion of graft and collateral circulation, and (right) its complete patency 3 weeks after discontinuance of arteriovenous fistula.

infrarenal segment of the inferior vena cava was bypassed as indicated in Figure 73-4. The materials used for the bypasses were Teflon, Dacron, and autogenous vein grafts. These bypass proceudres resulted in an overall patency rate ranging from 83% to 100% (Figs. 73-7 to 73-9). In a similar series of experiments *without* AV shunts carried out in my laboratory, the fate of such grafts was only moderately

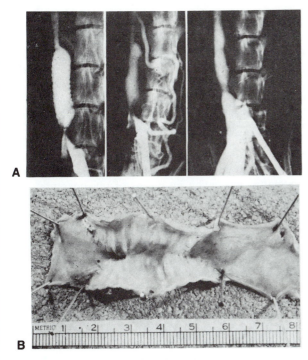

Figure 73-7. A. Teflon graft and adjacent host inferior vena cava after 163 days of implantation. Note smooth, thin, neointima of graft. **B.** Phlebogram of inferior vena cava showing Teflon bypass graft: (left) immediately after implantation, (center) its appearance 4 days later with partial occlusion of distal anastomosis with pressure of collateral circulation, and (right) 3 months later with complete patency and disappearance of collateral circulation.

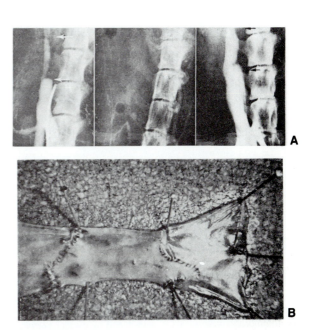

Figure 73-9. A. Autogenous jugular vein bypass graft and adjacent host inferior vena cava. **B.** Phlebogram of inferior vena cava, showing vein bypass graft: (left) immediately after implantation, (center) its complete occlusion 13 days later, and (right) its complete recanalization 2 months postoperatively. Note increased diameter of lumen of latter, in comparison with its original size.

improved by the use of anticoagulants; the patency rate was only 36.3% during a 4-month period of observation. This was true even when autogenous vein grafts were used.

The creation of an AV fistula results not only in pressure but primarily in flow increase. Shenk et al.[22] showed that in an acute AV fistula the proximal venous flow is enormously increased, although the pressure may become only slightly positive. Similarly, Stansel,[23] in his study on inferior vena cava replacement with synthetic grafts, showed only a moderate increase in pressure in spite of the distal AV fistula. Protection against thrombosis of a graft with a temporary AV fistula is primarily due to increased blood flow as the most important hemodynamic factor.

Although the effect of AV shunting on the patency of these grafts appears undeniable, an important question is whether the time necessary to achieve the desired protective effect of such a fistula can be determined. From the available evidence, both that reported in the literature and our personal observations, it appears that the first postoperative week is a crucial period during which thrombosis of the graft may occur. If, during this time, a neointima of fibrin is formed, the hazards of thrombosis may be avoided, all other factors being equal. The shortest duration of an AV fistula in our series was 22 days. Its discontinuation did not result in closure of the graft. Thus an evaluation of the critical period for an AV fistula is of practical significance.

The size of the graft is another important factor in determining the rate of patency.[24] Isodiametric synthetic grafts, because of the variable degrees of thickness or ulcer-

ation of the neointima, result in either marked narrowing or complete occlusion by thrombosis.

One of the important findings of studies in which either a synthetic graft or an autogenous vein graft was used with the temporary AV fistula is that, after a week or two, a perigraft fibrosis occurs that imparts to the conduit a certain degree of rigidity, which by itself maintains the patency of the lumen. This result can now be achieved by the use of a PTFE graft with external stenting, which provides resistance against the weight of the overlying tissues, thereby preventing collapse of the graft. The rings that encircle the standard PTFE graft provide an equivalent of perigraft fibrosis, which maintains the patency of the lumen. Because of the availability of the PTFE graft, the use of an AV fistula is questioned today in most cases. However, in some instances the use of an AV shunt might be necessary if the lumen is relatively narrow and greater flow is needed to maintain patency, especially in the absence of external stenting of the PTFE graft.[18]

Bypass of the inferior vena cava is indicated not only for vascular problems of the venous system or of the periphery but also for tumors, injuries, and congenital caval defects and when external pressure from other conditions impedes the flow of the venous blood though the inferior vena cava and leads to venous insufficiency of the lower extremities. Creating a bypass of this vessel has become much simpler than in the past, both as a result of the hemodynamic studies of AV fistula and because of the availability of PTFE grafts with stents.

Results: An Appraisal

The postoperative assessment of surgical results must be based on objective determination of symptoms and signs. Postoperative phlebography and noninvasive venous assessment are of great significance, however, in evaluating, as objectively as possible, the results obtained by the surgical procedure.

Husni et al.[25] have emphasized, on the basis of their experience, that in venous reconstructive procedures there is a great need for proper selection of patients and for postoperative evaluation by means of phlebography and ambulatory venous pressure studies.[25] Of a total of 119 cases of venous reconstruction for postphlebitic disease during a period of 15 years, 83 crossover procedures were carried out. The results without AV fistulas (71 cases) yielded a 72% success rate, whereas with AV fistulas (12 cases) 78% were successful.

Halliday et al.,[12] in a study of 42 of 47 patients available for review of long-term results of venous crossover graft procedures (the longest follow-up period being 18 years), found that the accumulated patency rates based on clinical assessment differed from those based on objective demonstration of patency by phlebography (Fig. 73-10). A total of 50 cases were evaluated clinically and 34 by phlebography. There seems to be an important difference between the two types of evaluation. At 5 years, 89% of the grafts were clinically determined to be patent, in comparison with 75% on the basis of phlebography. Ambulatory venous

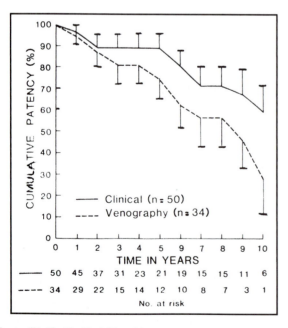

Figure 73-10. Modified life table showing cumulative patency of femorofemoral crossover grafts determined by clinical examination and by venography. Standard errors are shown on the curve. (*From Halliday P, Harris J, May J: Femoro-Femoral Crossover Grafts [Palma Operation]: A Long-Term Follow-Up Study, in Bergan JJ, Yao JST (eds): Surgery of the Veins. New York, Grune & Stratton, 1985.*)

pressure measurements may complement preoperative phlebography in the selection of patients suitable for this operation, but phlebography remains the best method for objectively proving graft patency. Halliday and his associates concluded that "femorofemoral bypass grafting should be considered early in the management of a patient with chronic unilateral postthrombotic iliac vein thrombosis, preferably before irreversible damage has occurred in the calf."

More recently, O'Donnell et al.,[14] in the face of uncertainty regarding conventional therapy results, concurred with those who believe that direct venous reconstruction may be superior in the long run. They based their observations and conclusions on clinical, hemodynamic, and anatomic follow-up of six patients with saphenous vein crossover bypass* (Palma procedure) and ten patients with axillary vein valve to popliteal vein transplants (PVTs). Late (>2 years) anatomic and functional assessment showed that in both groups—those with femoral bypass and those with PVTs—the veins were patent (the use of B-mode imaging of the deep veins has been of great diagnostic help postoperatively). O'Donnell et al. concluded that, although longer follow-up may be required, the methods used and the results achieved were a definite improvement over the conservative approach to management in cases of chronic venous insufficiency.

Valvuloplasty

In recent years, in addition to the procedures described above, valvuloplasty and normal vein interposition for chronic venous insufficiency have been introduced. These methods are not yet widely accepted.

Valvular incompetency after deep vein thrombosis is usually a consequence of recanalization of the veins. In such a process, the affected valves undergo morphologic damage, which leads to their insufficiency.

In the past decade, several investigators have reported encouraging results in their attempts to correct chronic venous insufficiency. Two methods have been used: (1) replacement of damaged valves and (2) interposition of a relatively short segment of vein as a graft containing normal valves.[26,27]

Surgical correction of incompetent valves has been reported by several investigators. Kistner's data, published originally in 1982 (as reported in 1985 in *Surgery of the Veins*[26]), was based on 46 cases in which good clinical results were achieved in 80%. Of 46 patients, 41 had postoperative descending phlebography. Kistner's concept is based on consideration of surgical replacement of incompetent valves as an adjunctive measure in highly selected cases only.

Taheri et al.[27] as of their 1985 report had provided vein valve transplant or valvuloplasty for 67 limbs (62 patients). Of the 48 follow-up patients, 43 had vein valve transplants, and improvement or complete relief was achieved in 32 (75%). The remaining five patients had valvuloplasty, and none improved.

Conclusions

The results reported above may appear encouraging, but controversy remains. Further experience is obviously necessary before indications for surgery, the long-term evolution of venous insufficiency, and the validity of the conceptual approach to the treatment of this ubiquitous problem can be defined. Thus the introductory remarks about the technical limitations of venous reconstructive procedures are apparently still valid in spite of the significant progress achieved in recent years. In comparison with the technologic gains made in arterial reconstruction, venous surgery has failed to reach the same level. The reasons for the difference between the two types of surgery have been amply explained in this chapter. There remains a great need for improvement, not only in diagnostic methods, but also in the proper selection of patients and the use of appropriate surgical techniques, because all of these elements influence the results of venous reconstructive treatment.

REFERENCES

1. Haimovici H, Hoffert PW, et al.: An experimental and clinical evaluation of grafts in the venous system. Surg Gynecol Obstet 131:1173, 1970.
2. Child CG: Eck's fistula. Surg Gynecol Obstet 96:375, 1953.
3. Clermont G: Suture laterale et circulaire des veines. Presse Med 1:229, 1901.
4. Payr E: Beitrage zur Technik der Blutgefasse und Nervennaht. Arch Klin Chir 62:67, 1904.
5. Carrel A: La technique operatoire des anastomoses vasculaires et la transplantation des visceres. Lyon Med 98:859, 1902.
6. Carrel A, Guthrie CC: Uniterminal and biterminal venous transplantation. Surg Gynecol Obstet 2:266, 1906.
7. Kunlin J, Kunlin A, et al.: Le retablissement de la circulation veineuse par greffe en cas d'obliteration traumatique ou thrombophlebitique. Mem Acad Chir 79:109, 1953.
8. Warren R, Thayer TB: Transplantation of the saphenous vein for postphlebitic stasis. Surgery 35:867, 1954.
9. Palma EC, Eperson R: Vein transplants and graft in the surgical treatment of postphlebitic syndrome. J Cardiovasc Surg 1:94, 1960.
10. Dale WA: Chronic iliofemoral venous occlusion including 7 cases of cross-over vein grafting. Surgery 59:117, 1966.
11. Raju S: Venous insufficiency of the lower limb and stasis ulceration: Changing concepts and management. Ann Surg 197:688, 1983.
12. Halliday P, Harris J, May J: Femoro-femoral crossover grafts (Palma operation): A long-term follow-up study, in Bergan JJ, Yao JST (eds): Surgery of the Veins. New York, Grune & Stratton, 1985, p 241.
13. Langsfeld M, Hershey FB, et al.: Duplex B-mode imaging for the diagnosis of deep venous thrombosis. Arch Surg 122:587, 1987.
14. O'Donnell TF, Mackey WC, et al.: Clinical, hemodynamic, and anatomic follow-up of direct venous reconstruction. Arch Surg 122:474, 1987.
15. Palma EC: Vein grafts for treatment of postphlebitic syndrome, in Haimovici H (ed): Vascular Surgery: Principles and Techniques, 2nd ed. Norwalk, Conn., Appleton-Century-Crofts, 1984, p 1049.
16. Soyer T, Lempinen M, et al.: A new venous prosthesis. Surgery 72:864, 1972.

---

* A procedure that O'Donnell calls saphenofemoral bypass.

17. Matsumoto H, Hasegawa T, et al.: A new vascular prosthesis for a small caliber artery. Surgery 74:519, 1973.

18. Vollmar J: Reconstruction of the iliac veins and inferior vena cava, in Hobbs JT (ed): The Treatment of Venous Disorders. Lancaster, Pa, MTP Press, 1977, p 320.

19. Dean RE, Read RC: Influence of increased blood flow on thrombosis in prosthetic grafts. Surgery 55:581, 1964.

20. Kunlin J: Les Greffes Veineuses. In 15 Congres de la Societe Internationale de Chirurgie, Lisbonne, 1953, p 875.

21. Steinman C, Alpert J, Haimovici H: Inferior vena cava bypass grafts: An experimental evaluation of a temporary arteriovenous fistula on their long-term patency. Arch Surg 93:747, 1966.

22. Schenk WG, et al.: Regional hemodynamics of chronic experimental arteriovenous fistulas. Surg Gynecol Obstet 110:44, 1960.

23. Stansel HC Jr: Synthetic inferior vena cava grafts. Arch Surg 89:1096, 1964.

24. Haimovici H, Zinicola H, et al.: Vein grafts in the venous system: An experimental evaluation of autogenous veins used as bypass implants. Arch Surg 87:542, 1963.

25. Husni EA: Reconstruction of veins: The need for objectivity. J Cardiovasc Surg 24:525, 1983.

26. Kistner RL: Venous valve surgery, in Bergan JJ, Yao JST (eds): Surgery of the Veins. New York, Grune & Stratton, 1985, p 205.

27. Taheri SA, Heffner R, et al.: Technique and results of venous valve transplantation, in Bergan JJ, Yao JST (eds): The Veins. New York, Grune & Stratton, 1985, p 219.

CHAPTER 74
Fasciotomy

Calvin B. Ernst, Bruce H. Brennaman, and Henry Haimovici

Fasciotomy is designed to decompress the neurovascular elements and the skeletal muscles encased in a rigid osteofascial compartment to prevent neuromuscular ischemia and necrosis. A variety of pathologic conditions may lead to vascular compromise of skeletal muscles and to ischemic impairment of neural function in such a closed system. The most common entities that may require decompressive fasciotomy are the revascularization procedures, especially those for severe acute ischemia and for severe traumatic lesions of the extremities of both an orthopedic and vascular nature.

Following the description by Volkmann[1] in 1881 of the traumatic ischemic contracture, a number of investigators reported similar clinical and pathologic findings resulting from acute arterial occlusions.[2,3] These reports dealt primarily with the morphologic effects of ischemic muscle damage, swelling of the muscle fibers leading sometimes to fibrosis, and resulting contracture.[3,4]

The pathogenic mechanism of Volkmann's contracture remained unclear, although Volkmann believed that it was due to skeletal muscle anoxemia. The first investigative work that brought this problem into proper focus was published by Jepson in 1926.[5] He demonstrated experimentally in dogs that considerable edema in the muscles can result from constriction of an extremity. Jepson found that drainage of edema from the intermuscular spaces relieved the muscle swelling and restored the extremity to a normal state. His experimental data suggested that intrinsic pressure was responsible for the ischemic condition, and he concluded that drainage of edema was essential for preventing the necrotic changes and contracture.

Jepson's contribution provided both the pathogenic mechanism, that is, the increased pressure of the compartment, and its management. However, this contribution was slow to gain recognition and make the necessary clinical impact. One of the earliest clinical applications of fasciotomy was reported by Dennis[6] in 1945 for acute massive deep venous thrombosis. In the same year, Horn[7] described the syndrome of acute ischemia of the anterior tibial compartment. Subsequently, fasciotomy was performed for arterial injuries in civilian and military practice, as well as for other vascular entities.[8,9] Recent investigations of the role of compartmental pressure and the need for a more comprehensive decompression of more than one compartment have provided better understanding of the pathogenesis of the compartmental syndrome and its treatment.[10,11]

CLINICAL AND PATHOLOGIC DATA

The main vascular and allied disorders for which fasciotomy is indicated are acute occlusive arterial diseases, massive venous thrombosis, functional anterior tibial syndrome, limb fractures, crush injuries, and replantation of limbs. With the use of more sophisticated and more readily available street weapons among the civilian population, the incidence of compartment compression syndromes secondary to severe soft-tissue injury without significant vascular damage appears to be increasing.

Arterial diseases that may require fasciotomy include all forms of acute occlusion likely to induce muscle edema and hematoma such as embolism, acute thrombosis, arterial reconstruction, and arterial injuries.[12] Venous diseases include phlegmasia cerulea dolens, venous gangrene,[13] acute injuries of major limb veins, and combined arterial and venous injuries. Crush injuries,[14] limb fractures, circumferential burns, and replantation of limbs are other conditions that frequently lead to muscle ischemia and edema. Another group of patients who must be closely observed for onset of compartment syndromes are those suffering from drug-induced coma or stupor and subsequent positional compression of an extremity.

Pathogenic Mechanism

Irrespective of the vascular lesion, compromise of blood supply is one of the main factors that may initiate a chain of hemodynamic events resulting in edematous muscle tamponade of the nutrient (capillary) bed. First there is a rise

995

in pressure in the compartment due to the increased muscle bulk resulting from edema. Then there is fluid retention and associated small hemorrhages, which in turn interfere further with the vascular supply, and a viscous positive-feedback cycle develops. If unrelieved by fasciotomy, the changes occurring in the compartment will lead to compression myopathy with ensuing necrosis. Occlusion of the arteries and veins or their injury does not fully explain the pathogenic mechanism of compartment syndrome, however, since it may occur in the absence of vascular injury or occlusion. Therefore other factor(s) must influence the development of the compartment syndrome.

Regardless of the injury or ischemic insult, the response of the muscles and their supporting vascular beds in any affected compartment is to develop edema, which is thought to be the result of an increase in capillary permeability in the nutrient bed of the muscle. The end results are an increase in muscle bulk within the restricted confines of the fascial compartment and a rise in compartmental pressure. With increased pressure, there is a relative decrease in nutrient-bed capillary perfusion and resulting ischemia. An increase in capillary permeability and a further increase in muscle bulk and intercompartmental pressure follow.

The pressure at which nutrient blood flow ceases approximates the critical closing pressure of the capillary bed and has been estimated to be about 35 to 40 mm Hg. At compartment pressures above the critical closing pressure, perfusion of muscle essentially ceases, leading to the above-mentioned chain of ischemic events. Decompressive fasciotomy breaks this self-perpetuating ischemic cycle and allows reperfusion of muscle by venting it.

At the cellular level, the changes occurring at the onset of the self-perpetuating compartment compression cycle may be related to ischemia-reperfusion phenomena. The exact mechanisms responsible for the increase in capillary permeability are unknown. However, certain biochemical processes have been identified that can partially account for the increase. The increase in capillary permeability seen in an ischemia-reperfusion model in dogs was closely associated with the generation of oxygen-derived free radicals $(0_2^-, OH\cdot)$.[15] Using both direct and indirect measurements of capillary permeability and capillary pressure, Korthuis[15] found that capillary permeability was significantly increased in the presence of oxygen-derived free radical scavengers. A pathway by which generation of free radicals may arise in the ischemia-reperfusion phenomenon was developed (Fig. 74-1).[15] Resistance or vulnerability to ischemia appears to be related to tissue content of xanthine dehydrogenase and speed of conversion of this enzyme to xanthine oxidase, the source of the superoxide radical. Superoxide species are toxic to the intercellular matrix and cell membranes. Thus, it appears that the use of oxygen-derived free radical scavengers such as allopurinol, mannitol, catalase, dimethylsulfoxide, and superoxide dismutase to suppress or eliminate cytotoxic oxygen metabolites would be potentially useful in the treatment of compartment syndrome.

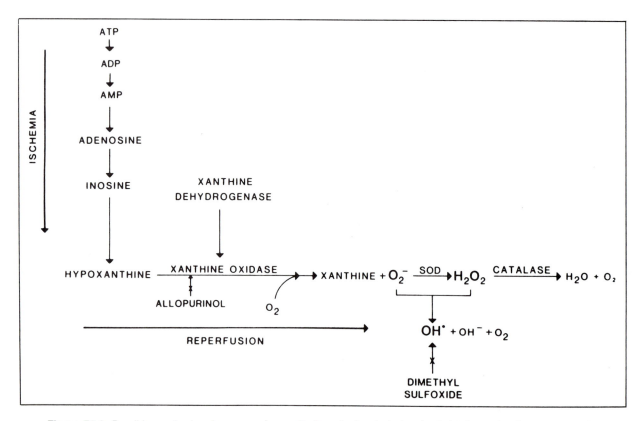

Figure 74-1. Possible mechanism for oxygen-free radical production in ischemic skeletal muscle. O_2 represents the superoxide anion; H_2O_2 respresents hydrogen peroxide; and OH^- represents the hydroxyl radical. (*From Korthuis RJ, Granger DN, et al.: Circ Res 57(4):599, 1985.*)

Further evidence for the presence of oxygen-derived free radicals in ischemia-reperfusion injury has been provided by Lee et al.[16] During episodes of ischemia, skeletal muscle sarcoplasmic reticulum has a depressed ability to transport intracellular calcium. Using this model in ischemic rat hindlimbs and later in reperfused limbs, Lee demonstrated that pretreatment with superoxide dismutase and catalase significantly increased calcium uptake by skeletal muscle sarcoplasmic reticulum when compared to untreated ischemic-reperfused controls. However, treatment with free radical scavengers did not return calcium uptake to a level consistent with nonischemic hindlimbs, suggesting that other mechanisms may be at play in the development of compartment syndrome.

Heppenstall et al.[17] investigated the biochemical and histologic changes that occurred in two models of skeletal muscle ischemia in dogs. They studied a tourniquet-induced ischemia-reperfusion model and a compartment syndrome model of ischemia-reperfusion. At the biochemical level, the compartment syndrome group demonstrated decreases in high-energy phosphate supply, with a significant delay in resynthesis of these high-energy phosphates. Also, intracellular pH measurements were significantly more acidotic in animals with compartment syndrome, and with slower return toward normal levels upon reperfusion. Ultrastructural damage to skeletal muscle cells was also noted to be more intense in the animals made ischemic by induction of compartment syndrome.

In summary, it would appear that the initiating events in the development of compartment syndrome revolve around an ischemia-reperfusion phenomenon and may be partially induced by the development of oxygen-derived free radicals. With the onset of intracompartment pressure elevation, a synergistic relationship may develop, resulting in more severe myopathy than seen with ischemia-reperfusion alone.

Clinically, it appears that oxygen-derived free radical scavengers may reduce the amount of muscle damage induced by the compartment syndrome. Compounds such as mannitol, allopurinol, catalase, dimethylsulfoxide, and superoxide dismutase have been used with success to reduce the damage caused by ischemia in the heart, intestine, pancreas, kidney, and brain.[18–20] Walker and associates[21,22] used contolled oxygen delivery alone and in combination with mannitol, superoxide dismutase, and catalase in a dog model of ischemia-reperfusion. Both methods were successful in significantly reducing the degree of muscle necrosis when compared with untreated ischemic controls. Although these studies are encouraging, further investigation will be required before the treatment of compartment syndrome will routinely include the use of free radical scavengers.

INDICATIONS

Early fasciotomy is essential to prevent irreversible changes. The compression myopathy of the forearm and the leg compartments displays varying degrees of impending ischemia. The course of this compartment syndrome may be divided into three stages:

Stage I: Pain, swelling, and paresthesias
Stage II: Neurologic deficit, absent pulses, and early focal necrosis of the muscles
Stage III: Advanced necrosis of the muscles and the overlying skin.

Clinical criteria for indications for fasciotomy, although well established, are still controversial because of their lack of reliability. Classically, there are six clinical findings that have been recognized in the diagnosis of compartment syndrome:

1. Pain in the affected extremity that generally is out of proportion to the injury or condition of the extremity
2. Pain induced by passive stretch of the muscles in the affected compartment
3. Paralysis or paresis of the muscles in the affected compartment
4. Hypesthesia or paresthesia in the cutaneous distribution of the nerves that traverse the affected compartment
5. Induration or inflammation or both of the affected compartment
6. Diminished or absent distal pulses

That clinical manifestations are sometimes inadequate to make the diagnosis of compartment compression is documented by the frequent finding of severe irreversible myonecrosis even when fasciotomy is performed soon after the onset of symptoms. This finding suggests that the clinical manifestations of the syndrome become manifest late in the course of the disease and emphasizes the need for early recognition and aggressive management.

The use of compartment pressure measurements has been suggested as a more reliable indicator of the need for decompressive fasciotomy.[11,23,24] Initial efforts in this area left much to be desired because of technical difficulties in obtaining accurate tissue pressure measurements.[25] Recent studies and technology have improved the reproducibility and reliability of compartment pressure measurement as a clinical indicator of the need for fasciotomy.[26–29] The use of compartment pressures is based on the concept of critical closing pressure. In the skeletal muscle bed, the critical closing pressure has been experimentally estimated in man to be about 40 mm Hg.[30,31] Based on this estimate, a net perfusion pressure of less than 40 mm Hg would result in near-total cessation of capillary bed perfusion in the affected compartment. Therefore tissue pressure measurements greater than 40 mm Hg strongly suggest need for fasciotomy. Other investigators have used a compartment pressure within 30 mm Hg of the patient's diastolic blood pressure as an indication for fasciotomy.[24,26] Still other investigators have used absolute compartmental pressure measurements ranging from 30 mm Hg to 45 mm Hg as an indicator to perform decompressive fasciotomy.[27,28] Lack of uniformity and the individual variations between patients have hampered the use of compartment pressures as a uniformly reliable indicator for fasciotomy.

Many different techniques for the measurement of compartment pressure have been described.[26–28,32] Different catheters have been developed for the continuous measurement of compartment pressures. Use of these catheters requires experience, and sophisticated measuring methods

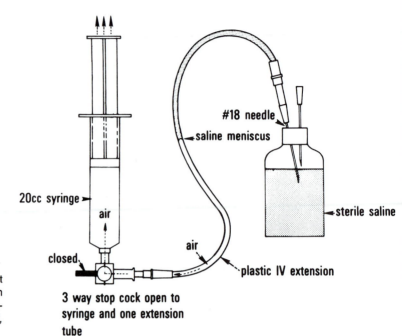

Figure 74-2. To measure compartment pressures, apparatus is assembled as shown to aspirate column of sterile saline in extension tubing. (*From Whitesides TE, Haney TC, et al.: Arch Surg 110:1311, 1975.*)

complicate evaluation. Whitesides et al.[32] reported a simplified technique for measurement of compartment pressures that can be performed with readily available equipment. The assembled system is shown in Figure 74-2. The 20 cc syringe is assembled with its plunger withdrawn to the 15 cc mark. The three-way stopcock is turned off to the needle before its insertion into the compartment. After insertion of the needle into the desired compartment, the system is modified as shown in Figure 74-3, and the stopcock is turned so as to open all three ports of the stopcock simulta-

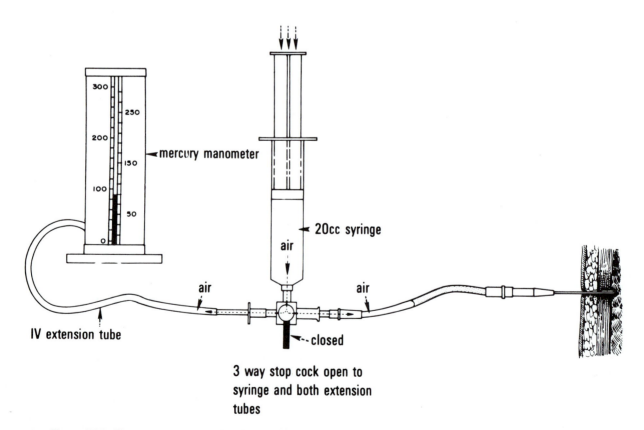

Figure 74-3. Tissue pressure is measured by determining the amount of air pressure within this closed system that is required to barely overcome the pressure within closed compartment and to inject very slowly a minute quantity of saline. (*From Whitesides TE, Haney TC, et al.: Arch Surg 110:1311, 1975.*)

neously. The syringe plunger is then *slowly* depressed, causing an observable rise in the mercury manometer. When the saline meniscus begins to move, the pressure is noted and recorded as the compartment pressure. This technique provides a simple method to assess compartment pressures in patients who do not show overt clinical signs of compartment syndrome.

The needle is inserted at about the junction of the upper one third and lower two thirds of the leg. The anterior compartment is entered at a point approximately one fingerbreadth lateral to the lateral border of the tibia. The lateral compartment is entered approximately three fingerbredths from the lateral border of the tibia. The deep posterior compartment is approached about one fingerbreadth posterior to the posterior border of the tibia on the medial surface of the leg, sliding the needle parallel to the patient's bed until it is just behind the tibia. The superficial posterior compartment pressure is measured as the needle is withdrawn from the deep posterior compartment. It is best to inject a small amount of saline (1 ml) when the catheter is placed to clear tissue from the end of the needle. Gentle pressure on the leg will give a small pressure wave if the catheter is clear and functioning well.

In summary, clinical diagnosis of compartment syndrome requires a high index of suspicion. Clinical signs and direct measurements of compartment pressure are not consistently diagnostic when used alone. Together, however, they are complimentary. The major complications of the compartment syndrome come from procrastination in performing fasciotomy, resulting in a ''too little and too late'' phenomenon.[10]

ANATOMY OF THE COMPARTMENTS

Any anatomic location in which muscles are enveloped in an osteofascial sheath has the potential to develop a compartment syndrome. The compartments of the leg and the forearm are of most interest to the vascular surgeon, with the former being most important. A brief anatomic description of only these compartments is given.

The forearm contains two clinically significant compartments: the volar and dorsal. The volar compartment includes the flexors of the wrist and fingers and has the radial and ulnar vasculature traversing the compartment. Its boundaries are the radius laterally and the ulna medially, with the intervening interosseous membrane as its deep border and the deep fascia of the forearm more superficially. The ulnar and median nerves traverse the compartment and provide innervation to its muscles, the intrinsic muscles of the hand, and the skin over the palmar surface of the hand.

The dorsal compartment contains the extensors of the wrist and fingers, with blood supply through the posterior interosseous artery and the muscular branches of the radial artery. The radial nerve traverses the compartment and innervates the skin of the dorsum of the hand and the muscles of the compartment. It is bounded by the radius, ulna, and interosseous membrane, as well as its own deep fascia.

The leg contains four osteofascial compartments: ante-

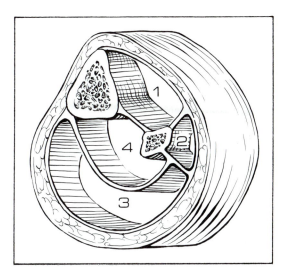

Figure 74-4. Cross section of the four compartments of the leg: *1*, anterior tibial; *2*, lateral peroneal; *3*, superficial posterior; and *4*, deep posterior.

rior tibial, lateral peroneal, superficial posterior, and deep posterior (Fig. 74-4).

The anterior tibial compartment includes the tibialis anterior, the extensor digitorum longus, the extensor hallicus longus, and the peroneus tertius muscles. Their functions are to evert and dorsiflex the foot and to extend the toes. The anterior tibial neurovascular bundle traverses the anterior compartment and lies on the interosseous membrane.

The lateral compartment contains the peroneus longus and peroneus brevis muscles. The lateral compartment also contains the deep peroneal nerve.

The superficial posterior compartment contains the gastrocnemius and soleus muscles. The deep posterior compartment contains the tibialis posterior, the flexor digitorum longus, and the flexor hallicus longus muscles. The posterior tibial and peroneal vessels and the posterior tibial nerve lie in the deep posterior compartment.

The enveloping fasciae of all these compartments, especially those of the anterior and lateral compartments, are quite rigid (Fig. 74-4). The most commonly affected compartment is the anterior tibial. The greater occurrence of the anterior tibial compartment syndrome can be explained by a combination of anatomic and physiologic factors. The arterial supply to the muscles of this compartment consists of end-type branches with very little collateral circulation.

TECHNIQUE

The major requirement for relief of the compartment syndrome is adequate decompression of all involved compartments. A variety of methods are described below, all of which, when performed properly, will provide the needed decompression of an involved compartment. The choice of technique is dependent on the suspected severity of the compartment syndrome and the number of compartments requiring decompression.

Anesthesia

Fasciotomy of an isolated compartment compression can usually be carried out using local anesthesia. If several compartments are involved, which is the usual case, it is best to perform decompression using an epidural or spinal or even general anesthesia.

Short Skin Incisions

This method of fasciotomy is suitable for an isolated compartment syndrome. Two short skin incisions are made at both ends of the compartment (Fig. 74-5) and are carried through the subcutaneous tissue down to and including the fascia. Straight scissors* are used for the incision of the fascia, and the procedure is performed subcutaneously between the two areas of exposure (Fig. 74-5A). As soon as the fascia is opened, the underlying muscle bulges through the incision. The muscle may appear as grayish or congested tissue and is sometimes pale, having a fish-flesh appearance. The fascia is left open, whereas the skin may be closed with a few interrupted stitches. Should there be a great amount of edema, the skin must be completely incised over the fascial incision by connecting the short skin incisions. Such a skin incision is left open and is closed secondarily 4 to 5 days later. In the event that difficulty is encountered in approximating the edges, a split-thickness skin graft is applied to the defect.

It must be emphasized that if adequacy of the decompression is questionable because of a limited fasciotomy, a more extensive skin incision is used without hesitation. Complete decompression of all involved compartments is necessary, especially in cases of unyielding phlegmasia cerula dolens and in posttraumatic compartment compression.

Long Skin Incision

Lower Extremity
The anterolateral compartment of the leg is entered through an extensive skin incision (Fig. 74-5D and E). The fascia is incised from below the knee to above the ankle. The muscles encountered at that level, namely, the extensor digitorum and the peroneal muscles, are separated to the level of the entry of the deep peroneal nerve into the lateral compartment. In localized muscle necrosis of the antero-lateral compartment, wide excision of its contents may be indicated, to be followed by skin grafting (Figs. 74-6 and 74-7).

The superficial posterior compartment is entered by a long incision (see Fig. 74-5D) placed somewhat medially and going through the gastrocnemius down to and including the soleus. For the deep posterior compartment, the incision is carried beyond the soleus and enters the deep group, including the tibialis posterior, the flexor digitorum longus, and the flexor hallicus longus. At that level one finds the neurovascular bundles, the posterior tibial and the peroneal arteries with two satellite veins and the posterior tibial nerve. It may be necessary in some cases also to split the posterior tibialis muscle down to the interosseous membrane.

Combined extensive fasciotomy in the thigh may sometimes be required, especially in patients with phlegmasia cerula dolens.[13] Such incisions are made on both the medial and lateral aspects of the thigh in the same direction as those in the leg (see Fig. 74-5E).

Upper Extremity
The incisions in the forearm are made from the elbow through the wrist, incising the fascia overlying the volar and dorsal compartments. Such incisions allow exploration of the vessels and the nerves, together with evaluation of the degree of muscle ischemia. As in the lower extremity, extensive fasciotomies of the arm are sometimes indicated, especially in patients with severe trauma or massive edema associated with phlegmasia cerulea dolens. The incisions are carried out on both the medial and lateral aspects from the shoulder down to the elbow.

Parafibular Four-Compartment Decompression

For parafibular four-compartment decompression a long lateral skin incision is made directly over the fibula and runs its length from just below its neck to a point 3 to 4 cm above the lateral malleolus.[24,25,35] The anterior compartment is opened by retracting the anterior skin flap, and it is opened over its entire length. Care is taken to avoid injury to the common peroneal nerve at the neck of the fibula and the superficial peroneal nerve at the lower level (junction of the upper two thirds and the lower one third of the leg).

The lateral compartment is opened directly beneath the skin incision, which is deepened to incise fascia overlying the peroneal muscles. The edge of the skin flap overlying the posterior compartment is retracted, and it is opened over its entire length. The superficial posterior compartment, after the fibular origin of the soleus muscle is detached, is thus exposed. The gastrocnemius-soleus group is then retracted posteriorly to expose the deep posterior compartment, which is opened over its entire length. In the deep compartment, care should be taken to avoid injury to the posterior tibial and peroneal vessels and the posterior tibial nerve. The wound is left open and is covered with fine-mesh gauze and a dry bulky dressing. Seven to fourteen days later, the wound may be closed, or delayed closure may be carried out by using a split-thickness skin graft within 1 to 2 weeks.

Four-Compartment Fasciotomy with Fibulectomy

Four-compartment fasciotomy with fibulectomy was used during the Vietnam conflict for vascular injuries.[10] Since

---

*Specifically designed instruments with a curved cutting edge have been described by Mozes et al.[33] and Rosato et al.[34]

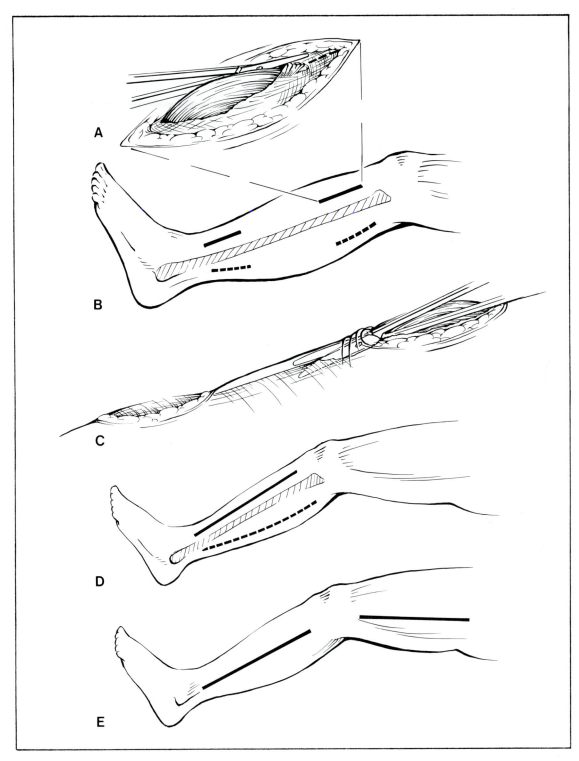

Figure 74-5. Skin incisions for different types of fasciotomies. **A.** Incision of fascia and bulging muscle through its aperture. **B.** Short skin incisions of the leg for the anterior (*continuous line*) and posterior (*broken line*) compartments. **C.** Fasciotomy performed with straight scissors subcutaneously between the two short skin openings. **D.** Long skin incisions of the leg for anterior (*continuous line*) and posterior (*broken line*) compartments. **E.** Long skin incision of the leg and thigh.

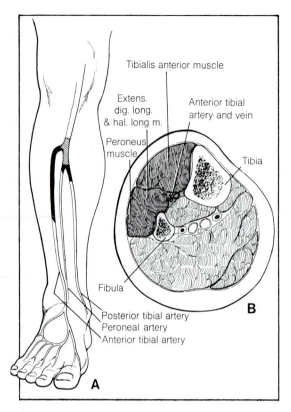

Figure 74-6. A. Embolic occlusion of the popliteal artery and its three branches. **B.** Cross section at the midleg level, indicating necrosis of the anterolateral compartment.

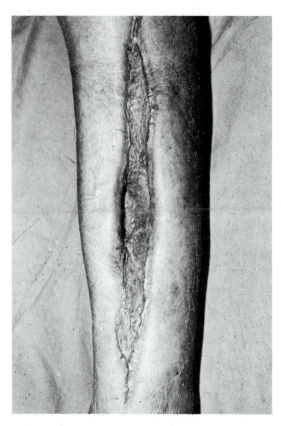

Figure 74-7. Healed leg in which the entire anterolateral compartment was excised because of muscle necrosis. Healing was completed through use of a skin graft.

the fibula has no weight-bearing function, its excision would result in few, if any, untoward effects. Only the distal fibula is essential because of its participation in providing stability of the ankle joint.

Exposure of the fibula and of the four compartments is identical to the preceding technique without fibulectomy (Fig. 74-8). With the introduction of the perifibular procedure, fibulectomy-fasciotomy has been used less frequently, since the former modality accomplishes the four-compartment fasciotomy without the bone resection. It is mentioned briefly here because of the rare need for its application.

The four-compartment decompression is useful in certain well-defined conditions. Its greatest value lies in its use for extensive vascular injuries with massive tissue damage rather than in other vascular entities affecting the leg compartments.

PITFALLS AND COMPLICATIONS

The most serious pitfall is delayed recognition of the leg and forearm compartment syndromes that require early

and urgent fasciotomies. Inadequate decompression by limited skin incisions in the presence of markedly swollen muscles may be a significant error. Likewise, partial debridement of damaged muscles may lead to further infection and secondary amputation. Long skin incisions, so necessary to decompress severely edematous muscles, with their edges left unapproximated for several days may leave neurovascular structures, vascular grafts, or tendons unprotected. Every effort must be made to cover these structures with either the adjacent tissues or a split-thickness skin graft when appropriate.[36]

If the muscle ischemia is too far advanced, fasciotomy may not always achieve its therapeutic goal. In cases of ischemic venous thrombosis with incipient gangrene, for example, results of fasciotomy may be mediocre because of protracted wound healing due to the delayed procedure and superimposed infection.

In the majority of the cases, however, in promptly recognized compartment syndromes, fasciotomy properly performed will reduce morbidity, save limbs, and have few, if any, complications.

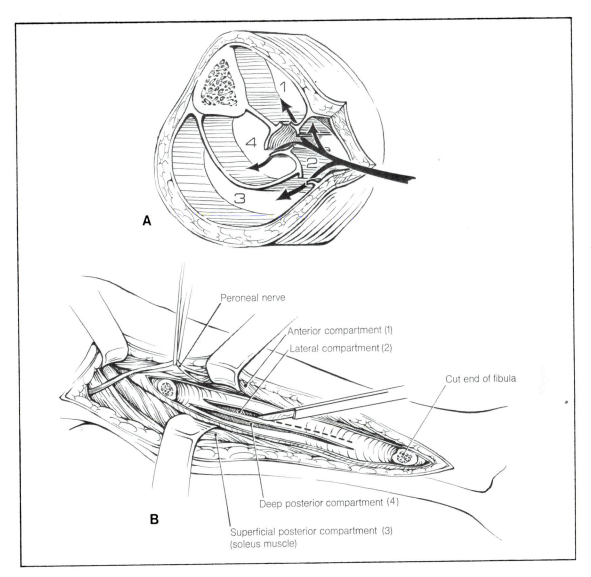

Peroneal nerve

Anterior compartment (1)

Lateral compartment (2)

Cut end of fibula

Deep posterior compartment (4)

Superficial posterior compartment (3)
(soleus muscle)

Figure 74-8. A. Cross section showing entrances for decompression of the four compartments of the leg: *1*, anterior tibial; *2*, lateral peroneal; *3*, superficial posterior; and *4*, deep posterior. **B.** Fibulectomy-fasciotomy technique (see text).

REFERENCES

1. Volkmann RV: Die ischaemischen muskellahmungen und kontrakturen. Zentralbl Chir 8:801, 1881.
2. Brooks B: Pathologic changes in muscle as a result of disturbances of circulation: An experimental study of Volkmann's ischemic paralysis. Arch Surg 5:188, 1922.
3. Griffiths DL: Volkmann's ischemic contracture. Br J Surg 28:239, 1940.
4. Jacobs AL: Arterial embolism in the limbs. Edinburgh, Churchill Livingstone, 1959, p 60.
5. Jepson PN: Ischemic contracture: Experimental study. Ann Surg 84:785, 1926.
6. Dennis C: Disaster following femoral vein ligation for thrombophlebitis; relief by fasciotomy; clinical case of renal impairment following crush injury. Surgery 17:265, 1945.
7. Horn CE: Acute ischemia of the anterior tibial muscle and the long extensor muscles of the toes. J Bone Joint Surg 27:615, 1945.

8. Chandler JG, Knapp RW: Early definitive treatment of vascular injuries inn the Viet Nam conflict. JAMA 202:136, 1967.
9. Patman RD, Thompson JE: Fasciotomy in peripheral vascular surgery. Report of 164 patients. Arch Surg 101:663, 1970.
10. Ernst CB, Kaufer H: Fibulectomy-fasciotomy. An important adjunct in the management of lower extremity arterial trauma. J Trauma 11:365, 1971.
11. Matsen FA, Krugmire RB: Compartmental syndromes. Surg Gynecol Obstet 147:943, 1978.
12. Haimovici H: Myopathic-nephrotic-metabolic syndrome associated with massive acute arterial occlusions. J Cardiovasc Surg 14:589, 1973.
13. Haimovici H: Phlegmasia cerulea dolens. Venous gangrene, in Ischemic Forms of Venous Thrombosis. Springfield, Ill, Charles C Thomas, Publisher, 1971.
14. Weeks RS: The crush syndrome. Surg Gynecol Obstet 127:369, 1968.
15. Korthuis RJ, Granger DN, et al.: The role of oxygen-derived free radicals in ischemia-induced increases in canine skeletal muscle vascular permeability. Circ Res 57(4):599, 1985.

16. Lee KR, Cronenwett JL, et al.: Effect of superoxide dismutase plus catalase on Ca^{2+} transport in ischemic and reperfused skeletal muscle. J Surg Res 42:24, 1987.

17. Heppenstall RB, Scott R, et al.: A comparative study of the tolerance of skeletal muscle to ischemia. J Bone Joint Surg 68A(6):820, 1986.

18. McCord JM: Oxygen-derived free radicals in post-ischemic tissue injury. N Engl J Med 312:159, 1985.

19. Parks DA, Buckley GB, Graiger DN: Role of oxygen-derived free radicals in digestive tract diseases. Surgery 94:415, 1983.

20. Saufey H, Bulkley GB, Cameron JL: The pathogenesis of acute pancreatitis: The source and role of oxygen-derived free radicals in three experimental models. Ann Surg 201:633, 1985.

21. Labbe R, Lindsay T, Walker PM: The extent and distribution of skeletal muscle necrosis after graded periods of complete ischemia. J Vasc Surg 6:152, 1987.

22. Walker PM, Lindsay TF, et al.: Salvage of skeletal muscle with free radical scavengers. J Vasc Surg 5:68, 1987.

23. Whitesides TE, Haney TC, et al.: A simple method for tissue pressure determination. Arch Surg 110:1311, 1975.

24. Mubarak SJ, Woen CA, et al.: Acute compartmental syndromes: Diagnosis and treatment with the aid of the Wick catheter. J Bone Joint Surg (Am) 60:1091, 1978.

25. Rollins DL, Bernhard VM, Towne JB: Fasciotomy. An appraisal of controversial issues. Arch Surg 116:1474, 1981.

26. Whitesides TE, Haney TC, et al.: Tissue pressure measurements as a determinant for the need of fasciotomy. Clin Orthop 113:43, 1975.

27. Russell WL, Apyan PM, Burns RP: Utilization and wide clinical implementation using the Wick catheter for compartment pressure measurement. Surg Gynecol Obstet 160(3):207, 1985.

28. Matsen FA, Winquist RA, Krugmire RB: Diagnosis and management of compartmental syndromes. J Bone Joint Surg 62A(2):286, 1980.

29. Allen MJ, Stirling AJ, et al.: Intracompartmental pressure monitoring of leg injuries. J Bone Joint Surg 67B(1):53, 1985.

30. Ashton H: Critical closure in human limbs. Br Med Bull 19(2):149, 1963.

31. Jennings AMC: Some observations of critical closing pressures in the peripheral circulation of anesthetized patients. Br J Anesth 36:683, 1964.

32. Whitesides TE, Haney TC, et al.: A simple method for tissue pressure determination. Arch Surg 110:1311, 1975.

33. Mozes M, Ramon Y, Jahr J: The anterior tibial syndrome. J Bone Joint Surg 44A:730, 1962.

34. Rosato FE, Barker CF, et al.: Subcutaneous fasciotomy—description of a new technique and instrument. Surgery 59:383, 1966.

35. Matsen FA: Compartmental Syndromes. New York, Grune & Stratton, Inc, 1980, p 163.

36. Ledgerwood AM, Lucas CE: Massive thigh injuries with vascular disruption. Role of porcine skin grafting of exposed arterial vein grafts. Arch Surg 107:201, 1973.

CHAPTER 75

Diagnosis and Management of Lymphedema

Thomas F. O'Donnell, Jr., and Anson Yeager

Lymphedema, the accumulation of excess amounts of water and protein within the subcutaneous tissue and skin, is caused by lack of lymphatic function. Lymphedema has been divided into two broad classifications based on the cause of the lymphatic dysfunction. Primary lymphedema results from in utero vascular dysplasia, which is associated most commonly with an insufficient number of lymphatic vessels and nodes, whereas secondary lymphedema occurs after destruction or extirpation of the lymphatic vessels or nodes or both.[1]

ETIOLOGY

Primary Lymphedema

There are several theories for the cause of primary lymphedema. Although the majority of experts agree that it is due to an in utero vascular dysplasia, two groups have favored an acquired cause of primary lymphedema. Calnan[2] argued that the female predominance of lymphedema and the predilection for involvement of the left leg favored an acquired cause for lymphedema. Kountz and Calnan[3] showed that venous obstruction may be associated with anatomic and functional changes in the lymphatics. They theorized that the location of the right iliac artery predisposed the underlying left lymphatic vessels and left iliac vein to compression. The partial venous obstruction associated with this arterial compression resulted in an initial elevation in venous pressure and also subsequent lymphatic abnormalities. Rigas et al.'s findings of increased femoral vein pressure in patients with primary lymphedema support Calnan's theory. Phlebography of the iliac venous system frequently shows compression of the left iliac vein by the overlying iliac artery. Indeed, several surgeons have reported series of vascular procedures to relieve this venous obstruction.

Since Negus et al.[5] had observed normal femoral venous pressures in a group of 12 patients with primary lymphedema who had undergone previous lymphography, they challenged the concept that iliac artery compression caused primary lymphedema. In addition, they performed postmortem studies by injecting acrylic to form casts of the left iliac vein, as well as carrying out a series of left femoral phlebograms to assess whether the iliac vein was compressed. These two studies revealed partial compression of the left iliac vein, but this narrowing was insufficient to cause significant hemodynamic obstruction. The fundamental weakness to the acquired theory for primary lymphedema is the observation that hypoplasia is the most common lymphographic pattern observed in primary lymphedema. The lymphographic pattern of a decreased number of lymphatic vessels would be difficult to rationalize on the basis of obstruction.

A second mechanism proposed as supporting evidence for the acquired cause of primary lymphedema is based on the inflammatory changes that have been observed in lymphatic vessels or lymph nodes of patients with primary lymphedema. In a series of patients with primary lymphedema, Olszewski and colleagues[6] biopsied the lymphatic vessels and observed a normal number of lymphatic vessels, but these vessels had a hyperplastic and thickened intimal layer with an obstructed lumen. Olszewski felt that recurrent infection led to these histologic changes in the vessel wall and subsequent obliteration of the lymphatic vessels. Since the vessels would not opacify on ascending lymphography, hypoplasia or aplasia would be the anatomic finding on lymphography. A decade later, Fyfe et al.[7] observed fibrotic changes in the afferent portion of the lymph node rather than in the lymphatic vessels and believed that such changes were due to recurrent inflammation. Like Olszewski, Fyfe theorized that lymph flow would be obstructed and the lymphatic vessels might subsequently fibrose.

That in utero vascular dysplasia is the cause of primary lymphedema is consistent with the etiology of other vascular anomalies. Indeed, O'Donnell and Kinmonth[8] observed that lymphatic anomalies were often found in the same limb with arterial and venous dysplasia.

Secondary Lymphedema

Radiation to both lymph nodes and lymphatic vessels, planned surgical extirpation for the treatment of cancer, inadvertent surgical injury to the lymphatic vessels or nodes, or finally, recurrent infections may disrupt lymphatic function and cause secondary lymphedema (Table 75-1). An experimental model of lymphedema in which the skin, subcutaneous tissue, and lymphatic vessels were removed was accompanied by an initial transient edema in all experimental animals' limbs.[9] Although this edema had resolved by the second postoperative month, nearly one third of the animals had significant recurrence of lymphedema at 2 years postoperatively, and one half of the animals had developed marked lymphedema at 5 years. Serial ascending lymphograms obtained from these animals showed progressive dilatation of the lymphatic vessels, as well as a numerical hyperplasia, which was similar to the lymphographic pattern observed in a limb with postmastectomy lymphedema. Certainly, the most common cause of secondary lymphedema is neoplasia and its treatment. The removal of lymph nodes or accompanying lymphatic vessels may be followed by significant limb swelling in up to 30% of patients. In a series of patients after mastectomy, Kreel and George[10] performed lymphography and demonstrated that collateral lymphatic flow was established across the mastectomy site by 1 to 2 months postoperatively. In several instances the collateral network traversed to the opposite axilla. This work corroborated the previous pioneering study of Kinmonth and Taylor[11] who showed the importance of collateral lymphatic pathways after mastectomy. When the critical collateral networks such as those to the parasternal and supraclavicular nodes or the collateral vessels across the mastectomy site are destroyed by postirradiation fibrosis or by infection, lymphedema may ensue.

Recurrent pyogenic infections are the next major cause of secondary lymphedema. Although beta-streptococcus is the most frequently isolated bacterium in these infections, *Staphylococcus aureus* and Gram-negative aerobes have also been implicated. The infectious process causes an obliteration of the lymphatic vessels and fibrosis of the afferent

lymph nodes. Some of the edema observed in the post-thrombotic limb is related to obliteration of the lymphatics by repeated bouts of cellulitis and exemplifies the infectious cause of secondary lymphedema. Each successive episode of cellulitis causes fibrosis of the lymphatic vessel, with obstruction and enhancement of the underlying edema. For example, on lymphography the lymphatics may be obliterated in many of the limbs with severe postthrombotic changes. A rare cause of lymphedema in the continental United States is filarial infection, in which the worms cause obstruction of the lymphatics at the nodal level.[12]

DIAGNOSIS

The diagnosis of lymphedema can usually be made by a physician who is familiar with its rather typical clinical presentation and findings. The patient's history, as well as the appearance of the lymphedematous limb, are quite characteristic. Although the symptoms and physical findings are similar in primary and secondary lymphedema, the history usually differs.

History

The typical patient with primary lymphedema is a female who first notes the onset of mild-to-moderate foot and ankle edema, usually beginning around menarche. The left limb is more frequently involved than the right. Depending on the duration of lymphedema, the patient usually observes an insidious progression centripetally to involve the calf and lower thigh areas. Occasionally, patients may relate the onset of their lymphedema to minor trauma so that they may initially be seen by an orthopedic surgeon for evaluation of a possible ankle sprain.

In contrast, the typical patient with secondary lymphedema has usually undergone a surgical procedure 4 to 5 years previously and has possibly received concomitant radiation. In this patient, the recent onset of edema may be associated with a minor infection. It is important to establish the extent of the previous surgical procedure and the amount and sites of irradiation. Subsequent evaluation of this patient should rule out recurrence of the neoplasm, which is an unusual cause of edema. Alternatively, a history of recurrent cellulitis or trauma to the leg should be elicited.

Symptoms

The cosmetic deformity produced by limb swelling is usually the reason for seeking medical care and is the first symptom noted by a patient (Table 75-2). The edema usually involves the distal portion of the extremity initially and is worse at the end of the day after prolonged standing or use of the extremity. The edema may resolve with elevation of the limb at night. As the process becomes more severe, the level of the edema progresses to involve the more proximal portions of the limb so that the limb girth increases at both proximal and distal sites. As the lymphedema progresses,

TABLE 75-1. CAUSES OF SECONDARY LYMPHEDEMA

Cause	Pathophysiology	Lymphographic Pattern
Malignant disease	Obstruction of node by tumor	Obstruction with collateral circulation
Radiation	Obstruction of lymphatic trunks by extrinsic fibrosis at lymph node level	Obstruction
Surgery or trauma	Obstruction at lymphatic vessel level	Obstruction with collateral circulation
Filariasis	Obstruction at lymph node level	Obstruction; widened varicose lymphatics with reflux
Pyogenic infection	Obliteration of lymphatic trunks	Hypoplasia

addition to defining the status of the lymph nodes, CT shows the relative distribution of edema fluid within the extremity. A characteristic honeycomb appearance to the edema fluid within the subcutaneous tissue is diagnostic of lymphedema.

Lymphography

Lymphography is the most definitive method available for objectively documenting the presence of lymphedema. The studies of Kinmonth[16-18] of St. Thomas's Hospital have pioneered our understanding of lymphedema.

Primary Lymphedema

Kinmonth classified primary lymphedema based on the anatomic pattern described on lymphography. Patients were classified into those with aplasia (absence of any lymphatic vessels) (Fig. 75-3), those with hypoplasia (decreased number and size of lymphatic vessels and nodes) (Fig. 75-4), and finally, those with hyperplasia (increased number of vessels and nodes) (Fig. 75-5). As is shown in Table 75-3, most patients (approximately 90%) fall into the hypoplasia or aplasia group, a smaller proportion into the hyperplastic group. This observation is consistent with a dysplastic cause of primary lymphedema. In a review with Kinmonth, we assessed 20 lymphangiograms of patients

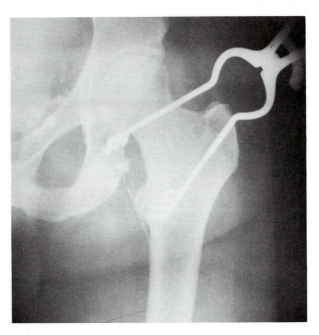

Figure 75-3. Because no lymphatic trunks were accessible on the dorsum of the foot, a lymph node was exposed in the groin. Infusion of ultra-Lipiodol directly into the lymph node reveals no lymphatic vessels except for a thin, wispy lymphatic collateral at the level of the trochanter.

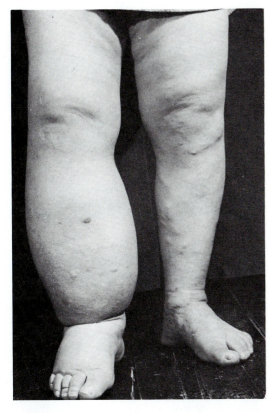

Figure 75-2. Anterior view of right leg with marked lymphedema. The lower thigh and entire calf are involved by the lymphedematous process. The ankle crease is absent because of the redundancy of lymphedematous calf tissue.

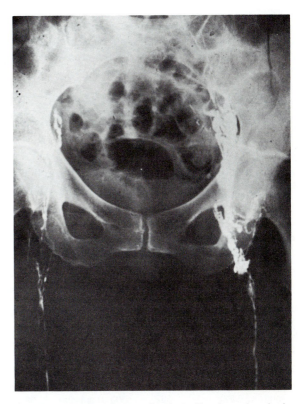

Figure 75-4. Lymphangiogram of patient with primary lymphedema and hypoplasia. The number of lymphatic trunk vessels at the thigh level are markedly reduced from the normal 10 to 15 vessels.

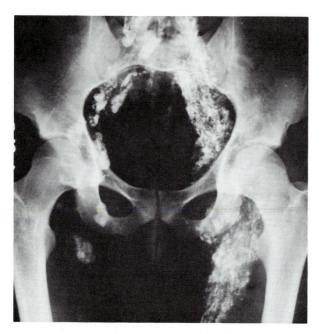

Figure 75-5. Lymphangiogram of patient with primary lymphedema and hyperplasia. Multiple trunks and lymph nodes are noted.

with lymphedema associated with mixed vascular deformities of either the veins alone or combined with the arteries.[8] Those patients with lymphatic hypoplasia had an average of 2.1 vessels at the upper thigh-inguinal area, with an average width of 0.6 ± 0.2 mm. At this level the normal lymphangiogram shows up to 12 lymphatic vessels, and the width of individual vessels are usually in excess of 1 mm. On the other hand, those patients with hyperplastic lymphatics showed an increased number, averaging 18.5 ± 3.5 vessels, with a width of nearly 2 mm at this level.

Secondary Lymphedema
As opposed to primary lymphedema, the lymphographic pattern in secondary lymphedema is predominantly one of increased width and number of lymphatic trunks, which is related to obstruction (Fig. 75-6). Kreel and George's[10] early study of postmastectomy patients with lymphedema showed marked hyperplasia of the lymphatics and dermal

TABLE 75-3. RESULTS OF LYMPHOGRAPHY IN PRIMARY LYMPHEDEMA

Series	No. of Cases	Hypoplasia/ Aplasia	Hyper- plasia
Buonocore and Young (1965)[65]	20	20	
Thompson[22] (1970)	50	47 (17 prox.*)	3
Kinmonth[13] (1972)	100	92 (5 aplasia)	8
Olszewski et al.[6] (1972)	120	111 (24 prox.*)	9
Saijo et al.[66] (1975)	12	7	5
Kinmonth[18] (1982)	562	506 (0 aplasia)	56
Total	864	783 (91%)	81 (9%)

* Proximal hypoplasia with an obstruction.

back flow. By contrast, patients with obliterative lymphangitis secondary to recurrent infections usually have a reduced number of lymphatic trunks but enlarged lymph nodes.

The edema that frequently occurs after arterial reconstruction, particularly after infrainguinal bypass, is due to interruption of the lymphatic vessels. Earlier it was theorized that fluid accumulation in the limb postoperatively was due to leakage of water and protein from the capillaries under the influence of improved perfusion pressure. Schmidt and associates[19] disproved this theory in their study of 37 patients who underwent lymphography after femoropopliteal bypass. Lymphangiograms were performed on the third and ninth postoperative day and revealed intact vessels at the knee and groin if edema was minimal. Mild lymphedema was present when at least three lymph vessels were preserved, whereas moderate-to-severe lymphedema was noted when all lymph vessels had been divided and no intact lymphatic vessel was visualized. Subsequent repeat revascularization procedures were associated with the greatest degree of lymphedema.

Lymphatic Function

For clinical purposes, transit time and radioactive albumin disappearance curves are the only two techniques that have

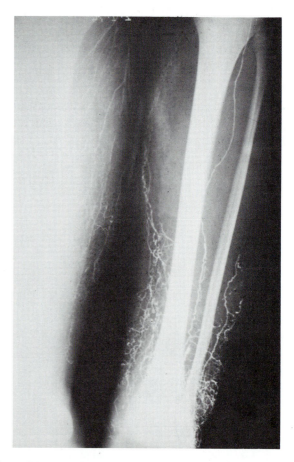

Figure 75-6. Lymphangiogram in patient with previous surgery to the lower extremity and secondary lymphedema. Markedly hyperplastic "steel wool" pattern of lymphatic vessels is observed.

had widespread use in the functional evaluation of lymphedema. Although measurement of the time taken by a column of contrast media to reach a specific site on the limb is a crude method and subject to many variables, a standardized lymphangiographic technique does afford the opportunity to quantitate lymphatic function. Lipiodol injected into the pedal lymphatics at a rate of 1 ml over 7 minutes will reach the inguinal nodes within 5 minutes and the sacroiliac joint within 35 minutes in a patient with a normal lymphatic system. Lymphatic stasis due to decreased vessel caliber (hypoplasia) or increased capacitance (numerical hyperplasia) may slow the transit time. An altered transit time may be the only evidence of lymphatic malfunction in some patients with mild edema and normal lymphatic anatomy by lymphography.[13]

One of the main functions of the lymphatic tree is to clear protein from the extravascular extracellular fluid space and return it to the intravascular space, so the rate at which labeled albumin is cleared from this site should assess lymphatic function. Indeed, ^{131}I-albumin disappearance curves are prolonged in the lymphedematous limb.[20] This delayed clearance may be related to trapping of albumin within the interstitial space and its subsequent pooling or to reversal of the ratio of normal subcutaneous tissue pressure to muscle compartment pressure. In lymphedema, interstitial fluid protein concentration is elevated, and subcutaneous pressure is higher than muscle compartment pressure. Despite this attractive physiologic rationale, however, measurements of disappearance curves have little value in the initial assessment of lymphedema.[21] This technique's greatest use is in determining the effects of various surgical procedures for treatment of lymphedema.[22]

Degree of Lymphedema

The two standard methods for assessing the degree of lymphedema are measurement of limb circumference at specific anatomic sites and measurement of limb volume by water displacement (see Table 75-2). The absolute increase in the amount of lymphedematous tissue is represented by the abnormal minus the normal dimension, whereas the degree of lymphedema (relative amount of lymphedematous tissue) is related to the ratio of the [(abnormal−normal)/normal]. Since there are no tables of normal values applicable to a wide range of limb dimensions, most clinicians use the contralateral limb as the control, or normal, value. These techniques are hampered by variation of technique, observer error from measurement to measurement, difference in normal limb size (especially in upper limbs), and lack of reproducibility.

Perhaps the most convenient method for circumferential measurements of girth are the premade measurement devices used for fitting elastic compression stockings, which consist of a series of paper tapes. In our experience this method of measuring limb girth avoids the variation in technique, observer error, and lack of reproducibility inherent in other methods.

For those physicians who see patients with lymphedema frequently, limb-volume measurement by water displacement provides objective estimates of total limb edema. The limb is immersed in a large cylinder fitted with a tap so that the excess volume of water that escapes through the tap can be volumetrically measured in another container. The volume displacement method does not identify the particular segment of the limb that has increased or decreased in dimension.

Soft-tissue x-ray examination or xeroradiography provides an objective means for measuring skin and subcutaneous thickness independently. In a series of 11 patients with secondary lymphedema, O'Donnell et al.[23] demonstrated a fourfold increase in skin thickness and a twofold increase in subcutaneous tissue width. Another important factor assessed by this method is the degree of subcutaneous fibrosis. The amount of subcutaneous scarring, or fibrosis, is related to tissue compliance and therefore provides a prediction of the limb's responsiveness to compression. Because of the radiation exposure inherent in this technique, we have limited its use to a yearly exposure.

Tissue tonometry measurement, which uses devices similar to those used in assessing glaucoma, is an alternative to xeroradiography for determining the degree of subcutaneous tissue fibrosis. This method is particularly important in assessing the effects of pharmacologic treatment of subcutaneous fibrosis. B-mode ultrasound provides excellent characterization of other vascular tissues and may have great promise as a noninvasive technique for assessing the degree of subcutaneous fibrosis.

TREATMENT

Nonsurgical Treatment

More than 90% of patients with lymphedema can be managed by nonsurgical means. Wolfe and Kinmonth[24] demonstrated that the extent of the disease could be assessed accurately within the first year of diagnosis by the response to therapy. The goals of therapy are to reduce limb size, preserve and improve the quality of the skin and subcutaneous tissue, and prevent infection (Table 75-4).

TABLE 75-4. TREATMENT OF LYMPHEDEMA

Nonsurgical	Surgical
Reduction in limb size	*Physiologic procedures*
Elevation	Buried dermal flap (Thompson)
Elastic compression	Lymphovenous shunt
Massage	Full-thickness skin bridge
External pneumatic compression	Omental transposition
	Subcutaneous tunnels
Improvement in skin quality	Lysis of fibrotic venous obstruction
Treatment of fungal and bacterial infections	Entertomesenteric bridge
Skin lotion	*Excisional procedures*
Benzopyrones	Skin and subcutaneous tissue excision with split-thickness skin graft coverage (Charles)
	Staged excision of subcutaneous tissue with vascularized local flaps (Homans)

Reduction in Limb Size

Initial treatment of mild lymphedema may require only elevation of the limb at night and the use of compression stockings during the day to maintain a reduced limb girth. Elevation of the extremity can be accomplished by placing blocks under the foot of the bed or by suspending the arm in a sling. Measurement of the extremity for compression stockings is carried out in the reduced state before reaccumulation of edema fluid because the elastic compression effect is related to the initial unstretched circumference. We use a 40 to 50 mm Hg gradient stocking (Sigvaris) for most patients. The length of the stocking should be matched to the extent of the disease. Below-knee stockings are more comfortable because they do not bind behind the knee and are easier to don and remove. This length is appropriate for patients with foot, ankle, and calf swelling. Thigh-length stockings or panty hose are preferable for patients with significant thigh edema.

In some of our younger patients, we have had success with the use of a double stocking to increase compressive pressure.[25] Two full-length 30 to 40 mm Hg elastic stockings are used initially. At 2 months the outer stocking is changed to 40 to 50 mm Hg, and at 4 months the inner stocking is increased to 40 to 50 mm Hg. At 6 months the outer stocking is increased to 50 to 60 mm Hg. In our studies digital plethysmography showed no adverse hemodynamic effect on distal arterial flow. Our initial trial included eight patients with limb girths measured sequentially at 10 constant points for the 10-month treatment period. No patient discontinued therapy, and all demonstrated a decrease in limb girth (Table 75-5). Some patients experienced an initial increase in thigh girth, but this decreased after 4 months of therapy. A double-compression stocking is a treatment option for younger patients who can tolerate the higher pressure and can manage the difficulty of putting on and removing the stockings.

Similar to the findings of Zeissler et al.[26] in more than 100 of our patients followed for 5 years, the conscientious use of elastic stockings maintained limb girth in a reduced state. We have not used the extubation technique of Van der Molen and Toth[27] whereby a soft rubber tube is wound around the leg, beginning at the toes and progressing proximally, developing 200 to 300 mm Hg pressure. Although they described "good results," general anesthesia was needed to apply their technique.

External Pneumatic Compression. Our initial experience with pneumatic compression involved a low-pressure unicell boot or sleeve inflated to 60 mm Hg for 12.5 seconds of compression followed by a 35-second rest period. Seventeen patients were included in our initial prospective study reported by Raines et al.[28] Nine patients with upper-extremity lymphedema showed a 50% reduction in hand girth, but forearm and upper arm reduction was less than 20%. The patients with lower extremity lymphedema showed a similar response pattern with less reduction of the ankle and calf than of the foot. We found that patients with a greater degree of subcutaneous fibrosis as measured by xeroradiography responded less well to pneumatic compression therapy than did patients with softer subcutaneous tissues.

We now use a high-pressure sequential pneumatic compression device, the Lympha Press, developed by Zelikovski.[29] The compression garment is constructed of multiple circumferential chambers that are pressurized to 110 to 150 mm Hg in a sequential centripetal fashion so that, in essence, the edema fluid is milked in the extremity distally to proximally. Because only a few chambers are fully pressurized at any one time, the higher pressures are much better tolerated by the patient than with the unicell design compression device, and the limb reduction is achieved more rapidly. Richmand et al.[30] reported our initial results in 25 patients treated in a prospective study (Table 75-6 and 75-7). Seven patients with upper-extremity lymphedema and 18 with lower-extremity lymphedema were treated for a 24-hour period. All extremities showed a decrease in circumferential girth. Lower-extremity leg volume was reduced an average of 45% with a midcalf circumference decrease of 47%. Immediately after treatment, patients were fitted with compression stockings at the new reduced girth. A second group of patients, many with milder disease, were followed for a mean of 27 months. The long-term results for 30 patients demonstrated a relative limb-girth reduction of 15.6% (absolute 2.7 cm) at the ankle and 18.1% (absolute 3.2 cm) at the low calf (see Table 75-6). Optimal results have been dependent on patient compliance and the condition of the subcutaneous tissue.

Skin Maintenance

Improvement and preservation of skin quality is the second goal of nonoperative therapy. Maintaining the skin in good condition is imperative to prevent serious sequelae and progression of the lymphedema process. The skin should be cleansed daily, and a water-based lotion such as polysorb hydrate should be applied twice daily. Minor trauma to the skin should be avoided. Pruritic skin should be treated with a steroid cream. Fungal infections should be treated and prevented by the use of antifungal agents. Bacterial infections are best prevented, but when they occur, they should be treated aggressively, oftentimes requiring intravenous therapy initially for at least 7 days, followed by a prolonged (2- to 4-week) course of oral antibiotics.

Subcutaneous Tissue

The hardening of the subcutaneous tissue in patients with advanced lymphedema is related to a fibrotic process that occurs as plasma proteins are deposited in the tissue. These proteins induce an inflammatory reaction. Experimentally produced lymphedema softens when treated with benzopyrones.[31] In Europe, warfarin (Coumadin), a benzopyrone,

TABLE 75-5. EFFECT OF DOUBLE COMPRESSION ELASTIC STOCKING ON LOWER EXTREMITY LYMPHEDEMA*

Girth	Meta-tarsal†	Malle-olar†	Low Calf†	Thigh
Precompression	25.1 ± 0.7	27 ± 1.6	35.5 ± 2.1	55.5 ± 1.1
Postcompression	21.2 ± 1.2	22.4 ± 1.3	31 ± 1.8	53 ± 2.2

* Girth measurements (mean centimeters ± SE).
† Significant difference to at least $P < .05$ by paired t test.

TABLE 75-6. REDUCTION IN LYMPHEDEMATOUS LOWER EXTREMITY LIMB GIRTH BY HIGH PRESSURE PNEUMATIC COMPRESSION

| | Acute Treatment Group (No. = 18) | | Long-term Treatment Group (No. = 30) | | |
	(Abs.* [cm])	(Rel.† [%])	Initial Treatment Session Results (Abs.* [cm])	Long-term Results (Abs.* [cm])	Pretreatment (Rel.† [%])
Ankle	8.4 ± 1.5	37 ± 6	2.7	2.7	15.6
Midcalf	8.1 ± 1.4	47 ± 5	2.0	2.9	14.6
Midthigh	1.5 ± 0.3	36 ± 7	0.7	1.9	3.7

* Absolute reduction = (Girth pretreatment − Girth posttreatment).
† Relative reduction = [(Abnormal girth − Normal girth)/Normal girth × 100].

has been used for this effect because, theoretically, the drug should enhance lysis of proteins by macrophages and reduce the fibrosis. Because of the potential side effects, however, we have not used this approach.

Infection

Recurrent lymphangitis, most commonly due to beta-hemolytic streptococci, is the main presenting symptom in 15 to 20% of patients with lymphedema. The sudden onset of infection with rapid progression, sometimes even leading to the development of shock, is related to the lack of the normal lymphatic immunologic barriers. Patients should be resuscitated and treated with intravenous penicillin or oxacillin, pending cultures. The source of bacterial invasion should be evaluated. Often the site of entry is due to tinea pedis, but it can also occur at hair follicles with no apparent break in the skin. Cultures can be obtained by saline aspiration of the cellulitic margin. We treat patients with an aggressive regimen of intravenous antibiotics for at least 7 days, followed by an additional 3-week course of oral antibiotics. Local fungal infections should be treated with antifungal creams. More invasive fungal infections may require oral griseofulvin treatment. Subsequent infection can be prevented with an antifungal powder. In patients with two or more bacterial infections a year, oral prophylaxis with penicillin (PEN-VEE-K 250 mg po bid) or erythromycin (250 mg po bid) can reduce the number of infectious episodes.

Surgical Treatment

Traditionally, the indications for surgical treatment of lymphedema have been *cosmetic*, to improve the size and shape of the limb; *functional*, to reduce limb weight and improve skin texture; and *preventive*, to decrease the number of infections or to prevent the occurrence of angiosarcoma, a lethal complication. A wide variety of surgical procedures have been described, consistent with the overall poor success rate. We exercise the surgical option in only that small percentage of patients with massive edema who appear most likely to benefit from a surgical procedure. Chilvers and Kinmonth[32] demonstrated that overall only 30% of patients undergoing reduction surgery (Thompson flap) retained long-term benefit. Most patients had returned to their preoperative girth 2 to 4 years after the original surgery. Only those patients with massive edema appeared to benefit. The surgical morbidity associated with the procedure, particularly skin-flap necrosis in nearly 25%, resulted in prolonged hospitalization and convalescence.

Patients with a severe functional disability due to marked skin change or with immobility secondary to massive edema unresponsive to compression are candidates for surgical treatment. Surgery should be avoided in patients with minimal edema (less than 3 cm circumferential difference between normal and affected limb), gross obesity, disease that is actively progressing, and in whom a firm diagnosis of lymphedema is not established as the cause of limb swelling.

Kinmonth[13] divided surgical treatment of lymphedema into two types: physiologic and excisional.

Physiologic Procedures

The goal of physiologic procedures is to promote drainage of lymph from the abnormal superficial subcutaneous lymphatics into either the normal lymphatics of the deep system (fascial lymphatics) or proximally or into the venous system (Table 75-8). Kondoleon[33] excised a wedge of fascia and subcutaneous tissue to promote lymphatic connections between superficial and deep lymphatics. Sistrunk[34] removed more subcutaneous tissue and had slightly better results, suggesting that it was the removal of subcutaneous tissue that was most beneficial in reducing limb girth.[34]

Handley[35] placed long silk threads into the subcutaneous tissue from hand to shoulder to create conduits to the normal shoulder lymphatics.[35] Variations of this procedure have been performed by several surgeons. O'Reilly[36] used nylon setons in two women with postmastectomy edema.[36] He noted encouraging physical results but no change in albumin removal. Silver and Puckett[37] created subcutaneous tunnels and claimed good results but lacked objective measurements to assess the procedure.[37]

TABLE 75-7. REDUCTION IN LYMPHEDEMATOUS UPPER-EXTREMITY GIRTH BY SEQUENTIAL HIGH PRESSURE PNEUMATIC COMPRESSION (NO. = 7)

	Absolute Reduction (cm)	Relative Reduction (%)
Wrist	0.9 ± 0.2	45 ± 14
Midforearm	1.9 ± 0.3	28 ± 7
Midupper arm	1.4 ± 0.3	25 ± 13

TABLE 75-8. PHYSIOLOGIC OPERATIONS FOR LYMPHEDEMA

Series	No. of Patients	Type*	Results† Good	Fair	Poor	Criteria	Length of Follow-up (Yr)
Buried dermal flap							
Thompson[22] (1970)	50	1	29	17	4	Circumference, clearance studies	1–10
Thompson[67] (1969)	23	2	14	8	1	Circumference, clearance studies	1–9
						Circumference, clearance studies	1
Sawney[53] (1974)	5	1	No change	5	0	Circumference, volume displacement	1
						Circumference, patient's and surgeon's evaluation	1
Bunchman and Lewis[68] (1974)	10	1	2	4	4		
Kinmonth et al.[69] (1975)	108	1	29	61	18		
Totals	196		74 (38%)	95 (48%)	27 (14%)		
Lymphovenous Anastomosis							
Politowski et al.[42] (1969)	16	1	8	6	2		
Milanov et al.[43] (1982)	50	2	15	28	7		
Krylov et al.[70] (1979)	73	2	25	46	2		
Gong Kang et al.[44] (1985)	71	2	72	15	40		3–24 mo
Totals	230		120 (52%)	95 (41%)	15 (6.5%)		
Omental Transposition						Size, function, frequency of cellulitis attacks	1–7
Goldsmith[47] (1974)	22	Mixed	10 (46%)	4 (18%)	8 (36%)		
Enteromesenteric bridge						Circumference, contrast lymphography, isotope lymphography	2.5–7
Hurst/Kinmonth et al.[50] (1985)	8	1	6		2		

* 1, Primary lymphedema; 2, secondary lymphedema.
† Author's interpretation of varied criteria for each series.

Lymphovenous Shunts. Kerstein and Licalzi[38] described the use of a direct lymph node–to–venous anastomosis in 1963. Nielubowicz and Olszewski[39] published the first clinical results of lymphovenous shunts. They reported on four patients with secondary lymphedema who had reduced limb size after a lymphovenous shunt. Three patients underwent lymphography and showed patent anastomoses. The fourth patient died of her primary disease, but postmortem examination showed patency in the medulary sinuses. This surgical approach suggested that a physiologic reconstruction was possible in patients with lymphedema and stimulated worldwide interest and research.

Lymphovenous anastomosis can be done in several ways. The lymph node can be sectioned sagittally and anastomosed to a vein. A direct microsurgical anastomosis can be performed between the vein and the lymph vessel. Finally, a specially constructed tube can be used to create the anastomosis.[40]

Long-term results for lymphovenous shunts are lacking. Experimental procedures in a canine model showed initial patency, but occlusion developed in 100% of the anastomoses by 1 month.[41] Politowski et al.[42] reported on 16 patients with primary lymphedema who had undergone the procedure described by Nielubowicz and Olszewski.[39] Follow-up of 6 to 18 months showed "good results" in eight patients, "fair results" in six, and "unsatisfactory results" in two. Milanov,[43] a Russian surgeon, reported on 50 patients who underwent lymphovenous anastomosis for postmastectomy lymphedema. "Good results" were noted in only 15 patients and "satisfactory results" in 28. Gong-Kang et al.[44] had 91 patients who had obstructive lower-extremity lymphedema treated by microlymphaticovenous anastomosis. "Excellent and good results" were noted in 79%, with an average limb circumference reduction of 6.4 cm. Fifty of these patients suffered from filariasis. Follow-up averaged 24 months. Of note is their opinion that long-standing obstructive lymphedema results in destruction of lymphatics and renders the patients unacceptable as candidates for microlymphaticovenous anastomosis. O'Brien and Das[45] showed that three or more anastomoses were needed to reduce limb size and emphasized that technical experience was an important factor in obtaining good results with microvascular surgery. Clodius et al. have also emphasized the problems associated with microvascular surgery. Fibrotic changes in the subcutaneous tissue associated with lymphedema result in a change in the lymphatic system, which may prevent reconstruction in patients with primary lymphedema. Thus lymphaticovenous anastomosis appears to be better suited to the treatment of obstructive forms of secondary lymphedema.

Omental Transposition. Goldsmith[47] attempted to bridge an area of lymphatic insufficiency by omental transposition. Long-term results were disappointing, and one patient died secondary to an incarcerated hernia along the tract of the omentum to the groin.

Full-thickness grafts have been tried to bypass lymphatic obstruction. Again, this procedure depends on bypassing a block with normal lymphatics above and below the site of obstruction. Various pedicle and myocutaneous flaps have been described, with a variety of problems resulting and variable success.

Enteromesenteric Bridge. Kinmonth experimented with ileum stripped of its mucosa, and transposing and anastomosing it with a bridge of mesentery to sectioned lymph nodes distal to an obstruction.[48] He reported the first clinical result in 1978 and the long-term follow-up in 1985.[49,50] In all, eight patients with iliac lymph node and vessel obstruction were treated. Follow-up was 2.5 to 7 years, and sustained clinical improvement was noted in six patients. Contrast lymphography performed during the first year postoperatively demonstrated function in five of the six successfully treated patients. A second lymphogram obtained for one patient 6.5 years after operation showed persistent function. Lymphoscintigraphy in four patients at late follow-up was normal in three of four patients tested. The two patients who failed to improve initially subsequently required a reducing operation.

Buried Dermal Flap. The most widely performed operation for lymphedema is the Thompson procedure.[51] The subcuta-

neous tissue is excised, and a posterior dermal flap is fixed to the deep fascia. The intent of the buried flap is to encourage spontaneous anastomoses between the superficial and deep fascial lymphatics. Thompson[22] and Harvey[52] used radioactive albumin disappearance curves to assess the results and showed increased removal of albumin. Sawney[53] found similar results and reduction of limb girth in the early postoperative period, but subsequent albumin studies no longer demonstrated the improvement.

Kinmonth performed lymphangiograms after the Thompson procedures but was unable to demonstrate any superficial to deep lymphaticolymphatic anastomoses. He concluded that the improvement after operation was due to the excision of the subcutaneous tissue and perhaps to a compressive massaging effect by the calf muscles on the lymphatics of the buried flap as demonstrated on cinelymphographic studies. Table 75-8 summarizes the results of several series of the Thompson procedure.

Excisional Procedures (Table 75-9)
Charles[54] worked in an area endemic for tropical elephantiasis and developed an operation that consisted of removing both skin and subcutaneous tissue. Split-thickness skin grafts were used to cover the exposed fascia. At present, the Charles procedure is restricted to those patients with severe skin changes that prevent the use of vascularized skin flaps or subcutaneous lipectomies. Unless the transition area in the thigh is tapered, a pantaloon appearance results. Hyperkeratotic skin, recurrent sepsis, graft failure, and condylomata development are late complications. Dellon and Hoopes[55] reported long-term results in 10 patients observed for as long as 20 years after a Charles procedure. No recurrence of lymphedema and excellent functional results were noted. Miller,[56] however, found less satisfactory results in five patients treated this way. Three of his patients eventually underwent amputation for severe skin changes or

TABLE 75-9. EXCISIONAL OPERATIONS FOR LYMPHEDEMA

Series	Types of Procedures	No. of Patients	Lymphedema Type*	Results		Criteria	Length of Follow-up (Yr)
				Good	Fair		
Fonkalsrud[60] (1979)	Subcutaneous lymphangiectomy	6	1	6	0	Cosmetic, functional	At least 1
Bunchman and Lewis[68] (1974)	Charles (complete excision of subcutaneous tissue and skin)	14	1	14†	0	—	5
Dellon and Hoopes[55] (1977)	Charles	12	1	12	0	Circumference	10½
Miller[58] (1975)	Staged subcutaneous excision	14	Mixed	0	14	Circumference	½–6 (6 for 4)
Miller[59] (1977)	Staged subcutaneous excision	21	Not specified	0	21	Circumference	1–4
Bunchman and Lewis[68] (1974)	Staged subcutaneous excision	5	1	5	0	—	1
Feins et al.[61] (1977)	Staged excisions (pediatric age group)	3	1	0	39	Patient interview	—

* 1, primary lymphedema; mixed, primary and secondary lymphedema.
† But undesirable pantaloon effect.

chronic cellulitis. He believed that the deformity caused by the skin graft was worse than the original lymphedema skin changes and warned against the widespread use of the procedure.

Homans[57] of Boston described a procedure in which subcutaneous tissue was excised in stages through the development of well-vascularized flaps. Large volumes of subcutaneous tissue can be excised and complications such as flap necrosis and sinus formation appear to occur less frequently than with the buried dermal flap. Miller[56,59] has reported his results for staged subcutaneous excision and believes that the procedure is associated with a consistent reduction in size and an improvement in function. Fonkalsrud[60] and Feins et al.[61] have reported results for pediatric patients and noted good results with minimal morbidity. Operation was restricted to patients with moderate-to-severe lymphedema. Fonkalsrud recommended that the procedure be deferred until after the age of 2 because of hypertrophic scarring.

Evaluation of follow-up data is difficult because of the lack of uniform objective measurements or criteria for assessing the degree of lymphedema preoperatively and the changes postoperatively. The follow-up period for many of the studies is short, resulting in a lack of long-term data by which to evaluate and compare results.

Venous Obstruction

Several authors have argued that relief of venous obstruction should be the primary target for intervention in cases of secondary lymphedema. Hughes and Patel[62] lysed the fibrotic encasement around the axillary vein in patients with postmastectomy lymphedema. They noted "good results" in 15 of 19 patients, as did Larsen and Crampton[63] in 4 of 8 patients undergoing a similar procedure.

As already noted, an element of lymphedema may exist in patients with congenital mixed vascular disorders. Treatment should be directed to the more prominent clinical problem in these patients, although elastic stocking support may be appropriate to both problems.[64]

REFERENCES

1. Allen EV, Barker NW, Hines EA: Peripheral Vascular Diseases. Philadelphia, WB Saunders Co, 1946.
2. Calnan J: Lymphoedema: The case for doubt. Br J Plast Surg 21:32, 1968.
3. Calnan J, Kountz SI: Effect of venous obstruction on lymphatics. Br J Surg 52:800, 1965.
4. Rigas A, Vomoyannis A, et al.: Measurement of the femoral vein pressure in edema of the lower extremities: Report of 50 cases. J Cardiovasc Surg 12:411, 1971.
5. Negus D, Edwards JM, Kinmonth JB: The iliac veins in relation to lymphedema. Br J Surg 56:481, 1969.
6. Olszewski W, Machowski Z, et al.: Clinical studies in primary lymphedema. Pol Med J 11:1560, 1972.
7. Fyfe NC, Rutt DC, et al.: Intralymphatic steroid therapy for lymphedema: Preliminary studies. Lymphology 15:23, 1982.
8. O'Donnell TF, Edwards JM, Kinmonth JB: Lymphography in the mixed vascular deformities of the lower extremities. J Cardiovasc Surg (Torino) 17:453, 1976.
9. Olszewski W; On the pathomechanism of development of post-surgical lymphedema. Lymphology 6:35, 1973.
10. Kreel L, George P: Post-mastectomy lymphangiography: Detection of metastases and edema. Ann Surg 163:470, 1966.
11. Kinmonth JB, Taylor GW: The lymphatic circulation in lymphedema. Ann Surg 139:129, 1954.
12. Gooneratne BWM: Lymphography of filarial infections. Lecture presented at St. Thomas Hospital, 1969.
13. Kinmonth JB: The Lymphatics: Diseases, Lymphography and Surgery. Baltimore, The Williams & Wilkins Co, 1972.
14. Milroy WF: An undescribed variety of hereditary oedema. NY State J Med p 505, 1892.
15. Shepard AD, Mackey WC, et al.: Light reflection rheography (LRR): A new non-invasive test of venous function. Bruit 8:266, 1984.
16. Eustace PW, Kinmouth JB: The normal lymphatic vessels of the inguinal and iliac areas with special emphasis on the efferent inguinal vessels. Lymphology 5:23, 1976.
17. Kinmonth JB: Primary lymphedemas: Classification and other studies based on oleolymphography and clinical features. J Cardiovasc Surg (Torino), Special Supplement for XVII Congress of European Society of Cardiovascular Surgeons, 1969.
18. Kinmonth JB: The Lymphatics: Surgery, Lymphography and Diseases of the Chyle and Lymph Systems. London, Edward Arnold, 1982.
19. Schmidt KR, Welter H, et al.: Lymphangiographische Untersuchungen zum Extremitatenodem nach rekonstruktiven Gefasseingriffen im Femoropoplitealbereich. Roefo 128:194, 1978.
20. Taylor GW, Kinmonth JB, et al.: Lymphatic circulation studied with radioactive plasma protein. Br Med J 5011:133, 1957.
21. Emmett AJ, Barron JN, Veall N: The use of I-131 albumin tissue clearance measurements and other physiological tests for the clinical assessment of patients with lymphoedema. Br J Plast Surg 20:1, 1967.
22. Thompson N: Buried dermal flap operation for chronic lymphedema of the extremities. Ten year survey of results in 79 cases. Plast Reconstr Surg 45:541, 1970.
23. O'Donnell TF, Kalisher L, et al.: Assessment of lymphedema by xeroradiography. Physiologist 19:3, 1976.
24. Wolfe JH, Kinmonth JB: The prognosis of primary lymphedema of the lower limbs. Arch Surg 116:1157, 1981.
25. O'Donnell TF: Abnormal peripheral lymphatics, in Clouse ME, Wallace S (eds): Lymphatic Imaging. Lymphography, Computed Tomography and Scintigraphy, 2nd ed. Baltimore, The Williams & Wilkins Co., 1985, p 142.
26. Zeissler RM, Rose G, Nelson PA: Postmastectomy lymphedema: Late results of treatment in 385 patients. Arch Phys Med Rehabil 53:159, 1972.
27. Van der Molen HR, Toth LM: The conservative treatment of lymphedema of the extremities. Angiology 25:470, 1974.
28. Raines JK, O'Donnell TF, et al.: Selection of patients with lymphedema for compression therapy. Am J Surg 133:430, 1977.
29. Zelikovski A, Manoach M, et al.: Lympha-press, a new pneumatic device for the treatment of lymphedema of the limbs. Lymphology 13:68, 1980.
30. Richmand DR, O'Donnell TF, Zelikowski A: Sequential pneumatic compression for lymphedema. A controlled trial. Arch Surg 120:1116, 1985.
31. Casley-Smith JR, Foldi-Borcsok E, Foldi M: A fine structural study of the removal of the effectiveness of benzo-pyrone treatment of lymphedema by the destruction of the macrophages by silica. Br J Exp Pathol 59:116, 1978.
32. Chilvers AS, Kinmonth JB: Operation for lymphedema of the lower limbs. A study of the results in 108 operations using vascularized dermal flaps. J Cardiovasc Surg 16:115, 1975.
33. Kondoleon E: Die Chirurgische behandlulnng der elephantiastischen oedeme. Munch Med Wochenschr 59:525, 1912.
34. Sistrunk WE: Modifications of the operation for elephantiasis. JAMA 71:800, 1918.

35. Handley WS: Lymphangioplasty. Lancet 1:783, 1908.
36. O'Reilly K: Treatment by nylon setons of lymphedema of the arm following radical mastectomy. Med J Aust 1:1269, 1972.
37. Silver D, Puckett J: Lymphangioplasty: A 10 year evaluation. Surgery 80:748, 1980.
38. Kerstein MD, Licalzi L: Microvascular procedures in the management of lymphedema. Vasc Surg 11:188, 1977.
39. Nielubowicz J, Olszewski W: Surgical lymphaticovenous shunts in patients with secondary lymphedema. Br J Surg 9:262, 1968.
40. Degni M: New techniques of lymphatic-venous anastomosis for the treatment of lymphedema. J Cardiovasc Surg 19:577, 1978.
41. Packett CL, Jacobs GR, et al.: Evaluation of lympho-venous anastomoses in obstructive lymphedema. Plast Reconstr Surg 66:116, 1980.
42. Politowski M, Bartowski S, Dynowski J: Treatment of lymphedema of the limbs by lymphatico-venous fistula. Surgery 66:639, 1969.
43. Milanov NO, Abalmasov KG, Lein AP: Correction of lymph flow disturbances following radical mastectomy. Vestn Khir 128:63, 1982.
44. Gong-Kang H, Ru-Qi H, et al.: Microlymphaticovenous anastomosis in the treatment of lower limb obstructive lymphedema: Analysis of 91 cases. Plast Reconstr Surg 76:671, 1985.
45. O'Brien BM, Das SK: Microlymphatic surgery in management of lymphoedema of the upper limb. Ann Acad Med Singapore 8:474, 1979.
46. Clodius L, Piller NB, Casley-Smith JR: The problems of lymphatic microsurgery for lymphedema. Lymphology 14:69, 1981.
47. Goldsmith HS: Long term results of omental transposition for chronic lymphoedema. Ann Surg 180:847, 1974.
48. Hurst PA, Kinmonth JB, Rutt DL: A mesenteric pedicle graft for bridging lymphatic obstruction. Br J Surg 65:358, 1978.
49. Kinmonth JB, Hurst PA, et al.: Relief of lymph obstruction by use of a bridge of mesentery and ileum. Br J Surg 5:829, 1978.
50. Hurst PA, Stewart G, et al.: Long term results of the entero-mesenteric bridge operation in the treatment of primary lymphoedema. Br J Surg 72:272, 1985.
51. Thompson N: The surgical treatment of chronic lymphoedema of the extremities. Surg Clin North Am 47:445, 1967.
52. Harvey RF: The use of 131-I labelled human serum albumin in the assessment of improved lymph flow following buried dermis flap operations in cases of post-mastectomy lymphedema of the arm. Br J Radiol 42:260, 1969.
53. Sawney CP: Evaluation of Thompson's buried dermal flap operation for lymphedema of the limbs: A clinical and radioisotopic study. Br J Plast Surg 27:278, 1974.
54. Charles RH: in Latham A, English TC (eds): A System of Treatment, vol 3. London, J & A Churchill Ltd, 1912, p 504.
55. Dellon AL, Hoopes JE: The Charles procedure for primary lymphedema. Long-term clinical results. Plast Reconstr Surg 60:589, 1977.
56. Miller TA: Charles procedure for lymphedema: A warning. Am J Surg 139:290, 1980.
57. Homans J: Treatment of elephantiasis of legs. N Engl J Med 215:1099, 1936.
58. Miller TA: Surgical management of lymphedema of the extremity. Plast Reconstr Surg 56:633, 1975.
59. Miller TA: A surgical approach to lymphedema. Am J Surg 134:191, 1977.
60. Fonkalsrud EW: Surgical management of congenital lymphedema in infants and children. Arch Surg 114:1133, 1979.
61. Feins NR, Rubin R, et al.: Surgical management of 39 children with lymphedema. J Pediatr Surg 12:471, 1977.
62. Hughes JH, Patel AR: Swelling of the arm following radical mastectomy. Br J Surg 53:4, 1966.
63. Larsen NE, Crampton AR: A surgical procedure for postmastectomy edema. Arch Surg 106:475, 1973.
64. O'Donnell TF: Congenital mixed vascular deformities of the lower extremities: The relevance of lymphatic abnormalities to their diagnosis and treatment. Ann J Surg 185:162, 1977.
65. Buonocore E, Young JR: Lymphangiographic evaluation of lymphedema and lymphatic flow. AJR 95:751, 1965.
66. Saijo M, Monroe IR, Mancer K: Lymphedema: A clinical review and follow-up study. Plast Reconstr Surg 56:513, 1975.
67. Thompson N: The surgical treatment of advanced postmastectomy lymphedema of the upper limb. With the later results of treatment by buried dermis flap operation. Scand J Plast Reconstr Surg 3:54, 1969.
68. Bunchman MM, Lewis SR: The treatment of lymphedema. Plast Reconstr Surg 54:64, 1974.
69. Kinmonth JB, Patrick JH, Chilvers AS: Comments on operations for lower limb lymphedema. Lymphology 8:56, 1975.
70. Krylov VS, Rabkin IE, et al.: Rol'limfografii pri opredelenii pokazanii k nalozheniiu priamogo limfovenoznogo anastomoza. Khirurgiia (Mosk) 9:3, 1979.

PART VIII
Amputations and Rehabilitation

CHAPTER 76
Amputation of Lower Extremity

Henry Haimovici

According to a 1966 census conducted by H. W. Glattly,[1] of the National Research Council, the total number of amputations in the United States was estimated at more than 30,000 a year, of which 85% were for the lower extremity. Of these, over 80% were necessary because of ischemic gangrene alone, the rest being for injury. In 1975, Kay and Newman[2] reported on 6000 new amputations and showed that 93% were performed in patients over 61 years old, for vascular disease, with a male/female ratio of approximately 9:1. These figures indicate the magnitude of the problem that the great number of patients afflicted with advanced vascular disease may face, in spite of the fact that, since the advent of the reconstructive arterial surgery era, the outlook for many of these patients has been radically improved. Indeed, today limb salvage, in the presence of even advanced ischemic changes, may be achieved in a fairly high percentage of cases. Before any level of limb amputation, evaluation for a possible reconstructive arterial procedure is being done in all patients.

Unfortunately, in spite of this progress, a relatively large number of patients, especially those with associated diabetes mellitus, still fall in the group with unsalvageable ischemic lesions of the lower extremity.

As a result of accumulating experience since the mid-1960s, new concepts in amputee management have emerged.[3-5] The main reasons for the recent progress are the availability of multidisciplinary services and a few basic guiding principles.

1. Amputation, as an operative act, should be considered in the context of preoperative and postoperative care. This can be achieved by the services of skilled teams, including vascular surgeons, rehabilitation personnel, prosthetists, and psychosocial guidance personnel.
2. Gentle, atraumatic handling of the tissues is essential to avoid failures, usually because of the critical wound healing of the ischemic tissues.
3. Amputation should not be looked on merely as synonym for cutting off a limb. It must be considered a plastic and reconstructive operation requiring great respect for tissues and careful wound management, with a view to early patient rehabilitation. Unfortunately, amputations in general are regarded as devoid of any challenge and are often relegated to the junior member of the staff, who is usually lacking in knowledge and experience.
4. Selection of a site for amputation is often a critical decision that requires proper evaluation of the degree of blood supply at this level.[6,7] It should be based not on the preconceived "safest" site for healing but on vascular assessment of tissue viability.

Although it is obvious that the first amputation must be the last, this principle should in no way substitute a safe judgment for a properly evaluated level of amputation. This attitude has much too often led the surgeon with little experience to do an above-knee amputation, the acknowledged safest site for early healing, when a more distal one should have been indicated. The detailed criteria for levels of amputation will be described below. Suffice it to state at this point that healing not only at the below-knee but also at the foot level may occur more often if the basic principles of evaluating arterial insufficiency and careful technique are observed rigorously.

PRINCIPLES OF CONSERVATIVE MANAGEMENT (NONSURGICAL)

In the presence of severe ischemia of the extremities characterized by rest pain and impending or frank gangrene, the scope of conservative nonsurgical management is necessarily limited. Its basic principles include (1) protection of the involved extremity, (2) meticulous treatment of the lesions, and (3) use of antibiotics, analgesics, and vasodilators.

Protective measures, such as bed rest and avoidance of any pressure or trauma to the affected extremity, are essential. Thus a cradle should be placed over the feet, and the patient's limb should rest on a pillow to prevent pressure on the toes and heel, the two areas most vulnerable to any degree of trauma.

Meticulous foot care is one of the prerequisites for successful conservative management. Soap-and-water footbaths should be followed by the application of local dressings consisting of antibiotic ointment or plain petrolatum gauze on the lesion. Special attention should be paid to the interdigital spaces, where ulcers or draining sinuses may be overlooked. The dressing should cover the entire involved area. Local debridement of lesions should be done only if there is evidence of their separation from the adjacent tissues and should not be carried beyond their demarcation line.

Antibiotics are essential, especially for the lesions associated with lymphangitis or cellulitis. In diabetic patients, fungal infection, mostly in the interdigital spaces, is quite prevalent. After the footbath, to which an antibacterial solution such as povidone-iodine has been added, the skin should be dried and a fungicidal powder applied.

Analgesics are required for severe rest pain, which usually prevents sleep. One may have to try the entire gamut of these medications, ranging from aspirin to opiates, before relieving this ischemic pain.

Smoking is to be avoided completely. It aggravates all arterial diseases.

Vasodilating drugs have been recommended in the management of chronic arterial disease, but they are of little or no value in the presence of advanced ischemic lesions.

AMPUTATIONS

Preoperative Management

The first step in the care of the patient with an ischemic foot and gangrene is bed rest. The major objectives in the preoperative phase are (1) avoidance of trauma, (2) control of infection, (3) control of pain, and (4) preservation of muscular strength and joint motion (rehabilitation).

Avoidance of Trauma
The patient should be in Fowler's position, with the limb slightly dependent, the leg and thigh being supported by a pillow to avoid any possible pressure on the heel. A lambskin mat placed under it may help to prevent decubitus pressure. A heel protector consisting of a 1- to 1½-inch thick foam pad secured to the heel may be more helpful. Overhead handles should be provided to enable the patient to turn over in bed without pushing with the feet and elbows. A cradle should be placed over the foot to avoid the weight of blankets on the toes.

Control of Infection
Foot care is an integral part of the preoperative treatment and should consist of (1) daily gentle washings of the foot and leg with lukewarm water and soap, (2) removal of all scabs, (3) debridement of calluses or corns under which an abscess is often present, (4) application of antibiotic ointment in the open ulcerations or in the necrotic lesions with denuded edges, and (5) systemic antibiotics.

Control of Pain
Control of pain is an important facet of the management, especially in patients who have dependency edema as a result of prolonged sitting during the day and often during the night because of rest pain. Use of analgesics is particularly necessary to enable the patient to sleep with the legs horizontal and thus to reduce edema so as to render the tissues more suitable for local surgery.

Rehabilitation
The patient's rehabilitation should be started before amputation, to prevent deterioration of function in the muscles and joints. An integrated program with the rehabilitation department is an important part of the preoperative and postoperative management of the amputee.

General Principles for Selection of Level of Amputation

Selection of the level of amputation depends on local and systemic factors. Among the local factors are the type of onset of the ischemia, which may be acute, progressive, or chronic, the extent of gangrene or ulceration, the degree of infection, the condition of adjacent areas, the degree of arterial impairment, and the severity of pain.

Gangrene
Acute ischemia is usually due to arterial embolism, thrombosis, or vascular injuries. The clinical features and treatment differ from those of the other two types of ischemia, especially the chronic. As described previously (Chapters 28, 29, and 31), in the presence of acute ischemia, with pregangrenous or frank gangrenous lesions not suitable for salvage procedures, the level of amputation in the majority of patients is above the knee. The timing of the amputation will depend on the degree of pain, systemic toxicity, presence of myoglobinuria due to myonecrosis, and renal toxicity (oliguria or anuria). These factors are characteristic of acute rhabdomyolosis and are not seen in progressive or chronic arterial occlusions. (For further information, see Chapter 28.) *Chronic* ischemia is most commonly due to arteriosclerosis (Chapters 35 and 36).

The extent of gangrene and the presence or absence of a demarcation line are important factors. Absence of a line of demarcation usually indicates a spreading process, which precludes a local conservative procedure. The presence of a demarcation line, on the other hand, implies that the gangrene has become localized and that vascularity proximal to this point is adequate. Unless the general condition of the patient contraindicates delay, it is always an advantage to wait for the development of a sharp line of demarcation.

Infection
Local infection associated with gangrene is often present in varying degree, especially in diabetic patients. Infection may become a major problem if spreading lymphangitis or cellulitis that cannot be checked is present. In such cases, and in the presence of suppuration, surgery cannot be de-

layed. Exclusive use of antibiotics may not be helpful and ultimately may prove disastrous in uncontrollable sepsis.

Condition of Adjacent Areas

Evaluation of the tissues proximal to the gangrenous area is essential when local surgery is contemplated. Color changes, trophic lesions of the skin, edema, and bone involvement are important criteria. Thus, cyanosis of the skin proximal to the gangrenous area that is not reversible on elevation of the limb usually indicates advanced ischemia of the tissues and contraindicates local surgery. Thin, shiny skin with marked loss of subcutaneous tissue suggests poor vascularity. Edema in the absence of venous obstruction or cardiorenal disease is generally due to dependency and can be eliminated by keeping the limb horizontal.

Degree of Arterial Impairment

For evaluating the degree of arterial insufficiency, noninvasive modalities (Chapter 2), arteriography (Chapter 33), and clinical criteria may provide most of the desired information. The acute or chronic mode of onset often determines not only the extent of the gangrene but also the level of amputation. The patency of major arteries is determined by palpation and should be checked with Doppler ultrasound, a pulse volume recorder (PVR), and an ankle/arm pulse index (Chapter 2). Although the presence of a popliteal or pedal pulse appears to ensure prompter healing of a toe or transmetatarsal amputation wound, absence of these pulses is not a contraindication to surgery at this level. This also holds true for the below-knee level. Use of xenon 133 for blood flow measurement has been advocated as another index (see Below-Knee amputation). Obviously, in the absence of functioning major arteries, it is axiomatic that the vascularization of the tissues depends on the degree of collateral circulation. Elevation-dependency tests and skin temperatures at different levels determined under basal conditions are helpful guides in assessing the collateral arterial supply. Rapid blanching of the toes and foot on elevation and marked rubor on dependency suggest poor collaterals. The presence of a sharp difference in skin temperature between the proximal and distal areas of the extremity indicates recent arterial occlusion. Under these circumstances, the level of amputation must be well above the cold area. Whenever possible, surgery is delayed in the hope that collateral circulation may develop and thereby permit a more distal amputation.

Pain

Pain is commonly associated with ischemic tissues and is more severe when gangrene is spreading. When pain radiates from the involved toes toward the ankle or leg and remains unrelieved by heavy sedation, it should be regarded as a contraindication to a toe or transmetatarsal procedure. A higher level for amputation is then indicated.

Systemic Factors

The general condition of the patient should always be evaluated as to age, severity of diabetes, toxicity, cardiac status, presence of hypertension, cerebrovascular accidents, renal function, and water-electrolyte balance. An attempt is made to *grade* each patient according to these factors. Although the local signs are the chief criteria determining the level of amputation, in some patients the poor or precarious general condition is important in guiding the choice of the surgical procedure.

Finally, in assessing both local and systemic factors, it is important to consider the duration of the lesions, the initiating cause, the effectiveness of previous treatments, and the condition of the other leg.

LEVELS OF AMPUTATION

There are six possible levels of amputation for ischemic gangrene: (1) toes, (2) transmetatarsal, (3) Syme, (4) supramalleolar, (5) midleg (below-knee), and (6) thigh (above-knee) (Fig. 76-1).

Toes

Two levels are available for amputation of toes: transphalangeal and transmetatarsal.

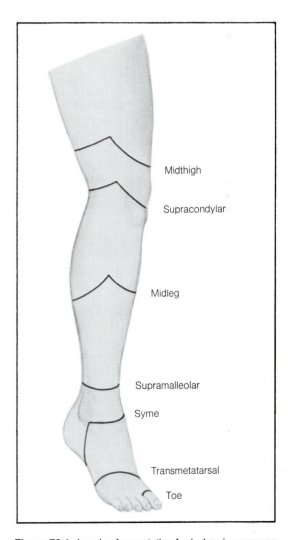

Figure 76-1. Levels of amputation for ischemic gangrene.

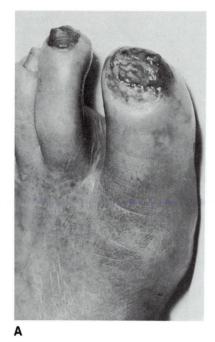
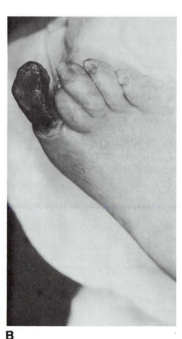

A   **B**

Figure 76-2. A. Ischemic ulcer of the great toe localized to the distal phalanx and involving the nail bed. **B.** Gangrene of the right great toe involving distal and half of proximal phalanges. Note demarcation line. Patient had a successful femoropopliteal bypass graft, which was instrumental in arresting gangrenous process. The toe was subsequently removed through demarcation line.

Transphalangeal

Transphalangeal amputations through the proximal phalanx are feasible only when the following *indications* are present: (1) localized and well-demarcated necrosis or (2) deep ulceration, with or without denuded bone or exposed tendon, of the distal end of the toes (Fig. 76-2A,B). This procedure may be performed on one or more toes simultaneously.

Contraindications to this level of amputation are (1) lack of a demarcation line, (2) lesions extending to the proximal phalanx, (3) uncontrolled infection, (4) dependency rubor of the toes, (5) sharp difference in skin temperature between toes and adjacent forefoot, and (6) severe rest pain affecting the toes and proximal foot as well.

Preoperative skin care, use of antibiotics, and extreme gentleness in handling the tissues during the amputation cannot be overemphasized.

Technique. The patient is placed in the supine position, with the foot slightly dependent. The skin preparation must be gentle and should include the interdigital spaces of all toes and extend to the entire foot up to the ankle.

Equal lateral flaps, in preference to dorsal–plantar ones, should be used (Fig. 76-3). The apex of the skin incisions must be just distal to the base of the proximal phalanx, which is distal to the metatarsophalangeal joint.

The incisions are carried down to the bones, the tendons are first stretched and then cut to allow them to retract proximally, and the phalanx is divided with a bone cutter. Bleeding arterioles are ligated.

The skin flaps are approximated without tension and are closed with a few wide interrupted sutures. In well-demarcated, distally located lesions, in the absence of cellulitis and edema, a closed amputation is the method of choice.

In the presence of uncontrollable infection, all the other factors being equal, the stump is left open. The operative technique is similar to that for a closed amputation, except that the incision may be extended proximally into the plantar or dorsal surfaces of the foot for drainage of associated infected tendon sheaths. The wound is gently packed open with ½-inch plain gauze placed in the wound. A continuous wet dressing, with plain normal saline solution or an antibiotic solution, is applied for a few days until the gross infection has subsided. Then one may switch to an antibiotic ointment, which is applied to the wound, the dressing being changed daily. Healing occurs by second intention and usually requires several weeks.

Transmetatarsal

Transmetatarsal amputations are most suitable for the first and fifth toes. If the lesions extend beyond the distal phalanx and affect the adjacent toes (second or fourth), a two-toe transmetatarsal amputation may be indicated. Contraindications to this type of amputation are the same as for the transphalangeal, especially if the lesions (necrosis and infection) extend into the interdigital webs and beyond.

The decision as to a one- or two-toe amputation, as opposed to a five-toe amputation, may sometimes be difficult to make. It is the author's experience that a transmetatarsal amputation of the foot is preferable to a two-toe amputation. Healing is usually prompter, and recurrent toe lesions are avoided.

Procedure. The procedure for the first or fifth toe is carried out with the patient in the supine position. Preparation of the skin is similar to that for the transphalangeal amputation.

A racquet-type skin incision is used, and a slightly longer plantar flap is fashioned so as to obtain a dorsal scar (Fig. 76-4A,B,C). In making the incision around the base of the toe, it is important not to cut through the skin of the base of the adjacent digit. A few millimeters of skin

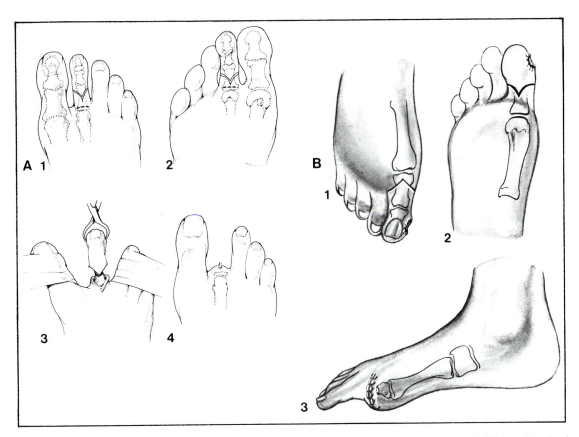

Figure 76-3. A. Technique of transphalangeal amputation of second toe. Note use of lateral flaps and division of proximal phalanx at its base. 1. Dorsal view. 2. Plantar view. 3. Dorsal view of the skin flaps. 4. Closure of the stump. **B.** Transphalangeal amputation of great toe. 1. Skin incision of flaps, dorsal view. 2. Plantar view of same. 3. Suture of stump.

of the proximal phalanx of the amputated toe should be left to facilitate the closure of the angle.

The tip of the toe is then held with a towel clip. The toe is disarticulated, great care being taken not to open the joint of the adjacent toe.

Flaps are developed without removing the subcutaneous tissue. The head of the metatarsal and the neck are freed of the soft tissues by carrying out the deboning close to the metatarsal. A Gigli saw is used for dividing the bone. Its end should be beveled to avoid a sharp angle on the skin. The removal of sesamoids is optional. Excess skin flap should be trimmed, care being taken to achieve closure without tension.

A drain (¼-inch Penrose) may be used through a stab wound of the plantar flap at the most dependent position, if oozing is present.

Postoperative care is similar to that of other foot amputations (toes or transmetatarsals).

Transmetatarsal Amputation of the Foot

Transmetatarsal amputation was first reported in 1949 by McKittrick et al.[7] and consists of removal of all the toes and metatarsal heads, thus creating a short foot. In the majority of cases, the procedure is carried out for diabetic patients, who are more liable than nondiabetics to develop necrotic lesions of the toes.[8]

Indication for a transmetatarsal amputation is gangrene or ulceration of one or several toes (Fig. 76-5). A sharp line demarcating the lesions is a favorable sign, whereas absence of a line of demarcation, usually indicating a spreading process, is a contraindication. Considerable experience and judgment are necessary to formulate the correct indications for this operation. In cases of recent gangrene, for instance, it is important to wait for the development of a sharp line of demarcation before the level of amputation can be safely decided on. In some selected cases, involving the first or fifth toe, as pointed out above, single-toe amputation may be carried out with a reasonable chance of success. However, our experience, as well as that of others, suggests that it is always safer to perform a transmetatarsal amputation of all the toes, especially when more than one is involved.[8]

Local infection, frequently associated with gangrenous or ulcerated lesions, should be controlled before surgery, either by antibiotics alone or in combination with adequate drainage. After the infection has been brought under control, a closed amputation can be performed safely. However, in cases without control of infection due to invasive deep sepsis, an open procedure is more expedient and safer. It is usually necessary to wait 2 to 3 weeks before operation to accomplish a good result. After this period of bed rest and local treatment, the patient should be free of ischemic pain and the infection should be arrested.

The index of tissue viability on the dorsum and plantar

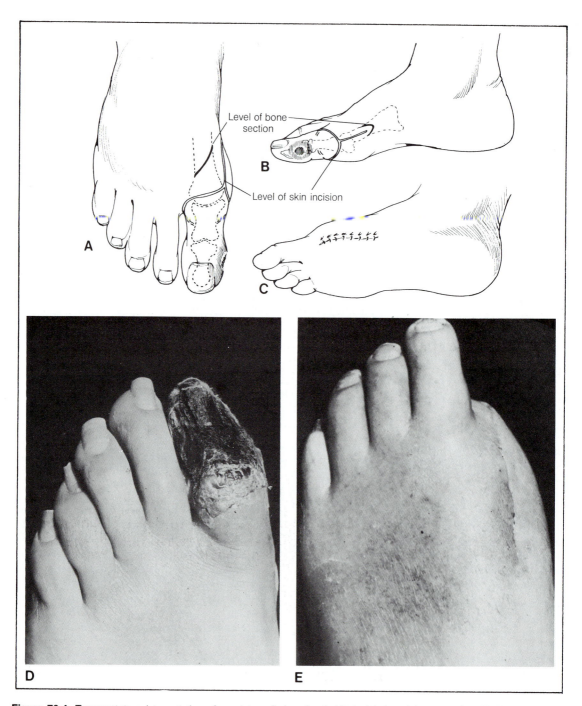

Figure 76-4. Transmetatarsal amputation of great toe. **A.** Levels of skin incision and bone section. **B.** Medial view of same. **C.** Skin closure. **D.** Gangrenous lesion of the great toe. **E.** Healed transmetatarsal amputation of great toe.

flaps should be assessed both clinically and, if possible, arteriographically. Clinically, the area should be free of dependent rubor, and the venous filling time on the dorsum of the foot should not be unduly prolonged (not more than 12 to 20 seconds).

Contraindications are permanent cyanosis and shiny, thin skin with marked loss of subcutaneous tissue. Extension of gangrene from the toe toward the dorsum or ball of the foot is indicative of poor prognosis.

Local edema due to dependency and osteomyelitis of the metatarsal bones do not always preclude a successful outcome. However, it is essential that dependency edema be eliminated by the horizontal position of the lower extremity before operation. The presence of osteomyelitis despite the use of antibiotics may necessitate an open amputation. Local pain radiating toward the ankle or leg, often unrelieved by narcotics, should be regarded as a contraindication.

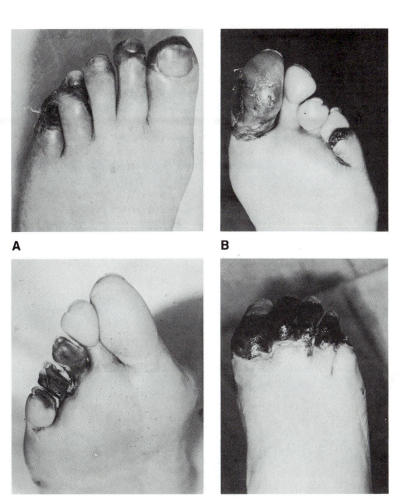

A

B

C

D

Figure 76-5. A to **D.** Gangrenous toe lesions treated with transmetatarsal amputation of foot.

Technique

Preoperative Care. Successful outcome of a transmetatarsal amputation requires careful preoperative asepsis of the foot, a fact that cannot be too strongly emphasized. Washing the skin once or twice daily with surgical soap and water, especially the interdigital webs, for a period of about a week is strongly recommended in all cases.

Anesthesia. Spinal or epidural anesthesia is most suitable for these patients.

Position. The patient is placed in a supine position with the foot and lower half of the leg prepared and draped in the usual fashion. The gangrenous toes are covered with an occlusive dressing.

Skin Incisions. The *dorsal* incision is made in a coronal shape at the midshaft level of the metatarsals, extending from the edge of the plantar surface of the foot on one side across to the edge of the plantar surface on the other side just posterior to the narrowest portion of the metatarsals.

The *plantar* incision extends from the previous one at a right angle along its edge to within 1 cm of the flexion area between the base of the toes and the ball of the foot. It is a curved and parallel incision at the level of the metatarsal heads. Incision is carried down to the metatarsophalangeal joints. By dorsiflexion of the toes, the incision can very easily reach these joints and start their separation. All the toes are disarticulated at the metatarsophalangeal joints.

Flaps. A plantar flap (Fig. 76-6) is then developed through the cleavage spaces in an attempt to avoid any unnecessary trauma. The metatarsals and the adjacent tendons are thus separated from the plantar flap. The latter is dissected proximally up to the proposed site of division of the metatarsals.

Division of Metatarsals. First the metatarsals are separated by dividing the intrinsic muscles with straight scissors, to the level of the dorsal flap retraction, and then transected individually by means of a Gigli saw. The head of the metatarsal is held with a bone holder, the dorsal flap is retracted gently by the assistant, and the Gigli saw is positioned as proximally as possible without injuring any of the soft tissues. After division of the metatarsals, further shortening of their ends by means of a rongeur may sometimes be necessary.

The loose tendons and any traumatized tissue are ex-

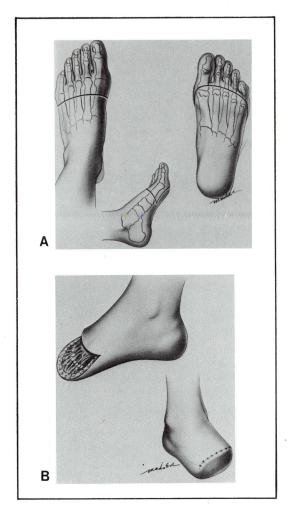

Figure 76-6. A. Drawings depicting lines of skin incisions for fashioning dorsal and plantar flaps. **B.** Plantar flap and closure of amputation stump.

cised and carefully trimmed away. Since primary healing is not always certain, the skin flaps must be handled with great gentleness. Dissecting forceps for holding the flaps must be avoided. It cannot be overemphasized that in these ischemic tissues, the margin between success and failure may be very slight.

Closure. Before closure of the amputation is carried out, the wound is irrigated with an antibiotic solution (kanamycin). The flaps are then approximated without tension by means of nonabsorbable silk or synthetic fibers or fine stainless steel wire. A drain is unnecessary in most instances, except when oozing is uncontrollable. In such cases, a ½-inch Penrose drain is placed between the flaps, to be removed within 48 to 72 hours.

Postoperative Care. The dressing consists of a layer of petrolatum gauze placed on the suture line and a wide gauze dressing applied over the entire foot up to the ankle and secured in place with a 3- to 4-inch gauze bandage.

The foot is placed on a foam rubber pillow in a slightly dependent position. A cradle is placed over it to protect the stump from any trauma. Administration of antibiotics

is continued for 10 to 14 days or longer if necessary. Sutures are removed 14 to 21 days postoperatively.

After healing of the stump, resumption of weight bearing is delayed by about 2 more weeks. The patient is then instructed to use properly fitted shoes and cautious ambulation. The patient may use his or her ordinary shoes in which the fore part is blocked with a foam rubber piece tailored to replace the missing toes. A metal shank may be placed in the sole of the shoe to prevent curling up.

Amputations proximal to the head of the metatarsals involve the loss of the normal weight-bearing mechanism of the forefoot. If the stump contracts in an equinovarus position, an orthopedic shoe may be necessary to correct this deformity. This has rarely occurred in my experience.

Transmetatarsal Amputation with Wedge Excision of Plantar Flap

Chronic ulceration of the ball of the foot frequently develops in patients with occlusive arterial disease and diabetes. These lesions usually involve the plantar surface under a metatarsal head and appear as an open, infected area surrounded by thick callus leading to a denuded tendon or joint. Although such lesions often heal with bed rest and local dressings, the associated diabetic neuropathic condition and the occasional underlying osteomyelitis of the

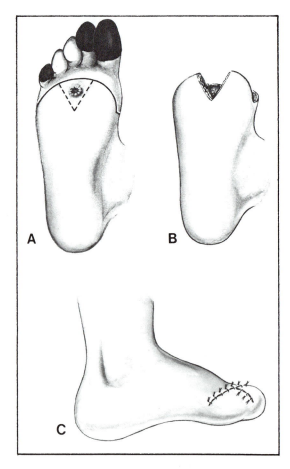

Figure 76-7. Drawing depicting transmetatarsal amputation with plantar wedge excision.

metatarsal head appear to be responsible for their great tendency to recur. In these cases, I recommend a modified transmetatarsal amputation.[9,10]

After a standard technique is carried out as described above, the plantar flap is revised at the level of the chronic ulceration. This consists of a wedge excision of the plantar flap involving the entire ulceration, the base of the wedge being distal and its tip proximal, as indicated in Figure 76-7. After excision of the involved area, the two segments of the plantar flap are approximated with a few interrupted sutures. The stump is then closed in the usual fashion by coapting the plantar and the dorsal flaps. A drain is placed across the foot between the two flaps and is left in place for 48 to 72 hours.

Postoperative care is guided by the same principles as in the standard procedure. In these cases, however, it is necessary to irrigate the stump through the drain with an antibiotic solution for a few days. Healing of the stump may be delayed by 1 or 2 weeks.

Open Transmetatarsal Amputation of Toes

Indications

The indications for open transmetatarsal amputation are a combination of the following: (1) gangrene of one or more toes associated with cellulitis and undrained infection ex-tending into adjacent metatarsal areas, usually occurring in patients with diabetic neuropathy having loss of pain sensation, or (2) ulcerated and infected calluses, including toe lesions. In all these cases, usually one or both pedal pulses are present.

Contraindications

Rarely do nondiabetic patients have a foot neuropathy with preservation of pedal pulses associated with gangrene of toes and sepsis. If severe ischemia is part of the findings, an open procedure usually fails and a higher level of amputation is required. In such cases, if arterial reconstruction is not feasible or successful, a primary amputation should be above the foot.

Procedure

In the presence of suppurative infection involving one or two toes in a neuropathic diabetic foot, the surgical treatment may be carried out in two stages.

In the *first stage*, a drainage amputation through the metatarsal of one or both toes is performed, provided there is evidence of good circulation in the foot (Fig. 76-8).

Before the procedure is undertaken, it is important to assess the extent of the infection, the presence of tenderness along the tendon sheaths, and the production of purulent or mixed purulent–necrotic tissue drainage by applying methodical pressure over the plantar and dorsal areas. Active

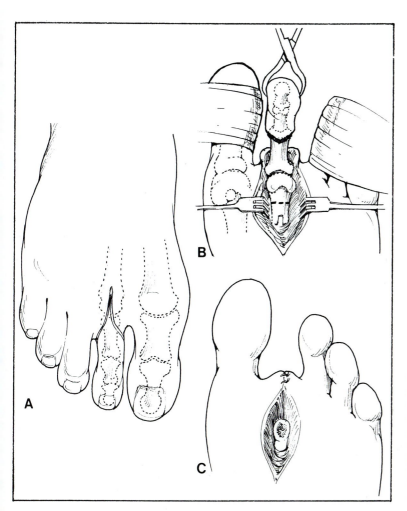

Figure 76.8. Drainage amputation. **A.** Skin incision of the second toe, dorsal view. **B.** Exposure of proximal phalanx and second metatarsal, plantar view. Note bone division proximal to metatarsal head. **C.** Reroofing of wound cavity and open plantar wound cavity and open plantar wound for drainage purposes. (*Adapted from Warren R, Record EE: Lower Extremity Amputations for Arterial Insufficiency. Boston, Little, Brown, 1967.*)

and passive movement of the toes is helpful in promoting drainage from the open lesions.

The operation at this stage consists of an *open transmetatarsal amputation* of toes. Amputation of the *first* and *fifth* toe is carried out as indicated in Figure 76-4A,B,C. Amputation of a middle toe is depicted in Figure 76-3A.

A plantar incision is carried out around the base of the toe and then is extended over the metatarsal area. The toe is disarticulated, and the metatarsal is divided through the midshaft. The flexor tendon is shortened. Reroofing of the toe stump with two or three sutures is often feasible. The plantar area over the divided metatarsal is left open for drainage (Fig. 76-8). If the infection extends along the flexor tendons, the length of the incision should extend slightly beyond, up to the level of normal-appearing tissue. Adequate drainage is essential.

Wet dressings with a topical antibiotic solution are applied for a few days until local drainage and infection are brought under control.

As mentioned earlier, in the performance of these amputations it is important to avoid entering the joints of adjacent toes. Sesamoid bones of the first toe are removed, and the wound cavity is left open for drainage.

Once the local sepsis and necrosis are cleared up and there is a good prospect for rehabilitation, further surgery may not be necessary. However, should there be residual gangrenous or ulcerative lesions of the other toes, a formal transmetatarsal amputation of the foot may be carried out as a *second stage*.

Open Transmetatarsal Amputation of the Foot

Indications for this procedure are the same as for single open-toe amputations. The technique for an open amputation is identical to the closed procedure, except that the stump is handled differently. Partial approximation of the flaps, with irrigation of the foot through a drain placed across the foot, is often sufficient to bring this condition under control. After 7 to 10 days, the local infection may subside. After removal of drains, the two flaps are approximated with a foot dressing.

In the presence of necrosis and infection, the stump is left wide open. Daily irrigations and dressings are continued until the wound is clean and granulating. Healing by second intention may occur within 2 to 3 months (Fig. 76-9).

Results

Successful outcome of a closed or open transmetatarsal amputation of the foot depends on strict adherence to several factors, indicated above.

The advantages of this procedure cannot be overemphasized, especially in elderly patients in whom a higher amputation may often result in prolonged rehabilitation or even permanent invalidism. Although the hospital stay of many of these patients is relatively long, use of their own limb fully justifies the efforts involved in their management (Fig. 76-10).

Rehabilitation of these patients is rather simple. Usually no special shoe is required: the toe of the regular shoe is

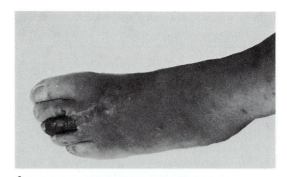

A

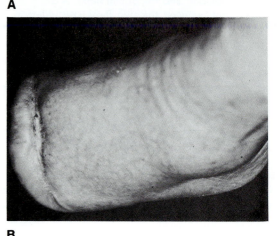

B

Figure 76-9. A. Gangrene of third toe and of adjacent two toes (lesion of fourth toe not visible on photograph). Note blister and underlying necrotic lesion of dorsum at level of third toe. These lesions were associated with deep invasive infection uncontrollable by antibiotics. The patient was diabetic and had severe sensory loss because of neuropathy but with excellent pedal pulses. An open transmetatarsal procedure was performed. **B.** Result of stump healing of open transmetatarsal amputations 3½ months later. This surgery was performed for lesions shown in **A.**

filled with cotton or with a foam rubber piece. At times, it is necessary to incorporate in the sole of the shoe a metal shank or a spring steel to prevent the curling up of the toe of the shoe. If a patient develops an ulcer or a callus on the stump, a tarsal bar added on the shoe may be helpful in preventing recurrence.

The immediate results of stump healing are slightly better in nondiabetic patients. In the open procedure, the rate of healing is less favorable than in the closed technique. The overall incidence of healing, based on our personal experience, is 66%. In the failures, a reamputation below the knee was carried out successfully in the majority of cases.

Follow-up results in these patients indicate that about 10% of them may require further amputations within 18 to 26 months after the original healing.[8,10] These results are similar to those reported by Wheelock,[11] who showed that 60 to 74% of his patients remained healed for 2 or more years after the amputation.

It should be pointed out again that prior revascularization by either bypass grafts (Fig. 76-11) or lumbar sympa-

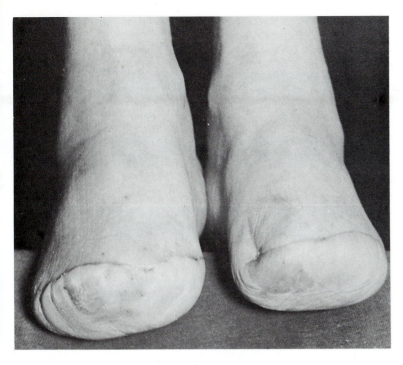

Figure 76-10. Healed bilateral transmetatarsal amputation stumps.

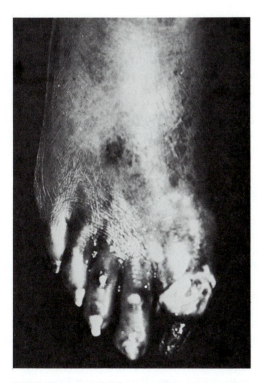

Figure 76-11. Gangrene of right great toe in process of separation after a femoropopliteal bypass. The bypass was carried out 1 week earlier for a spreading necrotic process associated with occlusion of the superficial femoral and anterior tibial arteries. Eventually the lesion was removed through proximal phalanx, and the toe healed by secondary intention.

thectomy may be helpful by providing a more adequate collateral circulation and thus increasing substantially the rate of success of transmetatarsal amputations.[12,13]

DIABETIC FOOT LESIONS

The ischemic lesions of the foot in a diabetic are frequently associated with, and sometimes dominated by, two other important clinical manifestations: diabetic neuropathy and local infection. Their association, in varying degrees, lends to the lesions a truly characteristic clinical picture, often referred to as the "diabetic foot." Because of their quasi-specificity, these lesions justify a separate description.[14]

The clinical manifestations may be classified under the following four headings: (1) arteriosclerosis obliterans, (2) peripheral neuropathy, (3) infection, and (4) combined lesions. Only the management of manifestations 2 and 3 will be considered in this section.

Peripheral Neuropathy

Peripheral diabetic neuropathy is perhaps one of the most significant and characteristic abnormalities encountered in diabetic patients. It may occur without arteriosclerosis obliterans, or the diabetic patient may develop this condition in combination with it. Despite a wide literature on this subject, these complications of diabetes often go unrecognized. Awareness of their presence is, however, essential for the proper management of the patient who displays trophic disorders of the lower extremities.

The major clinical manifestations include sensory disturbances, autonomic nerve involvement, trophic skin lesions with plantar ulcers, and degenerative arthropathy.

Infection

It is a well-established fact that diabetic patients are very vulnerable to infection. Any breaks in the continuity of the skin may act as a port of entry and a nidus for the growth of bacteria. In diabetes, pyogenic organisms are often associated with a mycotic infection, especially with epidermophytosis. It should be emphasized that foot sepsis usually starts as a mycotic infection, leading to the development of maceration. This may result in interdigital fissures or ulcerations that may become secondarily infected with bacteria. As a result of circulatory impairment, infection in diabetic patients is likely to lead readily to lymphangitis, cellulitis, deep tissue abscess, osteomyelitis, and ultimately gangrene. The loss of tissue can often be traced to an initial infection in subungual or interdigital ulcers, fissures of the heel, traumatic lesions of the foot, or ill-advised surgery for ingrown toenails or calluses and corns.

Clinically, the pedal pulses (dorsalis pedis and posterior tibial) are palpable, there is loss of pain sensation, and often there are callosities, usually ulcerated or displaying an infected hematoma under them. Frequently, the patients have an ingrowing toenail with subungual infection but little or no associated pain. Although the major arteries of the foot appear to be patent, the small arterioles are often occluded, the skin is usually warm, and the subcutaneous tissue appears well nourished.

The main *indications* for surgery in these patients with a diabetic foot are suppurative infection extending most often beyond the subcutaneous tissue into the subfascial plane of the foot and involving not uncommonly the adjacent joints.

Treatment of these various conditions varies according to the degree and extent of the infection and possible associated gangrene.

Infection of the nail groove or *nail bed* is due to either an ingrown toenail or an infected subungual hematoma or osteomyelitis of the phalanx. Decompression of these areas is essential to prevent further extension of tissue damage. Wedge excision of the nail is achieved without anesthesia in most patients. If anesthesia is necessary, a procaine block of the common peroneal nerve at the level of the neck of the fibula, near its emergence from the popliteal space, may be adequate to handle an ingrown nail of the great toe.

Infected heel fissures are best treated by bed rest, saline solution applications, and antibiotic ointment. Gentle lifting and excision of the thickened skin edges will free the underlying necrosis and provide drainage for the septic material. After debriding these lesions, a heel protector or a foam pad should be wrapped around the foot and ankle.

Superficial *lymphangitis* and *cellulitis*, not responding promptly to systemic antibiotics, most often mask underlying abscesses either of the subcutaneous tissue or of the subfascial layer. As a rule, the infection and necrosis are more extensive than the appearance of the skin would allow one to suspect. It is therefore essential not to procrastinate with the use of antibiotics and to proceed promptly with incision and drainage of these lesions.

In *superficial abscesses*, incision and debridement with wide drainage followed by continuous wet dressings with an antibiotic solution for 7 to 10 days may suffice to arrest the septic process.

Subfascial abscesses of the deep plantar surface are often more difficult to diagnose because of the presence of edema and absence of fluctuation. A mixture of pus and necrotic tissue is confined in the subfascial space with no spontaneous drainage. In most cases, one finds an associated gangrenous toe, an infected callus or bunion, or an infection in the web space between the toes, all of which may account for the invasive sepsis of the flexor tendon sheaths leading to the plantar space.

Surgical Management

The role of surgery in the management of deep plantar space infection depends on the extent of the infection and the associated lesions. Involvement of one toe is handled by (1) an open amputation, either through the proximal phalanx or through the metatarsal, and (2) subfascial incision of the adjacent plantar region with excision of the flexor tendons and necrotic tissue (Fig. 76-8). An additional dorsal incision may be necessary in some cases. Toe amputation, complete excision of devitalized tissues, and adequate drainage are required for successful treatment of these lesions (Fig. 76-8). This amputation-drainage procedure must be followed by daily wet wound packing, appropriate antibiotics, protective measures for the foot, and systemic supportive management.

The duration of the postoperative management may vary according to (1) the control of local sepsis and necrosis, and the necessity of further local debridement, and (2) the degree of associated ischemia.

In the presence of a popliteal and one pedal pulse the prognosis is usually good. After infection has subsided, the wound is left to close by secondary intention, or a revision of the amputation with primary closure may be carried out. A more formal proximal amputation may also have to be considered in some cases. A split-thickness skin graft can be used, especially in dorsal areas. In general, this type of treatment is prolonged and taxes the skill and patience of the surgeon and the nursing staff.

Syme Amputation

This operation, first described by Syme in 1842, is the classic amputation in the region of the ankle and until recently was used for nonvascular conditions only. The merits of this amputation for ischemic lesions of the forefoot appear to be limited. However, under certain defined circumstances, it may be a useful procedure.[15,16]

Indications are (1) well-demarcated gangrenous or ulcerated lesions of the foot beyond the metatarsal heads, involving the dorsum as well as the plantar aspect at the level of the ball of the foot, and (2) failure of a transmetatarsal amputation.

Contraindications are (1) gangrenous lesions of the heel or on the dorsum of the foot near the ankle and (2) obvious ischemic changes, as disclosed by rubor on dependency or a sharp decrease in skin temperature as compared with the proximal leg.

Clinical, thermometric, noninvasive, and arteriographic

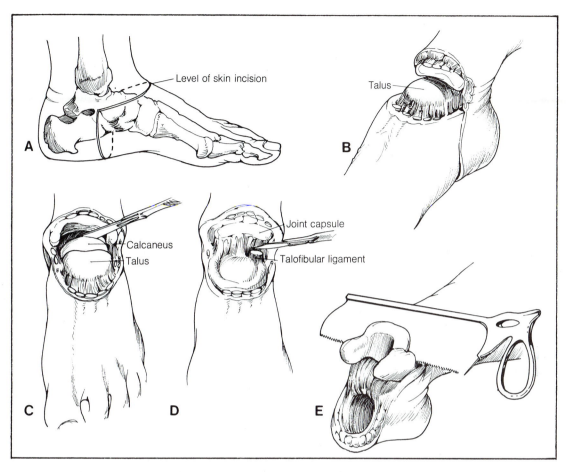

Figure 76-12. Syme amputation. **A.** Skin incision. **B.** Deepening of anterior incision. **C.** Further dissection of plantar flap by cleaning fascia from calcaneus. **D.** Division of talofibular ligament. **E.** Division of tibia and fibula above malleoli.

assessments of the circulation of the ankle and distal part of the foot are essential to determine the indications for the Syme amputation. Usually the ankle pulses are absent, although a popliteal pulse may be present. However, the collateral circulation at the level of the amputation site is the determining factor and cannot be properly evaluated by the measures described above. Prior lumbar sympathectomy or reconstructive arterial surgery by increasing the collateral circulation may, in certain instances, lower the amputation site from the midleg to the Syme level.

Surgical Technique

The patient is placed in the supine position. The surgeon stands at the end of the operating table facing the foot, which hangs over the table or is raised by a hard-rolled sheet placed under the lower third of the leg. The incision, shown in Figures 76-12 and 76-13, is made on the anteroinferior edge of the medial malleolus, extending around the sole of the foot coronally with the longitudinal axis, then to the anteroinferior border of the external malleolus, and finally around the anterior aspect of the ankle joint to meet the beginning of the incision. The ankle is disarticulated. It is first opened by division of its anterior ligament. Then the lateral ligaments are cut from within outward, and the foot is dislocated in a plantar direction.

The next step, which is the most important, consists

in the division of the posterior ligament of the joint, the detachment of the insertion of the tendo calcaneus, and the dissection of the calcaneum out of the heel flap. During these stages of the operation, the plantar dislocation of

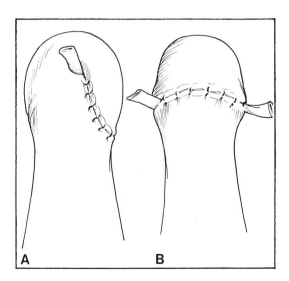

Figure 76-13. Syme amputation (continued). Stump with subfascial drain. **A.** Lateral view. **B.** Anterior view.

the foot is steadily increased. There is great danger of wounding the posterior tibial and peroneal arteries when the posterior ligament is cut, because both arteries are closely applied to the back of the ligament. Their branches, which supply the skin of the heel, are also in danger when the calcaneum is being dissected out of the flap. To avoid such accidents, which may result in sloughing of the flap, the surgeon keeps the knife closely applied to the bone throughout these stages of the operation. The anterior tibial artery, the medial and lateral plantar arteries, and the two saphenous veins are the main vessels that require ligation. Because the stump is to be an end-bearing one, particular attention should be paid to the shortening of the nerve trunks, so that these do not become involved in scar tissue at the end of the stump.

The tibia and fibula are divided across and perpendicular to the axis to remove the cartilage of the ankle joint. All the devitalized tissues are removed. The heel flap is folded over the bone ends and is sutured in position after being trimmed as required. Drainage is provided by a Penrose tube left in place for 48 to 72 hours.

Warren and Record[17] recommend a dressing consisting of a narrow flat sponge to be laid around the suture line. Because of the tendency of the heel flap to slip, they emphasize the need for a bridle as an essential part of the dressing, despite the fact that it will need frequent renewal for 3 weeks. The patient is not allowed to lower the stump before 2 weeks and thereafter only if tolerated. No prosthesis is attempted before 6 weeks.

Results

The resulting stump is a somewhat bulbous prominence in the ankle region. Most of the patients operated on were male. Understandably, this procedure is not popular with women because the prosthesis is also unsightly; most of them prefer a below-knee amputation.

The long-term observation of these stumps disclosed that, as a rule, they hold up well to the end-bearing pressure. Recurrent blistering and areas of necrosis occurring around the stump are due either to an ischemic flap or to misuse of the prosthesis. Although the few reports on the Syme amputation for ischemic lesions of the foot have been encouraging, this procedure has not been accepted widely by the majority of vascular surgeons. The successful outcome of this amputation may depend in large part on careful selection of the patients and meticulous postoperative care and proper use of the orthopedic shoe.

Supramalleolar or Lower-Third-of-Leg Amputation

Gangrene of the foot and spreading infection are serious surgical problems in patients in poor general condition. Despite the use of antibiotics and blood transfusions as well as other general measures, a major amputation still represents a great surgical risk in these cases. An open guillotine amputation through the lower third of the leg, just above the malleoli, offers great advantages in such desperate cases. Its rapid execution and minimal surgical trauma are its chief assets. This amputation may be performed either as a definitive procedure in cases of intractable

heart failure or malignant disease or as a preliminary step before an operation at the site of election becomes feasible. After supramalleolar amputation, the toxemia subsides, the general condition improves quickly, and diabetes becomes readily controlled. A midleg or thigh amputation with primary closure can then be done with much less risk.

Operative Technique

The patient is placed in the supine position. The foot is isolated carefully from the site of the amputation by an occlusive dressing just at the level of the malleoli. A tourniquet is not applied.

The skin incision is made about $1\frac{1}{2}$ to 2 inches above the malleoli at the narrowest part of the ankle (Fig. 76-14). The incision is carried through the skin, subcutaneous tissue, and fascia. At the site of retraction fascia, the muscles are divided down to the bones. The major vessels are clamped and divided. Both tibia and fibula are then sawed with a handsaw or electric saw at the site of retraction of the skin. The wound is irrigated with warm saline solution, and additional hemostasis is carried out as needed. A dressing consisting of a nonadherent petrolatum gauze is applied. Gauze dressing and a bandage are wrapped around the stump and leg. A posterior molded splint is then applied to maintain the knee straight.

If the procedure is performed as a preliminary to an elective higher amputation, the wound is left open. When sepsis is controlled, the proximal amputation may be carried out 7 to 10 days later.

If the procedure is performed as a definitive amputation, it is possible in certain instances to close the stump in two layers. The fascia is closed with interrupted 3–0 plain catgut and the skin with 4–0 silk sutures. A $\frac{1}{4}$-inch Penrose drain may be placed in the subfascial space for 48 to 72 hours. Antibiotics are administered as needed.

Results

In a series of 22 patients with supramalleolar amputations,[6] 14 of the amputations were done as a definitive procedure and the remainder as a preliminary to midleg amputation for 7 patients and midthigh amputation for 1 patient. Of those with the definitive procedure, 6 patients improved and their wounds healed (Fig. 76-15). Eight patients died in the hospital from visceral malignancy or intractable heart disease.

The major scope of this amputation remains one of eliminating uncontrollable infection or as a rapid guillotine in desperately ill patients with intractable cardiac disease or in those with metastatic malignancy.

Below-Knee[*] Amputation

In a 1968 survey of lower-extremity amputations for ischemia performed in 14 Veterans Administration hospitals,

---

[*]In previous editions, "midleg" was used instead of "below-knee amputation." The former specifically indicates the middle of the leg, whereas the latter may refer to the leg and foot as well. Because of usage, however, the term "below-knee" is the accepted term, with the understanding that it means an area 6 to 8 inches distal to the patella.

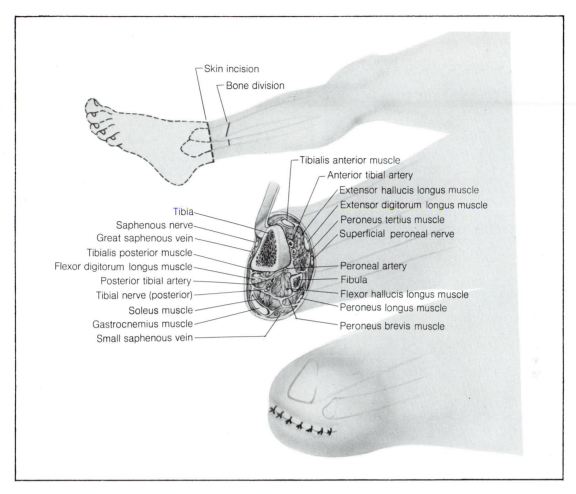

Figure 76-14. Supramalleolar amputation technique.

Warren and Kihn[18] found that the majority are still done above the knee joint. Before the antibiotic era, the reluctance of both general and vascular surgeons to perform below-knee amputations was somewhat understandable, but this attitude, still prevailing in some centers, is no longer justifiable. Since 1945, Silbert and I[19] have been advocating the below-knee (or midleg, the term used by us) amputation and have proved it to be feasible and highly successful. Since the mid-1950s, the trend from above-knee to below-knee amputation has been increasingly accepted, thus reflecting a changing concept in the management of gangrenous lesions of the foot.

Indications for this level of amputation are (1) gangrene of several toes, extending to or beyond the adjacent metatarsal lesion and showing no tendency to demarcate, (2) spreading gangrene of the foot, with or without associated gangrene of the heel or ankle, (3) spreading gangrene of several toes, associated with uncontrollable infection of the foot, and (4) failure of a transmetatarsal or Syme amputation.

Contraindications to this level of amputation are (1) extensive gangrene and infection of the leg, with absence of the femoral pulse at the groin, (2) gangrene of the foot associated with irreducible flexion contracture of the knee joint, and (3) recent acute occlusion of the femoral or iliac artery with inadequate collateral supply at below-knee level. In such instances it is not safe to amputate below the knee unless there has been an interval of at least 2 to 3 months after the arterial occlusion. This appears to be the necessary time for an adequate collateral circulation to develop to midleg level.

Clinical criteria include objective blood flow measurements at the proposed level of amputation, which may be helpful in cases in which doubt exists about the viability of the skin and underlying muscles. Several radioisotope clearances in the skin and muscle have therefore been advocated. Thus Moore[20] used xenon 133 by local injection of the skin to determine blood flow measurements at the site of the proposed amputation level. The critical flow rate for skin healing was estimated to be about 2 ml/100 g of tissue per minute. This and similar tests based on clearance of radioisotopic substances are less decisive in determining the level of amputation. Noninvasive tests and arteriography offer more direct information about the collateral circulation.

Ankle systolic blood pressure measurements, when compared with the brachial systolic pressure, provide an index (a/b) that is a better guide to the local vascularity

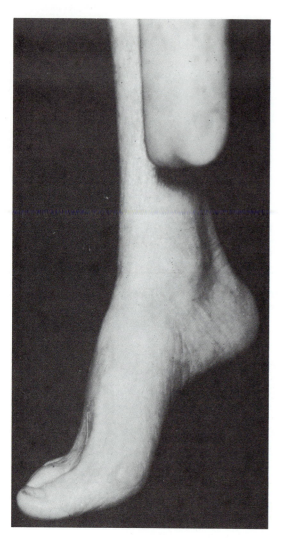

Figure 76-15. Healed open supramalleolar amputation in an 80-year-old woman who had gangrene and sepsis of the foot and heart failure.

(see Chapter 2.) However, the usefulness of the index in providing a criterion for amputation at the toe or metatarsal level is not always entirely accepted. Arteriography, although important in mapping the lesions of the major arteries and indicating the amount of collateral flow, may not always indicate the extent and adequacy of blood flow to the skin or muscle. Therefore, it is usually necessary to rely on combined clinical, noninvasive, and arteriographic findings for determining the level of amputation.

Because the below-knee level of amputation is critical in a dysvascular patient, strict adherence to principles of tissue, bone, vessel, and nerve management is essential for (1) providing a stump that will heal by first intention and (2) saving the knee joint. In the past few decades, great strides have been achieved both technically and in postamputation management.

Four below-knee amputation procedures are available, and choosing one of them depends on the specific case and on the surgeon's personal experience. The important features of these procedures are as follows: (1) use of anterior and posterior myocutaneous flaps, either unequal or equal, (2) use of long posterior myocutaneous flaps, (3) use of equal medial and lateral flaps, and (4) use of osteomyoplasty.

Use of Unequal Anterior and Posterior Myocutaneous Flaps

I have used unequal anterior and posterior flaps in certain below-knee amputation procedures for over three decades. The myocutaneous flaps are fashioned in two stages and joined at the closing of the stump, to form a myocutaneous flap. This procedure has been used only in the dysvascular cases. The flaps are always designed at a level where the vascularity of the skin appeared adequate. The posterior flap is slightly longer than the anterior. The muscles are divided after the skin flaps are fashioned. The two bones are divided at an appropriate proximal level, so as to prevent any possible tension or pressure on the skin and muscles at the closure of the stump. Furthermore, the tibial crest is removed by proper beveling of the tibial end. All the steps are detailed in the following description.

Operative Technique. Low spinal or epidural anesthesia is preferred in the majority of cases. Inhalation anesthesia may be employed whenever a spinal is contraindicated.

POSITION OF PATIENT. The patient may be placed in either the prone or the supine position. Placing the patient in the *prone position* offers great advantages in that it permits flexion of the leg and makes the operation much simpler (Fig. 76-16). Objection to this position, however, arises when a patient has severe cardiorespiratory problems. A tourniquet is not used, because it may seriously jeopardize an already precarious arterial supply to the leg.

LENGTH OF STUMP. The *ideal length* of the below-knee amputation stump ranges between $5\frac{1}{2}$ and 7 inches, depending on the height of the patient and the length of the leg. The procedure is carried out through the middle third, known as the "site of election." Although a shorter stump is not desirable in certain patients because of advanced proximal ischemia of the tissues, it is much preferable to have a short stump than an above-knee amputation.

SKIN FLAPS (Fig. 76-17). For the *posterior flap*, a curved incision is made on the posterior surface of the leg about 8 inches below the patella. The incision curves caudad, in a convex fashion, across the calf and then proceeds toward the lateral surface of the fibula. For the *anterior flap*, the leg is then flexed at a right angle and a shorter skin flap is made on the anterior surface of the leg. This incision extends almost across from the ends of the previously created posterior flap.

MUSCLE SECTION AND TREATMENT OF POSTERIOR NEUROVASCULAR BUNDLES. The leg is replaced in the horizontal position. At the level of skin retraction, the gastrocnemius, the plantaris tendon, and the soleus are divided. Section of the soleus muscle must be carried out carefully because of numerous avalvular veins in its body. The muscles are

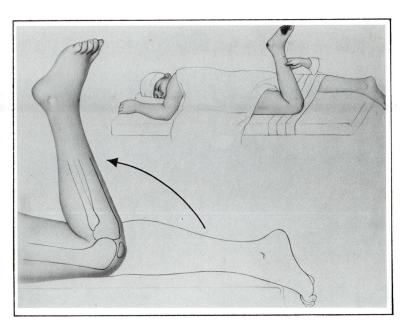

Figure 76-16. Prone position of patient for below-knee amputation.

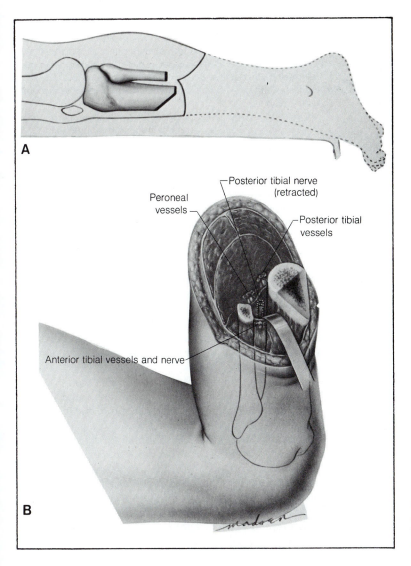

Figure 76-17. A. Skin incisions for anterior and posterior flaps. **B.** Below-knee amputation completed. Note bevel of tibia and slightly shorter fibula.

beveled cephalad. A thin fascia separates the superficial group of muscles from the deep ones, and below this fascia are the posterior tibial and peroneal vessels, all of which are mobilized and divided. The posterior tibial nerve is also mobilized and stretched distalward. Before the nerve is clamped and divided with a sharp knife, it is injected with 10 ml of 1% lidocaine.

ANTEROLATERAL MUSCLES AND ANTERIOR TIBIAL NEUROVAS-CULAR BUNDLE. The leg is then flexed at a right angle. The tibialis anterior, the extensor digitorum longus, and the extensor hallucis longus are divided between the tibia and the fibula. After division of the muscles, the neurovascular bundle is exposed on the anterior surface of the interosseous membrane and then mobilized, clamped, and divided. The leg is then placed again in the horizontal position, and the deep group of muscles is divided.

DIVISION OF BONES. After the bones are freed from the muscle and interosseous membrane attachments, the fibula is sawed by means of Gigli saw and a hand-driven or mechanically driven saw is used for the tibia. The crest is beveled, and then the two bones are divided across at the same level about 1½ inches above the skin incision.

COMPLETION OF PROCEDURE. After *irrigation* of the wound with antibiotic solution, the stump is closed, the posterior group of muscles is attached to the muscles of the anterior tibial compartment, and the fascia is attached in a similar fashion between the two edges.

Careful handling of the *skin* is of the utmost importance. Either loosely tied sutures or strips of adhesive tape are used for closure. Skin traction is not applied (Fig. 76-18).

Subfascial *drains* are used rarely except in cases where infection might be suspected.

Dressing and splinting, as well as postoperative care, will be described below in conjunction with the other techniques.

Use of Equal Anterior and Posterior Myocutaneous Flaps

McCullough et al.,[21] in their discussion of below-knee amputation, give the following description of the procedure:

If adequate bleeding occurs from the skin, the incision is at once carried through the skin, subcutaneous tissue, fascia, and muscle around the circumference of the leg following the outlined flaps. If the skin does not bleed, more proximal flaps are designed. Posteriorly, the incision is carried just deep to the gastrocnemius fascia, but anteriorly, it is carried through the anterior tibial compartment muscles obliquely, superiorly, and posteriorly. The vessels are clamped and ligated following section. The periosteum of the tibia and fibula is incised transversally and a periosteal elevator is used to elevate the tibial and fibular periosteum proximally with the anterior myocutaneous flap to a distance of approximately 2.5 cm above the apex of the previously designed flaps. At this point, the fibula is transected with a Gigli's saw. The tibia is similarly transected at the same level but in such a manner that the Gigli's saw is pulled proximally to give a bevel as it approaches the anterior cortex. If preferred, as stated in the previous method, a power saw may be used. It is most important that the soft tissue be gently retracted adequately to prevent injury during this stage. An amputation knife is then inserted between the ends of the

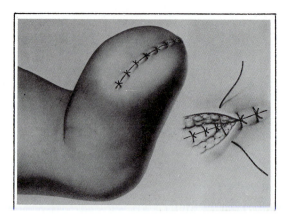

Figure 76-18. Closure of fascia and skin, and appearance of stump after complete closure.

divided bones and the entire posterior compartment is divided with a cut that passes obliquely distally and posteriorly to merge at the previous level of incision in the gastrocnemius fascia. Vessels are clamped and ligated following section, and the posterior tibial nerve is drawn down, ligated, severed sharply with a knife, and allowed to retract. If a tourniquet has been used, it is released at this time, and meticulous hemostasis is achieved [I have been against the use of any type of tourniquet because one deals with dysvascular tissues, and even a short period of tourniquet application may further aggravate the ischemia of the tissues]. The sharp corners of the beveled tibia and fibula are then smoothed carefully with a rasp.

The muscles and fascia of the anterior tibial compartment are then approximated to the posterior compartment musculature. Excess muscle has to be trimmed in order to avoid a bulbous stump.

The long posterior flap is attached to the anterior tibial compartment muscles. . . . This is a myoplastic closure, the subcutaneous tissue being carefully approximated so that minimal tension is required on the skin sutures. The skin is carefully approximated with fine sutures to gain accurate apposition of skin edges, which is particularly important, especially in the dysvascular patient.

Two comments can be made regarding the statements presented above. First, the use of the amount of bleeding of incised skin as a criterion for determining the level of amputation is not consistent with present preoperative vascular evaluation methods, for which several hemodynamic and noninvasive tests are available. Second, careful design of skin flap incisions will prevent the creation of "dog ears," which are undesirable for a properly fashioned stump.

Use of Long Posterior Myocutaneous Flaps

Because the posterior muscle compartment and the skin of the dysvascular limb are generally more adequately vascularized than the anterior, it is desirable to use a long posterior flap as described by Ghormley[22] and subsequently popularized by Burgess.[23] This procedure aims at compensating, as much as possible, the less vascularized anterior flap. Although it is claimed that the long posterior flap necessitates some sacrifice in stump length, this may be avoided by prior evaluation of the degree of vascularity.[24] This procedure, then, appears to be the proper choice in the absence of advanced arterial involvement of the flaps.

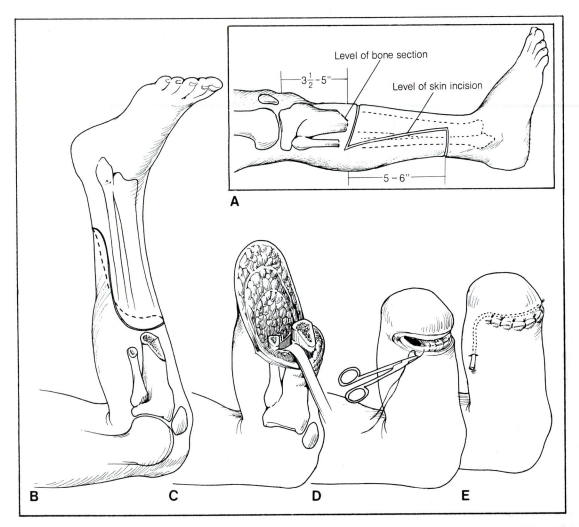

Figure 76-19. Below-knee amputation technique, using a long posterior musculocutaneous flap. **A.** Outline of skin incision and level of bone section. (*Redrawn from Burgess EM: Major amputations, in Nora PF (ed): Operative Surgery. Philadelphia, Lea & Febiger, 1972.*) **B.** Prone position with leg flexed at right angle, indicating skin incisions for the flaps. **C.** Amputation completed, indicating length of posterior flap. **D.** Closure of fascia with interrupted absorbable sutures. **E.** Closed stump with suture line placed anteriorly and a subfascial drain (broken lines).

Operative Technique. The below-knee amputation procedure with a long posterior flap is carried out as follows.

POSITION OF PATIENT. The supine position on the operating table requires knee and hip flexion and support of the knee and leg. The supine position may have its greatest indication in patients with cardiorespiratory problems, which make lying on the chest somewhat hazardous.

INCISION FOR MYOCUTANEOUS FLAPS. A circular skin incision at the site of election is recommended by some to avoid fashioning of flaps. The implied fear of hazardous complications associated with flaps is not justified in view of the good results in almost all cases in which they are used.

A long posterior flap (Fig. 76-19) is recommended because of its usually better blood supply, as mentioned above, than that of the anterior flap. Use of a longer anterior flap, especially by orthopedic surgeons, is undesirable for pa-

tients with vascular insufficiency because of the frequency of necrosis of the stump and because problems related to below-knee amputation are likely to increase. Thus the use of a longer posterior flap, as recommended by Ghormley,[22] is desirable whenever possible, especially if the anterior tibial compartment is severely ischemic.

The fashioning of the posterior flap is carried out with the patient in the supine position after the fibula and tibia are divided. This maneuver is accomplished by inserting a sharp amputation knife posterior to the tibia and sweeping it distally, following the skin incision of the posterior flap. Thus the calf muscles are transected and amputation is completed. In this technique, hemostasis is accomplished by putting pressure on the popliteal space and posterior aspect of the calf and then tying the vessels after the specimen has been removed. If the posterior flap is slightly longer, the excess can always be tailored to provide adequate stump length.

MUSCLE STABILIZATION. The long posterior myocutaneous flap of the gastrocnemius-soleus mass is brought forward and sutured to the deep fascia of the anterior muscle compartment and to the periosteum at the level of the end of the tibia (this step is called myoplasty). Suture of muscle to bone holes, achieved by means of a screw drill in a procedure called myodesis (formerly recommended by some), is no longer used by the majority of surgeons.

According to some reports, however, the muscles and even the fascia were not reattached. This omission is considered serious. I prefer to close the fascia and bring the muscles over the end of the bones, suturing them directly to the anterior compartment muscle and fascia and to the periosteum of the tibia if possible. The ultimate result is functionally satisfactory. Myoplasty appears to preserve the proprioceptive reflexes and is said to lessen postoperative muscle atrophy.

DRAINS. Use of subfascial drains is optional. Some surgeons believe that a drain may be a pathway by which bacteria gain access to the wound. However, in certain cases, in which oozing appears uncontrollable or infection may be feared, drains offer great advantages if left in place for 24 or 48 hours.

Postoperative Care. The postoperative care will depend on the type of prosthesis applied. If the patient has a rigid dressing consisting of plaster (see Chapter 77), the patient is seen by the rehabilitation department for early exercise and ambulation.

PROSTHETIC REGIMEN. Immediate postsurgical care involves the use of a rigid-dressing prosthetic regimen, which has been adopted by most vascular surgeons. My experience recommends it highly. It facilitates early ambulation, often lessens postoperative pain, and promotes wound healing. A more detailed discussion follows.

DRESSING AND SPLINTING. In the majority of cases, immediate postoperative use of a rigid prosthesis is indicated, as mentioned. However, if immediate prosthesis cannot be used or is not available, the following is recommended. Two or three layers of petrolatum gauze are applied over the suture line, and a six- to eight-layer gauze dressing is placed over the entire stump and the knee. The dressing is maintained with a snugly applied 4-inch-wide gauze bandage. A well-padded molded plaster splint, 6 inches wide, is applied over the posterior aspect of the stump and the lower part of the thigh to prevent flexion contracture of the knee joint. The splint, secured in place with a snugly applied 4-inch elastic bandage, is necessary to prevent postoperative pain and breakdown of the end of the stump (Fig. 76-20).

SOFT DRESSING. An alternative to this application of a splint and in the absence of a rigid dressing, a soft dressing consisting of an Unna boot bandage is applied over the stump and extending to the lower half of the thigh. This provides better immobilization of the wound and allows inspection of the latter should there be any drainage to the wound.

Equal Medial and Lateral Flaps (Sagittal Incision)

The distance from the anterior and posterior apices of the incision to the most distal end of the flap should not exceed 3 cm in cases of vascular insufficiency. The incision is deepened through the subcutaneous tissue and muscle, with no dissection between the layers, so as to form a myocutaneous flap. As the incision is deepened through the muscle layers, the knife is directed somewhat proximally so as to produce a beveled muscle flap. The tibia and fibula are divided after periosteum is elevated from these bones to a level slightly superior to the original anterior apex of the skin incision. As in the previous methods, the tibia is beveled. It is important to make a very oblique bevel, because failure to do so may result in a tibial prominence in the line of the anterior portion of the incision. After removal of the specimens, subcutaneous tissues are carefully approximated so as to reduce the tension on the skin sutures, and the skin is closed with an interrupted fine suture. The amputation is then completed in a fashion similar to that for the previous procedure.

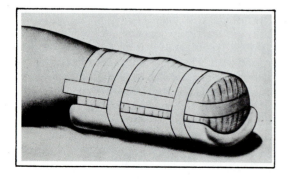

Figure 76-20. Posterior molded splint applied to posterior aspect of stump and lower half of thigh.

Results

Although the results of below-knee amputations may vary somewhat from one procedure to another, in my own experience the use of anterior and posterior myocutaneous flaps and the use of long posterior myocutaneous flaps have resulted in excellent healing of the stump. Thus, in a series of 400 cases in which the anterior and posterior flaps were used, primary healing occurred in 76.5% and delayed healing, requiring several more weeks beyond the normal 2- to 3-week period, occurred in 20.2% (Fig. 76-21). Reamputation above the knee was required in 3.3% of these delayed-healing cases (Fig. 76-22). Of the 400 patients in the series, 80% had arteriosclerosis and diabetes, only 20% were not diabetic. Unfortunately, the majority of patients with ischemic and gangrenous lesions of the foot also have arteriosclerosis and diabetes. Many of them have, in addition to diabetes, an accompanying infection that further complicates local treatment before and during the procedure.

Hospital Mortality Rates. Every death that occurred before complete healing of the stump in the series described above was regarded as a surgical death, even though the cause was entirely unrelated to the surgical procedure. The overall mortality rate in our series was 4.5%. The cause of death was acute coronary thrombosis and heart failure in the majority of cases. Pulmonary embolism, sepsis and decubi-

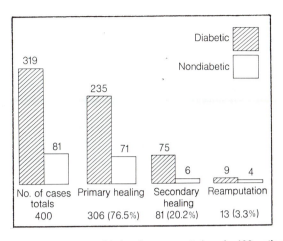

Figure 76-22. Results of below-knee amputations in 400 patients.

tus ulcers, toxemia, secondary thigh amputation, and uremia were the other common causes of surgical death.[25]

Advantages of Below-Knee Versus Above-Knee Amputations. Midleg amputations have three major advantages over thigh amputations: (1) lower mortality rates, (2) preservation of the knee joint with better prospect of rehabilitation, and (3) minimal or no stump pain.

Above-Knee (Thigh) Amputation

Indications for primary thigh amputation are restricted to those cases in which a below-knee procedure does not meet the criteria for a successful outcome. Although since the mid-1950s the percentage of below-knee amputations has steadily increased, the ratio of below- to above-knee still ranges from 1:2 to 1:4, as attested by recent publications on this subject. In our experience, indications for above-knee amputations are essentially (1) extensive gangrene and infection of the foot extending above the ankle, (2) associated painful flexion contracture of the knee joint, and (3) recent acute occlusion of the femoral or iliac artery (Figs. 76-23 and 76-24).

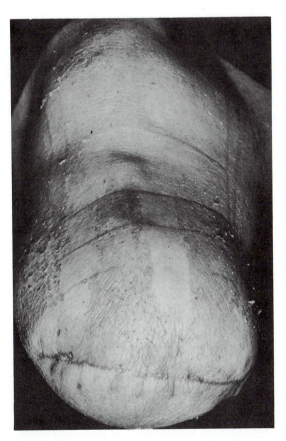

Figure 76-21. Healed below-knee amputation stump.

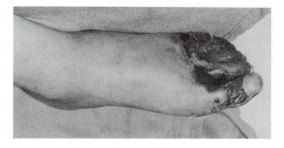

Figure 76-23. Gangrene involving distal portion of the foot, caused by acute thrombosis of popliteal and tibial arteries. Both foot and leg were cold. An above-knee amputation was carried out.

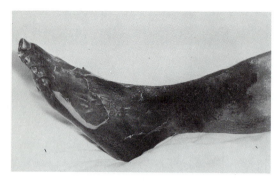

Figure 76-24. Massive gangrene involving foot and half of leg, caused by acute thrombosis of femoral artery and necessitating a midthigh amputation.

Anatomic Review

A brief review of the anatomic structures may be helpful in undertaking the different types of amputations through the thigh (Fig. 76-25).

There are three groups of *muscles* in the thigh. The anterolateral group consists of the sartorius and quadriceps femoris. The quadriceps is formed by the rectus femoris and the three vasti, which combine to form the patellar tendon. The vasti surround the shaft of the femur on its lateral, anterior, and medial surfaces.

The medial group consists of the gracilis and the three adductors. The adductor magnus, by far the largest of the group, extends down as far as the adductor tubercle.

The posterior group (hamstrings) are the biceps and the semitendinosus and semimembranosus. The biceps muscle is inserted into the head of the fibula. The other two muscles both pass to the medial side of the upper end of the tibia.

The *vessels* of the thigh include the femoral and the popliteal. The femoral artery lies along the upper two thirds of a line drawn from the midinguinal point to the adductor tubercle when the thigh is slightly flexed. In the upper third of the thigh, the artery is medial to the sartorius. In the subsartorial canal, which is the middle third, it is posterolateral. At the junction of the middle and lower third, it passes through the opening of the adductor magnus to become the popliteal artery, which is closely applied to the femur. The femoral vein in its lower part is posteromedial to its artery. The profunda vessels lie deep on the anterior surface of the adductor magnus. The long saphenous vein ascends in the superficial fascia on the medial side.

The *femoral nerve* breaks up into branches immediately below the inguinal ligament. The only branch of the latter to be recognized in an amputation of the thigh is the saphenous nerve, which accompanies the femoral artery as far as the opening of the adductor magnus. The *sciatic nerve,* the largest nerve of the body, divides at a varying level in the thigh into medial and lateral popliteal nerves, the former still being called the posterior tibial and the latter called the peroneal nerve. They lie on the posterior surface of the adductor magnus, the peroneal nerve passing under cover of the biceps.

Surgical Techniques

The literature on thigh amputation includes discussions of a great variety of techniques. These techniques are classified into two groups: (1) the end-bearing and (2) the ischial-bearing. The level of division of the extremity between the knee joint and the supracondylar region is an end-bearing amputation, whereas the one carried out above the junction of the middle and lower thirds of the femur is ischial-bearing. Both the end-bearing and the ischial-bearing amputations are satisfactory, provided the technical performance of the procedure and the application of the prosthesis are carried out properly. With few exceptions, vascular surgeons employ either the supracondylar or the mid-thigh amputation. Indications for these two levels differ to some extent according to the type of vascular abnormality.

The *end-bearing* amputations are usually classified into three groups: (1) disarticulation of the knee, (2) osteoplastic, and (3) tendinoplastic.

Disarticulation of Knee. The knee joint disarticulation may be used either as a preliminary guillotine amputation or as a definitive procedure. It is used very rarely in the United States and is applied primarily by orthopedic surgeons to nonischemic conditions.

Osteoplastic Procedure. The *Gritti-Stokes amputation* is an osteoplastic procedure. It appears to have the favor of vascular surgeons in Great Britain and Canada because of its good end-bearing features. Martin and Wickham[26] believe that in advanced arterial occlusive disease with gangrene of the foot, this procedure results in a stump that is functional at an early date. In this technique (Fig. 76-26), the femur is divided at the supracondylar level, and the posterior surface of the patella is sawed away and fixed to the end of the femur. These authors reported that, of the 75 patients of a group of 80 who survived the operation, the stumps healed by first intention in 58 and there was delayed healing in 17. The average time of healing was 14 days for patients with arteriosclerosis, whereas in those with diabetes the average time was 32 days.

Tendinoplastic Amputation. Several techniques have been described for tendinoplastic amputations (Fig. 76-27): the aperiosteal supracondylar tendinoplastic amputation of Kirk, the rounded epicondylar tendinoplastic amputation of Slocum, and the Callander amputation. The first two techniques are used primarily for nonvascular conditions, whereas the third is designed to be used in the presence of vascular disease. It is a supracondylar amputation with long anterior and posterior flaps, the section of the muscles being performed through the tendinous insertions.

These three techniques of amputation provide a stump that is sufficiently broad for end-bearing. Thus the weight is borne in a more normal fashion through the hip joint instead of being transmitted to the ischial tuberosity. Because of the length of the stump, there are some difficulties in fitting the best type of mechanical knee joint. Such amputations are used mostly by orthopedic surgeons and find little favor with the majority of vascular surgeons.

Ischial-bearing amputations are performed through the lower or middle third of the thigh. These two levels of amputations are most widely used for vascular conditions.

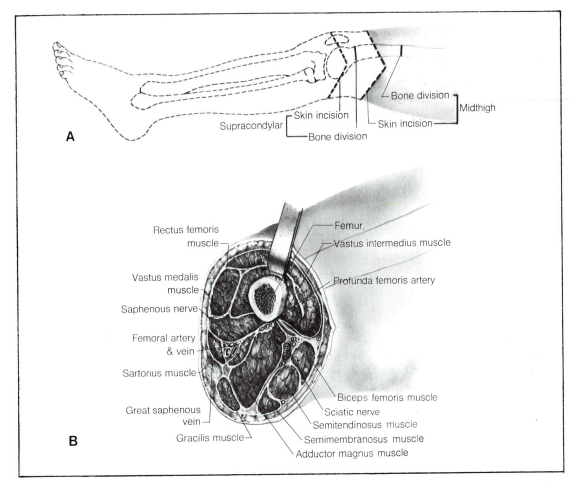

Figure 76-25. A. Drawing indicating levels of skin incision and bone division for supracondylar and midthigh amputations. **B.** Cross section of midthigh.

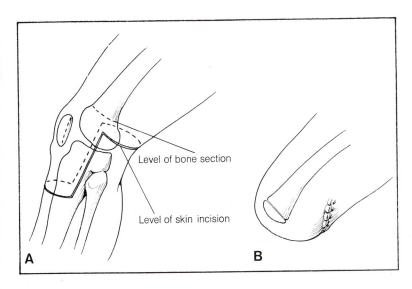

Figure 76-26. Gritti-Stokes amputation. **A.** Diagram showing levels of skin incision and bone section. **B.** Closed stump showing suture line.

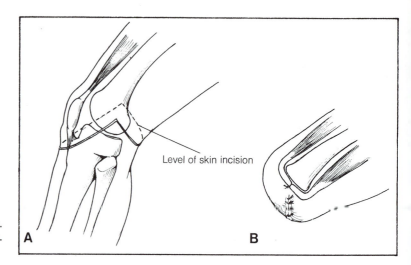

Figure 76-27. Tendinoplastic amputation.
A. Diagram showing level of skin incision.
B. Closed stump showing suture line.

Amputations Through Lower Third

The operation is performed with the patient in a supine position. Although a circular incision may be used, our preference is for anterior and posterior flaps, the anterior being slightly longer (Fig. 76-28). The distal anterior incision is just above the proximal border of the patella. The posterior flap is slightly shorter. The quadriceps tendon is divided at the level of the anterior incision and is raised in the flap.

After the skin incision has been completed, the posterior group of muscles is divided as indicated in Figure 76-

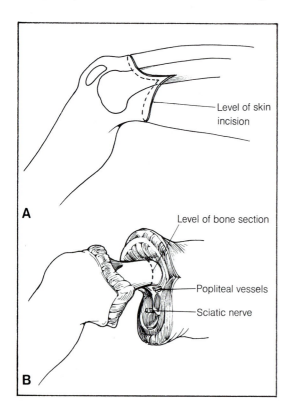

Figure 76-28. Amputation through lower third of thigh, indicating level of skin incision **(A)** and level of bone section **(B)**.

28. The femoral vessels are identified as they pass through the adductor magnus foramen. The popliteal vessels that are present at this lower-third level are divided individually near the junction with the femoral and are doubly ligated with absorbable sutures. The sciatic nerve, found on the back of the adductor magnus, is mobilized and injected with 10 ml of 1% lidocaine before being transected with a sharp knife. A ligature applied gently without too much tension is placed around the nerve. Before its division, the nerve is pulled downward. Then, after its transection, it retracts under the posterior group of muscles. The femur is then sawed transversely at the junction between the middle and lower thirds. The stump is irrigated with an antibiotic solution of kanamycin and bacitracin. The quadriceps tendon is turned over the bone stump, and the fascia is sutured with interrupted absorbable suture material.

Drainage for 48 hours may be advisable as a precautionary measure, but it is not mandatory unless oozing cannot be controlled. The skin is closed with simple sutures. A layer or two of petrolatum gauze is applied on the suture line, a gauze dressing is placed over the end of the stump and held in place with gauze bandages, and a stockinet covering over the entire area is secured around the root of the extremity.

Postoperatively, the patient is encouraged to extend his stump, which demonstrates the ability to hyperextend the hip joint spontaneously. It is not necessary to place the stump on a pillow, since this may have a tendency to produce some degree of flexion contracture. The patient is out of bed the next day.

The immediate postoperative use of a prosthesis, when indicated, is described in Chapter 77.

Amputations Through Middle Third

Indications for the midthigh amputation are the presence of acute occlusion of the femoral or iliac artery and poor collateral circulation due to involvement of the profunda femoris. In such cases, it is inadvisable to perform a more distal amputation because of the inadequate vascularity at that level, which would often result in breakdown of the stump. Furthermore, for patients who are debilitated and

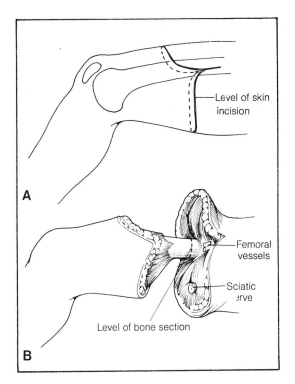

Figure 76-29. Amputation through middle third of thigh, indicating level of skin incision (**A**) and level of bone section (**B**).

whose prospects for rehabilitation with a prosthesis are remote, it is safer to divide the femur at its middle third.

The technique used is depicted in Figure 76-29. The femoral and profunda arteries are dealt with in the same fashion as in the previously described technique. The sciatic nerve is usually represented by an undivided trunk at this level. The flaps are approximated in a fashion similar to that in the previous method. Drainage may be used more frequently in this case because of the larger area of cut muscle, from which considerable oozing may occur.

In our experience with the above-knee amputation in the elderly patient with advanced ischemic changes, primary healing occurred in 95% of the cases. Breakdown of the suture line has been minimal in the majority of cases and has necessitated only a minor delay in the discharge of the patient from the hospital.

The disadvantages of thigh amputation versus below-knee amputation have already been mentioned. The postoperative mortality rate is much higher in this group of cases, according to most statistical studies, including our own. Rehabilitation of above-knee amputees is less effective than that of the below-knee group. Recent developments in the immediate postoperative stump fitting, however, have improved the outlook even of the above-knee amputee.

Failed Grafts and Level of Amputation

The fate of an extremity after graft failure is not always predictable, and a variety of factors, singly or in combination, may account for this uncertainty. Thus, whereas late

graft failure (i.e., beyond 1 year) does not necessarily lead to recurrence of the pregraft level of ischemia, early graft thrombosis (within days or 4 to 6 weeks) may seriously compromise the viability of the extremity. For example, early implantation failure of a graft may result in gangrene and major amputation. The incidence of this complication is variously reported, but at issue is the controversy that revolves around the level of amputation and the rate of revision procedures after grafts failure. In an attempt to determine the incidence of the effects of graft failures, a few series of primary amputations without prior revascularization procedures were compared,[27] the published statistics differed widely. Although a few centers reported that only a few limbs were worse after occlusion of femoral popliteal or infrapopliteal grafts,[28-30] others found that in 60 to 70% of the patients, amputations had been carried out higher than would have been the case otherwise.[31-34]

To gain some insight into the underlying reasons for the wide range of results, one may find it desirable to compare series of limb amputations after graft failures with series of primary amputations without prior revascularization procedures. Although it is well recognized that no two series of patients are entirely comparable, analysis of the overall results of the two groups may nevertheless shed some light on the incidence of the respective procedures and their relative significance in the postgraft failures. Thus, Warren and Record,[17] in a series of 802 cases collected from the literature found healing occured in 86% of below-knee amputations, of which 73% healed by primary and 27% by secondary intention. In a series of 400 cases of below-knee amputations collected from the Montefiore Vascular Service (more than 50% were my patients), healing occurred in 96.7% of cases, of which 76.5% healed by primary and 20.2% by secondary intention. Healing of amputation to the above-knee level occurred in 13 (3.3%) of cases. Of these patients, 75% had a nonpalpable popliteal artery as disclosed by oscillometry and in many instances by arteriography. In addition, 80% of these patients had arteriosclerosis and diabetes. The overall hospital mortality rate was 4.5%. Burgess and Marsden[28] reported on 140 patients with primary amputation in whom healing at the below-knee level occurred in 113 patients, or 80% of the cases.

Admittedly, it is sometimes difficult to predict which of the patients who finally had higher amputations would have had a more distal one if it had been a primary procedure. Nevertheless, there is little doubt that the effects of sudden and early graft closure may affect negatively the already compromised circulatory status of the grafted limb. The notion that, if the graft fails, rarely, if ever, is anything lost may be self-deluding. As Warren[35] stated in commenting editorially on the article by Burgess and Marsden,[28] "Few vascular surgeons fail to remember at least one patient whose limb became more ischemic after closure of a graft." Unfortunately, both the surgeon and the patient must be aware of such a possibility, even though it may be rare. These facts should eliminate the optimistic interpretation that if a graft fails, no more of the limb will be lost than would otherwise have been lost. Nevertheless, reconstructive arterial procedures in the presence of threatening ischemia of the limb are of immense value.

PITFALLS

Pitfalls of amputation include a variety of factors, most important of which are (1) wrong level of amputation, (2) technical errors, (3) delayed or inadequate prophylaxis against infection, (4) unrecognized venous thrombosis, and (5) failure to immobilize the stump postoperatively.

The *wrong level of amputation* may result from inadequate assessment of the optimum area of possible healing. Indeed, if a toe or a transmetatarsal amputation is carried out through borderline or poorly vascularized tissues, with failure of the stump to heal, higher amputation becomes unavoidable. If, on the other hand, the amputation is carried out above the knee because it is the so-called safest site for healing, adequate rehabilitation without the knee joint may be hampered, especially in an elderly individual. It cannot be too strongly reemphasized that selection of the level of amputation should be carried out with great care.

Technical errors may encompass excessive length of bones, redundancy of the soft tissues, inadequacy of hemostasis, and poor approximation of the skin edges.

Excessive length of bones will cause tension of the soft tissues and will inevitably lead to their breakdown. Therefore, before one attempts to close, it is important to approximate the flaps, and if there is the slightest tension, shortening of the bones should be carried out at this time.

Redundancy of the soft tissues, on the other hand, can result in an unsightly stump that may cause pain and be difficult to fit with a prosthesis. If noted at the time of closure, tailoring of the flaps should be done to match the length of bones with that of the musculocutaneous tissues.

Inadequacy of hemostasis may result in a hematoma, which in turn will produce pressure from inside, leading to ischemic changes of the skin. If oozing is present, a drain must be inserted in the subfascial space and left in place for 24 to 48 hours.

Closure of the skin edges should be done with extreme care to avoid puckering or scalloping. Poor matching of the edges leads to delayed healing of the scar. Skin approximation should be accomplished by single-loop monofilament interrupted sutures just tight enough to hold the edges together. Mattress sutures, unless applied without tension, should be avoided, because they have a tendency to strangulate the tissues.

Delayed or inadequate prophylaxis against infection, especially in diabetic patients, may lead to sepsis of the wound. Antibiotics should be used routinely for 7 to 10 days postoperatively. Before the stump is closed, irrigation of the tissues with an antibiotic solution should be done routinely.

Venous thrombosis in an extremity with a gangrenous foot of several weeks' duration is not an unusual finding. The popliteal, tibial, peroneal, or sural veins may contain fresh or organized thrombi, the potential source of pulmonary emboli. The surgeon is then faced with a dilemma of whether to ligate the femoral or just institute anticoagulation. Although it is difficult to formulate a definitive policy in the presence of these findings, ligation of the superficial femoral at this time may be seriously considered. As an alternative, anticoagulants should be instituted within 12 hours postoperatively, and the patient should be carefully monitored for possible chest pain. If such a condition develops, the proximal venous ligation should be carried out without delay.

Failure to immobilize a below-knee amputation may result in serious complications. The natural tendency of the patient to bend the knee and press the end of the stump against the bed mattress may injure the stump and result in severe pain. Immobilization of the stump is essential whether an immediate postoperative prosthesis or a posterior splint is used. The knee should remain straight for 2 to 3 weeks to allow healing without flexion contracture, pain, and breakdown.

Ischemic muscles may be encountered at the level of amputation, especially in the soleus and in the anterior tibial compartment. If focal necrosis or discoloration is found, the muscle should be excised until normal-appearing tissue is obtained.

COMPLICATIONS

Postoperative complications may be divided into early and late. The *early* complications include infection, delayed wound healing, painful stump, phantom sensations, and pressure sores related to the cast or splint application. *Late* complications include phantom pain, flexion contracture, and gangrene of the stump.

Early Complications

Infection
Before the advent of the antibiotic era, one of the dreadful aspects of gangrene was the vulnerability of the patient, especially the diabetic, to bacterial invasion of the tissues from the necrotic area. Since then, the incidence of morbidity and death due to infection has decreased markedly. In patients with infected gangrene of the toes or foot, antibiotics should be used before and after surgery. In patients with dry gangrene who are undergoing elective amputation, antibiotics should be administered for a period of 7 to 10 days postoperatively. The decision as to the type of drug to be used should be based on bacterial cultures of tissue specimens and the susceptibility of the bacteria to antibiotics. Although these tests may facilitate a logical choice of drug, it is not always advisable to wait for the laboratory results. A broad-spectrum antibiotic is then used routinely. Adherence to this policy should result in very little postoperative infection of the stump.

However, if an abscess develops in the stump, early and adequate drainage is mandatory. Fever and leukocytosis are indicative of possible local infection, and the stump should be examined for this possibility. If a superficial extrafascial infection is present, removal of a few sutures and the use of wet dressings, changed twice daily and closely supervised, may suffice to control this sepsis. However, should there be a subfascial infection, the stump must be opened, preferably in the operating room, and the wound irrigated, drains placed in the stump, and a proper antibiotic solution used topically. Prompt recognition of this complication may prevent further damage and obviate the need for high revision of the amputation site. However, in diabetic patients, in spite of all the measures, the infectious process may spread subfascially, and additional counterincisions may be necessary for control of the sepsis. This complication will prolong morbidity and delay rehabilitation of the patient.

Delayed Stump Healing
Delayed stump healing is seen mostly in transmetatarsal and below-knee amputations, although it is not unusual in an above-knee amputation. As a rule, the delay in wound healing is due to marginal necrosis of the skin edges and less frequently to involvement of the subfascial tissues.

Treatment of the necrotic lesions must be carried out with extreme care. One should not attempt to excise the necrotic edge of the skin until there is evidence of separation of the lesions. Daily dressings with wet saline applications or use of an enzymatic debriding agent may be helpful.

If the necrotic lesions are superficial, revision of the stump may not be necessary. However, if necrosis is extensive, revision of the stump, either at the same level or above the proximal joint, may be indicated. Indeed, in the latter event, early reamputation at a higher level must be considered to prevent prolonged illness and bed rest. In the absence of infection, primary closure of the wound is usually desirable and feasible.

Painful Stump; Phantom Sensations
The early postoperative pain is located in the stump or consists of phantom sensations and is most common in below-knee and above-knee amputations.

The stump pain, when unrelated to infection or marginal necrosis, represents a normal course of events in the healing process. Should the pain be unusually severe and persistent, a different explanation for the painful syndrome should be looked for.

The phantom sensations, consisting of the patient's perception of the missing distal portion of the limb, usually without actual pain, occurs in the early postamputation period. This is a self-limiting phenomenon, and the patient should be reassured about it.

The *pressure sores* caused by a tight cast or splint application may result in severe pain. The cast or the splint should be removed without delay to prevent any further damage to the skin, either at the end of the stump or around the patella. If the lesions resulting from the pressure due to the cast or splint are superficial, reapplication is permissible, provided the lesions are reviewed periodically. Should there be a deep pressure sore, it is preferable to delay reapplication of the splint or cast, and treatment of the lesions should be undertaken vigorously.

Unfortunately, especially in a debilitated individual or in a diabetic patient with marked diabetic neuropathy, the necrosis of the skin is sometimes unaccompanied by any clinical signs, and the lesions are discovered only at the routine removal of the cast. Local treatment of the necrotic area must be carried out without delay, and obviously reapplication of the cast is to be omitted.

Late Complications

Phantom Limb Pain
Unlike the phantom sensations, phantom limb pain occurs 2 to 3 months after the amputation or even later. Phantom pain is more frequently noted and is more severe in above-knee amputations. It usually occurs when the amputation was delayed, with the patient having had severe pain due to gangrene. The cause of the persistent excruciating pain is not well understood. Neuroma of the cut end of the nerve has often been incriminated as a cause of phantom pain.

In the past, prefrontal lobotomy was used for control of this type of pain. Alternatives to this radical procedure are section of the sciatic nerve proximal to the stump, lumbar sympathectomy, and cordotomy. They have not always been successful in relieving this dreadful complication, although sciatic nerve section, in our experience, has produced gratifying results.

It has been suggested that a better psychologic adjustment of the patient to the loss of the extremity, with a greater effort in rehabilitating the patient, may be helpful in preventing this phantom pain.

Flexion Contracture
Flexion contracture of the knee joint or of the hip joint may occur often as a result of stump or phantom pain or as a result of persistent ischemia of the stump or a combination of the two. It is likely that, in some cases, the level of amputation was too distal.

Gangrene of the Stump
In some patients, after a period of a few weeks or months, the arterial disease of the affected limb may progress to the point of inducing superimposed ischemia, leading to necrosis of the stump. Under those circumstances, a higher amputation is unavoidable.

In connection with the progression of the arteriosclerotic process in the amputated limb, it is well to point out that in diabetic patients, the remaining limb may also progress to gangrene and necessitate, within a period of 3 years, amputation of this limb in about 30 to 40% of the cases. It is therefore important to evaluate the arterial tree of the remaining limb in the hope that a bypass graft or a lumbar sympathectomy may be possible as a prophylactic measure.

REFERENCES

1. Glattly HW: Aging and amputations. Artif Limbs 10:1, 1966.
2. Kay HW, Newman JD: Relative incidence of new amputations: Statistical comparisons of 6000 new amputations. Orthot Prosthet 29:3, 1975.
3. Berlemont M: Notre expérience de l'appareillage precoce des amputés des membres inférieurs aux Établissements Héliomarins de Berck. Ann Med Physique 4:213, 1961.
4. Weiss M: The Prosthesis on the Operating Table from the Neurophysiological Point of View. Report of the Workshop Panel on Lower Extremity Prosthetic Fitting, National Academy of Sciences, Committee on Prosthetics Research and Development, February, 1966.

5. Burgess EM, Romano RL: The management of lower extremity amputees using immediate postsurgical prosthesis. Clin Orthop 57:137, 1968.

6. Silbert S, Haimovici H: Criteria for the selection of the level of amputation for ischemic gangrene. JAMA 155:1554, 1954.

7. McKittrick LE, McKittrick JB, Risley TS: Transmetatarsal amputation for infection or gangrene in patients with diabetes mellitus. Ann Surg 130:826, 1949.

8. Haimovici H: Criteria for and results of transmetatarsal amputation for ischemic gangrene. Arch Surg 70:45, 1955.

9. Haimovici H: Peripheral arterial disease in diabetes. NY State J Med 61:2988, 1961.

10. Haimovici H: Amputations for ischemic gangrene: Selection of level and results, in Haimovici H (ed): The Surgical Management of Vascular Diseases. Philadelphia, Lippincott, 1970, pp 147–157.

11. Wheelock FC Jr: Transmetatarsal amputations and arterial surgery in diabetic patients. N Engl J Med 264:316, 1961.

12. Haimovici H: Unpublished data.

13. Wheelock FC Jr, Filtzer HS: Femoral grafts in diabetics: Resulting conservative amputations. Arch Surg 99:776, 1969.

14. Haimovici H: Peripheral arterial disease in diabetes, in Ellenberg M, Rifkin H (eds): Diabetes Mellitus: Theory and Practice. New York, McGraw-Hill, 1970, pp 890–911.

15. Warren R, Thayer TR, et al.: The Syme amputation in peripheral arterial disease. Surgery 37:156, 1955.

16. Dale GM: Syme's amputation for gangrene from peripheral vascular disease. Artif Limbs 6:44, 1961–1962.

17. Warren R, Record EE: Lower Extremity Amputations for Arterial Insufficiency. Boston, Little, Brown, 1967.

18. Warren R, Kihn RB: A survey of lower extremity amputations for ischemia. Surgery 63:107, 1968.

19. Silbert S, Haimovici H: Results of midleg amputations for gangrene in diabetics. JAMA 144:454, 1950.

20. Moore WS: Determination of amputation level: Measurement of skin blood flow with xenon 133. Arch Surg 107:798, 1973.

21. McCollough NC, Harris AR, Hampton FL: Below-knee amputation, in Atlas of Limb Prosthetics. St. Louis, CV Mosby, 1981.

22. Ghormley RK: Amputation in occlusive vascular disease, in Allen EV, Barker ND, Hines EA Jr (eds): Peripheral Vascular Diseases. Philadelphia, WB Saunders, 1946, pp 783–795.

23. Burgess EM: The stabilization of muscles in lower extremity amputations. J Bone Joint Surg (Am) 50A:1486, 1487, 1968.

24. Dean RH, Yao JS, Thompson RG, Bergan JJ: Predictive value of ultrasonically derived arterial pressure in determination of amputation level. Am J Surg 41:731, 1975.

25. Haimovici H: Results of below-knee amputation in 400 cases without reconstructive arterial surgery. Unpublished data.

26. Martin P, Wickham JE: Gritti-Stokes amputation for atherosclerotic gangrene. Lancet 2:16, 1962.

27. Haimovici H: Failed grafts and level of amputation [Editorial]. J Vasc Surg 2(3):371, 1985.

28. Burgess, EM, Marsden FW: Major lower extremity amputations following arterial reconstruction. Arch Surg 108:655, 1976.

29. Sumner DS, Strandness DE Jr: Hemodynamic studies before and after bypass grafts to the tibial and peroneal arteries. Surgery 86:442, 1979.

30. Samson RH, Gupta SK, et al.: Level of amputation after failure of limb salvage procedures. Surg Gynecol Obstet 154:56, 1982.

31. Stoney RJ: Ultimate salvage for the patient with limbs threatening ischemia. Am J Surg 136:228, 1978.

32. Szilagyi DE, Hagemann JH, et al.: Autogenous vein grafting in femoropopliteal atherosclerosis. Surgery 86:836, 1979.

33. Ramsburgh SR, Lindenauer SM, et al.: Femoropopliteal bypass for limb salvage surgery. Surgery 81:453, 1977.

34. Kagmers M, Satiami B, Evans WE: Amputation level following successful distal limb salvage operations. Surgery 87:683, 1980.

35. Warren R: Editorial comment on paper by Burgess and Marsden (Ref. 31). Arch Surg 108:660, 1974.

CHAPTER 77
Immediate Postoperative Prosthetic Fitting and Rehabilitation

† Allen S. Russek

PRINCIPLES

The objective of a surgeon who does a major amputation of the lower extremity is to achieve the greatest functional performance in the shortest possible time after surgery. The surgeon, therefore, must be aware of his total role in the overall management of the amputee and that his responsibility does not terminate with healing of the wound.

It is necessary to concentrate on two major factors for improving the ultimate function of the individual who loses a lower extremity by elective amputation. The first is to reestablish physiologic and neuromuscular conditions as close as possible to the preamputation state. The second factor is to reduce the time during which there is a disturbance in weightbearing.

HISTORICAL DATA

The concept of applying a prosthetic device intraoperatively after lower extremity amputation is today a well-accepted procedure. The primary objective was the speed of rehabilitation claimed by the proponents of this technique.

The introduction of this procedure is credited to a French orthopedic surgeon, Berlemont.[1] His early work managing ward patients who were secondarily healing various levels of traumatic amputation led to his development of the technique. To expedite healing time, Berlemont devised a temporary prosthesis to be put over the healing amputation stump so that preliminary trussing could be initiated. To his surprise, this technique not only permitted earlier ambulation but also appeared to accelerate the secondary healing process. Berlemont's results encouraged Marion Weiss,[2] of Poland, to apply this technique to stumps healing primarily. This test proved highly successful. It stimulated several investigators worldwide.[3] In the United States, E. Burgess,[4] an orthopedic surgeon in Seattle, Washington, applied this prosthetic design for immediate postoperative amputations of the lower extremity. The techniques appeared most applicable to below-knee amputation, although all amputation levels have been fitted with a prosthesis immediately after surgery. Most vascular centers that adopted the technique of immediate postoperative prosthesis reported excellent results with many advantages, for example, protection of the stump wound from external trauma, stump immobilization, prevention of joint flexion contracture, and edema control, all of which contributed to relatively fast healing and ambulation. In contrast, few reports showed traumatic lesions and multiple disadvantages connected with this technique.[4] However, in general, the proponents of this method reported more than 80% of excellent to good results.[5–8]

Immediate fitting has been performed following conventional amputation with no participation by the surgeon. However, these phases are (1) preoperative preparations, (2) surgical phase, (3) prosthetic phase, and (4) training phase.

PREOPERATIVE PREPARATIONS

It is estimated that 75% of patients having lower extremity amputations are of advanced age. The largest group falls between ages 55 and 65. Of these, 80% of the amputations are for the ischemic extremity, and more than half the patients have diabetes. This is a difficult group to rehabilitate after amputation. They require the efforts of more than one person in their comprehensive management. Every surgeon who does amputations should arrange to do them in a hospital with adequate personnel and facilities. Essentially he should be the principal member of a team; he should have a satisfactory working relationship with a physiatrist, who with a rehabilitation staff participates in keeping the whole patient as well as the amputated limb in good physical condition, and with other specialists to maintain concomitant physical deficits under control in this older age group. It is most necessary to have a working relationship with an experienced prosthetist. Except in emergencies, every amputation should be planned. Where immediate fitting is anticipated, a preoperative conference is necessary 1 or 2 days in advance of surgery, if possible.

---

† Deceased. This chapter, which appeared in the second edition, was revised and updated by Henry Haimovici, editor.

1049

Its purpose is to permit the participants to exchange information relative to the patient and to prepare for the procedure so that each will know his role, including the patient. It allows the time necessary for the prosthetist to measure the patient and obtain the materials and components to be used.

SURGICAL PHASE

Amputation in the lower extremity when performed for ischemia should be based on a number of criteria.* Surveys made by the Committee on Prosthetic Research and Development of the National Research Council indicated that in the early 1950s amputation above the knee in vascular cases, particularly in diabetes, constituted more than 60% of those cases. By the late 1950s, it had dropped to about 50%. In the past 10 years it has fallen to less than 20%, according to investigators using the myoplastic amputation and immediate-fitting techniques.

The importance of preserving the knee cannot be overemphasized. The clinical examination taking into account the appearance, extent and character of gangrene, growth of hair, skin temperature, edema, pulses, and sensation all contribute to formulating a judgment. These can be reinforced by other objective observations, such as arteriography, thermography, plethysmography, the use of radioactive xenon 133, and Doppler recordings. Sometimes the final determination can truly be made only by direct observation after incision.

The operative plan should follow the principles of the surgical considerations previously described to provide a well-shaped, stable stump that can accommodate and tolerate immediate fitting. After closure of the stump, a silk or nylon dressing is placed over the wound and covered with a small amount of gauze fluffs over which the Orion Lycra sterile stump sock is rolled.

PROSTHETIC PHASE AND BELOW-KNEE AMPUTATION

Below-knee amputation comprises over 75% of amputations performed for vascular disease. The above-knee amputation is performed in up to 25% of cases. The immediate-fitting technique will be described in detail for these levels. This technique can be used for the less frequently performed Syme, knee disarticulation, and hip disarticulation procedures with modified components.

The rigid postoperative cast socket is applied by the prosthetist or by the surgeon if no prosthetist is available. In below-knee amputations the stump sock is drawn above the knee and held taut by an assistant throughout the procedure until the plaster sets (Fig. 77-1). If an assistant is not available, this can be accomplished by the prosthetist's applying an adequate shoulder suspension harness to put tension on the sock. The tension is maintained in the long

---

*See criteria for level of amputation in Chapter 76. By adhering to those criteria, it is possible in most cases to determine in advance the site of amputation.

axis of the limb so that the proximal portion of the sock is not lifted anteriorly, which would result in a loose cast. This is one of the most important steps in the entire procedure to avoid malfit or displacement of the felt relief pads when the plaster is rolled on. The relief pads are now cut to fit the stump. The medial pad is placed to occupy the hollow just below the medial condylar flare. It is trimmed to prevent the posterior extension from reaching the hamstring tendons. The anterior margin is beveled and rests $\frac{1}{4}$ inch from the sharp tibial crest and extends $\frac{3}{8}$ inch beyond the cut end of the tibia. The posterior margin is tapered feather-thin to blend with the stump contour so that no ridge is created when the stump is wrapped in the plaster. Any protruding edge or elevation may result in a pressure lesion. The lateral felt relief pad is cut the same length as the medial pad and placed opposite it $\frac{1}{4}$ inch from the tibia crest, with the beveled margin facing the medial pad. This creates a $\frac{1}{2}$ inch bridge of plaster over the tibial tubercle and crest. The lateral pad is skived to avoid a ridge posteriorly. A space of more than $\frac{1}{2}$ inch must be avoided. The patellar pad is then cut to fit over the entire patella. The circumference of the pad is skived and feathered to fit flush over the slightly flexed knee. When the pads are fitted and skived, the stump sock and backs of the pads are sprayed with Dow Corning medical adhesive, type B, and allowed a few seconds to become tacky. With the stump sock maintained under constant tension, the pads are carefully placed on the stump sock. The anterior margins of the pads should be parallel, not more than $\frac{1}{2}$ inch apart. They are drawn a bit closer when the cast is applied and adequately protect the anterior tibial crest from pressure (Fig. 77-2).

The proper size sterile reticulated polyurethane distal cap or pad is now applied over the end of the stump, covering as well the distal ends of the felt relief pads.

Application of Rigid Dressing

While continuous tension is maintained on the stump sock, elastic plaster bandages are used for the first wraps of the cast. This type of bandage is used because it conforms well to the contours of the stump and can provide the desired proximal compression on the stump. The experienced prosthetist or surgeon develops a specific pattern of application. The recommended pattern is to start the elastic plaster wrap at the distal lateral aspect of the stump, covering the proximal edge of the polyurethane distal cap and locking the bandage with $1\frac{3}{4}$ turns with very little tension. This fixes the distal cap and felt pads in position. The bandage is then brought up anterolaterally over the end of the stump with almost full tension and stretched to create proximal compression. When it is drawn medially over the anterior portion of the stump, the tension is rapidly reduced to avoid circular constriction. The bandage is then stretched and brought up anteromedially, the tension being released as the bandage passes over the front lateral aspect of the stump. These wraps are repeated and the bandage used up, with mild tension, reaching up to the knee. By this time there should be central proximal compression by the overlapped double layers of the bandage. Another elas-

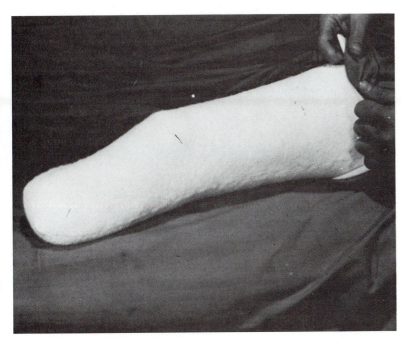

Figure 77-1. Stump sock is held taut by an assistant throughout the procedure.

tic bandage is then started, covering the upper portion of the first one and with circular turns and decreasing tension to no tension carried above midthigh with circular wraps. Care must be taken to avoid circular compression. The plaster bandage must lie flat in its complete width throughout. Any folding or reversing of the bandage will create traumatic ridges (Fig. 77-3).

The elastic plaster bandages are now reinforced with regular plaster splints in sugar-tong fashion anteroposteriorly and mediolaterally. The whole stump is then wrapped with a 4-inch regular plaster bandage past the midthigh. Before the cast is completed proximally, a 1½ inch suspension strap and buckle are incorporated in the wrap by placing two turns of the regular plaster over the strap. The strap is then folded back with the buckle up and wrapped with the remainder of the last bandage. As the plaster sets and while tension is still maintained on the stump sock, the cast is gently smoothed. Both hands are then placed above the femoral condyles with mild pressure to create a suspension factor. When the plaster has set, the tension on the stump sock may be released; a slit is now made in the stump sock, opposite the buckle; the buckle is pulled through and the sock folded over the top of the socket. The suspension belt is placed around the patient's waist, and the elastic webbing is pulled through the buckle (Fig. 77-4).

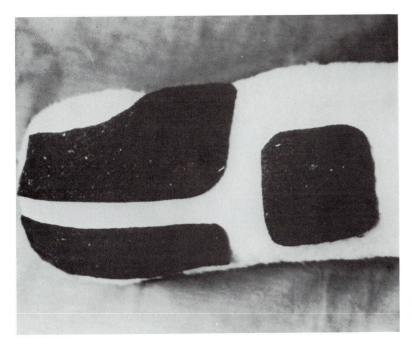

Figure 77-2. Measured, skived relief pads properly placed and adherent to the stump sock.

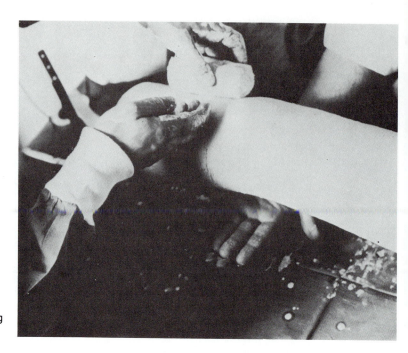

Figure 77-3. Extension of the rigid dressing without circular compression.

Application of Prosthetic Unit

With the patient's legs in neutral position and the knees about 2 inches apart, the metal straps of the socket attachment for the pylon are cut and shaped to the contours of the plaster socket (Fig. 77-5). With the stump raised about an inch off the table and the socket attachment in place, the attachment plate should be perpendicular to the table. The straps should be placed to allow for removal of the drain if one is used. The position of the straps is now marked on the socket with an indelible pencil when the center of the plate is offset $\frac{1}{2}$ inch medial to the anterior midline of the stump. Care must be taken not to allow the limb to rotate externally. The gap between the plate and socket is now filled with folded wet plaster bandage strips to avoid motion, slippage, or buckling of the straps on weightbearing. The straps are aligned with the pencil marks and the straps wrapped on to the socket with regular plaster bandages. The wraps should go down to the attachment plate, locking the plaster filling the distal gap (Fig. 77-6).

The prosthetic unit is then assembled. The pylon tube is cut to size, and the foot attached. The prosthetic foot is aligned with the opposite foot in a neutral position, allowing for a 1 inch heel. All bolts and tube clamp are tightened, and the adjustability of the unit is checked. At this point

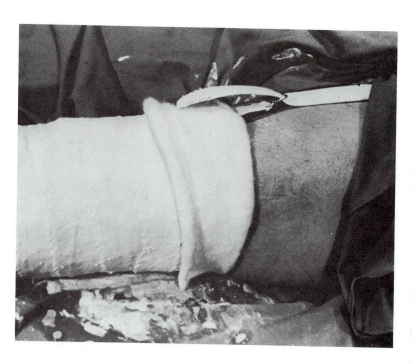

Figure 77-4. Completed rigid dressing and suspension.

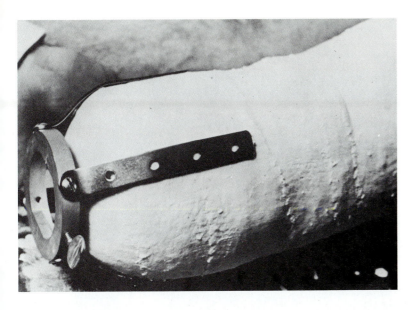

Figure 77-5. Fitting and alignment of supporting straps.

the plaster has set, but it is still soft enough to allow for relief of the patella. This is accomplished by cutting a window over the patella, holding a scalpel horizontally to avoid cutting the stump sock (Fig. 77-7). The window should be somewhat smaller than the patella pad. The plaster window is then removed and the felt relief pad pulled out. The socket now in contact with the anterior knee is properly flared to prevent pressure trauma to the patella (Fig. 77-8).

Application of Above-Knee Rigid Dressing or Cast Socket

After the sterile Orlon Lycra sock is rolled on, the patient is placed so that the buttock and amputation extend over the side of the operating table to have access to every aspect of the stump. The top of the stump sock is slit medially at the perineum, and the anterior, lateral, and posterior levels of the sock are pulled up 3 inches higher than that level. The top of the sock is folded back to spray the upper stump and buttock and inner surface of the sock with medical adhesive. The sock is then rolled up and held in tension proximally throughout the procedure by an assistant or shoulder harness. The tension on the sock is essential here, as it is in the application of the below-knee cast socket. A perineal apron is then applied, covering and adhering to the stump sock after the surfaces are sprayed with medical adhesive.

The end of the stump is then covered with a reticulated polyurethane distal pad of appropriate size with edges feathered to avoid a ridge (Fig. 77-9). Elastic plaster ban-

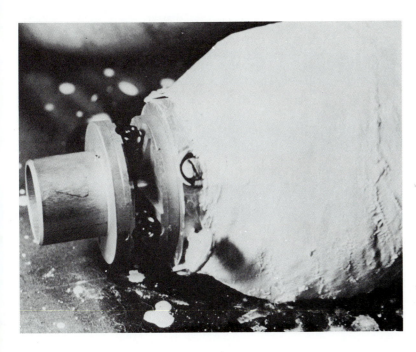

Figure 77-6. Plate firmly attached—no gaps.

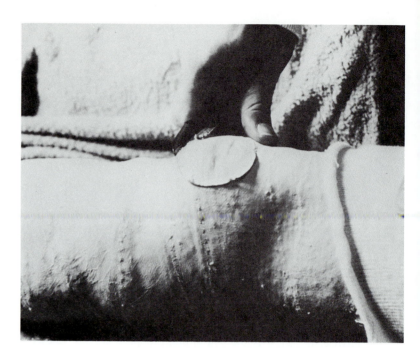

Figure 77-7. Cutting the patella relief window.

dages are then wrapped over the stump so that proximal pressure is developed by double wraps over the lateral, medial, and central aspects of the end of the stump. The bandages are kept flat, without wrinkles, reverses, or folding, letting up the tension whenever the possibility of circular constriction exists. Two bandages are usually used for this purpose. The cast socket is brought up to the perineum and 2 to 3 inches higher laterally and posteriorly, with little or no tension on the bandage proximally.

At this point the surgeon and prosthetist proceed along preplanned arrangements for shaping the socket. Many prefer the application of an adjustable casting fixture that,

when fitted over the wet plaster, forms a precise socket of modified quadrilateral shape (Fig. 77-10). The experienced surgeon or prosthetist can manually shape and mold the wet socket adequately. If there is time, there are several ways to incorporate the rigid dressing into a socket of appropriate specifications made the day before surgery. Although the socket formation is important, the suspension is critical. Many approaches have been tested to prevent the socket sliding down and even off the stump. The socket is fitted high anteriorly above Scarpa's triangle. This anterior rim is often pushed down when the patient sits up. One of the various modifications is used according to the length

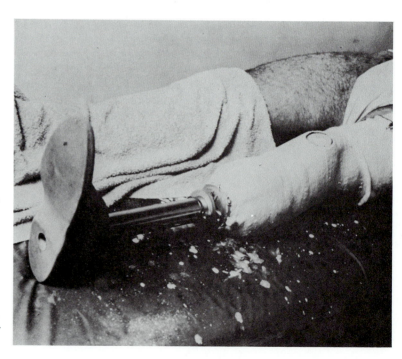

Figure 77-8. Completed immediate postoperative below-knee prosthesis.

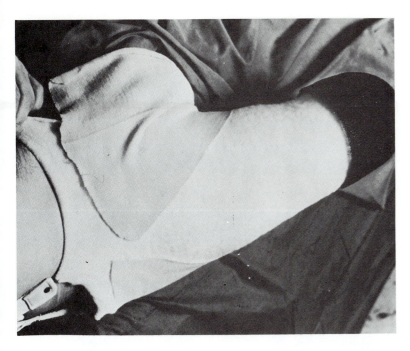

Figure 77-9. Application of the perineal apron and reticulated polyurethane distal pad.

of the stump, the adipose tissue, and general contours of the stump, pelvis, and abdomen. Whichever method is used, one can achieve a well-fitted, total-contact modified quadrilateral socket with the weight borne predominantly on the gluteal mass, avoiding focal pressure on bony points. The author prefers the manually shaped socket suspended by the broad waist belt and suspension cables developed by the Prosthetics Research Study sponsored by the Veterans Administration in Seattle, Washington.

Before the plaster socket sets, the upper rims are flared by gently pulling the stump sock to roll the sharp upper edges. When the socket is shaped, it is reinforced with regular plaster splints anteroposteriorly, mediolaterally,

and in the groin and upper rim (Fig. 77-11). A balsa wood block is now shaped and incorporated beyond the stump to give it continuity down to the level corresponding to the knee center desired. The straps of an attachment plate for an above-knee pylon are now cut and fitted to the stump and wrapped on to the cast with regular plaster. The alignment of this plate is important to minimize adjustments later. The plate should be parallel to the floor and vertical to the operating table with the stump in natural adduction and appropriate flexion, depending upon its length. The wood block must be attached without gaps by use of folded plaster splints firmly filling all spaces and molded into the general contour of a full thigh when laminated to the socket

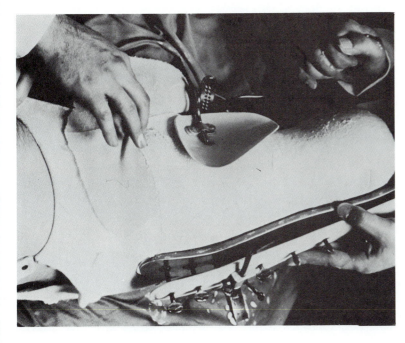

Figure 77-10. Casting fixture being applied to the wet cast to form a modified, adducted quadrilateral socket.

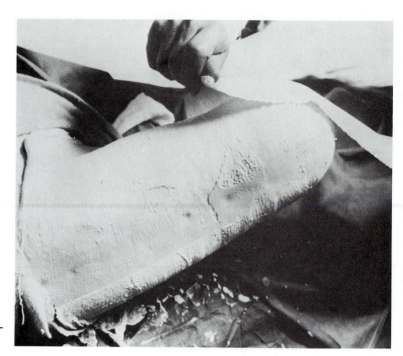

Figure 77-11. Reinforcement of the pre-shaped cast with regular plaster splints.

with the metal straps of the attachment plate. A pair of proper-size Bowden cables in a plastic housing is now placed on the socket and wrapped on with regular plaster so that the retainers are in position to hold the suspension straps of the waist belt (Fig. 77-12).

When all plaster is dry, the properly fitting belt is placed around the patient's waist, adjusted, and attached to the cables so that the patient can get 90° of flexion at the hips.

The adjusted prosthetic unit selected is now attached to the plate. The pylon tube with foot is fitted and cut to proper length, taking into account that the patient will wear a heel on the remaining foot (Fig. 77-13).

Postoperative and Training Phase

The postoperative course and training constitute an integrated continuous process. It varies with individual patients, but in general with the rigid dressing there is less pain and fewer complaints of phantom discomfort. Some patients have no pain at all, but most patients complain of pain of varying intensity for 3 or 4 days. The pain is usually accompanied by a feeling of general constriction of the amputation stump. This is no indication to do anything about the cast. If the patient complains of focal pain over a subcutaneous bony area, it should be relieved if it

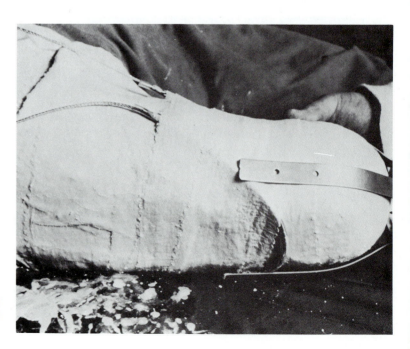

Figure 77-12. Wood block extension and Bowden cables in the cast; alignment and fitting of the prosthetic attachment plate.

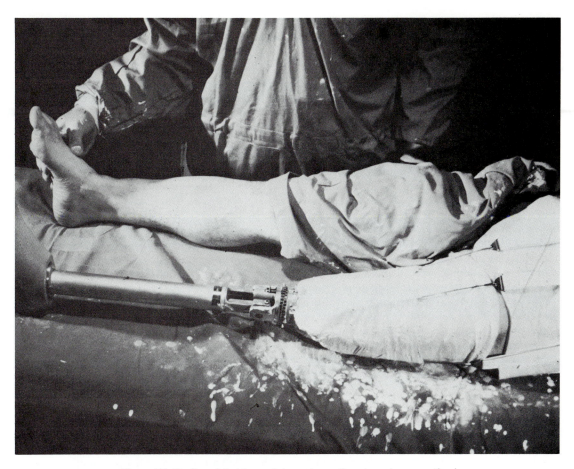

Figure 77-13. Completed immediate postoperative above-knee prosthesis.

persists. Relief is usually obtained by splitting the cast and taping it together wherever it separates. Persistent local pain over a bony point may require complete removal of the cast socket and reapplication with protection of the bony points. The reapplication must be done as soon as possible, since the stump has a tendency to swell in a very short time if the original cast is removed in the first 2 weeks.

On the first postoperative day the surgeon meets with the patient, the physiatrist, the prosthetist, and the physical therapist for aligning the prosthesis properly and working out a plan of training. A walker is placed in the patient's room so that the patient may stand. The pylon is attached to the rigid dressing in bed, and the patient is helped to sit up. If there are no orthostatic problems, he is allowed to stand with the support of the walker and to touch down with the prosthesis so that it can be adjusted. Five minutes of standing with contact of the prosthetic foot against the floor is all that is necessary. There is no advantage in placing any considerable weight into the prosthesis at that time. If the patient is not medically well or has a great deal of pain, it is advisable to postpone the initial standing for a few days. Control of the pain is achieved by the usual means of elevation of the amputated leg, the use of analgesics and narcotics when necessary, and encouragement of the patient.

Training with this type of postoperative prosthesis is not designed to achieve any great gait characteristics. The real objective is to reestablish proprioception and feedback by contact with the floor, which alerts the muscles and reestablishes the signaling system. Pain is also relieved by distal pressure on the stump by contact with the floor. If the patient has pain and is not standing, he may relieve the pain by placing a towel across the bottom of the cast socket with the pylon off and pulling on the towel to get proximal pressure against the end of the stump while in bed. It is inadvisable at this early stage to attempt to train the patient with a three-point gait, either between parallel bars or with crutches and the unamputated leg because the prosthesis has a tendency to fall off and will lose its compressive value. The patient is allowed to place more weight on the prosthesis progressively but never more than 15 to 20 pounds. This can be judged by having the patient stand on two scales each time he gets up to get the feeling of what 15 pounds of weight is like on the prosthetic side. Walking with the prosthesis is achieved progressively in parallel bars in the physical therapy department twice daily so that the patient does not have any long sessions of walking. It is never necessary for the patient to have his full weight on the prosthesis. This has been done by many patients without damage, but there is no real purpose in doing so until the definitive prosthesis is obtained.

Concomitant with the standing, balance, and limited

ambulation, the patient is also given exercises for the upper extremities and trunk, primarily to maintain a satisfactory degree of muscle power in the upper extremities and to ensure that he can maintain proper postural attitudes while standing and walking in the parallel bars. If a drain has been used, it should be removed through a window in the cast 48 hours after surgery. The window is replaced and held in place by plaster in order to avoid a weak spot in the closed cast socket. Daily training and exercises are carried out in the below-knee case for 14 days. If all goes well and there are no complications, the initial cast may be left on for 21 days. When the initial cast is removed at 14 days, it may be possible to remove all the sutures. In any case, those sutures that can be removed from healed areas should be removed. If any area does not appear to be completely healed, the sutures may remain. At that time another cast and pylon are applied as soon as possible. If healing is delayed and prolonged, it is still possible to keep the patient ambulatory with a temporary socket and pylon if there is no infection. The vertical position is one of the most effective means of improving the healing qualities of an amputation wound, particularly in the case of amputation for vascular impairment, since the isometric contraction of the muscles creates the so-called venous pump, which becomes much more efficient in the vertical than in the horizontal position.

In above-knee cases it may be necessary to remove the cast in 1 week and reapply another because of displacement of the amputation stump within the cast socket. It is difficult to maintain an undisturbed relationship between the stump and a cast socket in the above-knee case, since the socket has a tendency to fall off and usually is loose within a week. A new cast is then applied just as it was in the operating room, but it is somewhat easier with the patient awake. This is left on for 1 or 2 additional weeks while the patient is obtaining training in balance and ambulation. After 2 or 3 weeks of comfortable use, the second cast may be removed by splitting it and having the prosthetist take a cast from which to make a molded socket for a permanent prosthesis. The split cast is then reapplied, but if it does not conform closely to the stump and if it is not retained by the suspension, a new cast should be applied. When this is done, the permanent prosthesis should be delivered as soon as possible, that is, within only a few days, so that the patient is not without weightbearing at any time if the split cast cannot be used for that purpose.

After obtaining the permanent prosthesis, which is removable, the patient is required to wrap the amputation stump in a compressive dressing at night or whenever the prosthesis is not on in order to avoid swelling, which may occur even weeks after surgery if no rigid socket is applied. The training process requires supervision to the extent that the patient is not allowed to bear full weight on the prosthesis at any time. All of the walking, balancing, and standing are done in parallel bars and later with crutches. Full weightbearing is not really desirable until about 6 weeks after surgery, since connective tissues take that long to heal firmly and withstand the tensions of full weightbearing. With the permanent prosthesis, however, the gait characteristics of the patient must be taken into serious consideration, and then he is trained to walk with the best gait permitted by his amputation and his prosthesis. The length of time that the patient must stay in the hospital varies. Some patients may be discharged a week after surgery while wearing the postoperative prosthesis if no complications occur and if he does not have much pain. Most patients stay until the first cast change 2 to 3 weeks after surgery, after which they may remain at home and have the second cast removed and measurements for the permanent prosthesis made on an outpatient basis.

During this entire period the patient is seen daily by the physical therapist, who reports to the prosthetist and to the surgeon any variations from a normal course or the development of pain or malalignment or loosening of the prosthesis. In general, with this procedure the majority of patients are able to leave the hospital in an ambulatory state 1 month after amputation. In many cases the walking pylon is not applied to the cast socket because of the general condition of the patient or other contraindications. The rigid dressing, however, still retains its value in enhancing healing and diminishing the postoperative phantom pain. In those cases the cast is removed 2 or 3 weeks after surgery for the purpose of removing sutures, and the patient may then be measured for a temporary removable prosthesis.

This is the process of early ambulation, making it possible for the patient to walk 2 or 3 weeks after amputation with a temporary prosthesis with which he may be discharged to his home while being trained. In such cases the temporary prosthesis serves a useful purpose for 8 to 10 weeks, after which the patient may be measured for a permanent removable prosthesis. This applies to both above-knee and below-knee amputations. The usual relationship between above-knee and below-knee amputation on a time basis is that the above-knee amputation takes about one-third more time in each step for eventually being fitted with a permanent prosthesis than does the below-knee amputation.

ADVANTAGES OF IMMEDIATE POSTSURGICAL PROSTHESIS

It is the consensus among those who have experience with the rigid dressing and the application of an immediate postsurgical prosthesis for the purpose of allowing the patient to walk early that this is a great advance over conventional methods and the time it takes to fit a patient with a prosthesis. The rigid dressing itself provides tissue rest and increased comfort. With the amputation stump firmly fixed within a compressive cast socket, the patient can move about freely in bed without discomfort and can get up for the purpose of standing and balancing and ambulating without much pain. Nursing care is simplified in cases of this type. Moreover, the physiologic advantages are great. The stump matures much more rapidly. There is little threat of the development of a terminal hematoma in the amputation stump. The amputation stump is shaped better and heals faster. Most important of all, the method of myoplasty and the rigid dressing have demonstrated that the great majority of amputations for vascular impairment in the lower extremity can be made below the knee. Most statistics indicate that it is in the vicinity of 85%.

Secondary advantages are a shorter period of hospitalization and lower costs to the individual, a greater availability of hospital beds, diminished psychologic problems, and earlier return to productive activities, particularly for those who are still working. In terms of ambulation, a great many of the older patients who previously would have been considered poor candidates for practical ambulation do surprisingly well. The proprioceptive advantages of the stump properly shaped by myoplasty with its reestablishment of muscle function makes it possible for these elderly patients to have a much better feeling of security and control of the prosthesis than has followed conventional amputation and fitting with a permanent prosthesis after a significant loss of time and prolonged inactivity.

REFERENCES

1. Berlemont M: The Fitting of Amputees of the Lower Limbs with Prosthetic Devices on the Operating Table. Paper presented at the International Congress of Physical Medicine, Paris, 1964.
2. Weiss M, et al.: Myoplastic Amputation. Immediate Prosthesis and Early Ambulation. US Department of Health, Education, and Welfare, Public Health Services, National Institutes of Health, 1971.
3. Russek AS, Thompson WAL, et al.: Investigation of Immediate Prosthetic Fitting and Early Ambulation Following Amputation in the Lower Extremity, New York University, Institute of Rehabilitation Medicine, Rehabilitation Monograph XLI, Final Report, HEW Project No. RD-1958-M, April 30, 1969.
4. Burgess EM, Romano RL, Zettl JH: The Management of Lower Extremity Amputations. Surgery. Immediate Postsurgical Prosthetic Fitting. Patient Care. U.S. Government Printing Office, Washington, D.C. 1969.
5. Cohen SI, Goldman LD, et al.: The deleterious effect of immediate postoperative prosthesis in below-knee amputation for ischemic disease. Surgery 76:992, 1974.
6. Moore WS, Hall AD, Wylie EJ: Below-knee amputation for vascular insufficiency. Experience with immediate postoperative fitting of prosthesis. Arch Surg 97:886, 1968.
7. Sher MH: The air splint. An alternative to the immediate postoperative prosthesis. Arch Surg 108:746, 1974.
8. Warren R, James RC, et al.: The Boston interhospital amputation study. Experience with a community service in immediate postoperative amputation prosthetic fitting. Arch Surg 107:861, 1973.

CHAPTER 78
Immediate Postoperative Pneumatic Temporary Prosthesis for Below-Knee Amputees

Henry Haimovici

The benefits of a rigid dressing and the immediate postoperative temporary prosthesis, as described in Chapter 77, are well known and are reflected in the popularity of their use in the management of amputees.

The underlying concept for the immediate postoperative prosthesis is avoidance of edema of the stump, reduction of pain, achievement of accelerated healing of the amputation site, immediate postoperative mobility, narrowing of the gap between amputation and walking with a definitive prosthesis.

The method for applying an immediate postoperative plaster cast entails multidisciplinary services and requires above all a close cooperation among the surgeon, the physiatrist, and the physical therapist. The expertise of all concerned during the preoperative period, the immediate intraoperative application of the plaster cast, and the careful postoperative monitoring of the patient's local condition is essential for the successful outcome of this phase of management of the amputation stump.

While such multidisciplinary services can be found in most of the large medical centers, unfortunately their multiple services are not always available in community or small hospitals. As a result of the lack of such facilities or sometimes because of a lack of enthusiasm for a method that is not without hazards, and thus not universally acceptable, the search for an alternative method became necessary.

Little, of Sydney, Australia,[1] reported in 1971 the use of a pneumatic weightbearing prosthesis for below-knee amputees. His device is composed of two parts:

1. An inflatable plastic air-splint.
2. A rigid aluminum frame to which a solid ankle cushion heel (Sach) is attached. This allows the patient to use weightbearing and to ambulate postoperatively.

In 1974, Kerstein[2,3] and Sher[4] inspired by the use of a long air-splint in the emergency stabilization of long bone fractures, adopted a similar type of splint as an alternative to the immediate postoperative prosthesis. Sher reported[5] on a series of 44 patients treated between 1971 and 1980. The air-splint technique was applied in a total of 46 below-

knee amputees. While this procedure appears simple enough, few reports have appeared on its use so far. This chapter deals only with the type of equipment presently available in the USA.

DESCRIPTION OF EQUIPMENT

The equipment[*] includes three major components:

Air-splint. The air-splint, or pneumatic prosthesis, is designed to provide a protective cushion of air to achieve controlled counterpressure, which is uniformly exerted for the purpose of preventing stump edema. In addition, it helps avoid knee flexion contracture or faulty knee position and ultimately promotes stump shrinkage. There are three air-splint lengths: short (18 inches), medium (22 inches), and long (26 inches). The most commonly used is the medium size, which covers both the stump and half of the thigh. The air-splint is not used for weightbearing.

Rigid Brace. This component is a conical-shaped tube with its wider diameter at the proximal end (thigh) and the narrower one (foot) at the distal end. It is used in conjunction with the air-splint after inflation of the latter. There are three sizes of rigid braces to match the length of the air-splints.

The stump and the thigh up to the junction between the middle and upper thirds are enclosed in the air-splint, which is provided with an inflation stem that can be connected with the inflation pump.

Inflation System. The inflation system consists of three major components: a manometer or air pressure control unit, inflation pump, and connecting hose.

---

[*]For further information contact Jobst, Toledo, Ohio.

APPLICATION OF THE PROSTHESIS

This equipment is designed for (1) nonambulatory use for immediate postoperative prosthesis and (2) for ambulatory use.

Nonambulatory Use for Immediate Postoperative Prosthesis

At the completion of the below-knee operative procedure (see Chapter 77), a dressing consisting either of Owens silk or Xeroform gauze is applied directly on the suture line, which in turn is covered with an elastic gauze bandage or with an orlon lycra stump sock. Care should be taken to avoid a bulky dressing lest the air-splint be rendered ineffective in its role of uniform circumferential counterpressure.

An air-splint of appropriate size is then carefully placed around the limb, around both the BK stump and the distal half of the thigh. The splint extends beyond the end of the stump by about 4 inches. The unzipped and deflated air-splint is carefully positioned so that the zipper is placed on the anterior surface of the limb. Before starting the inflation, the splint must be fully closed.

Inflation of the Splint. The stem of the open inflation valve of the air-splint is connected to the hose of the manometer or air pressure control unit. The foot pump provides an easy way for checking and monitoring the degree of inflation. For nonambulatory use, a pressure range of 20 to 25 mm Hg is suggested. Higher pressures may cause pain in the stump or even breakage of the air-splint.

One of the pitfalls to be avoided is either overinflation or underinflation of the air prosthesis. If the patient experiences discomfort or pain, release of the air valve can be taught even to the patient. Use of the manometer provides a readily available guide. The pressure should be checked periodically and adjusted accordingly. The advantage of a transparent prosthesis is that it allows inspection of the dressing without removing the splint. In the event of drainage or stump infection, the removable splint provides easy access to the stump.

Ambulatory Use of the Prosthesis

The prosthesis in itself is not designed for weightbearing unless it is used in conjunction with the rigid brace. The pneumatic or air-splint is applied around the limb, zipped and closed, but not inflated. The rigid brace, of an appropriate size, is placed around the air-splint and limb. The rigid brace should be adjusted to the length of the patient's normal leg. The upper end of the air-splint should protrude approximately 4 inches above the top edge of the rigid brace so that the stem of the inflation valve is accessible to the hose of the manometer (Fig. 78-1).

At this point, the pneumatic splint is inflated through the inflation system as indicated previously. The pressure in the splint for ambulatory purpose ranges from 25 to 50 mm Hg. Again, overinflation above 50 mm Hg should be avoided. The exact pressure, however, varies with individual tolerance of the patient and personal experience. Ambulation with this device is advised to be used in conjunction with a walker or crutches. It is intended primarily for indoor use and not for street use.

Advantages. The advantages of this ambulatory device are several: (1) early postoperative ambulation, (2) early rehabilitation, and (3) its use before the stump is completely healed, which in itself is a great achievement similar to the one of the plaster cast, the difference being that the condition of the stump with borderline healing ability can be better monitored and controlled.

SUMMARY

The pneumatic splint for immediate postamputation use for below-knee amputees offers great advantages in terms of easy applicability and represents an acceptable alternative in the absence of a plaster cast. Wider experience is necessary to properly assess its indications and contraindications. Experience to date appears most encouraging.

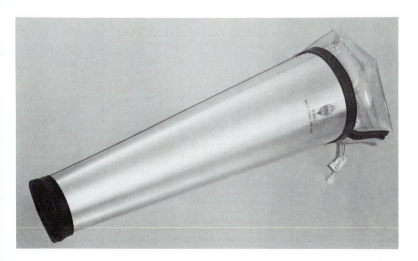

Figure 78-1. The rigid brace. Note the protruding air-splint above the proximal edge where the inflation valve of the splint is located.

REFERENCES

1. Little JM: A pneumatic weight-bearing temporary prosthesis for below-knee amputees. Lancet 1:271, 1971.
2. Kerstein MD: Utilization of an air-splint after below-knee amputation. Am J Phys Med 53:119, 1974.
3. Kerstein MD: A rigid dressing with a pneumatic prosthesis for below-knee amputees. Am Surgeon 40:373, 1974.
4. Sher MH: The air-splint: An alternative to the immediate postoperative prosthesis. Arch Surg 108:746, 1974.
5. Sher MH, Liebman P: The air-splint: A method of managing below-knee amputations. J Cardiovas Surg 23:497, 1982.

CHAPTER 79

Prosthetics for Lower-Limb Amputees

Jan J. Stokosa

Amputation is palliative. The amputation stump is a new limb that must serve the same function as the removed foot but with an anatomy not intended for such a purpose. It should be prepared for this new responsibility to ultimately potentiate medical and prosthetic rehabilitation. As technology advances the capabilities of prostheses, amputation surgery must reciprocate, and vice versa.

The goal of the prosthetist is to aid the amputee in reentering and regaining his place in society—working, playing, and engaging in a full range of human relationships. Progress in this endeavor is marked by the amputee's placing a diminishing emphasis on his amputation and his prosthesis. Ideally, the amputation and prosthesis will move outside the inner circle of the patient's life concerns. The prosthetist's role in this process, in the broadest terms, is to enhance the amputee's mobility and appearance, with maximum comfort.

The ultimate achievement of the prosthetist's goal is dependent on five factors:

1. The general physical and mental condition of the patient
2. The patient's understanding of the total rehabilitation process
3. The level of amputation
4. The quality of surgery and resultant physiology
5. The degree of mobility, comfort, and cosmesis afforded by the prosthetist

These five points can be achieved *only* through the cooperation of the essential participants: the patient, the surgeon, and the prosthetist. The physiatrist, nurse, physical therapist, rehabilitation counselor, family members, and others may also be productively involved.

PREOPERATIVE CONSIDERATIONS AND PREPARATION

It is generally agreed that the earliest possible explanation of why the surgery is necessary and of the entire process from preoperative preparation to prosthetic fitting and follow-up is of extreme benefit to the patient.[1-4] The development and presentation of this plan should involve at least the surgeon and the prosthetist; others should be involved based on the individual need and available resources. A visit from a mature person with a similar amputation history and similar characteristics is highly beneficial. Above all else, the entire orientation process should be realistic. Ranges of expectation, instead of the high points, should be communicated.

Unfortunately, even with the best of intentions and with considerable effort expended, this orientation process often fails. Patients consistently enter the prosthetic phase of their rehabilitation encumbered by misconceptions and unnecessary fears. Psychologic preparation of the patient is a fertile area for research and innovation.

In addition to general patient orientation, prosthetist and surgeon should collaborate on surgical objectives. The prosthetist will have a particular point of view that the surgeon should consider with his own. The prosthetist, along with the surgeon, will be concerned that the patient's general physical condition be maintained or improved, especially in regard to strength, balance, and range of motion of the hips and knees. The prosthetist will wish the stump to be as long as possible and free of pain, retaining as much of the physical and physiologic characteristics of the intact natural extremity as possible (Fig. 79-1). This will maximize weight-bearing surface and provide a long lever for more effective control of the prosthesis. Problems such as sharp bones, neuroma, and adherent tissue will, of course, be of great concern because they reduce the area of support and have a negative effect on the comfort and control of the prosthesis. The position of the scar, as long as it is nonadherent, thin, and flat, is not of importance.

Beyond these general considerations, surgeon and prosthetist must choose a specific postoperative management mode. There are four options: (1) rigid dressing, with or without weight bearing (immediate postsurgical fitting [IPSF]),[5] (2) semirigid dressing,[6,7] (3) controlled-environ-

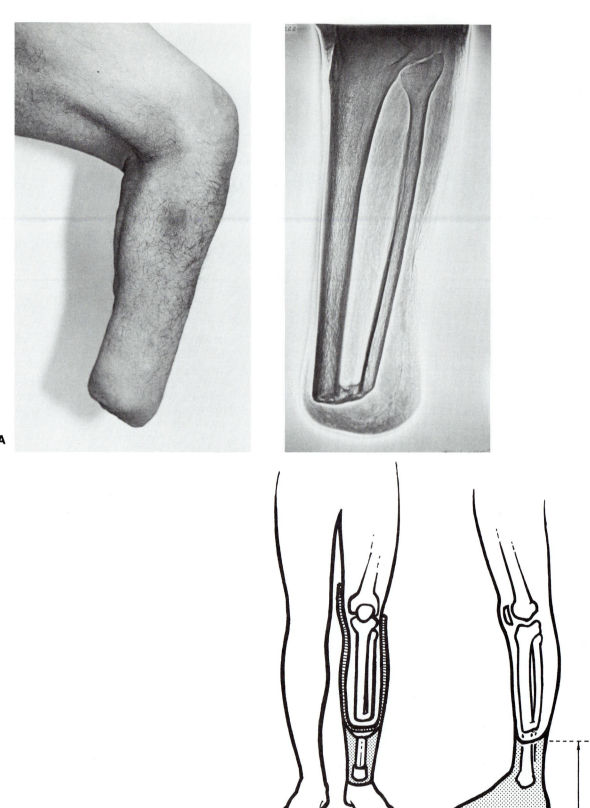

Figure 79-1. A. Xeroradiogram of ideal below-knee amputation stump. Space needed for prosthesis: 6¼ to 8⅝ inches.

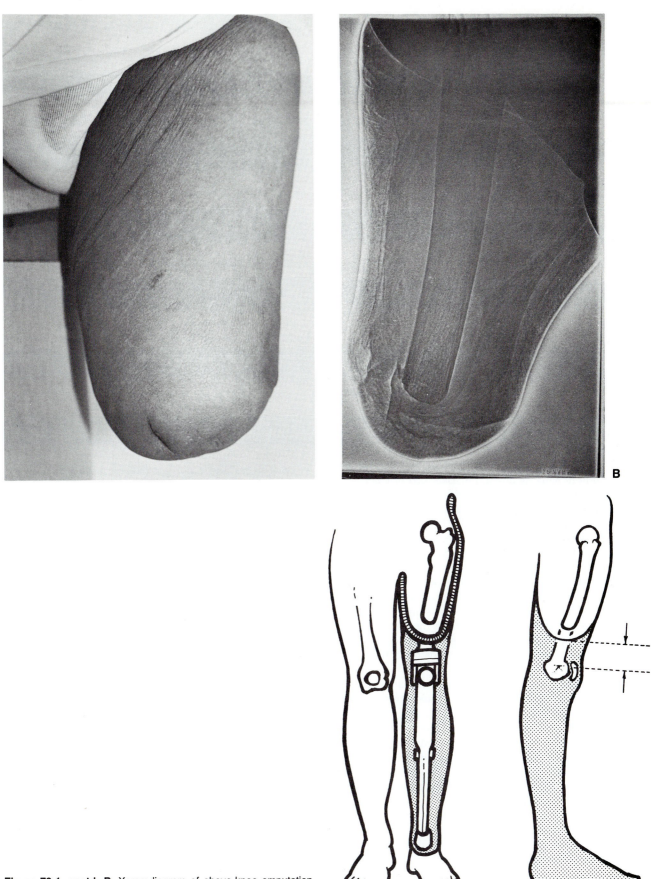

B

Figure 79-1, contd. B. Xeroradiogram of above-knee amputation stump. Space needed for prosthesis: 4 inches.

ment treatment (CET),[8] and (4) soft dressing.[9] The postoperative management mode may, of course, require modification if contraindications are discovered during surgery.

IPSF, semirigid dressing, and CET methods achieve highly positive results, both physical and psychologic, but are contraindicated unless specifically trained personnel are available for around-the-clock postoperative care.

IMMEDIATE POSTOPERATIVE CONSIDERATIONS

Postoperative treatment should, in the case of elective surgery, be a continuation of the preoperative plan. The plan should be reiterated in full to the patient. In the instance of emergency surgery, the plan, of course, must be established and communicated as soon as possible within the constraints of the situation.

The prosthetist will have a number of specific items to add to the surgeon's postoperative treatment plan. Most will involve physical therapy, intended to prevent nonuse degenerative processes. Generally, the plan should include the following:

1. To avoid knee-flexion and hip-flexion contractures, the patient should lie face down three to five times each day for 30 minutes or more, with the head turned away from the amputated side and both anterosuperior iliac spines in contact with the bed. The foot of the other leg should rest over the back edge of the bed or should be supported under its dorsal aspect.
2. The below-knee stump should always be supported in its entire length and should not be allowed to assume a position of hanging down, i.e., over bed or chair.
3. The stump should be wrapped with an elastic compression bandage to control postoperative edema. To assure adequate suspension, the wrap for the below-knee amputation should include the femoral condyles and should be above the superior border of the patella; for the above-knee amputation it should be wrapped around the waist at or above the iliac crests, using one continuous bandage (double, triple, and sometimes quadruple length bandages are necessary) (Fig. 79-2). The stump should be rewrapped three to five times during the day, and the wrapping should be left on overnight. Wrapping should be continued until well after the prosthesis has been fitted.
4. Physical therapy training to maintain or increase strength in the upper and lower extremities should begin as soon as possible.
5. When discharged from the hospital, the patient should be instructed about a home exercise program that will be monitored by a designated member of the rehabilitation team.
6. Weekly visits to the prosthetist should be scheduled to monitor stump fluid-volume changes.
7. Ambulation with or without the prosthesis should begin as soon as possible—the quicker the patient is restored to maximum function, the less likely it is that psychologic problems will arise.

When deep healing is achieved and stump fluid volume is stable, prosthetic fitting can begin.

A UNIFIED APPROACH[*]

In the design, fabrication, and fitting of any extremity prosthesis, comfort to the wearer must be an overriding concern. Discomfort to the wearer will result in rejection or improper use of the prosthesis, thwarting other benefits. The most sophisticated component part with the most accurate biomechanical alignment is of little value if walking causes pain or skin breakdown or both.

Comfort can be accomplished only if proper fitting[†] of the prosthetic socket[‡] to the amputation stump is achieved. Other comfort-enhancing aspects of the prosthesis and its alignment are subordinate to and dependent on proper socket fit. The amputation stump, together with the socket, forms a lever to control the prosthesis during the swing and stance phases of the walking cycle. The stump also must transmit the entire weight of the body to the prosthesis. The more accurately the socket fits the stump, the greater the comfort and efficiency.

The optimum-fitting socket is one that uses the entire skin surface of the amputation stump that is contained within the socket. Weight-bearing loads are distributed to benefit biomechanical efficiency and to maintain tolerable pressure levels on the skin and subdermal tissues. A loose-fitting socket reduces the overall proportionate pressures, thereby increasing stress on smaller areas. This of course results in pain and skin abrasions. An extremely tight-fitting socket causes the same problems as a loose-fitting socket and, in addition, may cause problems such as stump-edema syndrome, sebaceous cyst formation, and folliculitis.

In the optimum-fitting socket, most of the pressure of weight bearing is borne by direct vertical loading—of the tibia in the below-knee amputee and of the femur in the above-knee amputee. This result is more exceptional than routine. Usually the pressure of weight bearing is applied to the stump obliquely, as when a solid cone is forced into a hollow cone. An example of oblique pressure is the fitting condition brought about in a below-knee amputee when the fibula has been sectioned more than 1 inch above the distal tibia and the pretibial and posterior muscle groups have atrophied, resulting in a cone-shaped stump.

The entire design, fitting, and fabrication process consists of six basic steps: (1) initial mold; (2) cast reduction modification; (3) test socket fitting—static biomechanical analysis, dynamic biomechanical analysis, and alignment; (4) definitive prosthesis—fabrication and design theory; (5) definitive dynamic biomechanical alignment; and (6) final finishing. This process may take 8 to 16 visits to the prosthetist, with approximately 1½ hours per appointment. An additional 25 to 40 hours will be necessary for laboratory fabrication and preparation procedures.

---

[*]The prosthetic treatment of patients with other amputation levels (e.g., transmetatarsal, Syme's, upper-extremity) and with multiple amputations follows the same general course described in this section, with obvious differences in detail that are beyond the scope of this chapter.

[†]The term *fitting* refers to the shaping and contouring of the inner surface of the socket, with the goal of achieving a functional and comfortable union between prosthesis and amputation stump.

[‡]The term *socket* refers to the receptacle in which the amputation stump is contained.

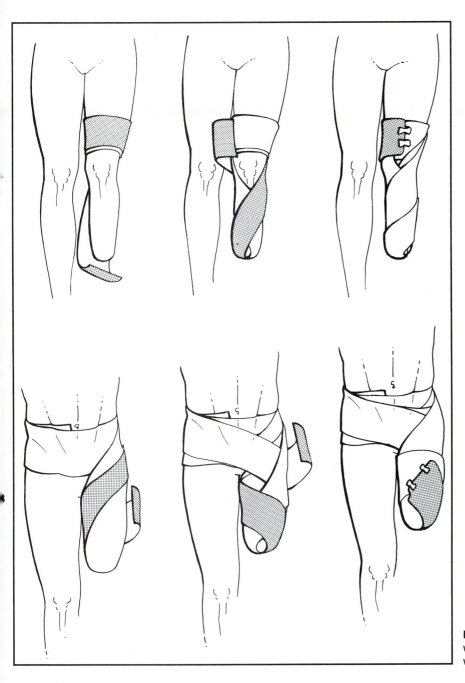

Figure 79-2. A. Below-knee compression wrapping. **B.** Above-knee compression wrapping.

Anatomic and Physiologic Considerations

The anatomy of the remaining portion of the limb after amputation is quantitatively and qualitatively different from the anatomy of an intact limb. The differences usually become manifest several months after surgery. Conventional amputation techniques render the greatest physiologic disturbance. Amputation techniques emphasizing a biologic approach such as in the Ertl technique result in a superior physiologic and biomechanical end organ. Ertl developed an osteoplastic flap to close the medullary cavity, thereby maintaining intramedullary pressure and concomitantly minimizing or eliminating bone hypersensitivity and im-

proved venous return. A standard procedure in this technique is the anchoring of the antagonstic muscle groups, myoplasty or myodesis. This procedure provides active muscle function, which in turn reduces atrophy and fatty degeneration.[10–13]

Of the numerous differences between the intact limb and the stump, the following are of particular importance to prosthetic fitting:

1. Cross-sectional area. Increased area provides reduced per-square-inch pressure (Fig. 79-3).
2. Capability of the bone(s) to bear weight in the long axis (Fig. 79-4). As more weight is borne though the long axis of the bone(s), tangential loads are reduced.

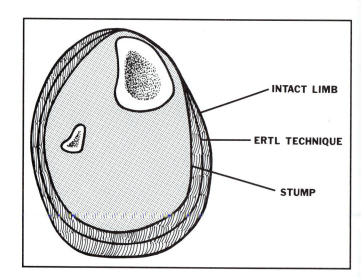

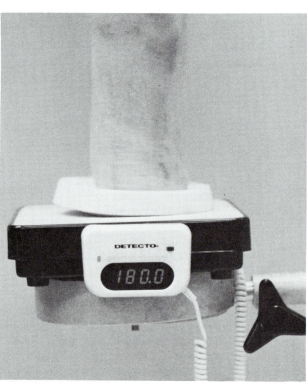

Figure 79-3. Cross-sectional comparison of intact limb: Ertl amputation stump and conventional amputation stump.

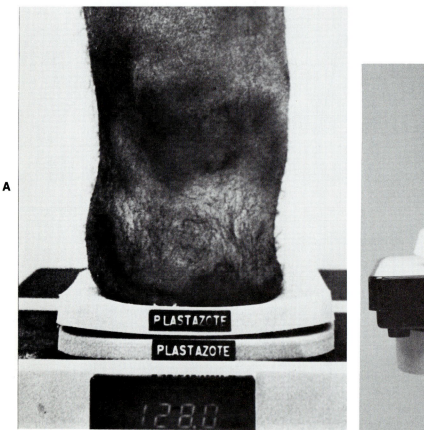

A

Figure 79-4. A. End-bearing capability of short amputation stump after osteoplastic-myoplastic (Ertl) procedure. **B.** End-bearing capability of long amputation stump after osteoplastic-myoplastic (Ertl) reconstructive surgery. Patient is insulin-dependent diabetic and also has a history of neuropathy in both legs and hands.

3. Circulatory condition.
4. Proprioceptive ability.

All points listed are positively influenced by osteoplastic myoplastic procedures.

An additional important consideration is the poor ability of the soft tissues of the stump to accept stresses necessarily imposed with prosthesis use.[14]

The stump shape that provides the best function is one that is more cylindrical. The cylindrical shape provides greater area and aids in rotational control of the prosthesis (see Fig. 79-1A).

Initial Mold

The initial mold is the first of three basic procedures (initial mold, cast reduction modification, test socket fitting—static and dynamic biomechanical analysis) that ultimately provide the model from which the total surface-bearing socket will be constructed.

Mindful of the patient's general physical condition, meticulous examination and palpation of the stump must be performed to discover conditions that may affect the fit of the prosthetic socket. Multiple-angle xeroradiograms should be used to observe the condition and quality of bone, muscle, and subcutaneous tissue.

The prosthetist must form a multidimensional mental image of what he perceives to be the optimal socket design and must choose the appropriate molding technique. It is essential that the prosthetist have in his repertoire a number of alternate molding approaches.

In selection of the molding approach, knowledge and experience are the best guides. Criteria can be delineated, but this process is the subject of a much longer work. Of the many different molding techniques, limited in the final analysis only by the innovativeness and expertise of the prosthetist, the molding techniques explained and illustrated herein are of good general use.

Below-Knee Molding

During the molding procedure, the patient with a below-knee amputation may be in the standing or sitting position. A mold-release cream is applied to the skin of the stump, and a sheer nylon sock is pulled over the stump and is held firmly in place by elastic suspension straps. The nylon sock contains and compresses the soft tissues of the stump, aiding the molding process. Anatomic landmarks may be marked with indelible pencil on the nylon (Fig. 79-5). These markings transfer automatically to the mold and subsequently to the cast.

An initial plaster splint is submerged in water and is applied to the anterior and pretibial surface of the stump from the tibial tubercle level distally. A wide elastic compression sling is then applied over the splint, wrapped around posteriorly, and held under tension. The wet plaster splint is deformed with the hands fully applied and with the fingers conforming to important anatomic landmarks, molding the plaster to the contours of the stump. Simultaneously, the patient performs a series of stump-muscle contractions to assist in forming the plaster (Fig. 79-6).

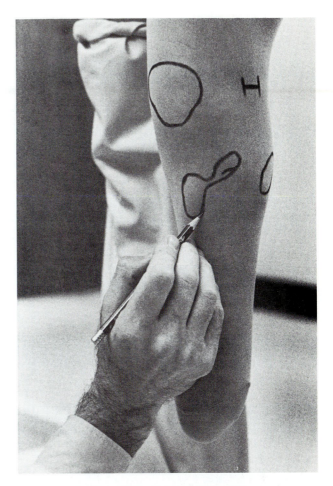

Figure 79-5. Outlining anatomic landmarks on below-knee stump.

After the initial plaster splint has hardened, a second splint is applied to the anterior proximal stump and knee area. The previously described procedure is followed to deform and contour the plaster.

The final step in the molding process is the application of a wet elasticized plaster bandage to compress the tissue of the stump posteriorly and distally (Fig. 79-7). As the plaster hardens, it is deformed and contoured by hand over the distal terminal tibial area—to provide maximal vertical loading—and the entire posterior aspect of the stump and knee areas. Again the patient simultaneously performs a series of muscle contractions, further deforming and contouring the plaster.

After the plaster has hardened, it is removed from the stump in one piece (Fig. 79-8). This is the mold—a hollow plaster replica of the stump, with markings indicating the anatomic landmarks of the stump indelibly transferred to its inner surface (Fig. 79-9).

Into this hollow mold, liquid plaster of Paris is poured (Fig. 79-10). This is the casting process. When the plaster of Paris hardens, the mold is stripped away (Fig. 79-11). A solid, three-dimensional cast of the stump as it is under slight compression and deformation remains. The indelible marks, indicating important anatomic landmarks, now ap-

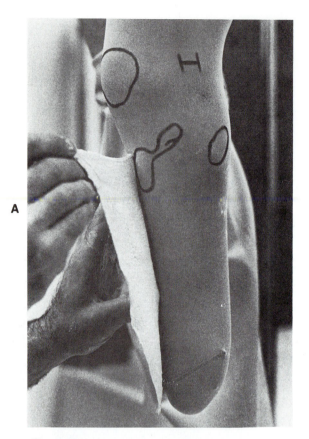

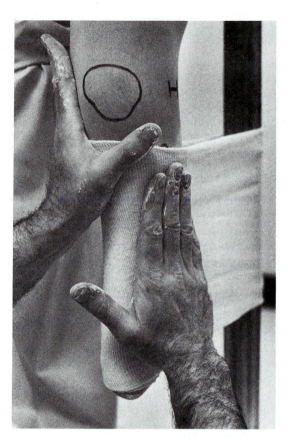

Figure 79-6. A. Application of plaster splint to below-knee stump. **B.** Deformation of plaster splint on below-knee stump.

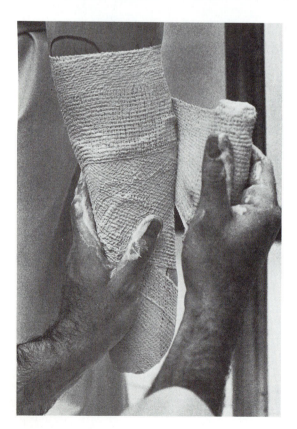

Figure 79-7. Application of elasticized plaster bandage to below-knee stump.

pear on the outside of the cast (Fig. 79-12). The cast is ready for modification.

Above-Knee Molding

Preparation of the above-knee mold is similar to that for the below-knee mold. With the patient in the weight-bearing position, anatomic landmarks may be identified.

Wet elasticized plaster bandages are applied to the entire surface of the stump and perineum, superior to the inguinal ligament and gluteal fold, and around the hips with considerable compression to ensure intimate contour. The wet plaster is hand molded to conform to the anatomy, enhancing areas for biomechanical advantage. When hardened, the mold is removed, and the cast is prepared as previously described.

Cast Reduction Modification

The cast is a three-dimensional representation of the amputation stump as it is under partial compression or stress. The purpose of cast modification is to create a model, necessarily subjective (i.e., based on observation and judgment as well as measurement), that is representative of the stump shape and volume under full stress of static and dynamic weight bearing (the shape and volume the stump would take as it transmits the weight of the body to the socket during standing and walking). This goal is accomplished by sculpting the cast (Fig. 79-13).

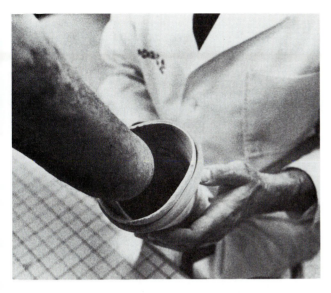

Figure 79-8. Removing the mold.

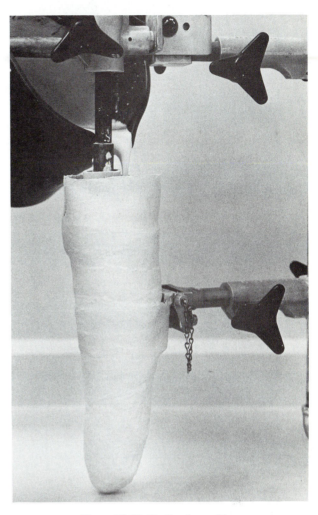

Figure 79-10. Casting the mold.

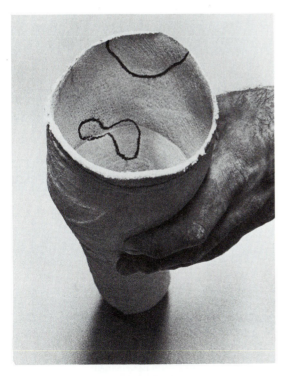

Figure 79-9. The mold.

The outer surface of the finished model will ultimately represent the inner surface of the socket. Shaving plaster from the cast will therefore increase pressure to the stump in that area; conversely, it reduces pressure in adjacent areas.

To achieve an optimum-fitting socket, a cast must be modified (1) to allow normal physiologic function, (2) to assure that pressure per unit area is within an acceptable pain threshold, with special care to assure maximum axial loading of the tibia in the below-knee stump, (3) to provide maximum rotational control of the prosthesis, (4) to distribute pressure over the *entire* surface of the stump, and (5) to achieve a geometric shape that will generate maximum biomechanical efficiency.

It has been reported that specific areas of the stump are not able to accept the pressures of weight bearing.[15] These areas are the head of the fibula, the tibial tubercle, the crest of the tibia, and the distal terminal tibia in the below-knee stump and the distal terminal femur in the above-knee stump. It has been shown, however, that these areas are able to bear significant pressures.[16,17] The total

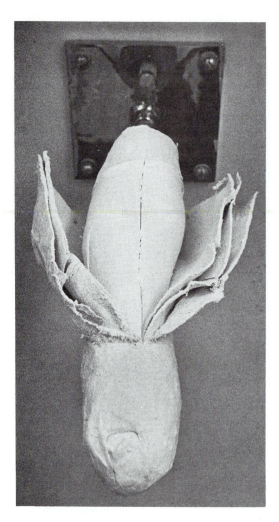

Figure 79-11. Separating the mold from the cast.

surface area available for pressure distribution may, of course, be reduced significantly by problem conditions such as exostotic bone, an adherent scar, and neuroma.

The completion of cast reduction modification results in a superior replication of the amputation stump (Fig. 79-14). The first test socket may now be made.

Test Socket Fitting—Static and Dynamic Biomechanical Analysis

A sheet of transparent plastic is vacuum-formed over the completed model to form the test socket. The purpose of the test socket(s) is to test the fit of the design and to provide diagnosotic information for use in achieving the optimum socket fit.

The test socket should first be fit under static, weight-bearing conditions. The lubricated stump is slid into the test socket, which is positioned and supported for standing by a static alignment fixture. The patient, standing in a comfortable posture, shifts his weight onto the stump (Fig. 79-15). The effects of pressure on the skin are observed through the plastic and empirically evaluated.

Fitting refinements are made in one of two ways: (1) direct modification to the test socket (grinding, heating and reshaping, or filling) or (2) rectification of the model and fabrication of another test socket. The degree of refinement required will dictate the modification procedure. It is not uncommon that fabrication and fitting of multiple test sockets are needed to achieve an acceptable fit.

When an acceptable fit is achieved under static weight-bearing conditions, the test socket can be readied for dynamic analysis. The necessary components (foot, ankle, knee) are attached to the socket with adjustable alignment couplings and a metal tube (Fig. 79-16). The suspension system, if not designed within the contours of the socket, is added at this time. Under close supervision, the patient dons the test prosthesis and begins walking between parallel bars.

The purpose of dynamic biomechanical analysis is to establish an efficient gait while maintaining comfort. The amputee provides valuable input beyond the prosthetist's ability to visualize deviations. Alignment couplings allow minute and infinite adjustments to be made (Fig. 79-17).

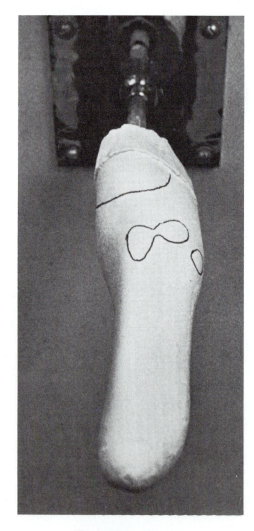

Figure 79-12. The cast.

Various foot, ankle, and, in the above-knee amputee, knee components are tested and evaluated by the amputee.

Walking imposes different and additional forces that may affect the comfort of the socket. The efficiency of alignment and the characteristics of the prosthetic foot also have significant influence on the comfort of the socket.

Fitting refinements are made as needed in the previously described way. Several alterations and sockets are usually required to optimize the fit. With each iteration, socket design is improved until an optimum level of comfort and function is reached.

Common errors in the use of test sockets are (1) not using transparent plastic, (2) using a plastic that is too flexible, allowing excessive plastic deformation under weight-bearing loads, (3) using multi-ply fitting socks between stump and test socket (I usually use a no fitting sock, affording maximum visual assessment), (4) restricting the number of test sockets (the number of test sockets required varies, based on the complexities of each case—I have used as few as one and as many as 30), and (5) confusing "total contact" with "total surface bearing."

Total contact is the condition that occurs when the entire surface of the stump is in complete contact with the socket, not necessarily under compression. Total surface

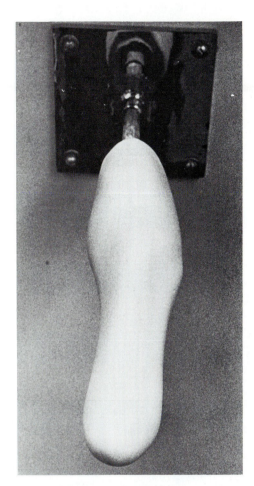

Figure 79-14. The model.

bearing is the condition that occurs when the entire surface of the stump is in complete contact with the socket while all unit areas are under compression to their proportionate tolerable level.

Total contact has become, in the minds of many, the ultimate goal and is often pursued as an end in itself. This pursuit is counterproductive because it is total surface bearing that should be the goal.

When optimum fit and biomechanical alignment are achieved in the test prosthesis, preparation is made for fabrication of the definitive prosthesis. The relative position of the test socket to the foot, ankle, and knee components must be precisely recorded and is usually accomplished by clamping the test prosthesis within a stationary measuring device designed specifically for this purpose. A final model of the amputation stump must then be made from the final test socket.

Definitive Prosthesis—Fabrication and Design Theory

The definitive prosthesis comprises a definitive plastic socket, the required mechanical foot, ankle, knee analog

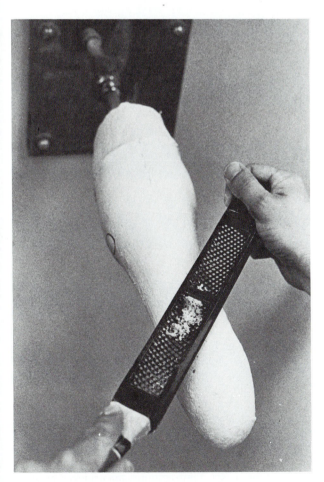

Figure 79-13. Cast reduction modification.

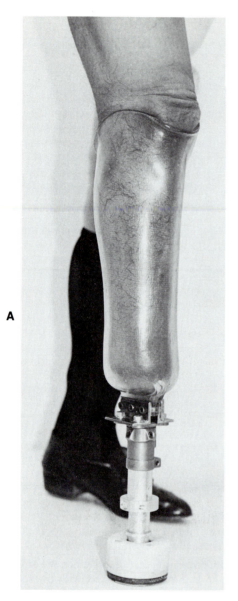

A

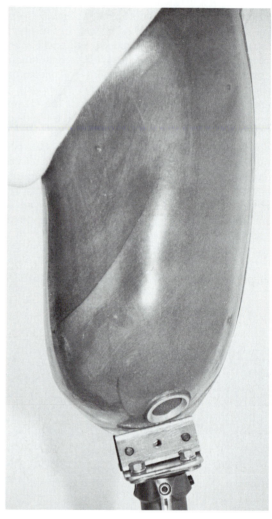

B

Figure 79-15. A. Static biomechanical analysis of below-knee test socket. **B.** Static biomechanical analysis of above-knee test socket.

component(s), and structural connections with anatomic external shape.

The definitive plastic socket is formed over the final model. This is accomplished by using either liquid lamination, impregnated lamination, or vacuum-formed sheet plastic. Various liquid resins can be used. The type and number of reinforcing materials and matrices can vary infinitely.

In most below-knee cases, a removable, soft insert liner is used between stump and socket to increase comfort. The liner is fabricated over the model, and the socket is made with the liner in place.

Most below-knee amputees wear prosthetic fitting socks. The socks vary in material (nylon, Orlon, Lycra, cotton, wool) and in ply, from a sheer nylon to a six-ply wool or cotton. When a fitting sock will be worn, it is placed over the model before the socket is made. Both liner and fitting sock are placed over the model before socket fabrication if use is planned for both.

The completed definitive socket must be attached to the selected foot, ankle, and knee components in one of the two ways—endoskeletal design or exoskeletal design.

In the endoskeletal design, components and socket are connected by a central metal tube. The metal tube-to-socket connection is achieved by bolting the tube to a plastic block, which is then glued to the socket. The entire apparatus is finally encased in a removable, soft, plastic-foam material that is shaped to imitate the missing limb.

In the exoskeletal design, components and socket are connected by wood or rigid plastic foam; which is bonded directly to the socket. Limb contours are achieved by shaping the external surface of the wood or plastic foam. Finally, socks) between the definitive prosthesis and the test prosthesis on which the existing dynamic analysis was based.

The patient should be encouraged to perform a full complement of activities, approximating activities he will perform in daily living. Special vocational or avocational activities should also be considered, with appropriate trials devised. When the patient and the prosthetist agree that optimum alignment has been reached, the prosthesis is ready for final finishing.

The adjustable alignment couplings remain within the prosthesis in the endoskeletal design. This feature sustains absolute fidelity of alignment. In the exoskeletal design the adjustable couplings must be removed before proceeding to the final finishing stage.

Final Finishing

The final step in the fabrication process is to give a cosmetically natural and agreeable appearance to the prosthesis (Figs. 79-18 and 79-19). In preparation for the actual shaping and finishing, careful circumference measurements, caliper measurements, tracings, and photographs are taken of the patient's intact limb.

A prefabricated, soft-foam cover is slipped over the endoskeletal componentry and socket. This cover is shaped to the measurements—converted left to right or right to left—of the patient's intact limb. Similar steps are followed in cosmetically finishing a prosthesis of exoskeletal design.

The patient dons the prosthesis and examines his appearance in a full-length mirror. Family members or other persons significant to the patient may often be productively involved in this final examination. After the patient has approved the appearance of his prosthesis, he is instructed in its proper care.

Postfitting Follow-up

Use of a prosthesis causes physical changes in the amputation stump—subcutaneous tissue shrinkage and either myoatrophy or myohypertrophia. No diagnostic apparatus is available to predict accurately the amount of change or when it will occur. Experience suggests, however, that systematic observation could produce a useful stump-change prediction formula. Salient variables effecting stump change are amputation surgical technique, somatotype, body weight and body weight fluctuation, phsyical activity (type, duration, and how consistently it is engaged in), and design of the prosthesis.

Changes in the amputation stump result in changes in the relationship between stump and socket. These changes may cause severe pain and skin breakdown if refitting adjustments are not made immediately.

The amputee himself makes initial refitting adjustments by altering the thickness of fitting socks. When this alteration no longer maintains comfort, the prosthetist may apply plastic filler or soft padding material to the inner surface of the socket to compensate for reduction in stump size, or he may remove plastic from the inner surface of the socket by grinding or sanding to compensate for an increase

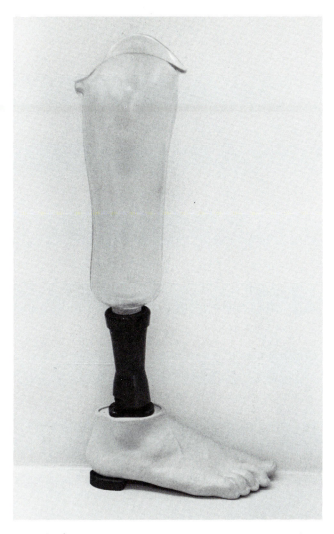

Figure 79-16. Below-knee test socket ready for dynamic biomechanical analysis.

a thin, rigid plastic lamination is made over the wood or plastic foam for structural integrity and cosmesis.

Endoskeletal-design prostheses normally have alignment adjustability. In addition, they have maximum modularity, allowing for quick and easy exchange of components. The exoskeletal-design prosthesis has no alignment adjustability and minimum modularity. The endoskeletal design is, however, more susceptible to scarring and tearing, especially in the kneeling position. This drawback is partially offset by the replaceability of the cover.

Definitive Dynamic Biomechanical Alignment

With the definitive socket attached to componentry, along with the adjustable alignment couplings, the prosthesis is returned to the measuring apparatus, and alignment based on early dynamic analysis is reestablished. With this accomplished, the patient dons the prosthesis and begins walking. Alignment and component refinements may be necessary because of subtle differences (e.g., material, weight, liners,

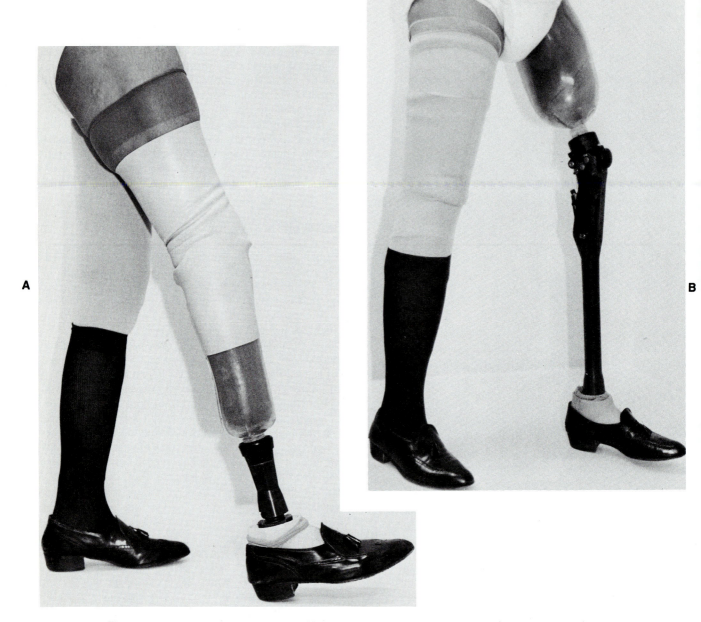

Figure 79-17. A. Below-knee dynamic biomechanical analysis. **B.** Above-knee dynamic biomechanical analysis.

in stump size or volume. The amount of adjustment that can be made in a socket is quite limited. When maximum refitting adjustments are reached, socket replacement is necessary.

The amputee should expect to experience periodic changes in stump size for the remainder of his life. A case in point is my experience with a World War I veteran in his 90s who still requires refitting adjustments as a result of soft-tissue shrinkage—even though he has been wearing a prosthesis for more than 70 years.

Excess modification and failure to refabricate new sockets when needed are among the most common prosthetist errors. This is far from a simple issue. The policies of third-party reimbursers often obstruct clinical decisions. I have found, however, that upon receiving a detailed written analysis of the clinical situation, most third-party reimbursers, with the exception of the Veterans Administration, accept charges for socket refabrication.

Occasional repair and replacement of worn or broken foot, ankle, or knee components will also be required on an ongoing basis.

COMMON STUMP PROBLEMS OF THE LOWER-EXTREMITY AMPUTEE

State-of-the-art amputation surgery and prosthetic care will eliminate a large share of the chronic pain and mobility problems suffered by many amputees.[18,19]

Beyond the issue of optimum vs. suboptimum care,

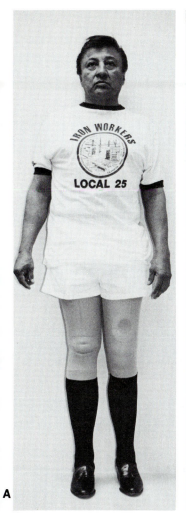
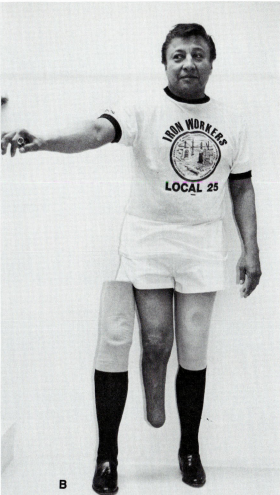
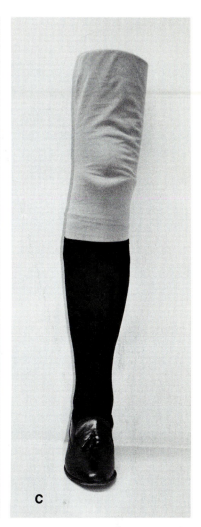

Figure 79-18. **A** to **C.** Endoskeletal below-knee prosthesis.

the amputee is subject to a variety of problem situations. The largest share of these problems concerns the amputation stump. Practitioners concerned with the amputee should be aware of several pathologic stump conditions that, if left untreated, can result in incapacitation.

Unfortunately, there is a dearth of information in the prosthetic-related literature regarding stump problems and their causes. Therefore, it is necessary to rely on clinical experience and judgment in much of this section.

Neuroma

Painful neuroma should not be a postoperative problem in the amputation stump if the nerve is treated properly during surgery.[20] However, if the nerve end is positioned over bone or adheres to bone or scar tissue, it may be irritated by pressure and traction from the prosthetic socket and may be a source of continual pain. Surgical intervention is the only complete solution to this problem.

Stump-Edema Syndrome

Initially in stump-edema syndrome (venous and lymphatic congestion of the distal stump), the stump appears cyanotic and edematous, and the patient may be only minimally uncomfortable. If the condition is allowed to persist, the distal stump skin becomes darkly pigmented, increasingly edematous, ulcerated, and painful. The cause of stump-edema syndrome is a prosthetic socket that is excessively tight circumferentially at its proximal border or that imposes excessive pressure over venous and lymphatic vessels. Recontouring the socket will correct the problem. Another cause is physical, requiring surgical revision.

Skin Lesions

Abrasions, blisters, sebaceous cysts, hair-root infections, furuncles, and cysts are almost exclusively caused by local-ized pressure and friction due to an ill-fitting prosthetic

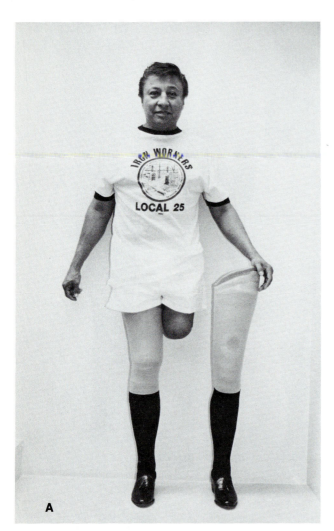

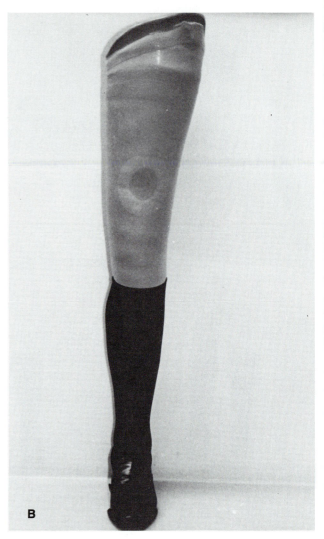

Figure 79-19. A, B. Endoskeletal above-knee prosthesis.

socket.[21] Skin lesions usually occur in areas on the stump that coincide with the proximal border of the socket where the potential for friction and localized pressure is great: inferior patellar and popliteal regions in the below-knee stump and inguinal, perineal, and gluteal fold areas in the above-knee stump. Limiting use of the prosthesis, allowing the skin lesion to heal, and performing socket correction will solve this problem. If the prosthesis is used when active lesions are present, the condition may be exacerbated to the degree that surgical intervention becomes necessary. In severe cases the problem may not be correctable.

Adherent Scar Tissue

Adherent scar tissue is unable to accept weight-bearing pressure. This condition, therefore, increases the per-unit pressure over the remaining skin surface. In most instances, surgical revision is necessary to correct this problem.

Sharp Bone

Sharp, distal bone terminations due to poor surgical technique or to exostosis reduce, in the same manner as adherent scar, the total surface area of support. Recontouring the socket in some instances will afford relief for the patient. More often surgical reconstruction is necessary.

Skin Grafts

With proper prosthetic fitting, adequately fashioned and healed skin grafts should not create problems.

General Comments

More sensitivity and attention to stump problems and more knowledge about them are needed on the part of both doctors and prosthetists. Unfortunately, the inability at present of many practitioners to deal effectively with stump problems results in patient neglect or mistaken psychiatric referrals.

HIGH TECHNOLOGY

The feasibility, even the existence, of high-technology prosthetic devices does not automatically lead to their application. The myoelectrically controlled below-elbow prosthesis, for example, has been available for more than 10 years and has yet to become commonly used. Another example is clear plastics, originally developed by the Veterans Administration in the late 1950s, which are today used by only a handful of practitioners.

Nothwithstanding the unencouraging history of high technology in prosthetics, the future is presented in the popular media as if it were already a reality. Computer-chip-controlled prosthetic devices and microelectronic brain implants wired to external prosthetic devices are examples.

It is, in my opinion, of extreme importance that prosthetists and related medical personnel not be seduced by misperceptions of the present or naive speculation about the future. Only by understanding the complex relationship of high technology to prosthetics can progress be effected.

Several fundamental obstacles stand in the way of rapid advancement in the use of high technology in prosthetics[22]:

1. Standard interface technology in prosthetics often will not accommodate technologic advances.
2. Current educational and training standards do not regularly produce prosthetists capable of applying technologic advances.
3. Sufficient markets do not exist to make highly specialized technologic advances feasible for mass production.
4. Most third-party reimbursers will not accept charges for new technology until it is in standard use.

VOCATIONAL AND AVOCATIONAL ADJUSTMENT

Adjustment is a word too often used by prosthetists to mean exclusively the acceptance of limitations. Acceptance of limitations is certainly a part of a mature understanding of what a person faces after the amputation of a limb but is *only* a part. The other aspect of the word "adjustment" is adaptation—the creative overcoming of limitations.

An open mind on the part of the prothetist can lead to innovations that open new worlds, both vocational and avocational, for the amputee. Three-track snow skiing provides an excellent example of what can be done.

The amputee, unless he is fortunate enough to locate and afford private rehabilitation counseling, depends primarily on the prosthetist for information, guidance, and often inspiration. Government programs are, for the most part, job-search services, offering little, if anything, else. The surgeon understandably has diminishing contact with the amputee after a successful operation. It is the prosthetist (and sometimes the family doctor) who is there when it comes time for the amputee to walk and rejoin the mainstream of life.

Prosthetists should, from their first contact with the amputee, provide information and counsel regarding the complex equation of genuine physical or technical limitations modified by the individual amputee's aspirations and will. "What is possible?" should always be an open question.

I have developed and use a mental formula in assessing what is possible for an individual amputee:

Objective physical capability + Available relevant technology + Prosthetist's ability and willingness to innovate × Amputee aspirations and will = What is possible.

High levels of amputee adjustment often involve increased costs. It is essential that these costs be placed in perspective—higher quality of life and reduced long-term disability expenditures vs. immediate outlay. Prosthetists and doctors must take the lead in educating third-party reimbursers, government policymakers, and the public in general about the long-term human benefits and monetary efficiencies of high-level amputee rehabilitation and adjustment.

ACKNOWLEDGMENTS

It is an extreme honor to be a contributor to *Haimovici's Vascular Surgery*. Thank you, Dr. Haimovici, for the opportunity to participate in such a prestigious project.

I am deeply grateful to my father, Walter J. Stokosa (1917-1971), who provided the foundation for my present level of knowledge; to my mother for her love and comforting support during those years; to the Honorable William G. Barr (1920-1987) for showing me the strength of spirit and perseverance.

Special thanks to Noreen Roeske Stokosa, friend and wife, for her loyal and dedicated support. Particular appreciation is given to Craig Starnaman for the excellent artwork provided. His ability to quickly and accurately grasp my word ideas and to transform them into creative illustrations is most respected. I am indebted to Ethel Huntwork for her shared concern in achieving the highest quality manuscript. I thank very much Dale Conlin, who came into the project late, under severe time constraints, and produced high-quality photographs of immeasurable value.

REFERENCES

1. Alldredge RH, Murphy EF: The influence of new developments on amputation surgery, in Klopsteg PA, Wilson PD, et al. (eds): Human Limbs and Their Substitutes. New York, McGraw-Hill Book Co, 1954, p 1112.
2. Vultee FE: Physical treatment and training of amputees, in Edwards JW (ed): Orthopaedic Appliances Atlas: vol. 2, Artificial Limbs. Ann Arbor, Mich, JW Edwards, 1960, p 313.
3. Friedman LW: The Surgical Rehabilitation of the Amputee. Springfield, Ill, Charles C Thomas, Publisher, 1978, p 88.
4. Hoffman CA, Bunch WH, Kestnbaum JS: Management of psychological problems, in Atlas of Limb Prosthetics: Surgical and Prosthetic Principles. St. Louis, The CV Mosby Co, 1981, p 483.
5. Burgess EM: Postoperative management, in Atlas of Limb

Prosthetics: Surgical and Prosthetic Principles. St. Louis, The CV Mosby Co, 1981, p 20.

6. Holliday PJ: Early postoperative care of the amputee, in Kostuik JP (ed): Amputation Surgery and Rehabilitation: The Toronto Experience. New York, Churchill Livingstone, Inc, 1981, p 219.

7. Kay HW: Wound dressings: Soft, rigid, or semirigid. Selected reading: A review of orthotics and prosthetics. Washington, DC, The American Orthotic and Prosthetic Assoc, 1980, p 41.

8. Burgess EM: Wound healing after amputation: Effect of controlled environment treatment: A preliminary study. J Bone Joint Surg 60A:245, 1978.

9. Baker WH, Barnes RW, Shurr DG: The healing of below-knee amputations, a comparison of soft and plaster dressings. Am J Surg 133:716, 1977.

10. Burgess EM, Romano RL, Zettl JH: The management of lower extremity amputations. Prosthetic and Sensory Aids Service, TR 10-6, Department of Medicine and Surgery, Veterans Administration, Washington, DC, Aug 1969, p 7.

11. Ertl J: Regeneration: Inre Anwendung in der Chirurgie. Leipzig, E Germany, Verlag Johann Ambrosius Barth, 1939.

12. Ertl W: Ertl amputation technique. Paper presented at the American Surgery Association, Sarasota, Fla, Oct 29, 1979.

13. Loon, HE: Biological and biomechanical principles in amputation surgery, in Prosthetics International, Proceedings of the Second International Prosthetics Course, Committee on Prostheses, Braces, and Technical Aids, International Society for the Welfare of Cripples, Copenhagen, 1960, p 46.

14. Murphy EF, Wilson AB Jr: Anatomical and physiological con-siderations in below-knee prosthetics. Selected Articles from Artificial Limbs, January 1954—Spring 1966. Huntington, NY, Krieger, 1970, p 283.

15. Quigley MJU: Prosthetic methods and materials, in Atlas of Limb Prosthetics: Surgical and Prosthetic Principles. St. Louis, The CV Mosby Co, 1981, p 53.

16. Katz KK, Susak Z, et al.: End-bearing characteristics of patellar-tendon-bearing prostheses—a preliminary report. Bull Pros Res 16:2, 1979.

17. Pritham CH: Newsletter—Prosthetics and Orthotics Clinic, vol. 6, nos. 1, 3, Winter, 1982.

18. Burgess EM: Postoperative management, in Atlas of Limb Prosthetics: Surgical and Prosthetic Principles. St. Louis, The CV Mosby Co, 1981, p 22.

19. McCullough NC III, Harris AR, Hampton FL: Below-knee amputation, in Atlas of Limb Prosthetics: Surgical and Prosthetic Principles. St. Louis, The CV Mosby Co, 1981, p 341.

20. Burgess EM, Romano RL, Zettl JH: The management of lower-extremity amputations. Prosthetic and Sensory Aids Service, TR 10-6, Department of Medicine and Surgery, Veterans Administration, Washington, DC, Aug 1969, p 18.

21. Harris WR: Common stump problems, in Kostuik JP (ed): Amputation Surgery and Rehabilitation: The Toronto Experience. New York, Churchill Livingstone, Inc, 1981, p 192.

22. Whipple L, Stokosa J: The not so simple ABC's of high technology. Disabled USA, Washington, DC, The President's Committee on Employment of the Handicapped, July 1983.

Index